PRIMER OF
Diagnostic Imaging

PRIMER OF *Diagnostic Imaging*

FIFTH EDITION

Ralph Weissleder, MD, PhD
Professor, Harvard Medical School
Radiologist, Massachusetts General Hospital
Boston, Massachusetts

Jack Wittenberg, MD
Professor, Harvard Medical School
Radiologist, Massachusetts General Hospital
Boston, Massachusetts

Mukesh G. Harisinghani, MD
Associate Professor, Harvard Medical School
Associate Radiologist, Massachusetts General Hospital
Boston, Massachusetts

John W. Chen, MD, PhD
Assistant Professor, Harvard Medical School
Assistant Radiologist, Massachusetts General Hospital
Boston, Massachusetts

ELSEVIER
MOSBY

ELSEVIER
MOSBY

3251 Riverport Lane
St. Louis, Missouri 63043

PRIMER OF DIAGNOSTIC IMAGING, FIFTH EDITION **ISBN: 978-0-323-06538-2**

Notices
Knowledge and best practice in this field are constantly changing. As new research and experience broaden our understanding, changes in research methods, professional practices, or medical treatment may become necessary.

Practitioners and researchers must always rely on their own experience and knowledge in evaluating and using any information, methods, compounds, or experiments described herein. In using such information or methods they should be mindful of their own safety and the safety of others, including parties for whom they have a professional responsibility.

With respect to any drug or pharmaceutical products identified, readers are advised to check the most current information provided (i) on procedures featured or (ii) by the manufacturer of each product to be administered, to verify the recommended dose or formula, the method and duration of administration, and contraindications. It is the responsibility of practitioners, relying on their own experience and knowledge of their patients, to make diagnoses, to determine dosages and the best treatment for each individual patient, and to take all appropriate safety precautions. To the fullest extent of the law, neither the Publisher nor the authors, contributors, or editors, assume any liability for any injury and/or damage to persons or property as a matter of products liability, negligence or otherwise, or from any use or operation of any methods, products, instructions, or ideas contained in the material herein.

Previous editions copyrighted 2007, 2003, 1997, 1994 by Mosby, Inc.

ISBN: 978-0-323-06538-2

Acquisitions Editor: Rebecca Gaertner
Developmental Editor: Arlene Chappelle
Publishing Services Manager: Patricia Tannian
Senior Project Manager: John Casey
Designer: Steven Stave

Printed in United States of America

Last digit is the print number: 9 8 7 6 5 4 3 2 1

To all of the radiologists whose
knowledge, research, and wisdom
contributed to this book

Reviewers

A number of present and former* staff members of the Department of Radiology, Massachusetts General Hospital, have reviewed and contributed to the different editions of *Primer of Diagnostic Imaging*. Jerry Glowniak, MD, Ross Titon, MD, and Arastoo Vossough, MD, PhD provided general comments on the entire content.

CHEST IMAGING
Meenakshi P. Bhalla, MD*
Theresa C. McLoud, MD
Jo-Anne O. Shepard, MD

CARDIAC IMAGING
Farouc Jaffer, MD
David Sosnovik, MD
Matthias Nahrendorf, MD
Stephen W. Miller, MD*

GASTROINTESTINAL IMAGING
Ashraf Thabet, MD
Peter R. Mueller, MD

GENITOURINARY IMAGING
Debra A. Gervais, MD
Michael J. Lee, MD*
Nicholas Papanicolaou, MD*

MUSCULOSKELETAL IMAGING
Felix S. Chew, MD*
Damian E. Dupuy, MD*
James T. Rhea, MD*

OBSTETRIC-GYNECOLOGIC IMAGING
Genevieve L. Bennett, MD*
Deborah A. Hall, MD
Mary Jane O'Neill*

BREAST IMAGING
Daniel B. Kopans, MD

NEURORADIOLOGY
Bradley R. Buchbinder, MD
Kenneth R. Davis, MD
R. Gilberto Gonzalez, MD, PhD
Michel H. Lev, MD
Javier Romero, MD
Pamela W. Schaefer, MD
David Schellingerhout, MD*

HEAD AND NECK IMAGING
Pearse Morris, MD*
David Schellingerhout, MD*
Daniel Silverstone, MD*
Alfred L. Weber, MD*

VASCULAR IMAGING
Stuart C. Geller, MD*
John A. Kaufman, MD*
Mark Rieumont, MD*

PEDIATRIC IMAGING
Johan G. Blickman, MD, PhD*
Robert T. Bramson, MD*
Susan Connolly, MD*

NUCLEAR MEDICINE
Edward E. Webster, PhD*
Edwin L. Palmer, MD

PHYSICS
Ronald J. Callahan, PhD
Edward E. Webster, PhD*
Umar Mahmood, PhD, MD

Preface

This fifth edition of the *Primer* functions both as a central learning system for residents and fellows, and a refresher text for faculty and practicing physicians. As in previous editions, the work presented within serves not only as the core curriculum for our fast-evolving specialty, but also as a contemporary reference text for practitioners. In it, we have strived to balance new information and older material required by the boards, with practical clinical utility. Since the preparation of the last edition, we have incorporated further advances in MR, PET, and CT imaging. We have thoroughly revised the new edition to reflect the numerous advancements in our specialty and, to the best of our knowledge, have corrected any inaccurate information. Furthermore, by continuing to have our successful graduates evaluate the content, we have ensured that the subject matter covers most information required by the American Board of Radiology examination. This year, we are particularly indebted to Dr. Ashraf Thabet for his extensive feedback. It is our hope that the *Primer* will continue to serve the next generation of radiologists, helping them navigate the stream of continuously emerging new information.

RALPH WEISSLEDER

JACK WITTENBERG

MUKESH G. HARISINGHANI

JOHN W. CHEN

Preface to the First Edition

The idea for this work began when one of us (RW) contemplated the enormity of material one needed to master during the radiology residency. A strategy was called for that would enhance retention of facts, techniques, and images and simplify their recall when, inevitably, they were forgotten. Thus was born the discipline at the end of each workday of computer processing important material, along with an accompanying sketch or two if sleep didn't intervene. At the very least it would be there in the computer for review those last 6 months before "Armageddon"; at the least it might help future Massachusetts General Hospital (MGH) residents. Five years later it all seems justified.

The MGH curriculum provides for rotations through all subspecialty divisions, 4 weeks at a time. A minimum of three staff and often several fellows comprise a subspecialty division, providing a wealth of educational resources. The information you find here is basically a distillation of teaching from these radiologists, supplemented by reading. Already you can recognize the potential for bias. Aside from the fellows who have trained elsewhere, much of what you will read in this book has the threat of being overly inbred. We have worked hard to avoid this pitfall. The decision as to what to include, emphasize, illustrate with a drawing, append as a pearl or two, is largely from a resident's point of view, although certainly influenced by the senior author. It's an eye on the average working day spent at a viewbox or passing needles and catheters, practical and functional. The emphasis is on the fundamentals, trying to give "low tech" its rightful place alongside the "high tech" of CT and MR. The more lengthy differential diagnostic lists and occasional appended esoterica come mostly from night and weekend refinements. By the third rotation in the fourth year, an organization of the assembled facts began to take place; the lean, bullet-type textual format served for a quick and efficient review. The leanness of the format was also gratefully received by divisional staff, who agreed to sacrifice precious summer hours to reassure us they had not been misquoted. The oft-repeated comment was, "It's like a record of my daily words being played back to me."

One of the unique strengths of this offering is the anatomic drawings, which one of us (JW) had nothing to contribute to other than sharpening pencils for the other (RW). Visuals are the critical other language of radiologic education. Unquestioned reliance on the specificity of an image suffers from the perils of an Aunt Minnie approach, but it's a good starting point to be able to recognize the variations in all her siblings. Furthermore, a drawing will never substitute for the hard copy. We hope that sort of companion tool will soon follow, perhaps in a suitable handy electronic form.

The format and size of the book are specifically designed to be a handy, readily available refresher of important signs, anatomic landmarks, common radiopathologic alterations, and practical differential diagnoses. It is not intended as a long-range substitute for the kind of sophisticated pathophysiologic, clinical information one needs to be the most effective radiologist. As the title indicates, we intend to prime the pump of intellectual curiosity. That quality of information comes from reading the more in-depth radiologic and other medical literature. Our judgment is that having mastered the information herein, you should certainly have enough information to intelligently and wisely discuss radiologic interpretation. However, a rich exchange with the internist, surgeon, neurologist, or obstetrician demands a mastering of much more material than you will find in this book.

It is critical that the authors be scrupulous in their acknowledgment of their sources of information. If we fail to do so with any of our resources, it is not out of immodesty or unintended claims of original material. The proffered information, while largely accumulated over 5 years, certainly represents a body of work (and therefore workers) that spans almost a century now. We have tried to filter out folklore and myths, but you know very well that much of what we all say, repeat, and defend is experiential and not always defensible on the basis of sensitivity, specificity, and accuracy of data. We have intended to describe information that we feel there are reasonable facts to support. If true data go unreferenced, however, we hope those authorities who recognize a little of their personal experience accept the unintended oversight as a mandate of the leanness and intent of our style.

It would be imprudent and graceless for us not to acknowledge some of the more local sources of major information. We are pretty sure that much of what we describe began with Drs. George Holmes and Aubrey Hampton; we recognize with clear certainty the leadership role in radiology of Drs. Laurence Robbins, Juan Taveras, and James Thrall. The most identifiable contributors are the present, often-quoted staff of our department. We are eternally grateful for their tireless daily educational tours de force and, in particular, thank those acknowledged contributors who took the time to review in detail the text we took from their lips. The many textbooks that served us particularly well in providing a bounty of useful information are listed in the Suggested Readings sections at the end of each chapter. These books were consulted, and information contained therein has been amalgamated with MGH teaching to provide a more seamless, complete, and less biased description of radiologic features. Lecture notes have been particularly helpful in distilling more complex information into readable text. After 5 years of compilation it is impossible to accurately trace each individual source of information.

RALPH WEISSLEDER

JACK WITTENBERG

Preface to the Second Edition

The second edition of the *Primer of Diagnostic Imaging* follows closely on the heels of the first to make up for our original gaps, omissions, and inconsistencies. In an attempt to provide as many fundamentals as possible the first time around, we emphasized certain modalities over others, but this time we have expanded on the newer modalities such as MRI and CT. We have also added new and updated graphics based on the positive feedback from the first edition. We hope these changes improve on our intent to provide a comprehensive review of radiology for residents, fellows, and possibly board-certified radiologists. The differential diagnosis sections now follow after each chapter rather than being aggregated at the end of the book. Finally, we have recruited a coeditor. Dr. Mark Rieumont, a recent ABR-minted radiologist and colleague, provides the balance of currency, perspective, focus, and feedback that sometimes eludes grizzled veterans.

What has fortunately not changed is the dedication of our MGH colleagues to peer review our material. We are extremely grateful to all of them for keeping us from making serious gaffes. Our lean style of bullet-like factual presentation persists to fill our perceived need for a comprehensive yet digestible source of information. While styles of curricula certainly vary among institutions, the basic fund of knowledge composing a curriculum should remain reasonably constant. A reminder of caution: this work should be viewed as a necessary infrastructure upon which we all must build a sophisticated superstructure of medical information.

RALPH WEISSLEDER

MARK RIEUMONT

JACK WITTENBERG

Preface to the Third Edition

Current, comprehensive, and clinically relevant. With these "C" words in mind, we offer our newest edition. Staying current is the major impetus, mindful that magnetic resonance imaging (MRI) is now nudging its way into many subspecialties other than neuroradiological and musculoskeletal imaging. We have made every effort to update information in these latter subspecialties and indicate where MRI is staking its toehold in the remainder. Since newer computed tomographic (CT) techniques have also affected our practice, additional information on the impact of multislice helical technology has been added. We recognize that the book is approaching the upper limits of portability but have deleted little in an effort to comply with our intention of the other "C" words.

We welcome Dr. Mukesh Harisinghani as our new coauthor. Dr. Harisinghani brings additional knowledge, careful review of content, and enthusiasm with him. He has an authoritative background in MRI and CT imaging. As before, many other colleagues in our and other departments have added comments and peer reviews. Their acknowledgment in the list of contributors always seems to fall short of the thanks we owe them.

We hope this new edition fulfills your every expectation.

RALPH WEISSLEDER

JACK WITTENBERG

MUKESH G. HARISINGHANI

Preface to the Fourth Edition

To spare those of you who bother to read prefaces, we refer you to prior ones, particularly the one to the third edition, because it is the shortest. Clearly, this text emphasizes subspecialty clinical and technical advances in CT and MRI, along with their updated protocols, and the emergence of PET.

Importantly, however, with this edition we have added some new talent. Our newest coauthor, John W. Chen, MD, PhD, adds his strong MRI multispecialty credentials and particular skills in neuroradiology. Because descriptive physics, particularly MRI, challenges the competency of most authors, we have included a dynamic CD version prepared by two of our creative senior residents, Stephen E. Jones, MD, PhD, and Jay W. Patti, MD.

We hope this new package contributes meaningfully to the care of your patients.

RALPH WEISSLEDER

JACK WITTENBERG

MUKESH G. HARISINGHANI

JOHN W. CHEN

Contents

Abbreviations

5-HIAA 5-hydroxyindoleacetic acid
AA aortic arch
A–a alveolar-arterial Po_2 difference
AAA abdominal aortic aneurysm
ABC aneurysmal bone cyst
ABPA allergic bronchopulmonary aspergillosis
ABS amniotic band syndrome
AC abdominal circumference; acromioclavicular; alternating current
ACA anterior cerebral artery
ACC agenesis of corpus callosum
ACL anterior cruciate ligament
ACLS advanced cardiac life support
ACOM anterior communicating (artery)
ACR American College of Radiology
ACT activated clotting time
ACTH adrenocorticotropic hormone
AD abdominal diameter; autosomal dominant; average distance
ADC apparent diffusion coefficient
ADEM acute disseminated encephalomyelitis
ADH antidiuretic hormone
AFB aortofemoral bypass
AFI amniotic fluid index
AFL air-fluid level
AFP alpha-fetoprotein
AFV amniotic fluid volume
AHA American Heart Association
AHD acquired heart disease
AI aortic insufficiency
AICA anterior inferior cerebellar artery
AICD automatic implantable cardioverter-defibrillator
AICV anterior intercostal vein
AIDS acquired immunodeficiency syndrome
AIP acute interstitial pneumonia
ALD adrenoleukodystrophy
ALS amyotrophic lateral sclerosis
AM abnormal motility
AMI acute myocardial infarction
AML angiomyolipoma; anterior mitral leaflet
amu atomic mass unit
ANCA antineutrophil cytoplasmic antibody
AP anteroposterior
APKD adult polycystic kidney disease
APUD amine precursor uptake and decarboxylation
AR autosomal recessive
ARDS acute respiratory distress syndrome
ARKD autosomal recessive kidney disease
ARPCKD autosomal recessive polycystic kidney disease
AS ankylosing spondylitis; aortic stenosis
ASA anterior spinal artery
ASD airspace disease; atrial septal defect
ASNR American Society of Neuroradiology
ATN acute tubular necrosis
AV arteriovenous; atrioventricular
AVF arteriovenous fistula
AVM arteriovenous malformation
AVN avascular necrosis
AZV azygos vein

BI Billroth I
BII Billroth II
BAC bronchoalveolar carcinoma
BAI basion-axial interval
BBB blood-brain barrier
BBBD blood-brain barrier disruption
BCDDP Breast Cancer Detection Demonstration Program
BCP basic calcium phosphate
BCS Budd-Chiari syndrome
BE barium enema
BF Bucky factor
BFM bronchopulmonary foregut malformation
BGO bismuth germanate
β-HCG beta-human chorionic gonadotropin
BIP bronchiolitis obliterans interstitial pneumonitis
BIRADS Breast Imaging Reporting and Data System
BLC benign lymphoepithelial cyst
BOOP bronchiolitis obliterans and organizing pneumonia
BP blood pressure
BPD biparietal diameter; bronchopulmonary dysplasia
BPF bronchopleural fistula
BPH benign prostatic hyperplasia
BPM beats per minute
BPOP bizarre parosteal osteochondromatous proliferation
BPP biophysical profile
Bq becquerel
BRBPR bright red blood per rectum

C-section cesarean section
C-spine cervical spine
CA carcinoma
CABG coronary artery bypass graft
CAD coronary artery disease
CAH chronic active hepatitis
CAPD chronic ambulatory peritoneal dialysis
CBD common bile duct
CBF cerebral blood flow
CBV cerebral blood volume
CC corneal clouding; craniocaudad; craniocaudal

CCA common carotid artery
CCAM congenital cystic adenoid malformation
CCF carotid-cavernous sinus fistula
CCK cholecystokinin
CPPD calcium pyrophosphate dihydrate
CCU coronary care unit
CD cystic duct
CD4 cluster designation 4 antigen
CDH congenital diaphragmatic hernia; congenital dislocation of the hip
CDI color Doppler imaging
CEA carcinoembryonic antigen
CECT contrast-enhanced computed tomography
CFA common femoral artery; cryptogenic fibrosing alveolitis
CHA calcium hydroxyapatite; common hepatic artery
CHD common hepatic duct; congenital heart disease
CHF congestive heart failure
Cho choline
CHP chronic hypersensitivity pneumonitis
CI cardiothoracic index
Ci Curie
CIDP chronic inflammatory demyelinating polyneuropathy
CLC corpus luteum cyst
CMC carpometacarpal (joint)
CMD corticomedullary differentiation
CMV cytomegalovirus
CN cranial nerve
CNS central nervous system
COP cryptogenic organizing pneumonia
COPD chronic obstructive pulmonary disease
CP cerebellopontine; choroid plexus
CPA cerebellopontine angle
CPAP continuous positive airway pressure
CPM central pontine myelinosis
cpm counts per minute
CPPD calcium pyrophosphate dihydrate
cps counts per second
Cr creatine/phosphocreatine
CREST calcinosis, Raynaud's, esophageal dysmotility, sclerodactyly, telangiectasia (syndrome)
CRL crown-rump length
CSF cerebrospinal fluid
CSP corrected sinusoidal pressure
CT computed tomography
CTA computed tomographic angiography
CTAP computed tomographic arterial portography
CTP computed tomographic perfusion
CTV computed tomographic venography
CU clinical unit
CVA cerebrovascular accident
CVS calcium volume score; chorionic villus sampling
CWP coal workers' pneumoconiosis
CXR chest radiograph

D dilatation
2D two-dimensional
3D three-dimensional
D-TGA complete transposition of great arteries
DA double arch
DAI diffuse axonal injury
DC direct current
DCIS ductal carcinoma in situ
DDH developmental dysplasia of the hip
DDX differential diagnosis
DES diethylstilbestrol; diffuse esophageal spasm
DFTN diffuse fold thickening with fine nodularity
DIC disseminated intravascular coagulation
DIP desquamative interstitial pneumonitis; distal interphalangeal (joint)
DISH diffuse idiopathic skeletal hyperostosis
DISI dorsal intercalated segment instability
DJD degenerative joint disease
DM diabetes mellitus
DNA deoxyribonucleic acid
DNET dysembryoplastic neuroepithelial tumor
DORV double-outlet right ventricle
DRE digital rectal examination
DSA digital subtraction angiography
DTPA diethylenetriaminepentaacetic acid
DU deep ulcer(s)
DVT deep vein thrombosis
DW Dandy-Walker
DWI diffusion-weighted imaging

E exposure
EA esophageal atresia
EAC external auditory canal
EBV Epstein-Barr virus
ECA external carotid artery
ECD endocardial cushion defect
ECF extracellular fluid
ECG electrocardiogram
ECMO extracorporeal membrane oxygenation
EDH epidural hematoma
EDV end-diastolic volume
EF ejection fraction
EFW estimated fetal weight
EG eosinophilic granuloma
EGA estimated gestational age
ENT ear, nose, throat
EPA Environmental Protection Agency
ERCP endoscopic retrograde cholangiopancreatography
ERPF effective renal plasma flow
ERV expiratory reserve volume
ESR erythrocyte sedimentation rate
ESV end-systolic volume
ET endotracheal tube
ETL echo train length
eV electron volt
EXP exponential

FAPS familial adenomatous polyposis syndrome
FCD fibrous cortical defect
FD filling defect
FDA Food and Drug Administration
FDG fluorodeoxyglucose
FEV forced expiratory volume

FIGO	International Federation of Gynecology and Obstetrics
FL	femur length
FLAIR	fluid-attenuated inversion recovery
FMC	focal myometrial contraction
FMD	fibromuscular dysplasia
FNA	fine-needle aspiration
FNH	focal nodular hyperplasia
FOD	focal spot–object distance
FOV	field of view
FRC	functional residual capacity
FS	focal spot; fractional shortening
FSE	fast spin echo
FSH	follicle-stimulating hormone
FTA-ABS	fluorescent treponemal antibody absorption (test)
FUO	fever of unknown origin
FWHM	full width at half maximum
Ga	gallium
GB	gallbladder
GBM	glioblastoma multiforme
GBPS	gated blood pool study
GCT	giant cell tumor
Gd	gadolinium
GDA	gastroduodenal artery
GE	gastroesophageal
GEJ	gastroesophageal junction
GFR	glomerular filtration rate
GH	growth hormone
GI	gastrointestinal
GIP	giant cell interstitial pneumonia
GIST	gastrointestinal stromal tumor
glut	glucose transporter
GM	gray matter
GnRH	gonadotropin-releasing hormone
GRE	gradient-recalled echo
GSD	genetically significant dose
GTD	gestational trophoblastic disease
GU	genitourinary
GVH	graft-versus-host (disease)
GWM	gray-white matter
H	height
HA	hepatic artery
HAZV	hemiazygos vein
Hb	hemoglobin
HbAS	sickle cell trait
HbSS	sickle cell disease
HC	head circumference
HCC	hepatocellular carcinoma
HCG	human chorionic gonadotropin
HD	Hurter and Driffield (curve)
HGH	human growth hormone
HIDA	hepatic iminodiacetic acid derivative
HIP	health insurance plan
HIV	human immunodeficiency virus
HLA	human leukocyte antigen
HLHS	hypoplastic left heart syndrome
HMD	hyaline membrane disease
HMDP	hydroxymethylene diphosphonate
HMPAO	hexamethylpropyleneamine oxime
HOCA	high-osmolar contrast agent
HPF	high-power field
HPO	hypertrophic pulmonary osteoarthropathy
HPS	hypertrophic pyloric stenosis
HPT	hyperparathyroidism
HR	heart rate
hr	hour
HRCT	high-resolution computed tomography
HS	hepatosplenomegaly
HSA	human serum albumin
HSG	hysterosalpingogram
HSV	herpes simplex virus
HTLV	human T-cell lymphotrophic virus
HTN	hypertension
HU	heat unit; Hounsfield unit
HVA	homovanillic acid
HVL	half-value layer
IA	intraarterial
IAA	interruption of aortic arch
IABP	intraaortic balloon pump
IAC	internal auditory canal
IBD	inflammatory bowel disease
ICA	internal carotid artery
ICRP	International Commission on Radiological Protection
ICU	intensive care unit
ICV	internal cerebral vein
ID	information density; inner diameter
IDA	iminodiacetic acid
IG	immunoglobulin
IgG	immunoglobulin G
IHF	immune hydrops fetalis
IHSS	idiopathic hypertrophic subaortic stenosis
IJV	internal jugular vein
IL-2	interleukin-2
ILO	International Labor Organization
ILT	inferolateral trunk
IMA	inferior mesenteric artery
IMV	internal mammary vein
INF	inferior
INH	isoniazid
INSS	International Neuroblastoma Staging System
IPF	idiopathic pulmonary fibrosis
IPH	idiopathic pulmonary hemorrhage
IPKD	infantile polycystic kidney disease
IPMT	intraductal papillary mucinous tumor
IQ	intelligence quotient
IRV	inspiratory reserve volume
IUD	intrauterine device
IUGR	intrauterine growth retardation
IUP	intrauterine pregnancy
IV	intravenous
IVC	inferior vena cava
IVDA	intravenous drug abuse(r)
IVP	intravenous pyelogram
IVS	interventricular septum
JRA	juvenile rheumatoid arthritis
keV	kilo electron volt
KS	Kaposi sarcoma

KUB	kidney, urethra, bladder
kVp	kilovolt (peak)
L	left; length
L-TGA	corrected transposition of great arteries
LA	left atrium
LAD	left anterior descending (artery)
LAE	left atrial enlargement
LAM	lymphangioleiomyomatosis
LAO	left anterior oblique
LATS	long-acting thyroid-stimulating (factor)
LBBB	left bundle branch block
LBWC	limb/body wall complex
LCA	left carotid artery; left coronary artery
LCIS	lobular carcinoma in situ
LCL	lateral collateral ligament
LCNEC	large cell neuroendocrine carcinoma
LCP	Legg-Calvé-Perthes (disease)
LCx	left circumflex (artery)
LD	lymphocyte depleted (Hodgkin lymphoma)
LD_{50}	lethal dose, 50%
LDH	lactate dehydrogenase
LEJV	left external jugular vein
LES	lower esophageal sphincter
LET	linear energy transfer
LFT	liver function test
LGA	large for gestational age; left gastric artery
LH	luteinizing hormone
LHA	left hepatic artery
LHD	left hepatic duct
LIJV	left internal jugular vein
LIMA	left internal mammary artery
LIMV	left internal mammary vein
LIP	lymphocytic interstitial pneumonia
LIQ	low intelligence quotient
LL	lower lobe
LLI	left lateral inferior
LLL	left lower lobe
LLS	left lateral superior
LM	lateromedial
LMB	left mainstem bronchus
LMI	left medial inferior
LMP	last menstrual period
LMS	left medial superior
LN	lymph node
LOCA	low-osmolar contrast agent
LP	lymphocyte predominant (Hodgkin lymphoma)
LPA	left pulmonary artery
LPM	anterolateral papillary muscle
LPO	left posterior oblique
LPV	left portal vein
L-R shunt	left-to-right shunt
LSA	left subclavian artery
LSCV	left subclavian vein
LSICV	left superior intercostal vein
LSMFT	liposclerosing myxofibrous tumor
LTV	lateral thoracic vein
LUL	left upper lobe
LUQ	left upper quadrant
LUS	lower uterine segment
LV	left ventricle
LVA	left vertebral artery
LVE	left ventricular enlargement
LVEF	left ventricular ejection fraction
LVH	left ventricular hypertrophy
mA	milliampere
MA	meconium aspiration; mesenteric adenopathy
MAA	macroaggregated albumin
MAb	monoclonal antibody
MAG	methyl-acetyl-gly
MAG3	methyl-acetyl-gly-gly-gly
MAI	*Mycobacterium avium-intracellulare*
MALT	mucosa-associated lymphoid tissue
MAOI	monoamine oxidase inhibitor
MAP	maximum-a-posteriori
mAs	milliampere second
MBq	megabecquerel
MC	mixed cellularity (Hodgkin lymphoma)
MCA	middle cerebral artery
MCD	medullary cystic disease
MCDK	multicystic dysplastic kidney
mCi	millicurie
∝Ci	microcurie
MCL	medial collateral ligament
MCTD	mixed connective tissue disease
MCV	middle cerebral vein
MD	monochorionic, diamniotic (twins)
MDA	metaphyseal-diaphyseal angle
MDCT	multidetector computed tomography
MDP	methylene diphosphonate
MELAS	mitochondrial myopathy, encephalopathy, lactic acidosis, strokelike episodes (syndrome)
MEN	multiple endocrine neoplasia
MERRF	myoclonic epilepsy with ragged red fibers (syndrome)
MeV	megaelectron volt
MFH	malignant fibrous histiocytoma
MGH	Massachusetts General Hospital
MI	myocardial infarction
MIBG	metaiodobenzylguanidine
MIBI	methoxyisobutyl isonitrile
MIP	maximum-intensity projection
ML	mediolateral
MLCN	multilocular cystic nephroma
MLD	maximum transverse diameter to the left from midline
MLEM	maximum likelihood expectation maximization
MLO	mediolateral oblique
MM	monoamniotic, monochorionic (twins)
MNG	multinodular goiter
mo	month
MOCE	multiple osteocartilaginous exostoses
MOM	multiples of median
MPA	main pulmonary artery
MPD	maximum permissible dose
MPM	posteromedial papillary muscle
MPV	main portal vein
mR	milliroentgen

MR	magnetic resonance
MRA	magnetic resonance angiography
MRCP	magnetic resonance cholangiopancreatography
MRD	maximum transverse diameter to the right from midline
MRI	magnetic resonance imaging
MRS	magnetic resonance spectroscopy
MRSA	methicillin-resistant *Staphylococcus aureus*
MRV	magnetic resonance venography
MS	multiple sclerosis
MSAFP	maternal serum alpha-fetoprotein
MSD	mean sac diameter
MT	magnetization transfer
MTB	*Mycobacterium tuberculosis*
MTF	modulation transfer function
MTP	metatarsal phalangeal (joint)
MTT	mean transit time
MVA	motor vehicle accident
MW	molecular weight
NAA	*N*-acetyl aspartate
nCi	nanocurie
NCRP	National Council on Radiation Protection
NEMA	National Electrical Manufacturers Association
NEMD	nonspecific esophageal motility disorder(s)
NEC	necrotizing enterocolitis
NEX	number of averages
NF	neurofibromatosis
NF1	neurofibromatosis type 1
NF2	neurofibromatosis type 2
NG	nasogastric
NH	nonhereditary
NHL	non-Hodgkin lymphoma
NIDDM	non-insulin-dependent diabetes mellitus
NIH	National Institutes of Health
NIHF	nonimmune hydrops fetalis
NOF	nonossifying fibroma
NOS	not otherwise specified
NP	neonatal pneumonia
NPH	normal-pressure hydrocephalus
NPO	nil per os (fasting)
NRC	Nuclear Regulatory Commission
NS	nodular sclerosing (Hodgkin lymphoma)
NSA	number of signals averaged
NSAID	nonsteroidal antiinflammatory drug
NSIP	nonspecific interstitial pneumonia
NTD	neural tube defect
NTMB	nontuberculous mycobacteria
OA	osteoarthritis
OC	oral contraceptive
OCH	Oriental cholangiohepatitis
OD	once daily; optical density; outer diameter
ODD	object-detector distance
OEIS	omphalocele, exstrophy, imperforate anus, special anomaly
OFD	occipitofrontal diameter
OI	osteogenesis imperfecta
OIC	osteogenesis imperfecta congenita
OIT	osteogenesis imperfecta tarda
OMC	osteomeatal complex
ORIF	open reduction and internal fixation
OSA	osteosarcoma
OSEM	ordered set expectation maximization
PA	posteroanterior; pulmonary artery
PAC	premature atrial contraction
PAH	pulmonary arterial hypertension
PAN	polyarteritis nodosa
PAPVC	partial anomalous pulmonary venous connection
PAVM	pulmonary arteriovenous malformation
PC	phase contrast
PCA	posterior cerebral artery
PCL	posterior cruciate ligament
PCN	percutaneous nephrostomy
PCNSL	primary central nervous system lymphoma
PCO	polycystic ovary
PCOM	posterior communicating (artery)
PCP	*Pneumocystis* pneumonia
PD	pancreatic duct
PDA	patent ductus arteriosus
PDW	proton density weighted
PE	photoelectric effect; pulmonary embolism
PEEP	positive end-expiratory pressure
PET	positron emission tomography
PFA	profunda femoral artery
PFC	persistent fetal circulation
PGE_1	prostaglandin E-1
PHA	pulse height analyzer
PHPV	persistent hyperplastic primary vitreous
PHS	pulse height selector
PI	pulsatility index
PICA	posterior inferior cerebellar artery
PICV	posterior intercostal vein
PID	pelvic inflammatory disease
PIE	pulmonary infiltrates with eosinophilia; pulmonary interstitial emphysema
PIOPED	prospective investigation of pulmonary embolus detection
PIP	postinflammatory polyp; proximal interphalangeal (joint)
PKU	phenylketonuria
PLN	projected length of needle
PLPN	projected length to pull back needle
PM	photomultiplier (tube)
PMC	pseudomembranous colitis
PMF	progressive massive fibrosis
PMHR	predicted maximum heart rate
PML	posterior mitral leaflet; progressive multifocal leukoencephalopathy
PMMA	polymethylmethacrylate
PMT	photomultiplier tube
PNET	primitive neuroectodermal tumor
PO	orally (per os)
Po_2	partial pressure of oxygen
post.	posterior
ppm	parts per million
PRF	pulse repetition frequency
PRL	prolactin
PROM	premature rupture of membranes
PSA	prostate-specific antigen

PSMA	prostate-specific membrane antigen
PSPMT	pulse spray pharmacomechanical thrombolysis
PSS	progressive systemic sclerosis
PT	prothrombin time
PTA	percutaneous transluminal angioplasty
PTCA	percutaneous transluminal coronary angioplasty
PTD	posttransplantation lymphoproliferative disorder
PTFE	polytetrafluoroethylene
PTH	parathormone
PTLD	posttransplantation lymphoproliferative disorder
PTT	partial thromboplastin time
PTU	propylthiouracil
PUD	peptic ulcer disease
PUL	percutaneous ureterolithotomy
PUV	posterior urethral valve
PV	portal vein
PVA	polyvinyl alcohol
PVC	premature ventricular contraction
PVH	pulmonary venous hypertension
PVNS	pigmented villonodular synovitis
PVOD	pulmonary venoocclusive disease
PVP	portal venous phase
PWI	perfusion-weighted imaging
PWMA	periventricular white matter abnormality
QA	quality assurance
qid	four times daily
R	range; right
RA	right atrium; rheumatoid arthritis
RAI	right anterior inferior
RAIU	radioactive iodine uptake
RAO	right anterior oblique
RAS	renal artery stenosis; right anterior superior
RB-ILD	respiratory bronchiolitis–associated interstitial lung disease
RBBB	right bundle branch block
RBC	red blood cell(s) (count)
RBE	relative biologic effectiveness
RCA	right carotid artery; right coronary artery
RCC	renal cell carcinoma
RCV	red cell volume
RDS	respiratory distress syndrome
REJV	right external jugular vein
RES	reticuloendothelial system
RF	radiofrequency; rheumatoid factor
RGA	right gastric artery
Rh	rhesus (factor)
RHA	right hepatic artery
RHD	right hepatic duct
RI	resistive index
RIJV	right internal jugular vein
RIMA	right internal mammary artery
RIMV	right internal mammary vein
RIND	reversible ischemic neurologic deficit
R-L shunt	right-to-left shunt
RLL	right lower lobe
RLQ	right lower quadrant
RMB	right mainstem bronchus
RML	right middle lobe
RNA	ribonucleic acid
ROI	range of interest
rPA	ratio of pulmonary artery diameter to aortic diameter
RPI	right posterior inferior
RPN	renal papillary necrosis
RPO	right posterior oblique
RPS	right posterior superior
RPV	right portal vein
RSA	right subclavian artery
RSCV	right subclavian vein
RSV	respiratory syncytial virus
RT	radiotherapy
RTA	renal tubular acidosis
RTV	right thoracic vein
r-tPA	recombinant tissue plasminogen activator
RUL	right upper lobe
RUQ	right upper quadrant
RV	reserve volume; right ventricle
RVA	right vertebral artery
RVEF	right ventricular ejection fraction
RVT	renal vein thrombosis
S/P	status post
SA	sinoatrial; subclavian artery
SAH	subarachnoid hemorrhage
SB	small bowel
SBFT	small bowel follow-through
SBO	small bowel obstruction
SC	subcutaneous
SCA	superior cerebellar artery
SCC	squamous cell carcinoma
SCFE	slipped capital femoral epiphysis
SCLS	small cell lung cancer
SD	standard deviation
SDAT	senile dementia, Alzheimer type
SDH	subdural hematoma
SE	spin echo
seg.	segment
SFA	superficial femoral artery
SGA	small for gestational age
SGOT	serum glutamic-oxaloacetic transaminase
SI	sacroiliac; signal intensity
SIN	salpingitis isthmica nodosa
SK	streptokinase
SL	sublingual
SLAC	scapholunate advanced collapse
SLE	systemic lupus erythematosus
SMA	superior mesenteric artery
SMV	superior mesenteric vein
SNR	signal-to-noise ratio
SPECT	single photon emission computed tomography
SPGR	spoiled gradient-echo
SPIO	superparamagnetic iron oxide
SSFSE	single-shot fast spin echo
ST	ST complex on ECG
STIR	short tau inversion recovery
STT	scaphotrapeziotrapezoid
SU	superficial ulcer(s)

sup.	superior
SUV	standardized uptake value
SVC	superior vena cava
T	tesla; thalamus; time
T1W	T1-weighted (images)
T2W	T2-weighted (images)
T3	triiodothyronine
T4	thyroxine
TA	truncus arteriosus
TAPVC	total anomalous pulmonary venous connection
TAPVR	total anomalous pulmonary venous return
TAR	thrombocytopenia-absent radius (syndrome)
TAS	transabdominal ultrasound
TB	tuberculosis
TBI	traumatic brain injury
TCC	transitional cell cancer
TD	tolerance dose
TDL	true depth of lesion
TDLU	terminal duct lobular unit
TE	echo time
TEE	transesophageal echocardiography
TEF	tracheoesophageal fistula
TF	thickened folds
TFA	tibiofemoral angle
TFCC	triangular fibrocartilage complex
TFN	thickened folds with nodularity
TGA	transposition of great arteries
TGC	time-gain compensator
THR	total hip replacement
TI	terminal ileum
TIPS	transjugular intrahepatic portosystemic shunt
TKR	total knee replacement
TLA	translumbar approach
TLC	total lung capacity
TLN	true length of needle
TLPN	true length to pull back needle
TM	tympanic membrane
TMC	toxic megacolon
TMJ	temporomandibular joint
TNM	tumor-node-metastases
TOA	tuboovarian abscess
TOF	time of flight
TORCH	toxoplasmosis, rubella, cytomegalovirus, herpes simplex virus (syndrome)
tPA	tissue plasminogen activator
TPN	total parenteral nutrition
TPO	tracheopathia osteoplastica
TR	repetition interval
TRAPS	twin reversal arterial perfusion sequence
TRUS	transrectal ultrasound
TSH	thyroid-stimulating hormone
TTN	transient tachypnea of the newborn
TURP	transurethral resection of prostate
TV	tidal volume; transvaginal
TVS	transvaginal sonography
UA	umbilical artery
UBC	unicameral bone cyst
UC	ulcerative colitis
UCD	uremic cystic disease
UGI	upper gastrointestinal
UIP	usual interstitial pneumonia
UK	urokinase
UL	upper lobe
UPJ	ureteropelvic junction
US	ultrasound
U.S.	United States
USPIO	ultrasmall superparamagnetic iron oxide
UTI	urinary tract infection
UV	ultraviolet; umbilical vein
UVJ	ureterovesical junction
VA	vertebral artery
VACTERL	vertebral body, anal, cardiovascular, tracheoesophageal, renal, limb anomalies (association)
VATS	video-assisted thoracoscopic surgery
VC	vital capacity
VCUG	voiding cystourethrogram
VDRL	Venereal Disease Research Laboratory
VHL	von Hippel-Lindau (disease)
VISI	volar intercalated segment instability
VMA	vanillylmandelic acid
VP	ventriculoperitoneal
$\dot{V}/\dot{Q}$	ventilation/perfusion
VR	Virchow-Robin (space)
VRE	vancomycin-resistant enterococcus
VSD	ventricular septal defect
VUR	vesicoureteral reflux
VZ	varicella zoster
W	width
WBC	white blood cell(s) (count)
WES	wall-echo-shadow (triad)
WHO	World Health Organization
WM	white matter
WPW	Wolf-Parkinson-White (syndrome)
w/w	weight (of solute) per weight (of total solvent)
XCCL	exaggerated craniocaudal
XGP	xanthogranulomatous pyelonephritis
yr	year
Z	atomic number

Please check entire *Primer* for additional abbreviations not listed above

Symbols

$<$	less (common) than
$\ll$	much less (common) than
$\leq$	less than or equal to
$>$	more (common) than
$\gg$	much more (common) than
$\geq$	greater than or equal to
$\rightarrow$	leads to
$\varnothing$	normal, unchanged
$\uparrow$	increased
$\downarrow$	decreased

CHAPTER 1

Chest Imaging

CHAPTER OUTLINE

Imaging Anatomy

GROSS LUNG ANATOMY

SEGMENTAL ANATOMY (Figs. 1-1 and 1-2)

Right Lung

Upper lobe	Apical	B1
	Anterior	B2
	Posterior	B3
Middle lobe	Lateral	B4
	Medial	B5
Lower lobe	Superior	B6
	Medial basal	B7
	Anterior basal	B8
	Lateral basal	B9
	Posterior basal	B10

Left Lung

Upper lobe		
Upper	Apicoposterior	B1, 3
	Anterior	B2
Lingula	Superior	B4
	Inferior	B5
Lower lobe	Superior	B6

Medial basal	B7
Anterior basal	B8
Lateral basal	B9
Posterior basal	B10

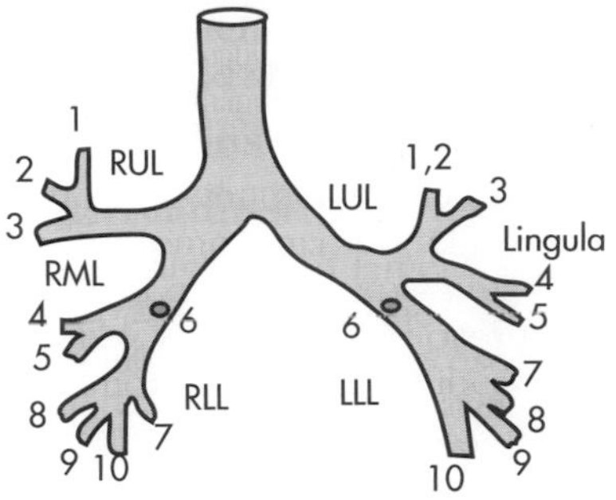

FIGURE 1-1

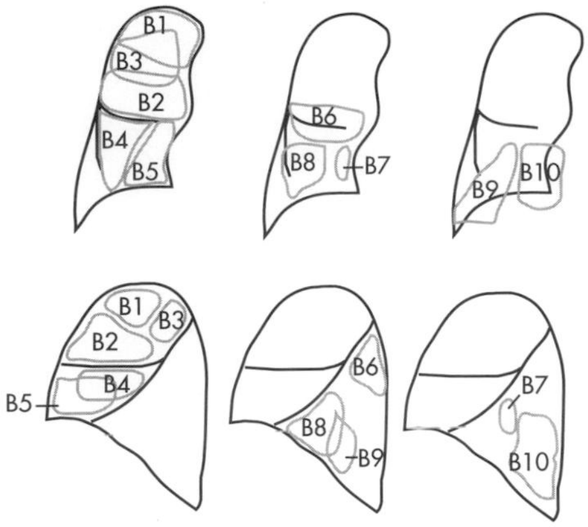

FIGURE 1-2

SEGMENTAL CT ANATOMY (Fig. 1-3)

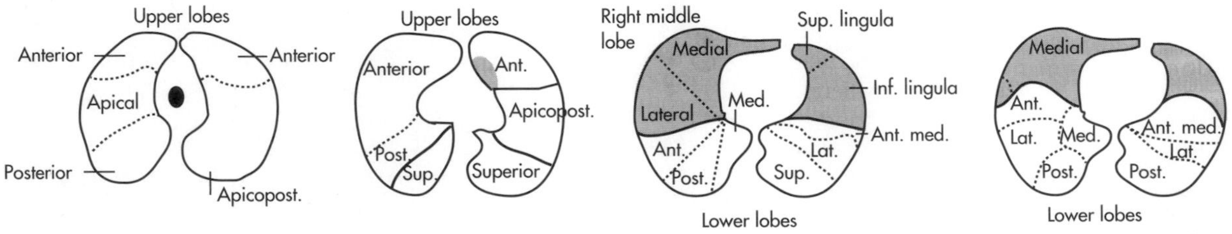

FIGURE 1-3

BRONCHIAL CT ANATOMY (Fig. 1-4)

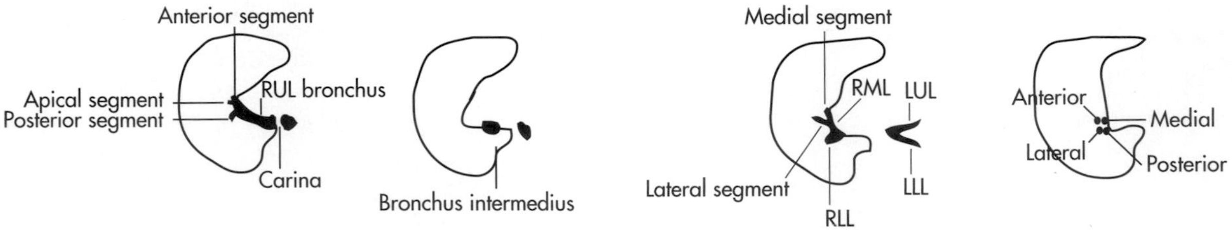

FIGURE 1-4

PLAIN FILM ANATOMIC LANDMARKS (Figs. 1-5 through 1-9)

Lines

- Anterior junction line: 2-mm linear line that projects over the trachea. Represents the anterior right and left pleura.
- Posterior junction line: extends above clavicles
- Azygoesophageal line: interface between RLL air and mediastinum
- Left paraspinal line: extends from aortic arch to diaphragm
- Right paraspinal line

Paratracheal Stripe

- Abnormal if >4 mm
- Never extends below right bronchus

Fissures

- Minor (horizontal) fissure
- Major (oblique) fissure
- Azygos fissure

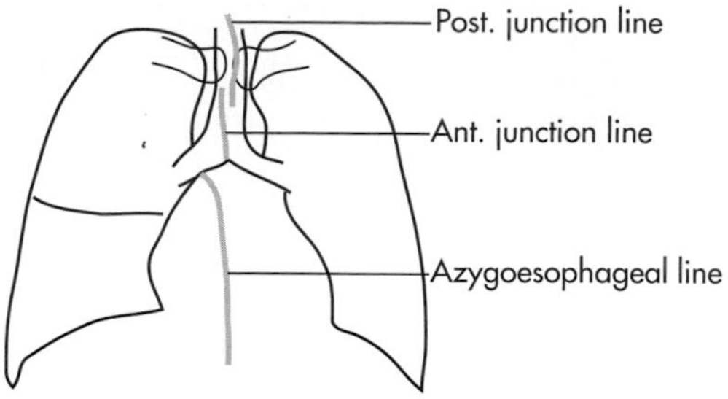

FIGURE 1-5

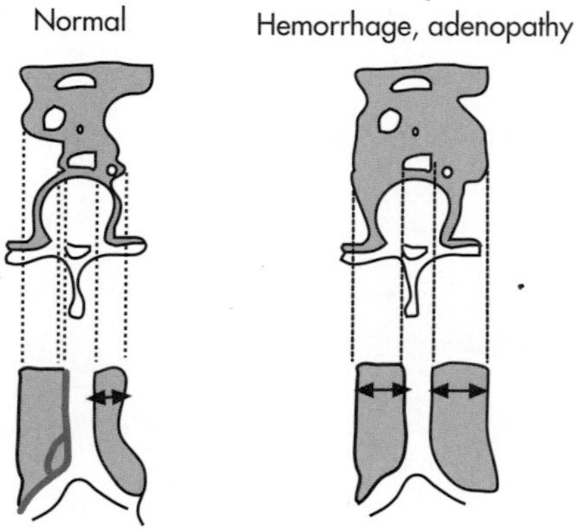

FIGURE 1-6

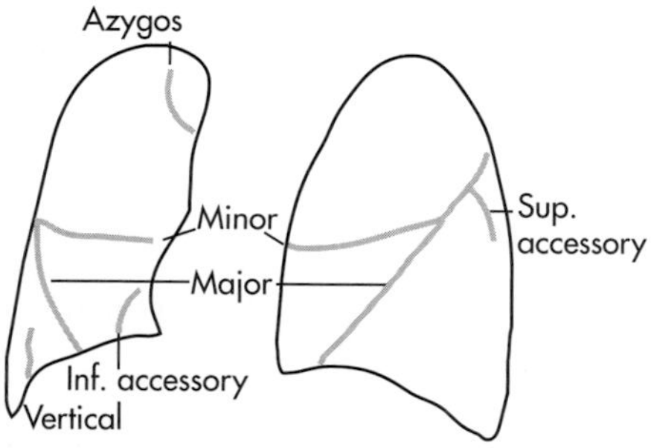

FIGURE 1-7

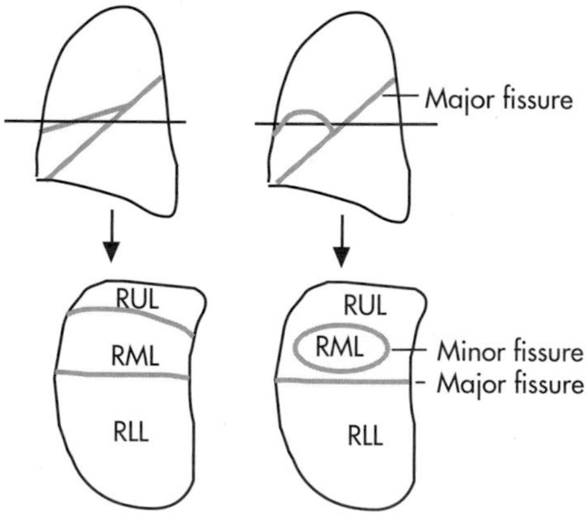

FIGURE 1-8

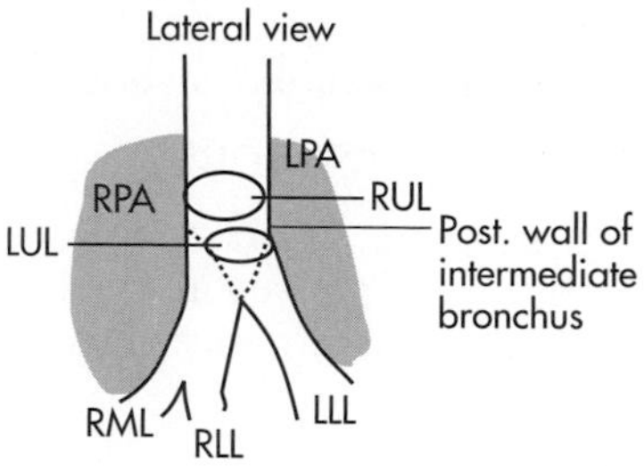

FIGURE 1-9

- Other fissures
  - Superior accessory lobe
  - Inferior accessory lobe

Upper Lobe Bronchi (Figs. 1-10 and 1-11)

- RUL bronchus always higher than LUL on lateral view
- Posterior wall of bronchus intermedius (right) normally <2 mm
- Tracheal bronchus (bronchus suis): 0.1% of population, arises from right wall of trachea (left much less common), supplies apical segment or occasionally entire right upper lobe
- Accessory cardiac bronchus: 0.1% of population, extends inferomedially from medial wall of bronchus intermedius or RLL bronchus toward mediastinum; may be blind ending

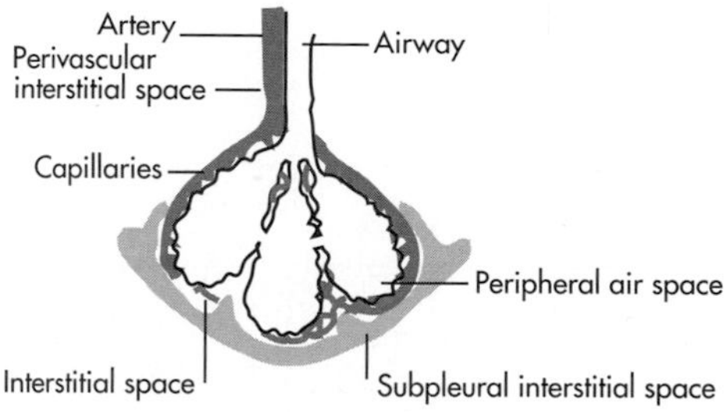

FIGURE 1-10

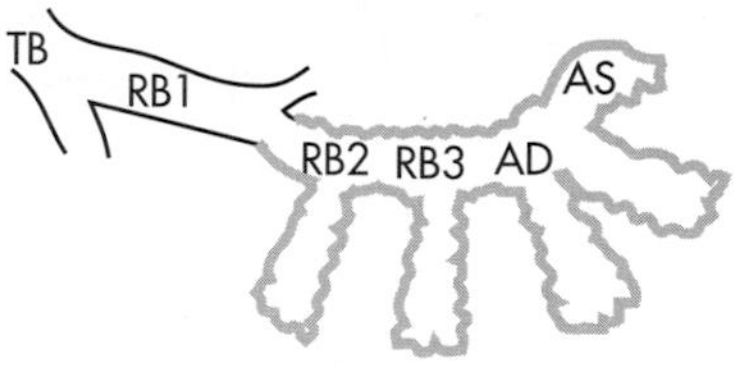

FIGURE 1-11

PARENCHYMAL ANATOMY

ACINUS

- Includes all structures distal to one terminal bronchiole. The terminal bronchiole is the last purely air-conducting structure.

- Acinus measures 7 mm
- Acinus contains about 400 alveoli

SECONDARY PULMONARY LOBULE

- Polygonal structure, 1.5 to 2 cm in diameter
- Three to five acini per secondary lobule
- Supplied by several terminal bronchioles

EPITHELIUM

The alveolar epithelium is made up of two cell types:

- Type 1 pneumocytes
- Type 2 pneumocytes: produce surfactant, have phagocytic ability, and regenerate

HIGH-RESOLUTION COMPUTED TOMOGRAPHY (HRCT) (Fig. 1-12)

Technique

- 1- to 1.5-mm thin collimation
- High spatial frequency reconstruction
- Optional
  - Increase in kVp or mA (140 kVp, 170 mA)
  - Targeted image reconstruction (one lung rather than both to improve spatial resolution)

HRCT Anatomy

The basic pulmonary unit visible by HRCT represents the secondary pulmonary lobule:

- Polyhedral 1.5-cm structure surrounded by connective tissue (interlobular septa)
- Central artery and bronchiole
- Peripheral pulmonary veins and lymphatics in septum

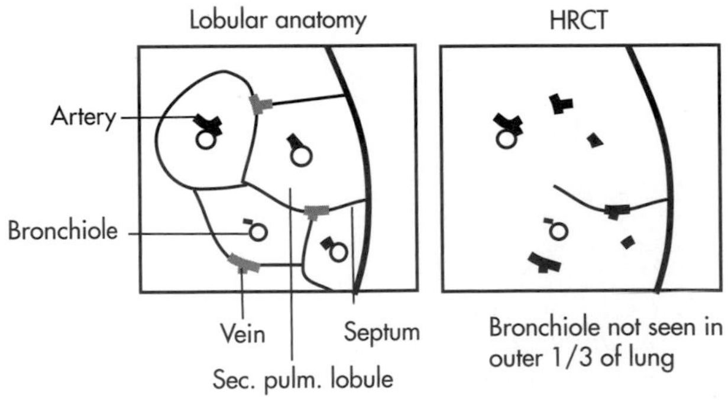

FIGURE 1-12

PULMONARY FUNCTION (Fig. 1-13)

LUNG VOLUMES, CAPACITIES, AND FLOW RATES

- Tidal volume (TV): normal respiratory cycle
- Vital capacity (VC): amount of air that can be expired with force after maximal inspiration

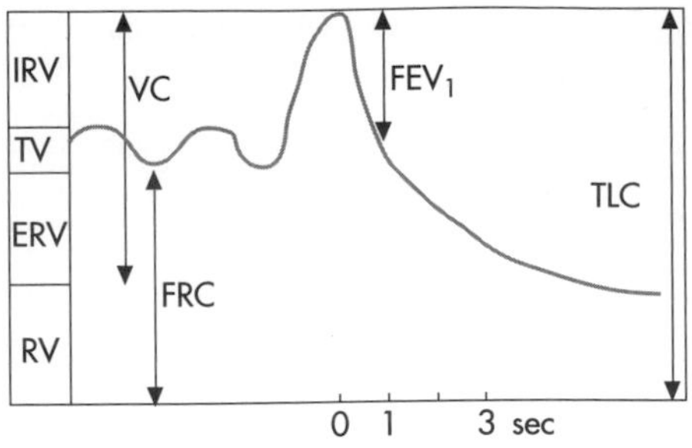

FIGURE 1-13

- Functional residual capacity (FRC): volume remaining in lung after quiet expiration
- Total lung capacity (TLC): volume contained in lung at maximum inspiration
- Forced expiratory volume (FEV): amount of air expired during 1 second (FEV_1)

MEDIASTINUM (Fig. 1-14)

- Superior mediastinum: plane above aortic arch; thoracic inlet structures
- Anterior mediastinum: contains thymus, lymph nodes, mesenchymal tissue; some classifications include the heart
- Middle mediastinum: contains heart, major vessels, bronchi, lymph nodes, and phrenic nerve
- Posterior mediastinum: starts at anterior margin of vertebral bodies; contains descending aorta, esophagus, thoracic duct, lymph nodes, nerves, and paravertebral areas

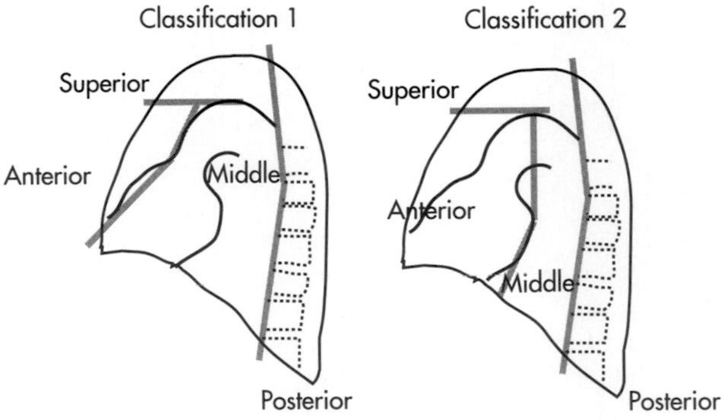

FIGURE 1-14

IMAGING PROTOCOLS

STANDARD CHEST CT PROTOCOL

Supine position. Scan in suspended inspiration at total lung capacity. Scan setup:

- 5- × 5-mm sections from apex of the lungs to the adrenals

- Six 1.25-mm high-resolution cuts throughout lung at 2.5-cm intervals
- 1-mm reconstructions through pulmonary nodules
- Number of different combinations of pitch and section thickness

In interstitial lung disease, the six cuts are repeated in prone position. Reconstruction is done with high-resolution bone algorithm.

Use of IV contrast:

- Evaluation of vascular structures, AVM, aortic dissection
- Evaluation of mediastinal tumors, enlarged lymph nodes
- Hilar masses
- Neck masses

PULMONARY EMBOLISM CT PROTOCOL

- Patient in supine position
- Scan range: adrenals to lung apex
- Injection of 140 mL of nonionic iodinated contrast at 3 mL/sec, with delay of 25 to 30 seconds. Scanning is performed with suspended respiration.
- Scans are retrospectively reconstructed from the dome of the diaphragm as 2.5-mm thick slices with 1-mm spacing.

DIAGNOSTIC RADIOLOGY REPORT (ACR)

An authenticated written interpretation should be performed on all radiologic procedures. The report should include the following items:

1. Name of patient and other identifier (e.g., birth date, Social Security number, or hospital or office identification number)
2. Name of the referring physician to provide more accurate routing of the report to one or more locations specified by the referring physician (e.g., hospital, office, clinic)
3. History
4. Name or type of examination
5. Dates of the examination and transcription
6. Time of the examination (for ICU/CCU patients) to identify multiple examinations (e.g., chest) that may be performed on a single day
7. Body of the report:
   - Procedures and materials

     Include in the report a description of the procedures performed and any contrast media (agent, concentration, volume and reaction, if any), medications, catheters, and devices.
   - Findings

     Use precise anatomic and radiologic terminology to describe the findings accurately.
   - Limitations

     Where appropriate, identify factors that can limit the sensitivity and specificity of the examination. Such factors might include technical factors, patient anatomy, limitations of the technique, incomplete bowel preparation, and wrist examination for carpal scaphoid.
   - Clinical issues

     The report should address or answer any pertinent clinical issues raised in the request for the imaging examination. For example, to rule out pneumothorax state "There is no evidence of pneumothorax"; or to rule out fracture, "There is no evidence of fracture." It is not advisable to use such universal disclaimers as "The mammography examination does not exclude the possibility of cancer."
   - Comparative data

     Comparisons with previous examinations and reports when possible are a part of the radiologic consultation and report and optionally may be part of the "impression" section.
8. Impression (conclusion or diagnosis)
   - Each examination should contain an "impression" section.
   - Give a precise diagnosis whenever possible.
   - Give a differential diagnosis when appropriate.
   - Recommend, only when appropriate, follow-up and additional diagnostic radiologic studies to clarify or confirm the impression.

Infection

GENERAL

PATHOGENS

Bacterial pneumonia

- *Streptococcus pneumoniae* (pneumococcus)
- *Staphylococcus*
- *Pseudomonas*
- *Klebsiella*
- *Nocardia*
- *Chlamydia*
- *Neisseria meningitides*
- *Haemophilus influenzae*
- Anaerobes
- *Legionella*
- *Mycoplasma pneumoniae*
- *Actinomyces israelii*
- *Mycobacterium tuberculosis*

Viral pneumonia (25% of community-acquired pneumonias)
- Influenza
- Varicella, herpes zoster
- Rubeola
- Cytomegalovirus (CMV)
- Coxsackievirus, parainfluenza virus, adenovirus, respiratory syncytial virus (RSV)

Fungal pneumonia
- Histoplasmosis
- Coccidioidomycosis
- Blastomycosis
- Aspergillosis
- Cryptococcosis
- Candidiasis
- Zygomycoses

Parasitic pneumonias
- *Pneumocystis jiroveci* Frenkel 1999 (formerly *Pneumocystis carinii)*
- *Toxoplasma gondii*

ACQUISITION OF PNEUMONIA

Community-acquired pneumonia
- *S. pneumoniae, Haemophilus*
- *Mycoplasma*

Hospital-acquired pneumonia (incidence 1%, mortality 35%): nosocomial infection
- Gram negatives: *Pseudomonas, Proteus, Escherichia coli, Enterobacter, Klebsiella*
- Methicillin-resistant *Staphylococcus aureus* (MRSA)
- Vancomycin-resistant enterococcus (VRE)

Pneumonia in immunosuppressed patients
- Bacterial pneumonia (gram negative) still most common
- Tuberculosis
- Fungal
- *Pneumocystis* pneumonia (PCP)

Endemic pneumonias
- Fungal: histoplasmosis, coccidioidomycosis, blastomycosis
- Viral

Aspiration-associated pneumonia (important)

RISK FACTORS

The radiographic appearance of pulmonary infections is variable depending on pathogen, underlying lung disease, risk factors, and prior or partial treatment.

COMMUNITY-ACQUIRED INFECTIONS

Risk Factor	Common Pathogens
Alcoholism	Gram negatives, *Streptococcus pneumoniae, M. tuberculosis*, aspiration (mouth flora)
Old age	*S. pneumoniae, Staphylococcus aureus*, aspiration
Aspiration	Mouth flora (anaerobes)
Cystic fibrosis	*Pseudomonas, S. aureus, Aspergillus*
Chronic bronchitis	*S. pneumoniae, H. influenzae*

Other risk factors for developing pneumonia:
- Bronchiectasis
- Coma, anesthesia, seizures (aspiration)
- Tracheotomy
- Antibiotic treatment
- Immunosuppression (renal failure, diabetes, cancer, steroids, AIDS)
- Chronic furunculosis *(Staphylococcus)*

RADIOGRAPHIC SPECTRUM OF PULMONARY INFECTIONS

SUMMARY

Type	Pathogen	Imaging
Lobar Pneumonia		
Infection primarily involves alveoli	*S. pneumoniae*	
Spread through pores of Kohn and canals of Lambert throughout a segment and ultimately an entire lobe	*K. pneumoniae*	
Bronchi are not primarily affected and remain air-filled; therefore:	Others	
	S. aureus	
Air bronchograms	*H. influenzae*	
No volume loss because airways are open	Fungal	
Nowadays uncommon due to early treatment		
Round pneumonia (children): *S. pneumoniae*		

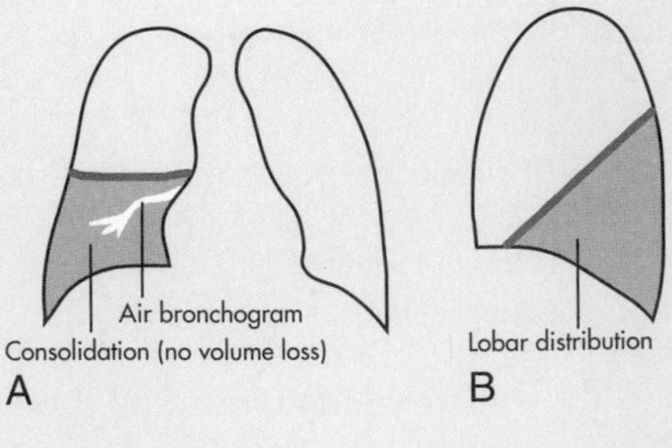

SUMMARY—cont'd

Type	Pathogen	Imaging
Bronchopneumonia Primarily affects the bronchi and adjacent alveoli Volume loss may be present as bronchi fill with exudate Bronchial spread results in multifocal patchy opacities	*S. aureus* Gram negatives Others *H. influenzae* *Mycoplasma*	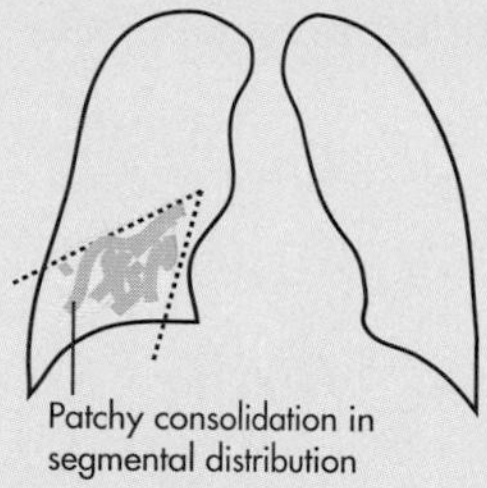
Nodules Variable in size Indistinct margins	Fungal *Histoplasma* *Aspergillus* *Cryptococcus* *Coccidioides* Bacterial *Legionella* *Nocardia* Septic emboli *S. aureus*	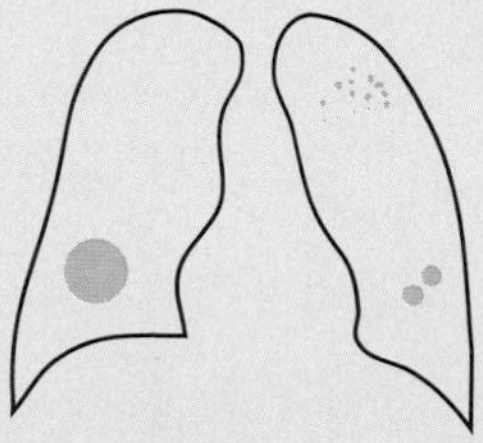
Cavitary Lesions Abscess: necrosis of lung parenchyma ± bronchial communication Fungus ball (air crescent sign) Pneumatoceles due to air leak into pulmonary interstitium *(S. aureus)*	Anaerobes Fungal TB	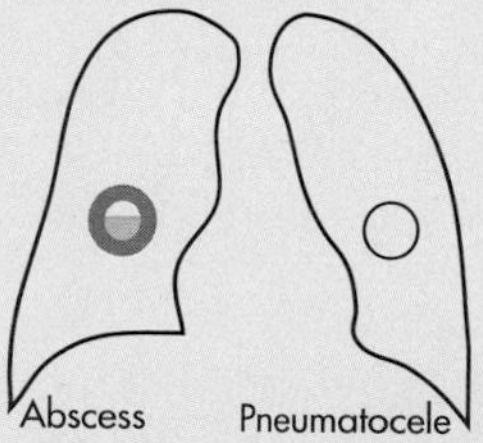
Diffuse Opacities Reticulonodular pattern: interstitial peribronchial areas of inflammation (viral) Alveolar location (PCP) Miliary pattern: hematogenous spread (TB)	Viral *Mycoplasma* PCP	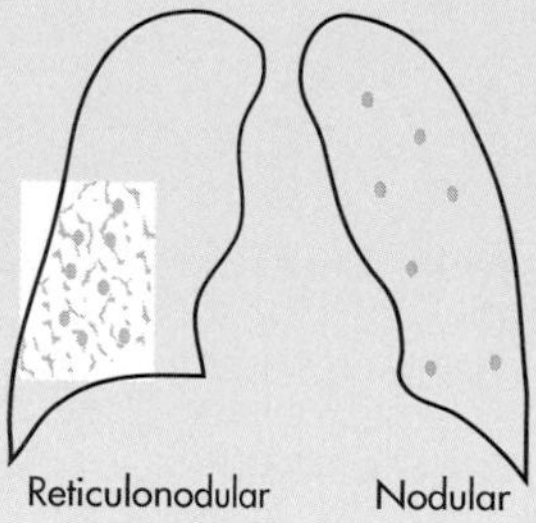

Complications of Pneumonia

- Parapneumonic effusion
  - Stage 1: exudation: free flowing
  - Stage 2: fibropurulent: loculated
  - Stage 3: organization, erosion into lung or chest wall
- Empyema
- Bronchopleural fistula (fistula between bronchus and pleural space) with eroding pleural-based fluid collections
- Bronchiectasis
- Pulmonary fibrosis, especially after necrotizing pneumonia or acute respiratory distress syndrome (ARDS)
- Adenopathy

RESOLUTION OF PNEUMONIA

- 80%-90% resolve within 4 weeks
- 5%-10% resolve within 4 to 8 weeks (usually in older or diabetic patients). Subsequent films should always show interval improvement compared with the prior films.
- Nonclearance
  - Antibiotic resistance
  - Consider other pathogen (e.g., *M. tuberculosis*)
  - Recurrent infection
  - Obstruction pneumonitis due to tumor

BACTERIAL INFECTIONS

GENERAL

Common Pathogens

- *S. pneumoniae*, 50% (40 to 60 years)
- *Mycoplasma*, 30%
- Anaerobes, 10%
- Gram negatives, 5%
- *Staphylococcus*, 5%
- *Haemophilus*, 3% (especially in infants and patients with COPD)

Clinical Findings

Pneumonic syndrome
- Fever
- Cough
- Pleuritic pain
- Sputum

Ancillary findings
- Headache, arthralgia, myalgia
- Diarrhea
- Hemoptysis

STREPTOCOCCAL PNEUMONIA

Radiographic Features

- Lobar or segmental pneumonia pattern
- Bronchopneumonia pattern
- Round pneumonia (in children)

STAPHYLOCOCCAL PNEUMONIA (Fig. 1-15)

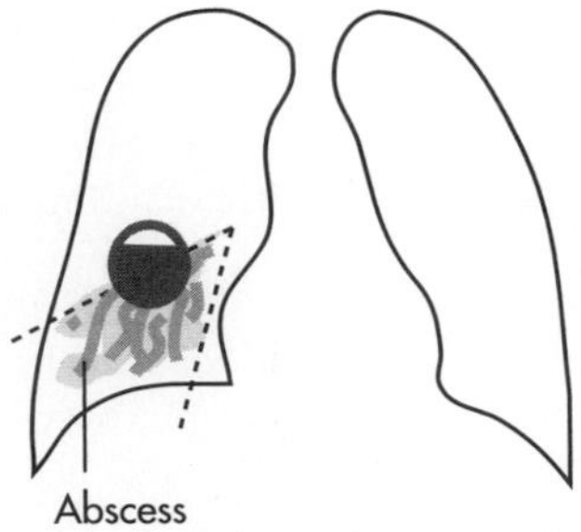

FIGURE 1-15

Radiographic Features

- Bronchopneumonia pattern
- Bilateral, >60%
- Abscess cavities, 25%-75%
- Pleural effusion, empyema, 50%
- Pneumatoceles, 50% (check valve obstruction), particularly in children
- Central lines
- Signs of endocarditis

PSEUDOMONAS PNEUMONIA

Typical Clinical Setting

- Hospital-acquired infection
- Ventilated patient
- Reduced host resistance
- Patients with cystic fibrosis

Radiographic Features

Three presentations:
- Extensive bilateral parenchymal consolidation (predilection for both lower lobes)
- Abscess formation
- Diffuse nodular disease (bacteremia with hematogenous spread; rare)

LEGIONNAIRES' DISEASE

Severe pulmonary infection caused by *Legionella pneumophila;* 35% require ventilation, 20% mortality. Most infections are community acquired. Patients have hyponatremia. Seroconversion for diagnosis takes 2 weeks.

Radiographic Features

Common features
- Initial presentation of peripheral patchy consolidation
- Bilateral severe disease
- Rapidly progressive
- Pleural effusions, <50%
- Lower lobe predilection

Uncommon features
- Abscess formation
- Lymph node enlargement

HAEMOPHILUS PNEUMONIA

Caused by *Haemophilus influenzae*. Occurs most commonly in children, immunocompromised adults, or patients with COPD. Often there is concomitant meningitis, epiglottitis, and bronchitis.

Radiographic Features

- Bronchopneumonia pattern
- Lower lobe predilection, often diffuse
- Empyema

MYCOPLASMA PNEUMONIA

Most common nonbacterial pneumonia (atypical pneumonia). Mild course. Age 5 to 20 years. Positive cold agglutinins, 60%.

Radiographic Features

- Reticular pattern
- Lower lobe predominance, often diffuse
- Consolidation, 50%

Complications

- Autoimmune hemolytic anemia
- Erythema nodosum, erythema multiforme
- Stevens-Johnson syndrome
- Meningoencephalitis

KLEBSIELLA (FRIEDLÄNDER) PNEUMONIA

Gram-negative organism. Often in debilitated patients and/or alcoholics.

Radiographic Features

- Consolidation appears similar to that of infection with *S. pneumoniae*
- Lobar expansion
- Cavitation, 30%-50%, typically multiple
- Massive necrosis (pulmonary gangrene)
- Pleural effusion uncommon

TUBERCULOSIS (TB) (Fig. 1-16)

Transmitted by inhalation of infected droplets of *Mycobacterium tuberculosis* or *M. bovis*. TB usually requires constant or repeated contact with sputum-positive patients because the tubercle does not easily grow in the immunocompetent human host. Target population includes:

- Patients of low socioeconomic scale (homeless)
- Alcoholics

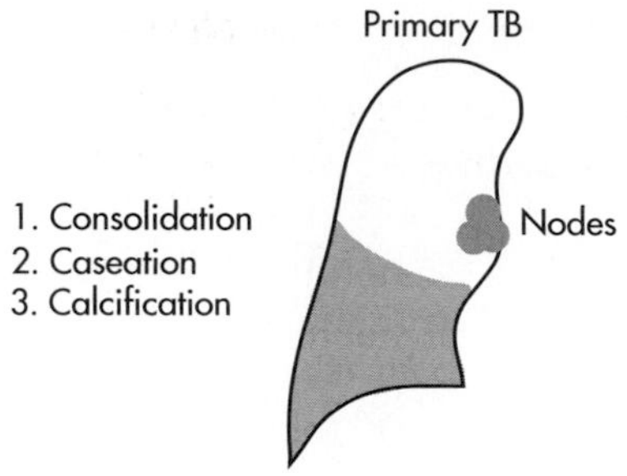

FIGURE 1-16

- Immigrants: Mexico, Philippines, Indochina, Haiti
- Elderly patients
- AIDS patients
- Prisoners

Primary Infection (Fig. 1-17)

Usually heals without complications. Sequence of events includes:

- Pulmonary consolidation (1 to 7 cm); cavitation is rare; lower lobe (60%) > upper lobes
- Caseous necrosis 2 to 10 weeks after infection
- Lymphadenopathy (hilar and paratracheal), 95%
- Pleural effusion, 10%
- Spread of a primary focus occurs primarily in children or immunosuppressed patients

Secondary Infection (Fig. 1-18)

Active disease in adults most commonly represents reactivation of a primary focus. However, primary disease is now also common in adults in developed

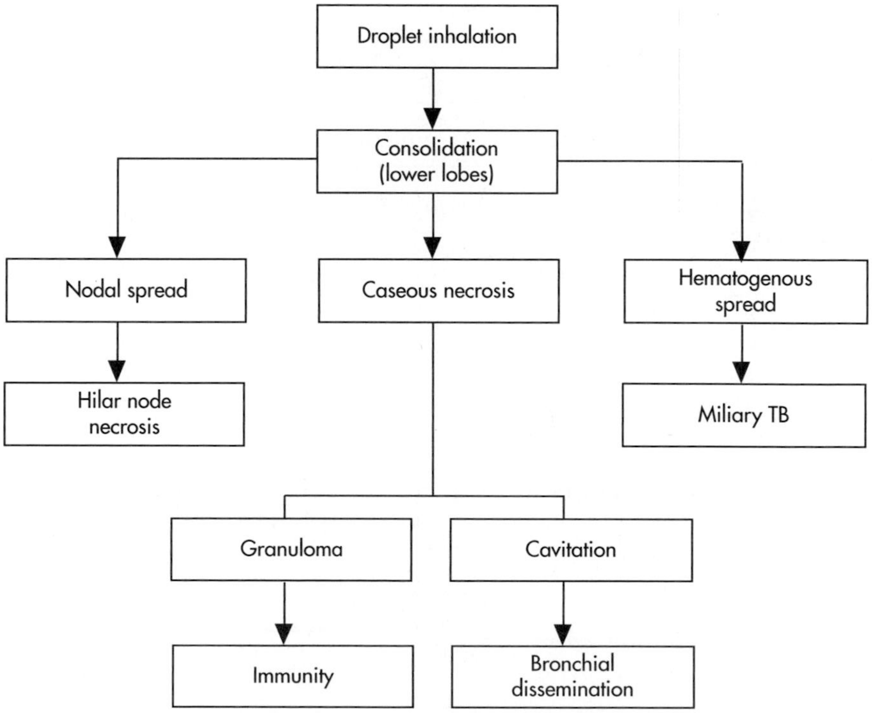

FIGURE 1-17

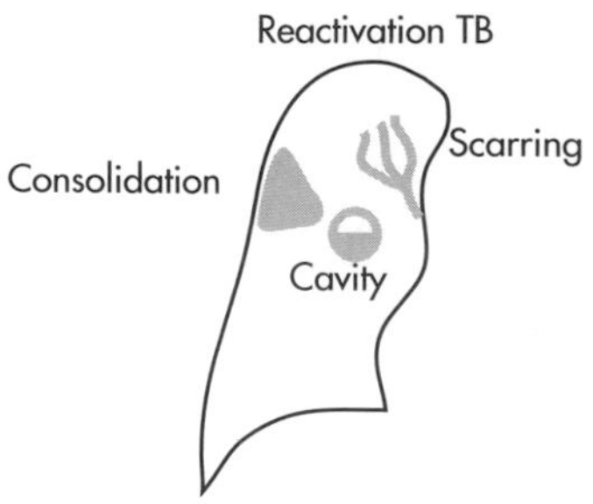

FIGURE 1-18

countries because there is no exposure in childhood. Distribution is as follows:

- Typically limited to apical and posterior segments of upper lobes or superior segments of lower lobes (because high Po_2?)
- Rarely in anterior segments of upper lobes (in contradistinction to histoplasmosis)

Radiographic Features

- Exudative tuberculosis
  Patchy or confluent airspace disease
  Adenopathy uncommon
- Fibrocalcific tuberculosis
  Sharply circumscribed linear densities radiating to hilum
- Cavitation, 40%

Complications (Fig. 1-19)

- Miliary TB may occur after primary or secondary hematogenous spread.
- Bronchogenic spread occurs after communication of the necrotic area with a bronchus; it produces an acinar pattern (irregular nodules approximately 5 mm in diameter).
- Tuberculoma (1 to 7 cm): nodule during primary or secondary TB; may contain calcification
- Effusions are often loculated.
- Bronchopleural fistula
- Pneumothorax

COMPARISON

	Primary TB	Reinfection TB
Location	Usually bases	Upper lobes, superior segment LL
Appearance	Focal	Patchy
Cavitation	No	Frequent
Adenopathy as only finding	Common	No
Effusion	Common	Uncommon
Miliary pattern	Yes	Yes

NONTUBERCULOUS MYCOBACTERIAL (NTMB) INFECTIONS

The two most common NTMB pathogens are *M. avium-intracellulare* and *M. kansasii* (less common: *M. xenopi, M. chelonei, M. gordonae, M. fortuitum* = "fast grower"). Unlike TB, NTMB infections are not acquired by human-human transmission but are a

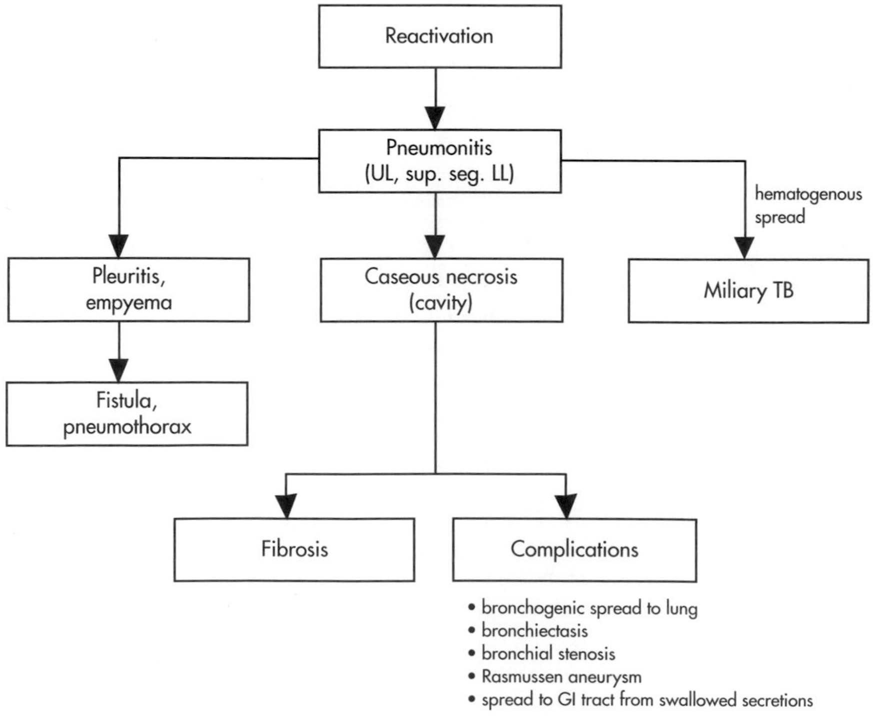

FIGURE 1-19

direct infection from soil or water. There is also no pattern of primary disease or reactivation: the infection is primary, although some may become chronic. The infection often occurs in elderly patients with COPD, older women in good health, and AIDS patients.

Radiographic Features

- NTMB infections may be indistinguishable from classic TB.
- Atypical features such as bronchiectasis and bronchial wall thickening are common.
- Nodules are common in older women.

CT FINDINGS

Findings	TB (%)	MAI %
Nodules <1 cm	80	95
Nodules 1-3 cm	40	30
Mass >3 cm	10	10
Consolidation	50	50
Cavity	30	30
Bronchiectasis	30	95
Bronchial wall thickening	40	95
Septal thickening	50	15
Emphysema	20	20
Calcified granuloma	15	5

NOCARDIA PNEUMONIA

Caused by *Nocardia asteroides,* worldwide distribution. Common opportunistic invader in:

- Lymphoma
- Steroid therapy; especially transplant patients
- Pulmonary alveolar proteinosis (common)

Radiographic Features

- Focal consolidation (more common)
- Cavitation
- Irregular nodules

ACTINOMYCOSIS

Actinomycosis is caused by *Actinomyces israelii,* a gram-positive normal saprophyte in oral cavity. Pulmonary disease develops from aspiration of organism (poor dentition) or from direct penetration into the thorax.

Radiographic Features

- Focal consolidation > cavitating mass
- Lymphadenopathy uncommon
- Extension into the chest wall and pleural thickening is less common today but still occurs and represents an important differential feature.

PULMONARY ABSCESS

The spectrum of anaerobic pulmonary infections includes:

- Abscess: single or multiple cavities >2 cm, usually with air-fluid level
- Necrotizing pneumonia: analogous to abscess but more diffuse and cavities <2 cm
- Empyema: suppurative infection of the pleural space, most commonly as a result of pneumonia

Predisposing Conditions

- Aspiration (e.g., alcoholism, neurologic disease, coma)
- Intubation
- Bronchiectasis, bronchial obstruction

Treatment

- Antibiotics, postural drainage
- Percutaneous drainage of empyema
- Drainage/resection of lung abscess only if medical therapy fails

SICKLE CELL ANEMIA

- Patients with sickle cell disease are at increased risk of pneumonia and infarction. These entities are difficult to differentiate, hence called *acute chest syndrome.*
- Pneumonias were originally due to pneumococci but now are due to viruses or *Mycoplasma.* Differential diagnosis includes atelectasis and infarct.
- Infarcts more frequent in adults than in children. Rare in children under 12 years of age.
- Consolidation is seen on chest films; resolves more slowly than in the general population, and tends to recur.

VIRAL PNEUMONIA

GENERAL

Classification

DNA viruses
- Unenveloped
  - Parvoviruses
  - Papovaviruses
  - Adenoviruses
  - Hepatitis viruses (hepatitis B)
- Enveloped
  - Herpesviruses (herpes simplex, Epstein-Barr, varicella zoster, CMV)
  - Poxviruses (variola, molluscum contagiosum)

RNA viruses
- Unenveloped
  - Picornaviruses (hepatitis A, coxsackievirus)

- Caliciviruses
- Reoviruses

Enveloped

- Retroviruses (HIV)
- Arenaviruses
- Coronaviruses
- Togaviruses
- Bunyaviruses
- Orthomyxoviruses (influenza)
- Paramyxoviruses (mumps, measles, RSV, parainfluenza)

Occurrence

Immunocompetent hosts
  Influenza
  Hantavirus
  Epstein-Barr
  Adenovirus
Immunocompromised hosts
  Herpes simplex
  Varicella-zoster
  Cytomegalovirus
  Adenovirus

Spectrum of Disease

- Acute interstitial pneumonia: diffuse or patchy interstitial pattern, thickening of bronchi, thickened interlobar septa
- Lobular inflammatory reaction: multiple nodular opacities 5 to 6 mm (varicella; late calcification)
- Hemorrhagic pulmonary edema: mimics bacterial lobar pneumonia
- Pleural effusion: usually absent or small
- Chronic interstitial fibrosis (bronchiolitis obliterans)

INFLUENZA PNEUMONIA

Influenza is very contagious and thus occurs in epidemics. Pneumonia, however, is uncommon.

Radiographic Features

- Acute phase: multiple acinar densities
- Coalescence of acinar densities to diffuse patchy airspace disease (bronchopneumonia type)

VARICELLA ZOSTER PNEUMONIA

Fifteen percent of infected patients have pneumonias; 90% are older than 20 years.

Radiographic Features

- Acute phase: multiple acinar opacities
- Coalescence of acinar opacities to diffuse patchy airspace disease
- 1- to 2-mm calcifications throughout lungs after healing

CMV PNEUMONIA

Occurs most commonly in neonates or immunosuppressed patients.

Radiographic Features

- Predominantly interstitial infection, multiple small nodules (common)
- Adenopathy may be present

SWINE-ORIGIN INFLUENZA A (H1N1) VIRUS (S-OIV) INFECTION

Epidemiologic data to date suggest that the newly emerged H1N1 virus, although transmissible from person to person, is of relatively low virulence. Chest radiographs are normal in more than half of patients. However, the disease can progress to bilateral extensive airspace disease in severely ill patients. These patients are also at a high risk for PE, which should be sought carefully on contrast enhanced CT scans.

FUNGAL INFECTIONS

GENERAL

Two broad categories:
  Endemic human mycoses (prevalent only in certain geographic areas):

- Histoplasmosis (Ohio, Mississippi, St. Lawrence River valleys)
- Coccidioidomycosis (San Joaquin Valley)
- Blastomycosis

Virus	Centrilobular Nodules	Lobar Ground-glass	Diffuse Ground-glass	Thickened Interlobular Septa	Consolidation
Influenza	+++	+++	+		+
Epstein-Barr	+	+	+		+
CMV	++	++	++	+	+
Varicella-zoster	+++	+	+		
Herpes simplex	+	+++	+		+++
Measles	++	+	+		+
Hantavirus			+++	+	++
Adenovirus	++	+			+++

Opportunistic mycoses (worldwide in distribution) occur primarily in immunocompromised patients (aspergillosis and cryptococcosis may also occur in immunocompetent hosts).
- Aspergillosis
- Candidiasis
- Cryptococcosis
- Mucormycosis

Radiographic Features
- Acute phase: pneumonic type of opacity (may be segmental, nonsegmental, or patchy); miliary (hematogenous) distribution in immunosuppressed patients
- Reparative phase: nodular lesions with or without cavitations and crescent sign
- Chronic phase: calcified lymph nodes or pulmonary focus with fungus (e.g., histoplasmosis)
- Disseminated disease (spread to other organs) occurs primarily in immunocompromised patients

HISTOPLASMOSIS (Fig. 1-20)

Histoplasma capsulatum is particularly prevalent in the Ohio, Mississippi, and St. Lawrence River valleys, although the agent is worldwide in distribution. The organism is most prevalent in soil that contains excrement of bats and birds (bat caves, chicken houses, old attics, or buildings).

Clinical Findings
Most patients are asymptomatic or have nonspecific respiratory symptoms, increased complement fixation titer, and positive *H. capsulatum* antigen.

Radiographic Features
Consolidation (primary histoplasmosis)
- Parenchymal consolidation
- Adenopathy is very common and may calcify heavily later on.

Nodular form (chronic histoplasmosis, reinfection)
- Histoplasmoma: usually solitary, sharply circumscribed nodule, most commonly in lower lobes
- Fibrocavitary disease in upper lobes indistinguishable from postprimary TB
- Cavitary nodules

Disseminated form (immunocompromised patients)
- Miliary nodules
- Calcifications in liver and spleen

Mediastinal Histoplasmosis
Mediastinal histoplasmosis may follow pulmonary histoplasmosis. Two distinct entities (which may not always be separable from each other):

Mediastinal granuloma
- Results from spread of *H. capsulatum* to lymph nodes
- Granulomas usually calcified

Mediastinal fibrosis (fibrosing mediastinitis)
- May cause superior vena cava syndrome, airway compression, PA occlusion, pericarditis
- Diffuse infiltration of mediastinum
- Multiple densely calcified nodes

COCCIDIOIDOMYCOSIS (Fig. 1-21)

Coccidioides immitis is endemic in the southwest United States (San Joaquin Valley, "valley fever") and in Central and South America. Infection occurs due to inhalation of spores in soil. Human-to-human infection does not occur.

Clinical Findings
Cutaneous manifestations common; 70% are asymptomatic.

Radiographic Features
Consolidation (primary form)
- "Fleeting" parenchymal consolidation, most commonly lower lobes
- Adenopathy in 20%

Nodular form (chronic form, 5%)
- 15% cavitate
  - 50% have thin-walled cavity (suggestive of diagnosis)
  - 50% have thick-walled cavity (i.e., nonspecific)
  - May present with pneumothorax
- Nodules rarely calcify.
- Hilar or paratracheal adenopathy

Disseminated form (immunocompromised patients; rare: 0.5% of all forms)
- Miliary nodules
- Extrapulmonary spread

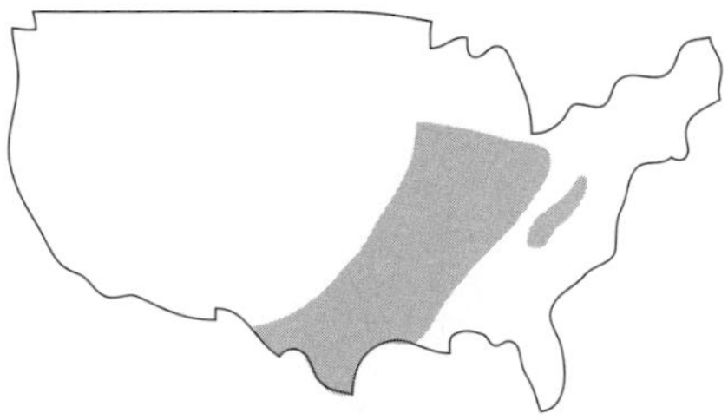

FIGURE 1-20

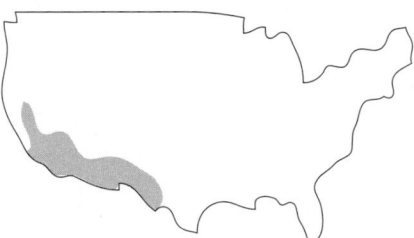

FIGURE 1-21

NORTH AMERICAN BLASTOMYCOSIS (Fig. 1-22)

- Caused by *Blastomyces dermatitidis;* uncommon infection. Most infections are self-limited.
- CXR is nonspecific: airspace disease > nodule (15% cavitate) or solitary mass > miliary spread.
- Focal blastomycosis typically occurs in paramediastinal location and has an air bronchogram, findings that may suggest the diagnosis.
- Satellite nodules around primary focus are common.
- Adenopathy, pleural effusions, and calcifications are very uncommon.
- Bone lesions, 25%
- Skin lesions are common.

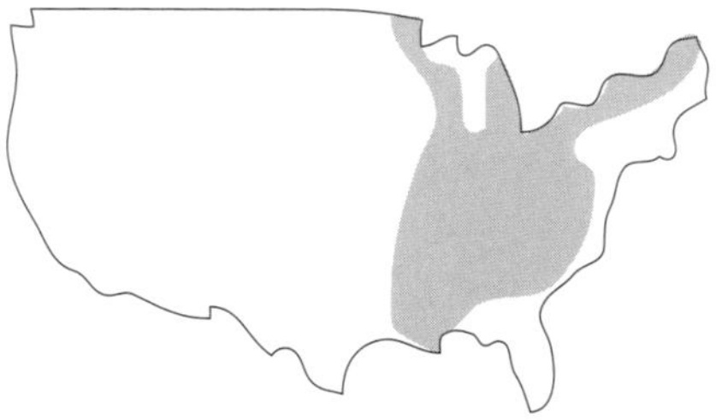

FIGURE 1-22

ASPERGILLOSIS (Fig. 1-23)

Aspergillus is a ubiquitous fungus that, when inhaled, leads to significant lung damage. The fungus grows in soil, water, decaying vegetation, and hospital air vents. Infection with *A. fumigatus* > *A. flavus, A. niger,* or *A. glaucus*. There are four unique forms of pulmonary aspergillosis, each associated with a specific immune status.

TYPES OF ASPERGILLOSIS

Type	Lung Structure	Immune Status	Pathology
Allergic (ABPA)	Normal	Hypersensitivity	Hypersensitivity → bronchiectasis, mucus plugging
Aspergilloma	Preexisting cavity	Normal	Saprophytic growth in preexisting cavity
Invasive	Normal	Severely impaired	Vascular invasion, parenchymal necrosis
Semi-invasive	Normal	Normal or impaired	Chronic local growth, local cavity formation

ALLERGIC BRONCHOPULMONARY ASPERGILLOSIS (ABPA)

ABPA represents a complex hypersensitivity reaction (type 1) to *Aspergillus,* occurring almost exclusively in patients with asthma and occasionally cystic fibrosis. The hypersensitivity initially causes bronchospasm and bronchial wall edema (IgE mediated); ultimately there is bronchial wall damage, bronchiectasis, and pulmonary fibrosis.

Clinical Findings

Elevated *Aspergillus*-specific IgE, elevated precipitating IgG against *Aspergillus,* peripheral eosinophilia, positive skin test. Treatment is with oral prednisone.

Radiographic Features

- Fleeting pulmonary alveolar opacities (common manifestation)
- Central, upper lobe saccular bronchiectasis (hallmark) (Fig. 1-24A)
- Mucus plugging ("finger-in-glove" appearance) (Fig. 1-24B) and bronchial wall thickening (common)
- Chronic disease may progress to pulmonary fibrosis predominantly in upper lobe (end stage).
- Cavitation, 10%

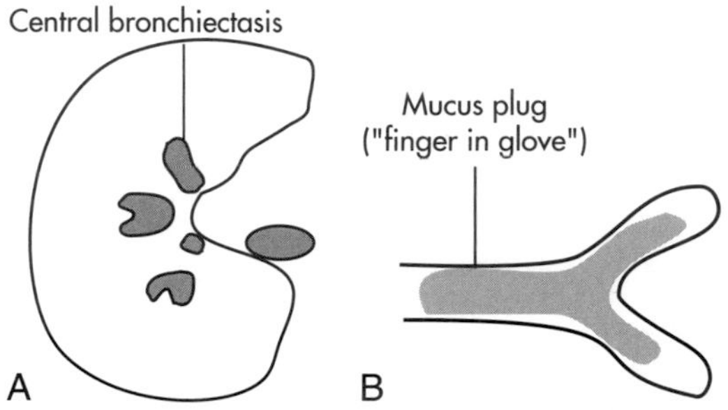

FIGURE 1-24

ASPERGILLOMA (MYCETOMA, FUNGUS BALL)

Represents a saprophytic infection in preexisting structural lung disease (cavitary or bulla from TB, end-stage sarcoid, emphysema). Commonly in upper lobes, solitary lesions. The fungus grows in the cavity, creating a "fungus ball" consisting of fungus, mucus, and inflammatory cells. Treatment is with

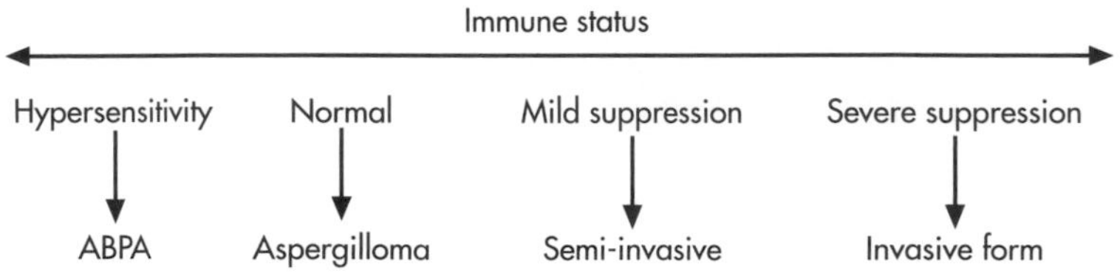

FIGURE 1-23

surgical resection and intracavitary administration of amphotericin.

Radiographic Features

- Focal intracavitary mass (3 to 6 cm), typically in upper lobes
- Air may surround the aspergilloma (Monod sign), mimicking the appearance of cavitation seen with invasive aspergillosis.
- Small area of consolidation around cavity is typical.
- Adjacent pleural thickening common
- Fungus ball moves with changing position

INVASIVE ASPERGILLOSIS

Invasive aspergillosis has a high mortality (70%-90%) and occurs mainly in severely immunocompromised patients (bone marrow transplants, leukemia). The infection starts with endobronchial fungal proliferation and then leads to vascular invasion with thrombosis and infarction of lung ("angioinvasive infection"). Additional sites of infection (in 30%) are brain, liver, kidney, GI tract. Treatment is with systemic and/or intracavitary administration of amphotericin.

Radiographic Features (Fig. 1-25)

- Multiple pulmonary nodules, 40%
- Nodules have a characteristic halo of ground-glass appearance (represents pulmonary hemorrhage)
- Within 2 weeks, 50% of nodules undergo cavitation, which results in the air crescent sign. The appearance of the air crescent sign indicates the recovery phase (increased granulocytic response). Note that the air crescent sign may also be seen in TB, actinomycosis, mucormycosis, septic emboli, and tumors. Do not confuse the air crescent sign with the Monod sign (clinical history helps to differentiate).
- Other manifestations:
  Peribronchial opacities
  Focal areas of consolidation

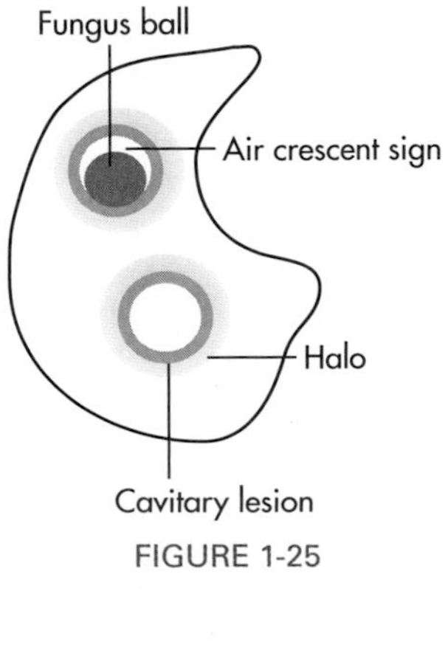

FIGURE 1-25

SEMI-INVASIVE ASPERGILLOSIS

This form of aspergillosis occurs in mildly immunocompromised patients and has a pathophysiology similar to that of invasive aspergillosis except that the disease progresses more chronically over months (mortality: 30%). Risk factors include diabetes, alcoholism, pneumoconiosis, malnutrition, and COPD. Treatment is with systemic and/or intracavitary administration of amphotericin.

Radiographic Features

- Appearance similar to that of invasive aspergillosis
- Cavitation occurs at 6 months after infection

CRYPTOCOCCOSIS

Caused by *Cryptococcus neoformans,* which is worldwide in distribution and ubiquitous in soil and pigeon excreta. Infection occurs through inhalation of contaminated dust.

Clinical Findings

Common in patients with lymphoma, steroid therapy, diabetes, and AIDS.

Radiographic Features

- Most common findings in lung are pulmonary mass, multiple nodules, or segmental or lobar consolidation.
- Cavitation, adenopathy, and effusions are rare.
- Disseminated form: CNS, other organs

CANDIDIASIS

Caused by *Candida albicans* > other *Candida* species.

Clinical Findings

Typically in patients with lymphoreticular malignancy; suspect pulmonary disease if associated with oral disease. Often there is disseminated fungemia.

Radiographic Features

- Plain film is nonspecific: opacities (lower lobe) > nodules
- Nodular disease in disseminated form
- Pleural effusion, 25%
- Cavitation and adenopathy are rare.

ZYGOMYCOSES

Group of severe opportunistic mycoses caused by fungi of the Zygomycetes class:

- Mucormycosis *(Mucor)*
- *Rhizopus*
- *Absidia*

Zygomycoses usually have two major clinical manifestations:

- Pulmonary mucormycosis
- Rhinocerebral mucormycosis

Zygomycoses are uncommon infections and occur primarily in immunocompromised patients (leukemia, AIDS, chronic steroid use, diabetes).

Radiographic Features

- Radiographic features similar to those of invasive aspergillosis because of angioinvasive behavior of fungi

AIDS

GENERAL

Acquired immunodeficiency syndrome is caused by HTLV type III (human T-cell lymphotrophic virus = HIV [human immunodeficiency virus]). HIV-1 and HIV-2 viruses are single-stranded RNA viruses that bind to CD4 present on T lymphocytes (other cells: glial cells, lung monocytes, dendritic cells in lymph nodes). The viral RNA genome is copied into DNA with the help of reverse transcriptase and integrated into the host cellular DNA.

EPIDEMIOLOGY

The U.S. Centers for Disease Control and Prevention (CDC) estimates that at the end of 2008, there were 682,668 people living with a diagnosis of HIV infection in the 50 states and five U.S.–dependent areas. However, the total number of people living with an HIV infection in the U.S. is thought to be more than 1 million. Groups at highest risk include:

- Homosexual males, bisexual males, 60%
- IV drug abusers (IVDAs), 25%
- Recipients of blood products, 3%
- Congenital from AIDS-positive mothers
- Heterosexual females: most rapidly growing group due to partners who are IVDAs

Known routes of HIV transmission:

- Blood and blood products
- Sexual activity
- In utero transmission
- During delivery

CLINICAL FINDINGS

- Lymphadenopathy
- Opportunistic infections
- Tumors: lymphoma, Kaposi sarcoma
- Other manifestations:
  - Lymphocytic interstitial pneumonia (LIP)
  - Spontaneous pneumothorax (development of cystic spaces, interstitial fibrosis related to PCP)
  - Septic emboli

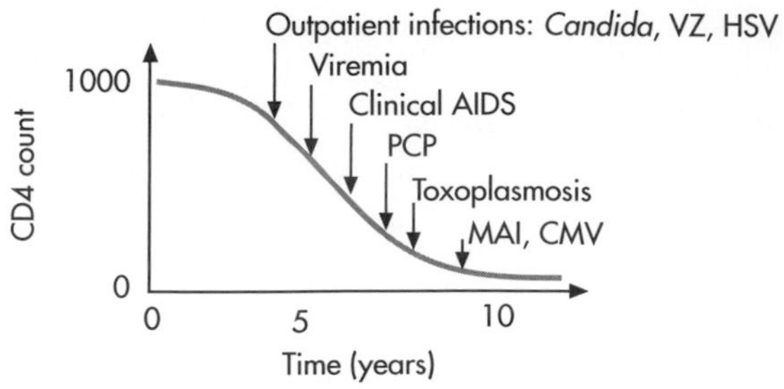

FIGURE 1-26

- Clinical findings supportive of AIDS: (Fig. 1-26)
  - CD4 count <200/mm^3; the dysfunction of the immune system is inversely related to the CD4 count; PCP: CD4 <200 cells/mm^3, MAI: CD4 <50 cells/mm^3
  - >1 case of bacterial pneumonia per year

Opportunistic Infections

- *Pneumocystis jiroveci* Frenkel 1999, 70%
- Mycobacterial infection, 20%; CD4 counts often <50 cells/mm^3
- Bacterial infection, 10% *(S. pneumoniae, Haemophilus)*
- Fungal infection (<5% of AIDS patients)
- *Nocardia,* <5%: cavitating pneumonia
- CMV pneumonia (common at autopsy)

CHEST

GENERAL

- 50% of all AIDS patients have pulmonary manifestations of infection or tumor.
- A normal CXR does not exclude the diagnosis of PCP.
- CMV is common at autopsy but does not cause significant morbidity or mortality; CMV antibody titers are present in virtually all patients with AIDS.
- Use of chest CT in AIDS patients:
  - Symptomatic patient with normal CXR; however, patients will commonly first undergo induced sputum or bronchoscopy or be put on empirical treatment for PCP.
  - To clarify confusing CXR
  - Workup of focal opacities, adenopathy, nodules

SPECTRUM OF CHEST MANIFESTATIONS (Fig. 1-27)

Nodules

- Kaposi sarcoma (usually associated with skin lesions)
- Septic infarcts (rapid size increase)
- Fungal: *Cryptococcus, Aspergillus*

Large opacity: consolidation, mass

- Hemorrhage
- NHL

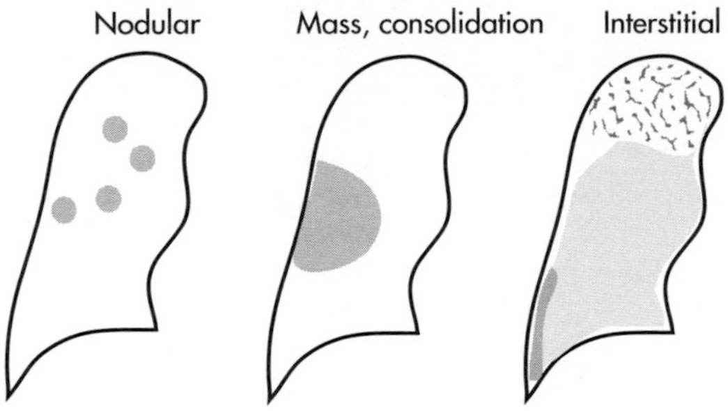

FIGURE 1-27

- Pneumonia
- Linear or interstitial opacities
- PCP
- Atypical mycobacteria
- Kaposi sarcoma

Lymphadenopathy

- Mycobacterial infections
- Kaposi sarcoma
- Lymphoma
- Reactive hyperplasia, rare in thorax

Pleural effusion

- Kaposi sarcoma
- Mycobacterial, fungal infection
- Pyogenic empyema

PCP infection (Figs. 1-28 through 1-30)

Radiographic Features

- Interstitial pattern, 80%
  - CXR: bilateral perihilar or diffuse
  - HRCT: ground-glass appearance, predominantly in upper lobe with cysts
- Progression to diffuse consolidation within days
- Normal CXR in the presence of pulmonary PCP infection, 10%
- Multiple upper lobe air-filled cysts or pneumatoceles (10%) causing:
  - Pneumothorax
  - Bronchopleural fistulas

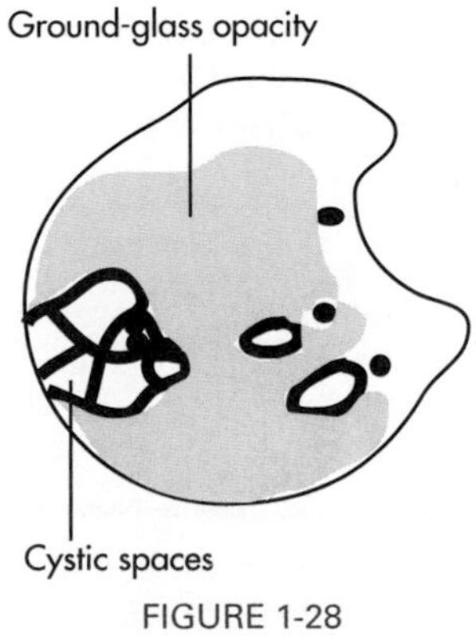

FIGURE 1-28

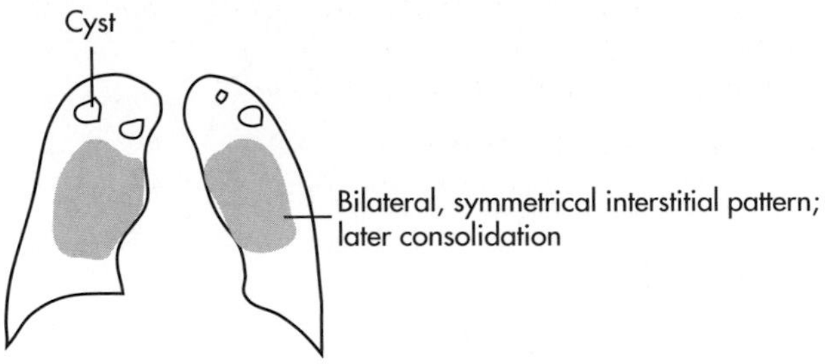

FIGURE 1-29

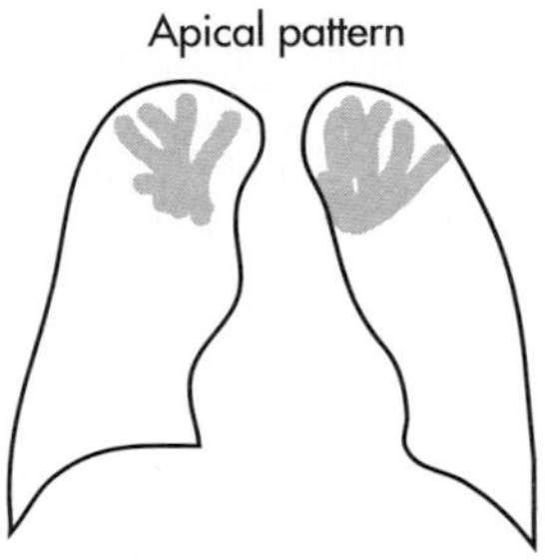

FIGURE 1-30

- Upper lobe PCP involvement is common, because aerosolized pentamidine may not get to upper lobes; upper lobe disease may mimic TB but the latter may have pleural effusions or lymphadenopathy, both of which are uncommon in PCP.
- Atypical patterns, 5%
  - Unilateral disease
  - Focal lesions, cavitary nodules
- PCP as a presenting manifestation of AIDS is decreasing because of effective prophylaxis.

MYCOBACTERIAL INFECTION

M. tuberculosis > *M. avium-intracellulare* (this pathogen usually causes extrathoracic disease). CD4 cell count usually <50 cells/mm^3.

Radiographic Features

- Hilar and mediastinal adenopathy common
  - Necrotic lymph nodes (TB) have a low attenuation center and only rim enhance with contrast.
  - MTB is more commonly associated with necrosis from MAI.
  - Adenopathy in Kaposi sarcoma or lymphoma enhances uniformly.
- Pleural effusion
- Other findings are similar to non-AIDS TB (upper lobe consolidations, cavitations)

FUNGAL INFECTIONS

Fungal infections in AIDS are uncommon (<5% of patients).

- Cryptococcosis (most common); 90% have CNS involvement.
- Histoplasmosis: nodular or miliary pattern most common; 35% have normal CXR.
- Coccidioidomycosis: diffuse interstitial pattern, thin-walled cavities

KAPOSI SARCOMA (Fig. 1-31)

The most common tumors in AIDS are:
- Kaposi sarcoma (15% of patients); incidence declining; M:F = 50:1.
- Lymphoma (<5% of patients)

Pulmonary manifestations of Kaposi sarcoma (almost always preceded by cutaneous/visceral involvement):
- Nodules
  - 1 to 3 cm
  - Single or multiple
  - Virtually always associated with skin lesions
- Coarse linear opacities emanating from hilum
- Pleural effusions (serosanguineous), 40%
- Adenopathy
- Lymphangitic tumor spread

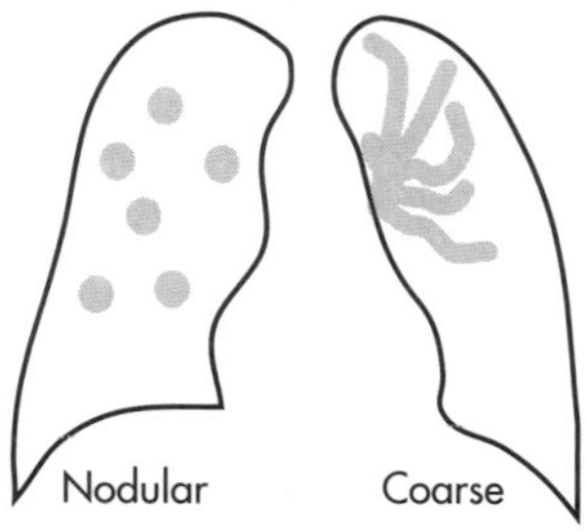

FIGURE 1-31

AIDS-RELATED LYMPHOMA

Non-Hodgkin lymphoma (usually aggressive B-cell type) > Hodgkin lymphoma.

Poor prognosis. Spectrum includes:
- Solitary or multiple pulmonary masses ± air bronchogram, 25%
- AIDS-related lymphoma is typically an extranodal disease (CNS, GI tract, liver, bone marrow): adenopathy not very prominent.
- Pleural effusions are common.

Neoplasm

GENERAL

LOCATION

Chest neoplasms are best categorized by their primary location:
- Lung tumors
- Pleural tumors
- Mediastinal tumors
- Tumors of the airway
- Chest wall tumors

CLASSIFICATION OF PULMONARY NEOPLASM

Malignant tumors
- Bronchogenic carcinoma
- Lymphoma
- Metastases
- Sarcomas, rare

Low-grade malignancies (previously bronchial adenoma)
- Carcinoid, 90%
- Adenoid cystic carcinoma (previously cylindroma, resembles salivary gland tumor), 6%
- Mucoepidermoid carcinoma, 3%
- Pleomorphic carcinoma, 1%

Benign tumors, rare
- Hamartoma
- Papilloma
- Leiomyoma
- Hemangioma
- Chemodectoma
- Pulmonary blastoma
- Chondroma
- Multiple pulmonary fibroleiomyomas
- Pseudolymphoma

PERCUTANEOVUS BIOPSY

The true positive rate of percutaneous lung biopsy is 90%-95%. False-negative results are usually due to poor needle placement, necrotic tissue, and so on. Tumor seeding is extremely uncommon (1:20,000).

Contraindications to biopsy are usually relative and include:
- Severe COPD
- Pulmonary hypertension
- Coagulopathy
- Contralateral pneumonectomy
- Suspected echinococcal cysts

Technique

1. Fluoroscopic or CT localization of nodule
2. Pass needle over superior border of rib to avoid intercostal vessels
3. Avoid passing through fissures
4. Coaxial needle system
   - 20-gauge outer needle
   - 22-gauge inner needle
5. Cytopathologist should be present to determine if sample is adequate and diagnostic.
6. Chest film after procedure to determine presence of pneumothorax

Complications

- Pneumothorax, 25%; 5%-10% require a chest tube (i.e., pneumothorax >25% or if patient is symptomatic)
- Hemoptysis, 3%

BRONCHOGENIC CARCINOMA

Bronchogenic carcinoma refers broadly to any carcinoma of the bronchus. However, the use of the term is usually restricted to the following entities:

CLASSIFICATION

Adenocarcinoma (most common), 40%
- Bronchoalveolar carcinoma (often PET negative)
- Papillary adenocarcinoma
- Acinar adenocarcinoma
- Solid adenocarcinoma with mucus formation

Squamous cell carcinoma, 30%
- Spindle cell carcinoma

Small cell carcinoma, 15%
- Oat cell
- Intermediate cell type
- Combined oat cell carcinoma

Large cell carcinoma, 1%
- Giant cell carcinoma
- Clear cell carcinoma

Adenosquamous tumor

RISK FACTORS FOR BRONCHOGENIC CARCINOMA

- Smoking: 98% of male patients and 87% of female patients with lung cancer smoke; 10% of heavy smokers will develop lung cancer. The strongest relationship between smoking and cancer has been established for SCC, followed by adenocarcinoma; the least common association is for bronchoalveolar carcinoma.
- Radiation, uranium miners
- Asbestos exposure
- Genetic predisposition (HLA-Bw44 associated?)

RADIOGRAPHIC SPECTRUM

Primary Signs of Malignancy (Fig. 1-32)
- Mass (>6 cm) or nodule (<6 cm) with spiculated, irregular borders

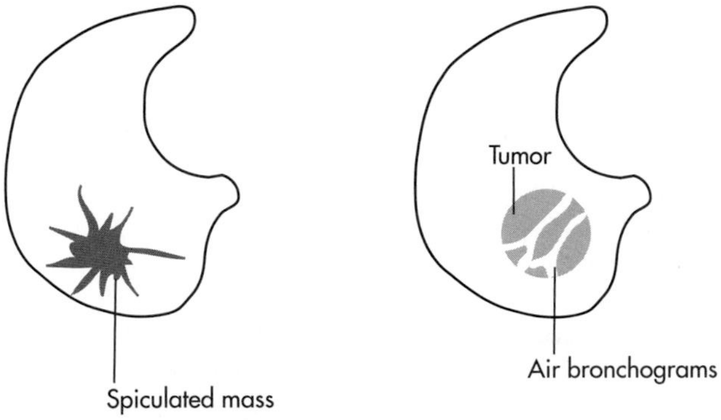

FIGURE 1-32

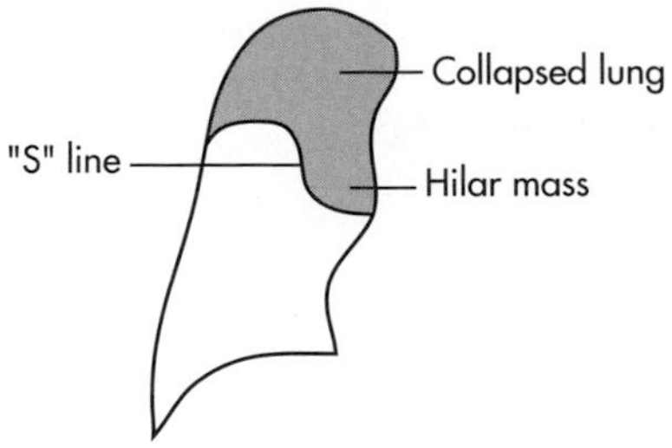

FIGURE 1-33

- Unilateral enlargement of hilum: mediastinal widening, hilar prominence
- Cavitation
  - Most common in upper lobes or superior segments of lower lobes
  - Wall thickness is indicative of malignancy.
  - <4 mm: 95% of cavitated lesions are benign.
  - >15 mm: 85% of cavitated lesions are malignant.
  - Cavitation is most common in SCC.
- Certain tumors may present as chronic airspace disease: bronchoalveolar carcinoma, lymphoma.
- Some air bronchograms are commonly seen by HRCT in adenocarcinoma.

Secondary Signs of Malignancy (Fig. 1-33)
- Atelectasis (Golden inverted "S" sign in RUL, LUL collapse)
- Obstructive pneumonia
- Pleural effusion
- Interstitial patterns: lymphangitic tumor spread
- Hilar and mediastinal adenopathy
- Metastases to ipsilateral, contralateral lung

LOCATIONS OF TUMORS

Tumor	Frequency	Location	Comments
Adenocarcinoma	40%	Peripheral	Scar carcinoma
Squamous cell carcinoma	30%	Central, peripheral*	Cavitation
Small cell carcinoma	15%	Central, peripheral*	Endocrine activity
Large cell carcinoma	1%	Central, peripheral	Large mass

*Rarely present as a resectable T1 lesion.

PARANEOPLASTIC SYNDROMES OF LUNG CANCER

Incidence: 2% of bronchogenic carcinoma

Metabolic
- Cushing syndrome (ACTH)
- Inappropriate antidiuresis (ADH)
- Carcinoid syndrome (serotonin, other vasoactive substances)
- Hypercalcemia (PTH, bone metastases)
- Hypoglycemia (insulin-like factor)

Musculoskeletal
- Neuromyopathies

- Clubbing of fingers (HPO)

Other

- Acanthosis nigricans
- Thrombophlebitis
- Anemia

RADIATION PNEUMONITIS

Radiation pneumonitis represents the acute phase of radiation damage and usually appears 3 weeks after treatment. Minimum radiation to induce pneumonitis is 30 Gy. The acute phase is typically asymptomatic but may be associated with fever and cough. Fibrosis usually occurs after 6 to 12 months.

Radiographic Features

- Diffuse opacities in radiation port
- HRCT allows better assessment of extent than plain film.

TUMOR STAGING (Fig. 1-34)

TNM STAGING SYSTEM, 7TH EDITION (NON–SMALL CELL LUNG CANCER)

Primary tumor (T)

T0 No evidence of a primary tumor

T1 <3 cm, limited to lung, not more proximal than lobar bronchus

T1a ≤ 2 cm

T1b >2 and ≤ 3 cm

T2 >3 cm but ≤ 7 cm;

- or invades parietal pleura
- or involves main bronchus ≥ 2 cm distal to carina
- or atelectasis/obstructive pneumonia extending to hilum but not involving entire lung

T2a >3 but ≤ 5 cm

T2b >5 but ≤ 7 cm

T3 >7 cm;

- or directly invades chest wall, diaphragm, phrenic nerve, mediastinal pleura, parietal pericardium
- or mainstem bronchus <2 cm distal to carina
- or atelectasis/obstructive pneumonia involving entire lung

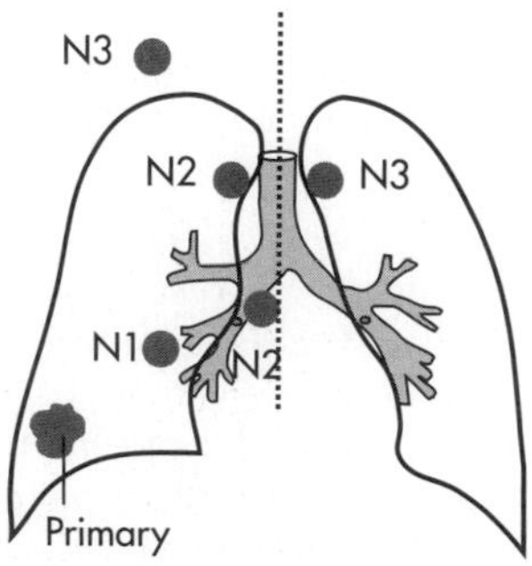

FIGURE 1-34

- or separate tumor nodules in a different ipsilateral lobe

T4 Heart, great vessels, trachea, recurrent laryngeal nerve, esophagus, vertebral body, or carina; or separate tumor nodules in a different ipsilateral lobe

Nodes (N)

N0 No lymph node involvement

N1 Ipsilateral hilar nodes

N2 Ipsilateral mediastinal or subcarinal nodes

N3 Contralateral hilar or mediastinal nodes; supraclavicular nodes

Metastases (M)

M0 No metastases

M1 Metastases

M1a Separate tumor nodules in contralateral lobe; or pleural nodules or malignant pleural dissemination

M1b Distant metastases

Unresectable Stages

- Tumors are unresectable if T4, N3, or M1 (stage 3b or 4)
- Stage 3b: N3, M0, any T; T4, M0, any N
- Stage 4: M1, any T, any N

5-YEAR SURVIVAL

Overall 5-year survival rate is 14%.

Stage 1: 57%-67%
Stage 2: 39%-55%
Stage 3a (limited disease): 23%
Stage 3b (T4): 7%
Stage 3b (N3): 3%
Stage 4: 1%

SMALL CELL CANCER STAGING

Although the TNM system can also be used for small cell cancer, it is often not used because of the presence of metastasis at the time of diagnosis. Instead, a two-stage system is used: “limited” and “extensive.” *Limited* stage means the cancer is confined to one lung with ipsilateral lymph node metastasis (can be encompassed by a single radiation port) and has better prognosis. *Extensive* stage means metastasis to contralateral lung and nodes or to distant organs (including the pleura). About two thirds of patients with small cell cancer are at the extensive stage at first diagnosis.

LYMPH NODE IMAGING

Anatomy (Fig. 1-35)

Anterior mediastinal nodes

- Parietal node group
  - Internal mammary nodes
  - Superior diaphragmatic nodes
- Prevascular node group (anterior to the great vessels)

Middle mediastinal nodes

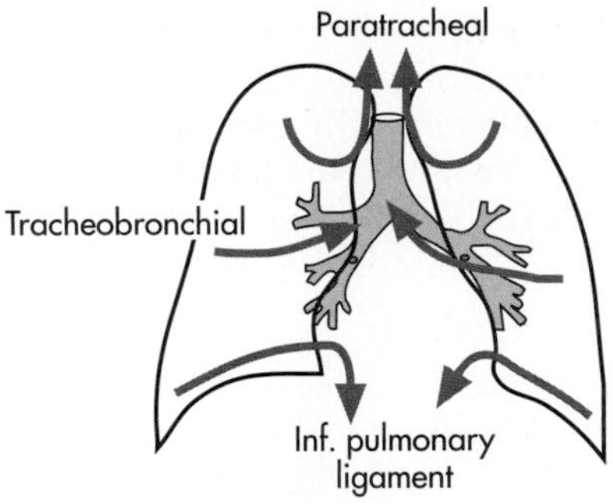

FIGURE 1-35

- Paratracheal*; the lowest node is the azygos node
- Subcarinal*: below bifurcation; drainage to right paratracheal nodes
- Subaortic; AP window node
- Tracheobronchial (pulmonary root, hilar)

Posterior mediastinal nodes
- Paraaortic
- Prevertebral
- Paraspinous: lateral to vertebral body

American Thoracic Society Classification (Fig. 1-36)

This classification system assigns numbers to regional lymph nodes:
- 2R, 2L: paratracheal
- 4R, 4L: superior tracheobronchial
- 5, 6: anterior mediastinal
- 7: subcarinal
- 8, 9: posterior mediastinal
- 10R, 10L: bronchopulmonary
- 11R, 11L: pulmonary
- 14: diaphragmatic

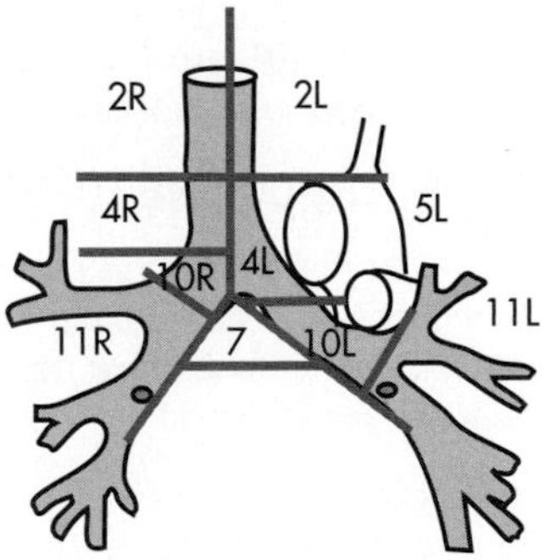

FIGURE 1-36

CT Criterion for Abnormal Nodes

Short-axis lymph node diameter >1 cm (60%-70% accuracy for differentiating between malignant and benign adenopathy)

*These nodes are best assessed by mediastinoscopy; the remainder of nodes are best assessed by CT.

CHEST WALL INVASION

Accuracy for detection of chest wall invasion by CT is 40%-60%.

Radiographic Features (Fig. 1-37)

Reliable signs
- Soft tissue mass in chest wall
- Bone destruction

Unreliable signs
- Obtuse angles at contact between tumor and pleura
- >3 cm of contact between tumor and pleura
- Pleural thickening
- Increased density of extrapleural fat

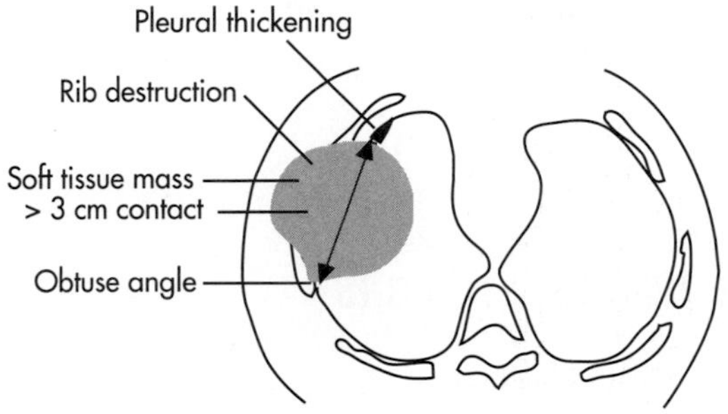

FIGURE 1-37

MEDIASTINAL INVASION

Contiguous invasion of mediastinal organs, heart, great vessels, aerodigestive tract, and vertebra indicates nonresectability.

Radiographic Features

- Diaphragmatic paralysis (phrenic nerve involvement)
- Mediastinal mass with encasement of mediastinal structures
- MRI may be useful to detect vascular invasion.

MALIGNANT PLEURAL EFFUSION

Development of pleural effusions usually indicates a poor prognosis. Presence of a documented malignant pleural effusion makes a tumor unresectable (M1). Incidence of pleural effusion:
- Bronchogenic carcinoma, 50%
- Metastases, 50%
- Lymphoma, 15%

Pathogenesis of Malignant Effusions

- Pleural invasion increases capillary permeability.
- Lymphatic or venous obstruction decreases clearance of pleural fluid.
- Bronchial obstruction → atelectasis → decrease in intrapleural pressure.

CENTRAL BRONCHIAL INVOLVEMENT

Tumors that involve a central bronchus usually cause lung collapse or consolidation. These tumors are considered unresectable (T4 tumors) only if they involve the carina.

METASTASES TO OTHER ORGANS

Lung tumors most frequently metastasize to:

Liver (common)

Adrenal glands (common)

- 30% of adrenal masses in patients with adenocarcinoma are adenomas.
- Most adrenal masses in patients with small cell carcinomas are metastases.
- Tumor may be present in a morphologically normal-appearing gland.

Other sites (especially small and large cell tumors)

- Brain (common)
- Bones
- Kidney

SPECIFIC LUNG TUMORS

ADENOCARCINOMA

Now the most frequent primary lung cancer. Typically presents as a multilobulated, peripheral mass. May arise in scar tissue: scar carcinoma.

BRONCHIOLOALVEOLAR CARCINOMA

Subtype of adenocarcinoma; slow growth. The characteristic radiographic presentations are:

- Morphologic type
  - Small peripheral nodule (solitary form), 25% (most common)
  - Multiple nodules
  - Chronic airspace disease
- Air bronchogram
- Absent adenopathy
- Cavitation may be seen by HRCT (Cheerio sign)

SQUAMOUS CELL CARCINOMA (SCC)

SCC is most directly linked with smoking. SCC carries the most favorable prognosis. The most characteristic radiographic appearances are:

- Cavitating lung mass, 30%
- Peripheral nodule, 30%
- Central obstructing lesion causing lobar collapse
- Chest wall invasion

PANCOAST TUMOR (SUPERIOR SULCUS TUMOR)

Tumor located in the lung apex that has extended into the adjacent chest wall. Histologically, Pancoast tumors are often SCC.

Clinical Findings

- Horner syndrome
- Pain radiating into arm (invasion of pleura, bone, brachial plexus, or subclavian vessels)

Radiographic Features (Fig. 1-38)

- Apical mass
- Chest wall invasion
- Involvement of subclavian vessels
- Brachial plexus involvement
- Bone involvement: rib, vertebral body

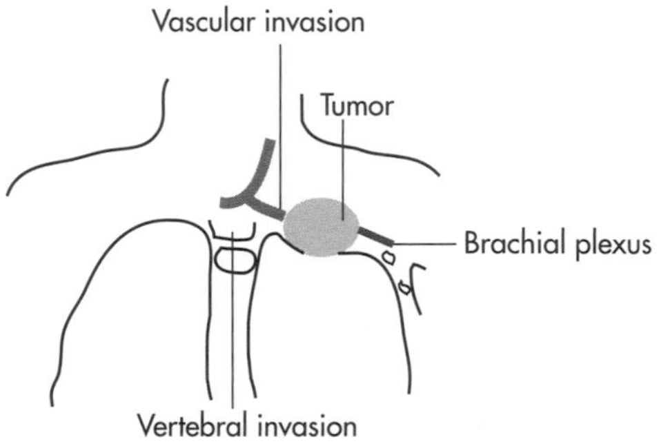

FIGURE 1-38

SMALL CELL CARCINOMA (NEUROENDOCRINE TUMOR, TYPE 3)

Most aggressive lung tumor with poor prognosis. At diagnosis, two thirds of patients already have extrathoracic spread:

- Typical initial presentation: massive bilateral lymphadenopathy
- With or without lobar collapse
- Brain metastases

LARGE CELL CARCINOMA

Usually presents as large (>70% are >4 cm at initial diagnosis) peripheral mass lesions. Overall uncommon tumor.

CARCINOID (NEUROENDOCRINE TUMOR, TYPES 1 AND 2)

Represent 90% of low-grade malignancy tumors of the lung. The 10-year survival with surgical treatment is 85%.

Types

- Typical carcinoid: local tumor (type 1)
- Atypical carcinoid (10%-20%): metastasizes to regional lymph nodes (type 2); liver metastases are very rare.

Radiographic Features

PET negative

Centrally located carcinoid, 80%

- Segmental or lobar collapse (most common finding)

- Periodic exacerbation of atelectasis
- Endobronchial mass

Peripherally located carcinoid, 20%
- Pulmonary nodule
- May enhance with contrast

COMPARISON OF CLINICAL, PATHOLOGIC, AND IMAGING FINDINGS IN NEUROENDOCRINE TUMORS OF THE LUNG

Findings	Typical Carcinoid	Atypical Carcinoid	LCNEC	SCLC
Demographic Features				
Mean patient age (yr)	40-49	50-59	60-69	70-79
Association with smoking	No	Yes	Yes	Yes
M:F ratio	1:1	2:1	>2.5:1	>2.5:1
Histopathologic Features				
Mitoses per 10 HPFs	<2	2-10	>10	>50
Necrosis	No	Yes	Yes	Yes
Imaging Findings				
Central to peripheral ratio	3:1	3:1	1:4	10-20:1
Calcification or ossification	30%	30%	9%	Up to 23%
Extrathoracic metastases	15%	15%	35%	60%-70%
Enhancement	High; central or rim	High; central or rim	High	High with necrosis
FDG uptake at PET	Low	Low	High	High

FDG, fluorodeoxyglucose; HPF, high-power field; LCNEC, large cell neuroendocrine carcinoma; SCLC, small cell lung cancer.

HAMARTOMA (Fig. 1-39)

Hamartomas are the most common benign tumors of the lung composed of cartilage (predominant component), connective tissue, muscle, fat, and bone. 90% are peripheral, 10% are endobronchial.

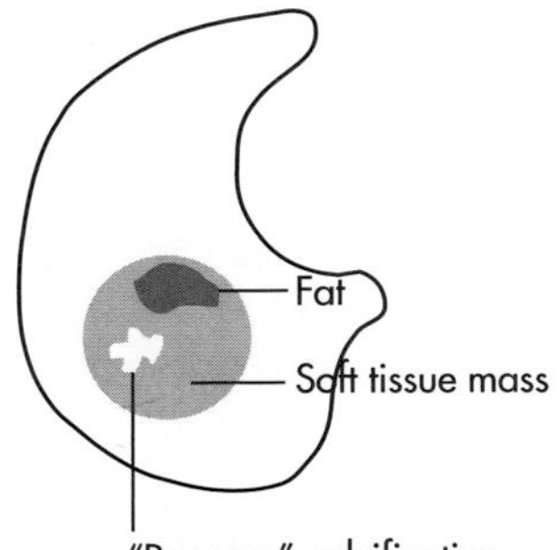

FIGURE 1-39

Radiographic Features
- Well-circumscribed solitary nodules
- Chondroid "popcorn" calcification is diagnostic but uncommon (<20%).
- Fat attenuation within a lesion by HRCT is pathognomonic.

CARNEY TRIAD

Predominant in Young Women
- Gastric smooth muscle tumors (epithelioid leiomyosarcoma)
- Functioning extraadrenal paraganglioma
- Pulmonary chondroma

TRACHEOBRONCHIAL PAPILLOMATOSIS

Radiographic Features
- Multiple, well demarcated nodules that can grow
- Cavitate with 2 to 3 mm thick walls
- Air fluid levels may develop
- Risk of squamous cell carcinoma 15 years after diagnosis

PULMONARY BLASTOMA

Predominant in Males, Poor Prognosis

Radiographic Features
- Large peripheral mass that is well circumscribed
- May show pleural invasion and may metastasize

LUNG METASTASES FROM OTHER PRIMARY LESIONS

GENERAL

Pathways of metastatic spread from a primary extrathoracic site to lungs (in order of frequency):
- Spread via pulmonary arteries
- Lymphatic spread (celiac nodes → posterior mediastinal nodes + paraesophageal nodes) and in lung parenchyma
- Direct extension
- Endobronchial spread

Neoplasms with rich vascular supply draining into systemic venous system:
- Renal cell carcinoma
- Sarcomas
- Trophoblastic tumors
- Testis
- Thyroid

Neoplasms with lymphatic dissemination:
- Breast (usually unilateral)
- Stomach (usually bilateral)

- Pancreas
- Larynx
- Cervix

Other neoplasms with high propensity to localize in lung:
- Colon
- Melanoma
- Sarcoma

Radiographic Features

- Multiple lesions, 95% > solitary lesion, 5%
- Lung bases > apices (related to blood flow)
- Peripheral, 90% > central, 10%
- Metastases typically have sharp margins.
- Fuzzy margins can result from peritumoral hemorrhage (choriocarcinoma, chemotherapy).
- Cavitations are common in SCCs from head and neck primary lesions.

CALCIFIED METASTASES

Calcifications in lung metastases are observed in:

Bone tumor metastases
- Osteosarcoma
- Chondrosarcoma

Mucinous tumors
- Ovarian
- Thyroid
- Pancreas
- Colon
- Stomach

Metastases after chemotherapy

GIANT METASTASES ("CANNON BALL" METASTASES) IN ASYMPTOMATIC PATIENT

- Head and neck cancer
- Testicular and ovarian cancer
- Soft tissue cancer
- Breast cancer
- Renal cancer
- Colon cancer

STERILE METASTASES

This term refers to pulmonary metastases under treatment that contain no viable tumor. Nodules typically consist of necrotic and/or fibrous tissue.

Chronic Lung Disease

IDIOPATHIC DISEASES

OVERVIEW OF IDIOPATHIC INTERSTITIAL PNEUMONIAS

Diagnosis	Clinical Findings	HRCT Features	Differential Diagnosis
UIP/IPF	40-70 years, M>F; >6 month dyspnea, cough, crackles, clubbing; poor response to steroids	Peripheral, basal, subpleural reticulation and honeycombing ± ground-glass opacity	Collagen vascular disease, asbestosis, CHP, scleroderma, drugs (bleomycin, methotrexate)
NSIP	40-50 years, M = F; dyspnea, cough, fatigue, crackles; may respond to steroids	Bilateral, patchy, subpleural ground-glass opacity, ± reticulation	Collagen vascular disease, CHP, DIP
RB-ILD	30-50 years, M > F; dyspnea, cough	Ground-glass, centrilobular nodules, ± centrilobular emphysema	Hypersensitivity pneumonitis
AIP/diffuse alveolar damage	Any age, M = F; acute-onset dyspnea, diffuse crackles and consolidation	Ground-glass consolidation, traction bronchiectasis and architectural distortion	ARDS, infection, edema, hemorrhage
COP	Mean 55 years, M = F; <3 month history of cough, dyspnea, fever; may respond to steroids	Subpleural and peribronchial consolidation ± nodules in lower zones; atoll sign (ring-shaped opacity)	Collagen vascular disease, infection, vasculitis, sarcoidosis, lymphoma, alveolar carcinoma
DIP	30-54 years, M > F; insidious onset weeks to months of dyspnea, cough	Ground-glass opacity, lower zone, peripheral	Hypersensitivity pneumonitis, NSIP
LIP	Any age, F > M	Ground-glass opacity, ± poorly defined centrilobular nodules, thin-walled cysts and air trapping	DIP, NSIP, hypersensitivity pneumonitis

AIP, acute interstitial pneumonia; CHP, chronic hypersensitivity pneumonitis; COP, cryptogenic organizing pneumonia; DIP, desquamative interstitial pneumonitis; IPF, idiopathic pulmonary fibrosis; LIP, lymphoid interstitial pneumonia; NSIP, nonspecific interstitial pneumonia; RB-ILD, respiratory bronchiolitis-associated interstitial lung disease; UIP, usual interstitial pneumonia.

USUAL INTERSTITIAL PNEUMONIA (UIP)

Multiple etiologies exist, which may produce a histologic pattern of UIP. Idiopathic pulmonary fibrosis (IPF) is the term used when no cause is identified; synonyms: cryptogenic fibrosing alveolitis (CFA, British term). Prognosis: mean survival 4 years (range 0.4 to 20 years). Lung biopsy is necessary for diagnosis. Treatment with steroids is useful in 50%, also cytotoxic agents.

Clinical Findings

- Clubbing, 60%
- Nonproductive cough, 50%
- Dyspnea
- Weight loss, 40%

Pathology

Pathologic changes are nonspecific and also occur in a variety of secondary disorders such as collagen vascular disease, drug reactions, pneumoconiosis, chronic hypersensitivity pneumonitis. Histology demonstrates alveolar fibrosis characterized by spatial and temporal heterogeneity, with architectural distortion.

Radiographic Features (Figs. 1-40 and 1-41)

Distribution
- IPF: Primarily in lower lung zones
- Peripheral subpleural involvement

HRCT pattern
- Early: ground-glass appearance
- Later: reticular pattern predominantly in lower lobes
- End stage: honeycombing
- Traction bronchiectasis indicates fibrosis.

Other
- Low lung volumes (fibrosis)
- Pulmonary hypertension with cardiomegaly (fibrosis), 30%
- Uncommon findings
  - Pleural thickening, 5%
  - Pneumothorax, 5%
  - Effusion, 5%

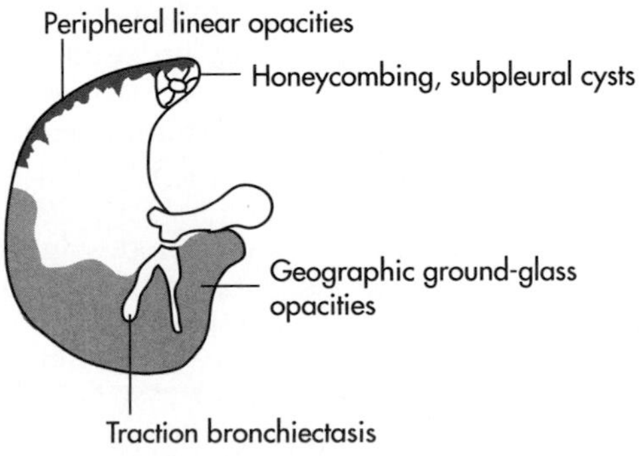

FIGURE 1-40

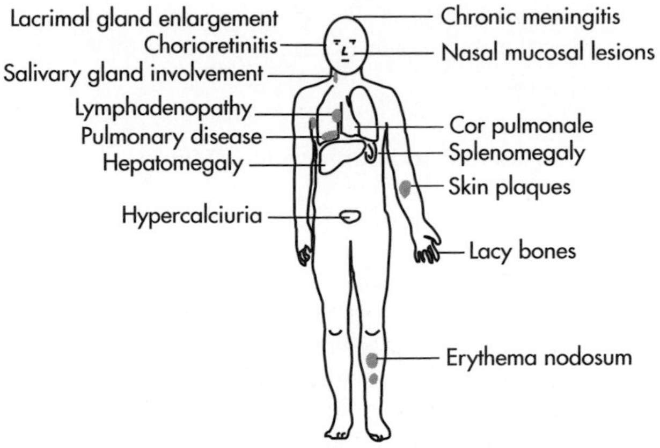

FIGURE 1-41

SARCOID

The term *sarcoid* (sarcoma-like) was first coined by Caesar Boeck in 1899 to describe one of the skin lesions of sarcoidosis because of its histologic resemblance to a sarcoma. Systemic granulomatous disease of unknown etiology (lung, 90% > skin, 25% > eye, 20% > hepatosplenomegaly, 15% > CNS, 5% > salivary glands > joints > heart). Treatment is with steroids.

Clinical Findings

Ten to 20 times more common in blacks than in whites, 30% are asymptomatic.

Prognosis

Adenopathy only: more benign course
- 75% regress to normal within 3 years
- 10% remain enlarged
- 15% progress to stages 2 and 3

Parenchymal abnormalities: 20% develop progressive pulmonary fibrosis

Associations

- Löfgren syndrome: acute febrile illness with bilateral hilar adenopathy and erythema nodosum in a patient with sarcoid. May also have uveitis or parotitis and arthralgias of large joints. These findings are associated with a favorable prognosis.
- Heerfordt syndrome: parotid gland enlargement, fever, uveitis, and cranial nerve palsies. The condition is usually self-limited and most commonly affects patients in the 2nd to 4th decades of life.
- Lupus pernio: violaceous (blue-purple) raised skin lesions on the cheeks and nose in a patient with sarcoid. Prognosis is poor.
- In HIV: A number of cases of new-onset sarcoid have been described in HIV patients after initiation of antiretroviral therapy with rise in CD4 count. This may be related to immune

restoration. The radiologic features are similar to those of sarcoid in non-HIV patients.

Diagnosis

Biopsy
- Bronchial and transbronchial biopsy (sensitivity 90%)
- Open lung biopsy (sensitivity 100%)
- Lymph node, parotid gland, or nasal mucosa biopsy (sensitivity 95%)
- Mediastinoscopy (sensitivity 95%)

Kveim test (sensitivity 70%-90%). Problems:
- Unavailability of validated tissue suspension (made from splenic tissue of infected patients)
- Lack of reactivity late in the disease
- Delay of 4 to 6 weeks before reactivity occurs

Radiographic Features (Figs. 1-42 and 1-43)

Stages (Siltzbach classification, plain film):

Stage 0: initial normal film, 10%

Stage 1: adenopathy, 50%
- Symmetrical hilar adenopathy
- Paratracheal, tracheobronchial, and azygos adenopathy are commonly associated with hilar adenopathy (Garland triad).
- Calcification, 5%

Stage 2: adenopathy with pulmonary opacities, 30%
- Reticulonodular pattern
- Acinar pattern may coalesce to consolidation.
- Large nodules >1 cm (2%)

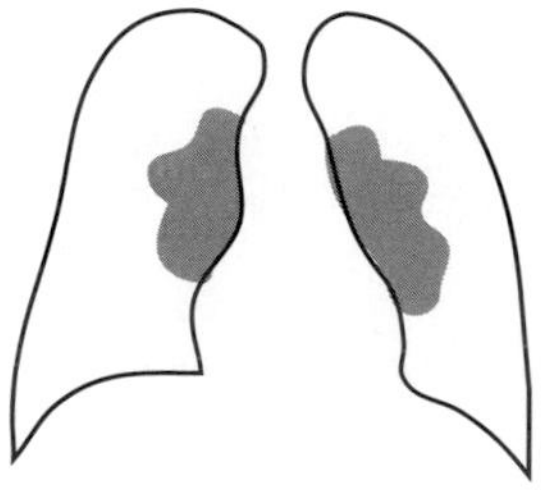

FIGURE 1-42

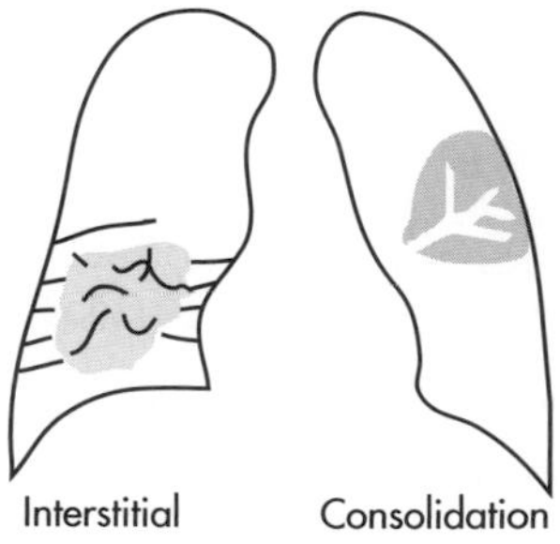

FIGURE 1-43

Stage 3: pulmonary opacities without hilar adenopathy, 10%

Stage 4: pulmonary fibrosis, upper lobes with bullae

Other less common plain film findings:
- Pleural effusion, 10%
- Unilateral hilar adenopathy, 1%-3%

- Eggshell calcification of lymph nodes
- Complications:
  - Pneumothorax (blebs, bullae)
  - *Aspergillus* with fungus ball: A complication of stage 4 disease. Pleural thickening may be the earliest indication of *Aspergillus* superinfection, occurring 2 to 3 years before appearance of an intracavitary fungus ball. The pleural thickening may achieve a thickness of 2 cm or more.
  - *Cardiac arrhythmias:* Early initiation of steroid therapy can help to prevent these arrhythmias.
  - Bronchostenosis with lobar/segmental collapse

CT Features

Lung parenchyma
- Nodules (90%), along lymphatic distribution (i.e., central or axial and subpleural)
- Linear pattern, 50%
- Ground-glass opacity, 25%
- Subpleural thickening, 25%
- Pseudoalveolar consolidation, 15%

Lymph nodes
- Adenopathy, 80%

Bronchi
- Wall abnormalities, 65%
- Luminal abnormalities, 25%
- Bronchiectasis, 10%

End stage
- Upper lobe fibrosis
- Bullae
- Traction bronchiectasis

^{67}Ga Scintigraphic Findings

Accumulation of ^{67}Ga is a sensitive but nonspecific indicator of active inflammation in patients with sarcoidosis. Gallium avidity cannot be used alone to establish a diagnosis of sarcoidosis. However, ^{67}Ga imaging is useful in identifying extrathoracic sites of involvement, detecting active alveolitis, and assessing response to treatment.

Gallium uptake in thoracic lymph nodes, lungs, and salivary and lacrimal glands is particularly suggestive of sarcoidosis. How well the extent of gallium uptake in the lung correlates with the degree of alveolitis is controversial. However, ^{67}Ga scans may be useful as a baseline study at the time of diagnosis. If results of ^{67}Ga scintigraphy are initially positive, negative findings from a subsequent ^{67}Ga scan obtained during the course of treatment suggest that alveolitis has resolved. In such a patient, gallium may be a useful marker for disease activity and response to therapy.

NONSPECIFIC INTERSTITIAL PNEUMONIA (NSIP)

Important to distinguish from UIP given a better response to steroids. Patients are typically younger than those with UIP and symptoms are milder. Associated with drug exposure hypersensitivity pneumonitis and collagen vascular disease.

Pathology

Histologically characterized by spatial and temporal homogeneity of interstitial inflammation with varying degrees of fibrosis. Limited fibrosis identifies the cellular NSIP subtype; however, the fibrotic NSIP subtype is more common.

HRCT Features

- Patchy ground-glass opacities, reticular opacities, micronodules
- Subpleural, symmetric, without the basilar predominance seen in UIP
- Honeycombing occasionally seen in fibrotic subtype

RESPIRATORY BRONCHIOLITIS-ASSOCIATED INTERSTITIAL PNEUMONIA (RB-ILD)

Smoking-related interstitial lung disease, representing a symptomatic form of the often incidentally detected respiratory bronchiolitis. Smoking cessation is key to treatment, although steroids may be helpful.

Pathology

Histologically characterized by respiratory bronchioles that are filled with macrophages.

HRCT Features

- Diffuse centrilobular nodules and ground-glass opacities
- Bronchial wall thickening
- Coexisting centrilobular emphysema may be noted

DESQUAMATIVE INTERSTITIAL PNEUMONIA (DIP)

Represents the most severe form of the continuum of smoking-related interstitial lung disease (RB, RB-ILD, DIP).

Pathology

Histologically characterized by alveolar spaces that are filled with macrophages.

HRCT Features

- Diffuse ground-glass opacities (versus centrilobular distribution in RB-ILD)
- Peripheral and basilar predominance
- Septal thickening
- Occasional small cystic spaces

CRYPTOGENIC ORGANIZING PNEUMONIA (COP)

Formerly termed bronchiolitis obliterans organizing pneumonia (BOOP). Histologic pattern may also be seen in collagen vascular disease, drug exposure, and infection. Patients present with cough, mild dyspnea, and fever over several months; there may be an antecedent history of respiratory infection.

Pathology

Intraalveolar proliferation of granulation tissue is seen, with temporal uniformity.

HRCT Features

- Patchy consolidation or ground-glass opacities
- Subpleural, peribronchial, lower > upper lung distribution
- May also see small centrilobular nodules or large irregularly shaped masses
- Atoll sign: crescent-shaped opacity

LYMPHOID INTERSTITIAL PNEUMONIA (LIP)

Women > men, associated with Sjögren syndrome, SLE, HIV infection; rarely idiopathic. Common in pediatric AIDS patients. Variable response to steroids. May progress to lymphoma in <20%. A localized form of LIP has been called "pseudolymphoma" because of histologic resemblance to lymphoma.

Pathology

Diffuse interstitial infiltrate composed of lymphocytes, plasma cells, and histiocytes.

HRCT Features

- Ground-glass opacities ± poorly defined centrilobular nodules
- Basilar distribution or diffuse
- Perivascular cysts
- Late honeycombing

ACUTE INTERSTITIAL PNEUMONIA (AIP)

Present with severe dyspnea requiring mechanical ventilation, usually several weeks after viral URI. Mortality, 50%. Men = women, supportive therapy although steroids may help. Formerly known as Hamman-Rich syndrome.

Pathology

Diffuse alveolar damage. Exudative phase demonstrates hyaline membranes and alveolar infiltration by lymphocytes. Progresses to organizing phase after 1 week, with alveolar wall thickening due to fibrosis.

HRCT Features

- Similar to ARDS, but often with a symmetric, posterior lower lobe distribution

- Exudative phase: ground-glass opacities, consolidation
- Organizing phase: architectural distortion, traction bronchiectasis, honeycombing

LYMPHOPROLIFERATIVE DISORDERS

Spectrum of lymphoid abnormalities in the chest characterized by accumulation of lymphocytes and plasma cells in the pulmonary interstitium or mediastinal/hilar lymph nodes. Believed to be due to stimulation of bronchus-associated lymphoid tissue by antigens.

Types

Nodal disorders
- Castleman disease (see Middle Mediastinal Tumors)
- Infectious mononucleosis
- Angioimmunoblastic lymphadenopathy: drug hypersensitivity

Pulmonary parenchymal disorders
- Plasma cell granuloma (inflammatory pseudotumor, histiocytoma)
- Pseudolymphoma
- Lymphocytic interstitial pneumonia (LIP)
- Lymphomatoid granulomatosis

OVERVIEW OF LYMPHOPROLIFERATIVE DISEASES

Diagnosis	Lung	Nodes	Effusion	Malignancy
Nodes				
Castleman disease	Unaffected	Yes	No	No
Infectious mononucleosis	Mediastinal adenopathy	Yes	No	No
Angioimmunoblastic lymphadenopathy	Interstitial and alveolar opacity	Yes	10%	30%
Parenchymal				
Plasma cell granuloma	Solitary pulmonary mass	No	No	No
Pseudolymphoma	Single or multiple parenchymal masses, air bronchograms	No	No	20%
LIP	Bilateral interstitial disease	No	No	<20%
Lymphomatoid granulomatosis	Multiple pulmonary nodules, frequent cavitation	Rare	35%	30%

DIFFERENTIATION OF LYMPHOMA AND LYMPHOPROLIFERATIVE DISEASE

Parameter	Lymphoproliferative Disorder	Lymphoma
Location	Parenchyma *or* lymph nodes but not both	Parenchyma *and* lymph nodes
Lymphoid population	Polyclonal	Monoclonal
Onset	Young patients (<30 years)	Old patients (>50 years)
Prognosis	Usually benign or low-grade malignancy	Malignant

PLASMA CELL GRANULOMA

Local cellular proliferation of spindle cells, plasma cells, lymphocytes, and histiocytes in lung. Most common tumor-like pulmonary abnormality in children <15 years. Treatment is resection.

Radiographic Features (Fig. 1-44)
- Solitary lung mass 1 to 12 cm
- No or very slow growth
- Cavitation and calcification uncommon

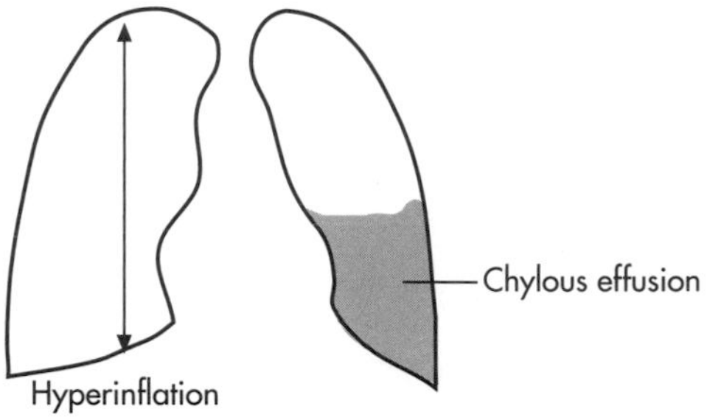

FIGURE 1-44

LYMPHANGIOLEIOMYOMATOSIS (LAM)

Proliferation of smooth muscle cells along lymphatics in lung, thorax, and abdomen. Unknown etiology. Rare.

Clinical Findings

Young women presenting with spontaneous pneumothorax, chylothorax, hemoptysis, slowly progressive dyspnea. Ten-year survival 75%. Similar lesions may be seen in tuberous sclerosis (LAM has been dubbed a *forme fruste* of tuberous sclerosis).

Extrapulmonary LAM is rare.

Radiographic Features

Plain film/HRCT (Fig. 1-45)
- Numerous cystic spaces, 90%
  - Size of cysts usually <5 to 10 mm
  - Thin walled
  - Surrounded by normal lung

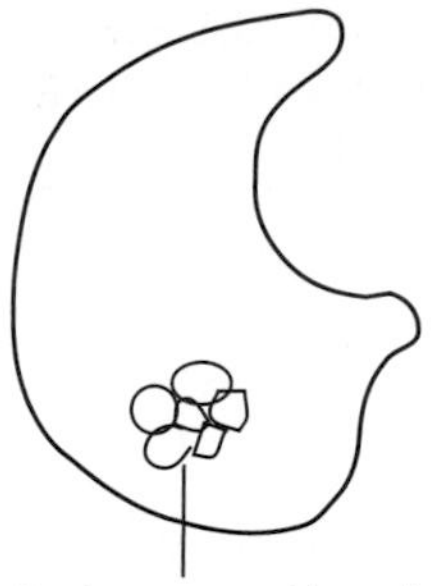

FIGURE 1-45

- Recurrent pneumothorax, 70%
- Chylous pleural effusions, 25%
- Plain film: overinflation, irregular opacities, cysts
- Occasionally multiple nodules: multifocal micronodular pneumocyte hyperplasia

Lymphangiography
- Obstruction of lymphatic flow at multiple levels
- Dilated lymphatics
- Increased number of lymphatics
- Renal angiomyolipomas, which are often small and asymptomatic
- Chylous ascites (in up to one third of patients), uterine leiomyomas, and lymphaticoureteral and lymphaticovenous communications
- Abdominal and pelvic lymph angioleiomyomas
- Abdominal lymph nodes

TUBEROUS SCLEROSIS

Identical lesions as in LAM

COLLAGEN VASCULAR DISEASES

Collagen vascular diseases have a common pathogenesis in the lung: immune response → inflammation (interstitial pattern, granuloma) → vasculitis → obstruction (e.g., respiratory insufficiency, PA hypertension).

Pearls
- Lower lungs are more frequently affected (higher blood flow).
- Vasculitides of large arteries (e.g., periarteritis nodosa) cause pulmonary hypertension.
- Most common complication is infection (secondary to immunosuppressive medications).

RHEUMATOID ARTHRITIS (RA)

There are seven forms of pleuropulmonary disease associated with RA:

Rheumatoid lung nodules, 20% (necrobiotic)
- Usually multiple
- Nodules may change in size rapidly or disappear completely.
- Association between cutaneous and pulmonary nodules

Pleural effusion and pleuritis
- Clinically, pleuritis is the most common pulmonary feature of RA.
- Effusions are bilateral in the majority of patients.
- Proportionately more common in men
- Fluid has low pH and low glucose.
- Effusions are usually unilateral.

Caplan syndrome
- Nodular rheumatoid lung disease associated with pneumoconiosis fibrosing alveolitis

Constrictive bronchiolitis

Lymphoid hyperplasia

Pulmonary hypertension

Radiographic Features
- Bibasilar patchy alveolar opacities are early findings.
- Dense reticulonodular pattern is most frequent
- Pleural involvement, 20%
- End stage: honeycombing, PAH

ANKYLOSING SPONDYLITIS (AS)

- Pulmonary fibrocystic changes in 1%-10%
- Upper lobe fibrotic scarring, infiltration, cystic airspaces
- Ancillary findings:
  - Ossification of spinal ligaments, sacroiliitis
  - Cardiomyopathy

SYSTEMIC LUPUS ERYTHEMATOSUS (SLE)

Pleural abnormalities are the most common findings.
- Pleural thickening
- Recurrent pleural effusions
- Pleuritis is thought to be pathogenetically similar to polyserositis affecting joints.
- Glucose level of pleural effusion is normal (decreased in RA).

Pulmonary disease: wide spectrum of findings, but the usual presentation is as acute lupus pneumonitis:
- Acute lupus pneumonitis: vasculitis and hemorrhage resulting in focal opacities at the lung bases
- Alveolar opacities, which may progress to ARDS
- Fibrosing alveolitis, rare
- Elevating diaphragm, atelectasis at bases (shown to be due to diaphragmatic dysfunction)
- Lupus-like disease can also be seen with drugs such as hydralazine and procainamide.

OTHER COLLAGEN VASCULAR DISEASES WITH PULMONARY MANIFESTATIONS

- Progressive systemic sclerosis (PSS) exists in two forms:
  - PSS with scleroderma
    - After esophagus, lung is the second most common site.
    - Interstitial fibrosis is the most common pulmonary manifestation.
    - Pulmonary vascular and pleural changes are less common.
  - PSS with CREST (calcinosis, Raynaud, esophageal dysmotility, sclerodactyly, telangiectasia)
    - Usually in older women
    - Long history of PSS with swollen fingers
    - Mild disease, slowly progressive, greater life expectancy
- Polymyositis, dermatomyositis
- Mixed connective tissue disease (MCTD)

VASCULITIS AND GRANULOMATOSES

CLINICORADIOLOGIC FEATURES SUGGESTIVE OF VASCULITIS

- Deforming of ulcerating upper airway lesions
- Palpable purpura
- Peripheral neuropathy
- Rapidly progressive glomerulonephritis
- Pulmonary renal syndrome
- Chest imaging showing nodular or cavitary disease
- Diffuse alveolar hemorrhage

WEGENER GRANULOMATOSIS

Systemic granulomatous process with destructive angiitis involving lung, upper respiratory tract, and kidney (necrotizing glomerulonephritis); type IV immune mechanism. The upper respiratory tract is affected in almost all patients, with lungs and kidneys involved in 90% and 80% of patients, respectively.

Radiographic Features (Fig. 1-46)

- Multiple nodules with cavitation (common)
- Interstitial, reticulonodular opacities at lung bases (earliest finding)

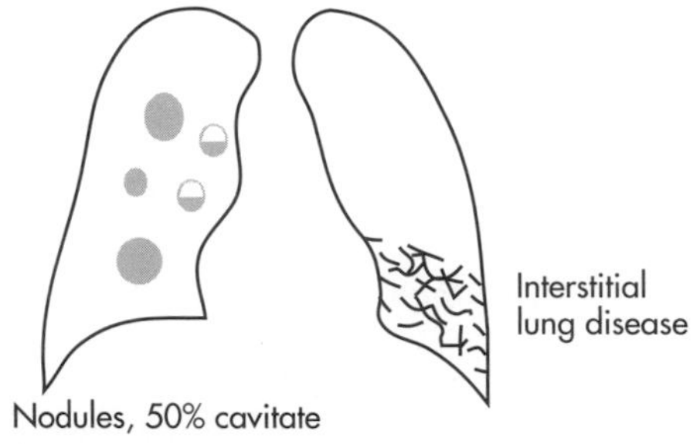

FIGURE 1-46

- Diffuse opacities (common) are due to:
  - Atelectasis: bronchoconstriction
  - Confluent nodules and masses
  - Pulmonary hemorrhage
  - Superimposed infection
- Other findings:
  - Pleural effusions, 25%
  - Adenopathy (rare)

LYMPHOMATOID GRANULOMATOSIS

Now considered a B-cell lymphoma. Men > women. The multiple nodules are smaller than those in Wegener. Nodules are not numerous and tend to cavitate.

CHURG-STRAUSS—ALLERGIC ANGIITIS AND GRANULOMATOSIS

Similar to polyarteritis nodosa, but patients have pulmonary diseases and asthma. Affects skin, kidneys, lung, heart, and CNS; eosinophilia.

Radiographic Features

- Patchy peripheral areas of consolidation
- Fleeting opacities
- Multiple nodules

BEHÇET DISEASE

Chronic multisystem vasculitis, characterized by:

- Recurrent oral and genital ulcerations
- Uveitis
- Additional clinical manifestations in multiple organ systems

Radiographic Features

- Pulmonary arterial aneurysm: fusiform to saccular, commonly multiple and bilateral, located in the lower lobe or main pulmonary arteries
- Thickening of the aorta and SVC (vasculitis)
- Subpleural alveolar infiltrates, and wedge-shaped or rounded areas of increased density, which represent focal vasculitis and thrombosis resulting in infarction, hemorrhage, and focal atelectasis

OTHER CHRONIC DISORDERS

LANGERHANS CELL HISTIOCYTOSIS (EOSINOPHILIC GRANULOMA)

Langerhans cell histiocytosis consists of three clinical syndromes:

- Letterer-Siwe: acute disseminated form
- Hand-Schüller-Christian: chronic disseminated form
- Eosinophilic granuloma:
  - Solitary bone lesion
  - Small cystic spaces in lung parenchyma
  - 3- to 10-mm pulmonary nodules
  - Apical reticulonodular pattern
  - Pneumothorax, 30%

IDIOPATHIC PULMONARY HEMORRHAGE (IPH)

Recurrent pulmonary hemorrhage, which may result in interstitial fibrosis. Age usually <10 years.

Radiographic Features

- Diffuse airspace pattern (radiographic appearance similar to Goodpasture syndrome)
- Hilar adenopathy

AMYLOID

Extracellular deposition of protein derived from light chains of monoclonal Ig.

Classification

- Primary amyloid: heart, lung (70%), skin, tongue, nerves
- Amyloid associated with multiple myeloma (carpal tunnel syndrome, common)
- Secondary amyloid (liver, spleen, kidney) in:
  - Chronic infections
  - Chronic inflammations
  - Neoplasm
- Heredofamilial amyloidosis (familial Mediterranean fever; other syndromes)
- Local amyloidosis in isolated organs
- Amyloid associated with aging

Radiographic Features

- Adenopathy and calcifications are common.
- Plain film findings are nonspecific, with multiple nodules or diffuse linear patterns.
- Pulmonary involvement can be either diffuse or focal.
- Diagnosis requires biopsy.

NEUROFIBROMATOSIS

Twenty percent of patients with neurofibromatosis have pulmonary involvement:

- Progressive pulmonary fibrosis
- Bullae in upper lobes and chest wall
- Chest wall and mediastinal neurofibromas
- Intrathoracic meningoceles
- Ribbon deformities of the ribs

PULMONARY ALVEOLAR MICROLITHIASIS

Tiny calculi within alveoli. Unknown cause (hereditary). Rare.

Radiographic Features

- Sandlike microcalcifications of lung (black pleura sign)
- Bilateral, symmetrical involvement
- Pulmonary activity on bone scan

ALVEOLAR PROTEINOSIS

Proteinaceous, lipid-rich surfactant from type II pneumocytes accumulates in alveoli. Unknown etiology (may be associated with lymphoma or acute silicosis). Extensive sputum production (liters/day). Diagnosed with biopsy, sputum electron microscopy for alveolar phospholipids. Prognosis: Some people with pulmonary alveolar proteinosis suffer from shortness of breath for their entire lifetime. However, this lung disorder is rarely fatal as long as patients undergo regular lung washings. Complications include nocardiosis, aspergillosis, cryptococcosis, and lymphoma. Treatment is with aerosolized proteolytic agents and bronchoscopic lung lavage with 10 to 20 L saline (therapy of choice).

Radiographic Features

- Bilateral, symmetrical airspace disease (butterfly, batwing pattern)
- Acinar pattern may become confluent (consolidation)
- CT: multifocal, panlobular, ground-glass, and airspace opacities with septal thickening ("crazy paving")
- Other findings from superimposed opportunistic infection

DRUG-INDUCED LUNG DISEASE

A large number of therapeutic drugs can cause lung toxicity. Because the findings are often nonspecific, a high index of suspicion is required. The most common abnormalities are:

Diffuse interstitial opacities
- Cytotoxic agents: bleomycin, methotrexate, carmustine, cyclophosphamide
- Gold salts

Pulmonary nodules (uncommon)
- Cyclosporine
- Oil aspiration

Focal ASD
- Amiodarone accumulates in lysosomes of phagocytes; high iodine content results in increased CT density of affected lung and liver

Diffuse ASD (pulmonary edema, hemorrhage)
- Cytotoxic agents: cytarabine, IL-2, OKT3
- Tricyclic antidepressants
- Salicylates
- Penicillamine
- Anticoagulants

Adenopathy
- Phenytoin (Dilantin)
- Cytotoxic agents: cyclosporine, methotrexate

Pleural effusions
- Drug-induced SLE
- Bromocriptine
- Methysergide, ergotamine tartrate

Inhalational Lung Disease

PNEUMOCONIOSIS

Pneumoconioses are caused by inhalation of inorganic dust particles that overwhelm the normal clearance mechanism of the respiratory tract.

Types

Benign pneumoconiosis: radiographic abnormalities are present while there are no symptoms or only minimal symptoms (not fibrogenic):

- Tin = stannosis
- Barium = baritosis
- Iron = siderosis

Fibrogenic pneumoconiosis (symptomatic)

- Silica = silicosis
- Asbestos = asbestosis
- Coal workers' pneumoconiosis (CWP)

INTERNATIONAL LABOR ORGANIZATION (ILO) CLASSIFICATION (Fig. 1-47)

The ILO classification can be used to classify or follow pneumoconioses. All pneumoconioses have similar radiographic features that range from few tiny nodules to end-stage lung disease.

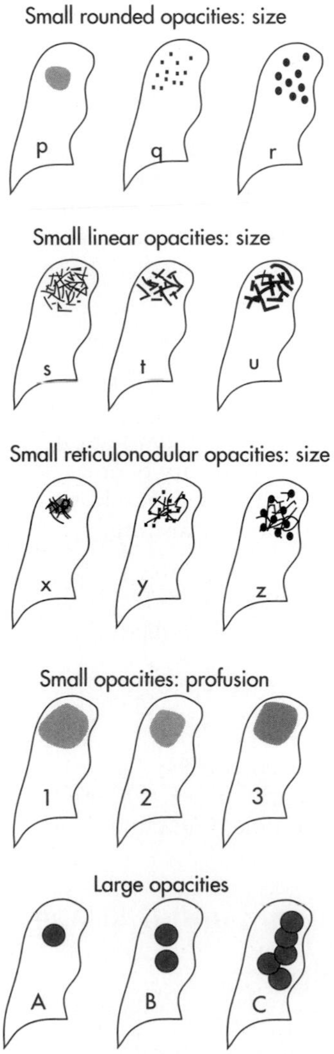

FIGURE 1-47

Small opacities

Size:

- Nodules: p = <1.5 mm, q = <3 mm, r = >3 to 10 mm
- Reticular: s = fine, t = medium, u = coarse
- Reticulonodular: x = fine, y = medium, z = coarse (this is not part of ILO classification)

Location ("zone"): upper middle and lower zone of each lung field

How many (profusion = concentration): category 1 = few nodules, category 2 = lung markings still visible, category 3 = lung markings obscured

Large opacities

Size: A = <5 cm, B = half of upper lung zone affected, C = > half of upper lung zone affected

Other features

Pleural thickening, plaques

Pleural calcification, diffuse

SILICOSIS

Causative agent is silicone dioxide (SiO_2) in quartz, cristobalite, and tridymite. The severity of disease is related to the total amount of inhaled dust. Inhaled particles need to be <5 µm in diameter because larger particles are removed by upper airways. Treatment is to stop exposure; however, in contrast to CWP, silicosis may be progressive despite removal from a dust environment. Isoniazid (INH) chemoprophylaxis is advised. Occupations most at risk (only 5% of patients with >20 years' exposure will develop a complicated form of pneumoconiosis) are:

- Mining (gold, tin, copper, mica)
- Quarrying (quartz)
- Sandblasting

Pathology

- Silica is phagocytosed by pulmonary macrophages.
- Cytotoxic reaction causes formation of noncaseating granuloma.
- Granulomas develop into silicotic nodules (2 to 3 mm in diameter).
- Pulmonary fibrosis develops as nodules coalesce.

Clinical Findings (Fig. 1-48)

Chronic silicosis

- 20 to 40 years of exposure
- Predominantly affects upper lobes
- Rarely develops into massive fibrosis

Accelerated silicosis

- 5 to 15 years of heavy exposure
- Middle and lower lobes are also affected.

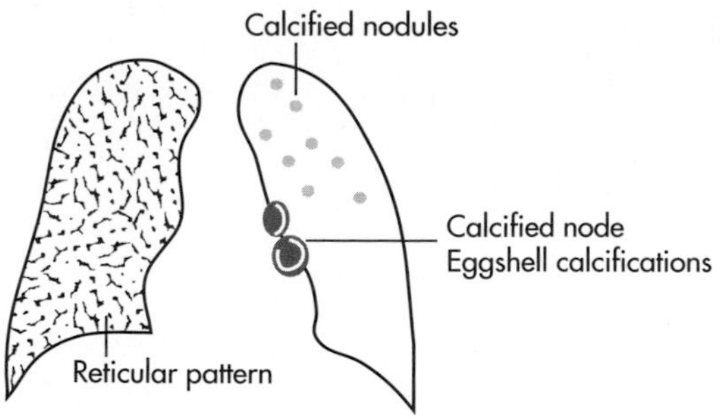

FIGURE 1-48

- Radiographic appearance is similar to that of alveolar proteinosis.
- Concomitant diseases:
  - TB, 25% (silicotuberculosis)
  - Collagen vascular disease, 10% (scleroderma, RA, SLE, Caplan syndrome)

Acute silicosis (silicoproteinosis)
- <3 years of exposure
- Fulminant course: diffuse multifocal ground-glass or airspace consolidations
- TB, 25%

Caplan syndrome
- RA
- Lung disease:
  - Silicosis (less common) or CWP (more common)
  - Rheumatoid nodules

Radiographic Features

Nodular pattern (common)
- Nodules: 1 to 10 mm
- Calcific nodules, 20%
- Upper lobe > lower lobe
- Coalescent nodules cause areas of conglomerate opacities.

Reticular pattern (may precede or be associated with the nodular pattern)

Hilar adenopathy
- Common
- Eggshell calcification, 5%

Progressive massive fibrosis (PMF)
- Masses (>1 cm) formed by coalescent nodules
- Usually in posterior segment of upper lobes
- Vertical orientation
- Cavitation due to ischemia or superinfection from TB
- Often bilateral
- Retracts hila superiorly
- Main differential diagnosis: neoplasm, TB, fungus

Concomitant TB

COAL WORKERS' PNEUMOCONIOSIS (CWP)

Development of pneumoconiosis depends on the kind of inhaled coal: anthracite (50% incidence of pneumoconiosis) > bituminous > lignite (10% incidence).

Pathology: coal macule around respiratory bronchioli with associated focal dust (centrilobular emphysema).

Radiographic Features

Radiographically indistinguishable from silicosis
- Simple (reticulonodular) pneumoconiosis
  - Upper and middle lobe predominance
  - Nodules: 1 to 5 mm
  - Centriacinar emphysema surrounds nodules.
- Complicated pneumoconiosis with progressive massive fibrosis
  - Usually evolves from simple CWP
  - Mass lesions >1 cm in diameter

ASBESTOS

Asbestos exposure causes a variety of manifestations:

Pleura
- Pleural plaques (hyalinized collagen)
- Diffuse thickening
- Benign pleural effusion (most common manifestation)
- Pleural calcification

Lung
- Interstitial fibrosis (asbestosis)
- Rounded atelectasis with comet tail sign of vessel leading to atelectatic lung
- Fibrous masses

Malignancy
- Malignant mesothelioma
- Bronchogenic carcinoma
- Carcinoma of the larynx
- GI malignancies

Pathogenicity of fibers: crocidolite (South Africa) > amosite > chrysotile (Canada).

High-risk professions:
- Construction, demolition
- Insulation
- Pipefitting and shipbuilding
- Asbestos mining

ASBESTOS-RELATED PLEURAL DISEASE

Focal Pleural Plaques

Hyalinized collagen in submesothelial layer of parietal pleura. Focal interrupted areas of pleural thickening.
- Pleural plaques have no functional significance.
- Most common manifestation of asbestos exposure
- Preferred location: bilateral, posterolateral mid and lower chest
- Only 15% of pleural plaques are visible by CXR.

Diffuse Pleural Thickening

- Less frequent than focal plaques
- Unlike focal plaques, diffuse thickening may cause respiratory symptoms (abnormal pulmonary function test results)
- Thickening of interlobar fissures
- May be associated with round atelectasis

Pleural Calcifications

Pleural calcification in the absence of other histories (hemothorax, empyema, TB, previous surgery) is pathognomonic of asbestos exposure.

- Calcium may form in center of plaques.
- Contains uncoated asbestos fibers but no asbestos bodies
- Usually requires >20 years to develop

Benign Pleural Effusions

Early sign of asbestos-related disease. Usually sterile, serous exudate. The diagnosis is one of exclusion: rule out other causes of pleural effusion:

- Malignant mesothelioma
- Bronchogenic carcinoma
- TB

Round Atelectasis

Round-appearing peripheral atelectasis associated with pleural thickening. Although not unique to asbestos exposure, round atelectasis is common in patients with asbestos exposure and pleural thickening. Most commonly in posterior part of lower lobe.

Radiographic Features (Fig. 1-49)

- Round mass in lung periphery
- Thickened pleura (due to asbestos-related disease)
- Mass is most dense at its periphery.
- Mass is never completely surrounded by lung.
- Atelectasis forms an acute angle with pleura.
- Comet sign: bronchi and vessels curve toward the mass.
- Signs of volume loss: displaced fissure

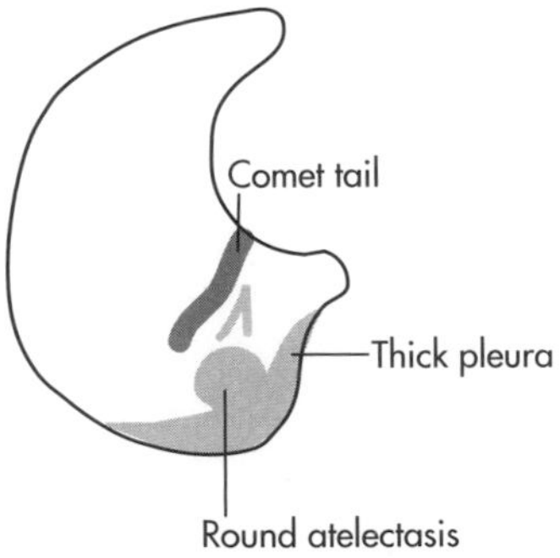

FIGURE 1-49

ASBESTOSIS

Refers exclusively to asbestos-related interstitial pulmonary fibrosis.

Radiographic Features

- Reticular, linear patterns
- Initial subpleural location
- Progression from bases to apices
- Honeycombing occurring later in the disease
- No hilar adenopathy

MALIGNANCY IN ASBESTOS-RELATED DISEASE

- 7000-fold increase of mesothelioma (10% risk during lifetime; latency >30 years after exposure)
- 7-fold increase of bronchogenic carcinoma
- 3-fold increase of GI neoplasm

ANTIGEN-ANTIBODY–MEDIATED LUNG DISEASE

Allergic reactions in lung can cause one of four patterns of disease:

- Granulomatous alveolitis
  - Hypersensitivity alveolitis
  - Chronic beryllium disease
- Pulmonary eosinophilia (pulmonary infiltrations with eosinophilia [PIE])
- Asthma
- Goodpasture syndrome

HYPERSENSITIVITY PNEUMONITIS (EXTRINSIC ALLERGIC ALVEOLITIS)

Granulomatous inflammation of bronchioles and alveoli caused by immunologic response to inhaled organic material. Type III (Ag-Ab complex mediated) and type IV (cell mediated) hypersensitivity reactions. Antigens are often fungal spores or avian-related antigens.

HYPERSENSITIVITY ALVEOLITIS

Disease	Antigen Source	Antigen
Farmer's lung	Moldy hay	*Micropolyspora faeni*
Bird fancier's lung (pigeons, parakeets)	Avian excreta	Avian serum proteins
Humidifier lung	Contaminated air conditioners	Thermophilic *Actinomyces*
Bagassosis	Moldy bagasse dust	*Thermoactinomyces sacchari*
Malt worker's lung	Moldy malt	*Aspergillus clavatus*
Maple bark stripper's lung	Moldy maple bark	*Cryptostroma corticale*
Mushroom worker's lung	Spores from mushrooms	Thermophilic *Actinomyces*

Radiographic Features

Acute, reversible changes

- Diffuse ground-glass pattern
- Reticulonodular interstitial pattern
- Patchy areas of consolidation (rare)

Chronic, irreversible changes

- Progressive interstitial fibrosis (often upper lobe predominance) with honeycombing
- Pulmonary hypertension

CHRONIC BERYLLIUM DISEASE

T-cell–dependent granulomatous response to inhaled beryllium (beryllium copper alloy, fluorescent strip lighting). Now a rare disease.

Radiographic Features

Many similarities to sarcoidosis:

- Reticulonodular pattern → fibrosis
- Bilateral hilar lymph node enlargement

Distinction between berylliosis and sarcoidosis:

- History of exposure to beryllium
- Positive beryllium transformation test
- Increased concentration of beryllium in lung or lymph nodes
- Negative Kveim test

PULMONARY INFILTRATES WITH EOSINOPHILIA (PIE)

Group of diseases characterized by transient pulmonary opacities and eosinophilia (>500/mm^3).

Types

Löffler syndrome (Simple pulmonary eosinophilia, SPE)

- Idiopathic origin
- Benign transient pulmonary opacities
- Minimally symptomatic, self-limited
- Rare

Acute eosinophilic pneumonia

- Acute febrile illness <5 days
- Hypoxemia
- Diffuse alveolar or mixed alveolar-interstitial opacities
- Response to steroids with no relapse after discontinuation of steroids
- >25% in BAL fluid

Chronic eosinophilic pneumonia (idiopathic origin)

- Severe, chronic pneumonia
- Predominantly nonsegmental peripheral opacities

Pneumonias of known origin:

- Allergic bronchopulmonary mycoses (type 1 + 2 hypersensitivity)
  - *Aspergillus* (ABPA is the most important one)
  - Rare: *Candida, Curvularia lunata, Drechslera hawaiiensis, Helminthosporium, Stemphylium lanuginosum*
- Helminth infection (nodular opacities, very high eosinophilia count, high IgE):
  - *Ascaris*
  - Schistosomiasis; 50% with pulmonary involvement
  - *Toxocara canis*
  - Microfiliariasis
- Drugs
  - Penicillin, tetracycline, sulfonamides
  - Salicylates
  - Chlorpropamide, imipramine
  - Nitrofurantoin (causes chronic interstitial eosinophilic alveolitis with progression to fibrosis)

GOODPASTURE SYNDROME

Three main features: pulmonary hemorrhage, iron-deficiency anemia, and glomerulonephritis. Binding of circulating antibodies to glomerular and alveolar basement membranes. Symptoms include hemoptysis and renal failure. Diagnosis is made by antiglomerular basement membrane antibody, immunofluorescence of antibody, and renal biopsy.

Radiographic Features

- Pulmonary hemorrhage: consolidation with air bronchogram
- Clearing of pulmonary hemorrhage in 1 to 2 weeks
- Repeated hemorrhage leads to hemosiderosis and pulmonary fibrosis → interstitial reticular pattern
- Renal findings

TOXIN-INDUCED INTERSTITIAL PNEUMONITIS/FIBROSIS

DRUG-INDUCED PULMONARY TOXICITY

Chemotherapeutic drugs

- Bleomycin
- BCNU
- Cyclophosphamide
- Methotrexate
- Procarbazine

Other drugs

- Amiodarone
- Nitrofurantoin
- Gold
- Carbamazepine

SILO FILLER DISEASE

- Due to NO_2 production (yellow gas) in silos
- NO_2 forms nitric acid (HNO_3) in lungs, causing pulmonary edema and later COP.
- Silo filler disease only occurs in September and October, when silos are being filled.
- Safe NO_2 levels below 5 ppm

Airway Disease

TRACHEA

MALIGNANT TRACHEAL NEOPLASM

Ninety percent of all tracheobronchial tumors are malignant.

Types

Primary malignancies
- SCC (most common)
- Adenoid cystic carcinoma (second most common)
- Mucoepidermoid (less common)
- Carcinoid (less common; strong contrast enhancement, octreotide uptake)

Metastases
- Local extension (common)
  - Thyroid cancer
  - Esophageal cancer
  - Lung cancer
- Hematogenous metastases (rare)
  - Melanoma
  - Breast cancer

BENIGN NEOPLASM

Only 10% of tracheobronchial tumors are benign. Benign tumors are typically <2 cm.

Types

Papilloma
- Common laryngeal tumors in children, rare in adults, often multiple
- May cause lung nodules
- Malignant potential-SCC. (These lesions are caused by the human papillomavirus and are benign but may degenerate into malignancies.)

Hamartoma
- Fat density is diagnostic.
- Often calcified (popcorn pattern)

Adenoma
- Rare

SABER-SHEATH TRACHEA

Reduced coronal diameter (< of sagittal diameter). Only affects the intrathoracic trachea; the extrathoracic trachea appears normal.
- 95% of patients have COPD
- More common in male patients
- Tracheal ring calcification is common.

TRACHEOPATHIA OSTEOPLASTICA (TPO)

Foci of cartilage and bone develop in the submucosa of the tracheobronchial tree. Benign, rare condition. Most cases are discovered incidentally at autopsy.

Clinical Findings
- Dyspnea, hoarseness, expiratory wheeze/stridor (airway obstruction)
- Hemoptysis (mucosal ulceration)
- Cough and sputum production
- Rarely: atelectasis, pneumonia

Radiographic Features
- Calcified tracheobronchial tree, nodules, osteocartilaginous growth
- Thickening of tracheal cartilage
- Sparing of the posterior membranous portion
- Narrowed lumen
- Distal three fourths of the trachea and the proximal bronchi are most commonly involved.

RELAPSING POLYCHONDRITIS

Collagen vascular disease characterized by inflammation and progressive destruction of cartilage throughout the body (ribs, trachea, earlobes, nose, joints). Rare.

Diagnostic Criteria (>3 needed)
- Recurrent chondritis of auricles (painful ear)
- Inflammation of ocular structures (e.g., conjunctivitis, scleritis, keratitis)
- Chondritis (painful) of laryngeal/tracheal cartilage
- Cochlear or vestibular damage

Radiographic Features

Trachea
- Diffuse narrowing (slitlike lumen)
- Thickening of tracheal wall

Location
- Ear, 90%
- Joints, 80%
- Nose, 70%
- Eye, 65%
- Respiratory tract, 55%
- Inner ear, 45%
- Other: cardiovascular, 25%; skin, 15%

TRACHEOBRONCHOMALACIA

Refers to weakening of tracheal and bronchial walls.

Primary (uncommon)
- Occurs in children
- May be associated with laryngomalacia

Secondary (more common)
- Intubation
- COPD
- Less common causes: recurrent infections, trauma, relapsing polychondritis
- Compression of trachea by vessels or mediastinal mass

Radiographic Features
- Collapsed walls of trachea and bronchi
- Recurrent pneumonia

TRACHEOBRONCHOMEGALY (MOUNIER-KÜHN DISEASE)

Atrophy and dysplasia of trachea and proximal bronchi. Associated with Ehlers-Danlos syndrome. The trachea measures >3 cm, and/or bronchi measure >2.4 cm. Tracheal diverticula.

CONGENITAL BRONCHIAL ATRESIA

Narrowing or obliteration of a subsegmental, segmental, or lobar bronchus.

- LUL > RUL > RML > RLL, LLL
- Mucus plugging of dilated distal bronchus
- Collateral ventilation distal to obstruction with air trapping → distal lung is hyperlucent

CHRONIC BRONCHIAL DISEASE

Group of diseases characterized by increased airway resistance and reduction in expiratory flow. Entities include chronic bronchitis, emphysema, asthma, bronchiectasis, and cystic fibrosis. The most common combination is chronic bronchitis and emphysema, often referred to as chronic obstructive pulmonary disease.

CHRONIC OBSTRUCTIVE PULMONARY DISEASE (COPD)

COPD is characterized by progressive obstruction to airflow. Two components:

- Chronic bronchitis is a clinical diagnosis: excessive mucus formation and cough for >3 months during 2 consecutive years; all other causes of expectoration have to be ruled out. The diagnosis of chronic bronchitis is based on clinical history; chest films add little information except to exclude other underlying abnormalities.
- Emphysema is a pathologic diagnosis: abnormal enlargement of airspace distal to the terminal nonrespiratory bronchiole.

The exact etiology of COPD is unknown:

- Tobacco smoke
- Industrial air pollution
- α_1-Antitrypsin deficiency (autodigestion)

Clinical Syndromes

Blue bloaters

- Bronchitis, tussive type of COPD
- Episodic dyspnea due to exacerbation of bronchitis
- Young patients

Pink puffers

- Emphysematous type of COPD
- Progressive exertional dyspnea due to the emphysema
- Elderly patients

Radiographic Features

Features are nonspecific:

Tubular shadows (thickened bronchial walls)

- Parallel shadows if bronchiole is imaged in longitudinal section
- Thickening of bronchi imaged in axial section.
- Increased lung markings ("dirty chest")
- Accentuation of linear opacities throughout the lung
- Very subjective finding

EMPHYSEMA

Abnormal enlargement of distal airspaces with destruction of alveolar walls with or without fibrosis. Underlying cause: imbalance of proteases and antiproteases.

Clinical Findings

- Chronic airflow obstruction
- Decreased FEV_1

TYPES OF EMPHYSEMA*

	Panacinar	Centroacinar	Paraseptal
Predominant location	Lower lobes	Upper lobes	Along septal lines (periphery of lung and branch points of vessels)
Distribution	Homogeneous	Patchy	Peripheral
Associations	α_1-Antitrypsin deficiency, smoking	Chronic bronchitis, smoking	Smoking
Involvement	All components of acinus homogeneously involved	Center of pulmonary acinus involved	Usually entire secondary pulmonary lobule
Imaging	Panlobular emphysema 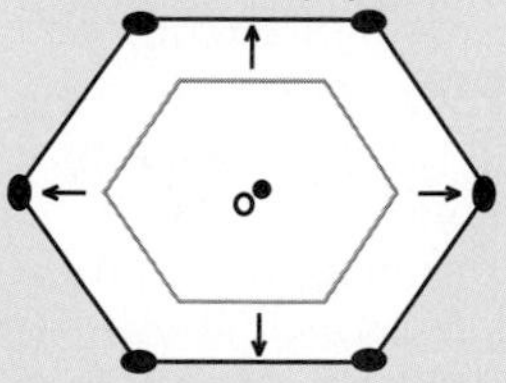	Normal pulmonary lobule 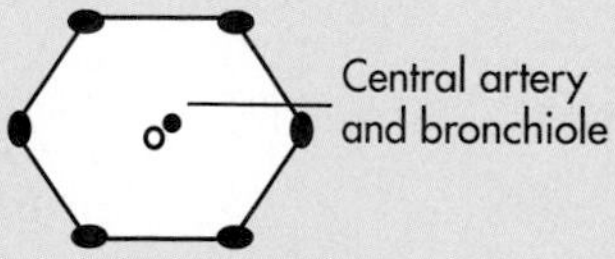 Centrilobular emphysema 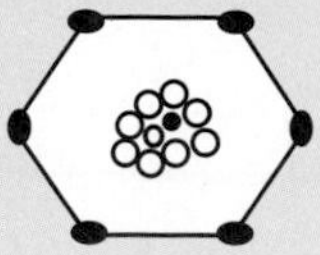	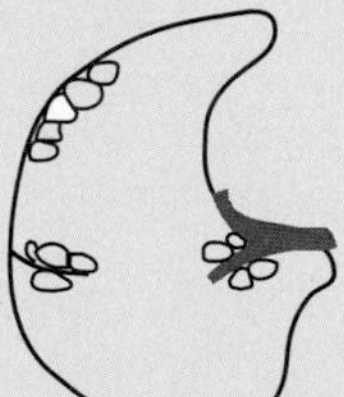

*The designations "lobular" and "acinai" refer to the number of acini affected (a few acini make up a lobule).

Radiographic Features (Fig. 1-50)

Overinflation
- Flattening of hemidiaphragms (reliable sign): highest level of the dome is <1.5 cm above a straight line drawn between the costophrenic and the vertebrophrenic junctions.
- Tenting of diaphragm (invagination of thickened visceral pleura attached to septa between basal bullae)
- Saber-sheath trachea
- Other, less reliable signs:
  - Increase of retrosternal airspace >3 cm measured at level 3 cm below the sternomanubrial junction
  - Craniocaudal diameter of lung >27 cm
  - Anterior bowing of sternum
  - Accentuated kyphosis
  - Widely spaced ribs

Vascular abnormalities
- Decreased number of vessels in areas of abnormal lung
- Absence of peripheral pulmonary vessels
- Fewer arterial branches
- Central pulmonary artery increased in size

Emphysema
- Decreased attenuation of abnormal lung
- An air-fluid level indicates infection of a bulla.

HRCT
- Centriacinar (centrilobular): the central portion of the pulmonary lobule is involved.
- Panacinar (panlobular): the whole acinus is involved, and central arteries and bronchioles can be seen (usually at apices).
- Paraseptal: emphysematous changes adjacent to septal lines in periphery and along fissures

Pearls
- As emphysema becomes more severe with time, the CT differentiation of the three types of emphysema becomes more difficult.

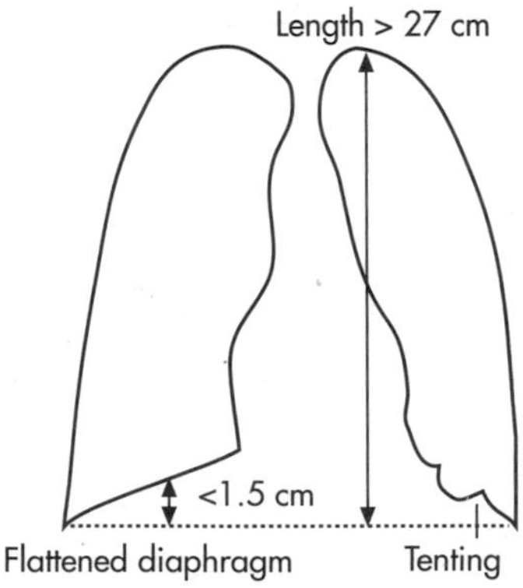

FIGURE 1-50

- Different types of emphysema may coexist.
- Moderate to severe emphysema can be detected on CXR; for the detection of mild forms HRCT is usually required.
- HRCT is currently the most sensitive method to detect emphysema; however, normal HRCT does not rule out the diagnosis of emphysema.
- Always look at CXR before interpreting HRCT; occasionally, CXR changes of emphysema are more evident than HRCT changes (e.g., hyperinflation).
- 20% of patients with emphysema have normal HRCT.
- 40% of patients with abnormal HRCT have normal pulmonary function tests.
- Bullous lung disease is a severe form of emphysema that is highly localized and >1 cm in size.

ASTHMA

Hyperirritability of airways causes reversible airway obstruction (bronchial smooth muscle contraction, mucosal edema, hypersecretion of bronchial secretory cells: bronchospasm). The etiology is unknown (IgE participation).

Types

Extrinsic, allergic form
- Childhood asthma
- Immunologically mediated hypersensitivity to inhaled antigens

Intrinsic asthma
- Adults
- No immediate hypersensitivity

Radiographic Features

Normal CXR in majority of patients

Severe or chronic asthma:
- Air trapping, hyperinflation: flattened diaphragm, increased retrosternal airspace
- Limited diaphragmatic excursion

Bronchial wall thickening (tramlines), a nonspecific finding, is also seen in chronic bronchitis, cystic fibrosis, bronchiectasis, and pulmonary edema.

Complications
- Acute pulmonary infection
- Mucus plugs
- Allergic bronchopulmonary aspergillosis (ABPA)
- Tracheal or bronchial obstruction
- Pneumomediastinum/pneumothorax

BRONCHIECTASIS

Irreversible dilatation of bronchi (reversible bronchial dilatation may be seen in viral and bacterial pneumonia). Recurrent pneumonias and/or hemoptysis

MORPHOLOGIC CLASSIFICATION OF BRONCHIECTASIS

	Cylindrical	Varicose	Cystic
Terminal divisions*	20	18	4
Pathology	Not end stage	Destroyed lung	Destroyed lung
CXR, HRCT	Fusiform dilatation, tramlines, signet signs	Tortuous dilatation rare	Saccular dilatation, "string of cysts," AFL common
	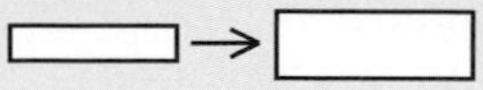	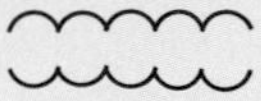	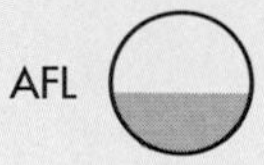

*Normal tracheobronchial tree has 23 to 24 divisions.

occur. HRCT is now the method of choice for workup of bronchiectasis.

Types

Congenital (rare)
- Abnormal secretions: cystic fibrosis
- Bronchial cartilage deficiency: Williams-Campbell syndrome
- Abnormal mucociliary transport: Kartagener syndrome
- Pulmonary sequestration

Postinfectious (common)
- Childhood infection
- Chronic granulomatous infection
- ABPA
- Measles

Bronchial obstruction
- Neoplasm
- Inflammatory nodes
- Foreign body
- Aspiration

Radiographic Features

Plain film
- Tramline: horizontal, parallel lines corresponding to thickened, dilated bronchi
- Bronchial wall thickening (best seen end-on)
- Indistinctness of central vessels due to peribronchovascular inflammation
- Atelectasis

HRCT (Fig. 1-51)
- Conspicuous bronchi
  Bronchi can be seen in outer third of lung.
  Bronchi appear larger than accompanying vessels.
- Bronchial walls
  Thickened walls
  Signet ring sign: focally thickened bronchial wall adjacent to pulmonary artery branch

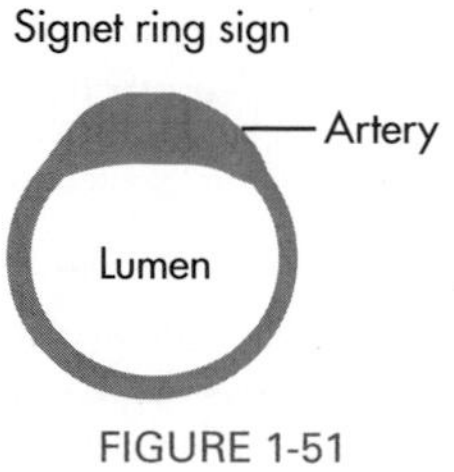

FIGURE 1-51

Pearls

- Bronchography may be indicated if clinical suspicion of bronchiectasis is high and CT is negative; CT has a low positive predictive value for mild forms of bronchiectasis. Bronchography is rarely performed alone.
- Differentiation of cystic bronchiectasis and cystic spaces in IPF (honeycombing) is difficult; bronchiectasis usually involves lower lobes; honeycombing is not associated with air-fluid levels.
- To distinguish emphysema from bronchiectasis, expiratory scans will show air trapping in bullae; cystic bronchiectasis will collapse.

CYSTIC FIBROSIS

Caused by an abnormality in the cystic fibrosis transmembrane conductance regulator protein, which regulates the passage of ions through membranes of mucus-producing cells. Autosomal recessive disease (incidence 1:2000).

Pathophysiology

- Dysfunction of exocrine glands causing thick, tenacious mucus that accumulates and causes bronchitis and pneumonia
- Reduced mucociliary transport: airway obstruction with massive mucus plugging

Spectrum of disease

Pulmonary, 100%
- Chronic cough
- Recurrent pulmonary infections: colonization of plugged airways by *Staphylococcus* and *Pseudomonas*
- Progressive respiratory failure
- Finger clubbing: hypertrophic osteoarthropathy from hypoxemia

GI tract
- Pancreatic insufficiency, 85%: steatorrhea, malabsorption
- Liver cirrhosis
- Rectal prolapse
- Neonates: meconium ileus, meconium peritonitis, intussusception

Other
- Sinusitis: hypoplastic frontal sinus, opacification of other sinuses
- Infertility in males

Radiographic Features

Severity of bronchiectasis
- Mild: lumen equal to adjacent blood vessels
- Moderate: lumen 2 to 3 times the size of adjacent blood vessels
- Severe: lumen >3 times the size of adjacent blood vessels

Peribronchial thickening
- Wall thickness ≥ the diameter of adjacent blood vessels

Mucus plugging
- Determine number of pulmonary segments involved
- Air trapping → increased lung volumes
- Collapse, consolidation
- Bullae

Location: predominantly upper lobes and superior segments of lower lobes

Other
- Reticular, cystic pattern of lung fibrosis
- Prominent hila:
  - Adenopathy
  - Large pulmonary arteries (PAH)
- Recurrent pneumonias

Complications

Early
- Lobar atelectasis (especially RUL)
- Pneumonia

Late
- Respiratory insufficiency, hypertrophic osteoarthropathy
- Recurrent pneumothorax (rupture of bullae or blebs)
- Cor pulmonale and pulmonary arterial hypertension
- Hemoptysis
- *Aspergillus* superinfection

BRONCHIOLITIS OBLITERANS

Bronchiolitis obliterans (Swyer-James syndrome, unilateral emphysema) refers to unilateral air trapping caused by obstruction of distal bronchioles.

Etiology of Adult Bronchiolitis

Obliterative
- Exposure to toxic fumes
- Bone marrow transplant
- Viral infections
- Drugs

Proliferative
- Acute infectious
- Respiratory bronchiolitis
- COP
- COPD
  - Asthma
  - Chronic bronchitis

CT Features

- Nodules with branching opacities: tree-in-bud appearance
- Ground-glass attenuation and consolidation
- Mosaic pattern
  - Seen with obliterative bronchiolitis
  - Mosaic pattern due to hypoxic vasoconstriction in areas of bronchiolar obstruction with redistribution to normal areas
  - Decreased size and number of vessels in affected lung with air trapping on inspiration/expiration CT; thus the apparent ground-glass-appearing lung is normal.
- Other nonspecific findings
  - Bronchiectasis
  - Bronchial wall thickening

Lung Injury

TRAUMA

Four major mechanisms of injury:
1. Direct impact
2. Sudden deceleration (motor vehicle accident): sudden torsion at interfaces of fixed (e.g., paraspinal) and mobile (e.g., lung) components
3. Spallation: broad kinetic shock wave, which is partially reflected at a liquid-gas interface, leading to local disruption of alveoli and supporting structures
4. Implosion: low-pressure afterwave that causes rebound overexpansion of gas bubbles

Other mechanisms of chest trauma include:
- Posttraumatic aspiration
- Inhalation injury
- Increased capillary permeability: fat emboli, oligemic shock, neurogenic pulmonary edema

Pearls

- Radiographic and clinical evidence of lung trauma is often absent in the first 2 to 3 hours after trauma.
- There is no consistent relationship between external chest wall injury and underlying lung injury, especially in children.
- Radiographic studies usually underestimate the true extent of pulmonary trauma.

PNEUMOTHORAX (Fig. 1-52)

Common causes:

- Iatrogenic
  - Percutaneous biopsy, 20%
  - Barotrauma, ventilator, 20%
- Trauma
  - Lung laceration
  - Tracheobronchial rupture
- Cystic lung disease
  - Bulla, bleb: often in healthy young men; 30% recurrence
  - Emphysema, asthma
  - PCP
  - Honeycombing: end-stage interstitial lung disease
  - Lymphangioleiomyomatosis (pneumothorax in 75% of cases)
  - Eosinophilic granuloma (pneumothorax in 20% of cases)
- Parenchymal necrosis
  - Lung abscess, necrotic pneumonia, septic emboli, fungal disease, TB
  - Cavitating neoplasm, osteogenic sarcoma
  - Radiation necrosis
- Other
  - Catamenial: recurrent spontaneous pneumothorax during menstruation, associated with endometriosis of pleura

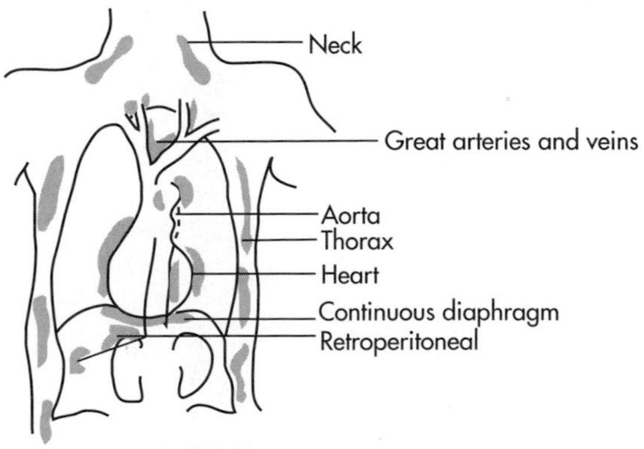

FIGURE 1-52

RADIOGRAPHIC FEATURES (Figs. 1-53 and 1-54)

Appearance

- Upright position
  - Air in pleural space is radiolucent.
  - White line of the visceral pleura is distinctly visible.
  - Volume loss of underlying lung
  - Supine position
  - Deep sulcus sign: anterior costophrenic angle sharply delineated

Detection

- Lateral decubitus (suspected side should be up, whereas it should be down for fluid); 5 mL of air detectable
- Upright expiration film
- CT most sensitive

Size of pneumothorax can be estimated but is rarely of practical use

- Average distance (AD in cm) = (A + B + C)/3
- % Pneumothorax ≈ AD (in cm) x 10, e.g.:
  - AD of 1 cm corresponds to a 10% pneumothorax
  - AD of 4 cm corresponds to a 40% pneumothorax

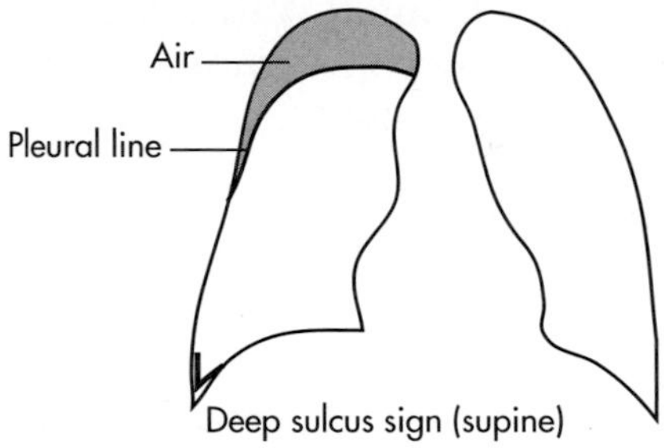

FIGURE 1-53

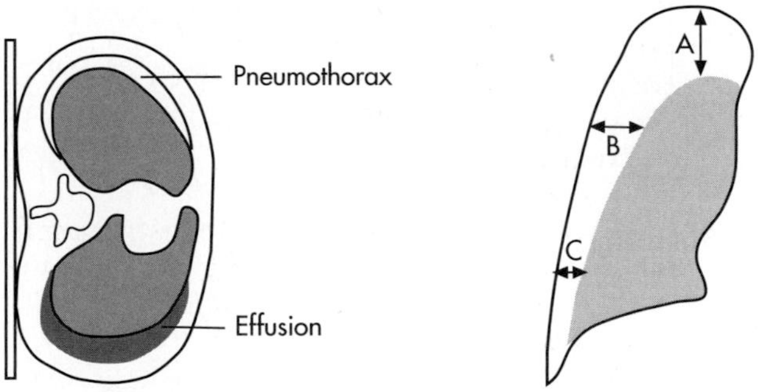

FIGURE 1-54

TENSION PNEUMOTHORAX (Fig. 1-55)

Valve effect during inspiration/expiration leads to progressive air accumulation in thoracic cavity. The increased pressure causes shift of mediastinum and ultimately vascular compromise. Treatment is with emergency chest tube placement.

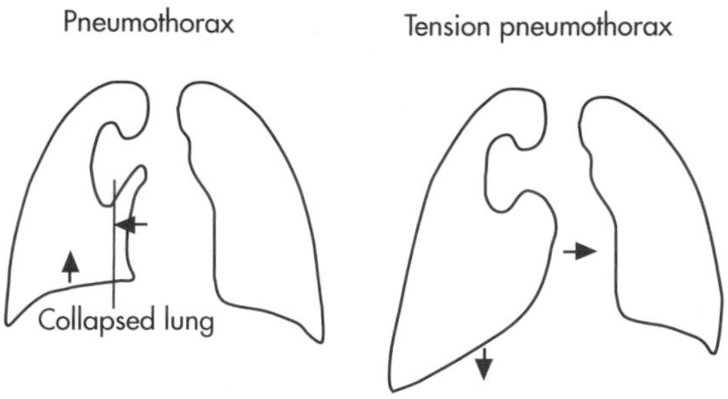

FIGURE 1-55

Radiographic Features

- Overexpanded lung
- Depressed diaphragm
- Shift of mediastinum and heart to contralateral side

PERCUTANEOUS CHEST TUBE PLACEMENT FOR PNEUMOTHORAX

Indication

- All symptomatic pneumothoraces

Technique for Heimlich Valve Placement (for Biopsy-Induced Pneumothorax)

1. Entry: midclavicular line, 2nd to 4th anterior intercostal space
2. Aspirate air with 50-mL syringe.
3. Use small drainage kit that includes a Heimlich valve (one-way airflow system). During expiration, positive intrapleural pressure causes air to escape through the valve.

Technique for Chest Tube Placement (Any Pneumothorax)

1. Entry: posterior or lateral or region of largest pneumothorax as defined by CT
2. Local anesthesia
3. Place 12- to 16-Fr drainage catheter using trocar technique.
4. Put catheter to wall suction.
5. Catheter can be removed if there is no pneumothorax 24 hours after clamping of the catheter.

CONTUSION

Endothelial damage causes extravasation of blood into interstitium and alveoli.

Occurs mainly in lung adjacent to solid structures (e.g., ribs, vertebrae, heart, liver).

Appears 6 to 24 hours after injury. Hemoptysis is present in 50%. Mortality rate of 15%-40%.

Radiographic Features

- Pulmonary opacities are due to hemorrhage and edema.
- Air bronchograms are commonly seen by CT but are not always present if there is associated bronchial obstruction.
- Contusions usually appear 6 to 24 hours after trauma and resolve by 7 to 10 days.
- Opacities that do not resolve by 7 to 10 days may represent:
  - Postlaceration hematoma
  - Aspiration
  - Hospital-acquired pneumonia
  - Atelectasis
  - ARDS

LUNG LACERATION (Fig. 1-56)

Produced by sharp trauma (rib fractures), deceleration, shearing, or implosion. Pathogenetically, there is a linear tear (may be radiographically visible) that becomes round or ovoid (pneumatocele) with time. Usually accompanied by hemoptysis and pleural and parenchymal hemorrhage. Bronchopleural fistulas are a common complication. Detection of a laceration is clinically important as lacerations can become secondarily infected and also lead to bronchopleural fistula, requiring prolonged chest tube drainage.

TYPES OF PULMONARY LACERATIONS

Type	Location	Pneumothorax	Mechanism
1	Midlung	Variable	Shear between parenchyma and tracheobronchial tree
2	Paraspinal	Uncommon	Shear due to sudden herniation of lower lobe parenchyma in front of vertebral column
3	Subpleural	Usual	Puncture by displaced rib fracture
4	Subpleural	Usual	Shear at site of transpleural adhesion

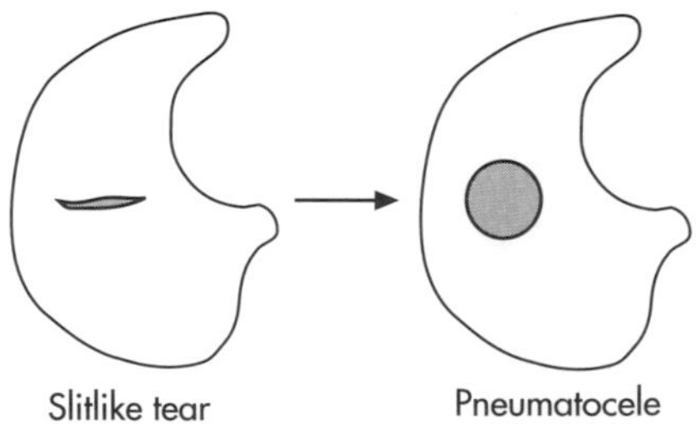

FIGURE 1-56

FAT EMBOLISM

Lipid emboli from bone marrow enter pulmonary and systemic circulation. When complicated by ARDS, fat embolism has high mortality. Frequently CNS is also affected.

Radiographic Features

- Subject in patients with initially clear lungs, sudden onset of dyspnea, and multiple fractures.
- Interstitial and alveolar hemorrhagic edema produces a varied radiographic appearance.
- Radiographic opacities induced by fat embolism become evident only 48 hours after the incident ("delayed onset").
- Opacities clear in 3 to 7 days.

TRACHEOBRONCHIAL TEAR

High mortality (30%). Requires early bronchoscopy for early detection to avoid later bronchostenosis. Two presentations:

- Tear of right mainstem and distal left bronchus: pneumothorax not relieved by chest tube placement. Most common locations are main bronchi (R > L); 75% occur within 2 cm of tracheal carina.
- Tear of trachea and left mainstem bronchus: air leaks are usually confined to mediastinum and subcutaneous tissues.

DIAPHRAGMATIC TEAR

Ninety percent of tears occur on the left side, 90% of clinically significant hemidiaphragm ruptures are overlooked initially, and 90% of strangulated diaphragmatic hernias are of traumatic etiology.

Radiographic Features (Fig. 1-57)

- Air-fluid levels or abnormal air collection above diaphragm
- Abnormal elevation of left hemidiaphragm with or without herniated gastric fundus or colon
- Contralateral tension displacement of mediastinum
- Abnormal location of NG tube
- Confirmation of tear by coronal MRI

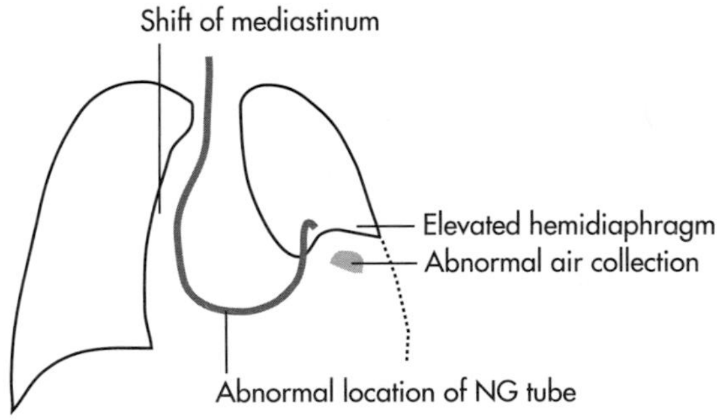

FIGURE 1-57

ESOPHAGEAL TEAR

- Esophageal tear (thoracic inlet, gastroesophageal junction)
- Blunt injuries usually seen in phrenic ampulla and cervical esophagus, whereas penetrating injuries can occur anywhere.
- Chest radiographs are nonspecific and usually show wide mediastinum, left pleural effusion, or hydropneumothorax.
- Pneumomediastinum is common but is a nonspecific finding.
- Pleural effusion has low pH and high amylase levels.

OTHER INJURIES

- Aortic injury
- Hemothorax
- Chylothorax
- Cardiac injury
- Fractures: rib, spine

POSTOPERATIVE CHEST

COMPLICATIONS OF SURGICAL PROCEDURES

Mediastinoscopy

Complication rate, <2%:

- Mediastinal bleeding
- Pneumothorax
- Vocal cord paralysis (recurrent nerve injury)

Bronchoscopy

- Injury to teeth, aspiration
- Transient pulmonary opacities, 5%
- Fever, 15%
- Transbronchial biopsy:
  - Pneumothorax, 15%
  - Hemorrhage (>50 mL), 1%

Wedge Resection

- Air leaks (common)
- Contusion
- Recurrence of tumor

Median Sternotomy Complications

Complication rate, 1%-5%:

- Mediastinal hemorrhage
- Mediastinitis (focal fluid collection)
- Sternal dehiscence
- False aneurysm
- Phrenic nerve paralysis
- Osteomyelitis of sternum

Chest Tube Placement

- Horner syndrome (pressure on sympathetic ganglion)
- False aortic aneurysm

PNEUMONECTOMY (Fig. 1-58)

Radiographic Features

- Two thirds of the hemithorax fills with fluid in 4 to 7 days; it is important that successive films demonstrate gradual fill-in and that the residual

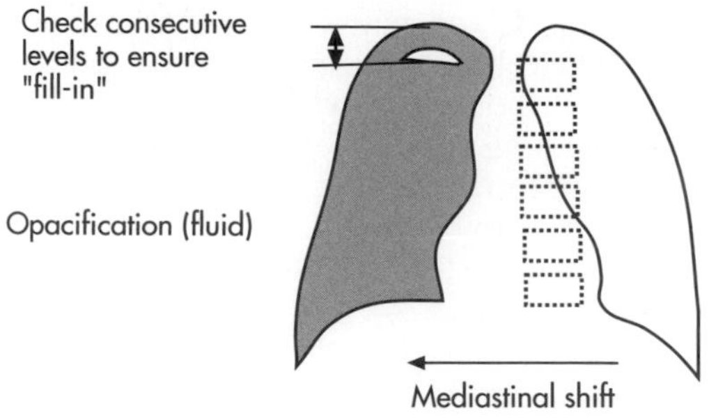

FIGURE 1-58

air bubble does not get bigger; an air bubble increasing in size is suggestive of a bronchopleural fistula.
- Gradual shift of the mediastinum and heart toward the pneumonectomy side
- Contralateral lung may normally be herniated toward the pneumonectomy side at the apex and mimic the presence of a residual lung.

Lobectomy
- Remaining lobes expand to fill the void; splaying of vessels
- Slight shift of mediastinum, elevation of hemidiaphragm

(Sub)segmental Resection
- Little or no parenchymal rearrangement
- Postoperative opacities (hemorrhage, confusion, edema) common

POSTPNEUMONECTOMY SYNDROME

This rare syndrome refers to airway obstruction that occurs after pulmonary resections and is due to an extreme shift of the mediastinum or rotation of hilar structures. Occurs most often after right pneumonectomy or after left pneumonectomy when a right arch is present.

Radiographic Features (Fig. 1-59)

Airway obstruction
- Air trapping: hyperinflated lung
- Recurrent pneumonia, bronchiectasis

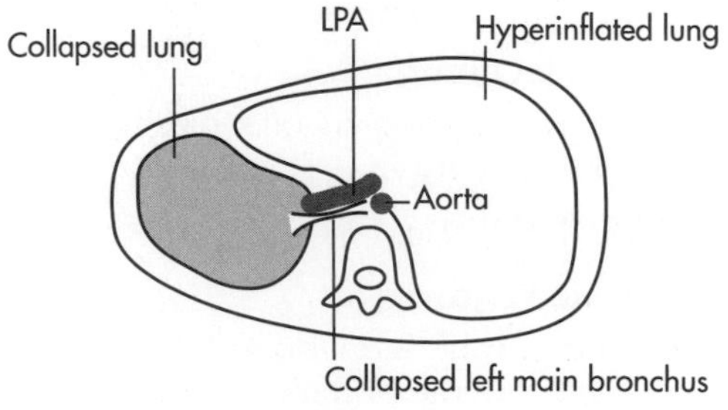

FIGURE 1-59

Narrowing of bronchi or trachea, bronchomalacia
Postsurgical changes
- Hyperinflation of contralateral lung
- Marked shift of mediastinum

BRONCHOPLEURAL FISTULA (BPF)

A fistula between bronchus and pleural space develops in 2%-4% of pneumonectomy patients; with large fistulas, the fluid in the pneumonectomy cavity may drown the opposite healthy lung. Factors that predispose to BPF include:
- Active inflammation (TB), necrotizing infection
- Tumor in bronchial margin
- Devascularized bronchial stump, poor vascular supply
- Preoperative irradiation
- Contamination of the pleural space

Radiographic Features

Plain film
- Persistent or progressive pneumothorax
- Sudden shift of mediastinum to the normal side

Nuclear medicine
- Xenon leak

Sinography with nonionic contrast material
- Examination of choice to define the size of a pleural cavity and bronchial communication
- Alternatively, thin section CT may show communication.

TORSION

Lobar Torsion

A prerequisite for torsion is the presence of complete fissures. Predisposing factors include masses, pleural effusion, pneumothorax, pneumonia, and surgical resection of inferior pulmonary ligament. Rare.
- Most commonly the right middle lobe (RML) rotates on its bronchovascular pedicle.
- Obstruction of venous flow, ischemia, and necrosis result.
- Plain film: mobile opacity at different locations on different views

Cardiac Herniation

Rare. 50%-100% mortality. Most often occurs after a right pneumonectomy requiring intrapericardial dissection.

Radiographic Features (Fig. 1-60)
- Heart is rotated to the right
- Cardiac herniation through pericardial sac results in intrapericardial air, which originates from the postpneumonectomy space
- Presence of a notch
- Intracardiac catheters are kinked
- "Snow cone" appearance of heart border

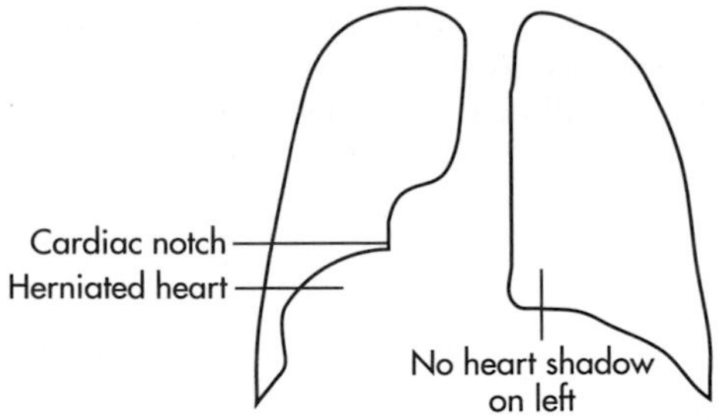

FIGURE 1-60

LUNG TRANSPLANTATION

Transplantation of the left lung is technically easier because of the longer left bronchus.

Radiographic Features

Reimplantation response
- Diffuse alveolar pattern of noncardiogenic pulmonary edema develops within 4 to 5 days in the transplanted lung owing to capillary leak. It never develops later.
- The alveolar pattern lasts 1 to several weeks.

Rejection
- Acute rejection is most commonly detected by biopsy when there are no associated radiographic findings; when radiographic findings are present, they include:
  - Diffuse interstitial pattern in peribronchovascular distribution
  - Septal thickening
  - Pleural effusion
  - Alveolar edema
- Chronic rejection
  - Bronchiolitis obliterans (air trapping on expiratory scans)
  - Bronchiectasis

Infections, 50% of patients
- Infections usually involve the transplanted lung, not the native lung, because of poor mucociliary clearance and/or lymphatic interruption.
- Pathogens: *Pseudomonas, Staphylococcus* > other bacterial, viral, fungal infections

Airways
- Leaks at bronchial anastomosis site are the most common abnormality and usually present as pneumomediastinum and/or pneumothorax in the perioperative period.
- Operations to prevent leaks
  - Omental flap around anastomosis
  - Telescope-type anastomosis
- Bronchial strictures may require stenting

Lymphoproliferative disorder
- Multiple or solitary pulmonary nodules or lymphadenopathy

Pulmonary Vasculature

PULMONARY ARTERY HYPERTENSION

GENERAL

PAH is defined as P_{sys} >30 mm Hg or P_{mean} >25 mm Hg.
Normal pulmonary arterial pressures in adult:
- P_{sys}: 20 mm Hg
- P_{dias}: 10 mm Hg
- P_{mean}: 14 mm Hg
- Capillary wedge pressure: 5 mm Hg

Causes of PAH

Primary PAH (females 10 to 40 years; rare)

Secondary PAH (more common)
- Eisenmenger syndrome
- Chronic PE
- Emphysema, pulmonary fibrosis
- Schistosomiasis (most common cause worldwide)

Classification

Precapillary hypertension

Vascular
- Increased flow: L-R shunts
- Chronic PE
- Vasculitis
- Drugs
- Idiopathic

Pulmonary
- Emphysema
- Interstitial fibrosis
- Fibrothorax, chest wall deformities
- Alveolar hypoventilation

Postcapillary hypertension
- Cardiac
  - LV failure
  - Mitral stenosis
  - Atrial tumor
- Pulmonary venous
  - Idiopathic venoocclusive disease
  - Thrombosis

Radiographic Features

- Enlarged main PA (diameter correlates with pressure): >29 mm is indicative of PAH.
- Rapid tapering of PA toward the periphery
- Decreased velocity of pulmonary flow by MRA
- Calcification of the pulmonary arteries is pathognomonic but occurs late in the disease.
- Cardiomegaly (cor pulmonale)
- If the ratio of pulmonary artery diameter to aortic diameter is greater than 1 (rPA >1) by CT, there is a strong correlation with elevated mean PA pressure, particularly in patients <50 years of age.

TYPES OF PULMONARY EDEMA

Signs	Cardiac	Renal	Lung Injury
Heart size	Enlarged	Normal	Normal
Blood flow	Inverted	Balanced	Normal
Kerley lines	Common	Common	Absent
Edema	Basilar	Central: butterfly	Diffuse
Air bronchograms	Not common	Not common	Very common
Pleural effusions	Very common	Common	Not common
	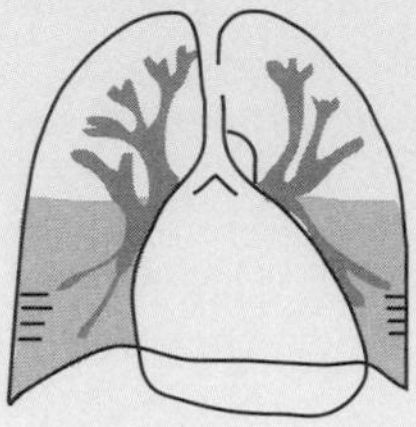	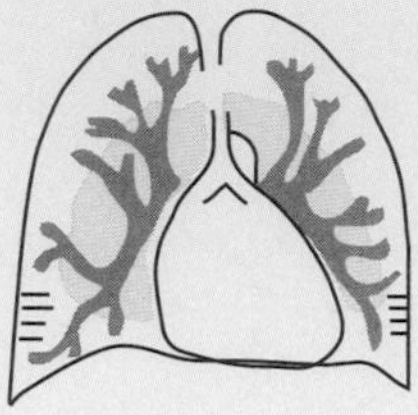	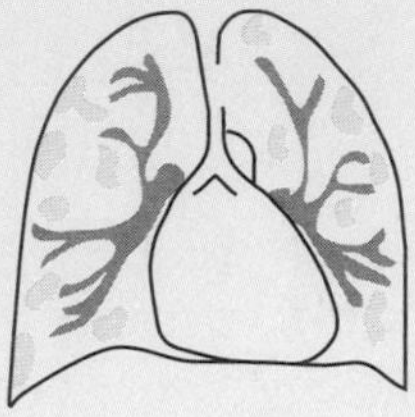

- By HRCT scans, both primary and secondary forms of pulmonary hypertension may produce a mosaic pattern of lung attenuation, a finding suggestive of regional variations in parenchymal perfusion. A vascular cause for the mosaic pattern is suggested when areas of high attenuation contain larger-caliber vessels and areas of low attenuation contain vessels of diminished size.

PULMONARY EDEMA

Causes of Pulmonary Edema

Cardiogenic
- Adults
  - Left ventricular (LV) failure from CAD (most common)
  - Mitral regurgitation (common)
  - Ruptured chordae
  - Endocarditis
- Neonates
  - TAPVC below diaphragm
  - Hypoplastic left side of heart
  - Cor triatriatum

Renal
- Renal failure
- Volume overload

Lung injury (increased permeability: capillary leak)
- Septic shock, neurogenic shock
- Fat embolism
- Inhalation: SO_2, O_2, Cl_2, NO_2
- Aspiration, drowning

GRADING OF CARDIOGENIC PULMONARY EDEMA (Figs. 1-61 through 1-63)

Fluid accumulation in the lung due to cardiogenic causes (CHF; pulmonary venous hypertension) follows a defined pattern:

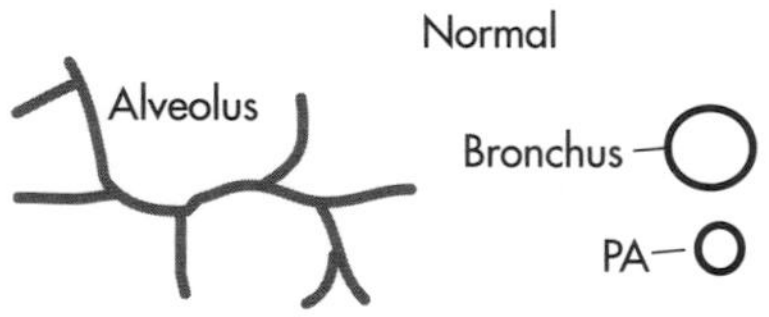

FIGURE 1-61

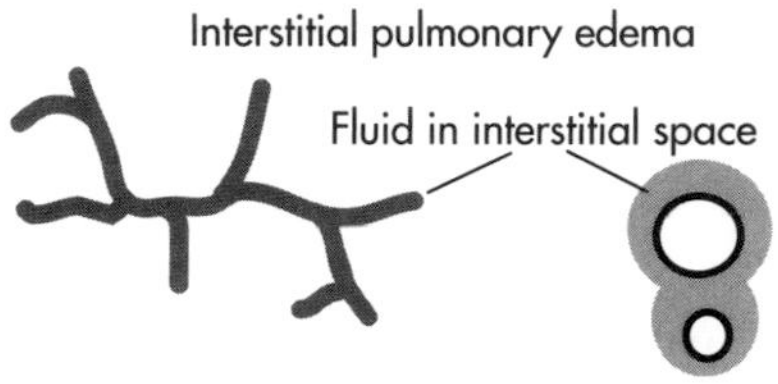

FIGURE 1-62

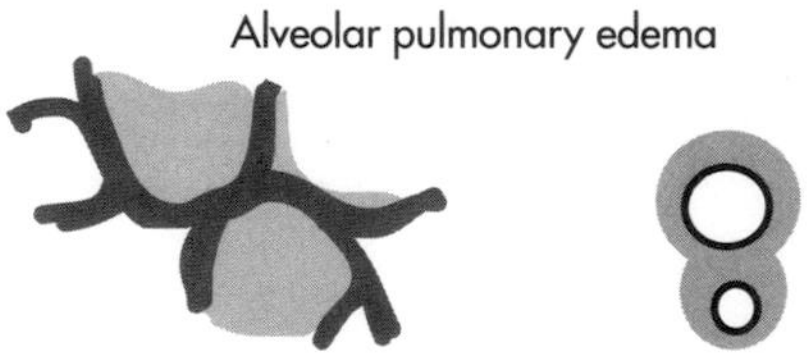

FIGURE 1-63

Grade 1: vascular redistribution (10 to 17 mm Hg)
- Diameter of upper lobe vessels equal to or increased over diameter of lower lobe vessels at comparable distance from hilum
- Pulmonary veins in first intercostal space >3 mm in diameter

Grade 2: interstitial edema (18 to 25 mm Hg)
- Peribronchovascular cuffing, perihilar haziness
- Kerley lines (differential diagnosis: chronic fibrosis from edema, hemosiderin, tumor, etc.)

- Unsharp central pulmonary vessels (perivascular edema)
- Pleural effusion

Grade 3: alveolar edema (>25 mm Hg)

- Airspace disease: patchy consolidation, air bronchograms

ASYMMETRICAL PULMONARY EDEMA

- Gravitational (most common)
- Underlying COPD (common)
- Unilateral obstruction of pulmonary artery: PE
- Unilateral obstruction of lobar pulmonary vein: tumor

PULMONARY EMBOLISM

Acute pulmonary embolism (PE) is associated with significant morbidity and mortality, causing 120,000 deaths/year in the United States.

Types

- Incomplete infarct: hemorrhagic pulmonary edema without tissue necrosis; resolution within days
- Complete infarct: tissue necrosis; healing by scar formation

Risk Factors

- Immobilization >72 hours (55% of patients with proved PE have this risk factor)
- Recent hip surgery, 40%
- Cardiac disease, 30%
- Malignancy, 20%
- Estrogen use (prostate cancer, contraceptives), 6%
- Prior deep vein thrombosis (DVT), 20%; risk factors:
  - Myocardial infarction
  - Thoracoabdominal surgery
  - Permanent pacemaker
  - Venous catheters

Clinical Findings

- Chest pain, 90%
- Tachypnea (>16 breaths/min), 90%
- Dyspnea, 85%
- Rales, 60%
- Cough, 55%
- Tachycardia, 40%
- Hemoptysis, 30%
- Fever, 45%
- Diaphoresis, 25%
- Cardiac gallop, 30%
- Syncope, 15%
- Phlebitis, 35%

Radiographic Features

Radiographic signs are nonspecific and are present only if a significant infarction occurs

Imaging Algorithm

- CT pulmonary angiography with axial CT of the inferior vena cava and the iliac, femoral, and popliteal veins is the mainstay of PE evaluation. If the findings are equivocal and clinical suspicion remains high, additional imaging is required ($\dot{V}/\dot{Q}$ scan, pulmonary angiography).
- $\dot{V}/\dot{Q}$ scan is preferred if iodinated contrast is contraindicated in the context of renal insufficiency or history of severe allergic reaction.
- Patients who have symptoms of deep vein thrombosis but not of pulmonary embolism initially undergo US, which is a less expensive alternative. If the findings are negative, imaging is usually discontinued; if they are positive, the patient is evaluated for pulmonary embolism at the discretion of the referring physician.
- In pregnant patients, CTA may be performed if there is high suspicion for PE and sonography fails to demonstrate lower extremity DVT. Axial CT of the IVC and the iliac, femoral, and popliteal veins is omitted.

Plain Film

- Westermark sign: localized pulmonary oligemia (rare)
- Hampton hump: triangular peripheral cone of infarct = blood in secondary pulmonary lobules (rare); does not grow → should reduce in size on successive radiographs
- Fleischner sign: increased diameter of pulmonary artery (>16 mm) seen in acute PE. It usually disappears within a few days.
- Cor pulmonale: sudden increase in size of RV, RA
- Pulmonary edema, atelectasis, pleural effusion, 50%

CT Findings in PE

- Adequately performed CT studies are essentially >90% sensitive and specific for large central emboli.
- Intraluminal filling defect surrounded by contrast
- Expanded unopacified vessel
- Eccentric filling defect
- Peripheral wedge-shaped consolidation
- Pleural effusion
- Allows evaluation of the inferior vena cava and the lower extremity veins to the knee
- Anatomic pitfalls in CT diagnosis of acute PE: lymph nodes, impacted bronchi, pulmonary veins, pulmonary arterial catheters, and pulmonary artery sarcomas.
- Technical pitfalls: respiratory or cardiac motion, poor bolus timing, quantum mottle, and edge-enhancing reconstruction algorithms

Scintigraphy

- Ventilation-perfusion mismatch

Angiography
- Constant intraluminal filling defects in PA
- Complete cut-off of PA or its branches
- Prolongation of the arterial phase; delayed filling and emptying of venous phase

VASCULITIS

OVERVIEW OF PULMONARY VASCULITIDES

Syndrome	Pathology	Other Affected Vessels
Polyarteritis nodosa	Necrotizing vasculitis	Renal, hepatic, and visceral aneurysm
Allergic granulomatous angiitis (Churg-Strauss syndrome)	Granulomatous vasculitis	Allergic history, eosinophilia
Hypersensitivity vasculitis	Leukocytoclastic vasculitis	Skin (common)
Henoch-Schönlein purpura vasculitis	Leukocytoclastic	Skin, GI, renal involvement usual
Takayasu arteritis	Giant cell arteritis	Aortic arch
Temporal arteritis	Giant cell arteritis	Carotid branches
Wegener granulomatosis	Necrotizing granulomatous vasculitis	Upper and lower respiratory tracts, glomerulonephritis

VENOUS ABNORMALITIES

PULMONARY ARTERIOVENOUS MALFORMATION (AVM)

Abnormal communication between pulmonary artery and veins. A communication between systemic arteries and pulmonary veins is much less common (<5%).

Types

Congenital, 60%
- Osler-Weber-Rendu disease (hereditary hemorrhagic telangiectasia)

Acquired, 40%
- Iatrogenic
- Infection
- Tumor

Radiographic Features
- Location: lower lobes, 70% > middle lobe > upper lobes
- Feeding artery, draining veins
- Sharply defined mass
- Strong enhancement
- Change in size with Valsalva/Mueller procedure

Complications
- Stroke, 20%
- Abscess, 10% (AVM acts as a systemic shunt)
- Rupture: hemothorax, hemoptysis, 10%

PULMONARY VARICES

Uncommon lesions that are typically asymptomatic and do not require treatment. Usually discovered incidentally.

Radiographic Features
- Dilated vein
- Usually near left atrium

Aortic Nipple

Normal variant (10% of population) caused by the left superior intercostal vein seen adjacent to the aortic arch. Maximum diameter of vein: 4 mm

PULMONARY VENOOCCLUSIVE DISEASE (PVOD)

In the typical form there is occlusion of small pulmonary veins. The proposed initial insult in PVOD is venous thrombosis, possibly initiated by infection, toxic exposure, or immune complex deposition.

Radiographic Features
- Edema without cephalization
- Pleural effusions
- Cardiomegaly
- CT findings
    - Secondary pulmonary arterial hypertension
    - Markedly small central pulmonary veins
    - Central and gravity-dependent ground-glass lung attenuation
    - Smoothly thickened interlobular septa
    - Normal-sized left atrium
    - Centrilobular nodules

Pleura

GENERAL

NORMAL PLEURAL ANATOMY
- Visceral pleura: covers lung
- Parietal pleura: covers rib (costal pleura), diaphragm (diaphragmatic pleura), mediastinum (mediastinal pleura)

Visceral and parietal pleura are continued at the pulmonary hilum and continue inferiorly as the inferior pulmonary ligament. Normal pleura (0.2 to 0.4 mm) is not visible by CT. Pleural thickening is present when a stripe of soft tissue is seen internal to a rib.

DIAGNOSTIC THORACENTESIS

Success rate 97%. Pneumothorax 1%-3% (<with blind thoracentesis).

Indication
- Suspected malignancy
- Suspected infection

Technique

1. Use US to determine skin entry site.
2. Anesthetize skin and subcutaneous and deep tissues.
3. Advance 18- to 22-gauge spinal needle into collection, going over the superior border of the rib to avoid the neurovascular bundle.
4. Aspirate 20 to 100 mL.

THERAPEUTIC THORACENTESIS

Success rate, 95%. Pneumothorax 7%.

Indication

- Respiratory compromise from large pleural effusions

Technique

1. Perform diagnostic thoracentesis
2. Skin nick
3. Place 7- to 10-Fr catheters for therapeutic thoracentesis. Remove catheter.
4. Obtain CXR to check for pneumothorax.

Expansion Pulmonary Edema

Pulmonary edema may occur as a result of rapid evacuation of large amounts of pleural effusion. We routinely evacuate 2 to 3 L without complications. Do not aspirate both lungs in the same sitting because of the risk of expansion pulmonary edema and/or bilateral pneumothoraces.

Vacuthorax

If the lung parenchyma is abnormally stiff (fibrosis), it cannot reexpand and fill the pleural space, resulting in a "vacuthorax." The patient is unlikely to benefit from thoracentesis in this circumstance.

PNEUMOTHORAX MANAGEMENT

Success rate, >90%.

Indication for Intervention

- Symptomatic pneumothorax
- Pneumothorax, >20%
- Enlarging pneumothorax on subsequent CXR
- Tension pneumothorax
- Poor lung function of contralateral lung disease

Technique

1. Two approaches
   - 2nd to 4th anterior intercostal space, midclavicular line
   - 6th to 8th intercostal space, midaxillary line or posterior
2. Local anesthesia, skin nick
3. Place 8- to 12-Fr catheters using a trocar technique. For the anterior approach, small Heimlich valve sets may be used.
4. After the lung is fully reexpanded for 24 hours, the catheter is placed on water seal for 6 hours and then removed if there is no pneumothorax.

Persistent Pneumothorax in Patient with Chest Catheter

- Persistent leak from airways (bronchial injury, lung laceration)
- Loculated pneumothorax
- Anterior pneumothorax
- Obstructed catheter

EMPYEMA DRAINAGE

Success rate, 80%. Complications (hemorrhage, lung injury), 2%.

Indication

- Pus on diagnostic thoracentesis
- Positive Gram stain
- Positive culture

Technique

1. Choose entry site adjacent to largest collection using US or CT.
2. Local anesthesia
3. Diagnostic tap with 18-gauge needle. Send specimen for bacteriologic testing.
4. Choice of drainage catheters
   - 10- to 16-Fr pigtail catheter for liquid effusions (usually placed by trocar technique)
   - 24-Fr catheter for thick collections (usually placed by Seldinger technique); dilators: 8, 10, 12, 14, 16, 20, etc.
5. Put catheter to suction.
6. Intrapleural tPA may be necessary for loculated effusions. tPA, 4-6 mg, is administered in up to 50 mL saline twice daily. Each administration consists of a clamping the tube and a dwell time of 30 minutes, after which the tube is placed back on suction.

Complications

- Technical catheter problems (clogging: change for larger catheter)
- Nonclearance of collection: surgical removal

FLUID COLLECTIONS

PLEURAL EFFUSIONS

Excess fluid in the pleural space. There are two generic types: transudates and exudates:

- Transudate: ultrafiltrate of plasma; highly fluid, low in protein, devoid of inflammatory cells

- Exudate: increased permeability of microcirculation; rich in protein, cells, and debris

DIFFERENTIATION BETWEEN TRANSUDATE AND EXUDATE

	Transudate	Exudate
Protein	<3 g/dL	>3 g/dL
Protein (plasma/fluid)	<0.5	>0.5
LDH	<200 IU <70% of serum level	>200 IU >70% of serum level
Common causes	CHF, renal failure cirrhosis	Infection (parapneumonic), tumor, embolism

Causes

Tumor
- Bronchogenic carcinoma
- Pleural metastases
- Malignant mesothelioma
- Lymphoma

Inflammation
- Pneumonia, TB, empyema
- Collagen vascular disease
- Abdominal disease
  - Pancreatitis
  - Subphrenic abscess
  - Boerhaave syndrome
  - Meigs syndrome (benign ovarian fibroma)

Cardiovascular
- Congestive heart failure
- Pulmonary embolism
- Renal failure

Congenital
- Hydrops (neonate)

Metabolic
- Hypoproteinemia

Trauma

Radiographic Features (Fig. 1-64)

Lateral decubitus films
- Most sensitive: may detect as little as 25 mL

PA, lateral films: blunting of costophrenic angles
- Posterior costophrenic angle (>75 mL required)
- Lateral costophrenic angles (>175 mL required)

Large effusions
- All cardiophrenic angles obliterated
- Mediastinal shift
- Elevated diaphragm

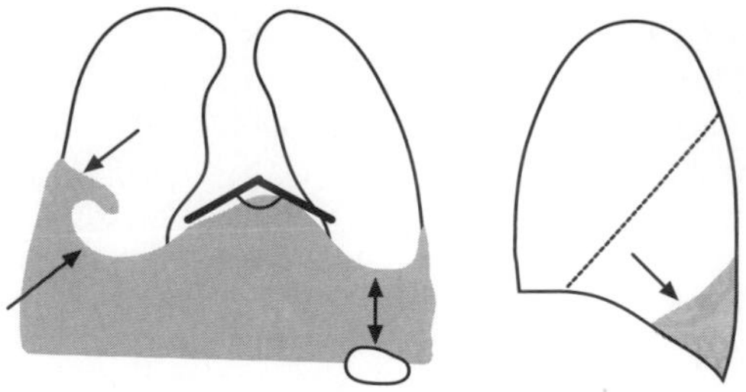

FIGURE 1-64

Split pleura sign (CT, MRI): loculated fluid between visceral and parietal pleura with thickening of pleura. Thickened pleura may enhance with IV contrast.

EMPYEMA

Empyema refers to either pus in the pleural space or an exudate that contains organism on a Gram stain (polymicrobial anaerobe, 35%; mixed aerobe/anaerobe, 40%; culture negative, 20%). There are three stages in the development of an empyema.

OVERVIEW

Parameter	Stage 1	Stage 2	Stage 3
Pathology	Exudative	Fibrinopurulent	Fibrinous
WBC count	Normal	>15,000/cm^3	>15,000/cm^3
pH	Normal	<7	<7
Glucose	Normal	<40 mg/dL	<40 mg/dL
LDH	>200 IU/L	>200 IU/L	>200 IU/L
Protein	>3 g/L	>3 g/L	>3 g/L
Treatment	Antibiotics	Percutaneous drainage	Surgery

Causes

- Postinfection (parapneumonic), 60%
- Postsurgical, 20%
- Posttraumatic, 20%

Radiographic Features

- Pleural fluid collection
- Thick pleura
- Pleural enhancement
- Gas in empyema collection may be due to:
  - BPF (common)
  - Gas-forming organism (rare)
- Empyema necessitans: spontaneous extension of empyema into chest wall, forming a subcutaneous abscess that may eventually open to skin and form a fistula. Causes: TB (70%), Actinomyces, Nocardia

DIFFERENTIATION BETWEEN EMPYEMA AND ABSCESS

	Abscess	Empyema
Cause	Necrotizing pneumonia (anaerobes, fungus)	Abscess extends to pleura; trauma, surgery
Shape	Round	Elliptical along chest wall
Air-fluid level	A=B	A≠B
Margins	Sharp or irregular	Sharp
Wall	Thick	Thin
Lung	Normal position	Displaced
Pleura	Not seen	Split
Vessel/ bronchi	Within	Displaced
Treatment	Antibiotics, postural drainage, percutaneous drainage in nonresponders	Percutaneous drainage

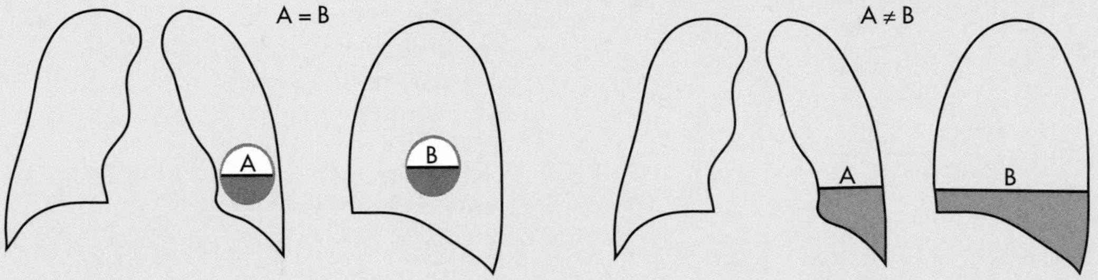

CHYLOTHORAX

Chylothorax is caused by disruption of the thoracic duct. Daily chyle production of 1.5 to 2.5L. Chyle contains chylomicrons from intestinal lymphatics and appears milky.

Causes

Tumor, 55% (especially lymphoma)
Trauma, 25%
- Iatrogenic duct laceration
- Sharp, blunt trauma

Idiopathic, 15%
Rare causes
- Lymphangioleiomyomatosis
- Filariasis

PLEURAL TUMORS

FIBROUS TUMOR OF THE PLEURA

Unifocal tumor of the pleura. No relation to asbestos exposure. Fibrous tumors originate from visceral (70%) or parietal (30%) pleura, usually on a pedicle.

Clinical Findings

- Respiratory symptoms
- HPO, 15%
- Hypoglycemia, 5%

Types

- Benign, 80% (previously classified as benign mesothelioma)
- Invasive, 20% (unlike malignant mesothelioma, this tumor grows only locally)

Radiographic Features

- Well-delineated, solitary pleural-based mass; often lobulated
- Pedunculated, 30%; mass may flop into different locations from film to film.
- Chest wall invasion may be seen in the invasive form, absent in benign form.
- Tumor may grow in fissure and simulate the appearance of a solitary pulmonary nodule.
- Recurrence rate after surgical resection, 10%
- May have associated pleural effusion, necrosis

MALIGNANT MESOTHELIOMA

Incidence is 500 new cases/year in the United States. Risk is 300 times larger in asbestos workers than in general population. Highest rates are in Seattle (shipyard industry) and St. Louis. Twenty to 40 years between asbestos exposure and tumor development. Three histologic variants (diagnosis usually requires an open pleural biopsy):
- Epithelial: difficult to differentiate from adenocarcinoma
- Mesenchymal
- Mixed

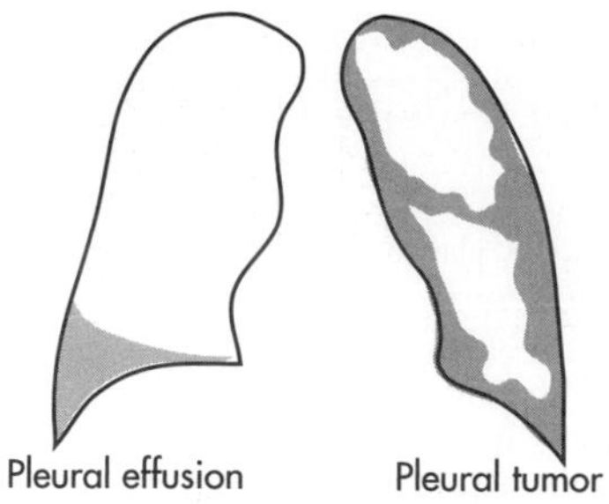

FIGURE 1-65

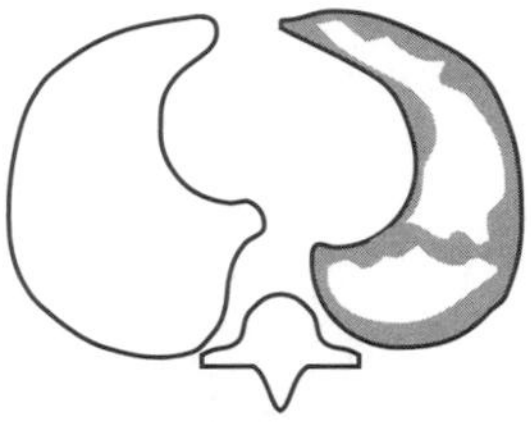
FIGURE 1-66

Radiographic Features (Figs. 1-65 and 1-66)
- Pleural thickening together with effusion, 60%
  - Isolated pleural thickening, 25%
  - Isolated pleural effusion, 15%
- Hemithoracic contraction, 25%
- Pleural calcification, 5%
- CT best shows full extent of disease:
  - Contralateral involvement
  - Chest wall and mediastinal involvement, 10%; diaphragm and abdominal extension
  - Pericardial involvement
  - Pulmonary metastases
- MRI useful to show chest wall or diaphragmatic extent

OTHER

DIAPHRAGMATIC PARALYSIS

Paralysis of the diaphragm can be unilateral or bilateral.

Clinical Findings (Fig. 1-67)
- Unilateral paralysis is usually asymptomatic.
- Bilateral paralysis results in respiratory symptoms.

Causes

Phrenic nerve paralysis
- Bronchogenic carcinoma
- Neuropathies, postinfectious, nutritional
- Spinal cord injury, myelitis
- CNS injury: stroke

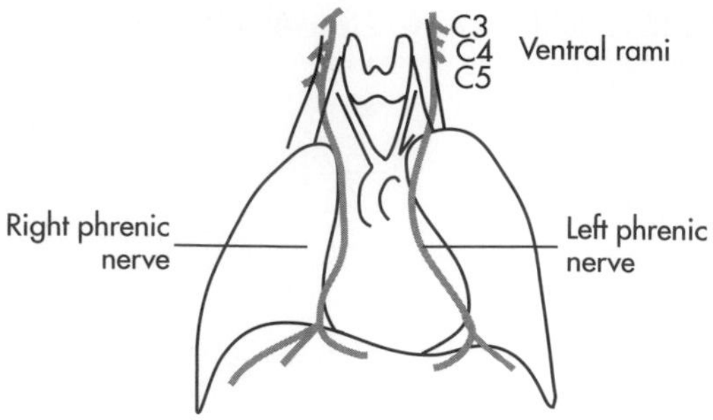

FIGURE 1-67

- Cardiac surgery
- Erb palsy (birth trauma)

Muscular disorders
- Myasthenia
- Polymyositis
- Muscular dystrophy

Idiopathic, 70%

Radiographic Features
- Elevated hemidiaphragm
- No motion of hemidiaphragm by fluoroscopy
- Paradoxical motion of hemidiaphragm using "sniff test"
- Reduced lung volume

Mediastinum

GENERAL

APPROACH TO MEDIASTINAL MASSES

- Location
  - Anterior mediastinum
  - Superior mediastinum
  - Middle mediastinum
  - Posterior mediastinum
- Invasive or noninvasive mass
- Content: fat, cystic, solid, enhancement

DIFFERENTIATION BETWEEN MEDIASTINAL AND PULMONARY MASSES

Mediastinal Mass	Pulmonary Mass
Epicenter in mediastinum	Epicenter in lung
Obtuse angles with the lung	Acute angles
No air bronchograms	Air bronchograms possible
Smooth and sharp margins	Irregular margins
Movement with swallowing	Movement with respiration
Bilateral	Unilateral

NORMAL VARIANTS CAUSING A WIDE MEDIASTINUM

- Anteroposterior (AP) projection instead of posteroanterior (PA) projection
- Mediastinal fat: obesity, steroid therapy
- Vascular tortuosity: elderly patients
- Low inspiratory supine position

ANTERIOR MEDIASTINAL TUMORS

THYMOMA

Thymoma is the most common anterior mediastinal tumor in the adult (very rare in children). Thirty percent are invasive (malignant thymoma). Parathymic syndromes are present in 40% of patients:

- 35% of thymoma patients have myasthenia gravis (15% of myasthenia gravis patients have thymoma).
- Aplastic anemia (50% have thymoma)
- Hypogammaglobulinemia (15% have thymoma)
- Red cell aplasia

Pathology

Benign thymoma, 75%
- Common in patients with myasthenia

Malignant thymoma, 25%
- Local spread into pleura but no hematogenous metastases
- More common in patients without myasthenia

Radiographic Features (Fig. 1-68)

- Anterior mediastinal soft tissue mass
  - Asymmetrical location on one side
  - Homogeneous density and signal intensity
  - Some have cystic components
  - Contrast medium enhancement
- Invasive thymomas show growth through capsule into adjacent tissue. Drop metastases into pleural space are common.
- Calcifications, 20%

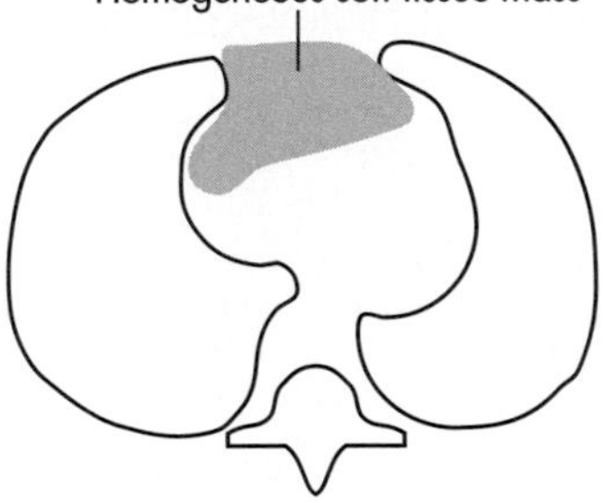

FIGURE 1-68

THYMOLIPOMA

Thymolipomas are benign, encapsulated mediastinal tumors that contain both thymic and adipose tissue. The tumor occurs most frequently in children and young adults. Tumors usually grow to large sizes (75% are >500 g) with few or no symptoms.

Associations

- Myasthenia gravis (in 3% of thymolipomas)
- Aplastic anemia
- Graves disease
- Hypogammaglobulinemia
- Lipomas in thyroid, pharynx

Radiographic Features

- Anterior mediastinal mass contains fatty and soft tissue elements.
- The mass is usually large and displaces mediastinal structures and/or lungs.
- Small tumors may be difficult to detect.
- Large tumors mimic liposarcoma.

BENIGN THYMIC HYPERPLASIA

Causes

- Myasthenia
- Thyrotoxicosis, Graves disease, Hashimoto thyroiditis
- Collagen vascular diseases:
  - SLE
  - Scleroderma
  - Rheumatoid arthritis
  - Behçet disease
- Rebound thymic hyperplasia:
  - Chemotherapy (hyperplasia is often a good prognostic indicator)
  - Addison disease
  - Acromegaly

Radiographic Features

- Enlarged thymus without focal masses; fat interspersed in parenchyma
- Size and morphology of normal thymus:
  - >20 years of age: <13 mm
  - >30 years of age: convex margins are abnormal
- No increase in size over time
- If clinical suspicion for malignancy is high, a biopsy should be performed.

THYROID MASSES

Thyroid masses that extend into the mediastinum: goiter > adenoma, carcinoma, lymphoma. Location of goiters within mediastinum:

- Anterior to brachiocephalic vessels, 80%
- Posterior to brachiocephalic vessels, 20%

Radiographic Features

Goiters

- Thoracic inlet masses (thymomas are lower in the anterior mediastinum)
- Mass is contiguous with cervical thyroid and is well defined.
- Heterogeneous density by CT: calcium, iodine (70 to 120 HU), colloid cysts
- Tracheal displacement is the most common finding by CXR.
- CT: marked and prolonged contrast enhancement
- Nuclear scan with either ^{99m}Tc or ^{123}I confirms the diagnosis (see Chapter 12).

Other

- Thyroid carcinoma has irregular borders.
- Thyroid lymphomas generally show little enhancement.

GERM CELL TUMORS

Tumors arise from rests of primitive cells and are of variable malignant potential. Mnemonic: "SECTE":

- **S**eminoma
- **E**mbryonal cell carcinoma
- **C**horiocarcinoma
- **T**eratoma (70% of germ cell tumors), teratocarcinoma
- **E**ndodermal sinus tumors (yolk sac tumors)

Teratoma (Fig. 1-69)

- 20% are malignant; therefore all mediastinal teratomas should be surgically removed.
- Teratomas typically present as large mass lesions.
- Variable tissue contents:
  - Calcification, 30%
  - Fat, fat-fluid levels
  - Cystic areas
  - Soft tissue

Seminoma

- Rarely infiltrative
- Large, unencapsulated lesions
- Occasionally associated with testicular atrophy

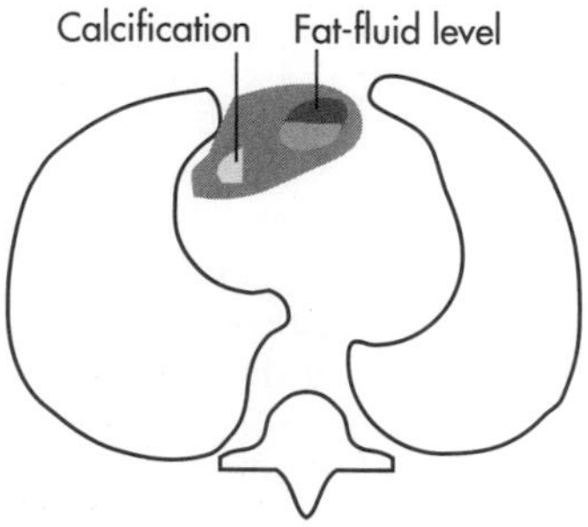

FIGURE 1-69

Embryonal Cell Carcinoma

- Mediastinal invasion is the rule: poor prognosis (mean survival time <10 months).
- Elevated AFP and human chorionic gonadotropin (HCG)

HODGKIN LYMPHOMA

The pathologic diagnosis is based on the presence of Reed-Sternberg cells. The cell of origin is the antigen-presenting interdigitating cells in the paracortical regions of the lymph node (not B or T cells). Ninety percent originate in the lymph nodes; 10% originate in extranodal lymphoid tissues of parenchymal organs (lung, GI tract, skin). Incidence is 1:50,000. Bimodal age distribution with peaks at 30 and 70 years.

TYPES OF HODGKIN LYMPHOMA

Type	Frequency	Prognosis
Lymphocyte predominant (LP)	<5% (young patients)	Most favorable
Nodular sclerosing (NS)	70%	Less favorable than LP
Mixed cellularity (MC)	25% (old patients)	Less favorable than NS
Lymphocyte depleted (LD)	<5%	Worst prognosis

STAGING (ANN ARBOR)

Stage*	Involvement
I	Single node group or region
IE	Single extranodal site
II	Two or more nodes on same side of diaphragm
IIE	Localized disease in an organ and node on same side of diaphragm
III	Node groups on both sides of diaphragm
IIIE	Above diaphragm + localized extralymphatic
IIIS	Above diaphragm + spleen
IV	Extension beyond above limit

*Constitutional symptoms (classification B) are present in 25%: fever, night sweats, weight loss.

Radiographic Features (Fig. 1-70)

- Superior mediastinal nodal (prevascular, paratracheal) involvement, 95%
- Contiguous progression from one lymph node group to the next
- Lung involvement, 15%
  - Pulmonary mass lesion, air bronchograms
  - Direct extension into lung from involved nodes (most common)
- Pleural effusions, 15%

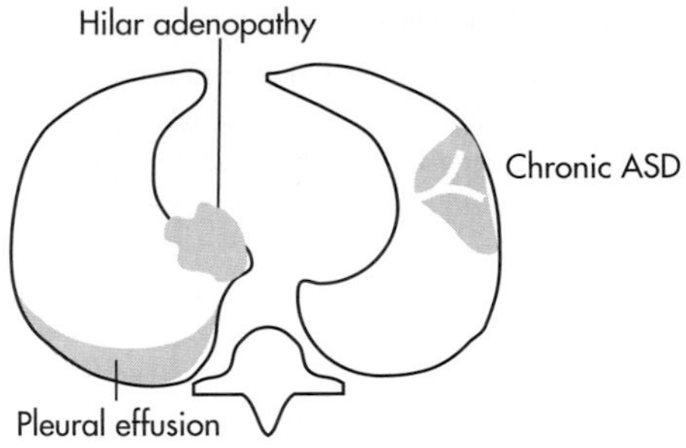

FIGURE 1-70

- Posttherapeutic mediastinal changes common
  - Thymic cysts
  - Thymic hyperplasia
  - Persistent mediastinal masses may be present without representing active disease: ^{67}Ga, PET scanning may be helpful for differentiation.

Pearls

- Recurrence of lymphoma
  - Radiation treatment: recurrence usually occurs outside the treatment field (commonly paracardiac region).
  - No radiation: recurrence usually in sites of previous involvement
- 5% of treated Hodgkin patients will develop aggressive leukemias
- Radiation pneumonitis occurs 6 to 8 weeks after completion of the radiation and evolves to mature fibrosis by 1 year.

NON-HODGKIN LYMPHOMA (NHL)

Sixty percent of cases originate in lymph nodes and 40% in extranodal sites. Eighty-five percent arise from B cells and 15% from T cells. Occurs in all age groups (mean age, 50 years). Increased incidence in patients with altered immune status:

- Transplant patients
- AIDS
- Congenital immunodeficiency
- Collagen vascular diseases: RA, SLE

CLASSIFICATIONS OF NON-HODGKIN LYMPHOMA*

Working Formulation	Rappaport	Comment
Low Grade		
Small, lymphocytic	Lymphocytic, well differentiated	Uncommon
Follicular, small cleaved	Nodular, poorly differentiated	Most frequent type
Follicular, mixed cells	Nodular, mixed	
Intermediate Grade		
Follicular, large cells	Nodular, histiocytic	
Diffuse, small cleaved	Diffuse, lymphocytic	
Diffuse, mixed cell	Diffuse, mixed	
Diffuse, large cell	Diffuse, histiocytic	GI involvement, 25%
High Grade		
Immunoblastic	Diffuse, histiocytic	GI involvement, 25%
Lymphoblastic	Lymphoblastic	Mediastinal mass, young patient
Small, noncleaved	Diffuse undifferentiated (Burkitt and non-Burkitt)	Abdominal form (North America), craniofacial (Africa)

*Constitutional symptoms are more common than in Hodgkin disease.

Radiographic Features

- Mediastinal and hilar adenopathy
  - Often generalized at presentation
  - Adenopathy may be noncontiguous.
- Lung involvement
  - May occur without adenopathy
  - Patterns: mass, chronic ASD
- Extrathoracic spread
  - Nasooropharynx
  - GI tract
  - Spread to unusual sites common

MIDDLE MEDIASTINAL TUMORS

BRONCHOPULMONARY FOREGUT MALFORMATIONS (Fig. 1-71)

Abnormalities in budding and differentiation of the primitive foregut. Depending on type, duplication cysts are also classified as posterior mediastinal masses. The lining of the cyst wall determines the cyst type:

- Bronchogenic cysts: ventral defects containing respiratory epithelium

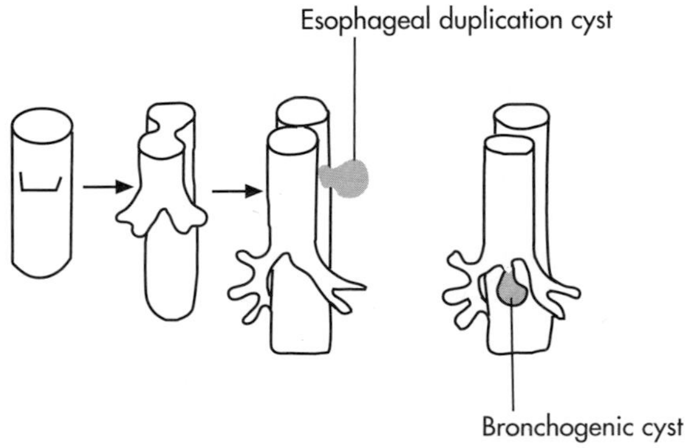

FIGURE 1-71

- Enteric cysts: posterior defects containing gastrointestinal epithelium (gastric mucosa > esophageal mucosa > small bowel mucosa > pancreatic tissue)

DIFFERENTIATION BETWEEN BRONCHOGENIC AND ENTERIC CYSTS

	Bronchogenic Cyst	Enteric Cyst
Location	Ventral	Dorsal
Level	Subcarinal	Supracarinal
Cyst wall	Imperceptible	Thick wall
Symptoms	Asymptomatic unless there is mass effect; usually as an incidental finding	Symptomatic: peptic ulceration, distention
Other imaging findings	May contain calcification	Vertebral body anomalies
	Associated rib anomalies	Hemivertebra
	CT: no contrast enhancement	Scoliosis
	T2 hypointense	Spina bifida

Radiographic Features (Fig. 1-72)
- Round mass of water/protein density
- Location
  - Bronchogenic cysts are mediastinal (75%) or pulmonary (25%). Mediastinal locations: subcarinal, 50%; paratracheal, 20%; hilar, paracardiac, 30%. Esophageal duplication cysts are located along the course of the esophagus.
- High CT density (40%) may be due to debris, hemorrhage, infection
- Calcifications in wall (rare finding)

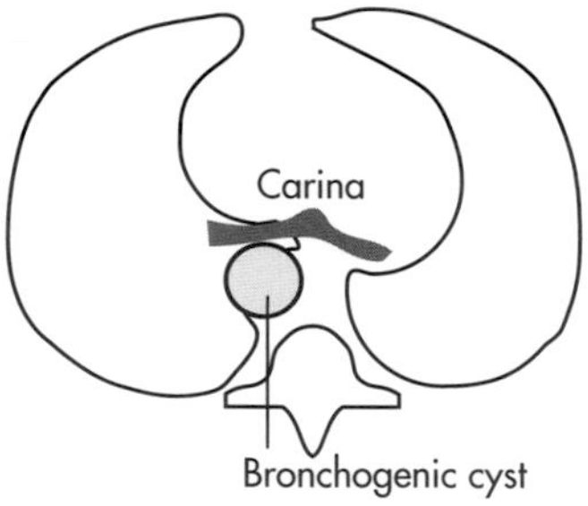

FIGURE 1-72

CASTLEMAN DISEASE (GIANT BENIGN LYMPH NODE HYPERPLASIA)

Large, benign mediastinal lymph node masses. Rare. Etiology is unknown (nodal hyperplasia vs. benign tumor). Two histologic types: hyaline vascular, 90%; plasma cell, 10% (associated with general symptoms: night sweats, fever, etc.). Age <30 years, 70%. Treatment is surgical excision. Includes hyaline vascular and plasma cell types.

Radiographic Features
- Bulky mediastinal mass lesion (3 to 12 cm): anterior > middle > posterior mediastinum
- Dense homogeneous contrast enhancement is the key feature ("vascular lesions")
- Nodal calcification may be present.
- Involvement of lymph nodes in neck, axillae, and pelvis is rare.
- Slow growth

FIBROSING MEDIASTINITIS

Cause is mediastinal histoplasmosis; may be idiopathic. May result in obstruction of pulmonary artery, veins, bronchi. Calcified lymph nodes.

POSTERIOR MEDIASTINAL TUMORS

NEURAL TUMORS

Posterior mediastinal neural tumors arise from:
- Peripheral nerves, 45% benign
  - Schwannoma (arise from nerve sheath)
  - Neurofibroma (contain all elements of nerve)
- Sympathetic ganglia (varying malignant potential)
  - Ganglioneuroma (benign)
  - Ganglioneuroblastoma
  - Neuroblastoma (malignant)
- Paraganglion cells, 2%
  - Paraganglioma (chemodectoma, histologically similar to pheochromocytoma): functional tumors, may secrete catecholamines. Intense contrast enhancement. Found in AP window.

Radiographic Features (Fig. 1-73)
- Schwannoma, neurofibroma
  - Arise posteriorly, frequently in neural foramina
  - May cause widening and erosion of neural foramina
  - Usually round or oval and <2 vertebral bodies long
  - Enhancement with contrast
  - T2-weighted (T2W) very hyperintense

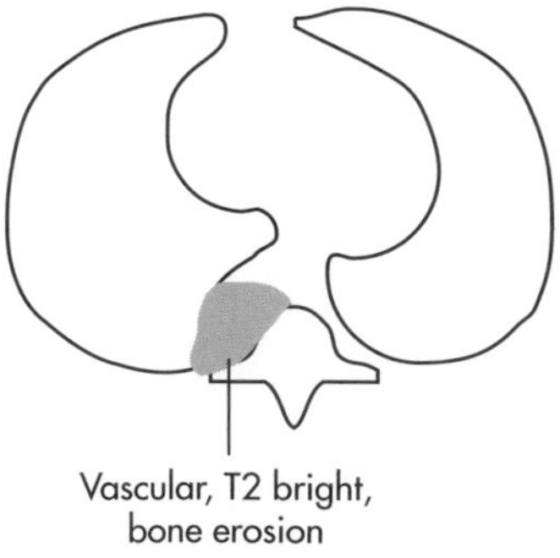

FIGURE 1-73

Sympathetic ganglia tumors
- Arise anterolaterally (more conspicuous on plain film)
- Usually elongated and fusiform (resembling sympathetic chain) and >2 vertebral bodies long

EXTRAMEDULLARY HEMATOPOIESIS

Paravertebral masses represent bone marrow extruded through cortical defects of vertebral bodies. Seen in congenital anemias (e.g., thalassemia). Suspect diagnosis if:
- Multiple bilateral posterior mediastinal masses
- Cortical bone changes by CT
- Clinical history of anemia
- Marked contrast enhancement

OTHER MEDIASTINAL DISORDERS

PNEUMOMEDIASTINUM

Sources of mediastinal air:

Intrathoracic
- Trachea and major bronchi
- Esophagus
- Lung
- Pleural space

Extrathoracic
- Head and neck
- Intraperitoneum and retroperitoneum

Radiographic Features
- Subcutaneous emphysema
- Elevated thymus: thymic sail sign
- Air anterior to pericardium: pneumopericardium
- Air around pulmonary artery and main branches: ring around artery sign
- Air outlining major aortic branches: tubular artery sign
- Air outlining bronchial wall: double bronchial wall sign
- Continuous diaphragm sign: due to air trapped posterior to pericardium
- Air between parietal pleura and diaphragm: extrapleural sign
- Air in pulmonary ligament

Differential Diagnosis

GENERAL

APPROACH TO CXR (Fig. 1-74)

1. Lungs
    - Focal or diffuse abnormalities
    - Lung volumes
        - Increased or decreased
        - Right/left difference in density
    - Hypolucent areas

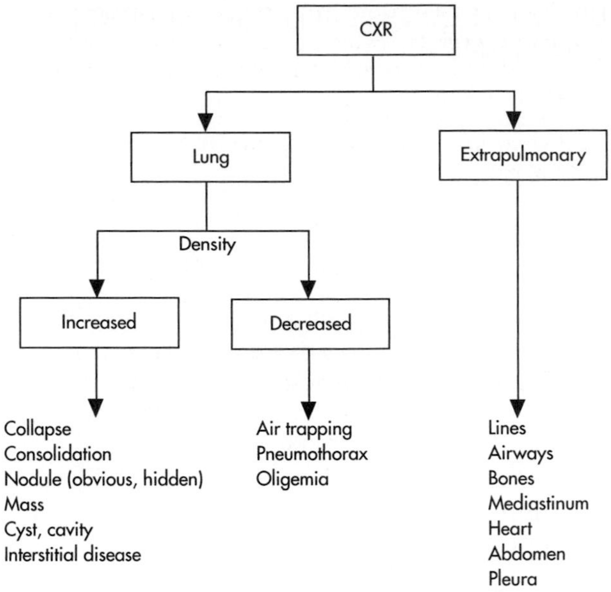

FIGURE 1-74

2. Trachea and bronchi
3. Mediastinal lines
    - Paratracheal stripe
    - AP window
    - Azygoesophageal recess
    - Paraspinal lines
    - Other lines
        - Anterior and posterior junction line
        - Posterior wall of intermediate bronchus
4. Hila and cardiac contour
5. Pleura, fissures
6. Bones
    - Focal metastases
    - Rib notching
    - Clavicles

APPROACH TO ICU FILMS

1. Lines (check position)
2. Pneumothorax, pneumomediastinum
3. Focal parenchymal opacities
    - Atelectasis
    - Pneumonia
    - Aspiration
    - Hemorrhage
    - Contusion
4. Diffuse parenchymal opacities
    - ARDS
    - Pneumonia
    - Edema
    - Less common:
        - Aspiration
        - Hemorrhage

DIRECTED SEARCH IN APPARENTLY NORMAL CHEST FILMS

Lungs
- Hidden nodules
- Subtle interstitial disease
- Differences in lung density
- Retrocardiac disease
- Bronchiectasis
- Pulmonary embolism

Mediastinum
- Posterior mediastinal mass
- Tracheal lesions, deviation
- Subtle hilar mass lesions

Bones
- Lytic, sclerotic lesions
- Rib notching

GENERIC APPROACHES TO FILM INTERPRETATION

The "4 Ds"
- Detection
- Description
- Differential diagnosis
- Decision about management

Lesion Description
- Location
- Extent
- Characteristics
  - Signal intensity, density, echogenicity, etc.
  - Behavior after administration of contrast material
- Differential diagnosis

UNIVERSAL DIFFERENTIAL DIAGNOSIS

Mnemonic: "TIC MTV:"
- **T**umor
- **I**nflammation
  - Infectious
  - Noninfectious causes
- **C**ongenital
- **M**etabolic
- **T**rauma, iatrogenic
- **V**ascular

ATELECTASIS

LOBAR, SEGMENTAL ATELECTASIS (Fig. 1-75)

Endobronchial lesion

Extrinsic bronchial compression
- Tumor
- Lymphadenopathy
  - Malignant
  - Benign adenopathy (i.e., sarcoid rarely causes lobar collapse])

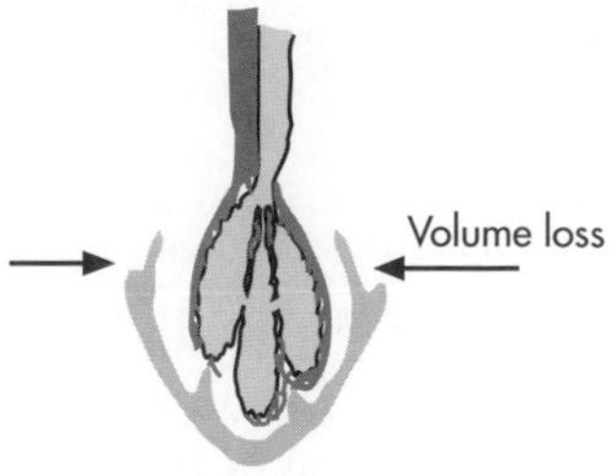

FIGURE 1-75

Rare causes

Bronchial torsion

SIGNS OF LOBAR ATELECTASIS

Direct signs
- Displacement of interlobar fissures (lobar collapse)
- Increase in opacity of the involved segment or lobe

Indirect signs
- Displacement of hila
- Mediastinal displacement
- Elevation of hemidiaphragm
- Overinflation of remaining normal lung
- Approximation of ribs

RUL Collapse (Figs. 1-76 through 1-78)
- Elevation of minor fissure
- Shift of trachea to right
- Elevation of hilum
- Thickening of right paratracheal in complete collapse

RML Collapse
- Best seen on lordotic views
- RML syndrome: recurrent atelectasis despite an open orifice:

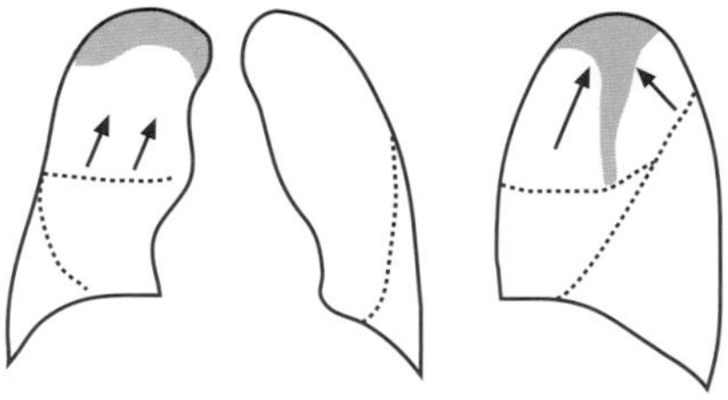

FIGURE 1-76

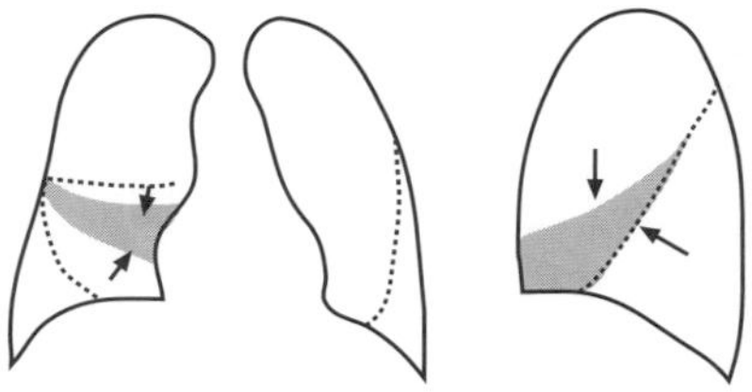

FIGURE 1-77

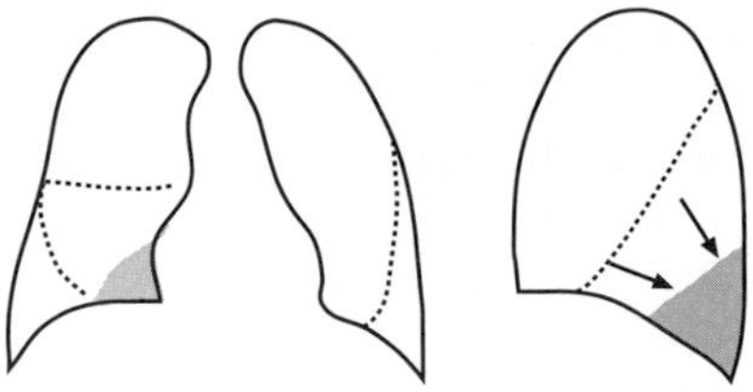

FIGURE 1-78

Absent collateral ventilation
Bronchus is surrounded by enlarged lymph nodes (TB)
May have coexistent bronchiectasis

RLL Collapse

- Triangular opacity in right retrocardiac region on PA film with obliteration of diaphragm
- Posterior displacement of right margin
- Opacity over the spine

LUL Collapse (Fig. 1-79)

- May be difficult to see: hazy density can be easily confused with loculated pleural effusion on PA film
- "Luftsichel": radiolucency in upper lung zone that results from upward migration of superior segment of the left lower lobe (LLL)
- Anterior displacement of major fissure on lateral view

LLL Collapse

- Left retrocardiac triangular opacity on PA film
- Posterior displacement of left major fissure on lateral film

CT Findings of Lobar Collapse (Figs. 1-80 and 1-81)

- Increased density of collapsed lobe
- See figure for patterns.

TYPES OF PERIPHERAL ATELECTASIS

Relaxation
- Pleural effusion
- Pneumothorax
- Bullous disease

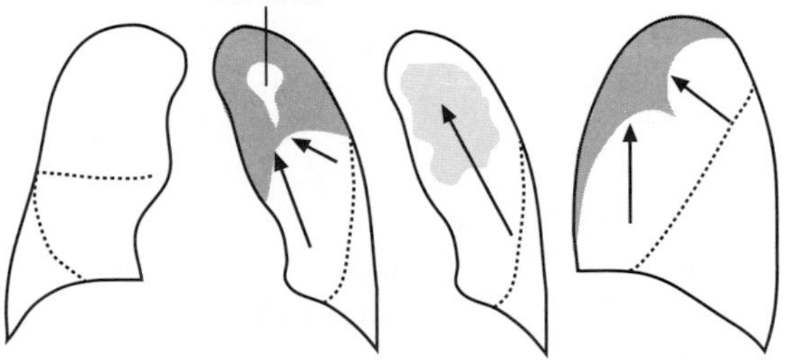

FIGURE 1-79

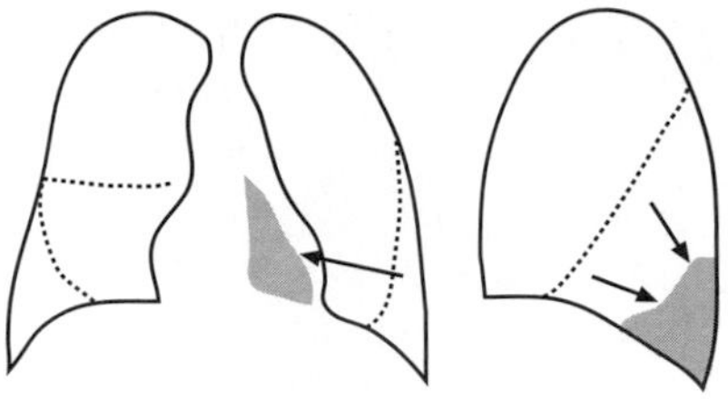

FIGURE 1-80

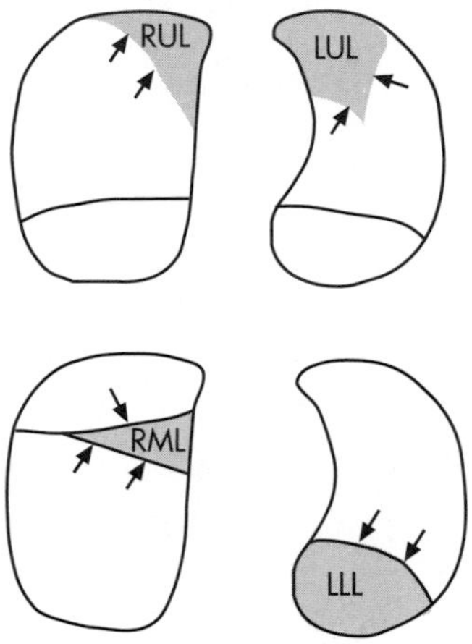

FIGURE 1-81

Atelectasis associated with fibrosis
- Granulomatous infections
- Pneumoconiosis
- Sarcoid

Resorptive atelectasis secondary to obstruction
- Platelike, discoid atelectasis

Depletion of surfactant (adhesive atelectasis; airways patent)
- ARDS of the newborn
- Radiation injury

Rounded atelectasis
- Due to pleural disease

CONSOLIDATION

Radiographic Features (Figs. 1-82 and 1-83)

Acinar shadow
- Air in acini (7 mm in diameter) is replaced by fluid or tissue
- May be confluence to form patchy densities

Air bronchogram
- Represents aerated airways in consolidated lung
- Air bronchogram may also be seen in some forms of collapse.

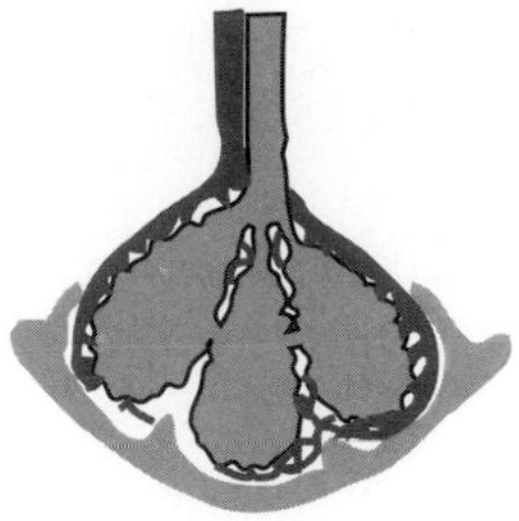

FIGURE 1-82

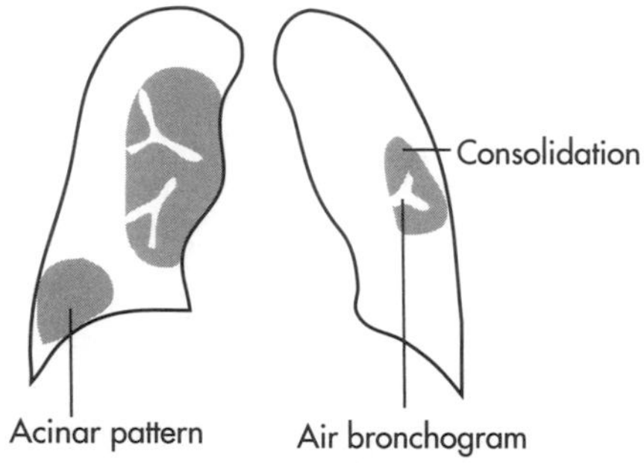

FIGURE 1-83

Absence of volume loss
- No displaced fissures
- No elevation of diaphragm

Nonsegmental distribution
- Intersegmental spread is common because channels of interalveolar communication (channels of collateral drift) allow passage of air and fluid
- Channels of collateral drift include:
  - Pores of Kohn (interalveolar openings)
  - Channels of Lambert (bronchioalveolar communications)
  - Direct airway anastomosis, 120 μm in diameter

CAUSES OF CONSOLIDATION

Fluid in Acini

Water (edema)
- Cardiac pulmonary edema
- Renal pulmonary edema
- Lung injury, pulmonary edema

Blood
- Trauma (most common)
- Bleeding disorder: anticoagulation, etc.
- Type II antigen-antibody reaction
- Goodpasture syndrome
- Henoch-Schönlein purpura
- Pulmonary infarct (Hampton hump)
- Vasculitis

Proteinaceous fluid
- Alveolar proteinosis

Inflammatory Exudate in Acini

Infection
- Bacterial infections (pus)
- *Nocardia,* actinomycosis, TB

Noninfectious
- Allergic hypersensitivity alveolitis
- Chronic eosinophilic pneumonia
- COP
- Pulmonary infiltration with eosinophilia
  - Loeffler syndrome
  - Chronic eosinophilic pneumonia
  - Pneumonitis
  - ABPA
  - Drugs: penicillin
- Aspiration of lipid material
- Sarcoid (resides only in interstitial space but encroaches on airspace to produce a pattern that mimics ASD)

Tumor in Acini

Bronchioalveolar carcinoma
Lymphoma

PULMONARY RENAL SYNDROMES

These syndromes are characterized by pulmonary hemorrhage and nephritis.

Pulmonary findings usually present as consolidation on CXR.
- Goodpasture syndrome (anti-GBM positive)
- Wegener disease (ANCA positive; nodules are more common than ASD)
- SLE
- Henoch-Schönlein purpura
- Polyarteritis nodosa
- Penicillamine hypersensitivity

ACUTE RESPIRATORY DISTRESS SYNDROME (ARDS)

Clinical syndrome characterized by sudden onset of triad:
- Respiratory distress
- Hypoxemia
- Opaque, stiff lungs

After an incipient catastrophic event, mediators of injury are activated → inflammatory response → endothelial damage → injury, pulmonary edema (ARDS): ARDS runs independent course from initiating disease.

Radiographic Features

- Diffuse alveolar consolidation, commonly indistinguishable from pneumonia or pulmonary edema
- End stage
- Interstitial fibrosis and scarring

Causes

- Massive pneumonia
- Trauma
- Shock
- Sepsis
- Pancreatitis
- Drug overdose
- Near-drowning
- Aspiration

CHRONIC AIRSPACE DISEASE

Tumors
- Bronchioalveolar carcinoma
- Lymphoma

Inflammation
- Tuberculosis, fungus
- Eosinophilic pneumonia
- Pneumonitis, BOOP/COP
- Alveolar sarcoid (mimics ASD)

Other causes
- Alveolar proteinosis
- Pulmonary hemorrhage
- Lipoid pneumonia, chronic aspiration

PULMONARY MASSES

APPROACH TO SOLITARY PULMONARY NODULE (Fig. 1-84)

DIFFERENTIATION BETWEEN BENIGN AND MALIGNANT NODULES

	Benign	Malignant
Shape	Round	Irregular
Size	<3 cm	>3 cm
Spiculations	No	Yes
Edge	Well defined	Ill defined
Satellite lesions	Yes	No
Cavitation	No	Yes
Doubling time (in volume)	<1 month or >2 years	>1 month or <2 years

The above-listed criteria *do not* allow reliable differentiation of a solitary pulmonary nodule. There are only *three* criteria by which a solitary pulmonary nodule can be judged benign:
- Fat density
- Specific types of benign calcifications (diffuse, central, popcorn, concentric):
  - >10% of a nodule consists of calcium with HU >200
  - Large or homogeneous calcification throughout nodule (exceptions: multiple metastases from osteosarcoma, thyroid carcinoma, etc.)
- Old films show no interval growth within a 2-year period

CT Workup

<4 mm: 99% benign if no known primary tumor
- Follow-up CT in 12 and 24 months; if no growth after 24 months, nodule is assumed benign.
- Follow-up CT in 3, 6, 12, and 24 months if clinical suspicion.

<4 to 8 mm: 94% benign if no known primary
- Follow-up at 3, 6, 12, and 24 months
- Consider PET or biopsy if high clinical suspicion

>8 mm: 50% malignant
- Percutaneous biopsy
- Other options: PET and surgical removal (VATS)

FIGURE 1-84

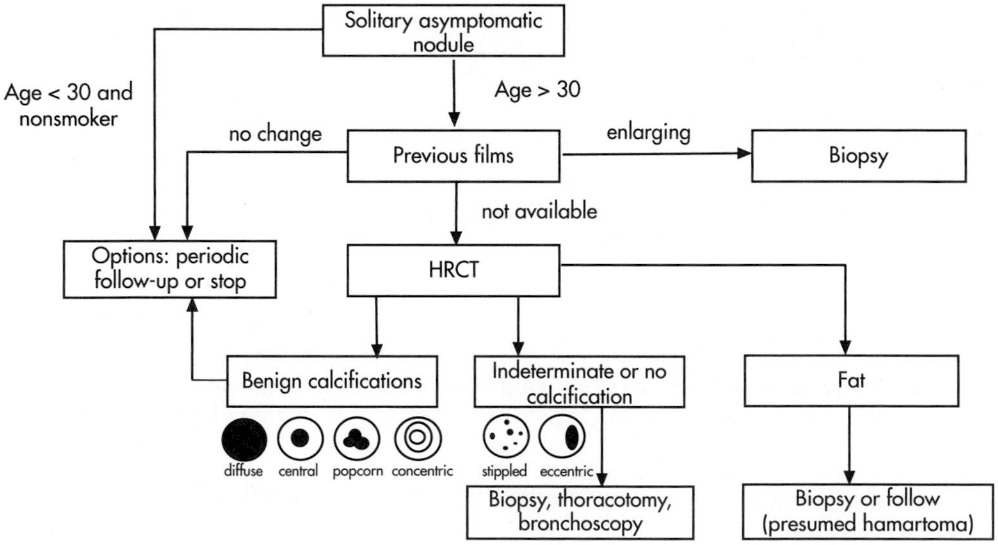

Pearls

- Always get a second imaging modality (CT > MR > angiogram) before sampling a solitary pulmonary nodule to exclude AV malformations. However, remember that 97% of all solitary nodules are either granulomas or primary carcinomas.
- Extrapulmonary densities may mimic pulmonary lesions.
  - Artifact (nipple, skin, electrodes)
  - Pseudotumor (fluid in fissure)
  - Pleural mass or plaque
  - Rib fracture
- Solitary pulmonary metastases seen on CXR will be truly solitary in only 50% of the cases.
- Any solitary pulmonary nodule in cancer patients requires further workup:
  - Comparison with old films
  - Percutaneous biopsy if large enough
  - Close follow-up (usually 3-month intervals)
- HRCT for nodule densitometry
  - Perform only in nodules <3.0 cm in diameter.
  - Densities of >200 HU indicate presence of calcification.

HIDDEN ZONES (Fig. 1-85)

Subtle pulmonary nodules are often missed if <3 cm and located in:

- Upper lobes (apices)
- Central, paramediastinal
- Superimposed onto ribs and clavicle

An effort should be made to perform a directed search in these regions to detect subtle lung cancer. This zone has also been called the lawyer zone. The threshold of lesion detection by plain film is approximately 9 mm.

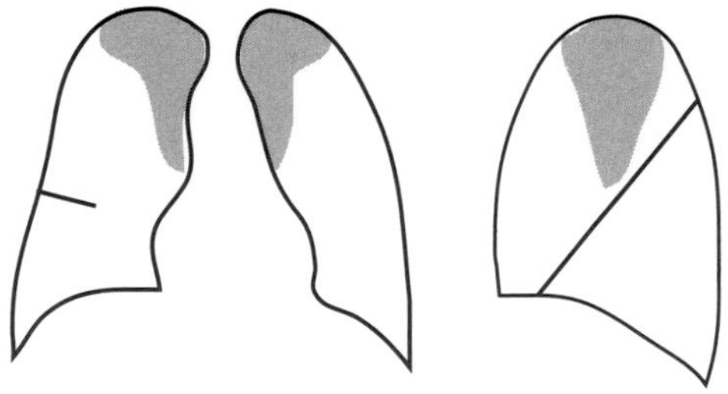

FIGURE 1-85

SOLITARY NODULE

Criteria: <6 cm. May be smooth, lobulated, discrete, circumscribed, calcified, cavitated, or have satellite lesions.

Tumor (45%)
- Primary carcinoma, 70%
- Hamartoma, 15%
- Solitary metastasis, 10%

Inflammation (53%); regional variations
- Histoplasmoma
- Tuberculoma
- Coccidioidomycosis

Other (2%)
- Vascular, 15%
  - AV fistula
  - Pulmonary varix (dilated pulmonary vein)
  - Infarct, embolism
- Congenital, 30%
  - Sequestration
  - Bronchial cyst
- Miscellaneous, 45%
  - Round pneumonia
  - Loculated effusion in fissure
  - Mucus plug
  - Enlarged subpleural lymph node
  - Silicosis (usually multiple nodules)

MULTIPLE NODULES

Multiplicity of pulmonary nodules often indicates hematogenous dissemination.

Causes

Metastases

Abscess
- Pyogenic: *Staphylococcus* > *Klebsiella* > *Streptococcus*
- Immunocompromised patient: *Nocardia, Legionella*

Granulomatous lung diseases
- Infectious
  - TB
  - Fungus: *Aspergillus, Histoplasma*
- Noninfectious
  - Sarcoid
  - Rheumatoid nodules
  - Silicosis
  - Wegener disease
  - Necrotizing granulomatous vasculitis
  - Histiocytosis

Unilateral pulmonary embolism

MILIARY PATTERN (Fig. 1-86)

Special pattern of multiple pulmonary nodules characterized by small size and diffuse bilateral distribution (too numerous to count). If the nodules are small enough, also consider the differential diagnosis for nodular interstitial disease.

Causes

- Hematogenous infection: TB, histoplasmosis
- Hematogenous tumor seeding:
  - Metastases: thyroid, melanoma, breast, choriocarcinoma
  - Eosinophilic granuloma
  - Bronchioalveolar cancer

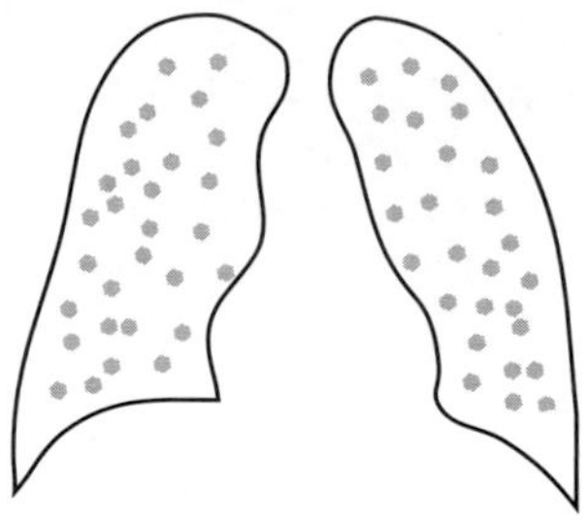

FIGURE 1-86

- Silicosis
- Sarcoid

CALCIFIED LUNG NODULES

Larger (>1 mm)
- Tumor
  - Metastases from medullary thyroid cancer
  - Mucinous or osteogenic metastases
- Infection
  - Previous varicella pneumonia
  - Histoplasmosis, coccidioidomycosis, TB
  - Parasites: schistosomiasis
- Other
  - Silicosis, CWP

Very small (0.1 to 1 mm; sandlike)
- Alveolar microlithiasis
- Chronic pulmonary venous hypertension
- "Metastatic" calcification from severe renal disease

LARGE (>6 CM) THORACIC MASS

Pulmonary
- Tumor
  - Bronchogenic carcinoma
  - Metastases (SCC from head and neck)
- Abscess
- Round atelectasis
- Intrapulmonary sequestration
- Hydatid disease

Extrapulmonary
- Fibrous tumor of the pleura
- Loculated pleural effusion
- Torsed pulmonary lobe
- Chest wall tumors (Askin tumor)
- AAA
- Mediastinal masses

UPPER LUNG ZONE OPACITIES WITH CALCIFIED ADENOPATHY

- Silicosis
- Sarcoidosis
- Berylliosis
- CWP
- TB

INFECTION THAT CAN CAUSE CHEST WALL INVASION

- *Actinomyces*
- *Nocardia*
- TB
- *Blastomyces*
- *Aspergillus*
- *Mucor*

INFECTION WITH LYMPHADENOPATHY

- TB
- Histoplasmosis (fungal)
- EBV (viral)

CYSTIC AND CAVITARY LESIONS (Fig. 1-87)

APPROACH

The wall thickness and morphology are helpful (but not definitive) to determine if a cavitary lesion is benign or malignant.

Thickness (not always reliable)
- <2 mm, benign in 95%
- 2 to 15 mm, malignant in 50%
- >15 mm, malignant in >95%

Morphology (not reliable)

Eccentric cavity: suggests malignancy
- Shaggy internal margins: suggests malignancy

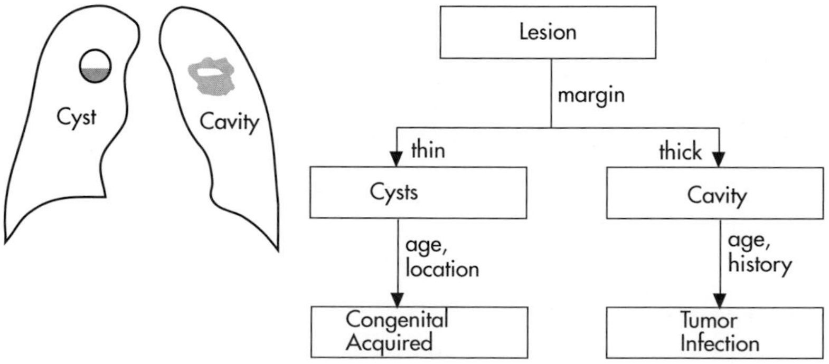

FIGURE 1-87

CYSTS (Figs. 1-88 and 1-89)

Parenchyma-lined space, filled with air or fluid

- Pneumatocele (posttraumatic, postinfectious): common
- Bulla (located within lung parenchyma), bleb (located within the nine histologic layers of the visceral pleura)
- Cystic bronchiectasis
- Langerhans cell histiocytosis
- Lymphocytic interstitial pneumonia
- Lymphangioleiomyomatosis
- Metastases
- Neurofibromatosis type 1
- Tracheobronchial papillomatosis
- *Pneumocystis jiroveci* pneumonia
- Congenital cysts
    - Intrapulmonary bronchogenic cysts (rib and vertebral body anomalies common)
    - Cystic adenomatoid malformation (multiple lesions)
    - Sequestration
- Hydatid cyst (onion skin appearance)

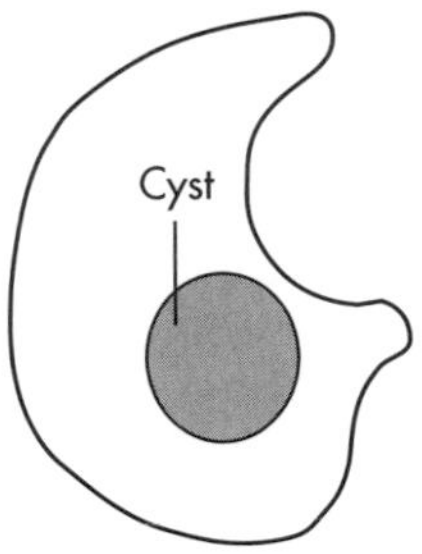

FIGURE 1-88

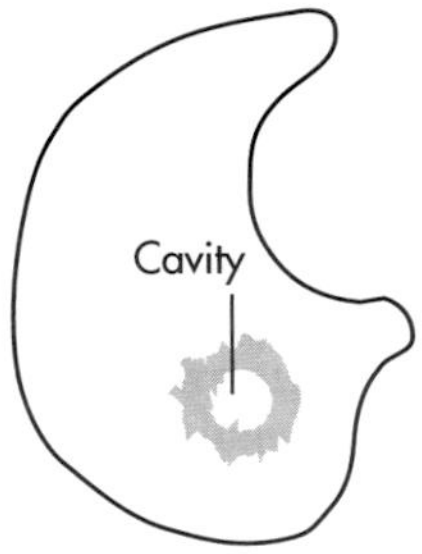

FIGURE 1-89

CAVITY

Parenchymal necrosis due to inflammation (benign) or tumor (malignant)

Abscess
- Pyogenic: *Staphylococcus* > *Klebsiella* > *Streptococcus*
- Immunocompromised patient: *Nocardia, Legionella*

Cavitated tumor
- SCC (primary SCC > head and neck SCC > sarcoma metastases)
- Sarcoma
- Lymphoma
- TCC of the bladder

Cavitated granulomatous mass (often multiple)
- Fungus: *Aspergillus,* coccidioidomycosis (thin wall)
- TB
- Sarcoid, Wegener disease, rheumatoid nodules
- Necrotizing granulomatous vasculitis

Cavitated posttraumatic hematoma

AIR CRESCENT SIGN IN CAVITY

This sign was originally described in aspergillosis and is most commonly seen there.

More recently, the sign has also been described with other entities:
- Mucormycosis
- Actinomycosis
- Septic emboli
- *Klebsiella pneumoniae* infection
- TB
- Tumors

SMALL CYSTIC DISEASE (Fig. 1-90)

True cyst wall
- Eosinophilic granuloma
- Lymphangioleiomyomatosis
- Cystic form of PCP
- Honeycombing in any end-stage interstitial disease
- LIP

No cyst wall
- Emphysema

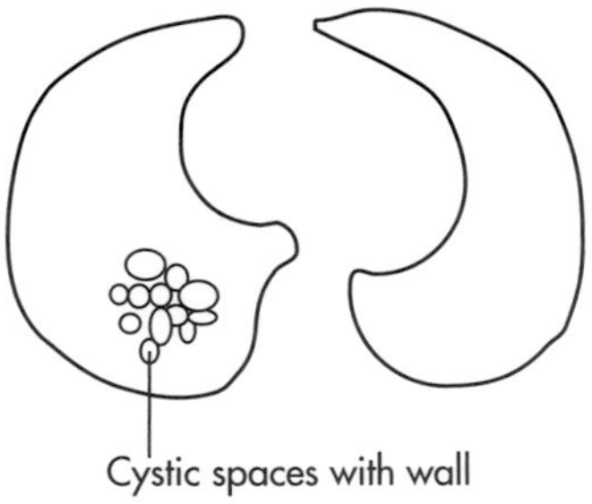

FIGURE 1-90

INTERSTITIAL LUNG DISEASE

RADIOGRAPHIC PATTERNS OF INTERSTITIAL DISEASE

Types of Densities

- Linear or reticular densities: thickened interlobular septa, fibrosis
- Reticulonodular densities: inflammation in peribronchovascular interstitium
- Nodular densities: granulomas

- Ground-glass opacity: usually represents acute interstitial disease (occasionally seen with chronic fibrosis)
    - Hazy increase in lung density
    - Vessels can be clearly seen through haze
- Honeycombing: ring shadows 2 to 10 mm; end-stage lung disease

Kerley Lines (Linear Densities) (Fig. 1-91)

Kerley B lines, peripherally located in interlobular septa:
- <2 cm long
- Peripheral
- Perpendicular to pleura

Kerley A lines:
- 2 to 6 cm long
- Central
- No relationship to bronchioarterial bundles

Kerley C lines
- Fine network caused by superimposition of Kerley B lines

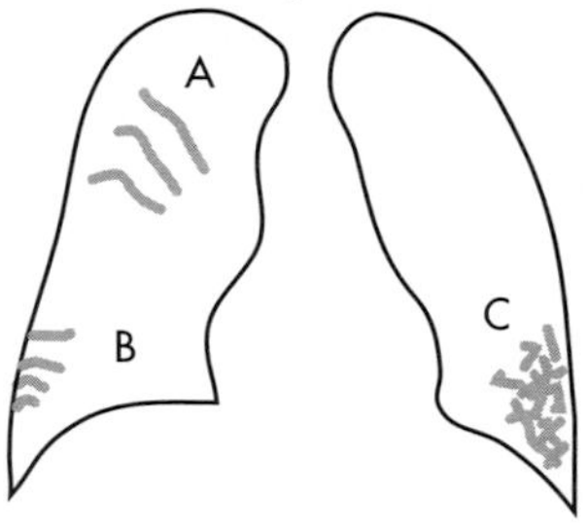

FIGURE 1-91

APPROACH

Define the following parameters:
- Type of pattern
- Distribution
- Lung volumes
- Evolution
- Pleural disease
- Lymph nodes

Generic Approach

Interstitial disease is due to thickening of interlobular septa (lymphatics, veins, or infiltration by cells), alveolar walls, and interstitium. Causes of thickening include

Fluid
- Water
    - Pulmonary edema
    - Venous obstruction (thrombosis)
- Proteinaceous material
    - Congenital pulmonary lymphangiectasia (very rare)

Inflammation
- Infectious (interstitial pneumonias)
    - Viral
    - Granulomatous (TB, fungal)
    - PCP
- Idiopathic
    - IPF
    - Sarcoid
- Collagen vascular disease
    - RA
    - Scleroderma
    - Ankylosing spondylitis
- Extrinsic agents
    - Pneumoconiosis (asbestos, silicosis, CWP)
    - Drugs

Tumor
- Interstitial tumors
    - Eosinophilic granuloma
- Lymphangitic tumor spread
- Desmoplastic reaction to tumor

MNEMONIC APPROACH TO DIFFERENTIAL DIAGNOSIS

Examples of Common Entities	
Distribution	
Upper lobes ("CASSET P")	**C**ystic fibrosis (not an interstitial disease)
	Ankylosing spondylitis
	Silicosis
	Sarcoid
	Eosinophilic granuloma (sparing of costophrenic angles)
	Tuberculosis
	***P**neumocystis carinii*
Lower lobes ("BADAS")	**B**ronchiectasis (not an interstitial disease)
	Aspiration
	Drugs, DIP
	Asbestosis
	Scleroderma, other collagen vascular diseases
Evolution	
Acute ("HELP")	**H**ypersensitivity (allergic alveolitis)
	Edema
	Lymphoproliferative
	Pneumonitis, viral
Chronic ("LIFE")	**L**ymphangitic spread
	Inflammation, infection
	Fibrosis
	Edema

Continued

MNEMONIC APPROACH TO DIFFERENTIAL DIAGNOSIS—cont'd

Lung Volumes	
Increased	Cystic fibrosis (associated with this pattern but not an interstitial disease)
	Eosinophilic granuloma (pneumothorax, 20%)
	Lymphangioleiomyomatosis (pneumothorax)
Decreased	Idiopathic pulmonary fibrosis
	Scleroderma
Pleural Disease	
Pleural plaques	Asbestosis
Pleural effusion	CHF
	Lymphangitic carcinomatosis
	Rheumatoid disease
Lymph Nodes	
Enlarged	Malignant adenopathy
	TB, fungus
	Sarcoid
Calcified	Silicosis

Nodular Opacities		
1- to 2-mm interstitial nodules	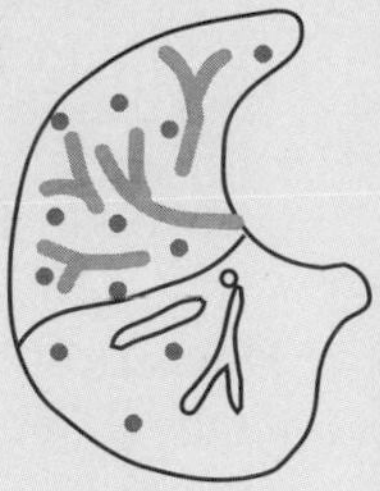	Hematogenous infection
Often associated with reticular opacities		Hematogenous metastases
		Sarcoid
		Pneumoconiosis
		Silicosis
		CWP
		Histiocytosis (EG, also cysts)
Cystic Spaces		
With or without walls	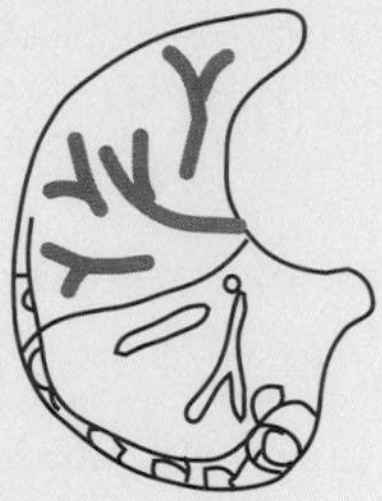	Lymphangioleiomyomatosis
		Cystic PCP
		Histiocytosis
		Honeycombing
		IPF
		LIP
		Any end-stage interstitial disease

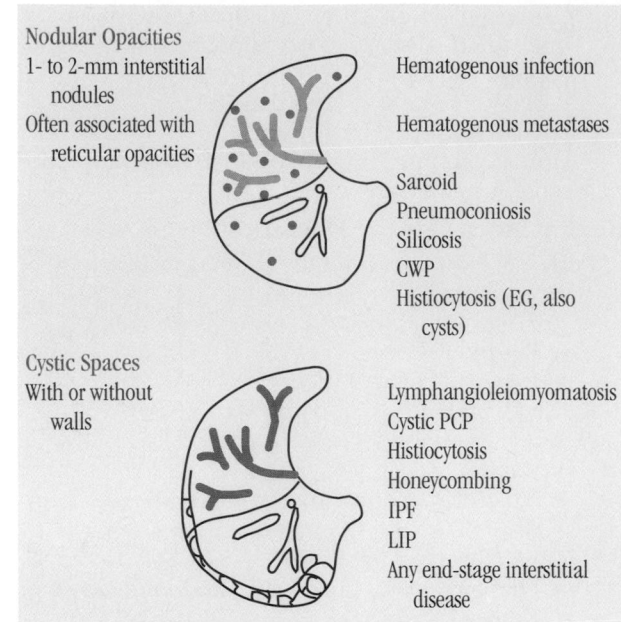

HRCT PATTERNS OF INTERSTITIAL LUNG DISEASE

	Imaging	Causes
Ground-Glass Opacity		
Increased haze	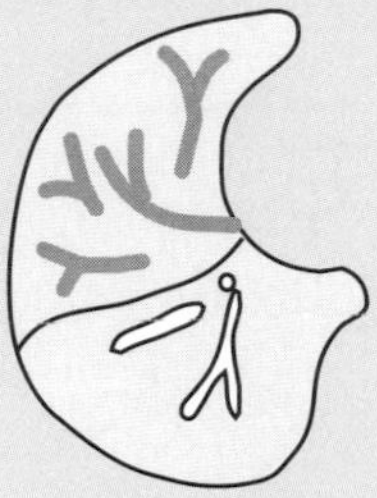	Allergic hypersensitivity
All acute interstitial diseases		All acute interstitial disease
		DIP
		Active IPF
		Viral
		PCP
		BOOP/COP
		Eosinophilic pneumonia
		Pulmonary edema
Reticulonodular Opacities		
Peribronchovascular thickening (peribronchial cuffing on CXR)	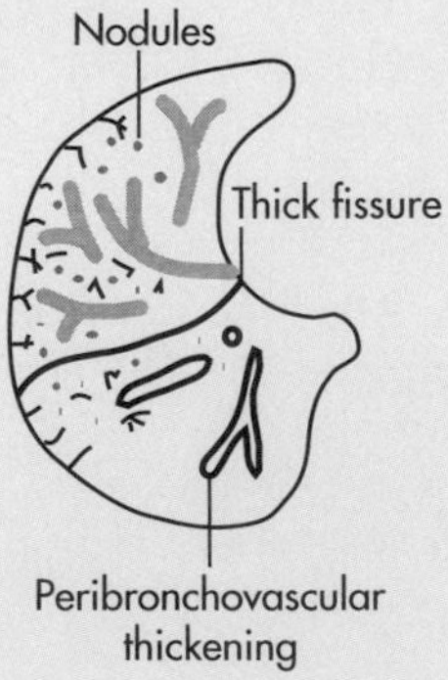	Pulmonary edema
Thickening of interlobular septa (Kerley lines)		Viral, mycoplasmal pneumonia, and PCP
		Lymphangitic tumor spread
		Pulmonary fibrosis
		IPF
		Secondary fibrosis
		Drugs
		Radiation
		Collagen vascular disease
		Hemosiderosis
		Asbestosis

CRAZY-PAVING APPEARANCE ON HRCT

Ground-glass opacity with overlying geometric structures formed by thickened interlobular septa and intraseptal lines

- Pulmonary alveolar proteinosis
- ARDS
- PCP
- Lipoid pneumonia
- Hemorrhage
- Bronchoalveolar carcinoma (BAC)
- Pulmonary edema

PULMONARY HEMORRHAGE

Focal
- PE
- Trauma (contusion)
- AVM
- Cancer (BAC)

Diffuse
- Wegener
- Goodpasture (resolves in days to weeks, can result in fibrosis)
- Idiopathic (children)
- Bone marrow transplant

HALO PATTERN OF GROUND-GLASS OPACITY

- Early invasive aspergillosis in a leukemic patient: ground glass around a nodule of consolidation
- Hemorrhage around a neoplasm
- Postbiopsy pseudonodule

PERIPHERAL GROUND-GLASS OPACITY AND CONSOLIDATION

- COP
- Infarcts
- Septic emboli
- Collagen vascular disease
- Contusion
- DIP
- Drug toxicity
- Eosinophilic pneumonia
- Fibrosis
- Sarcoidosis

HONEYCOMBING PATTERN ON HRCT

- UIP (idiopathic pulmonary fibrosis)
- Scleroderma/RA
- Asbestosis
- Chronic hypersensitivity pneumonitis
- Sarcoidosis
- Silicosis
- EG
- Drug toxicity: bleomycin

DISEASES SPREADING ALONG BRONCHOVASCULAR BUNDLE

- Sarcoidosis
- Lymphoma
- Lymphangitic spread of tumor
- TB
- Kaposi sarcoma

TREE-IN-BUD APPEARANCE

Infection
- TB
- Bronchopneumonia
- Fungal
- Asian panbronchiolitis
- Viral pneumonias

Bronchial disease
- Bronchiolitis

Congenital disorders
- Cystic fibrosis
- Dyskinetic cilia syndrome

Other
- Allergic bronchopulmonary aspergillosis
- Lymphangitic carcinomatosis
- EG

ABNORMAL DENSITY

HYPERLUCENT LUNG

Hyperlucency may be lobar, segmental, subsegmental, or generalized. Hyperlucency may or may not be associated with overexpansion of lungs.

Causes

Airways
- Obstruction of airways (air trapping); inspiratory/expiratory films may be of use to accentuate the hyperlucency
  - Emphysema, bullae
  - Large airway obstruction: asthma, mucus plug
  - Small airway obstruction (bronchioli): Swyer-James syndrome (bronchiolitis obliterans)
  - Compensatory hyperexpansion of residual lung after: surgical lobectomy, chronic lobar collapse
- Cysts
- Congenital
  - Hypogenetic lung syndrome
  - Congenital lobar emphysema

Vascular (hyperlucency caused by oligemia)
- PE
- Pulmonary artery stenosis

Chest wall abnormalities
- Mastectomy
- Poland syndrome (congenital absence of pectoralis muscle)

Pleural
- Pneumothorax

SMALL LUNG (FIG. 1-92)

May be associated with either decreased or increased density
- Hypogenetic lung syndrome
- Agenesis of pulmonary artery
- Chronic atelectasis
- Bronchiolitis obliterans (Swyer-James syndrome)

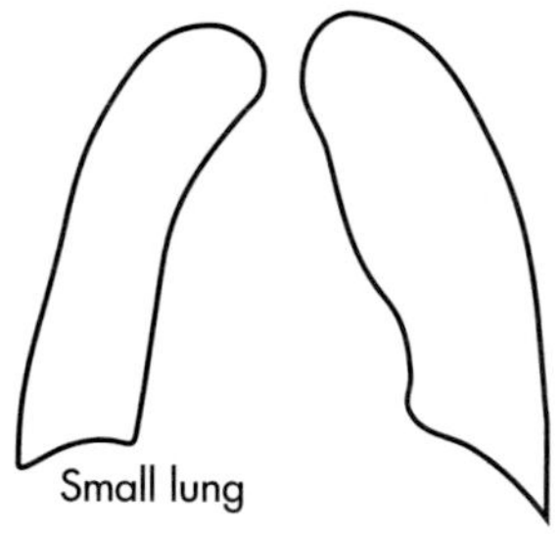

FIGURE 1-92

TRACHEOBRONCHIAL LESIONS

ENDOBRONCHIAL LESIONS

Focal bronchial abnormality

Causes

Tumors, 80%
- Malignancy, 70%:
  - SCC (most common)

Low-grade malignancies
Adenocystic carcinoma
Mucoepidermoid carcinoma
Small cell carcinoma
Carcinoid

- Metastases, 5%: RCC, melanoma, colon, breast, thyroid
- Other: hamartoma, mucoepidermoid carcinoma, hemangioma

Inflammatory disease, 20%

- TB

Other

- Mucus plug
- Foreign body (fishbone, dental)
- Trauma
- Broncholith

DIFFUSE TRACHEAL LUMINAL ABNORMALITIES

Increased diameter

- Tracheobronchomegaly (Mounier-Kuhn syndrome)
- Pulmonary fibrosis
- Tracheomalacia

Decreased diameter

- Saber-sheath trachea (most common cause)
- Tracheopathia osteochondroplastica
- Tracheomalacia (decreased diameter on expiration)
- Relapsing polychondritis
- Amyloidosis
- Sarcoidosis
- Wegener disease
- Tuberculous and fungal stenosis

BRONCHIECTASIS

Postinfectious (most common)

- Any childhood infection
- Recurrent aspiration
- ABPA: central bronchiectasis
- Chronic granulomatous infection
- Pertussis

Bronchial obstruction

- Neoplasm
- Foreign body

Congenital

- Cystic fibrosis (abnormal secretions)
- Bronchial cartilage deficiency: Williams-Campbell syndrome
- Abnormal mucociliary transport: Kartagener syndrome

UPPER LOBE BRONCHIECTASIS (Fig. 1-93)

- Cystic fibrosis
- TB
- Radiation
- ABPA (most commonly central)

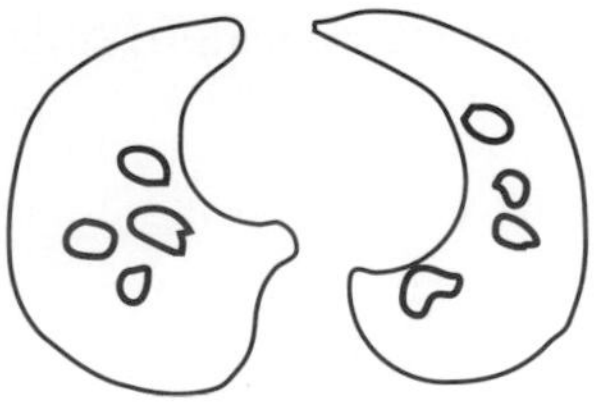

FIGURE 1-93

- Mounier-Kuhn syndrome
- Agammaglobulinemia
- Kartagener syndrome

MUCOID (BRONCHIAL) IMPACTION

Criteria: bronchus filled with soft tissue density (inspissated mucus); bronchi may be enlarged (bronchocele) or of normal size. No contrast enhancement.

Causes

- Asthma
- Cystic fibrosis
- ABPA
- Congenital bronchial atresia

PLEURAL DISEASE

PLEURAL-BASED MASS (Fig. 1-94)

Soft tissue mass along the chest wall; obtuse angles with chest wall.

Tumor

- Mesothelioma (malignant): multifocal, diffuse
- Fibrous tumor of the pleura (benign); unifocal may be locally invasive
- Malignant thymoma and lymphoma often have appearance similar to that of mesothelioma
- Metastases: breast, lung, prostate, thyroid, renal
- Lipoma (most common benign tumor)
- Extrapleural tumors

  Rib tumors
  Children: EG, ABC, Ewing sarcoma, neuroblastoma

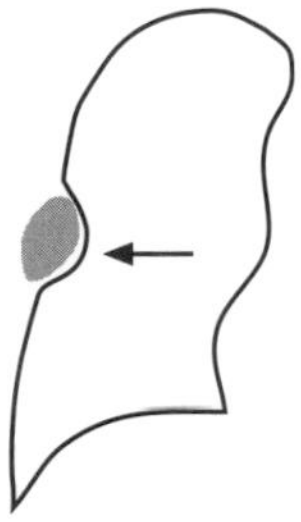

FIGURE 1-94

Adults: metastases > multiple myeloma > Paget disease, fibrous dysplasia
Plexiform neurofibromas in neurofibromatosis (bilateral)

Inflammatory
- Infectious: TB
- Asbestos related
- Actinomycosis (rib destruction)

Trauma, surgery, chest tubes

CALCIFIED PLEURAL PLAQUES

The most common causes of calcified pleural plaques (mnemonic: "TAFT") are:
- **T**uberculosis (usually diffuse plaques)
- **A**sbestos-related plaques (usually focal plaques)
- **F**luid (empyema, hematoma)
- **T**alc

ELEVATED HEMIDIAPHRAGM (Fig. 1-95)

Phrenic nerve paralysis
- Tumor
- Surgery
- Birth defect: Erb paralysis

Immobility because of pain
- Rib fractures
- Pleuritis, pneumonia
- PE
- Mass lesions
- Abdominal masses, subphrenic collection, abscess
- Diaphragmatic hernia
- Pleural tumors
- Subpulmonic effusion (apparent elevation of hemidiaphragm)

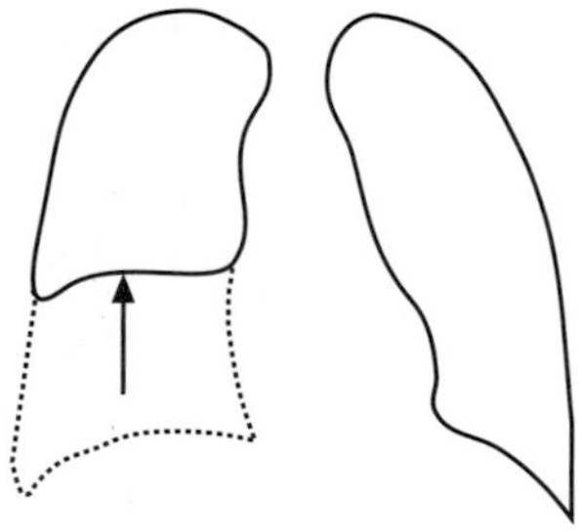

FIGURE 1-95

MEDIASTINUM (Fig. 1-96)

ANTERIOR MEDIASTINAL MASSES

Thymic masses
- Thymic cyst
- Thymolipoma
- Thymoma
  - Cystic
  - Benign (noninvasive) thymoma
  - Malignant (invasive) thymoma

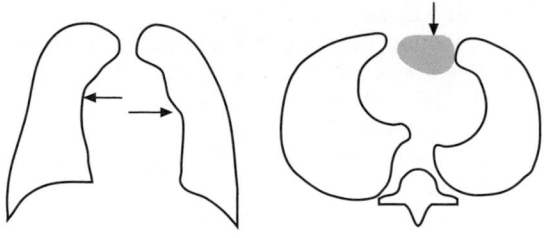

FIGURE 1-96

- Thymic carcinoma
- Thymic carcinoid
- Thymic lymphoma

Germ cell tumors (male > female)
- Seminoma
- Embryonal cell carcinoma
- Choriocarcinoma
- Teratoma

Lymphadenopathy: lymphoma, sarcoid, TB, etc.
Aneurysm and vascular abnormalities (involve both the anterior and superior mediastinal compartments)

Mnemonic for anterior mediastinal masses: the "4 Ts":
- Thymoma (most common anterior mediastinal mass) + other thymic lesions
- Thyroid lesions
- T-cell lymphoma (Hodgkin disease and NHL)
- Teratoma and other germ cell tumors (seminoma, choriocarcinoma), 10%

Cystic Anterior Mediastinal Mass

- Thymic cyst (3rd pharyngeal pouch remnant)
- Cystic thymoma (contains solid components besides cysts)
- Teratoma
- Bronchogenic cysts (usually located in middle mediastinum)
- Pericardial cyst

SUPERIOR MEDIASTINAL MASS

Descending through thoracic inlet
- Thyroid masses
- Adenopathy (primary head and neck tumors)
- Lymphatic cysts, cystic hygroma

Ascending through thoracic inlet
- Small cell carcinoma of the lung

Lymphoma

Aneurysm and vascular anomalies may involve both the anterior and superior mediastinal compartments.

MIDDLE MEDIASTINAL MASS

Adenopathy (often bilateral)
- Benign: sarcoid, TB, fungal infection, chronic beryllium exposure
- Malignant: metastases, lymphoma, leukemia

Congenital cysts
- Bronchogenic cysts (subcarinal, anterior trachea)
- Pericardial cysts

Aneurysm
- Aorta, aortic branches
- Pulmonary artery

Esophagus
- Hiatal hernia (common)
- Neoplasm
- Diverticula
- Megaesophagus: achalasia, hiatal hernia, colonic interposition

Other
- Mediastinal hemorrhage
- Mediastinal lipomatosis
- Bronchogenic cancer arising adjacent to mediastinum
- Aberrant RSA with diverticulum
- Varices
- Neurinoma from recurrent laryngeal nerve
- Malignancy of trachea
- Pancreatic pseudocyst

ADENOPATHY

Low-attenuation lymph nodes
- TB and fungal infections in AIDS (ring enhancement)
- Necrotic metastases (aggressive neoplasm)
- Lymphoma (occasionally)

Vascularized lymph nodes
- Castleman disease (giant benign nodal hyperplasia)
- Vascular metastases: renal cell, thyroid, small cell, melanoma

Calcified lymph nodes
- TB
- Histoplasmosis, other fungus
- Sarcoidosis
- Silicosis
- Radiation therapy

POSTERIOR MEDIASTINAL MASS (Fig. 1-97)

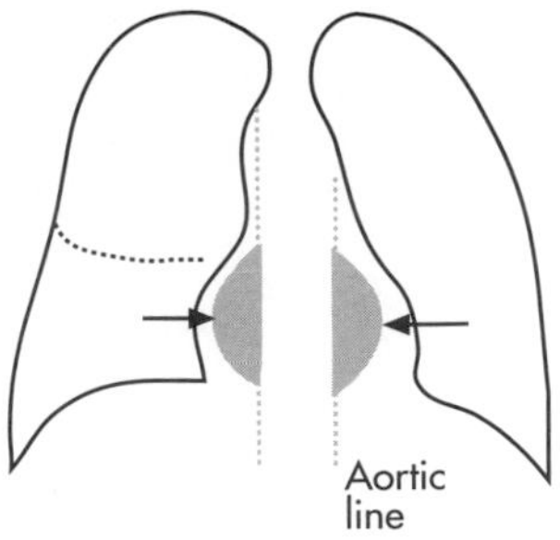

FIGURE 1-97

Neurogenic, 90%
- Peripheral nerves (20 to 40 years; <2 vertebral bodies long): schwannoma and neurofibroma, 45%
- Sympathetic ganglia (<20 years; >2 vertebral bodies long): ganglioneuroma, neuroblastoma, sympathicoblastoma
- Paraganglionic cells: pheochromocytoma, paraganglioma (least common)
- Lateral meningomyelocele

Thoracic spine
- Neoplasm
- Hematoma
- Extramedullary hematopoiesis (bilateral)
- Diskitis

Vascular
- Aneurysm
- Azygos continuation (congenital absence of IVC with dilated azygos and hemiazygos veins)

CARDIOPHRENIC ANGLE MASS

- Fat pad (most common cause)
- Diaphragmatic hernia (second most common)
  - Morgagni (anterior; 90% on right side)
  - Bochdalek (posterior; more common on left; not a true cardiophrenic mass)
- Pericardial cyst
- Cardiophrenic angle nodes (lymphoma usually recurrent, status postradiation)
- Aneurysm
- Dilated right atrium
- Anterior mediastinal mass
- Primary lung or pleural mass

FATTY MEDIASTINAL LESIONS

Purely fatty lesions
- Mediastinal lipomatosis
- Morgagni hernia (omentum)
- Bochdalek hernia (omentum)
- Periesophageal fat herniation

Tumors with fatty components
- Lipoma
- Liposarcoma
- Thymolipoma (children and young adults, lesions are usually very large)
- Germ cell tumors (also contain calcifications and cystic and solid regions)

HIGH-DENSITY MEDIASTINAL LESIONS (NONCONTRAST CT)

Calcified lymph nodes

Calcified primary mass
- Tumor
- Goiter
- Aneurysm

Hemorrhage

DENSELY ENHANCING MEDIASTINAL MASS

Vascular
- Aneurysm
- Vascular abnormalities
- Esophageal varices

Hypervascular tumors: paraganglioma, metastasis from thyroid cancer, RCC

Goiter

Castleman disease

RETROCRURAL ADENOPATHY

Inflammation
- Sarcoidosis
- LAM
- Amyloidosis

Infection
- AIDS
- TB
- *M. avium*

Lymphoma

Mets

PROMINENT HILA (Fig. 1-98)

Tumors
- Central bronchogenic carcinoma
- Lymphoma

Adenopathy
- Infectious: TB, fungi, histoplasmosis
- Inflammatory: sarcoid, silicosis
- Tumor: commonly oat cell, lymphoma, metastases

Pulmonary artery enlargement

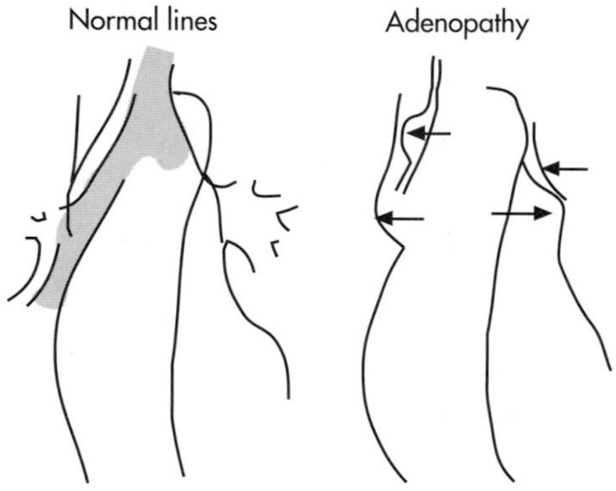

FIGURE 1-98

EGGSHELL CALCIFICATION IN HILAR NODES

- Silicosis, CWP
- Treated lymphoma
- Granulomatous disease such as histoplasmosis rarely contains eggshell calcification; diffuse calcifications are more common.
- Sarcoid (rare and late in disease)

PNEUMOMEDIASTINUM

Pulmonary
- Asthma (common)
- Barotrauma (intubation, diver)
- Childbirth
- Pneumothorax

Mediastinum
- Tracheobronchial laceration
- Esophageal perforation
- Mediastinal surgery
- Boerhaave syndrome

Abdomen
- Intraperitoneal or retroperitoneal bowel perforation
- Retroperitoneal surgery

Head and neck
- Esophageal rupture
- Facial fractures
- Dental or retropharyngeal infection, mediastinitis

Suggested Readings

Detterbeck FC, Boffa DJ, Tanoue LT. The new lung cancer staging system. *Chest*. 2009;136:260–271.
Felson B. *Chest Roentgenology*. Philadelphia: WB Saunders; 1999.
Fraser RG, Paré JAP, Paré PD, et al. *Diagnosis of Disease of the Chest*. 4th ed. Philadelphia: WB Saunders; 1999.
Freundlich IM, Bragg D. *A Radiologic Approach to Diseases of the Chest*. Baltimore: Williams & Wilkins; 1996.
Goodman LR, Putnam CE. *Critical Care Imaging*. 3rd ed. Philadelphia: WB Saunders; 1992.
Hansell DM, Armstrong P, Lynch DA, McAdams HP. *Imaging of Diseases of the Chest*. St. Louis: Mosby; 2005.
McLoud TC. *Thoracic Radiology: The Requisites*. St. Louis: Mosby; 1998.
Miller WT. *Diagnostic Thoracic Radiology*. New York: McGraw-Hill Professional; 2006.
Muller NL, ed. *The Radiologic Clinics of North America: Imaging of Diffuse Lung Disease*. Philadelphia: WB Saunders; 1991.
Muller N, Fraser R, Colman N, Pare E. *Radiologic Diagnosis of Diseases of the Chest*. Philadelphia: WB Saunders; 2001.
Naidich DP, Zerhouni EA, Siegelman SS. *Computed Tomography and Magnetic Resonance of the Thorax*. New York: Lippincott Williams & Wilkins; 1999.
Newell J, Tarver R. *Thoracic Radiology*. New York: Lippincott Williams & Wilkins; 1993.
Pare JAP, Fraser RG. *Synopsis of Diseases of the Chest*. Philadelphia: WB Saunders; 1993.
Reed JC. *Chest Radiology: Plain Film Patterns and Differential Diagnosis*. St. Louis: Mosby; 2003.
Webb RW, Higgins CB. *Thoracic Imaging: Pulmonary and Cardiovascular Radiology*. New York: Lippincott Williams & Wilkins; 2005.

CHAPTER 2

Cardiac Imaging

CHAPTER OUTLINE

Cardiac Imaging Techniques

PLAIN FILM INTERPRETATION

NORMAL PLAIN FILM ANATOMY

Posteroanterior (PA) View (Fig. 2-1)

Right cardiac margin has three segments:
- Superior vena cava (SVC)
- Right atrium (RA)
- Inferior vena cava (IVC)

Left cardiac margin has four segments:
- Aortic arch (AA) (more prominent with age)
- Main pulmonary artery (PA) at level of left main stem bronchus
- Left atrial appendage (may not be visible in normal hearts)
- Left ventricle (LV)
- RV is usually not seen in frontal projection

Lateral View (Fig. 2-2)

Anterior cardiac margin has three segments:
- Right ventricle (RV) is in apparent contact with sternum
- Main PA
- Ascending aorta

Posterior cardiac margin has two segments:
- LV
- Left atrium (LA)

Other anatomic landmarks:
- Trachea, bronchi
- Right PA en face anterior to carina
- Aortopulmonary window (triangle between aorta and PA)

Oblique Views (Fig. 2-3, A and B)

Right anterior oblique (RAO) and left anterior oblique (LAO) views are mainly used in coronary angiography and ventriculography. These views rarely add

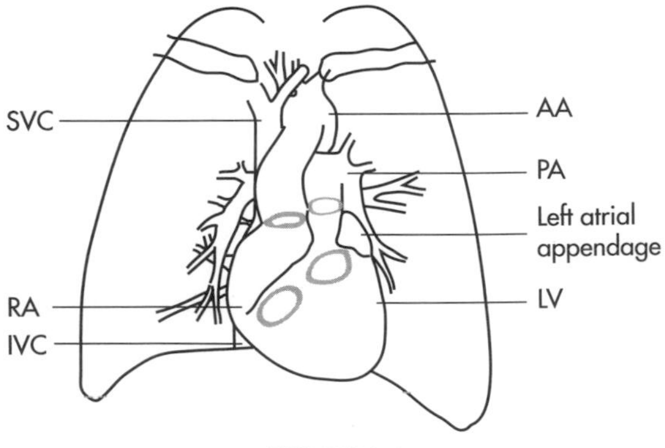

FIGURE 2-1

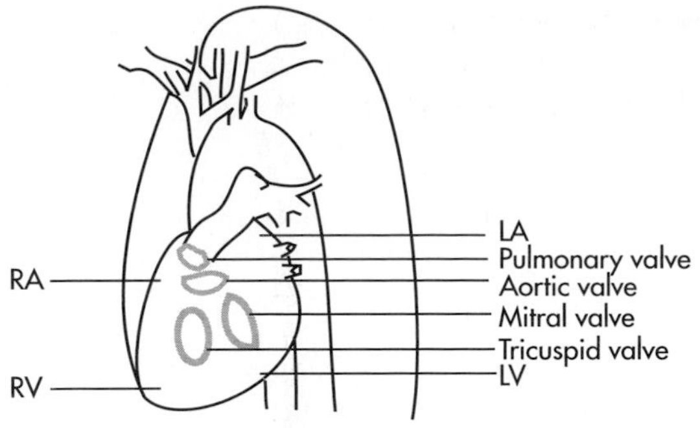

FIGURE 2-2

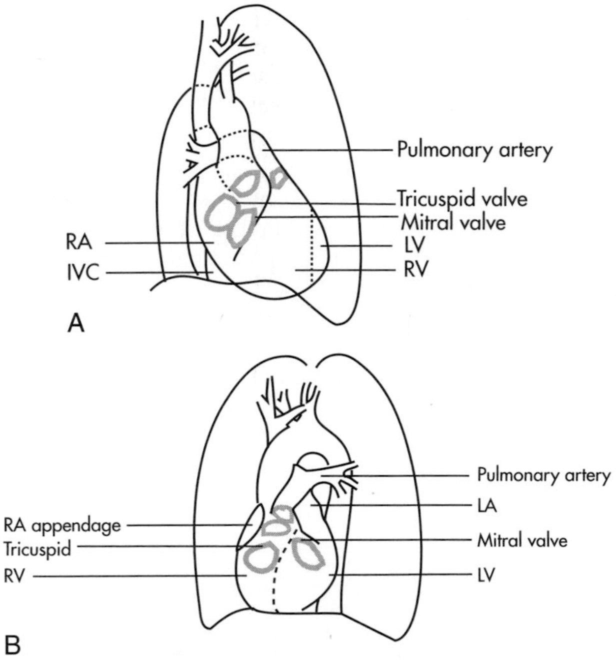

FIGURE 2-3

any diagnostic information in routine clinical practice. RAO view does not show calcified mitral or tricuspid valve.

RADIOGRAPHIC APPROACH TO INTENSIVE CARE UNIT (ICU) FILMS

1. Patient data present?
2. Date and time of examination are essential to report.
3. Postsurgical? If so, what type of surgery?
4. Appliances: intravascular, catheters, endotracheal tube, tubes, drains, etc. New appliances? Any catheters removed or repositioned?
5. Cardiac, mediastinal size and shape?
6. Pneumothorax present?
7. Lung disease: progression/regression?
8. Most important: any change from previous film?

Pearls

- Always obtain end-inspiratory films; varying lung volumes in inspiratory films will change the apparent extent and distribution of alveolar fluid.
- Positive end-expiratory pressure (PEEP) ventilation may underestimate airspace consolidation. PEEP decreases vascular mediastinal width.
- Quality of portable film is often suboptimal because:
  - Exposure time is longer than with routine films; this, along with the inability to often suspend respiration, causes indistinct vascular margins, which should not be mistaken as interstitial edema.
  - Patient positioning suboptimal
  - Anteroposterior (AP), not PA, position
  - Patient semierect
    - Small pleural effusions not readily detectable
    - Pulmonary vascularity may be "cephalized"
    - Varying tube-film distance
    - Varying cardiac/mediastinal silhouette
- Technique
  - Lower (80 to 90) peak kilovolt (kVp) than normal (120 to 140)
  - Variable daily density (exposure occurs at toe of HD curve): inadequate display of retrocardiac and mediastinal structures

ENDOTRACHEAL TUBE (ET)

Inflated cuff should not bulge tracheal wall. Tip of ET should be above the carina and below thoracic inlet:

- Neutral neck: 4 to 6 cm above carina
- Flexed neck: moves tip inferiorly by 2 cm
- Extended neck: moves tip superiorly by 2 cm

Complications of ET placement:

- Misplacement: atelectasis secondary to bronchial obstruction
- Tracheomalacia occurs above cuff pressures of 25 cm H_2O
- Tracheal rupture; radiographic findings include:
  - Pneumothorax
  - Pneumomediastinum
  - Subcutaneous emphysema
- Tracheal stenosis
- Dislodged teeth
- Laceration of nasoorophary nx

NASOGASTRIC TUBE

Tip with end holes should be located in stomach.

Complications

- Placement in airway
- Gastric and/or duodenal erosion

SWAN-GANZ CATHETER

Tip should be located in left or right PA, within 1 cm of hilum. There should be no loops in RA, RV (may cause arrhythmias).

Types

- Swan-Ganz catheter for measurement of wedge pressure
- Swan-Ganz catheter with integrated pacemaker (metallic bands visible)

Complications

- Pulmonary infarct
- Pulmonary hemorrhage
- Pulmonary artery pseudoaneurysm
- Infection

INTRAAORTIC BALLOON PUMP (IABP)

Tip should be located just distal to the takeoff of the left subclavian artery (LSA) and be 2 to 4 cm below aortic knob. Inflation may be seen during diastole.

Complications

- CVA (position too high)
- Renal or mesenteric ischemia (position too low)
- Aortic dissection
- Limb ischemia
- Infection
- Note initial positions of electrodes as they may migrate

EPICARDIAL PACING WIRE (Fig. 2-4)

Wires are typically anchored in the anterior myocardium; some slack may be left in pericardium. Multiple wires may be present. Wires exit through anterior chest wall.

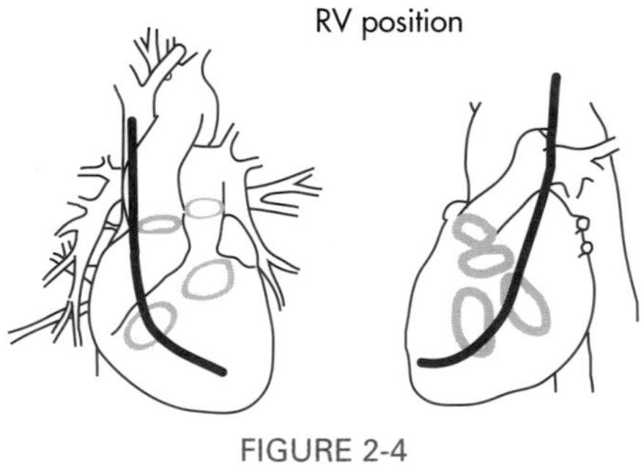

FIGURE 2-4

AUTOMATIC INTRACARDIAC DEFIBRILLATION DEVICE

Older systems: rectangular or ovoid antenna around RV and LV; newer systems: intraventricular electrodes.

Types of AICDs

- New models have pin sensors.
- Old models have spring.

CENTRAL VENOUS LINES

Tip should end in the SVC below the anterior first rib. Always rule out pneumothorax. Signs of impending catheter perforation (hemothorax, pneumothorax) include:

- Position of the tip against the vessel wall
- Sharply curved catheter tip
- Infection, thrombosis

PACEMAKER (Fig. 2-5)

Typical location is in apex of RV. May be located in atrial appendage for atrial pacing and in coronary sinus for atrial left ventricular pacing.

Complications

- Displacement of electrodes
- Broken wires (rare with modern pacemakers)
- Twiddler syndrome: rotation of pulse generator due to manipulation in a large pacemaker pocket
- Perforation
- Infection
- Venous thrombosis, vascular obstruction

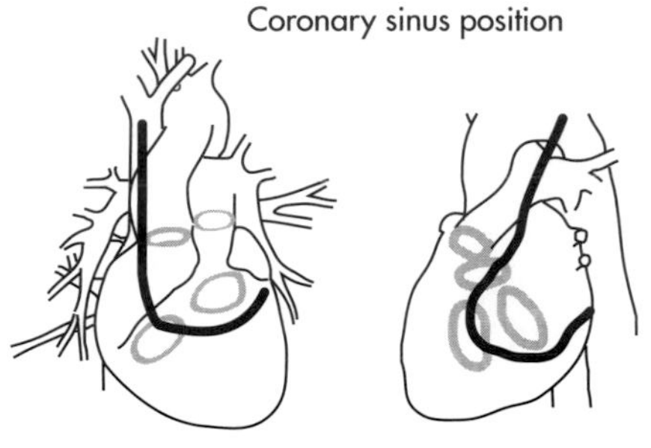

FIGURE 2-5

CHEST TUBES

Side port (interruption of radiodense band) has to be within thoracic cavity, otherwise there may be a leak. The tip of the tube should not abut the mediastinum.

Complications

- Residual pneumothorax
- Side port outside the thoracic wall

PROSTHETIC CARDIAC VALVES

Tissue Valves

No anticoagulation necessary; early breakdown

Heterografts

Porcine valves

- Carpentier-Edwards valve
- Hancock valve

Bovine valves
- Ionescu-Shiley valve (presently not used)

Homografts
Aortic in setting of endocarditis

Autografts
Native pulmonary valve, aortic valve

Mechanical Valves (Fig. 2-6)

More durable than tissue valves but require anticoagulation

Caged ball
- Starr-Edwards valve (presently not used)
- McGovern-Cromie (presently not used)
- Smeloff-Cutter valve (presently not used)

Caged disk
- Beal valve (presently not used)

Tilting disk
- Bileaflet—St. Jude Medical valve
- Single leaflet—Björk-Shiley valve (presently not used)
- Medtronic-Hall
- Lillehei-Kaster—later becomes Omniscience

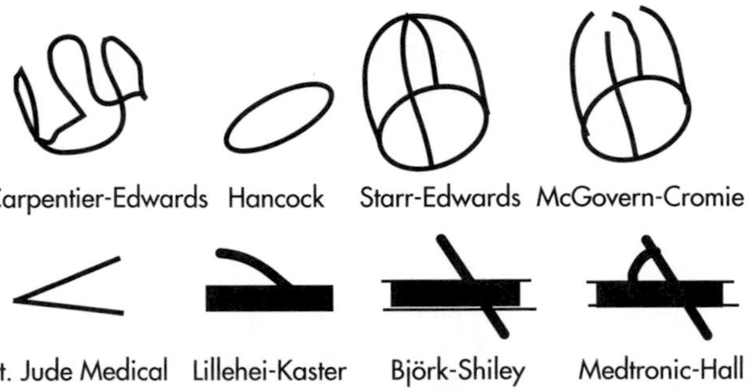

FIGURE 2-6

ANGIOGRAPHY

CARDIAC ANGIOGRAPHY

Technique for Left Ventriculography

- Femoral approach (sometimes radial artery)
- Pigtail for ventricular injections
- Straight end-hole catheter for pressure measurements
- 36 to 45 mL (3- to 4-second injection) at 15 mL/sec

Evaluation

1. Cardiac chamber size
2. Wall motion
3. Ejection fraction (EF)
4. Valvular stenosis, regurgitation, or shunts

Ejection Fraction

$$EF = \frac{(EDV - ESV)}{EDV} = \frac{\text{stroke volume}}{EDV} \quad \text{(Eq 2-1)}$$

where EDV = end-diastolic volume, ESV = end-systolic volume

Wall Motion Abnormalities (Fig. 2-7)
- Hypokinesis
- Akinesis
- Dyskinesis

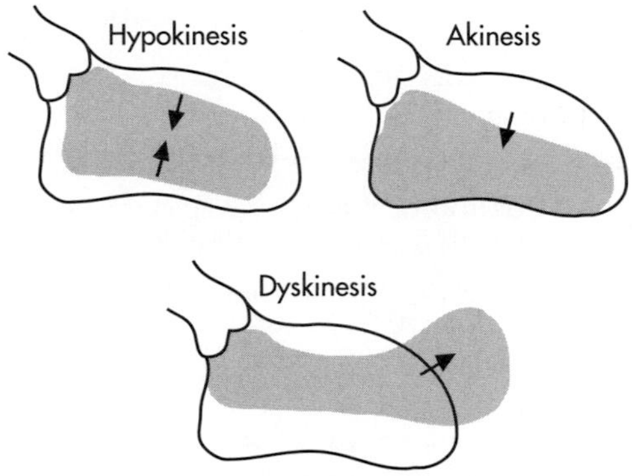

FIGURE 2-7

CORONARY ANGIOGRAPHY (Fig. 2-8)

Judkins catheters (6 Fr, groin) are the most commonly used catheters. Right and left Judkins catheters have different shapes.

Contrast Medium

- Hand injection: 7 to 9 mL for left coronary artery (LCA), 4 to 6 mL for right coronary artery (RCA)
- Low-osmolar contrast agents are usually used.
- Hyperosmolarity leads to electrocardiographic (ECG) changes.
- Citrate in contrast medium may cause hypocalcemia.
- 3000 U heparin IV; reversed by 350 mg of protamine

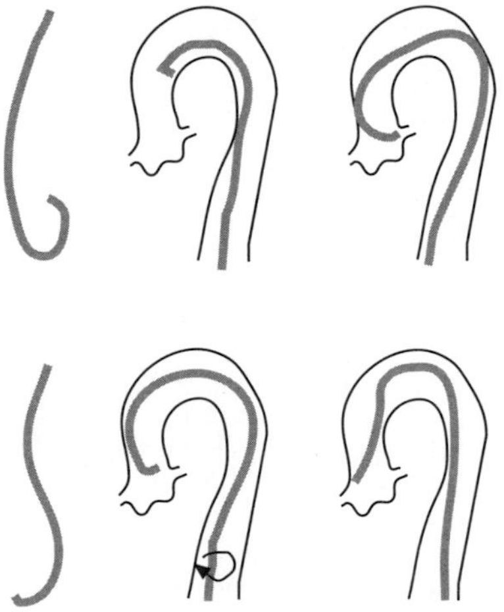

FIGURE 2-8

Complications

- Hematoma
- Arrhythmia
- Vasovagal reaction
- Contrast reaction/renal failure
- Acute myocardial infarction (AMI) <1%
- Stroke <1%
- Coronary air embolus
- Coronary artery dissection
- Perforation/dissection of aorta
- Femoral artery aneurysms

Interpretation

Steps in evaluation of coronary angiograms:

1. Which artery is being opacified?
2. Which projection (LAO or RAO)?
3. Stenosis present? If yes, grading of stenosis
4. Ventriculogram; analyze:
   - Wall motion
   - Ejection fraction
   - Presence of mitral regurgitation?

CORONARY ANGIOGRAM (Fig. 2-9, A–D)

RCA

- Conus artery
  First branch of RCA
  Runs anteriorly
- Sinoatrial (SA) nodal artery
  Branch of RCA in 40%-55%
- Muscular branches
- Acute marginal branch
- Posterior descending artery
- Atrioventricular (AV) nodal artery
  Branch of RCA in 90%
- Posterolateral ventricular branches

LCA

- Left anterior descending (LAD)
  Longest vessel
  Only vessel that extends to apex
  Septal branches
  Diagonal branches
- Left circumflex artery (LCx)
  Left atrial circumflex
  Marginal branches

Projections (Fig. 2-10)

LAO view projects the spine to the *left* (relative to the heart [i.e., on the right side of the image]). RAO projects the spine to the *right* (relative to the heart [i.e., to the left side of the image]).

Different projections (LAO, RAO) and angulations (caudal, cranial) are required to visualize all portions of the coronary arteries. Most commonly, the following projections are obtained:

- LAO with cranial angulation
- AP cranial or caudal angulation
- RAO cranial or caudal angulation
- Lateral (rarely used)

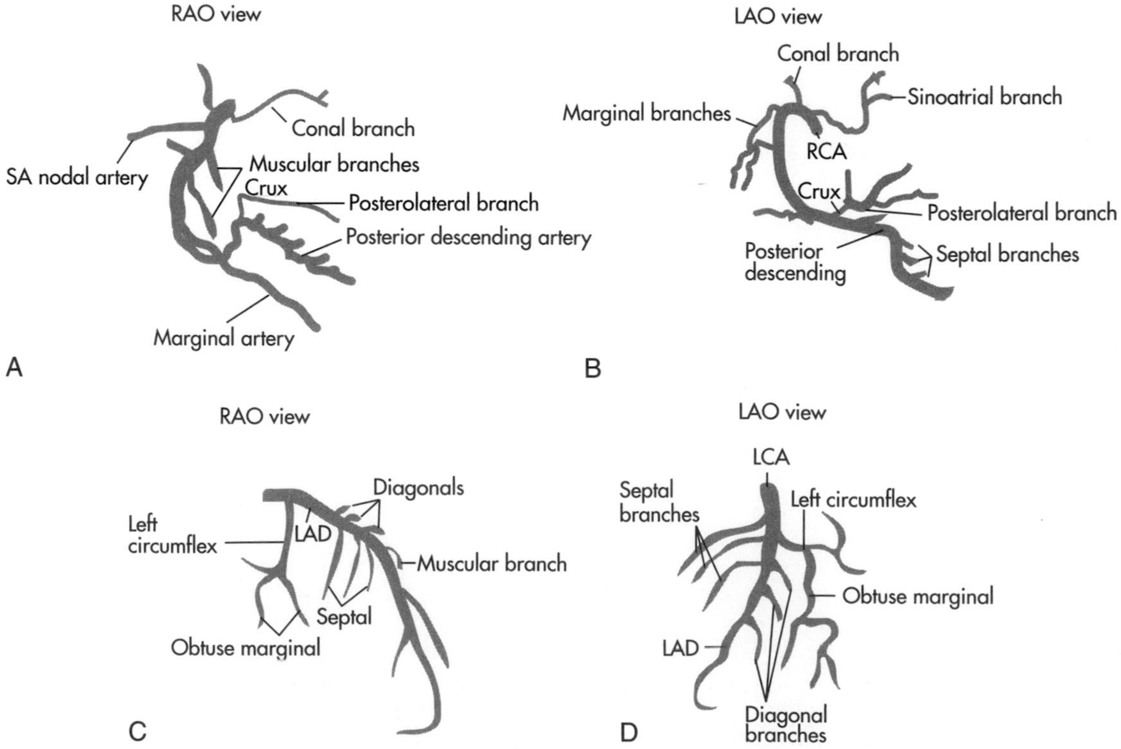

FIGURE 2-9

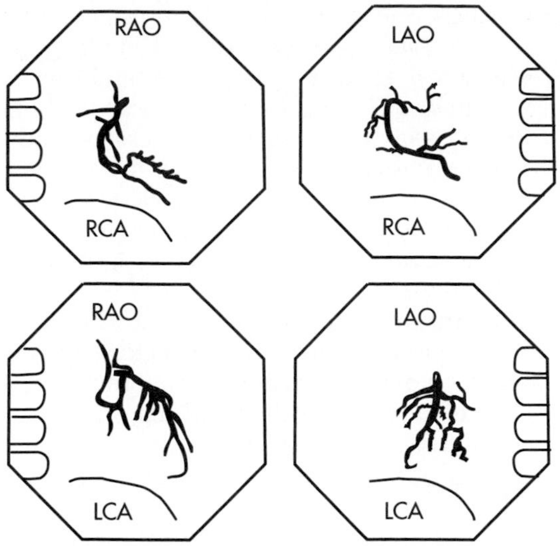

FIGURE 2-10

Although AP views are good for visualizing left main arteries, they are not as useful as RAO and LAO views because arteries overlie the spine.

Dominance

This refers to the artery that ultimately supplies the diaphragmatic aspect of the interventricular septum (IVS) and the LV.

- 85% of patients have right-sided dominance: RCA is larger than LCA and gives rise to the AV nodal artery.
- 10% of patients have left-sided dominance: LCA is larger than RCA and gives rise to the AV nodal artery.
- 5% of patients have a balanced coronary artery tree (codominant): two posterior descending arteries are present, one from the left circumflex and one from the RCA.

Pitfalls

- Intramyocardial bridge: LAD enters deep into the myocardium and may be compressed during systole; appears normal in diastole.
- Spasm of coronary arteries may be catheter induced (spasm can be provoked with ergot derivatives during angiography).
- Totally occluded arteries/bypasses may escape detection.
- Orifice stenoses can be missed if aortic injection not performed.
- Inadequate opacification—need to see contrast reflux into aorta.

Veins

- Epicardial veins accompany arteries and drain into coronary sinus.
- Thebesian venous system drains directly into all heart chambers.

MAGNETIC RESONANCE IMAGING

Cardiac MR is Tailored Extensively Depending on the Indication

- "White blood"—gradient echo (SSFP/FIESTA); Balanced Steady State Free Precession (SSFP) is optimal for cine cardiac imaging. Advantages of SSFP include highest SNR efficiency, high blood myocardial contrast, very fast, and can be gated. Signal depends on T2/T1, hence fluid and blood appear bright
- "Black blood"— double inversion recovery fast spin echo (HASTE/SSFSE), nulls signal from flowing blood
- ECG-gated bright-blood cine imaging: wall and valve motion, and gold standard method for volumetry – stack of short axis slices (EDV, ESV, EF)
- Delayed enhancement cardiac MRI (DE-CMRI): 10 to 30 minute delay after Gd, assessment of myocardial viability, inflammation, fibrosis
  - First pass perfusion imaging: modality with highest spatial resolution perfusion imaging, often done at rest and with dobutamine/adenosine stress
  - Dobutamine stress cine MRI detects hypokinesia and akinesia comparable to echo, but with higher resolution and diagnostic accuracy; also as real-time technique (using parallel imaging for acceleration) that does not require ECG gating;
  - T2 imaging to detect myocardial edema
- MR venogram: pulmonary vein ablation planning for atrial fibrillation
- Flow quantification: phase contrast sequences
- Arrhythmogenic right ventricular dysplasia: "black blood" fast spin echo images, fat-suppression techniques to confirm fat infiltration
- Standard axes:
  Short-axis: RV, LV
  Horizontal long-axis (4-chamber): RA, RV, LA, LV
  Vertical long-axis (2-chamber): LA, LV
- Other views:
  LVOT/Aortic root: ascending aorta, aortic valve
  3-chamber: LA, LV, RVOT, LVOT, aortic valve, mitral valve (rheumatic heart disease)

MR CORONARY ANGIOGRAPHY

Tremendous advances in magnetic resonance (MR) coronary angiography during the past decade have demonstrated promising potential for noninvasive diagnosis of coronary artery disease (CAD). The in-plane image resolution of current coronary artery MRI techniques is about 0.5 mm, which is sufficient for detection of stenoses in large coronary arteries and venous grafts after bypass surgery but inadequate for accurate detection of disease in smaller branches of the coronary vasculature.

- Fast gradient-echo sequences are commonly used (TR <10 msec, TE <3 msec)
- Multislice two-dimensional sequences are commonly used for breathhold sequences. Three-dimensional sequences are commonly used for nonbreathhold sequences (using navigator correction for respiratory motion).
- Fat saturation is used to suppress epicardial coronary fat.
- Newer phased-array, parallel imaging coils have increased signal-to-noise ratio (SNR).
- The scans are triggered to overcome cardiac motion, and this is done in one of three ways:
  - Prospective triggering: the QRS complex "triggers" the execution of the next imaging sequence. The search for the next trigger event is initiated after completion of the sequence part. Consequently, a single measurement can cover more than one cardiac cycle, and this can prolong the total acquisition time.
  - Retrospective gating: data are acquired continuously during the cardiac cycle. This is the method of choice for studies of cardiac function, because the complete heart cycle is covered during data acquisition. During the measurement, each acquired raw data line receives a time stamp. The trigger event is used to reset the time stamp to 0. At the end of the measurement, raw data can be resorted based on the time stamps, and images are reconstructed with a user-definable temporal resolution (by temporal interpolation). Additionally, arrhythmia rejection can be enabled excluding data acquired outside a user-definable heart cycle range.
  - Pulse-triggering: due to the delay of the pulse wave with respect to the ventricular contraction and due to its wider signal peak, pulse-triggering is not as reliable as the ECG. Usually the data are acquired over multiple heart cycles. This requires a breathhold to avoid blurring. To acquire data without breathhold, so-called navigator techniques are available that monitor the motion of the diaphragm, thus allowing for data acquisition in a particular phase of the respiratory cycle.
- Gated, segmented k-space acquisition is commonly used.
- Spiral imaging is an alternative imaging modality that samples k space along trajectories that start at the center of k space and spiral outward. This scheme is a more natural sampling pattern that has high sampling densities near the center of k space, where the power spectrum of the image is generally highest.
- Low-dose nitrate (coronary vasodilatation) or β-blocker pretreatment (to slow down heart rate) is still used.
- Currently, cardiac MRI is used in the clinical setting for the following purposes:
  - Assessment of anatomy in congenital malformations
  - Imaging of intracardiac masses such as thrombi and tumors (e.g., atrial myxoma, rhabdomyosarcoma, metastatic disease)
  - Assessment of morphology and wall motion in cases when echocardiography is not diagnostic (20% of echocardiography is not diagnostic owing to insufficient image quality [e.g., in obese patients or patients with emphysema])
  - First-pass perfusion measurements for assessment of myocardial ischemia. Myocardial viability: late enhancement MRI (10 to 30 minutes after gadolinium injection); "bright is dead"
  - Dobutamine stress cine-MRI to detect stress-induced ischemia

VENDOR-SPECIFIC SEQUENCE NOMENCLATURE

Sequence Type	Siemens	GE	Philips	Hitachi	Toshiba
Spin echo	SE	SE	SE	SE	SE
Turbo/fast spin echo	TSE	FSE	TSE	FSE	FSE
Single-shot TSE/FSE	HASTE	Single-shot FSE	Single-shot FSE	Single-shot FSE	FASE
Gradient echo	GRE	GRE	FFE (fast field echo)	FE	Field echo
Spoiled GRE	FLASH	SPGR	T1-FFE	RF spoiled SARGE, RSSG	Field echo
Coherent GRE	FISP	GRASS	FEE	Re-phased SARGE	Field echo
Steady-state free precession	PSIF	SSFP	T2-FFE	Time-reversed SARGE	
True FISP	True FISP	FIESTA	Balanced FFE	Balanced SARGE	True SSFP

FASE, fast advanced spin echo; FE, fast echo; FFE, fast field echo; FIESTA, fast imaging employing steady-state acquisition; FISP, fast imaging with steady-state precession; FLASH, fast low-angle shot; FSE, fast spin echo; GRASS, gradient-recalled acquisition in steady state; GRE, gradient echo; HASTE, half Fourier acquisition single-shot turbo spin echo; PSIF, reverse fast imaging with steady-state precession; RF, radiofrequency; RSSG, radiofrequency-labeled SARGE; SARGE, spoiled steady-state acquisition rewinded gradient echo; SE, spin echo; SPGR, spoiled gradient recalled; SSFP, steady-state free precession; TSE, turbo spin echo.

- A combined diagnostic session of cine-MRI for morphology and function, first-pass perfusion MRI, and late-enhancement MRI to assess viability is feasible in less than 1 hour and answers the most relevant clinical questions.

COMPUTED TOMOGRAPHY

CT ANGIOGRAPHY OF CORONARY ARTERIES

Cardiac cycle is approximately 1 second; ideal temporal resolution for imaging should be <50 msec. Temporal resolution is defined as the window within the cardiac period where CT data is acquired. Acquisition may occur during a single heartbeat or multiple heartbeats, with gantry rotation being the primary determinant. The high temporal resolution of multidetector CT makes it useful for cardiac imaging, including coronary calcium scoring and functional assessment of the heart.

Technique

As the number of slices increased from 4 to 16 slices to 40 to 64 slices, major changes have occurred within the detector geometry and the necessary postprocessing algorithms. Based on oblique x-ray projections of thin collimated slices, gantry design necessitates the use of special three-dimensional back-projection algorithms to correct for artifacts arising from the cone beam geometry. Whereas 16-slice scanners acquire 16 parallel projections within a single rotation, new multidetector CT allows either for 64 parallel slices based on newly designed and widened detector arrays or for overlapping projections based on flying focal spots along the z-axis. This improves spatial resolution and reduces image artifacts. Thin-slice collimations are now in the range of 0.5 to 0.625 mm at a maximum gantry rotation speed of 0.33 sec/360°. This further speed up in gantry rotation allows for a higher temporal resolution, which is of the essence in functional assessment of the heart and also in respect to image quality at different heart rates. (Fig. 2-11)

COMPARISON

	ECG Triggering	ECG Gating
Benefits	Pulsed radiation Low radiation exposure	Spiral acquisition Volumetric data set Full RR coverage Variable data reconstruction High reproducibility
Drawbacks	Sequential data acquisition Predefined timing necessary Partial RR interval covered	Continuous radiation High radiation exposure

Optimization of Image Quality

- Cardiac CT scans are ECG triggered. Similarly as in MRI, the triggering can be prospective or retrospective.
- Retrospectively, ECG-gated data acquisition provides coverage of the full cardiac cycle, which reduces artifacts. The choice of a +460% image reconstruction window is appropriate for calcium scoring.
- The image quality is inversely related to the heart rate (length of diastole shortens). The use of new faster gantry speeds up to 0.33 sec/360° now also provides better image quality at higher heart rates, although this might also be in systole.
- Insufficient breathholding or slightly different positions of the heart at subsequent heart beats are artifacts that can be more difficult to control.

CORONARY CT ANGIOGRAPHY

The improved spatial resolution of 64-slice scanners leads to less pronounced blooming artifacts of coronary calcifications and coronary stents (especially along the z-axis). This allows for an improved delineation of calcified and noncalcified plaques.

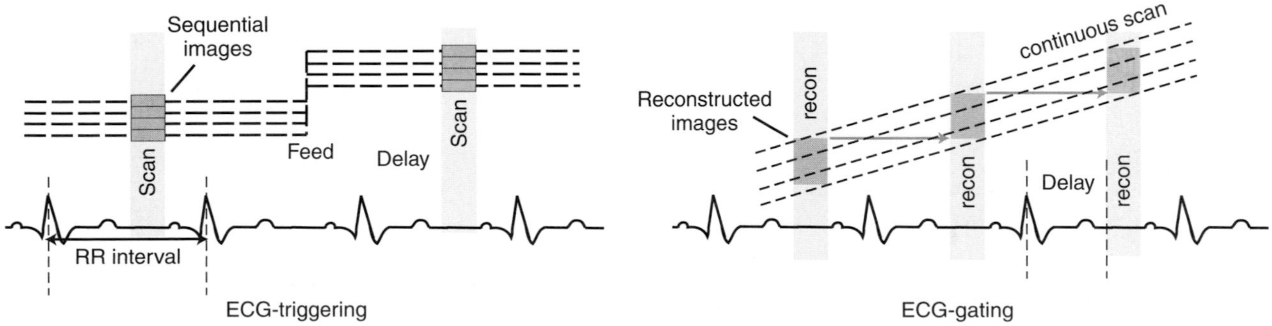

FIGURE 2-11

COMPARISON OF SCAN PROTOCOL PROPOSALS ON DIFFERENT-GENERATION CT SCANNERS

Rows	4 Slice	16 Slice	64 Slice
Collimation	4 × 1 mm	16 × 0.75 mm	64 × 0.6mm
Speed	0.5 sec	0.37 sec	0.33 sec
Scan time	~40 sec	~20 sec	~10 sec
Slice	1.3 mm	1 mm	0.75 mm
Increment	0.7 mm	0.5 mm	0.4 mm
Contrast	~120 at 3.5 mL/sec	~100 at 4 mL/sec	~80 at 5 mL/sec
Delay	4 sec	6 sec	6 sec

Contrast volume = (delay + scan time) × flow rate.

CORONARY CALCIUM SCORING

- CT examinations are performed without contrast agent administration and therefore display only calcified components of plaque.
- Tissue densities ≥ 130 HU are set as the attenuation level corresponding to calcified plaque (traditional Agatston calcium score).
- An alternative and preferred method of determining the calcium score is by quantifying the actual volume of plaque (total calcium volume score, CVS).
- Both calcium scoring algorithms can be applied to fast multidetector CT images and provide a measure of total coronary plaque burden.
- Quantitative assessment of coronary artery calcifications is still performed using 3-mm slices according to definition, although modern MDCT scanners scan at much thinner collimations.

RADIATION EXPOSURE

- Cardiac CT for coronary imaging is not recommended by AHA guidelines because of radiation
- Overall radiation exposure may be reduced by ECG-pulsing: while data acquisition is still retrospectively gated, the tube current is ramped down to a minimal level in systole while it is at 100% of the predefined value during diastole.
- Exposure can be reduced by 40%-50% with the above method during calcium scoring.
- Using alternative kVp levels is another method for reducing exposure. However, prospective tube current modulation is susceptible to artifacts arising from ectopic heartbeats or other arrhythmias. Stable sinus rhythm is therefore considered a prerequisite for the use of these techniques.

ULTRASOUND

M-MODE ULTRASOUND (Fig. 2-12)

M-mode = motion mode = one-dimensional echocardiography. Part of routine cardiac echo. It is more exact than two-dimensional imaging because of higher

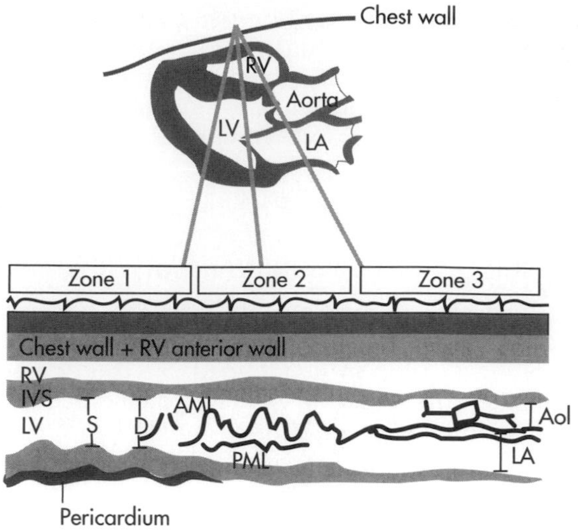

FIGURE 2-12

resolution and sampling rates. Pitfalls: sometimes it is difficult to get the transducer exactly in a 90° angle to long axis, mandatory for LV dimensions. Structures with broad surfaces perpendicular to the beam reflect well. The transducer is swept through three zones:

Zone 1

- Measurement of systolic and end-diastolic LV diameter allows calculation of fractional shortening (FS), which is an approximation of the EF and estimates LV function.
- Measurement of LV wall and IVS wall thickness
- Pericardial effusion may be detected and quantified.

Zone 2 (Fig. 2-13)

- Anterior (AML) and posterior mitral leaflets (PML) are identified.
- Mitral valve (MV) excursion (measured from D to E) is an index of MV mobility and inflow volume.
- EF slope: represents the rate of mid-diastolic posterior excursion of the AML; the EF slope is an index of mitral valve inflow.

Zone 3

- Aorta and aortic valve (rhomboid structure) are seen.
- Measurement of LA

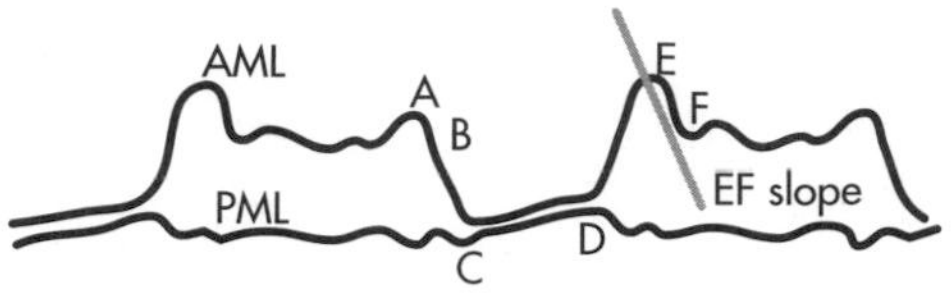

FIGURE 2-13

Two-Dimensional Cardiac Ultrasound

There are four common views: (Fig. 2-14)
- Long-axis view
- Short-axis view
- Apical view
- Suprasternal notch view

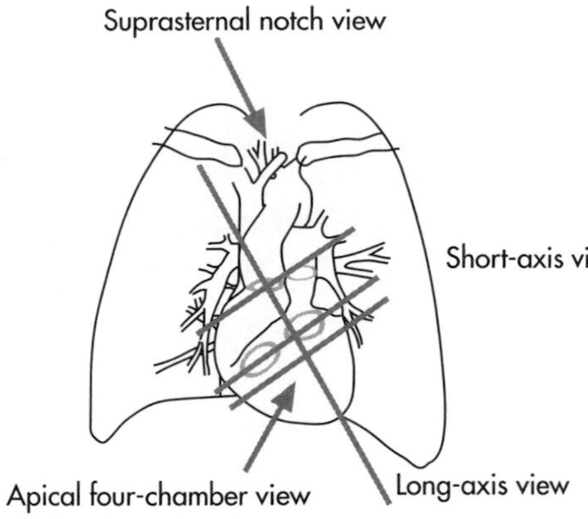

FIGURE 2-14

Long-Axis View (Fig. 2-15)

Transducer is in the 3rd or 4th intercostal space so that the beam is parallel to a line from the right shoulder to the left flank. Image is oriented so that the LA and LV are posterior and LA and aorta are left.

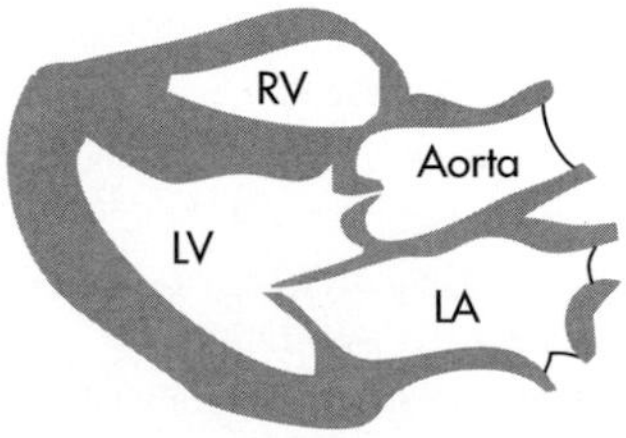

FIGURE 2-15

Short-Axis View (Fig. 2-16)

Transducer is in the 3rd or 4th intercostal space, but the beam is perpendicular to the long-axis view. Several levels are usually scanned, from cephalad to caudad: great arteries, plane of MV, and plane of papillary muscles (MPM = posteromedial papillary muscle; LPM = anterolateral papillary muscle). Image is oriented so that MPM is at 8 o'clock and LPM is at 4 o'clock.

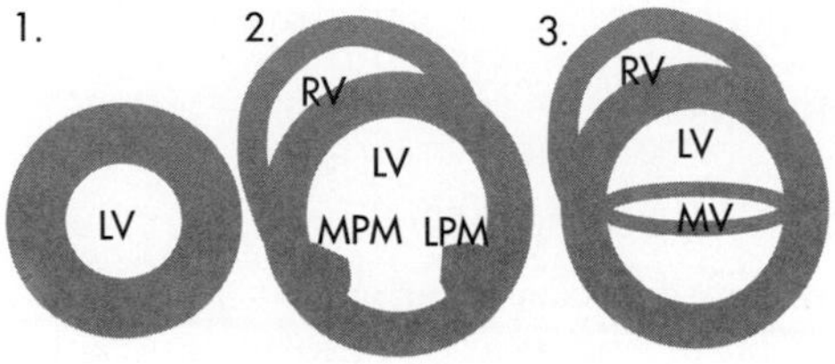

FIGURE 2-16

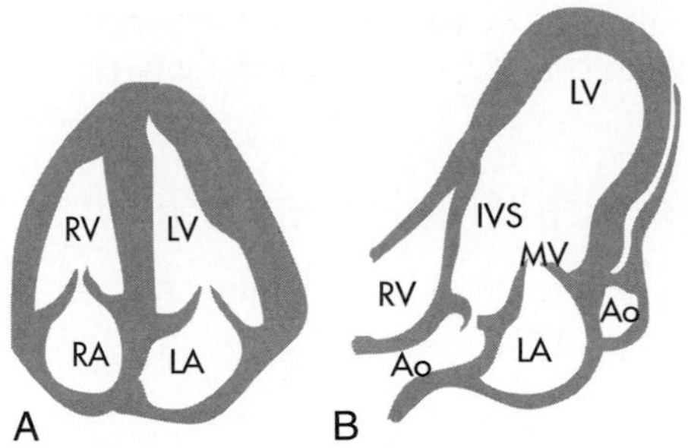

FIGURE 2-17

Apical View (Fig. 2-17, A and B)

Apical four-chamber view

Patient is in left lateral decubitus position. Transducer is at maximum point of impulse. Image is oriented so that RV and LV are anterior and LV and LA are on the right.

Apical Two-Chamber View (RAO View of the LV) (Fig. 2-18)

Transducer is at maximum point of impulse and directed in a plane parallel to the IVS. Image is oriented so that LV is anterior.

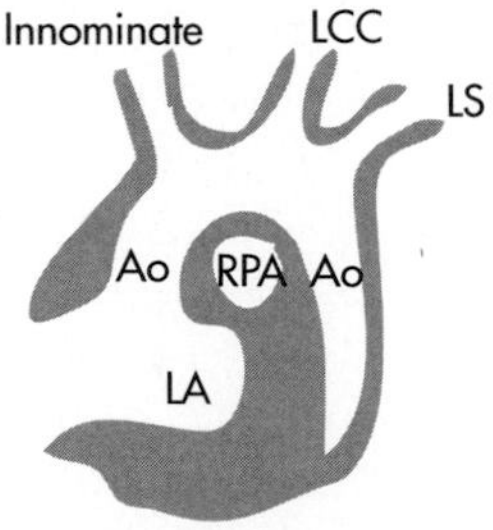

FIGURE 2-18

Suprasternal Notch View

Transducer is in the suprasternal notch with inferior and posterior beam angulation. Image is oriented so that the ascending aorta is on the left and the descending aorta is on the right.

DOPPLER

Continuous wave and pulsed wave Doppler are frequently used to assess stenosis or insufficiency of valves. One example is to decide if aortic stenosis requires surgery (cut off pressure gradient 50 mm Hg). Another important application for Doppler is evaluation of diastolic dysfunction.

COLOR DOPPLER

Capitalizing on the Doppler effect, Doppler echocardiography displays the direction and velocity of blood flow. It facilitates assessment of stenotic and insufficient valves and cardiac shunts (ASD, VSD) and estimation of pressure gradients across stenotic valves.

Congenital Heart Disease

GENERAL

INCIDENCE

Overall incidence of all anomalies is approximately 1% of newborns. The most common structural defects are bicuspid aortic valve and mitral valve prolapse (MVP), most of which are asymptomatic.

INCIDENCE OF SYMPTOMATIC CONGENITAL HEART DISEASE

	Frequency
Most Common Congenital Anomalies (All Age Groups; Bicuspid Aortic Valve and MVP Excluded)	
Ventricular septal defect (VSD)	30%
Atrial septal defect (ASD)	10%
Tetralogy of Fallot	10%
Patent ductus arteriosus (PDA)	10%
Coarctation of aorta	7%
Transposition of great arteries (TGA)	5%
First Month of Life (Serious Clinical Problems, High Mortality)	
Hypoplastic left heart	35%
TGA	25%
Coarctation	20%
Multiple serious defects	15%
Pulmonary atresia/stenosis	10%
Severe tetralogy of Fallot	10%

APPROACH (Fig. 2-19)

Evaluate five structures on the chest radiograph:
- Pulmonary vascularity
- Chamber enlargement

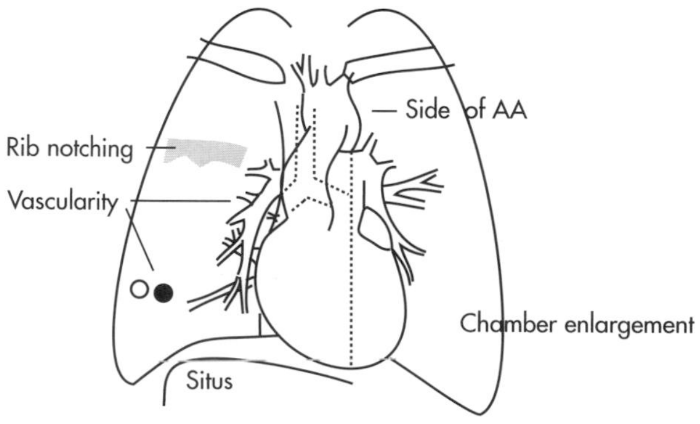

FIGURE 2-19

- Situs
- Side of AA
- Bone and soft tissue changes

Pulmonary Vascularity

Normal vascularity
- Right main PA = same size as trachea at level of AA
- Peripheral arteries (seen on end) = same size as adjacent bronchus

Pulmonary arterial overcirculation (shunt vascularity): common in CHD, less common in acquired heart disease (AHD)

Pulmonary venous hypertension (PVH) (edema) grades:
- Grade 1: vascular redistribution (10 to 17 mm Hg)
- Grade 2: interstitial edema (18 to 25 mm Hg)
- Grade 3: alveolar edema (>25 mm Hg)

Pulmonary arterial hypertension (PAH)
- Large main PA
- Usually normal hilar arteries

Eisenmenger pulmonary vasculature
- Combination of shunt and PAH
- Aneurysmal hilar arteries
- Calcified vessels (rare)

Cyanosis: there are no definitive signs to predict cyanosis by plain film; however, as a rule of thumb, cyanotic patients (right-to-left shunt) have small pulmonary arteries, and the main PA segment may not be visible or is concave.

Chamber Enlargement

Lateral view is more helpful in young children:
- LA enlargement
  - Posterior displacement of esophagus during barium swallow
  - Posterior displacement of left mainstem bronchus (LMB)
- LV enlargement: posterior displacement behind IVC
- RV enlargement: filling of retrosternal clear space

PA view; criteria for cardiomegaly:
- Cardiothoracic index >0.55

Situs

- Liver or IVC determines on which side the RA is located.
- Tracheobronchial tree: right mainstem bronchus (RMB) has a more acute angle than LMB.
- Incidence of CHD in situs inversus: 5%

ALGORITHM

CLASSIFICATION (Fig. 2-20)

The radiographic classification of CHD relies mainly on clinical information (cyanosis) and plain film information (pulmonary vascularity).

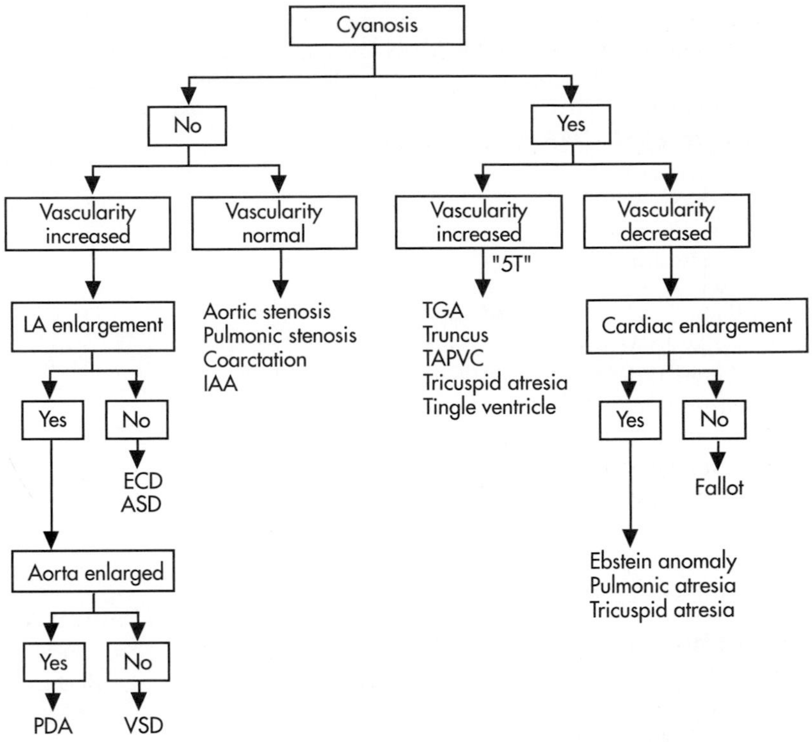

FIGURE 2-20

Acyanotic CHD with Increased Pulmonary Vascularity

Common: L-R shunt where pulmonary flow is greater than aortic flow; the shunt can be located in:

IVS
- Ventricular septal defect (VSD)

Atrium
- Atrial septal defect (ASD)

Large vessels
- Patent ductus arteriosus (PDA)
- Aorticopulmonary window (uncommon)

Other
- Endocardial cushion defect (ECD)
- Partial anomalous pulmonary venous connection (PAPVC)

Acyanotic CHD with Normal Pulmonary Vascularity

Normal pulmonary vascularity is associated with either outflow obstruction or valvular insufficiency before onset of congestive heart failure (CHF):

Outflow obstruction
- Coarctation of aorta
- Interruption of aortic arch (IAA)
- Aortic stenosis
- Pulmonic stenosis

Valvular insufficiency (rarely congenital)

Corrected transposition of great arteries (L-TGA) (isolated)

Cyanotic CHD with Decreased Pulmonary Vascularity

Decreased pulmonary vascularity because of obstruction of pulmonary flow. In addition, there is a R-L shunt due to an intracardiac defect.

Normal heart size
- Tetralogy of Fallot
- Fallot variants
- Tricuspid atresia

Increased heart size
- Ebstein anomaly
- Pulmonary stenosis with ASD
- Pulmonary atresia

Cyanotic CHD with Increased Pulmonary Vascularity (Admixture Lesions)

Common denominator of these lesions is that there is an "admixture" of systemic and pulmonary venous blood (bidirectional shunting). The mixing of venous and systemic blood may occur at the level of:

Large veins
- Total anomalous pulmonary venous connection (TAPVC) (ASD is also present.)

Large arteries
- Truncus arteriosus (TA) (VSD is also present.)

Multiple
- Transposition of great arteries (TGA) (VSD, ASD, or PDA is also present.)

Ventricle
- Single ventricle (VSD is present.)
- Double-outlet right ventricle (DORV) (VSD is present.)

CHD with PVH/CHF

- Cor triatriatum
- Mitral stenosis
- Hypoplastic left heart syndrome
- Coarctation of the aorta
- Cardiomyopathy
- Primary endocardial fibroelastosis
- Anomalous ICA
- Obstructed TAPVC

Increased incidence in females: ASD, PDA, and Ebstein anomaly

Increased incidence in males: AS, coarctation, pulmonary/tricuspid atresia, hypoplastic left heart, TGA

USE OF IMAGING MODALITIES FOR EVALUATION OF CHD

Chest Film

- Determine to which of the four categories a CHD belongs (based on pulmonary vascularity and cardiac contour abnormalities).
- Abdomen: determine situs.
- Bones: certain CHDs are associated with osseous abnormalities such as 11 ribs or hypersegmented sternum (Down syndrome).

Ultrasound

- Often allows diagnosis of a specific disease entity

Angiography

- Confirmation of diagnosis
- Pressure measurements
- Oxygenation
- Intervention

Magnetic Resonance Imaging (MRI)

- Diagnostic test for anomalies in pulmonary arteries, aorta, and vena cava

ACYANOTIC CHD WITH INCREASED PULMONARY VASCULARITY

VENTRICULAR SEPTAL DEFECT (VSD) (Fig. 2-21)

Second most common congenital cardiac anomaly

Types

- Membranous, 80%
- Muscular, 10%
- AV, 5%
- Conal, 5% (mostly supracristal)

Clinical Findings

- Small to moderate defects are initially asymptomatic.
- Large defects lead to CHF at 2 to 3 months of age.

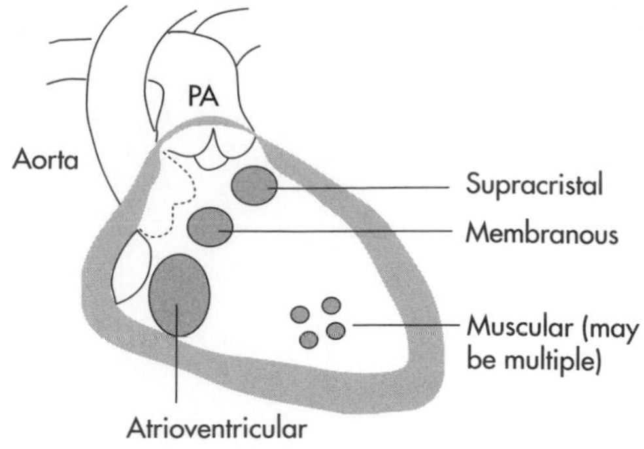

FIGURE 2-21

- 75% close spontaneously by age 10.
- 3% of patients develop infundibular stenosis.
- Eisenmenger syndrome (elevated pulmonary resistance leads to increased right-sided pressures) may develop in long-standing large defects; the end result is a R-L shunt with cyanosis.

Hemodynamics (Fig. 2-22)

- Blood flow from LV through IVS into RV
- Redundant flow: LV → VSD → RV → PA → LA → LV

Radiographic Features

Because of the variation in size of VSD, the radiographic features are variable and may range from normal cardiac size and pulmonary vessels to large RV, LV, and LA.

Chest film findings
- Small VSD: normal CXR
- Significant shunt (Q_{pulm}/Q_{aorta} >2): enlargement of heart, pulmonary arteries, and LA
- Eisenmenger physiology
  - Enlarged pulmonary arteries
  - Cardiac and LA enlargement may decrease RVH
  - Peripheral pulmonary arteries become constricted ("pruning")
  - Calcified PA (rare)

Ultrasound is the diagnostic method of choice.

Angiography is commonly performed preoperatively (pressure measurement, oxygenation).

Treatment

Expectant in small asymptomatic VSD because there is spontaneous closure in infancy, 30%

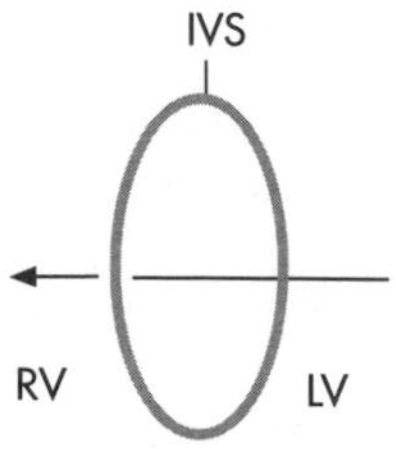

FIGURE 2-22

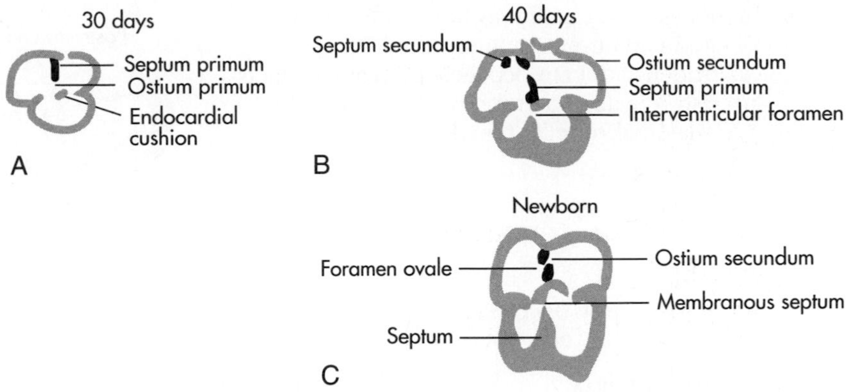

FIGURE 2-23

Surgical therapy (patch) in patients with CHF, pulmonary hypertension, or progressive worsening

ATRIAL SEPTAL DEFECT (ASD) (Fig. 2-23, A and B)

Most common congenital cardiac anomaly

Types (Fig. 2-23, C)

- Ostium secundum type: most common, 60%
- Ostium primum ASD: part of the ECD syndromes, 35%
- Sinus venosus defect (at entrance of SVC): always associated with PAPVC anomalous venous return, 5%

Associations (Fig. 2-24)

- Holt-Oram syndrome: ostium secundum defect
- Lutembacher syndrome: ASD and mitral stenosis
- Down syndrome: ostium primum defect

Clinical Findings

- May be asymptomatic for decades because of the low atrial pressure; even large defects are much better tolerated than VSD or PDA.
- Female preponderance
- May present with pulmonary hypertension

Hemodynamics

- Blood flows from LA to RA

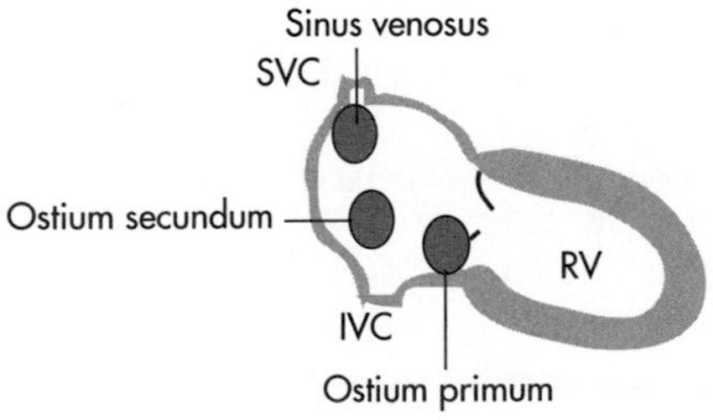

FIGURE 2-24

HEMODYNAMICS OF ASD

	Right Side	Left Side
Atrium	Enlarged	No change
Ventricle	Enlarged	No change
Vasculature	Increased	Aorta no change

Radiographic Features (Fig. 2-25)

Plain film

- RA, RV, and PA enlargement; no LA enlargement (different from VSD)
- The AA appears small (but in reality is normal) because of the prominent pulmonary trunk and clockwise rotation of heart (RV enlargement).

Ultrasound

- Imaging modality of choice for diagnosis

Angiography

- Useful for identifying associated anomalous pulmonary veins

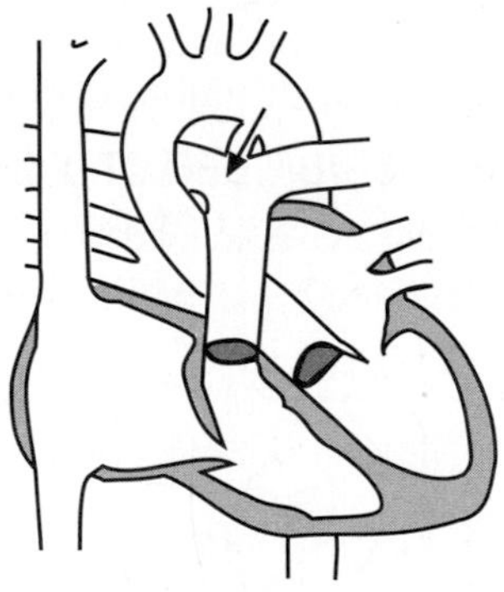

FIGURE 2-25

PATENT DUCTUS ARTERIOSUS (PDA)

In the fetus, a PDA represents a normal pathway of blood flow.

- Fetal circulation: flow from PA to aorta as intrauterine bypass of nonaerated lungs

- PDA closes functionally 48 hours after delivery.
- PDA closes anatomically after 4 weeks.

Highest incidence of PDA occurs in premature infants (especially if hyaline membrane disease is present) and in maternal rubella; females > males.

Clinical Findings

- Most are asymptomatic.
- Large defects lead to CHF at 2 to 3 months of age.

Hemodynamics

There is an L-R shunt because the pressure in the aorta is higher than in the pulmonary circulation.

HEMODYNAMICS OF PDA

	Right Side	Left Side
Atrium	No change	Enlarged
Ventricle	No change	Enlarged
Vasculature	Enlarged	Aorta enlarged

Radiographic Features

- Small PDA: normal CXR
- Increased pulmonary vascularity
- Enlargement of LA, LV
- Eisenmenger physiology may develop in long-standing, severe disease.

All the above features are identical to those seen in VSD; specific features to suggest PDA are:

- Unequal distribution of pulmonary arterial blood flow, especially sparing of left upper lobe
- Enlargement of aorta and AA
- PDA may be seen as faint linear density through the PA (occasionally calcifies).

Treatment

- Indomethacin (inhibits PGE_1, which is a potent dilator of the duct); successful in 60% of infants.
- Ligation of ductus through left thoracotomy
- Catheter closure with umbrella device

ENDOCARDIAL CUSHION DEFECT (ECD) (Fig. 2-26)

40% of ECD patients have trisomy 21 (Down syndrome).

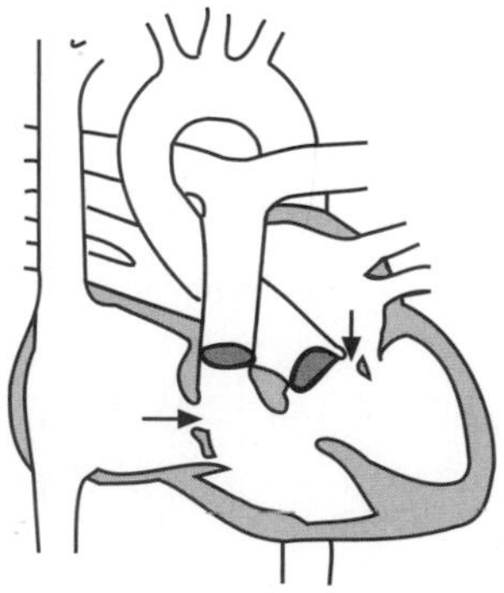

FIGURE 2-26

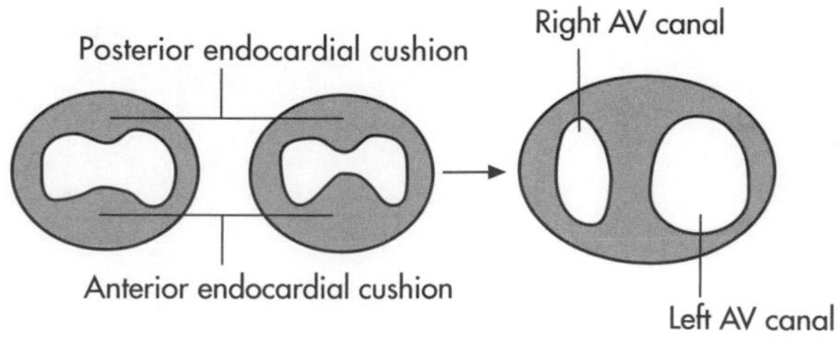

FIGURE 2-27

Types

- Partial AV canal (ostium primum defect ± cleft in anterior mitral or septal tricuspid leaflets)
- Transitional AV canal (ostium primum defect, cleft in both AV valves, defect in superior IVS)
- Complete AV canal (ostium primum defect, cleft in both AV valves, large defect in IVS: either common AV valve or separate mitral and tricuspid valves)

Clinical Findings (Fig. 2-27)

- Partial canals may be asymptomatic; both the degree of mitral insufficiency and the shunt through the ASD determine the clinical picture.
- Complete AV canal consists of large L-R shunts (ASD, VSD), mitral insufficiency, and CHF.

Embryology

Endocardial cushion tissue contributes to the formation of the ventricular septum, the lower atrial septum, and the septal leaflets of the MV and tricuspid valves. If the anterior and posterior endocardial cushions do not fuse, the AV valves (MV and tricuspid valves) do not develop properly.

Hemodynamics

HEMODYNAMICS OF ECD

	Right Side	Left Side
Atrium	Enlarged	Enlarged
Ventricle	Enlarged	Enlarged
Vasculature	Enlarged	Aorta no change

Radiographic Features (Fig. 2-28)

Plain film

- Cardiomegaly
- Increased pulmonary vascularity
- Screen for other trisomy 21 findings: 11 ribs, multiple manubrial ossification centers

Angiography

- Gooseneck deformity of left ventricular outflow tract on RAO view
- Abnormal prolapse of anterior MV leaflet in diastole

Treatment

- Primary surgical repair before age 2

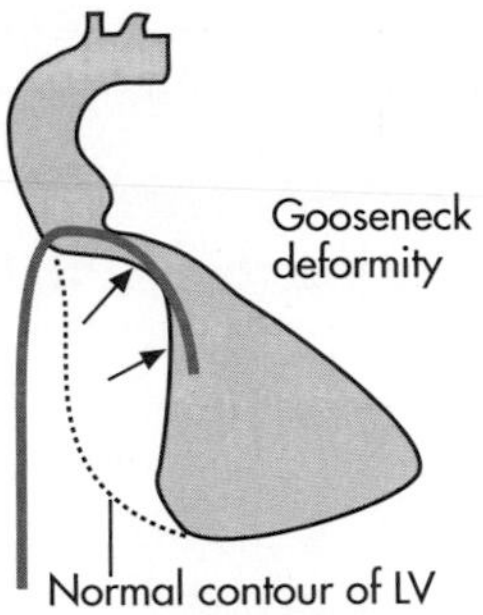

FIGURE 2-28

AORTOPULMONARY WINDOW (Fig. 2-29)

Synonyms: aortopulmonary septal defect, partial truncus arteriosus.

- Defect between ascending aorta and main or right PA
- L-R shunt
- Plain film findings are identical to those seen in PDA.
- Differentiation from truncus arteriosus:
  Two semilunar valves are present.
  No VSD
- Associated with PDA, 10%-15%
- Also associated with VSD and coarctation

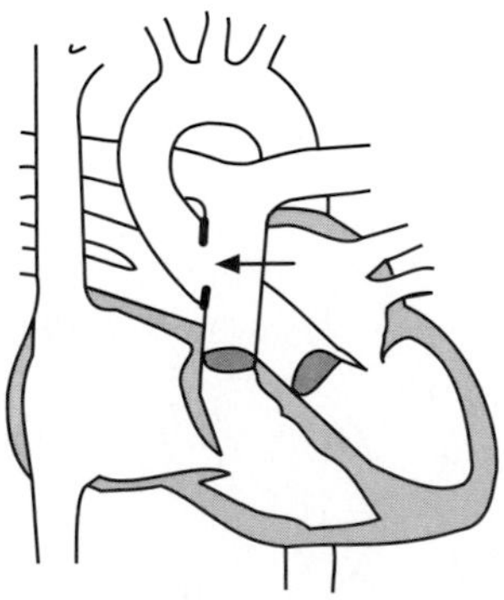

FIGURE 2-29

PARTIAL ANOMALOUS PULMONARY VENOUS CONNECTION (PAPVC)

Some but not all pulmonary veins drain to the systemic circulation rather than into the LA. Anomalous pulmonary venous connection is a L-R shunt. Pulmonary veins connect to RA or systemic veins. Cyanosis occurs because of Eisenmenger syndrome. PAPVC is not always cyanotic. Common connections of pulmonary veins include:

Supracardiac
- Right SVC (most common)
- Left SVC
- Azygos vein
- Innominate (via vertical vein)

Cardiac
- RA
- Coronary sinus

Intracardiac
- IVC (scimitar syndrome)
- Portal vein

Associations

ASD, 15% (especially the sinus venosus defect)

Radiographic Features

- Supracardiac and cardiac types resemble ASD findings.
- The anomalous vein of the infracardiac type looks like a Turkish scimitar (sword): scimitar sign.
- Infracardiac PAPVC is part of hypogenetic lung syndrome.

ACYANOTIC CHD WITH NORMAL PULMONARY VASCULARITY

VALVULAR PULMONARY STENOSIS (PS) (Fig. 2-30)

Clinical Findings

- Most patients are asymptomatic.
- Dysplastic type may show familial inheritance; also associated with Noonan syndrome (short stature, webbed neck, hypogonadism).

Types

- Dome-shaped type (95%): valve with a small orifice and three fused commissural raphes
- Dysplastic type (5%): thickened, redundant, immobile leaflets; commissures not fused

Hemodynamics

- Obstruction of right ventricular outflow

HEMODYNAMICS OF PS

	Right Side	Left Side
Atrium	No change	No change
Ventricle	Enlarged	No change
Vasculature	Poststenotic dilatation (only MPA and LPA)	Aorta no change

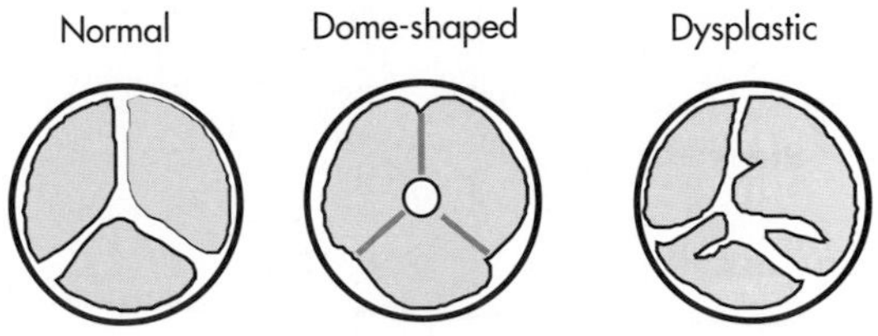

FIGURE 2-30

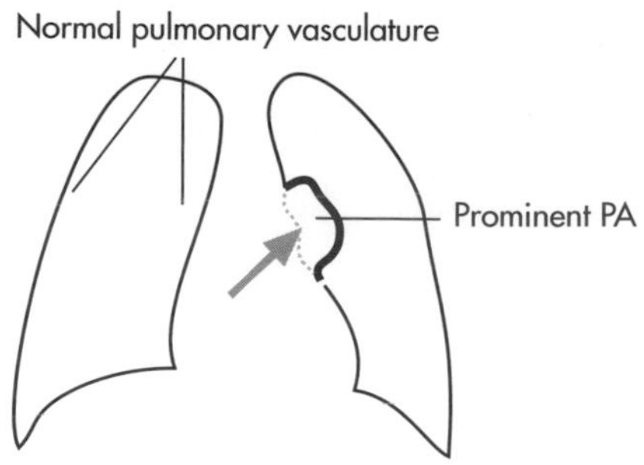

FIGURE 2-31

Radiographic Features (Fig. 2-31)

Plain film
- Poststenotic dilatation of main and/or left PA (jet through stenosed valve dilates PA)
- Right PA of normal size
- RV (hypertrophy)

Ultrasound
- Systolic doming of leaflets
- Thickened leaflets
- Doppler measurements

Treatment
- Most stenoses are amenable to balloon valvuloplasty.
- Surgical reconstruction may be necessary for dysplastic types.

CONGENITAL PERIPHERAL PULMONARY ARTERY STENOSIS

Causes
- Maternal rubella (common)
- Williams syndrome

Types (Fig. 2-32)
- Type 1: single, main PA stenosis
- Type 2: stenosis at bifurcation of right and left PA

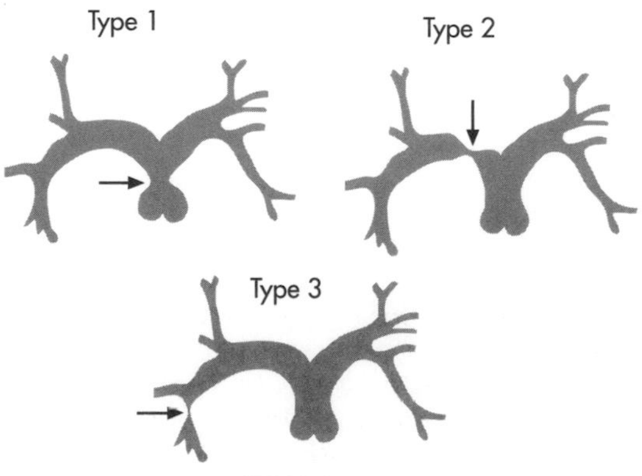

FIGURE 2-32

- Type 3: multiple peripheral stenosis
- Type 4: central and peripheral stenosis

Radiographic Features
- PA enlargement if associated valvular stenosis
- RV hypertrophy

CONGENITAL AORTIC STENOSIS

Clinical Findings
- Most are asymptomatic.
- Severe AS leads to CHF in infancy.
- Supravalvular type associated with Williams syndrome:
  - Mental retardation
  - Peripheral pulmonary stenoses
  - Diffuse aortic stenoses

Types

Subvalvular aortic stenosis
- Membranous subaortic stenosis
- Hypertrophic subaortic stenosis (fibromuscular tunnel)

Valvular aortic stenosis (most common) (Fig. 2-33)
- Bicuspid aortic valve (most common congenital heart anomaly)
- Unicommissural valve (single horseshoe-shaped valve)

Supravalvular aortic stenosis
- Localized
- Diffuse

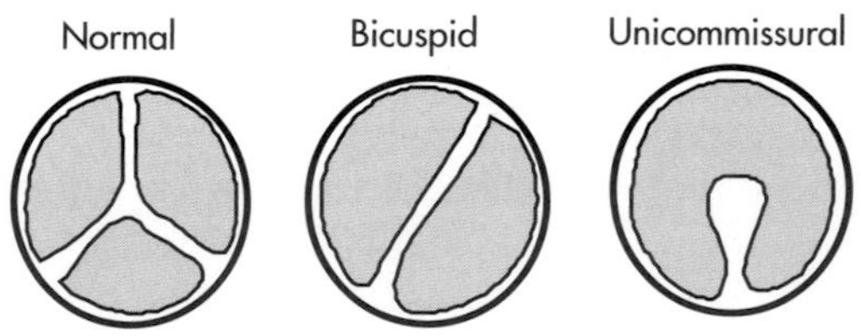

FIGURE 2-33

Radiographic Features

Plain film
- Cardiomegaly: LV hypertrophy
- Poststenotic dilatation of aorta is present only in valvular AS.
- CHF

Ultrasound and angiography
- Domed valve
- Jet through valve
- Hourglass deformity of ascending aorta (supravalvular AS)

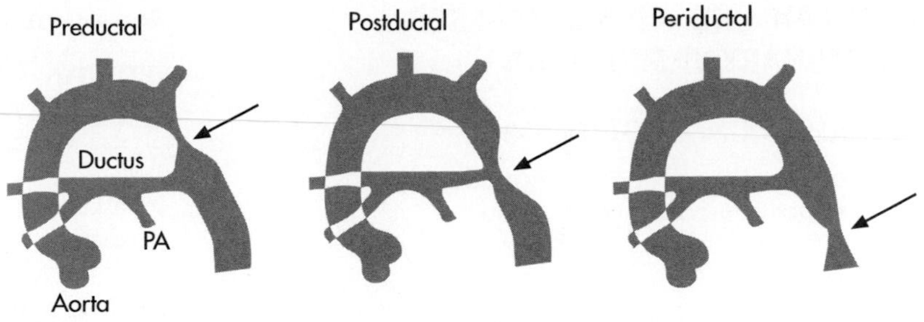

FIGURE 2-34

COARCTATION OF AORTA

Types (Fig. 2-34)

- Infantile type (diffuse type, preductal): tubular hypoplasia
- Adult type (localized type, postductal, periductal): short segment; common

Associations

- Coarctation syndrome: triad of coarctation, PDA, VSD
- In Turner syndrome, most common cardiac abnormality
- Bicuspid aortic valve, 50%
- Hypoplasia of the aortic isthmus (small arch)
- Circle of Willis aneurysms
- PDA aneurysm
- Intracardiac defects; occur in 50% with infantile type
- Marfan syndrome

Clinical Findings

- Blood pressure difference between arms and legs
- Diffuse type presents as neonatal CHF.
- Adult type is frequently asymptomatic; presents in young adult

Hemodynamics (Fig. 2-35)

- Preductal type has concomitant R-L shunting via PDA or VSD.
- Postductal coarctation has L-R flow through PDA.
- Collaterals to descending aorta
  - Internal mammary-intercostals
  - Periscapular arteries-intercostals

Radiographic Features

Plain film

- Aortic figure-3 configuration 50%:
  - Prestenotic dilatation of aorta proximal to coarctation
  - Indentation of aorta caused by the coarctation
  - Poststenotic dilatation
- Inferior rib notching:
  - Secondary to dilated intercostal arteries
  - Only ribs 3 to 8 involved
  - Only in children >8 years

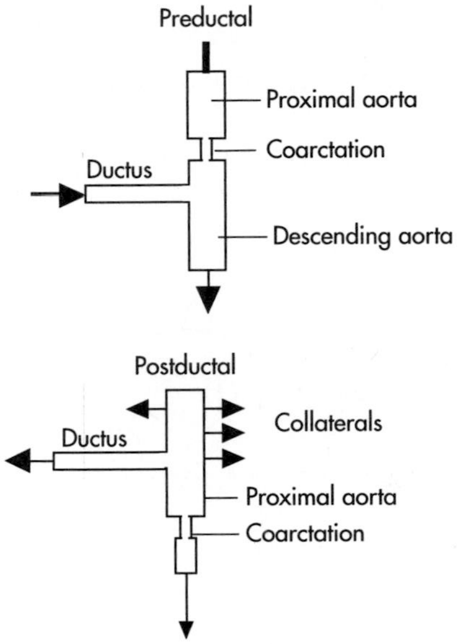

FIGURE 2-35

- Reverse-3 sign of barium-filled esophagus
- Prominent left cardiac border from left ventricular hypertrophy (LVH)
- Normal pulmonary vascularity

MRI

- Diagnostic study of choice
- Adequately shows site and length of coarctation
- Has replaced angiography (but angiography allows pressure measurements)
- Allows evaluation of collaterals

Treatment

- Resection of coarctation and end-to-end anastomosis
- Patch angioplasty: longitudinal incision with placement of a synthetic patch
- Subclavian patch: longitudinal incision of coarctation; division of subclavian artery and longitudinal opening to be used as a flap
- Percutaneous balloon angioplasty

CYANOTIC CHD WITH DECREASED PULMONARY VASCULARITY

TETRALOGY OF FALLOT (Fig. 2-36)

Most common cyanotic CHD of childhood Tetrad
- Obstructed RV outflow tract
- Right ventricular hypertrophy (RVH)
- VSD
- Aorta overriding the interventricular septum

Clinical Findings
- Squatting when fatigued (to increase pulmonary flow and thus O_2 saturation)
- Episodic loss of consciousness
- Cyanosis by 3 to 4 months; time of presentation depends on degree of RV outflow obstruction.

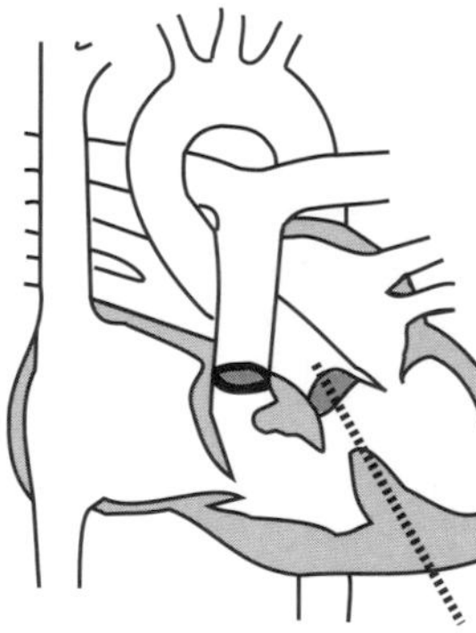

FIGURE 2-36

Associations (Fig. 2-37)
- Pulmonary infundibular or valve stenosis in most cases
- Right AA anomalies with aberrant vessels and vascular sling or rings, 25%
- Anomalies of coronary arteries, 5% (LAD from RCA, single RCA)
- Rare
  - Tracheoesophageal fistula
  - Rib anomalies, scoliosis

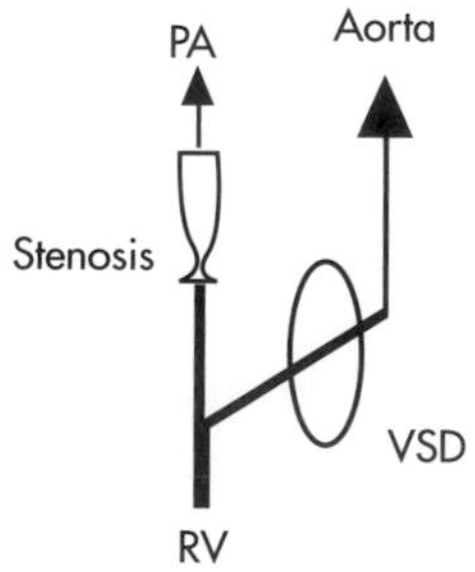

FIGURE 2-37

Hemodynamics

HEMODYNAMICS OF TETRALOGY OF FALLOT

	Right Side	Left Side
Atrium	No change	No change
Ventricle	Enlarged	No change
Vasculature	Decreased	Aorta normal

Radiographic Features (Fig. 2-38)

Plain film
- Boot-shaped heart (enlarged RV): coeur en sabot
- Right AA, 25%
- Small or concave PA

MRI
- Used to determine extent of systemic collateral vessels coming off the aorta

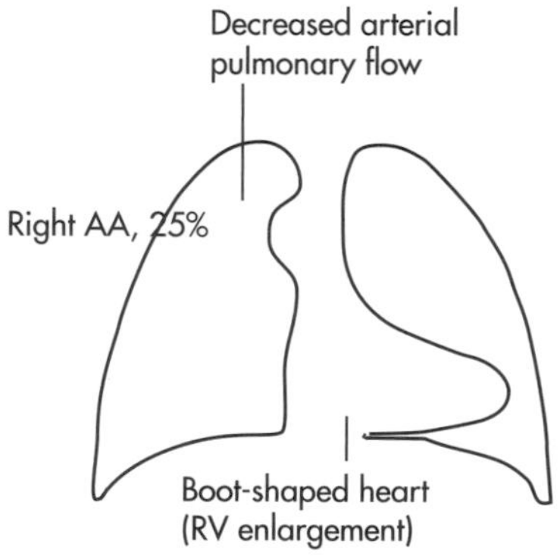

FIGURE 2-38

Treatment

Total corrective repair
- VSD closure and reconstruction of RV outflow tract
- Palliative shunts: systemic to PA shunt allows growth of pulmonary vessels.
- Blalock-Taussig shunt (subclavian artery → PA) is indicated in symptomatic patients who are poor surgical candidates (Fig. 2-39).

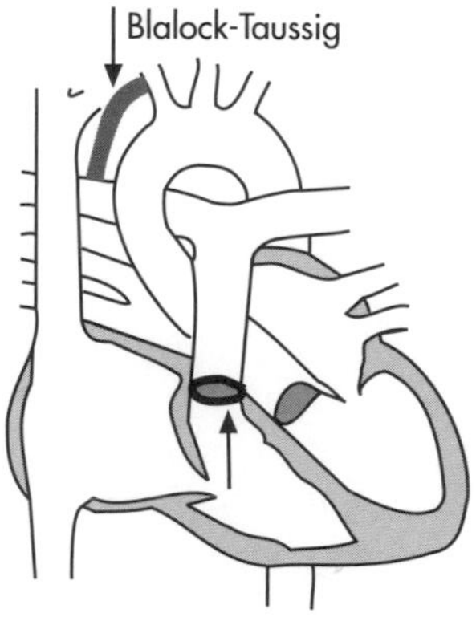

FIGURE 2-39

TETRALOGY VARIANTS

Pink Tetralogy
- VSD with mild pulmonic stenosis

Pentalogy of Fallot
- Tetralogy ± ASD

Trilogy of Fallot
- PA stenosis, RVH with patent foramen ovale

EBSTEIN ANOMALY (FIG. 2-40)

Deformity of the tricuspid valve with distal displacement of the tricuspid leaflets into the RV inflow tract; results in atrialization of superior RV.

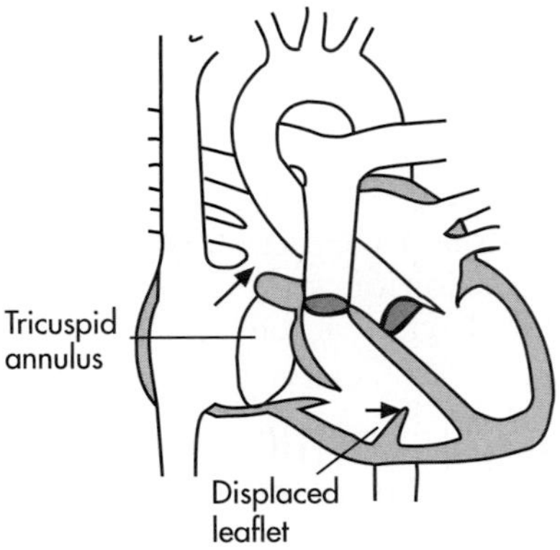

FIGURE 2-40

Associations
- Maternal lithium intake
- Patent foramen ovale or ASD nearly always present, 80%

Clinical Findings
- Tricuspid regurgitation and/or obstruction
- Arrhythmias (RBBB, WPW)
- 50% mortality in first year

Hemodynamics

HEMODYNAMICS OF EBSTEIN ANOMALY

	Right Side	Left Side
Atrium	Enlarged	No change
Ventricle	Enlarged	No change
Vasculature	No change	Aorta no change

Radiographic Features (Fig. 2-41)

Plain film
- Large squared heart (box-shaped heart) due to:
  Left side: horizontal position of RV outflow tract
  Right side: RA enlargement
- Decreased pulmonary vascularity

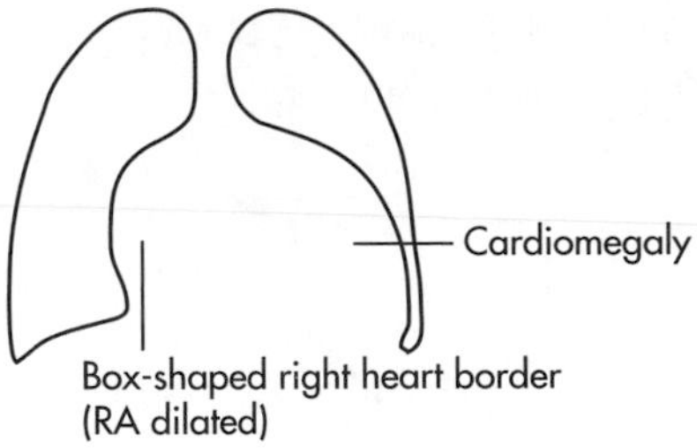

FIGURE 2-41

Ultrasound
- Displacement of tricuspid leaflets

Treatment
- Extracorporeal membrane oxygenation (ECMO) for temporization
- Tricuspid valve reconstruction
- Cardiac pacemaker for arrhythmias
- Bidirectional Glenn shunt (SVC-PA to increase pulmonary blood flow)

TRICUSPID ATRESIA (FIG. 2-42)

Complete agenesis of the tricuspid valve with no direct communication of the RA and RV

Associations
- Patent foramen ovale or ASD is always present.
- Complete transposition of great arteries (D-TGA), 35%
- VSD common
- Pulmonary atresia
- Hypoplastic right heart
- Extracardiac anomalies (GI, bone)

Hemodynamics

All blood crosses through a large ASD into the LA.

HEMODYNAMICS OF TRICUSPID ATRESIA

	Right Side	Left Side
Atrium	Enlarged	Enlarged
Ventricle	Decreased	Enlarged
Vasculature	Decreased	Aorta no change

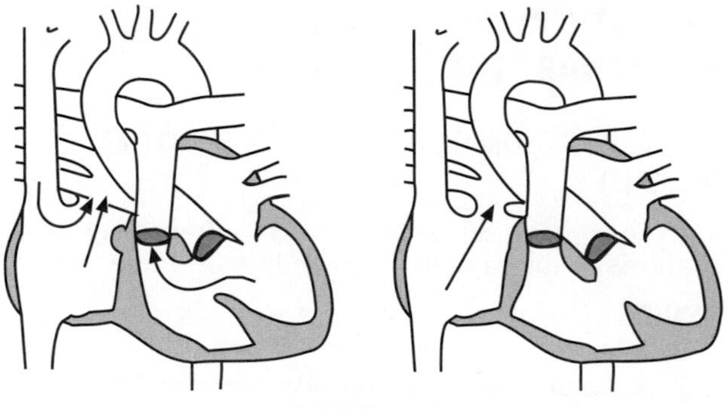
FIGURE 2-42

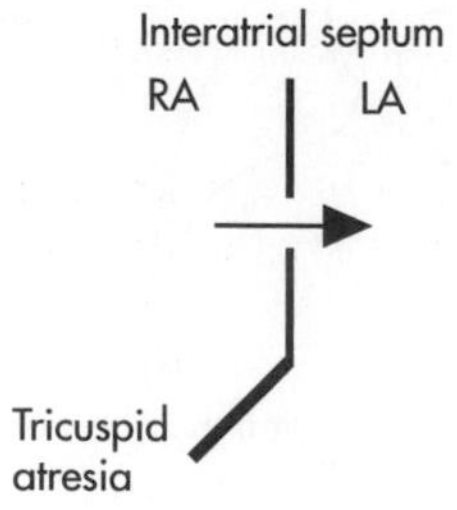

FIGURE 2-43

Radiographic Features (Fig.2-43)

Plain film
- May be normal
- No TGA: similar appearance as Fallot
- If TGA is present there is:
  - Increased pulmonary flow
  - Cardiomegaly
  - Narrow vascular pedicle

Treatment

Palliative
- Maintain patent PDA with prostaglandins.
- Blalock-Taussig
- Glenn anastomosis (SVC → PA)

Definitive (older patients)
- Fontan procedure: RA is connected to main PA. (Fig. 2-44)

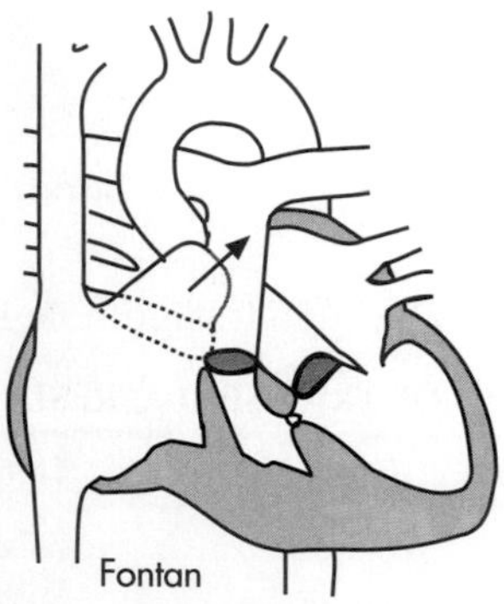

FIGURE 2-44

CYANOTIC CHD WITH INCREASED PULMONARY VASCULARITY

TRANSPOSITION OF GREAT ARTERIES (TGA) (Fig. 2-45)

TGA is the most common CHD presenting with cyanosis in the first 24 hours of life.

Types

D-TGA
- Aorta originates from RV.
- PA originates from LV.

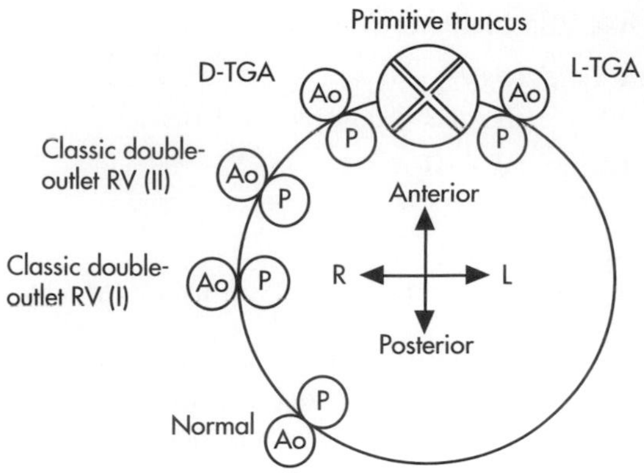

FIGURE 2-45

- Normal position of atria and ventricles: AV concordance

L-TGA
- Transposition of great arteries
- Inversion of ventricles: AV discordance

Relative position of aorta and PA can be derived from the diagram at the right.

COMPLETE TRANSPOSITION OF GREAT ARTERIES (D-TGA) (Fig. 2-46)

Two independent circulations exist:
- Blood returning from body → RV → blood delivered to body
- Blood returning from lung → LV → blood delivered to lung

This circulatory pattern is incompatible with life unless there are associated anomalies that permit mixing of the two circulations (e.g., ASD, VSD, or PDA).

Hemodynamics

Depend on the type of mixing of the two circulations

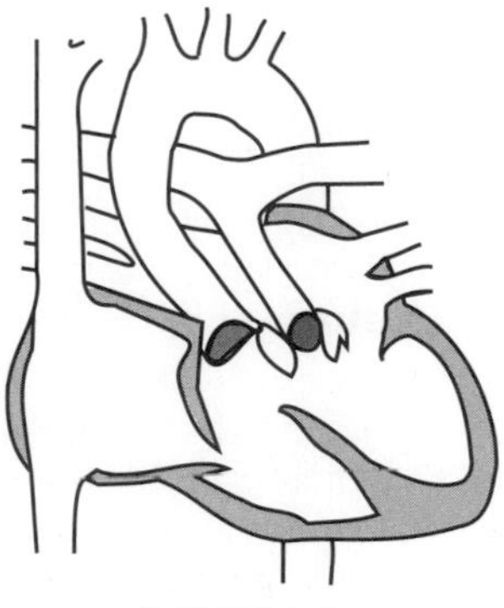
FIGURE 2-46

HEMODYNAMICS OF D-TGA

	Right Side	Left Side
Atrium	Normal, enlarged	No change
Ventricle	Normal, enlarged	No change
Vasculature	No change, enlarged	Aorta no change

Radiographic Features (Fig. 2-47)

Plain film
- "Egg-on-side" cardiac contour: narrow superior mediastinum secondary to hypoplastic thymus (unknown cause) and abnormal relationship of great vessels
- As pulmonary resistance decreases, pulmonary vascularity increases
- Right heart enlargement
- Pulmonary trunk not visible because of its posterior position

Ultrasound
- Aorta lies anterior, PA posterior.
- Transposition of arteries is obvious.

Treatment

PGE_1 is administered to prevent closure of PDA. Palliative measures include temporization methods before definitive repair. Corrective operation done during first year of life:
- Correct reattachment of large vessels (Jatene arterial switch procedure)
- Creation of an atrial baffle (Mustard, Senning, or Schumaker procedure)
- Rashkind procedure: atrial septostomy with balloon catheter
- Blalock-Hanlon: surgical creation of atrial defect

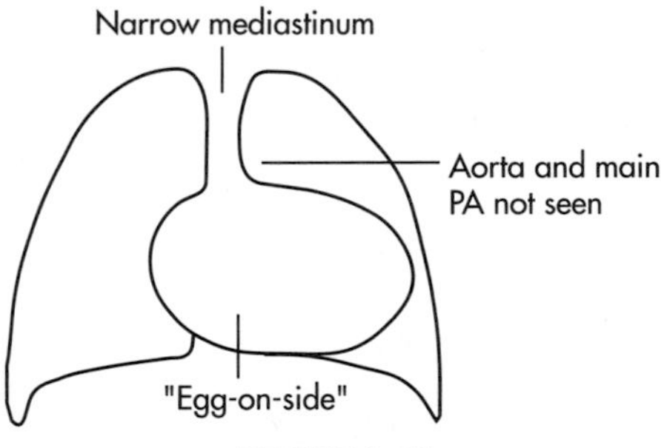

FIGURE 2-47

TAUSSIG-BING COMPLEX (DORV II)

Represents a partial transposition. Aorta connected to RV, PA arises from both LV and RV, and supracristal VSD. Radiographic appearance similar to that of D-TGA.

CORRECTED TRANSPOSITION OF GREAT ARTERIES (L-TGA)

Large vessels and ventricles are transposed (AV discordance and ventriculoarterial discordance). Poor prognosis because of associated cardiac anomalies. If isolated, this is an acyanotic lesion.

Associations
- Perimembranous VSD, >50%
- Pulmonic stenosis, 50%
- Anomaly of tricuspid valve
- Dextrocardia

Radiographic Features (Fig. 2-48)

Plain film
- Pulmonary trunk and aorta are not apparent because of their posterior position.
- LA enlargement
- Abnormal AA contour because of the leftward position of the arch
- Right pulmonary hilus elevated over left pulmonary hilus

Ultrasound
- Anatomic LV on right side
- Anatomic RV on left side

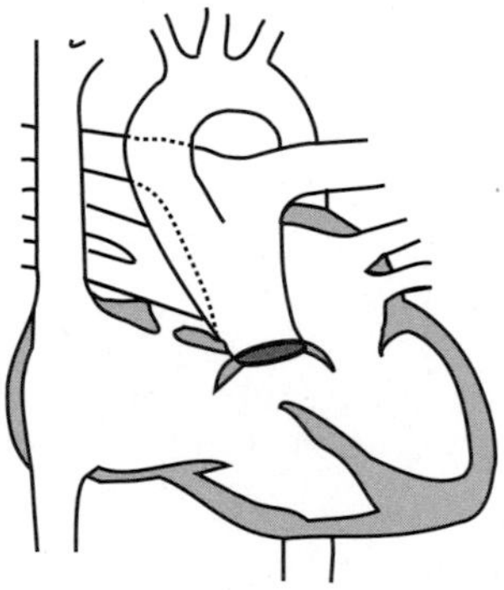

FIGURE 2-48

TRUNCUS ARTERIOSUS

Results from failure of formation of the spiral septum within the truncus arteriosus. As a result, a single vessel (truncus) leaves the heart and gives rise to systemic, pulmonary, and coronary circulation. The truncus has 2 to 6 cusps and sits over a high VSD.

Associations
- All patients have an associated high VSD.
- Right AA, 35%

Types (Figs. 2-49 and 2-50)
- Type 1: (most common): short main PA from truncus
- Type 2: two separate PAs from truncus (posterior origin)

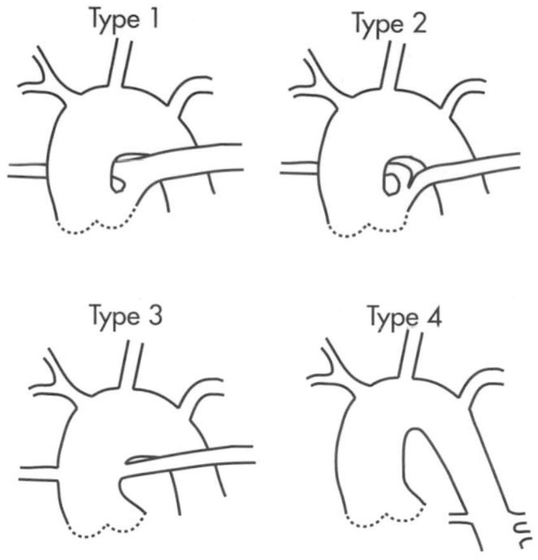

FIGURE 2-49

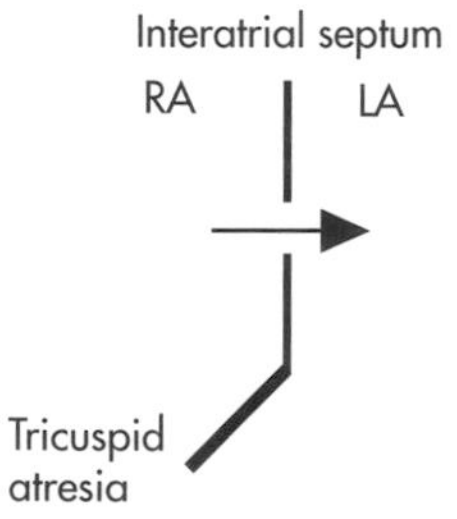

FIGURE 2-50

- Type 3: (least common): two separate PAs from truncus (lateral origin)
- Type 4: (pseudotruncus) PA from descending aorta = pulmonary atresia with VSD; findings of a tetralogy of Fallot combined with pulmonary atresia

Hemodynamics

Admixture lesion with both L-R (truncus → PA) shunt and R-L (RV → VSD → overriding aorta) shunt.

HEMODYNAMICS OF TRUNCUS ARTERIOSUS

	Right Side	Left Side
Atrium	No change	No change
Ventricle	Enlarged	Enlarged
Vasculature	Enlarged	Aorta enlarged

Radiographic Features

Plain film
- Enlargement of aortic shadow (which actually represents the truncus)
- Cardiomegaly due to increased LV volume
- Increased pulmonary vascularity
- Pulmonary edema, occasionally present
- Right AA, 35%

Ultrasound, MRI, angiography to determine type

Treatment

Three-step surgical procedure:
1. Closure of VSD so that LV alone empties into truncus
2. Pulmonary arteries removed from truncus and RV-PA conduit placed
3. Insertion of a valve between the RV and PA

TOTAL ANOMALOUS PULMONARY VENOUS CONNECTION (TAPVC) (Fig. 2-51)

Pulmonary veins connect to systemic veins or the RA rather than to the LA. TAPVC exists when all pulmonary veins connect anomalously. The anomalous venous return may be obstructed or nonobstructed.

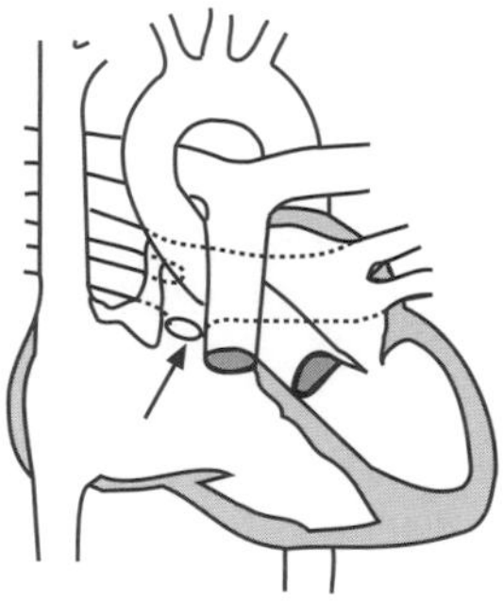
FIGURE 2-51

Types

Supracardiac connection (50%)

Supracardiac TAPVC is the most common type; infrequently associated with obstruction.
- Left vertical vein
- SVC
- Azygos vein

Cardiac connection (30%) (Fig. 2-52)
- RA
- Coronary sinus
- Persistent sinus venosus

Infracardiac connection (15%); majority are obstructed.

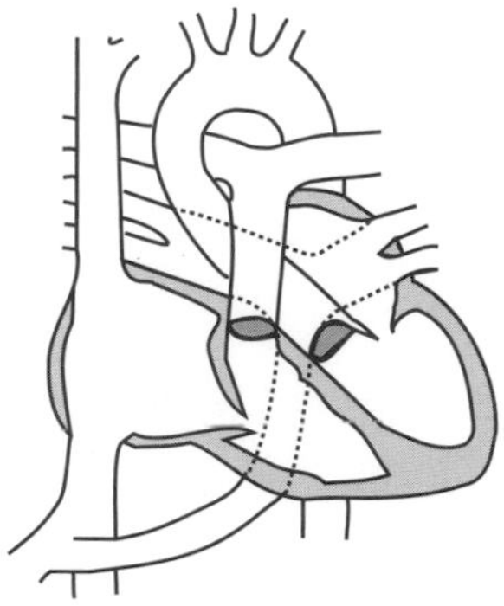
FIGURE 2-52

- Portal vein
- Persistent ductus venosus
- IVC (caudal to hepatic veins)
  - Gastric veins
  - Hepatic veins

Mixed types (5%)

Associations

- Patent foramen ovale, ASD (necessary to sustain life)
- Heterotaxy syndrome (asplenia more common)
- Cat's eye syndrome

Clinical Findings (Fig. 2-53)

- Symptomatology depends on presence or absence of obstruction.
- Obstructed: pulmonary edema within several days after birth
- Nonobstructed: asymptomatic at birth. CHF develops during first month.
- 80% mortality by first year

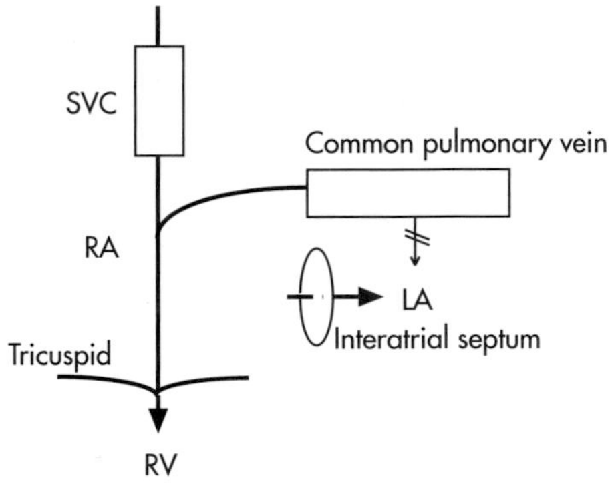

FIGURE 2-53

Hemodynamics

Unobstructed Pulmonary Vein

TAPVC causes a complete L-R shunt at the atrial level; therefore to sustain life, an obligatory R-L shunt must be present. Pulmonary flow is greatly increased, leading to dilatation of RA, RV, and PA.

HEMODYNAMICS OF UNOBSTRUCTED TAPVC

	Right Side	Left Side
Atrium	Enlarged	No change, decreased
Ventricle	Enlarged	No change, decreased
Vasculature	Enlarged	Aorta no change

OBSTRUCTED PULMONARY VEIN

Obstruction Has Three Consequences:

1. Pulmonary venous hypertension (PVH) and pulmonary arterial hypertension (PAH)
2. Pulmonary edema
3. Diminished pulmonary return to the heart, which results in low cardiac output

HEMODYNAMICS OF OBSTRUCTED TAPVC

	Right Side	Left Side
Atrium	No change	Decreased
Ventricle	No change, increased	Decreased
Vasculature	No change	Aorta decrease

Radiographic Features (Fig. 2-54)

Plain film of nonobstructed TAPVC

- Snowman heart (figure-of-eight heart) in supracardiac type; the supracardiac shadow results from dilated right SVC, vertical vein, and innominate vein.
- Snowman configuration (Fig. 2-55) not seen with other types
- Increased pulmonary vascularity

Plain film of obstructed TAPVC

- Pulmonary edema
- Small heart

RADIOGRAPHIC FEATURES OF TAPVC

Feature	Obstructed TAPVC	Nonobstructed TAPVC
Heart size	Normal	Enlarged
Pulmonary artery size	Normal	Enlarged
Pulmonary edema	Present early	Absent
Prominent venous density (snowman)	Rare (only in obstructed supracardiac TAPVC)	Frequent (especially in supracardiac forms of TAPVC)

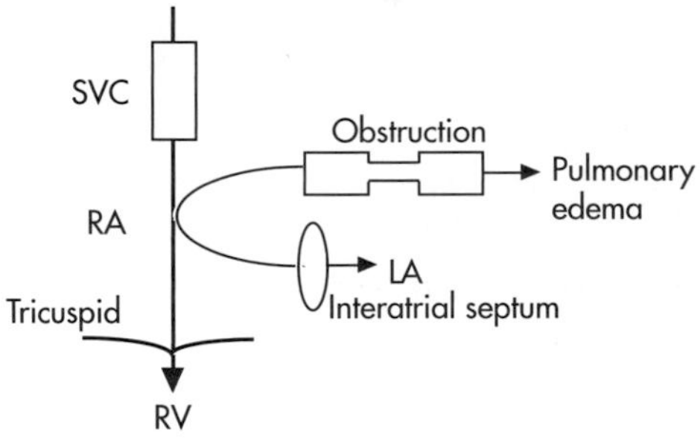

FIGURE 2-54

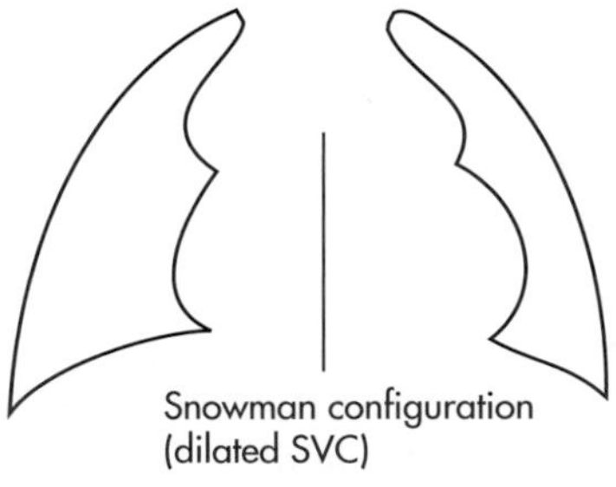

FIGURE 2-55

Treatment

Consists of a three-step procedure:

- Creation of an opening between the confluence of pulmonary veins and the LA
- Closure of the ASD
- Ligation of veins connecting to the systemic venous system

SINGLE VENTRICLE

Most commonly, the single ventricle has LV morphology and there is a rudimentary RV. The great arteries may originate both from the dominant ventricle or one may originate from the small ventricle. Rare anomaly with high morbidity. Common ventricle: absence of the interventricular septum.

Association

- Malposition of the great vessels is usually present.

Radiographic Features

- Variable appearance: depends on associated lesions
- Pulmonary circulation may be normal depending on the degree of associated pulmonic stenosis.

DOUBLE-OUTLET RIGHT VENTRICLE (DORV)

The great vessels originate from the RV. A VSD is always present; other malformations are common. Rare anomaly. Radiographic features are similar to those of other admixture lesions and depend on concomitant anomalies.

AORTA

PSEUDOCOARCTATION

Asymptomatic variant of coarctation: no pressure gradient across lesion (aortic kinking)

Associations

- Bicuspid aortic valve (common)
- Many other CHDs

Radiographic Features

- Figure-3 sign
- No rib notching
- Usually worked up because of superior mediastinal widening (especially on left) on CXR

INTERRUPTION OF AORTIC ARCH

Types

- Type A: occluded after LSA similar to coarctation
- Type B: occluded between LCA and LSA
- Type C: occluded between brachiocephalic artery and LCA

Associations

- Usually associated with VSD and PDA
- DORV and subpulmonic VSD (Taussig-Bing malformation)
- Subaortic stenosis

Radiographic Features

- Neonatal pulmonary edema
- No aortic knob; large PA

AORTIC ARCH ANOMALIES (Figs. 2-56 and 2-57)

Normal Development (Fig. 2-58, A-C)

- Right subclavian: arch IV (proximal) and 7th intersegmental artery
- Left subclavian: 7th intersegmental artery
- AA: arch IV (in part)
- Pulmonary arteries: arch VI
- Distal internal carotid artery ICA: primitive dorsal aorta
- Proximal ICA: arch III
- Common carotid: arch III

Pearls

- A large number of AA anomalies exist; however, only three are common:
  - L arch with an aberrant right subclavian artery (RSA) (asymptomatic)
  - R arch with an aberrant retroesophageal LSA (asymptomatic)
  - Double arch (symptomatic)
- Most significant abnormalities occur in tetralogy of Fallot.
- Normal lateral esophagram excludes significant arch anomalies and sling.

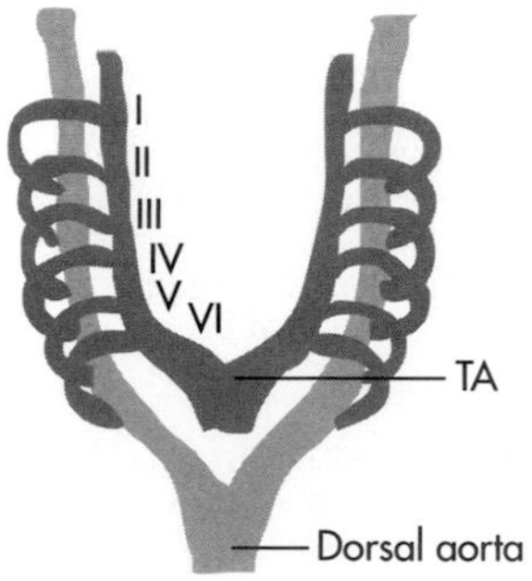

FIGURE 2-56

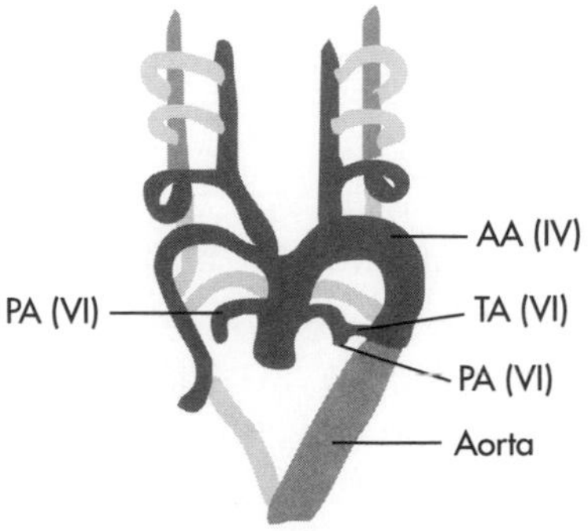

FIGURE 2-57

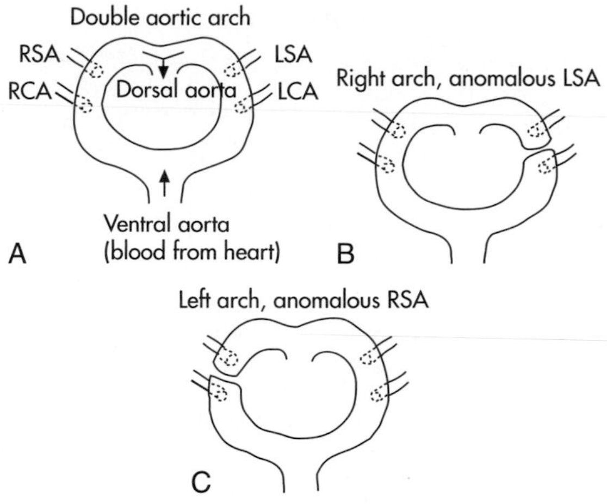

FIGURE 2-58

- Fluoroscopy of trachea may be helpful for classification.
- AP esophagram distinguishes double arch (bilateral esophageal indentations) from right arch.
- MRI is helpful to delineate vascular anatomy.

LEFT AORTIC ARCH WITH ABERRANT RIGHT SUBCLAVIAN ARTERY (Fig. 2-59)

Most common congenital AA anomaly (interruption #4 on diagram).

Asymptomatic, not a vascular ring.

Radiographic Features

- Left arch
- Abnormal course of RSA
  - Behind esophagus, 80% = retroesophageal indentation
  - Between esophagus and trachea, 15%
  - Anterior to trachea, 5%

Associations

- Absent recurrent right laryngeal nerve

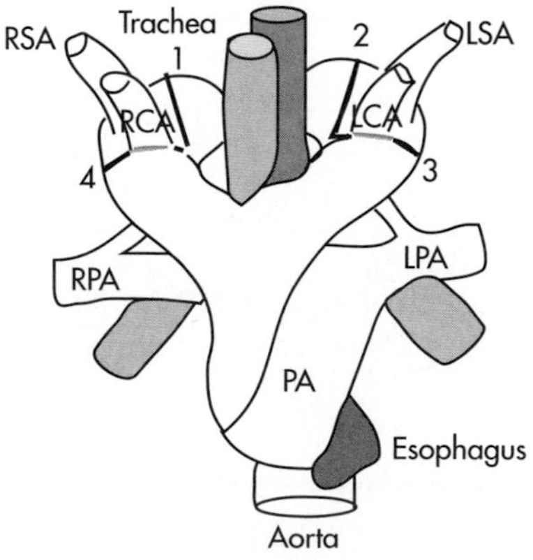

FIGURE 2-59

RIGHT AORTIC ARCH WITH ABERRANT LEFT SUBCLAVIAN ARTERY

Interruption #3 on above diagram. Only 5% have symptoms secondary to airway or esophageal compression.

Radiographic Features

- Right arch
- Retroesophageal indentation
- Diverticulum of Kommerell: aortic diverticulum at origin of aberrant subclavian artery

Associations

- CHD in 10%
- Tetralogy of Fallot, 70%
- ASD, VSD
- Coarctation

RIGHT AORTIC ARCH WITH MIRROR IMAGE BRANCHING (Fig. 2-60)

Interruption #2 on previous diagram. No vascular ring symptoms.

Radiographic Features

- Right AA
- No posterior indentation of esophagus

Associations

- Cyanotic heart disease in 98%
- Tetralogy of Fallot, 90%
- TA, 30%
- Multiple defects

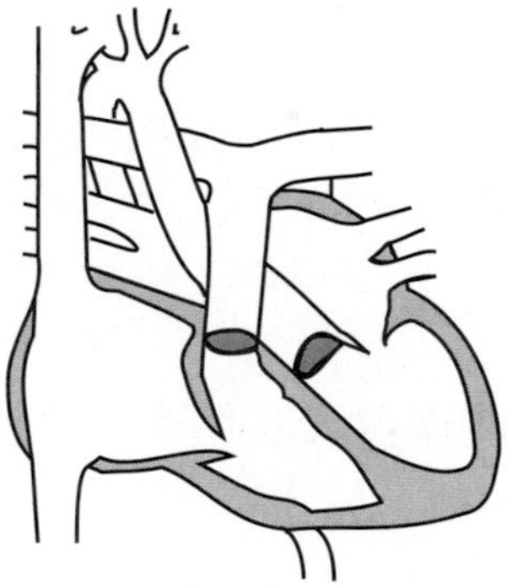

FIGURE 2-60

RIGHT ARCH WITH ISOLATED LEFT SUBCLAVIAN ARTERY

LSA attached to left PA via ductus arteriosus. The LSA is isolated from aorta and obtains blood supply from left vertebral artery; produces congenital subclavian steal. Interruptions near #2 and at #3.

Radiographic Features

- Right arch
- No posterior esophageal indentation

Associations

- Almost all are associated with tetralogy of Fallot.

DOUBLE AORTIC ARCH

Persistence of both fetal arches; concomitant CHD is rare. Most common type of vascular ring. Most symptomatic of vascular rings.

Radiographic Features

- Right arch is higher and larger than the left arch.
- Widening of the superior mediastinum
- Posterior indentation of the esophagus on lateral view
- Bilateral indentations of the esophagus on AP view

PULMONARY ARTERY

PULMONARY SLING (Fig. 2-61)

Aberrant left PA arises from the right PA and passes between the trachea (T) and esophagus (E). Compresses both trachea and esophagus. Tracheobronchiomalacia and/or stenosis occurs in 50%.

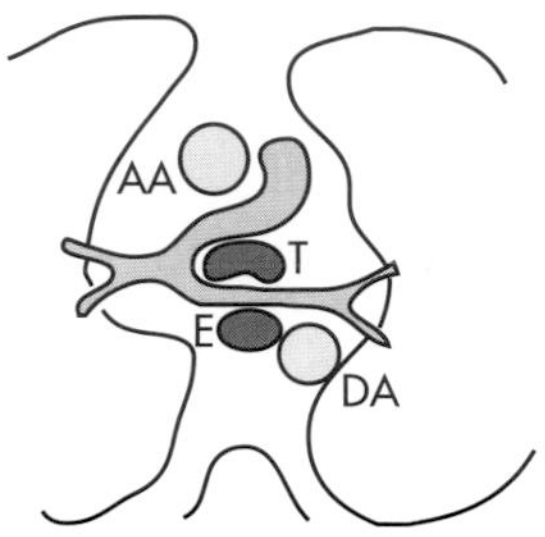

FIGURE 2-61

VASCULAR RINGS AND SLINGS (Fig. 2-62, A and B)

Vascular rings and slings are anomalies in which there is complete encirclement of the trachea and esophagus by the AA and its branches or PA. Symptoms are usually due to tracheal compression (stridor, respiratory distress, tachypnea); esophageal symptomatology is less common.

Types

Symptomatic (require surgery)
- Double AA
- Right arch + aberrant LSA + PDA (common)
- Pulmonary sling

Asymptomatic
- Anomalous innominate artery
- Anomalous left common carotid

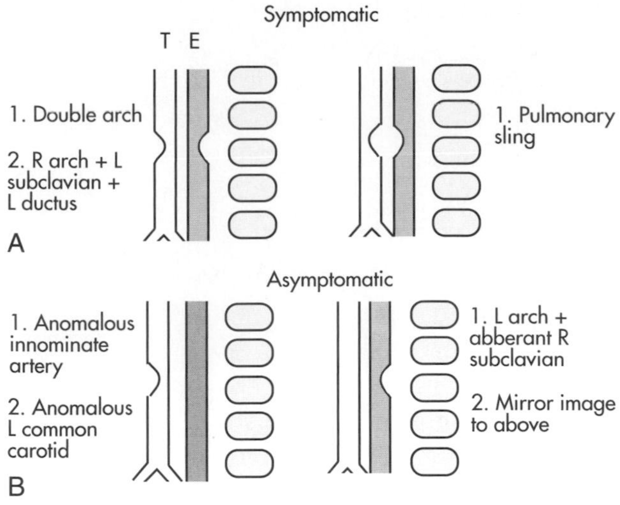

FIGURE 2-62

- Left arch + aberrant RSA
- Right arch + aberrant LSA (mirror image to above)

SITUS ANOMALIES

GENERAL

Abdominal Situs (Fig. 2-63)

Refers to position of liver and stomach:
- Abdominal situs solitus: liver on right, stomach on left (normal)
- Abdominal situs inversus: liver on left, stomach on right
- Abdominal situs ambiguous: symmetrical liver, midline stomach

Thoracic Situs (Fig. 2-64)

Refers to position of the tracheobronchial tree:
- Thoracic situs solitus (normal):
  LMB longer than

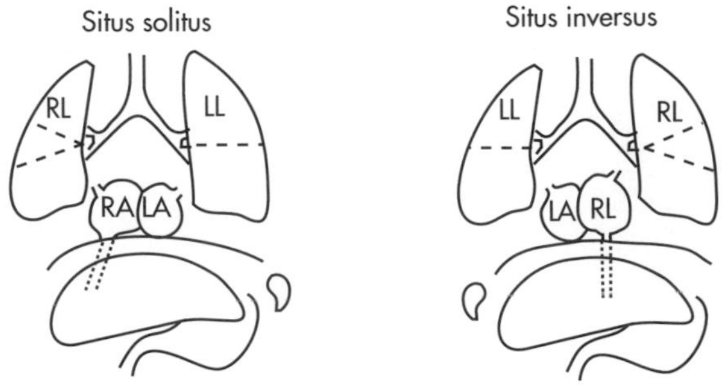

FIGURE 2-63

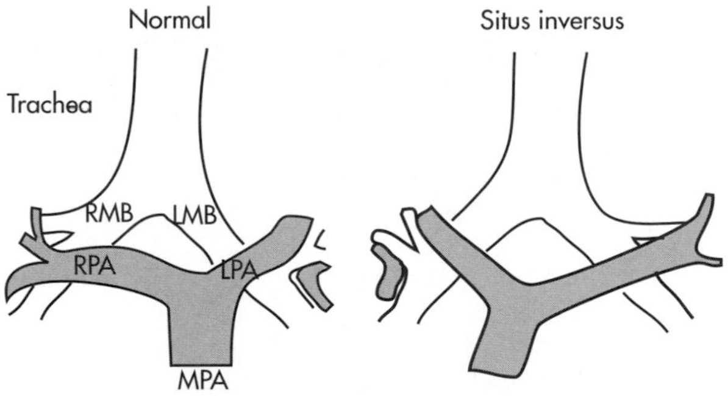

FIGURE 2-64

RMB Left upper lobe bronchus inferior to left PA (hyparterial bronchus)
Right upper lobe bronchus superior to right PA (eparterial bronchus)

- Thoracic situs inversus:
  Opposite of above
- Isomerism: refers to symmetrical development of heart or lungs:
  Left isomerism: 2 left lungs or 2 LA
  Right isomerism: 2 right lungs or 2 RA
- AV connections: refers to relation of atria to ventricles:
  Concordant: correct atrium with its ventricle (e.g., RA → RV)
  Discordant: mismatch of atrium and ventricle (e.g., RA → LV)
- Version: refers to position of an asymmetrical anatomic structure:
  Dextroversion: dextrocardia and situs solitus
  Levoversion: levocardia and situs inversus
- Position of bronchi:
  Eparterial: bronchus above PA (normally on right)
  Hyparterial: bronchus below PA (normally on left)
- Cardia: refers to position of heart on chest film. May have nothing to do with situs or cardiac structure:
  Levocardia (normal): heart on left side of chest
  Dextrocardia: heart on right side of chest (e.g., shift of mediastinum)

FREQUENCY OF CHD IN SITUS ANOMALIES

Situs	Frequency
Situs solitus/levocardia (normal)	1%
Situs solitus/dextrocardia	98% (corrected TGA with L-TGA)
Situs inversus/dextrocardia	4% (L-TGA)
Situs inversus/levocardia	100%

CARDIOSPLENIC SYNDROMES

Abnormal relationship between heart and abdominal organs and isomerism. Always consider polysplenia/asplenia when the cardiac apex and situs are discordant. The tracheobronchial anatomy is the best indicator of situs.

CARDIOSPLENIC SYNDROMES

	Asplenia (Right Isomerism)	Polysplenia (Left Isomerism)
Radiographic Findings		
Pulmonary vascularity	Decreased (obstructed flow)	Increased (overcirculation)
Bronchi	Eparterial	Hyparterial
Minor fissure	Bilateral	None, normal
Heart	Cardiomegaly/complex CHD	Cardiomegaly/moderate CHD
Atrium	Common atrium	ASD
Single ventricle	50%	DORV
Pulmonary veins	TAPVC	PAPVC
Great vessels	TGA 70%	Normal
SVC	Bilateral 50%	Bilateral 30%
Bowel	Malrotation	Malrotation
Spleen	Absent	Multiple
Abdominal situs	Ambiguous/inversus	Ambiguous/inversus
IVC/azygos	Normal	Azygous continuation

CARDIOSPLENIC SYNDROMES—cont'd

	Asplenia (Right Isomerism)	Polysplenia (Left Isomerism)
	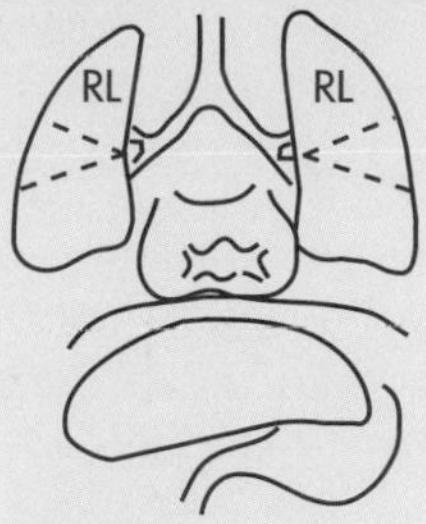	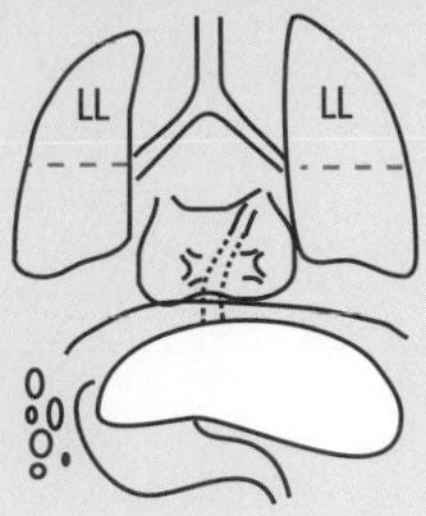
	Severe Disease	**Milder Disease**
Clinical Findings		
Age	Neonates	Infant
Cyanosis	Yes	No
Common problem	Infections (asplenia)	No infections
Prognosis	Poor	Good
CHD	L-TGA, pulmonary stenosis, single ventricle	PAPVC, ASD,VSD
Blood smear	Heinz and Howell-Jolly bodies	

OTHER

HYPOPLASTIC LEFT HEART (SHONE SYNDROME)

Spectrum of cardiac anomalies characterized by underdevelopment of LA, LV, MV, aortic valve, and aorta. Survival requires a large ASD and PDA with R-L and L-R shunting.

Clinical Findings

- Neonatal CHF within several days after birth
- Most infants die within first week as PDA closes.
- Cardiogenic shock; metabolic acidosis

Radiographic Features

- Increased pulmonary vascularity
- Severe pulmonary edema
- Prominent right heart, especially RA

Treatment

- Norwood procedure: PA-descending aorta conduit, followed by PA banding; palliative
- Heart transplant: curative attempt

COR TRIATRIATUM (Fig. 2-65)

Incomplete incorporation of pulmonary veins into LA, causing obstruction to pulmonary venous return; very rare.

Radiographic Features

- Mimics congenital mitral stenosis
- LA size usually normal

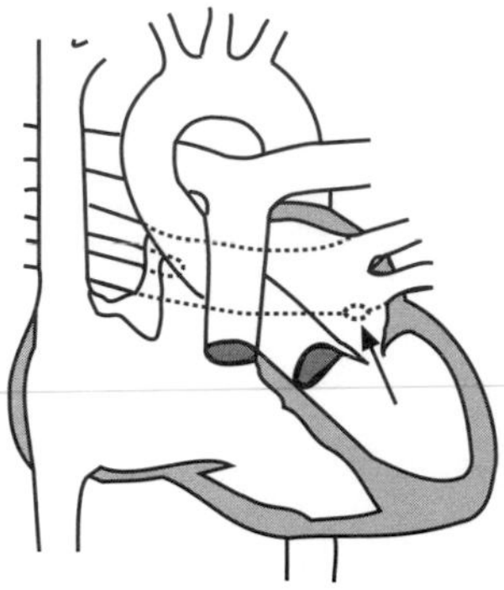

FIGURE 2-65

- Associated lesions:
  - Parachute mitral valve
  - Mitral web
- PVH and CHF

PERSISTENT FETAL CIRCULATION

Refers to persistent severe pulmonary hypertension in the neonate and consequent R-L shunting via a patent PDA. Treatment is with ECMO.

Causes of Neonatal Pulmonary Hypertension

- Idiopathic
- Meconium aspiration
- Neonatal pneumonia
- Diaphragmatic hernia
- Hypoxemia

AZYGOS CONTINUATION OF THE IVC (Fig. 2-66)

Developmental failure of the hepatic and/or infrahepatic IVC. Associated with polysplenia.

Radiographic Features

- Enlarged azygos vein
- Enlarged hemiazygos vein
- Absent IVC

DOWN SYNDROME

- ECD, 25%
- ASD
- VSD
- PDA
- Cleft MV
- AV communis
- 11 rib pairs, 25%
- Hypersegmented manubrium, 90%

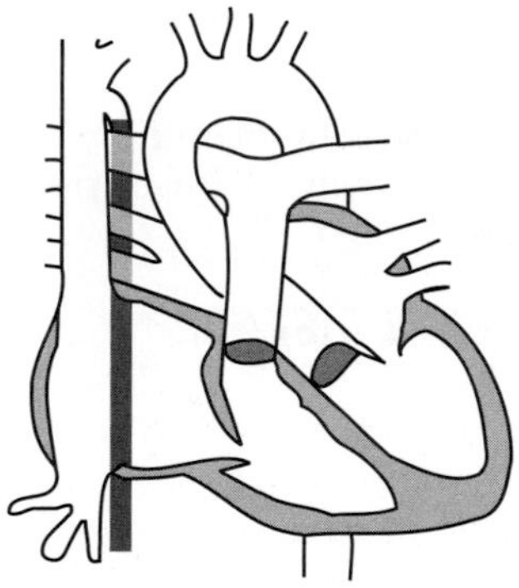

FIGURE 2-66

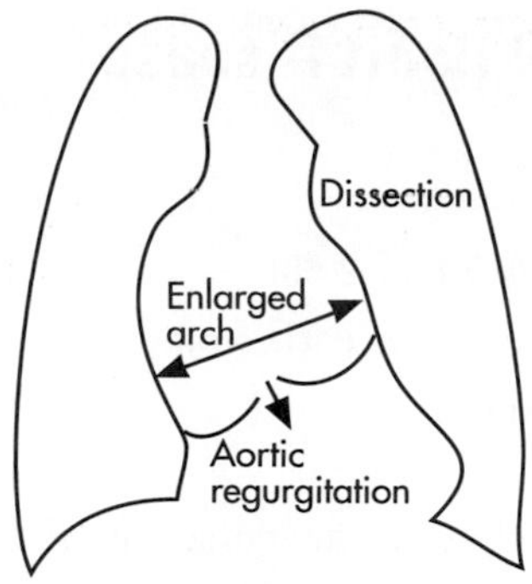

FIGURE 2-67

MARFAN SYNDROME (Fig. 2-67)

Autosomal dominant connective tissue disease (arachnodactyly) with cardiac abnormalities in 60%:

- Ascending aorta
  - Aneurysm
  - Aortic regurgitation (common)
  - Dissection
- Mitral valve
  - Prolapse (myxomatous degeneration)
  - Mitral regurgitation
- Coarctation
- Chest deformity, kyphosis
- Arachnodactyly
- Excessive limb length

TURNER SYNDROME

- Coarctation, 15%
- Bicuspid aortic valve

SURGICAL PROCEDURES FOR CONGENITAL HEART DISEASE

Procedure	Indication	Connection
Fontan	Tricuspid atresia Single ventricle Hypoplastic right ventricle Complex CHD	RA to PA conduit or anastomosis
Glenn	Tricuspid atresia Hypoplastic RV Pulmonary atresia	SVC to right PA anastomosis (bidirectional provides flow to both pulmonary arteries)
Rastelli	Pulmonary atresia	RV to PA conduit
Mustard-Senning	D-Transposition of the great arteries	Atrial rerouting of venous blood flow
Arterial switch procedure (Jatene)	D-Transposition of the great arteries	Switch of aorta and PA with reanastomosis of coronary arteries
Norwood	Hypoplastic right ventricle	First stage: use of main PA as ascending aorta, enlargement of aortic arch, systemic shunt to distal PA Second stage: modified Fontan
Blalock-Taussig shunt	Palliative shunt for obstruction of pulmonary blood flow (TOF, pulmonary atresia, tricuspid atresia)	Subclavian artery to PA graft
Waterston-Cooley	Palliative shunt for obstruction of pulmonary blood flow	Ascending aorta to right PA anastomosis
Potts	Palliative shunt for obstruction of pulmonary blood flow	Descending aorta to right PA anastomosis
PA banding	Left to right shunting	Band around PA

Acquired Heart Disease

GENERAL

CARDIOMEGALY (Fig. 2-68)

Global cardiomegaly leads to increased CI.

$$CI = \frac{MRD + MLD}{ID} \quad \text{(Eq 2-2)}$$

MRD = maximum transverse diameter to the right from midline

MLD = maximum transverse diameter to the left from midline

ID = internal diameter of the thorax drawn through the tip of the dome of the right diaphragm

Causes

- Valvular disease
- Cardiomyopathy
- CHD
- Pericardial effusion
- Mass lesions

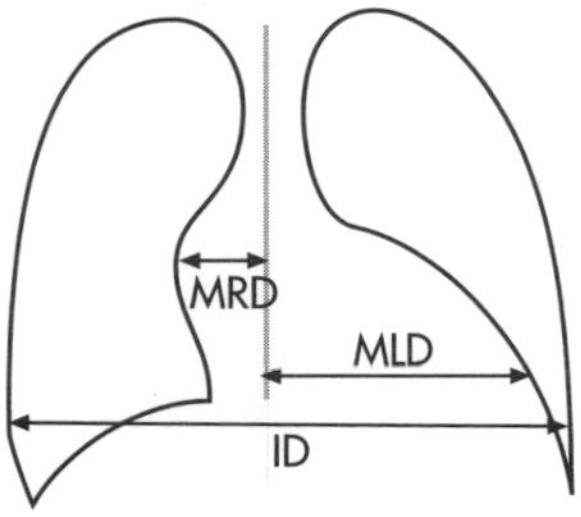

FIGURE 2-68

CHAMBER ENLARGEMENT

LA Enlargement (Fig. 2-69, A and B)

- LA measurement (right LA border to LMB >7 cm)
- Barium-filled esophagus is displaced posteriorly (lateral view).
- Double density along right cardiac border; a similar appearance may also be found in:
  - Patients with normal-sized LA
  - Confluence of pulmonary veins
- Bulging of LA appendage
- Widening of the angle of the carina (>60°)

LV Enlargement (Fig. 2-69, C and D)

- Left downward displacement of the apex (elongation of ventricular outflow tract)
- Round left cardiac border

RV Enlargement

- Rounding and elevation of cardiac apex

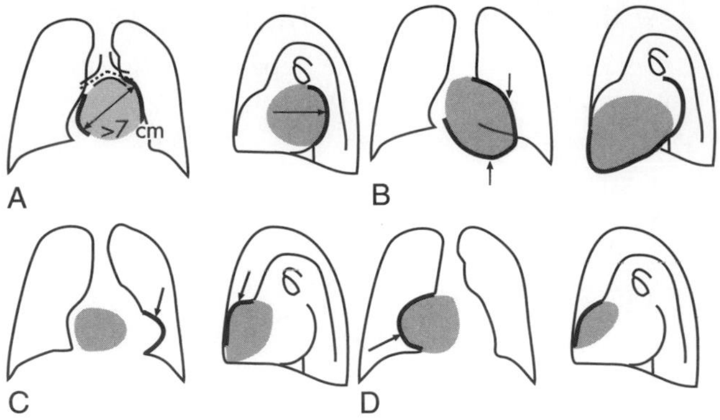

FIGURE 2-69

- Obliteration of retrosternal space on lateral view; normally, > one third of the distance from anterior costophrenic angle to the angle of Louis (manubriosternal junction)

RA Enlargement

- Difficult to assess by plain film
- Increased convexity of lower right heart border on PA view

VALVULAR HEART DISEASE

Mitral and aortic valves are the most commonly affected valves. Rheumatic fever is the leading cause of acquired valve disease.

MITRAL STENOSIS

Causes

- Rheumatic fever (most common)
- Bacterial endocarditis and thrombi
- Prolapse of LA myxoma

Clinical Findings

- Dyspnea on exertion and later at rest
- Atrial fibrillation and mural thrombus
- Episodes of recurrent arterial embolization
  - Neurologic deficit
  - Abdominal and flank pain (renal, splanchnic emboli)

Hemodynamics

MITRAL VALVE

Condition	Valve Area	LA Pressure
Normal	4 to 6 cm^2	<10 mm Hg
Symptomatic during exercise	1 to 4 cm^2	>20 mm Hg
Symptomatic at rest	<1 cm^2	>35 mm Hg

Radiographic Features (Fig. 2-70)

Plain film
- PVH in nearly all patients
- Normal overall heart size (pressure overload) but enlargement of LA
- Severe stenosis
  - Increase in pulmonary arterial pressure leads to RVH
  - Pulmonary hemosiderosis (ossified densities in lower lung fields)

Calcification of LA wall (laminated clot)

Ultrasound (Fig. 2-71)
- Increased LA dimensions (normal LV)
- RV enlargement if pulmonary hypertension is present
- Multiple echoes on MV leaflets (calcifications, vegetations)
- Doming of leaflets
- Doppler: velocity measurements

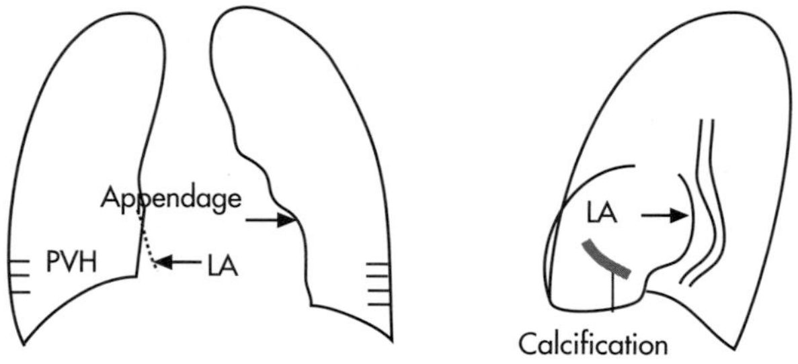

FIGURE 2-70

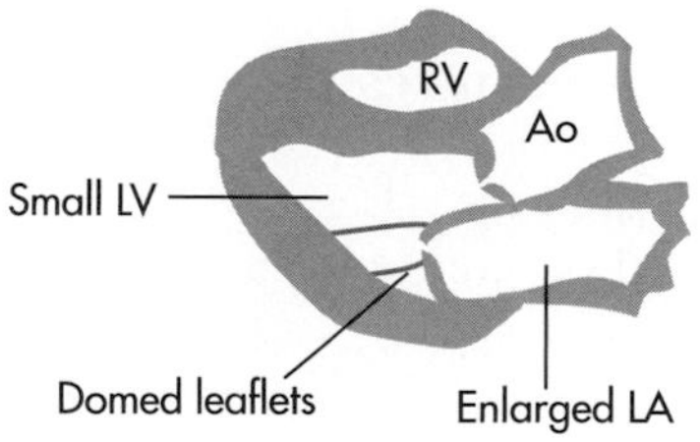

FIGURE 2-71

MITRAL REGURGITATION (Fig. 2-72)

Causes
- Rheumatic fever
- MVP (Barlow syndrome)
- Rupture of papillary muscle (secondary to MI, bacterial endocarditis)
- Marfan syndrome
- Bacterial endocarditis
- Rupture of chordae

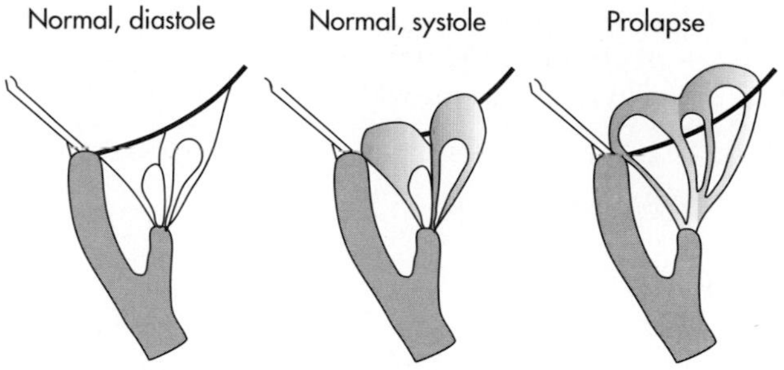

FIGURE 2-72

Clinical Findings
- Often well tolerated for many years
- Decompensation by sudden onset of pulmonary hypertension
- Acute presentation: MI, endocarditis

Hemodynamics
- MVP: movement of leaflet of MV into LA during systole

Radiographic Features (Figs. 2-73 and 2-74)

Plain film
- "Big heart disease" (volume overload, cardiomegaly)
- Enlarged chambers: LA + LV
- PVH (usually less severe than in mitral stenosis)

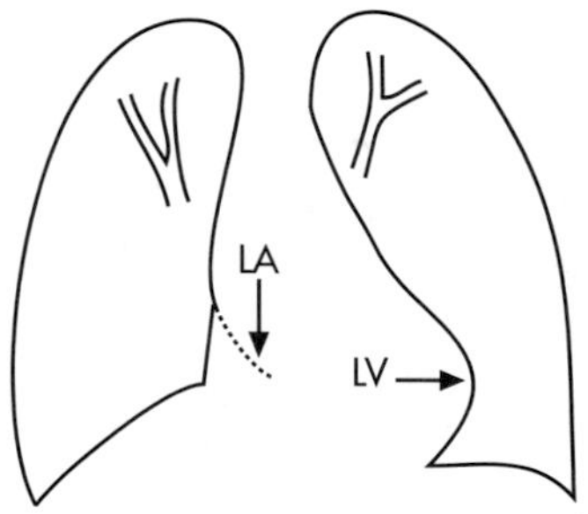

FIGURE 2-73

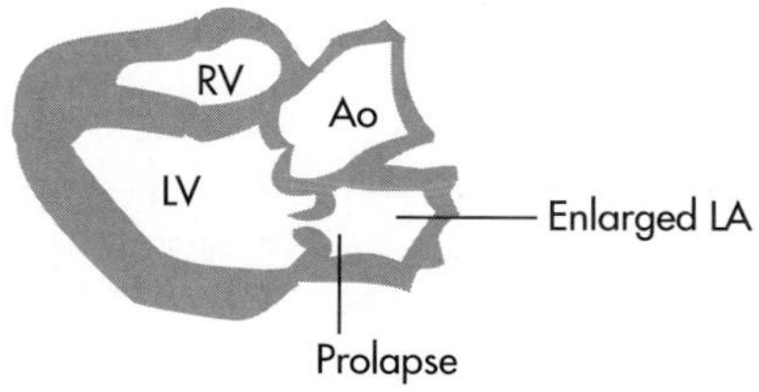

FIGURE 2-74

- Calcification of mitral annulus: may have J-, C-, or O-configuration
- Often coexistent with mitral stenosis

Ultrasound

- MVP
- Enlarged LA, LV

AORTIC STENOSIS

Types

Valvular: 60%-70%, most common form

- Degenerative leaflets in patients >70 years
- Bicuspid
- Rheumatic

Subvalvular, 15%-30%

- Idiopathic hypertrophic subaortic stenosis (IHSS); 50% are autosomal dominant
- Congenital (membranous, fibromuscular tunnel)

Supravalvular (rare)

- Williams syndrome
- Rubella

Clinical Findings

- Symptoms of LV failure (common)
- Angina, 50%; many patients also have underlying CAD.
- Syncope (in severe stenosis)
- Sudden death in children, 5%

AORTIC VALVE

Condition	Valve Area
Normal	2.0 to 4.0 cm^2
Symptomatic at exercise	<1.0 cm^2
Symptomatic at rest	<0.75 cm^2

Radiographic Features (Fig. 2-75)

Plain film

- Often difficult to detect abnormalities by plain film (usually no chamber enlargement)
- Enlargement of ascending aorta (does not occur with supravalvular AS)
- Calcification of aortic valve: rare before age 40

Ultrasound (Fig. 2-76)

- Multiple aortic valve echoes
- Poststenotic dilatation of aorta
- Doming of the aortic valve
- LVH
- Doppler: velocity measurements

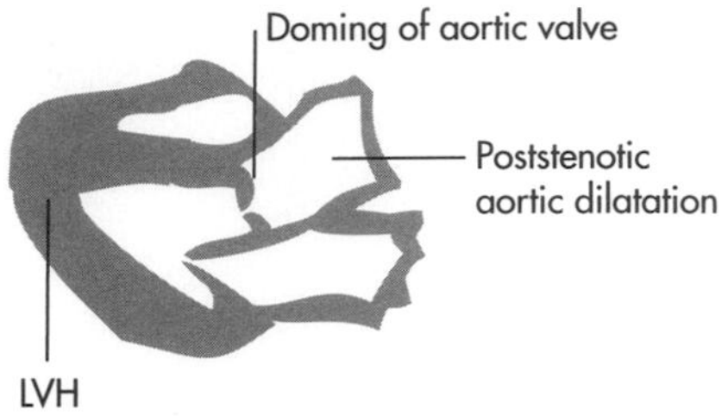

FIGURE 2-76

AORTIC REGURGITATION (Fig. 2-77)

Causes

- Rheumatic fever
- Systemic hypertension (may lead to dilatation of the aortic root)
- Aortic dissection
- Endocarditis
- Rare causes: Marfan syndrome, syphilitic aortitis, trauma, collagen vascular diseases (ankylosing spondylitis)

Radiographic Features

Plain film

- Cardiomegaly
- Dilated structures: LV, aorta

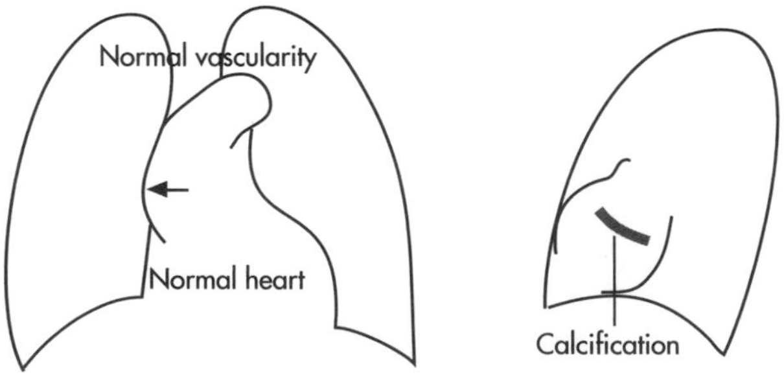

FIGURE 2-75

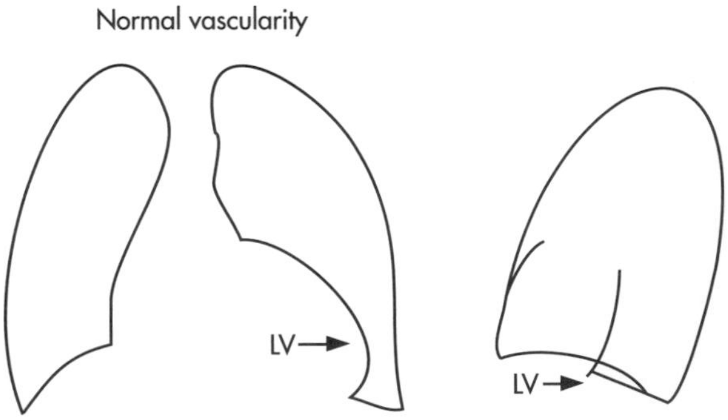

FIGURE 2-77

Ultrasound
- Dilation of LV and aorta
- Atypical valve leaflets
- High-frequency vibrations of the anterior mitral leaflet

MYOCARDIUM

DELAYED-ENHANCEMENT CARDIAC MRI (DE-CMRI)

Technique: DE-CMRI involves the administration of gadolinium (Gd) and subsequent T1-weighted gradient-recalled echo imaging 10 to 30 minutes later with an inversion recovery preparatory pulse that nulls normal myocardial signal; enhancement characteristics, wall motion, wall thickness, and chamber size.

Ischemia
- Delayed enhancement in acute and chronic ischemia involves the subendocardium, but may extend to involve a variable amount of thickness of the myocardium (transmural)
- Enhancement is seen within a typical territory of a coronary artery
- Enhancement affecting greater than 50% thickness of the myocardium associated with unlikely recovery after revascularization

Nonischemic cardiomyopathies
- Enhancement is not restricted to coronary artery distribution
- Myocarditis: predominantly subepicardial but may be transmural, may see increased T2-signal
- Diffuse subendocardial enhancement in LV may be seen with amyloidosis, systemic sclerosis, and postcardiac transplant
- Mesocardial (midinterventricular septum)
  - Hypertrophic cardiomyopathy: wall thickening, no chamber dilatation, enhancement may be diffuse or focal, systolic anterior motion of the mitral valve
  - Dilated cardiomyopathy: Reduced EF, chamber enlargement

ACUTE MYOCARDIAL INFARCTION (AMI)

Diagnosis of AMI is made by clinical history, ECG, and serum enzymes; role of imaging studies is ancillary:

Angiography
- Evaluate CAD
- Therapeutic angioplasty

Plain film
- Monitoring of pulmonary edema

Thallium
- Evaluate for segmental ischemia and scar tissue.

Gated blood pool study
- Wall motion kinetics
- Determination of ejection fraction

MRI
- Wall motion abnormalities, viability assessed with Gd
- Imaging of complications (false, true aneurysm, thrombus)

Complications of AMI

- Papillary muscle rupture: acute mitral regurgitation
- Septum perforation (VSD): volume overload
- Pericardial tamponade from free wall rupture (death)
- Aneurysm formation (true, false)
- LV thrombus
- Arrhythmia

Myocardial Disease	Pathology	First Pass MR findings	Delayed MR Findings	Significance
Acute infarct with reperfusion	Necrosis	Normal	High signal in affected artery (delayed washout)	Increased transmurality of delayed enhancement indicates poor prognosis
Acute infarct with no reperfusion	Necrosis, microvascular obstruction	Low signal in the infarct core	High signal in affected artery (delayed washout)	Increased complications such as heart failure, recurrent infarct
Stunned myocardium (acute infarction)	Normal perfusion but decreased function	Normal	Normal	Good prognosis
Chronic infarct	Fibrous tissue	Normal to slightly delayed perfusion	High signal in affected artery (delayed washout)	Poor prognosis in areas with enhancement in >50% of the wall thickness
Hibernating myocardium (high grade chronic CAD)	Noninfarcted myocardium with decreased function and blood flow	Normal	Normal	Good prognosis after revascularization

ANEURYSM

TYPES OF ANEURYSM

	True Aneurysm	False Aneurysm
Parameter		
Myocardial wall	Intact (fibrous)	Ruptured wall
Angiography	Dyskinetic/akinetic bulge in wall	Neck, delayed emptying
Location	Apical, anterolateral	Posterior, diaphragmatic
Aneurysm neck	Wide neck, >50%	Narrow neck, <50%
Cause	Transmural MI (most common) Congenital (Ravitch syndrome) Congenital (Chagas disease) Myocarditis	MI Trauma
Complications	Low risk of rupture Mural thrombus; embolization CHF Arrhythmias	High risk of rupture
	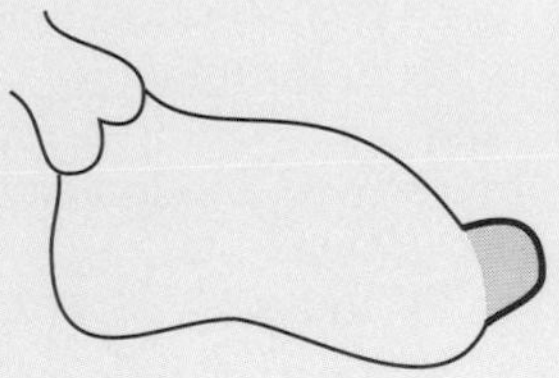	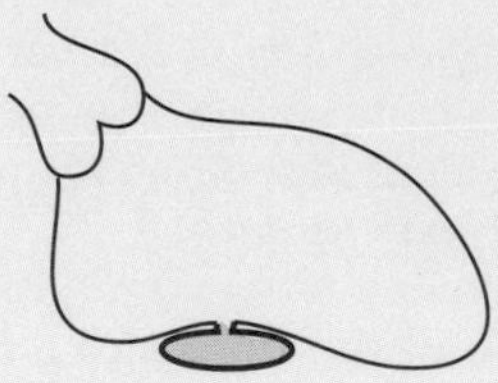

CARDIOMYOPATHIES

Causes

Hypertrophic cardiomyopathy (obstructed LV outflow segment)
- Familial: autosomal dominant, 50%
- Sporadic

Dilated cardiomyopathy (congested; unable to contract effectively during systole)
- Idiopathic (most frequent, unknown cause, familial association)
- Infectious (mostly virus)
- Metabolic (hyperthyroidism)
- Toxic: alcohol, doxorubicin (Adriamycin)
- Collagen vascular disease

Restrictive cardiomyopathy (unable to dilate effectively during diastole: impaired distensibility)
- Amyloid
- Sarcoidosis
- Löffler eosinophilic endocarditis
- Hemochromatosis

Pearls

- Restrictive cardiomyopathy and constrictive pericarditis have similar physiologic features.
- CT and MRI may be helpful.
  - 50% of patients with constrictive pericarditis have calcified pericardium easily detected by CT.
  - Thickened pericardium can be easily detected by MRI.

LIPOMATOUS HYPERTROPHY OF THE INTERATRIAL SEPTUM

Benign proliferation of fat in the interatrial septum sparing fossa ovalis (dumbbell shape) with thickness >2 cm. May be FDG-avid on PET. Typically in elderly obese patients. May cause arrhythmia.

ARRHYTHMOGENIC RIGHT VENTRICULAR DYSPLASIA (ARVD)

Inherited, progressive condition characterized by fatty infiltration of the right ventricle. Can cause life-threatening cardiac arrhythmias and sudden cardiac death in young people. Prevalence is 1 in 5000. Presents as symptomatic sustained ventricular tachycardia. ECG shows LBBB pattern. MRI: Fat signal in RV myocardium, RV hypokinesis, RV enlargement. Treatment is with a defibrillator and antiarrhythmic agents.

MYOCARDIAL NONCOMPACTION

Congenital cardiomyopathy leading to two-layered ventricular myocardium with prominent trabeculations. Ratio of noncompacted to compacted LV myocardium >2.3. May observe delayed enhancement by DE-CMRI. Associated with thromboembolism, CHF, and arrhythmia.

TAKOTSUBO CARDIOMYOPATHY

Transient left ventricular apical ballooning syndrome is a rare entity found more commonly in postmenopausal women after emotional stress. No coronary artery disease on cardiac catheterization. MRI may demonstrate apical ballooning with akinesis or hypokinesis and no delayed enhancement.

CORONARY ARTERIES

VARIANTS/ANOMALIES OF CORONARY ARTERIES

- Anomalous origin of LCA from PA
  - Venous blood flows through LCA, resulting in myocardial ischemia.
  - 15% of patients survive into adulthood because of collaterals.
- Anomalous origin of both coronary arteries from right sinus of Valsalva
  - Ectopic LCA takes an acute angle behind PA.
  - 30% sudden death (infarction)
- Anomalous origin of both coronary arteries from left sinus of Valsalva
  - RCA is ectopic.
- Congenital coronary AV fistula
  - Both arteries are orthotopic.
  - Venous side of fistula originates in RA, coronary sinus, or RV.
- RCA terminates at crux: 10%.
- SA nodal artery is a branch of the proximal RCA in >50%; less commonly, the SA nodal artery arises from the proximal left circumflex.
- Kugel's artery: collateral that connects the SA nodal artery and the AV nodal artery (anastomotic artery magnum)
- Vieussens' ring: collateral branches from right conus artery to LAD.

ATHEROSCLEROTIC CORONARY ARTERY DISEASE (CAD) (Fig. 2-78)

Now recognized as an inflammatory condition with established cascade of events. Three stages:

- Intimal fatty streaks (nonobstructive, clinically silent)
- Development of active inflammation with monocyte recruitment, macrophages (foam cells), fibrous plaques during adulthood (narrowing of lumen: angina)
- Late occlusive disease: calcifications, hemorrhage (angina, AMI)

Risk Factors

Strong correlation
- Elevated CRP, LDL
- Family members with atherosclerotic disease
- Smoking

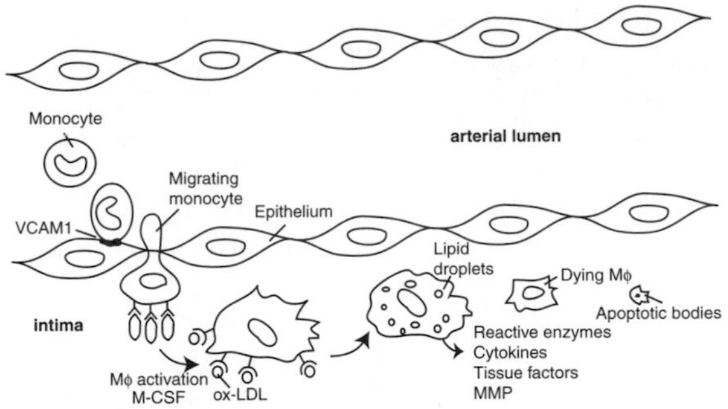

FIGURE 2-78

- Hypertension
- Hyperlipidemia
- Diabetes
- Male

Weaker correlation
- Obesity
- Stress
- Sedentary life

Treatment

- Reversal of risk factors (diet, smoking cessation)
- Medication (statins)
- Transluminal coronary angioplasty, coronary stents
- Surgery
  - Saphenous vein aortocoronary bypass
  - Left internal mammary coronary bypass

Annual Mortality

- 1 vessel disease: 2%-3%
- 2 vessel disease: 3%-7%
- 3 vessel disease: 6%-11%
- Low ejection fraction, doubles mortality
- Abnormal wall motion, doubles mortality

Radiographic Features

Plain film
- Calcification of coronary arteries are the most reliable plain film sign of CAD (90% specificity in symptomatic patients), but calcified coronary arteries are not necessarily stenotic.
- LV aneurysm is the second most reliable plain film sign of CAD. It develops in 20% MI.
- Location
  - Anteroapical wall: 70%
  - Inferior wall: 20%
  - Posterior wall: 10%
- CHF causing:
  - Pulmonary edema
  - Least reliable sign of CAD

Coronary CTA

Stenosis of >70% is considered significant in all coronary arteries except left main, in which threshold is 50%.

Coronary angiography
Stenosis occurs primarily in:
- Proximal portions of major arteries
- LAD>RCA>LCx

Collaterals develop if >90% of the coronary diameter is obstructed; two types of anastomosis:
- Connections between branches of the same coronary artery (homocoronary)
- Connections between the branches of the three major coronary arteries (intercoronary)

Common pathways of intercoronary anastomoses (Fig. 2-79) in descending order of frequency are:
1. Surface of apex
2. Surface of pulmonary conus
3. Between anterior and posterior septal branches
4. In the AV groove: LCx and distal RCA
5. On the surface of the RV wall
6. On the atrial wall around SA node

Left ventriculography
- RAO view most helpful
- Evaluate LV function, valvular insufficiency, shunts, mural thrombus.

Other techniques employed at cardiac catheterization:
- Transvalvular pressure measurements
- Cardiac output measurement
- O_2 saturation measurements: shunt detection
- Right-sided heart catheterization

GRADING OF STENOSIS

Type	Diameter
Not significant	<50% decrease
Significant	50%-75% decrease
Severe	>75% decrease

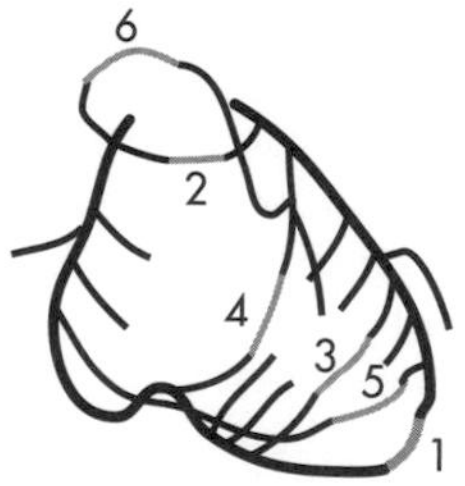

FIGURE 2-79

KAWASAKI DISEASE (MUCOCUTANEOUS LYMPH NODE SYNDROME)

Idiopathic acute febrile multisystem disease in children. Most cases are self-limited and without complications. Mortality from AMI: 3%. Treatment is with aspirin and gamma globulin.

Clinical Findings
- Fever and cervical lymphadenopathy
- Desquamating rash on palms/soles
- Vasculitis of coronary arteries

Radiographic Features
- Spectrum of coronary disease
  - Aneurysm: present in 25% (most are multiple when present)
  - Stenoses
  - Occlusion
  - Rupture
- Coronary artery aneurysms: usually in proximal segments and detectable by US
- Transient gallbladder hydrops

PERICARDIUM

NORMAL ANATOMY

Pericardium consists of two layers:
- External fibrous pericardium
- Internal serous epicardium

The normal pericardial cavity has 10 to 50 mL of clear serous fluid. Normal structures:
- Fat stripe: fat on surface of heart beneath pericardium seen on lateral chest film
- Superior pericardial recess (commonly seen by CT or MRI)

CONGENITAL ABSENCE OF THE PERICARDIUM

May be total or partial. Partial absence is more common, occurs mainly on the left, and is usually asymptomatic. Large defects may cause cardiac strangulation. Small defects are usually asymptomatic.

Radiographic Features

Total absence of the pericardium
- Mimics the appearance of the large silhouette seen in pericardial effusions

Partial absence of the pericardium
- Heart is shifted and rotated into left pleural cavity.
- PA view looks like an RAO view.
- Heart is separated from the sternum on cross-table lateral view.
- Left hilar mass: herniated left atrial appendage and pulmonary trunk

PERICARDIAL CYSTS

Pericardial cysts represent congenital malformations (persistent coelom).
- 90% unilocular, 10% multilocular
- 75% are asymptomatic; occur at all ages
- If there is communication with pericardial cavity, the entity is termed *pericardial diverticulum*.

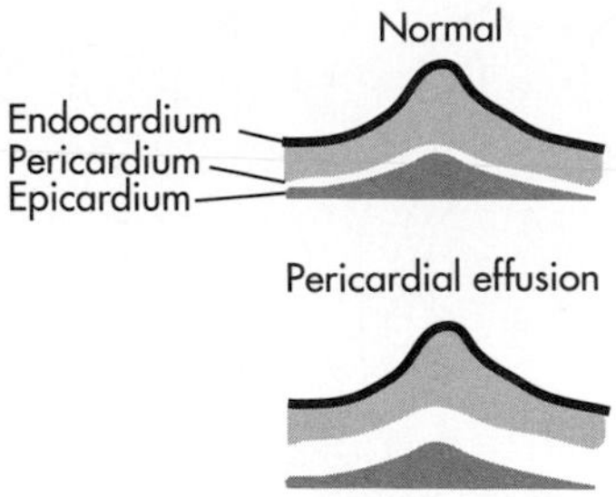

FIGURE 2-80

Radiographic Features (Fig. 2-80)
- Well-defined, rounded soft tissue density on plain film
- Most common location: cardiophrenic angles
- Other locations: anterior and middle mediastinum
- CT is helpful in establishing diagnosis.
- MRI: T1-variable, T2-bright, nonenhancing

PERICARDIAL EFFUSION

Causes

Tumor
- Metastases (melanoma, breast, lung)

Inflammatory/idiopathic
- Rheumatic heart disease
- Collagen vascular disease
- Dressier syndrome
- Postpericardiotomy syndrome
- Drug hypersensitivity

Infectious
- Viral
- Pyogenic
- Tuberculosis (TB)

Metabolic
- Uremia
- Myxedema

Trauma
- Hemopericardium
- Postoperative (frequently after pacemaker implantation and EP ablations)

Vascular
- Acute MI
- Aortic dissection
- Ventricular rupture

Radiographic Features

Plain film
- >250 mL is necessary to be detectable.
- Oreo cookie sign on lateral view: Subpericardial fat stripe measures >10 mm (a stripe 1 to 5 mm can be normal).
- Symmetrical enlargement of cardiac silhouette (water-bottle sign)
- Postsurgical loculated pericardial effusion may mimic an LV aneurysm.

Ultrasound
- Study of choice
- Echo-free space between epicardium and pericardium

CONSTRICTIVE PERICARDITIS

Causes
- TB (most common cause)
- Other infections (viral, pyogenic)
- Cardiac surgery
- Radiation injury

Radiographic Features
- Calcifications are common.
  - 50% of patients with calcification have constrictive pericarditis.
  - 90% of patients with constrictive pericarditis have pericardial calcification.
  - Pericardial calcification is more common in the atrioventricular grooves.
- Pericardial thickening >4 mm
- Pleural effusion, 60%
- PVH, 40%
- Elevated RV pressure: dilated SVC and azygos, 80%

CARDIAC MASSES

Benign
- Myxoma: most common benign adult cardiac tumor, left > right atrium, often originates from interatrial septum with stalk, may be mobile with prolapse through mitral valve (obstruction); T1- and T2-heterogeneous signal, heterogeneous or homogeneous enhancement.
- Rhabdomyoma: most common benign tumor in children, associated with tuberous sclerosis, T1-isointense, T2-hyperintense, hypoenhancement
- Lipoma: Second most common benign adult cardiac tumor, fat signal, no enhancement
- Fibroma: second most common benign cardiac tumor in children, right ventricular free wall, T1- and T2-hypointense, may or may not enhance
- Papillary fibroelastoma: most common tumor of valves, usually <1.5 cm, atrial surface of AV valves and aortic surface of aortic valve
- Hemangioma: capillary, cavernous, or AV malformation, may involve any chamber, T1-hypointense, T2-hyperintense, heterogeneous enhancement

Malignant
- Angiosarcoma: most common primary malignant tumor in adults, most commonly in the right atrium, T2-hyperintense with heterogeneous enhancement

- Rhabdomyosarcoma: most common primary malignant tumor in children, may be found in any chamber, associated with heart failure, may demonstrate homogeneous enhancement or necrosis
- Primary cardiac lymphoma: rare, usually immunocompromised, most commonly affects right atrium but may involve multiple chambers and pericardium, T2-hyperintense, heterogeneous enhancement
- Osteosarcoma: rare, dense calcifications better demonstrated on CT
- Metastases: most common malignant process involving heart, may occur via lymphatics (lung), hematogenous spread (melanoma), transvenous extension (RCC, hepatoma, adrenocortical carcinoma)
  - Lung > lymphoma, leukemia, breast, esophagus
  - Pericardium > myocardium
  - T1- hypointense (except melanoma) and T2-hyperintense, enhancement
  - Enhancement distinguishes tumor from bland thrombus

Tumor-like

- Thrombus: typically LA or LV, T1- and T2-hyperintense when acute, hypointense when chronic, no enhancement.
- Valvular vegetations (clinical endocarditis, valvular destruction)
- Normal anatomic structures
  - Eustachian valves (right atrium)
  - Crista terminalis (right atrium)
  - Moderator band (right ventricle)

Differential Diagnosis

CONGENITAL HEART DISEASE

ACYANOTIC HEART DISEASE (Figs. 2-81 through 2-84)

Increased Pulmonary Vascularity (L-R Shunt)

With LA enlargement (indicates that shunt is not in LA)

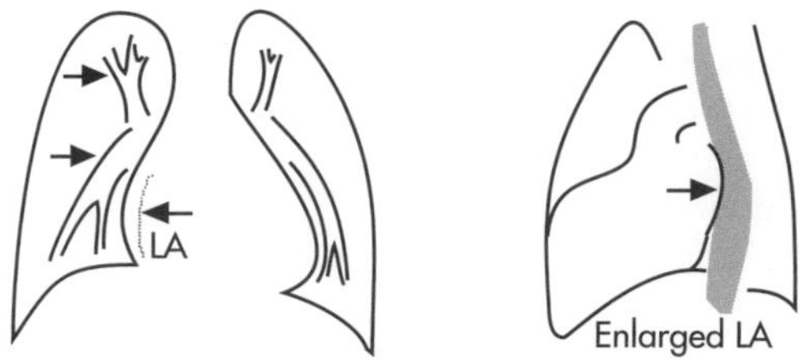

FIGURE 2-81

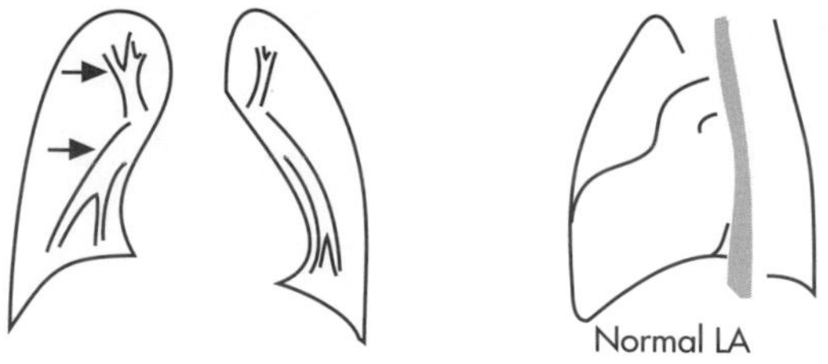

FIGURE 2-82

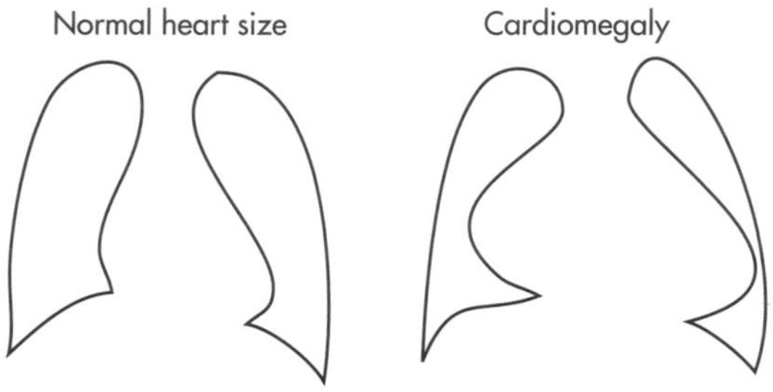

FIGURE 2-83

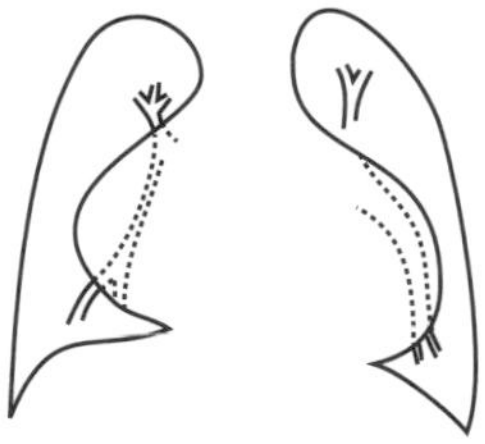

FIGURE 2-84

- VSD (normal AA)
- PDA (prominent AA)

With normal LA

- ASD
- BCD
- PAPVC and sinus venosus ASD

Normal Pulmonary Vascularity

- Aortic stenosis
- Coarctation
- Pulmonic stenosis

CYANOTIC HEART DISEASE

Normal or Decreased Pulmonary Vascularity

Normal heart size

- Tetralogy of Fallot (common)
- Fallot variants

Cardiomegaly (RA enlarged)

- Ebstein malformation
- Tricuspid atresia
- Pulmonic atresia

Pearls

Increased pulmonary vascularity (the "5 Ts"):

- TGA (most common)
- TA
- TAPVC
- Tricuspid atresia
- Tingle = single ventricle

PULMONARY EDEMA IN NEWBORNS

- Cardiac
  - Edema + large heart: hypoplastic RV or
  - LV Edema + normal heart: TAPVC below diaphragm
- Transient tachypnea of the newborn (TTN)
- Pulmonary lymphangiectasia
- Other rare CHD causing obstruction to pulmonary venous return:
  - Pulmonary vein atresia
  - Cor triatriatum
  - Supravalvular mitral ring
  - Parachute mitral valve

MASSIVE CARDIOMEGALY IN THE NEWBORN

- Box-shaped right heart (RA enlargement)
  - Ebstein anomaly
  - Uhl disease (focal or total absence of RV myocardium; very rare)
  - Tricuspid atresia
- Herniation of liver into pericardial sac
- Massive pericardial effusion

BOOT-SHAPED HEART

- Tetralogy of Fallot
- Adults
  - Loculated pleural effusion
  - Cardiac aneurysm
  - Pericardial cyst

CHD WITH NORMAL HEART SIZE AND NORMAL LUNGS

- Coarctation
- Tetralogy of Fallot

SKELETAL ABNORMALITIES AND HEART DISEASE

- Rib notching: coarctation
- Hypersegmented manubrium, 11 pairs of ribs: Down syndrome
- Pectus excavatum: prolapsed MV, Marfan syndrome
- Multiple sternal ossification centers: cyanotic CHD
- Bulging sternum: large L-R shunt
- Scoliosis: Marfan syndrome, tetralogy of Fallot

INFERIOR RIB NOTCHING

- Aortic obstruction
  - Coarctation
  - IAA
- Subclavian artery obstruction
  - Blalock-Taussig shunt (upper 2 ribs)
  - Takayasu disease (unilateral)
- Severely reduced pulmonary blood flow (very rare)
  - Tetralogy of Fallot
  - Pulmonary atresia
  - Ebstein anomaly
- SVC obstruction
- Vascular shunts
  - Arteriovenous malformation (AVM) of intercostals
- Intercostal neuroma
- Osseous abnormality (hyperparathyroidism)

SUPERIOR RIB NOTCHING

Abnormal osteoclastic activity

- Hyperparathyroidism (most common)
- Idiopathic

Abnormal osteoblastic activity

- Poliomyelitis
- Collagen vascular diseases such as rheumatoid arthritis, systemic lupus erythematosus
- Local pressure
- Osteogenesis imperfecta
- Marfan syndrome

DIFFERENTIAL DIAGNOSIS OF CHD BY AGE OF PRESENTATION

- 0 to 2 days: hypoplastic left heart, aortic atresia, TAPVC, "5 Ts"
- 7 to 14 days: coarctation, aortic stenosis, AVM, endocardial fibroelastosis
- Infants: VSD, PDA
- Adults: ASD

AORTA

RIGHT AORTIC ARCH AND CHD

Associations

Right aortic arches are associated with CHD in 5%.

- TA, 35%
- Tetralogy of Fallot, 30%
- Less common associations, 35%
  - TGA, 5%
  - Tricuspid atresia, 5%
  - Pulmonary atresia with VSD, 20%
  - DORV
  - Pseudotruncus
  - Asplenia
  - Pink tetralogy

ACQUIRED HEART DISEASE (FIG. 2-85)

APPROACH

- Pressure overload (stenosis, hypertension) causes hypertrophy: normal heart size
- Volume overload (regurgitation, shunt) causes dilatation: large heart size
- Wall abnormalities

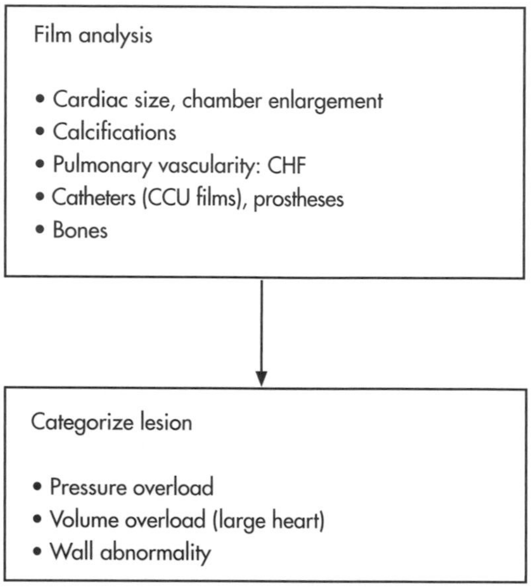
Film analysis
• Cardiac size, chamber enlargement
• Calcifications
• Pulmonary vascularity: CHF
• Catheters (CCU films), prostheses
• Bones
Categorize lesion
• Pressure overload
• Volume overload (large heart)
• Wall abnormality

FIGURE 2-85

ABNORMAL LEFT HEART CONTOUR

Pressure overload (normal heart size)
- Aortic or mitral stenosis
- Systemic hypertension
- Coarctation

Volume overload (large heart disease)
- Mitral or aortic regurgitation
- Shunts: ASD, VSD
- High-output states
- End-stage heart failure of any given cause

Wall abnormalities
- Aneurysm, infarct
- Cardiomyopathy

ABNORMAL RIGHT HEART CONTOUR

Pressure overload (normal heart size)
- PA hypertension
- Pulmonic stenosis (rarely isolated except in CHD)

Volume overload (large heart disease)
- Pulmonic or tricuspid regurgitation
- Shunts: ASD, VSD
- High-output states

Wall abnormalities
- Aneurysm, infarct
- Cardiomyopathy
- Uhl anomaly

SMALL HEART

- Normal variant (deep inspiration)
- Addison disease
- Anorexia nervosa/bulimia
- Dehydration
- Severe COPD

OVERVIEW OF PLAIN FILM FINDINGS

Lesion	Calcification	CHF	LAE	LVE
Mitral stenosis	+	+	+	−
Mitral regurgitation	−	−	++	+
Aortic stenosis	++	−	−	−
Aortic regurgitation	−	−	−	+

LAE, LA enlargement; LVE, LV enlargement; − usually absent; + present; ++ marked.

LEFT ATRIAL ENLARGEMENT

- Mitral regurgitation: LA and LV enlarged
- Mitral stenosis: LA enlarged, LV normal
- Rheumatic heart disease
- Atrial fibrillation
- Papillary muscle rupture (MI)

DELAYED MYOCARDIAL ENHANCEMENT (MRI)

- Subendocardial
  - Ischemic (coronary territory)
  - Amyloid (diffuse)
  - Cardiac transplant (diffuse)
  - Systemic sclerosis (diffuse)
  - Hypereosinophilic syndrome
- Mesocardial
  - Hypertrophic CM
  - Dilated CM
  - Chagas
- Transmural
  - Ischemia
  - Myocarditis
  - Sarcoid
- Subepicardial
  - Myocarditis
  - Sarcoid
  - Chagas
- Nodular/patchy enhancement
  - Amyloid
  - Myocarditis
  - Sarcoid

CARDIAC MASSES

- Thrombus
- Lipoma
- Infectious vegetation
- Metastases
- Atrial myxoma (left > right)
- Rhabdomyoma in infants (tuberous sclerosis)
- Pericardial cyst
- Angiosarcoma
- Rhabdomyosarcoma (children)
- Fibroma (children)
- Papillary fibroelastoma
- Lymphoma

T1 BRIGHT CARDIAC LESIONS

Benign
- Thrombus (no enhancement)
- Lipoma (T1 bright, use fat sat)
- Myxoma (T2 bright, variable enhancement)
- Lipomatous hypertrophy of the interatrial septum

Malignant (enhances)
- Angiosarcoma

PERICARDIAL EFFUSION (Fig. 2-86)

Transudate
- CHF
- AMI
- Postsurgical
- Autoimmune
- Renal failure

Infectious
- Viral

Tumor
- Pericardial metastases

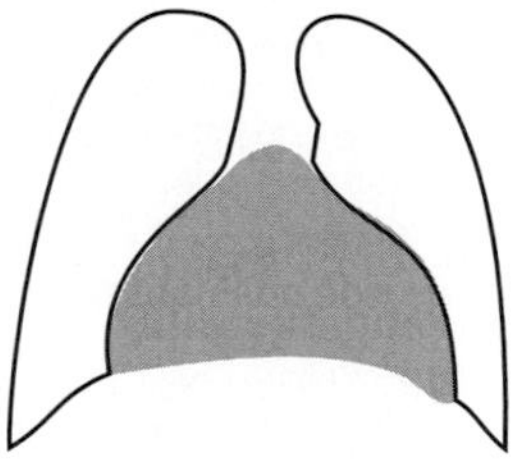

FIGURE 2-86

PNEUMOPERICARDIUM

- Iatrogenic/pericardiocentesis
- Barotrauma (children)
- Esophageal-pericardial fistula (malignancy)

HIGH-CARDIAC OUTPUT STATES

- Severe anemia
- Peripheral AVM
- Liver hemangioma
- Thyrotoxicosis
- Pregnancy

CHF

- High output failure (listed above) by age
- Premature: PDA
- First week: hypoplastic left heart syndrome (HLHS)
- 2nd week: coarctation
- Infant: VSD
- Child: ASD
- Increased heart size with normal vascularity
  - Pericardial effusion
  - Cardiomyopathy
  - Valvular disease

OVERVIEW

Type	Comments
Pericardial	
Pericarditis*	TB, uremia, AIDS, coxsackievirus, pyogenic
Pericardial cysts	In AMI
Myocardial	
Coronary arteries	Always significant in patients <40 years
Calcified infarct	Curvilinear calcification (necrosis)
Aneurysm	
Postmyocarditis	
Intracardiac	
Calcified valves	Indicates stenosis; most common: rheumatic fever
Calcified thrombus	In infarcts and aneurysm; 10% calcify
Tumors	Atrial myxoma is the most common calcified tumor.
Aorta	
Atherosclerosis	In >25% of patients >60 years
Syphilitic aortitis	In 20% of syphilis patients
Aneurysm	Predominantly in ascending aorta

*Follows fat distribution.
AIDS, acquired immunodeficiency syndrome.

PNEUMOPERICARDIUM

- Iatrogenic (aspiration, puncture)
- Cardiac surgery
- Barotrauma
- Fistula from bronchogenic or esophageal carcinoma

CORONARY ANEURYSM

- Atherosclerotic
- Congenital
- Periarteritis nodosa
- Kawasaki disease
- Mycotic

- Syphilis
- Trauma
- CABG (saphenous vein > IMA)

PULMONARY ARTERY

PULMONARY ARTERY ENLARGEMENT (Fig. 2-87)

PAH
- Primary PAH (young females, rare)
- Secondary PAH

PA stenosis
- Williams syndrome (infantile hypercalcemia)
- Rubella syndrome
- Takayasu disease
- Associated with CHD (especially tetralogy of Fallot)

PA dilatation
- Poststenotic jet
- AVM: Osler-Weber-Rendu disease

Aneurysm cystic medial necrosis
- Behçet syndrome
- Takayasu disease

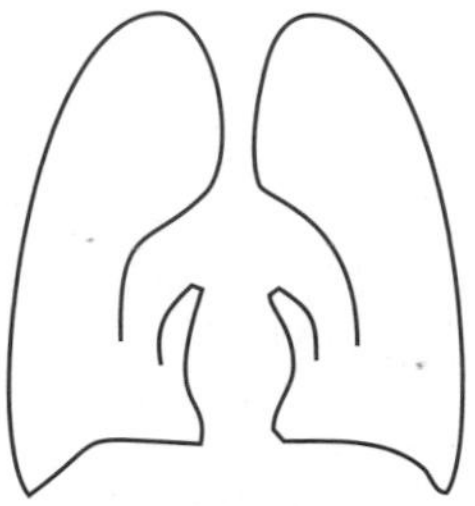

FIGURE 2-87

PULMONARY ARTERIAL HYPERTENSION (PAH)

P_{sys} >30 mm Hg

Classification

Precapillary hypertension
- Vascular
  - Increased flow: L-R shunts
  - Chronic PE
  - Vasculitis
  - Drugs
  - Idiopathic
- Pulmonary
  - Emphysema
  - Interstitial fibrosis
  - Fibrothorax, chest wall deformities
  - Alveolar hypoventilation

Postcapillary hypertension
- Cardiac
  - LV failure
  - Mitral stenosis
  - LA myxoma
- Pulmonary venous
  - Idiopathic venoocclusive disease
  - Thrombosis
  - Tumor

PULMONARY VENOUS HYPERTENSION (PVH)

P_{wedge} >12 mm Hg

LV dysfunction
- Ischemic heart disease: CAD
- Valvular heart disease
- CHD
- Cardiomyopathy

Left atrium
- Cor triatriatum: stenosis of pulmonary veins at entrance to LA
- LA myxoma

EISENMENGER PHYSIOLOGY

Chronic L-R shunt causes high pulmonary vascular resistance, which ultimately reverses the shunt (R-L shunt with cyanosis).

Causes
- VSD
- ASD
- PDA
- ECD

Suggested Readings

Braunwald E. *Heart Disease*. Philadelphia: WB Saunders; 2010.

Budoff MJ, Shinbane JS. *Cardiac CT Imaging: Diagnosis of Cardiovascular Disease*. New York: Springer; 2006.

Chen JT. *Essentials of Cardiac Roentgenology*. Philadelphia: Lippincott Williams & Wilkins; 1998.

Fink BW. *Congenital Heart Disease: A Deductive Approach to Its Diagnosis*. St. Louis: Mosby; 1991.

Higgins CB. *Essentials of Cardiac Radiology and Imaging*. Philadelphia: Lippincott Williams & Wilkins; 1992.

Hugo SF. *Radiology of the Heart: Cardiac Imaging in Infants, Children, and Adults*. New York: Springer-Verlag; 1985.

Kazerooni E, Gross BH. *Cardiopulmonary Imaging*. Philadelphia: Lippincott Williams & Wilkins; 2004.

Lardo AC, Fayad ZA, Chronos NA, Fuster V. *Cardiovascular Magnetic Resonance; Established and Emerging Application*. London: Taylor & Francis; 2004.

Miller SW. *Cardiac Angiography*. Boston: Little, Brown; 1984.

Miller SW. *Cardiac Radiology: The Requisites*. St. Louis: Elsevier Mosby; 2009.

Schoepf J. *CT of the Heart: Principles and Applications*. Totowa, NJ: Humana Press; 2005.

Thelen M, Erbel R, Kreitner K-F, Barkhausen J. *Cardiac Imaging: A Multimodality Approach*. New York: Thieme; 2009.

CHAPTER 3

Gastrointestinal Imaging

CHAPTER OUTLINE

Esophagus

GENERAL

ANATOMY

Normal Esophageal Contour Deformities (Fig. 3-1)
- Cricopharyngeus
- Postcricoid impressions (mucosal fold over vein)
- Aortic impression
- Left mainstem bronchus (LMB)
- Left atrium (LA)
- Diaphragm
- Peristaltic waves
- Mucosa: thin transient transverse folds: feline esophagus (versus thick folds in chronic reflux esophagitis); tiny nodules in elderly: glycogenic acanthosis

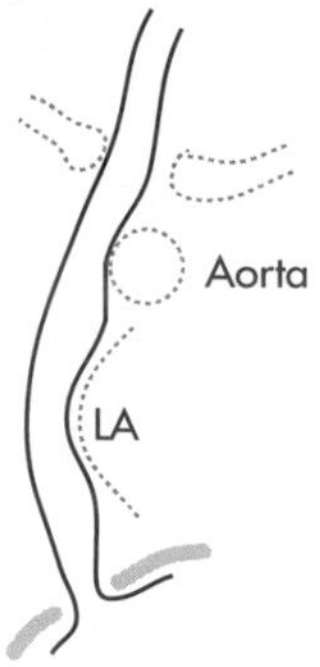

FIGURE 3-1

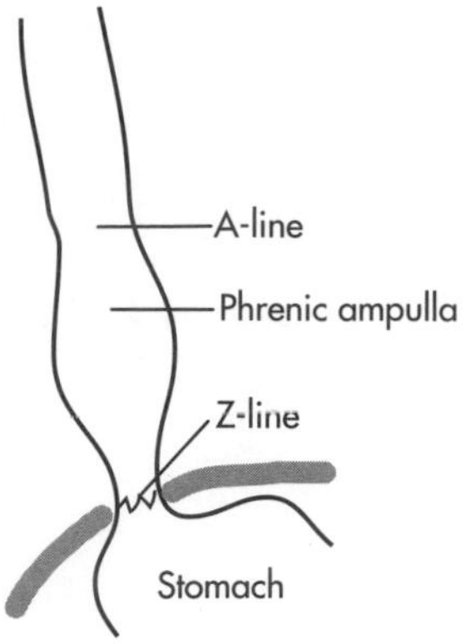

FIGURE 3-2

Gastroesophageal Junction (GEJ)

Anatomy (Fig. 3-2)

- Phrenic ampulla: normal expansion of the distal esophagus; does not contain gastric mucosa
- A-ring (for **a**bove; Wolf ring): indentation at upper boundary of the phrenic ampulla
- B-ring (for **b**elow): indentation at lower boundary of the phrenic ampulla; normally not seen radiologically unless there is a hiatal hernia
- Z-line (**z**igzag line): squamocolumnar mucosal junction between esophagus and stomach; not visible radiologically
- C-ring : diaphragmatic impression
- The esophagus lacks a serosa. Upper one third has striated muscle; lower two thirds have smooth muscle.

Peristaltic Waves

- Primary contractions: initiated by swallowing; distally progressive contraction waves strip the esophagus of its contents; propulsive wave
- Secondary contractions: anything not cleared from the esophagus by a primary wave may be cleared by a locally initiated wave; propulsive wave
- Tertiary contractions: nonpropulsive, uncoordinated contractions; these random contractions increase with age and are rarely of clinical significance in absence of symptoms of dysphagia; nonpropulsive wave; only peristaltic activity in achalasia

Peristalsis should always be evaluated fluoroscopically with the patient in a horizontal position. In the erect position the esophagus empties by gravity.

SWALLOWING (Fig. 3-3)

NORMAL SWALLOW

Swallowing Phase	Tongue	Palate	Larynx	Pharyngeal Constrictors
1. Oral	Dorsum controls bolus; base assumes vertical position	Resting	Resting	Resting
2. Early pharyngeal	Strips palate and moves dorsally	Velopharynx closure	Epiglottis deflects, larynx moves anterosuperiorly	Middle constrictors
3. Late pharyngeal	Meets relaxing palate	Begins descent	Vocal folds close, epiglottis retroflexes	Inferior constrictors
4. Esophageal	Returns to resting	Resting	Returns to resting	Completion of constriction, resting

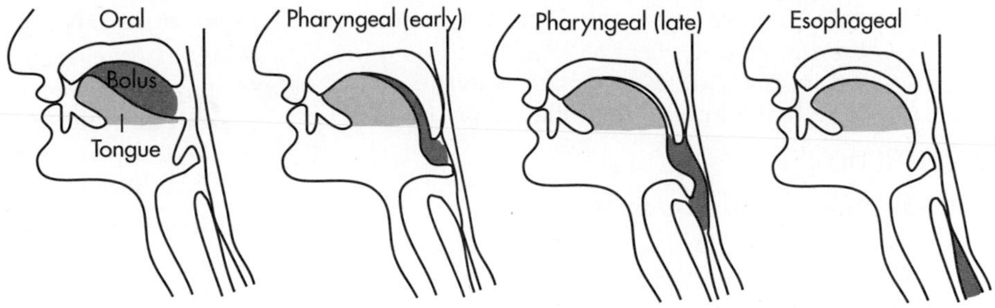

FIGURE 3-3

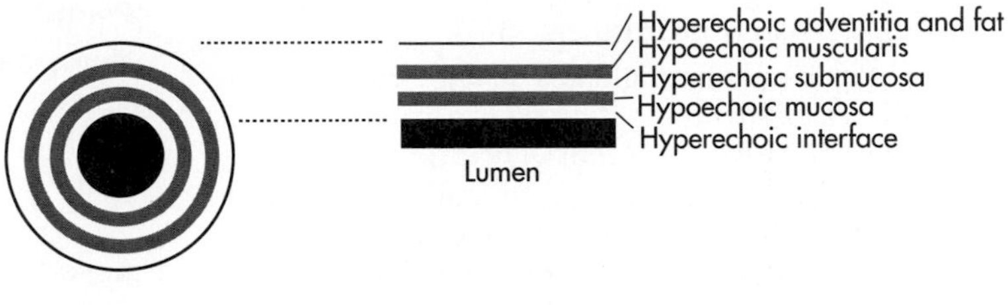

FIGURE 3-4

ESOPHAGEAL ULTRASOUND (Fig. 3-4)

Endoscopic esophageal transabdominal or gastric ultrasound (US) is performed mainly for staging of cancer or detection of early cancer. Most mass lesions and lymph nodes appear as hypoechoic structures disrupting the normal US "gut signature," consisting of different layers of hyperechogenic and hypoechogenic lines.

ESOPHAGEAL DISEASE

SCHATZKI'S RING

Thin annular symmetrical narrowing at junction of esophagus with stomach (B-ring level). Present in 10% of population, 30% of whom are symptomatic. Symptoms (dysphagia, heartburn) usually occur if rings cause esophageal narrowing of ≤ 12 mm. Now considered a consequence of reflux.

ESOPHAGEAL WEBS AND RINGS

Mucosal structures (web = asymmetrical, ring = symmetrical) may occur anywhere in the esophagus.

Associations

- Iron-deficiency anemia (cervical webs): Plummer Vinson syndrome
- Hypopharyngeal carcinoma

HIATAL HERNIA

There are two types:

Sliding hernia (axial type), 95%

- GEJ is above the diaphragm.
- Reflux is more likely with larger hernias.
- "Mixed" variant when hernia and esophagus are not in straight axis.

Paraesophageal hernia, 5%

- GEJ is in its normal position (i.e., below diaphragm).
- Part of the fundus is herniated above the diaphragm through esophageal hiatus and lies to the side of the esophagus.
- Reflux is not necessarily associated.
- More prone to mechanical complications; prophylactic surgery a consideration
- Usually nonreducible

Imaging Features (Fig. 3-5)

Criteria for diagnosing sliding hernia:

- Gastric folds above diaphragm
- Concentric indentation (B-line) above diaphragm
- Schatzki's ring above diaphragm

Associations

- Esophagitis, 25%
- Duodenal ulcers, 20%

Approach

- Maximally distend distal esophagus in horizontal position; distention can be achieved by sustained inspiratory effort
- Determine the type of hernia

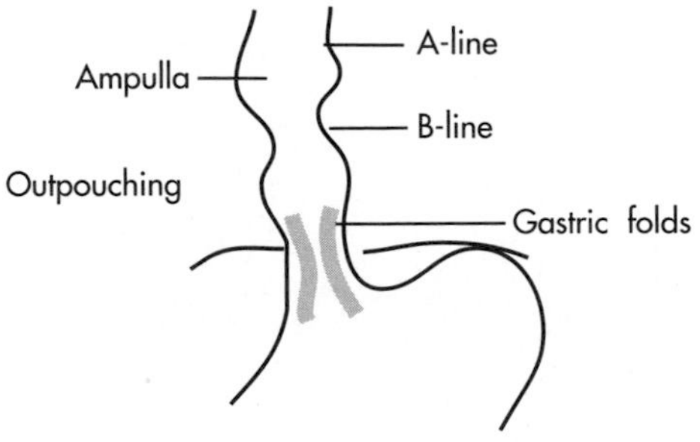

FIGURE 3-5

- Determine if there is reflux by Valsalva maneuver or Crummy water-siphon test (patient in supine RPO position continually drinks water to see if barium refluxes into midesophagus or above)

DIVERTICULA

Lateral Pharyngeal Pouches

AP esophagram at level of pharynx demonstrates lateral outpouchings through weakness in thyrohyoid membrane. Large in glassblowers and wind instrument players.

Zenker's Diverticulum (Fig. 3-6)

Pulsion diverticulum originates in the midline of the posterior wall of the hypopharynx at an anatomic weak point known as Killian's dehiscence (above cricopharyngeus at fiber divergence with inferior pharyngeal constrictor). During swallowing, increased intraluminal pressure forces mucosa to herniate through the wall. The etiology of Zenker's diverticulum is not firmly established, but premature contraction and/or motor incoordination of the cricopharyngeus muscle are thought to play a major role. Complications include:

- Aspiration
- Ulceration
- Carcinoma

Killian-Jamieson Diverticulum (Fig. 3-7)

- Below cricopharyngeus
- Off midline
- Lateral to cervical esophagus

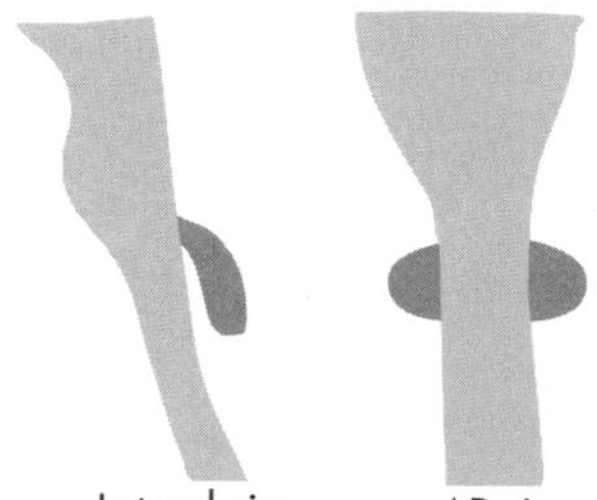

FIGURE 3-6

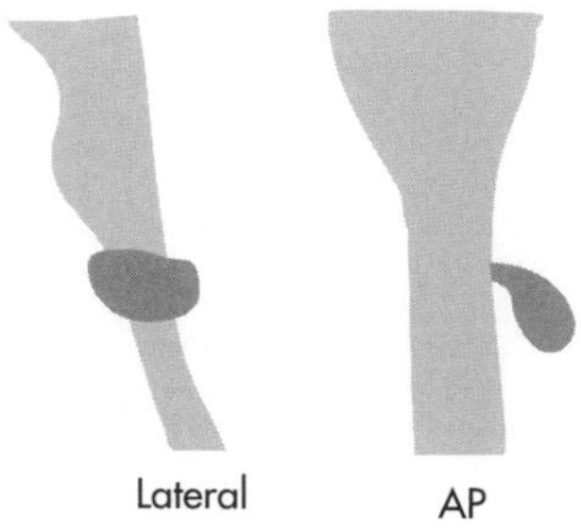

FIGURE 3-7

Epiphrenic Diverticulum

- May occasionally be recognized on chest radiographs by presence of soft tissue mass (often with air-fluid level) that mimics a hiatal hernia
- Large diverticulum can compress the true esophageal lumen, causing dysphagia.

Traction Diverticulum

- Outpouching of midesophagus due to adjacent inflammatory process (e.g., TB)
- Calcified mediastinal lymph nodes

Pseudodiverticulosis

Numerous small esophageal outpouchings representing dilated glands interior to the muscularis occur, usually after 50 years. Dysphagia is presenting symptom. Underlying diseases include candidiasis, alcoholism, and diabetes.

Associated Findings

- Esophageal stricture may occur above and/or below stricture.
- Esophagitis

Imaging Features

- Thin flask-shaped structures in longitudinal rows parallel to the long axis of the esophagus
- Diffuse distribution or localized clusters near peptic strictures
- Much smaller than true diverticula
- When viewed en face, the pseudodiverticula can sometimes be mistaken for ulcers. When viewed in profile, however, they often seem to be "floating" outside the esophageal wall with barely perceptible channel to the lumen; esophageal ulcers almost always visibly communicate with the lumen.

ESOPHAGITIS

Esophagitis may present with erosions, ulcers, and strictures and rarely with perforations and fistulas.

Types

Infectious (common in debilitated patients)
- Herpes
- Candidiasis
- Cytomegalovirus (CMV)

Chemical
- Reflux esophagitis
- Corrosives (lye)

Iatrogenic
- Radiotherapy
- Extended use of nasogastric tubes
- Drugs: tetracycline, antiinflammatory drugs, potassium, iron

Other
- HIV
- Scleroderma
- Crohn disease (rare)

- Dermatologic manifestations (pemphigoid, dermatomyositis bullosa)

Imaging Features

- Thickening, nodularity of esophageal folds
- Irregularity of mucosa: granularity, ulcerations
- Retraction, smooth, tapered luminal narrowing, stricture just above GE junction

Infectious Esophagitis (Fig. 3-8)

Herpes simplex
- Small ulcers, <5 mm
- Normal mucosa between ulcers
- More diffuse than reflux ulcers

Candidiasis
- Plaquelike, reticular
- Shaggy margins
- Often involve entire esophagus

CMV and HIV
- Typically elliptical large ulcers but may be tiny ulcers such as herpes
- Etiologic distinction between CMV and HIV ulcers is important because therapies are different.
- Behçet disease may have a similar appearance.

Mycobacterial
- Ulcers, sinus tracts

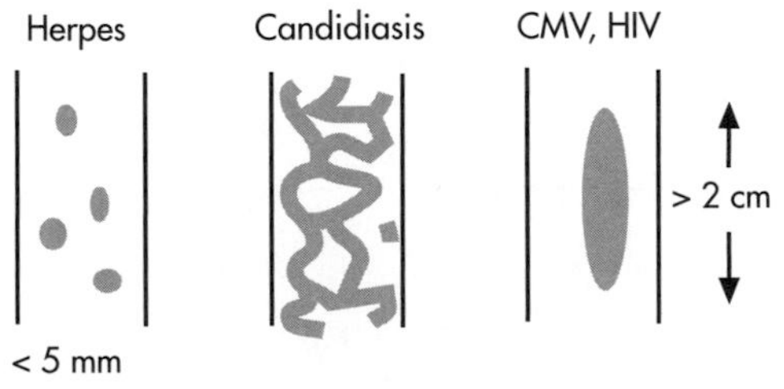

FIGURE 3-8

Inflammatory Eosinophilic Esophagitis

- Dysphagia may be chronic, history of allergies, eosinophilia
- Segmental proximal or midesophagus mild narrowing
- May involve entire esophagus
    - Increased risk of iatrogenic tear
- Responds to steroids

BARRETT'S ESOPHAGUS (Fig. 3-9)

Esophagus is abnormally lined with columnar, metaplastic acid-secreting gastric mucosa. It is usually due to chronic reflux esophagitis. Because there is an increased risk of esophageal cancer, close follow-up and repeated biopsies are recommended.

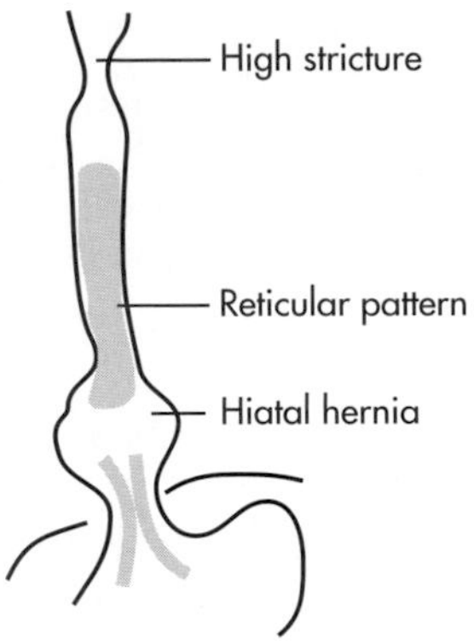

FIGURE 3-9

Imaging Features

- A reticular mucosal pattern, which may be discontinuous in the distal esophagus (short segment), is the most sensitive finding.
- Suspect the diagnosis if there is:
    - Upper or midesophageal stricture accompanied by reticular mucosal pattern below transition or ulcer
    - Low strictures: the majority cannot be differentiated from simple reflux esophagitis strictures, and biopsies are required

BOERHAAVE SYNDROME (Fig. 3-10)

Spontaneous perforation of the thoracic esophagus due to a sudden increase in intraluminal esophageal pressure. Severe epigastric pain. Treatment is with immediate thoracotomy. Mortality, 25%.

Imaging Features

- Pneumomediastinum
- Pleural effusion (left > right)
- Mediastinal hematoma
- Rupture immediately above diaphragm, usually on left posterolateral side (90%)

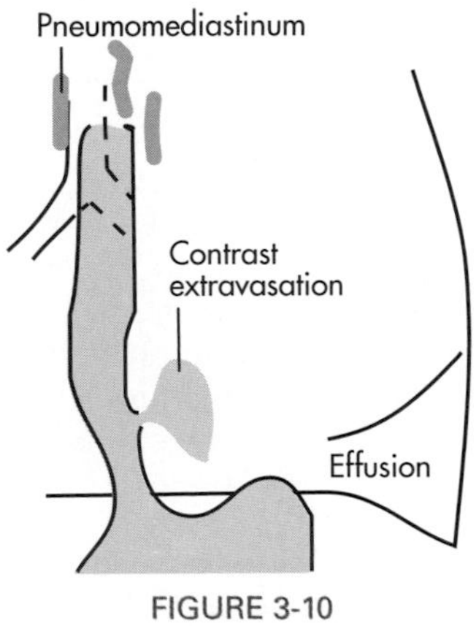

FIGURE 3-10

MALLORY-WEISS TEAR

Mucosal tear in proximal stomach, across GEJ, or in distal esophagus (10%), usually due to prolonged vomiting (alcoholics) or increased intraluminal pressure. Because the tear is not transmural, there is no pneumomediastinum.

Imaging Features

- Radiographs are usually normal.
- Intravasation rather than extravasation.
- There may be subtle mucosal irregularity.

ACHALASIA

The gastroesophageal sphincter fails to relax because of degeneration of Auerbach's plexus. The sphincter relaxes only when the hydrostatic pressure of the column of liquid or food exceeds that of the sphincter; emptying occurs more in the upright than in the horizontal position.

Types

- Primary (idiopathic)
- Secondary (destruction of myenteric plexus by tumor cells)
  - Metastases
  - Adenocarcinoma invasion from cardia
- Infectious: Chagas disease

Clinical Findings

- Primary occurs predominantly in young patients (in contradistinction to esophageal tumors); onset: 20 to 40 years
- Dysphagia, 100% to both liquids and solids when symptoms begin
- Weight loss, 90%

Diagnosis

- Need to exclude malignancy (fundal carcinoma and lymphoma destroying Auerbach's plexus), particularly in the elderly
- Need to exclude esophageal spasm
- Manometry is the most sensitive method to diagnose elevated lower esophageal sphincter (LES) pressure and incomplete relaxation.

Imaging Features (Fig. 3-11)

- Two diagnostic criteria must be met:
  - Primary and secondary peristalsis absent throughout esophagus
  - LES fails to relax in response to swallowing
- Dilated esophagus typically curves to right and then back to left when passing through diaphragm.
- There may be minimal esophageal dilation in the early stage of disease.
- Beaked tapering at GEJ
- Tertiary waves
- Air-fluid level in esophagus on plain film

DIFFERENTIATING SPASM FROM ACHALASIA

Parameter	Esophageal Spasm	Achalasia
Symptoms		
Dysphagia	Substernal	Xiphoid or suprasternal notch
Pain	Common	Rare
Weight loss	Rare	Common
Emotional	Common	Common
Motility		
Waves	Simultaneous	Tertiary
LES relaxation	Present	Absent
Imaging Features		
Esophageal contraction	Vigorous	Discoordinated
Esophageal emptying	Efficient	Poor
Response to Therapy		
Pneumostatic dilation	Not indicated	Good
Surgery	Long myotomy	Low cardioesophageal myotomy

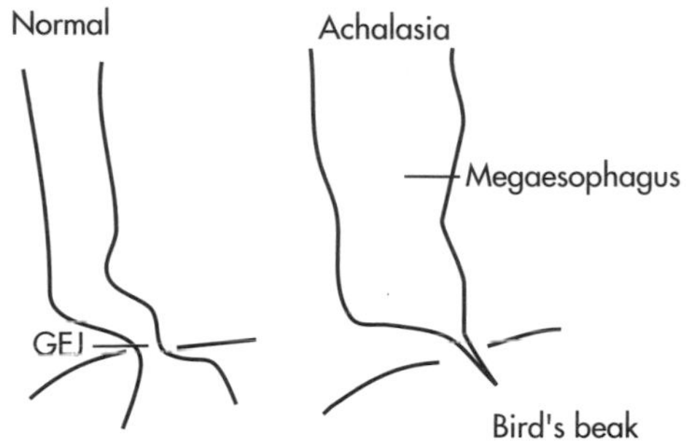

FIGURE 3-11

Complications

- Recurrent aspiration and pneumonias, 10%
- Increased incidence of esophageal cancer

Treatment

- Drugs: nitrates, β-adrenergic agonists, calcium blockers (effective in <50%)
- Balloon dilatation (effective in 70%)
- Myotomy: procedure of choice

SCLERODERMA (Fig. 3-12)

Collagen vascular disease that involves the smooth muscle of esophagus, stomach, and small bowel.

Imaging Features

- Lack of primary waves in distal two thirds
- GEJ patulous unless stricture supervenes

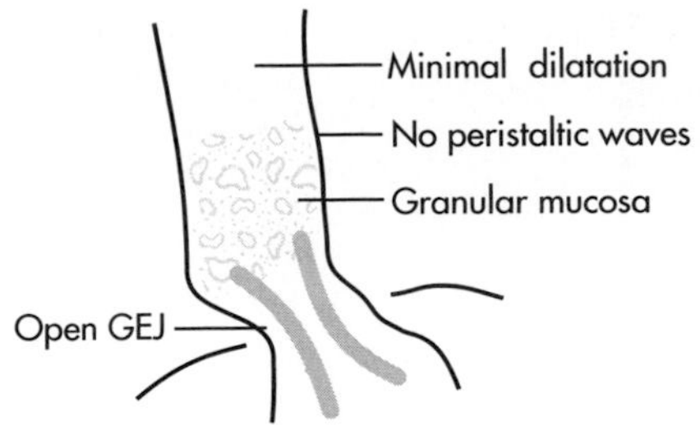

FIGURE 3-12

- Reflux esophagitis (common)
- Strictures occur late in disease
- Esophagus dilates most when stricture supervenes

DIFFERENTIATING ACHALASIA FROM SCLERODERMA

	Achalasia	Scleroderma
Esophagus	Massively dilated	Mildly dilated
GEJ	Closed, tapers to beak shape	Open; stricture late
Horizontal swallow	Tertiary contractions	Primary in proximal third, tertiary contraction in distal two thirds
Reflux	No	Yes
Complications	Aspiration pneumonia	Early: esophagitis Late: stricture, interstitial lung disease

DIFFUSE DYSMOTILITY (Fig. 3-13)

Characterized by intermittent chest pain, dysphagia, and forceful contractions. Diagnosis is diffuse esophageal spasm with manometry

Types

- Primary neurogenic abnormality (vagus)
- Secondary reflux esophagitis

Imaging Features

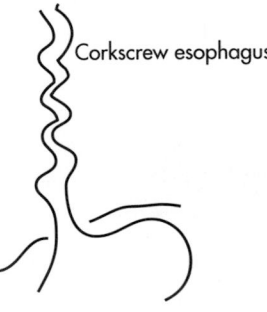

- Nutcracker corkscrew esophagus
- Nonspecific esophageal dysmotility disorders

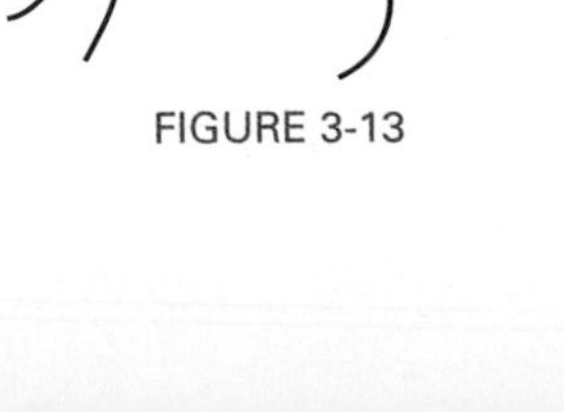

FIGURE 3-13

CHAGAS DISEASE (AMERICAN TRYPANOSOMIASIS)

Caused by *Trypanosoma cruzi,* which multiply in reticuloendothelial system (RES), muscle, and glia cells. When these cells rupture and organisms are destroyed, a neurotoxin is released that destroys ganglion cells in the myenteric plexus. Mortality, 5% (myocarditis, encephalitis).

Imaging Features

Esophagus
- Early findings: hypercontractility, distal muscular spasm; normal caliber
- Classic late findings (denervation): megaesophagus, aperistalsis, bird's beak appearance at GEJ (achalasia look-alike)
- Esophageal complications:
  - Ulcers, hemorrhage
  - Perforation into mediastinum, abscess formation; carcinoma, 7%

Colon
- Megacolon (anal sphincter neuropathy)
- Sigmoid volvulus, 10%

Heart
- Cardiomyopathy (cardiomegaly)
- Clear lungs, no pericardial effusions

Central nervous system (CNS)
- Encephalitis

BENIGN ESOPHAGEAL NEOPLASM

- Leiomyoma (may calcify) 50%
- Fibrovascular polyp (may be large and mobile attached to upper esophagus and may contain fat on CT), 25%
- Cysts, 10%
- Papilloma, 3%
- Fibroma, 3%
- Hemangioma, 2%

MALIGNANT ESOPHAGEAL NEOPLASM

Types

- Squamous cell carcinoma (most common worldwide)
- Adenocarcinoma, usually in distal esophagus at GEJ (in the United States, the incidence is now similar to squamous cell carcinoma)
- Lymphoma
- Leiomyosarcoma
- Metastasis

Associations

Squamous cell carcinomas are associated with:
- Head and neck cancers
- Smoking
- Alcohol
- Achalasia

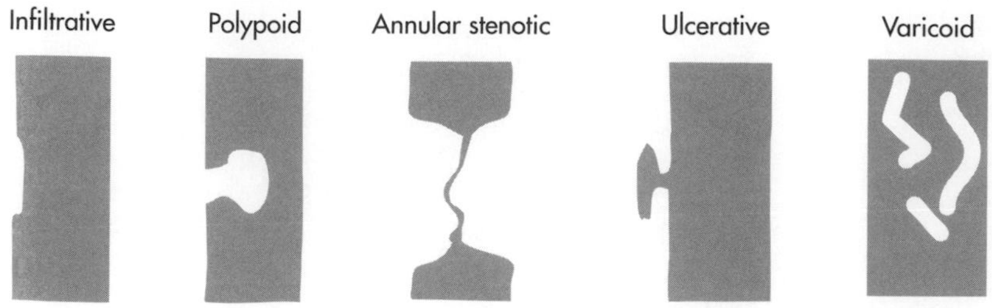

FIGURE 3-14

- Lye ingestion

Adenocarcinoma is associated with:

- Barrett's esophagus

Imaging Features (Fig. 3-14)

Staging (CT)

Invasion into mediastinum, aorta
Local lymph node enlargement
Metastases: liver, lung, lymphadenopathy, gastrohepatic ligament

Staging (endoscopic US)

- Extension through wall
- Lymph node metastases

Spectrum of appearance

- Infiltrative, shelflike margins
- Annular, constricting
- Polypoid
- Ulcerative
- Varicoid: does not change in configuration during fluoroscopy as do esophageal varices
- Unusual bulky forms: carcinosarcoma, fibrovascular polyp, leiomyosarcoma, metastases

LYMPHOMA

Because the esophagus and stomach do not normally have lymphocytes, primary lymphoma is rare unless present from inflammation. Secondary metastatic lymphoma is more common. Secondary esophageal lymphoma accounts for <2% of all gastrointestinal (GI) tract lymphomas (stomach > small bowel). Four radiographic presentations are infiltrative, ulcerating, polypoid, and endoexophytic.

ESOPHAGEAL FOREIGN BODY

Imaging Features

- Foreign body usually lodges in coronal orientation.
- It is important to exclude underlying Schatzki's ring or esophageal carcinoma once the foreign body is removed.

Stomach

TYPES OF BARIUM STUDIES

DOUBLE-VERSUS SINGLE-CONTRAST BARIUM STUDIES

	Single Contrast	Double Contrast
Contrast agent	Thin barium (40% w/w)	Thick barium (85% w/w) Effervescent granules
Differences	Opaque distention Compression is necessary to allow penetration of beam	Translucent distention ("see-through") Compression less important
	Fluoroscopy emphasized	Filming emphasized
Indication	Acute setting, uncooperative patient, obstruction	All elective barium studies

UPPER GASTROINTESTINAL SERIES

Patient Preparation

- Nothing by mouth for 8 hours before examination
- If a barium enema has been performed within the last 48 hours, give 4 tablespoons of milk of magnesia 12 hours before examination (cathartic).

Single-Contrast Technique (Fig. 3-15)

1. Patient is in upright position and drinks thin barium. Spot GEJ.
2. Prone position to observe esophageal motility. Spot GEJ, antrum, and bulb.

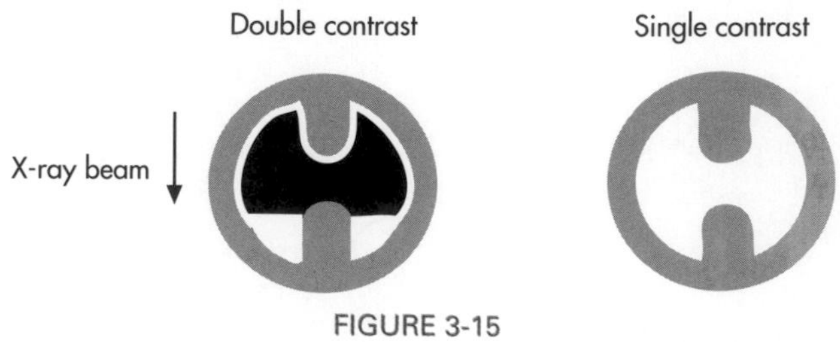

FIGURE 3-15

3. Turn supine under fluoroscopic control.
4. Turn LPO for air contrast of antrum, bulb. Evaluate duodenum and proximal small bowel.
5. Overhead films: LPO, RAO of stomach, PA of abdomen

Double-Contrast Technique

1. Patient upright in slight LPO position. Administer effervescent granules with 20 mL of water. Start patient drinking thick barium (120 mL) and obtain air-contrast spot films of esophagus.
2. Table down with patient in prone position (compression view may be obtained here). Patient rolls to supine position through the left side. Check mucosal coating: if not adequate, turn patient to prone again and back to supine position, roll to keep left side dependent (so that emptying of barium into the duodenum is delayed).
3. Obtain views of the stomach. This is generally the most important part of the study. The patient is turned to get air into different regions of the stomach.
   - Patient supine (for body of stomach)
   - Patient LPO (for antrum)
   - Patient RPO (for Schatzki's view for lesser curvature)
   - Patient RAO (for fundus)
4. Views of bulb in contrast and gas relief. First leave the patient in RAO view and then turn to LPO view. Include some C-loop.
5. Study of esophagus. Patient RAO drinking regular "thin" barium. Observe entire esophagus and evaluate motility. Take spot films (routinely of distended GEJ).
6. Overhead films (optional):
   - RAO, drinking esophagus
   - AP of abdomen
   - LPO and RAO stomach
7. Water-siphon test to exclude GE reflux, unless small bowel follow-through is simultaneously scheduled then done at end after swallowing additional barium

PERCUTANEOUS GASTROSTOMY

Success rate 95%, minor complications 1%-2%, and major complications 2%-4%.

Indications

- Decompression in terminally ill patients with gastric outlet or small bowel obstruction (SBO): gastrostomy is sufficient.
- Feeding: gastrojejunostomy preferred

Technique

1. Half cup of barium the night before to opacify colon. Nasogastric (NG) tube placement.
2. Distend stomach by insufflating air through NG tube; mark entry high in midbody pointing toward pylorus.
3. Anesthetic through four 25-gauge needles 1 to 2 cm away from insertion point. Leave needles in.
4. Gastropexy with T-tacks is not universally accepted. If they are placed, deploy them with 0.35-in ring wire under fluoroscopic guidance. Crimp T-tacks in place.
5. Place needle with guidewire into stomach through central insertion point.
6. Dilators 8, 10, 12, 14, 16 Fr; place 15-Fr peel-away sheath.
7. Place 14-Fr ultrathane gastrostomy catheter. Gastric decompression can be achieved with smaller-bore catheters (>10 Fr). Secure catheter in place.

Contraindications

- Organs overlying stomach: liver, colon, ribs (high position of stomach)
- Massive ascites (perform therapeutic paracentesis before gastrostomy)
- Abnormal gastric wall (ulcer, tumor): hemorrhage is common.
- Elevated bleeding time

NORMAL APPEARANCE

Anatomy (Fig. 3-16)

- Fundus
- Body
- Antrum
- Pylorus
- Curvatures: lesser, greater

Mucosal Relief

- Gastric rugae (prominent in body, proximal antrum): in double-contrast studies, rugae are more often effaced by gaseous distention.

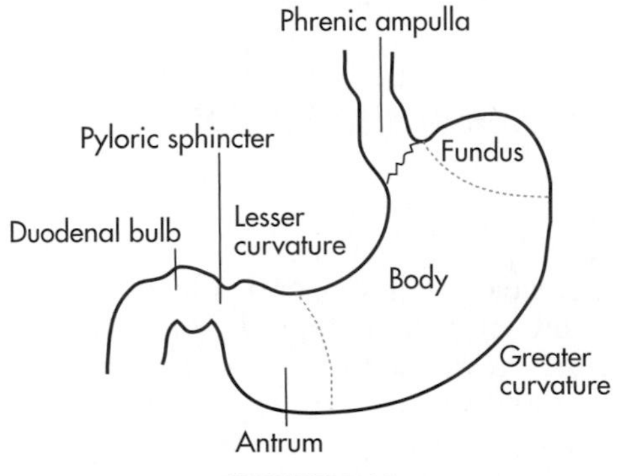

FIGURE 3-16

- Area gastricae (normal gastric mucosal pattern) is most prominent in antrum and body; ectopic duodenal area gastricae is present in 20%.

TYPES OF GASTRIC LESIONS

There are three morphologic types of lesions:
- Ulcer: abnormal accumulation of contrast media
- Polypoid lesion (masses): filling defect
- Coexistent pattern: ulcerated mass

The above lesions have different appearances depending on whether they are imaged with single- or double-contrast techniques, whether they exist on dependent or nondependent walls, and whether they are imaged in profile or en face.

Mucosal versus Extramucosal Location of Mass (Fig. 3-17)

The location of a lesion can be evaluated by observing the angle the lesion forms with the wall:

Acute angle (looks like an *a*): mucosal (polyp, cancer)

Obtuse angle (looks like an *o*): extramucosal (intramural or extramural)

Preservation of mucosal pattern is also a hint to location of lesions:
- Disruption of normal pattern: mucosal
- Presence of normal pattern: intramural or extramural location

Distinction of outline:
- Smooth, distinct: extramucosal
- Irregular, fuzzy: mucosal

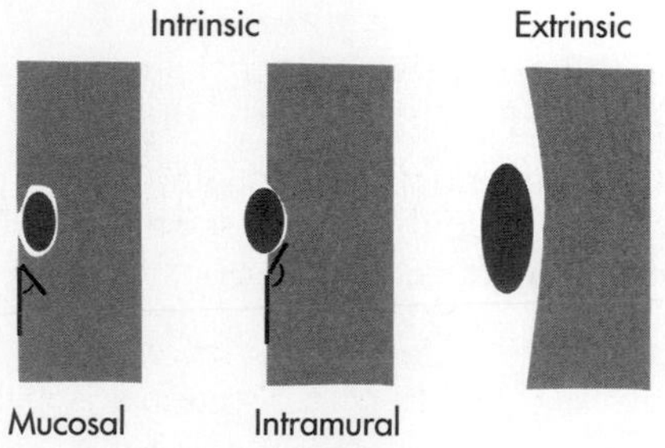

FIGURE 3-17

PEPTIC ULCER DISEASE (PUD)

Cause

Helicobacter pylori (gram negative) plays a major role in the development of peptic ulcer.
- Not all individuals with *H. pylori* will develop ulcers. Prevalence of *H. pylori:* 10% of population <30 years, 60% of population >60 years.
- Prevalence of *H. pylori* in duodenal and gastric ulcers: 80%-90%; risk factor for adenocarcinoma and lymphoma
- Approach:
  - Precaution against infection should be taken by all GI personnel.
  - *H. pylori* serology may become useful for diagnosis of PUD.
  - PUD heals faster with antibiotics and antacids than with antacids alone.
- Incidence markedly decreased

Detection

Detection rate of ulcers by double-contrast barium is 60%-80%.

Imaging Features (Fig. 3-18)

- Ulcer crater seen en face: distinct collection of barium that persists on different views; the collection is most often round but can be linear.
- Ulcer crater seen in profile: barium collection extends outside the projected margin of the gastric or duodenal wall.
- Double-contrast studies: the crater has a white center with surrounding black "collar."
- Greater curvature ulcers are commonly due to malignancy or NSAID ingestion. (Aspirin-induced ulcers are also called sump ulcers because of their typical location on greater curvature.)
- Multiple ulcers are usually due to NSAID ingestion.
- Signs of benign and malignant ulcers

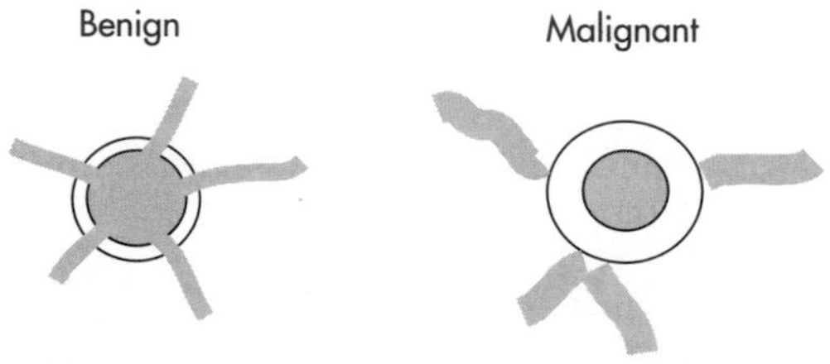

FIGURE 3-18

DIFFERENTIAL DIAGNOSIS OF ULCERS

Parameter	Benign Ulcer	Malignant Ulcer
Mucosal folds	Thin, regular, extend up to crater edge	Thick, irregular, do not extend through collar
Penetration	Margin of ulcer crater extends beyond projected luminal surface	Ulcers project within (projected) luminal surface; Carman's (meniscus) sign*
Location	Centrally within mound of edema	Eccentrically in tumor mound

DIFFERENTIAL DIAGNOSIS OF ULCERS—cont'd

Parameter	Benign Ulcer	Malignant Ulcer
Collar	Hampton's line: 1- to 2-mm lucent line around the ulcer[†]	Thick, nodular, irregular
Other	Normal peristalsis	Limited peristalsis
	Incisura: invagination of opposite wall	Limited distensibility
Gastrohepatic lymph nodes	Occasional	Common

*Results from the fluoroscopically induced apposition of rolled halves of the tumor margin forming the periphery of the ulcerated carcinoma; meniscus refers to meniscoid shape of ulcer.

[†]This line is caused by thin mucosa overhanging the crater mouth seen in tangent; it is a reliable sign of a benign ulcer, but present in very few patients.

GASTRITIS (95% OF ALL ULCERS)

Symptoms mimic PUD

Causes

- Nonsteroidal antiinflammatory drugs
- *H. pylori*
- Alcohol

Imaging Features

- Multiple tiny, aphthoid-like erosions throughout antrum, body
- Occurs on rugal folds
- Prominent area gastricae

Treatment

- Indentify and treat causal agent
- H2 blockers

Malignant Ulcers (5% of All Ulcers)

- Carcinoma, 90%
- Lymphoma, 5%
- Rare malignancies (sarcoma, carcinoid, metastases)

Complications of Gastric Ulcer (Fig. 3-19)

- Obstruction
- Posterior penetration of ulcer into pancreas
- Perforation
- Bleeding: filling defect in the ulcer crater may represent blood clots
- Gastroduodenal fistulas: double-channel pylorus

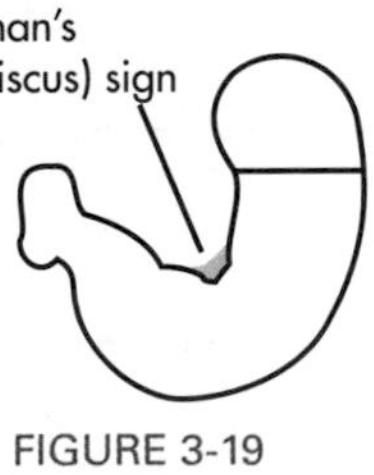

FIGURE 3-19

Pearls

- Categorize all gastric ulcers as definitely/probably benign or malignant.
- All patients, except for those with de novo definitely benign gastric ulcers, should proceed to endoscopy with biopsy.
- Benign ulcers decrease 50% in size within 3 weeks and show complete healing within 6 weeks with successful medical treatment.
- Benign ulcers may heal with local scarring.
- Ectopic pancreatic rest may contain a central umbilication that represents a rudimentary duct, not ulcer. Commonly located in antrum.
- Gastric diverticulum: commonly in posterior fundus; contains mucosal folds, neck, changes shape during fluoroscopy

MÉNÉTRIER DISEASE (GIANT HYPERTROPHIC GASTRITIS)

Large gastric rugal folds (hypertrophic gastritis) with protein-losing enteropathy. Clinical triad: achlorhydria, hypoproteinemia, edema. Typically occurs in middle-aged men. Complication: gastric carcinoma, 10%.

Imaging Features

- Giant gastric rugal folds, usually proximal half of stomach
- Hypersecretion: poor coating, dilution of barium
- Gastric wall thickening
- Small intestinal fold thickening due to hypoproteinemia
- Peptic ulcers are uncommon

EOSINOPHILIC GASTROENTERITIS

Inflammatory disease of unknown etiology characterized by focal or diffuse eosinophilic infiltration of the GI tract. An allergic or immunologic disorder is suspected because 50% of patients have another allergic disease (asthma, allergic rhinitis, hay fever). Only 300 cases have been reported to date. Treatment is with steroids.

Clinical Findings

- Abdominal pain, 90%
- Diarrhea, 40%
- Eosinophilia

Imaging Features

Stomach, 50%

- Tapered antral stenosis (common)
- Pyloric stenosis (common)
- Gastric fold thickening

Small bowel, 50%

- Fold thickening (common)
- Dilatation
- Luminal narrowing

GASTRODUODENAL CROHN DISEASE

- Aphthous ulcers, usually in antrum and duodenum
- Stricture: Pseudo-Billroth I appearance on barium studies
- Fistulization

ZOLLINGER-ELLISON SYNDROME

Syndrome caused by excessive gastrin production.

Clinical Findings

- Diarrhea
- Recurrent PUD
- Pain

Causes

Gastrinoma, 90%
- Islet cell tumor in pancreas or duodenal wall, 90%
- 50% of tumors are malignant
- 10% of tumors are associated with multiple endocrine neoplasia (MEN) type I

Antral G-cell hyperplasia, 10%

Imaging Features

- Ulcers
  Location: duodenal bulb > stomach > postbulbar duodenum
  Multiple ulcers, 10%
- Thickened gastric and duodenal folds
- Increased gastric secretions
- Reflux esophagitis

GASTRIC POLYPS

Gastric polyps are far less common than colonic polyps (2% of all patients with polyps)
- Hyperplastic polyps (80% of all gastric polyps; <1 cm, sessile; not premalignant)
  Associated with chronic atrophic gastritis
  Familial adenomatous polyposis (hyperplastic polyps in stomach, adenomatous polyps in colon)
  Typically similar size, multiple, and clustered in the fundus and body
  Synchronous gastric carcinoma in 5%-25% of patients
- Adenomatous polyps; infrequent, malignant degeneration very rare
  Solitary
  Malignant transformation in 50%
  Villous polyps (uncommon; cauliflower-like, sessile); strong malignant potential
  Hamartomatous polyps rare; Peutz-Jeghers; Cronkhite-Canada syndrome, juvenile polyposis

GASTRIC CARCINOMA

Third most common GI malignancy (colon > pancreas > stomach)

Risk Factors

- Pernicious anemia
- Adenomatous polyps
- Chronic atrophic gastritis
- Billroth II > Billroth I

Location

- Fundus/cardia, 40%
- Antrum, 30%
- Body, 30%

Staging

- T1: limited to mucosa, submucosa (5-year survival, 85%)
- T2: muscle, serosa involved (5-year survival, 50%)
- T3: penetration through serosa
- T4: adjacent organs invaded

Imaging Features (Fig. 3-20)

Features of early gastric cancers:
- Polypoid lesions (type 1)
  >0.5 cm (normal peristalsis does not pass through lesion)
  Difficult to detect radiographically
- Superficial lesions (type 2)
  2A: <0.5 cm
  2B: most difficult to diagnose (mucosal irregularity only)
  2C: 75% of all gastric carcinoma (folds tend to stop abruptly at lesion)
- Excavated lesion (type 3) = malignant ulcer

Features of advanced gastric cancer:
- Malignant ulcer: folds short of collar
- Ulcerated luminal mass

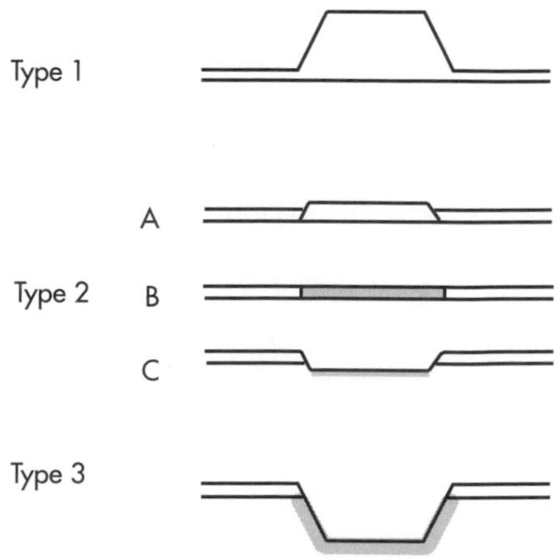

FIGURE 3-20

- Rigidity, diffuse narrowing: linitis plastica
- Thickened wall >1 cm by CT
- Lymphadenopathy
  - Gastrohepatic ligament
  - Gastrocolic ligament
  - Perigastric nodes
- Hepatic metastases

GASTRIC LYMPHOMA

3% of all gastric malignancies. Non-Hodgkin lymphoma (NHL) (common) > Hodgkin lymphoma (uncommon).

- Primary gastric lymphoma (arises from lymphatic tissue in lamina propria mucosae), 10%
- Secondary (gastric involvement in generalized lymphoma), 90%

Imaging Features

- Diffuse infiltrating disease

Normal gastric wall 2 to 5 mm (distended stomach) ≥ 6 mm is abnormal except at GEJ

- Thick folds
- Ulcerating mass
- More often than carcinoma, lymphomas spread across the pylorus into the duodenum.
- Hodgkin lymphoma of the stomach mimics scirrhous carcinoma (strong desmoplastic reaction).

GASTROINTESTINAL STROMAL TUMOR (GIST)

GIST is the most common mesenchymal neoplasm of the gastrointestinal tract and is defined by its expression of KIT (CD117), a tyrosine kinase growth factor receptor. The expression of KIT is important to distinguish GIST from other mesenchymal neoplasms such as leiomyomas, leiomyosarcomas, schwannomas, and neurofibromas. Pharmacologically targeting this receptor with a KIT tyrosine kinase inhibitor (STI-571, imatinib, Gleevec) has been shown to be of clinical usefulness. In the stomach, small intestine, colon, and anorectum, GIST accounts for almost all mesenchymal tumors, because leiomyomas and leiomyosarcomas in these sites are very rare. GIST most frequently occurs in the stomach (70% of cases), followed by the small intestine (20%-30%), anorectum (7%), colon, and esophagus. Patients with neurofibromatosis type 1 (NF1) have an increased prevalence of GIST, often multiple small GISTs.

Imaging Features

- Exophytic masses of stomach or small bowel that may ulcerate; obstruction rare despite size
- Heterogeneous contrast enhancement
- Crescent-shaped necrosis (Torricelli-Bernoulli sign) in large GIST
- 30% show aneurysm dilatation of enteric bowel.
- Liver is the most common site of metastases, followed by mesentery.
- Mesenteric metastases are smooth and multiple.
- Lymphadenopathy not common; if lymphadenopathy is present, consider alternate diagnosis of lymphoma.
- Good response to Gleevec (competitively binds to ATP binding site of tyrosine kinase, leading to cell death by apoptosis; areas of apoptosis appear as cystic spaces on CT or MRI)
- PET is a sensitive modality for follow-up of patients on therapy.

METASTASES

Contiguous Spread

- From colon (gastrocolic, gastrosplenic ligament)
- From liver (gastrohepatic ligament)
- From pancreas: direct invasion

Hematogenous Spread to Stomach (Target Lesions)

- Melanoma (most common)
- Breast
- Lung

Imaging Features

- Diffuse uniform thickening, no distensible, absent gastric folds, linitis plastica
- Multiple lesions with bull's eye appearance: sharply demarcated with central ulcer (much bigger than aphthoid ulcer)

CARNEY'S TRIAD (RARE)

- Gastric leiomyosarcoma
- Functioning extraadrenal paraganglioma
- Pulmonary chondroma

BENIGN TUMORS

Benign tumors are usually submucosal.

- Leiomyoma: most common benign tumor; may ulcerate, 10% malignant
- Lipoma, fibroma, schwannoma, hemangioma, lymphangioma
- Carcinoid (malignant transformation in 20%)

GASTRIC VOLVULUS

Abnormal rotation of stomach. Two types: (Fig. 3-21)

Organoaxial

- Rotation around the long axis of stomach
- Stomach rotates 180° so that greater curvature is cranially located; upside-down stomach
- Observed in adults with large hiatal hernia
- Complications rare

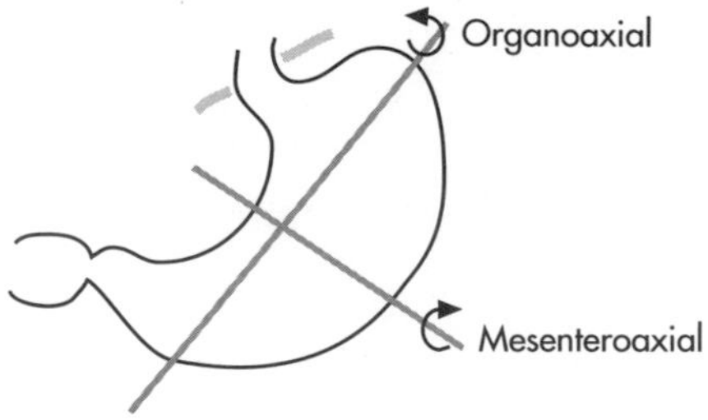

FIGURE 3-21

Mesenteroaxial
- Stomach rotates around its short axis (perpendicular to long axis)
- Fundus is caudal to antrum
- More common when large portions of stomach are above diaphragm (traumatic diaphragmatic rupture in children)
- Obstruction, ischemia likely

GASTRIC VARICES

Gastric varices represent dilated peripheral branches of short gastric and left gastric veins and appear as serpentine, nodular folds in body or fundus or as polypoid filling defects in the fundus.

Gastric varices are commonly associated with esophageal varices; the combination is often due to portal hypertension.

Gastric varices without esophageal varices are often caused by splenic vein obstruction and are most commonly secondary to pancreatitis or pancreatic carcinoma.

BENIGN GASTRIC EMPHYSEMA

Gas in wall of stomach is usually due to:
- Trauma from endoscopy, infection, ischemia, increased intraluminal pressure, vomiting, spontaneous or traumatic rupture of a pulmonary bulla into areolar tissue surrounding the esophagus
- No discernible underlying disease

Duodenum and Small Bowel

DUODENUM

NORMAL APPEARANCE

The duodenum has three segments: (Fig. 3-22)

Segment I
- Begins at pylorus and extends to the superior duodenal flexure
- Contains the duodenal bulb
- Intraperitoneal position: freely mobile

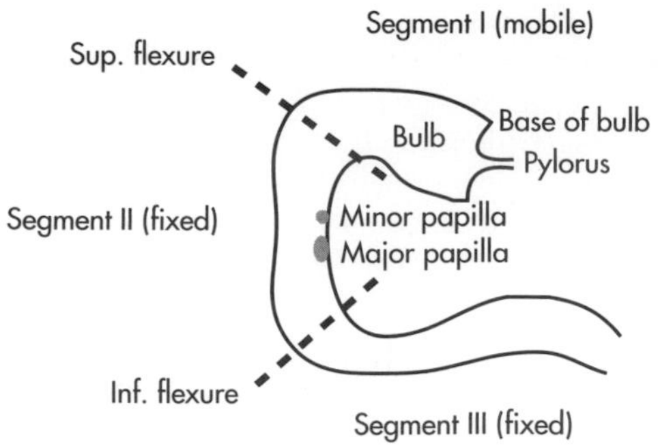

FIGURE 3-22

Segment II
- Begins at superior duodenal flexure and extends to inferior duodenal flexure
- Contains the major and minor papilla and the promontory
- Fixed retroperitoneal position

Segment III
- Extends from inferior duodenal flexure to ligament of Treitz
- Fixed retroperitoneal position

Mucosal Relief
- Folds in the duodenal bulb are longitudinally oriented.
- In the descending portion of the duodenum, Kerkring's folds are transversely oriented.
- These folds are usually visible despite complete duodenal distention.

Papilla (Fig. 3-23)

Major papilla (Vater's papilla): orifice for ducts
- Appears as round filling defect
- Located below the promontory
- 8 to 10 mm in length
- Abnormal if >15 mm

Minor papilla (accessory papilla, Santorini's papilla)
- Located superiorly and ventral to major papilla
- Mean distance from major papilla 20 mm
- Not usually visualized

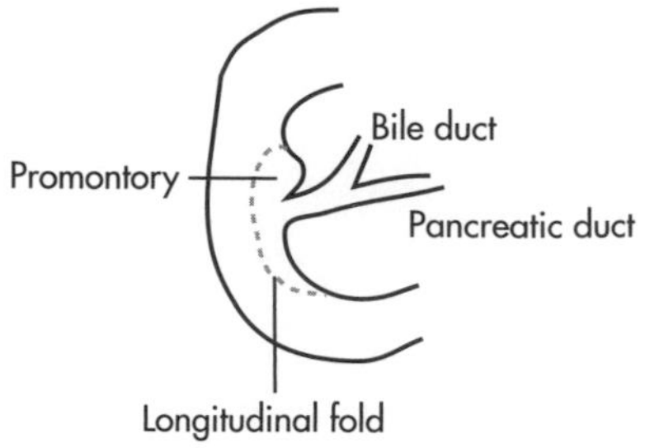

FIGURE 3-23

Promontory:
- Shoulder-like luminal projection along medial aspect of the second portion of the duodenum
- Begins superior to major papilla

DUODENAL ULCER (Fig. 3-24)

Duodenal ulcers are two to three times more common than gastric ulcers. All bulbar duodenal ulcers are considered benign. Postbulbar or multiple ulcers raise the suspicion for Zollinger-Ellison syndrome.

Bulbar, 95%
- Anterior wall: most common site, perforate
- Posterior wall: penetration into pancreas

Postbulbar, 5%

Predisposing Factors

- Chronic obstructive pulmonary disease
- Severe stress: injury, surgery, burn
- Steroids

Imaging Features

- Persistent round or elliptical collection; radiating folds, spasm
- Linear ulcers, 25%
- Kissing ulcers: 2 or more ulcers located opposite each other
- Giant ulcers
  - Crater is >2 cm.
  - Ulcer largely replaces the duodenal bulb.
  - A large ulcer crater may be mistaken for a deformed bulb but does not change shape during fluoroscopy.
- Duodenal ulcers often heal with a scar; this can lead to deformity and contraction of the duodenal bulb: cloverleaf deformity, or hourglass deformity.
- Postbulbar ulcers: any ulcer distal to the first portion of the duodenum should be considered to have underlying malignancy until proved otherwise (only 5% are benign ulcers, mostly secondary to Zollinger-Ellison syndrome).

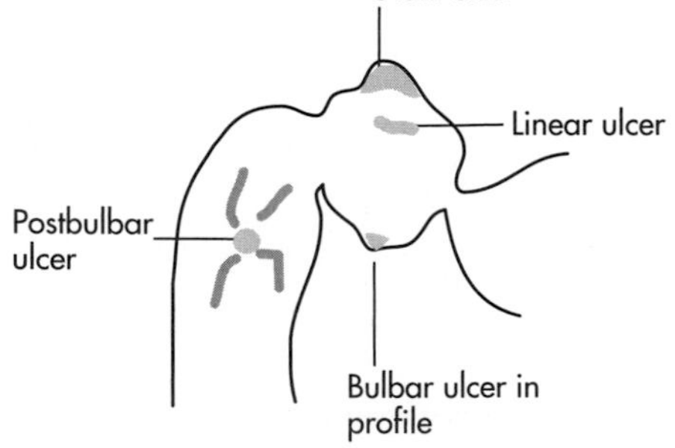

FIGURE 3-24

DUODENAL TRAUMA

Duodenal injuries are due either to penetrating (stab, gunshot) wounds or to blunt trauma (motor vehicle accident). Because the duodenum is immobile in retroperitoneum, most perforations occur there. Mortality of untreated duodenal rupture is 65%.

Location of Intestinal Trauma

- Duodenum/proximal jejunum, 95%
- Colon, 5%

Types of Injuries

- Perforation (requires surgery)
- Transection (requires surgery)
- Hematoma (nonsurgical treatment)

ORGAN INJURIES ASSOCIATED WITH DUODENAL TRAUMA

	Blunt Trauma (%)	Penetrating Trauma (%)
Liver	30	55
Pancreas	45	35
Spleen	25	2
Colon	15	10
Small bowel	10	25
Kidney	10	20

Imaging Features

Perforation:
- Extraluminal retroperitoneal gas
- Extravasation of oral contrast material

Perforation or hematoma:
- Thickening of duodenal wall or high density mass (clotted blood) can narrow the lumen
- Fluid in right anterior pararenal space or in the peritoneum
- Duodenal diverticula commonly project into head or uncinate process of pancreas and rarely present coming from lateral wall.

Surgical Treatment

- Simple repair
- Pyloric exclusion for complex injuries
- Whipple's procedure is rarely necessary.
- Surgical complications:
  - Intraabdominal abscess, 15%
  - Duodenal fistula, 4%
  - Duodenal dehiscence, 4%
  - Pancreatic fistula, 1%

BENIGN TUMORS

More common than malignant duodenal tumors.

Types

- Lipoma, leiomyoma (most common)
- Villous adenoma (cauliflower-like), adenomatous polyp
- Lymphoid hyperplasia
- Heterotopic gastric mucosa: Small angular filling defects in bulb, larger than nodules of lymphoid hyperplasia and smaller than Brunner's gland hyperplasia
- Brunner's gland hyperplasia
- Ectopic pancreas

ANTRAL MUCOSAL PROLAPSE

Anatomic variant characterized by movement of gastric mucosa bulging into the base of the duodenal bulb. No pathophysiologic significance.

Imaging Features

- Lobulated stellate filling defect in the duodenal bulb
- Filling defect in contiguity with antral rugal folds

MALIGNANT TUMORS

Infrequent. The most common locations of malignant tumors are in the periampullary and infraampullary areas.

Types

- Adenocarcinoma (most common)
- Leiomyosarcoma
- Lymphoma
- Metastases
- Benign tumors with malignant potential: villous and adenomatous polyps, carcinoid

UPPER GI SURGERY

Complications of Surgery (Fig. 3-25)

Immediate complications:
- Anastomotic leak
- Abscess
- Gastric outlet obstruction (edema)
- Bile reflux gastritis
- Ileus

Late complications:
- Bowel dysmotility: dumping, postvagotomy hypotonia
- Ulcer
- Bowel obstruction: outlet obstruction, adhesions, stricture
- Prolapse, intussusception
- Gastric carcinoma (in 5% of patients 15 years after surgery), Billroth II > Billroth I
- Metabolic effects: malabsorption
- Afferent loop syndrome
- Small pouch syndrome

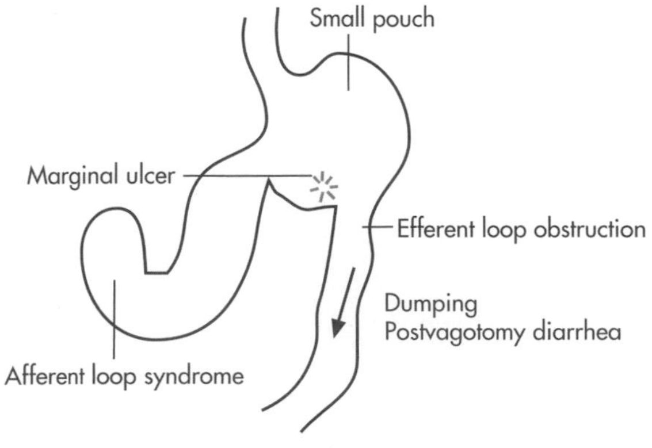

FIGURE 3-25

TYPES OF SURGERY

Type	Anastomosis/Surgery	Common Indication

Antireflux	Fundoplication (Nissen, Toupet, Belsey Mark IV)
	• Cuff of fundus surrounds distal esophagus
	• Distal esophagus smoothly narrowed for 2-4 cm
	• Soft tissue density (cuff) surrounds the narrowing
	• Complications:
	  • Distal esophagus too narrow
	  • Unraveling results in paraesophageal hernia
	  • Return of reflux
		Prevention of gastroesophageal reflux

Gastrectomy (Fig. 3-26, A)	Gastroduodenostomy (Billroth I)	Gastroduodenal ulcer
	Gastrojejunostomy (Billroth II)	Gastroduodenal ulcer
	Total gastrectomy	Gastric cancer
Vagotomy (Fig. 3-26, B)	Truncal vagotomy	
	Selective vagotomy	
	Parietal cell vagotomy	
	Drainage procedures	Facilitate gastric emptying after vagotomy
	Gastroenterostomy	
Palliative curative	Pancreaticoduodenectomy (Whipple) • Standard: Roux-en-Y choledochojejunostomy and pancreaticojejunostomy • Pylorus preserving	Pancreatic cancer

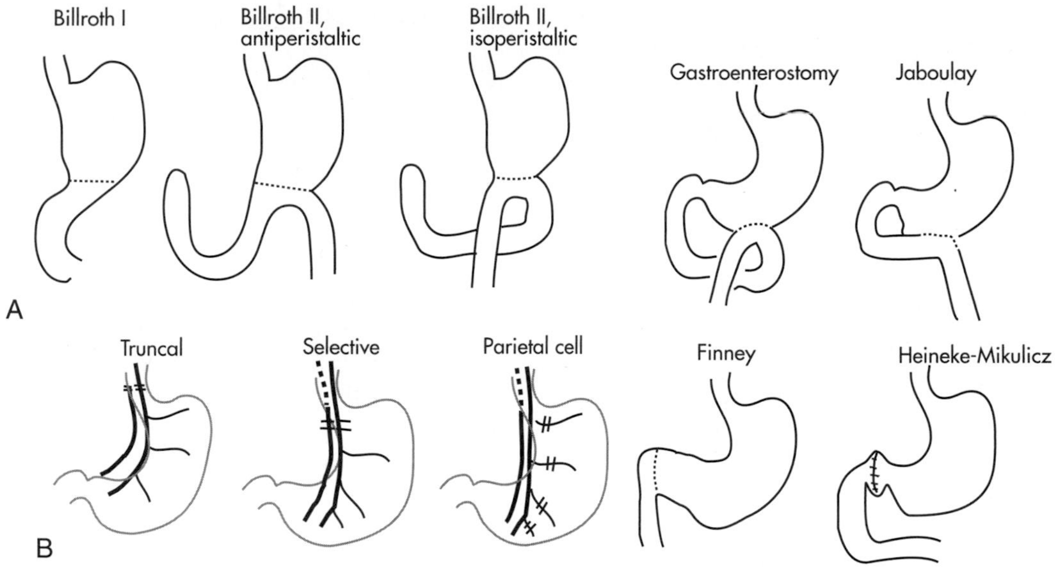

FIGURE 3-26

BARIATRIC SURGERY

Numerous bariatric surgical procedures exist, the most common being the Roux-en-Y gastric bypass. The laparoscopic approach to the Roux-en-Y gastric bypass is becoming the preferred method due to decreased hospital stays, faster recovery, and lower complications.

GASTRIC BYPASS (Fig. 3-27)

In gastric bypass surgery, a small gastric pouch (<30 mL) and a small gastrojejunostomy (<12 mm) are constructed (Roux-en-Y gastric bypass procedure). The remaining stomach is intact but functionally separate from food pathway. Currently, the Roux-en-Y gastric bypass combines restrictive and malabsorptive properties by creating a small gastric pouch and a Roux limb.

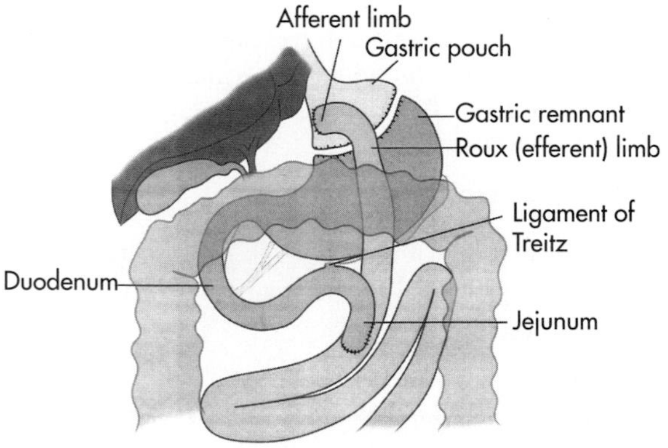

FIGURE 3-27

Complications

- Narrowing/stenosis
  - Immediate postsurgical narrowing is common and often subsides
  - Stenosis (lumen <6 mm) at >6 weeks after surgery is rare. Weight loss can be dramatic.
- Anastomotic leak
  - Incidence of leaks after Roux-en-Y bypass surgery is 1%-6%. More common after laparoscopic than open surgery.
  - The leak is commonly at the gastrojejunal anastomosis or at the enteroenteric anastomosis (both are life threatening).
  - Contrast material outside the confines of the gastric pouch and anastomosis indicates a leak. Although leaks from the enteroenteric anastomosis are rapidly clinically evident and severe, they are usually not diagnosed radiographically.
  - Immediate surgical exploration is needed
- Fistula
  - During surgery, the gastric pouch and remnant are surgically separated. Oral contrast should not directly enter the gastric remnant. The presence of oral contrast in the remnant thus indicates a gastro-gastric fistula.
  - Contrast may be seen in extruded stomach on SBFT by retrograde filling through the duodenum.
- Internal hernia: The most common herniation is the transmesenteric (or transmesocolonic) type, which occurs through the defect in the

transverse mesocolon. The herniated bowel is usually the Roux limb itself with a varying amount of additional small bowel loops. CT findings:
 Abnormal position of distended small bowel loops anterior to the pancreas and above the transverse colon; obstruction
 Inferior displacement of the transverse colon
 Crowding, engorgement, and deviation of mesenteric vessels
 The transition point is proximal to the jejunojejunostomy.
- Hernias may also occur in the small bowel mesenteric defect at the jejunojejunostomy site and in the space posterior to the Roux limb (Peterson type).
- Weight gain
  - Degradation of pouch restriction: very rapid passage of contrast through a patulous anastomosis degrades the restrictive properties of the laparoscopic Roux-en-Y gastric bypass, resulting in weight gain.

  Gastrogastric fistula. Although uncommon, a fistulous tract arising from the pouch may opacify the excluded stomach and is thought to be a result of the patient overeating

ADJUSTABLE GASTRIC BANDING

An adjustable band is laparoscopically placed around the proximal stomach, creating a small upper pouch 2 cm distal to the gastroesophageal junction. The cuff is connected to a reservoir placed in the anterior rectus sheath or subcutaneous tissues. The reservoir allows adjustment of band diameter percutaneously.

Complications:
 Band placed too low in stomach
 Band not placed around stomach
 Band placed around esophagus, which is undesirable because sensation of satiety lacking and risk of perforation
 Slippage of the band with upward herniation of stomach (late complication).

SLEEVE GASTRECTOMY

Left side (greater curvature and fundus) of stomach is surgically removed laparoscopically after staples are placed from the angle of His (angle formed as lateral border of esophagus meets the medial border of fundus) and the pylorus.

JEJUNUM AND ILEUM

NORMAL APPEARANCE

The small bowel can be examined by conventional small bowel follow-through (SBFT), enteroclysis, CT, or CT enteroclysis (the former two procedures are most common). The specific indications for enteroclysis are:
- Occult bleeding
- Recurrent obstructive symptoms
- Malabsorption
- To determine extent of Crohn disease

Normal Appearance of Small Bowel by SBFT

Luminal diameter
- >3 cm is abnormal

Fold thickness
- Valvulae conniventes measure 1 to 2 mm; more prominent in jejunum than ileum
- >3 mm is abnormal

Wall thickness
- Normal is 1 to 1.5 mm

Secretions
- There should normally be no appreciable fluid in small bowel.
- Excess secretions cause dilution of barium column.

CT

- Normal wall thickness: 1 to 1.5 mm
- Incomplete distention or luminal fluid may mimic abnormally thick wall; look for antidependent luminal gas collections to better assess wall thickness

JEJUNAL AND ILEAL DIVERTICULI

Jejunal and ileal outpouchings may predispose to bacterial overgrowth, vitamin B_{12} deficiency, and megoblastic anemia.

BLIND LOOP SYNDROME

Syndrome develops after bypassing small bowel by an enteroanastomosis with subsequent stagnation of bowel contents. Malabsorption in large diverticula may cause similar dynamics.

MALABSORPTION

Abnormal absorption of fat, water, protein, and carbohydrates from small bowel.

Imaging Features

- Dilatation of bowel loops
- Diluted barium (mixes with watery bowel content)

- Flocculated barium: barium aggregates into particles (mainly seen with older barium suspensions)
- Slow transit
- Segmentation of barium (lack of continuous column) rarely occurs with new agents
- Moulage pattern: featureless barium collection (rarely occurs with new agents)
- Hidebound pattern: valvulae thinner, closer together, wrinkled look
- Many of these features may no longer be seen with newer barium products.

Sprue

Three entities:

- Tropical sprue (unknown etiology; responds to antibiotics)
- Nontropical (adults; intolerance to gluten in wheat and other grains; HLA-DR3, IgA, IgM antibodies)
- Celiac disease (children)

Imaging Features

- Dilatation of small bowel is the most typical finding (caliber increases with severity of disease)
- Nodular changes in duodenum (bubbly duodenum)
- Reversal of jejunal and ileal fold patterns: "The jejunum looks like the ileum, the ileum looks like the jejunum, and the duodenum looks like hell."
- Segmentation
- Hypersecretion and mucosal atrophy cause the moulage sign (rare).
- Transient intussusception pattern (coiled spring) is typical.
- Increased secretions: flocculation with older barium suspensions
- Increased incidence of malignancy, aggressive lymphoma, carcinoma

Associated Disorders

- Dermatitis herpetiformis
- Selective immunoglobulin A deficiency
- Hyposplenism
- Adenopathy
- Cavitary mesenteric lymph node syndrome

Complications

- Ulcerative jejunoileitis: several segments of bowel wall thickening with irregularity and ulceration strictures may follow
- Enteropathy: associated T-cell lymphoma
- Increased incidence of cancers of esophagus, pharynx, duodenum, and rectum
- Sprue, small bowel obstruction, scleroderma (SOS): dilated, prolonged motility, normal folds

OTHER DISEASES CAUSING MALABSORPTION PATTERN*

Disease	Primary Pattern	Comment
Scleroderma	AM + D, hidebound folds	Muscularis replaced by fibrosis
Whipple	DFTN, adenopathy may occur	Intestinal lipodystrophy
Amyloidosis	DFTN	Tiny nodule filling defects
Lymphangiectasia	DFTN, MA	Dilated lymphatics in wall
Ig deficiencies	DFTN	Nodular lymphoid hyperplasia
Mastocytosis	DFTN	Hepatomegaly, PUD, dense bones
Eosinophilic gastroenteritis	Very thick folds (polypoid)	Food allergy, 70%
Graft-versus-host disease	Effaced folds (ribbon-like)	Bone marrow transplants
MAI infection	DFTN, MA, pseudo-Whipple	Immunocompromised host

*See also Infectious Enteritis.
AM, abnormal motility; D, dilatation; DFTN, diffuse fold thickening with fine nodularity; MA, mesenteric adenopathy; MAI, *Mycobacterium avium-intracellulare*.

MASTOCYTOSIS

Systemic mast cell proliferation in reticuloendothelial system (RES) (small bowel, liver, spleen, lymph nodes, bone marrow) and skin (95%) with histamine release.

Clinical Findings

- Diarrhea
- Steatorrhea
- Histamine effects (flushing, tachycardia, pruritus, PUD)

Imaging Features

Small bowel

- Irregular fold thickening
- Diffuse small nodules

Other

- Sclerotic bone lesions
- Hepatosplenomegaly
- Peptic ulcers (increased HCI secretion)

AMYLOIDOSIS

Heterogeneous group of disorders characterized by abnormal extracellular deposition of insoluble fibrillar protein material. Diagnosis is established by biopsy of affected organs (birefringence, staining with Congo red). Clinical amyloidosis syndromes include:

Systemic amyloidosis

- Immunocyte dyscrasia (myeloma, monoclonal gammopathy)
- Chronic/active disease (see below)
- Hereditary syndromes

Neuropathic form
Nephropathic form
Cardiomyopathic form
- Chronic hemodialysis
- Senile form

Localized amyloidosis
- Cerebral amyloid angiopathy (Alzheimer disease, senile dementia)
- Cutaneous form
- Ocular form
- Others

Common chronic/active diseases that are associated with systemic amyloidosis (there are many, less common causes):

Infections (recurrent and chronic)
- Tuberculosis (TB)
- Chronic osteomyelitis
- Decubitus ulcers
- Bronchiectasis
- Chronic pyelonephritis

Chronic inflammatory disease
- Rheumatoid arthritis (5%-20% of cases)
- Ankylosing spondylitis
- Crohn disease
- Reiter syndrome
- Psoriasis

Neoplasm
- Hodgkin disease (4% of cases)
- Renal cell carcinoma (3% of cases)

Imaging Features

Kidneys
- Nephrotic syndrome
- Renal insufficiency
- RTA
- Renal vein thrombosis

GI tract
- Diffuse thickening of small bowel folds
- Jejunization of ileum
- Small bowel dilatation
- Multiple nodular filling defects, >2 mm
- Hepatosplenomegaly
- Macroglossia
- Colonic pseudodiverticulosis (may be unilateral and large)

Heart
- Cardiomyopathy (restrictive)
- Rhythm abnormalities

Nervous system
- Signs of dementia
- Carpal tunnel syndrome
- Peripheral neuropathy

INTESTINAL LYMPHANGIECTASIA

Spectrum of lymphatic abnormality (dilated lymphatics in lamina propria of small bowel) that clinically results in protein-losing enteropathy.

Congenital (infantile) form presents with:
- Generalized lymphedema
- Chylous pleural effusions
- Diarrhea, steatorrhea
- Lymphocytopenia

Acquired (adult) form due to:
- Obstruction of thoracic duct (radiation, tumors, retroperitoneal fibrosis)
- Small bowel lymphoma
- Pancreatitis

Imaging Features

- Diffuse nodular thickening of folds in jejunum and ileum due to dilated lymphatics and hypoalbuminemic edema; mesenteric adenopathy on CT
- Dilution of contrast material due to hypersecretion
- Lymphographic studies
  - Hypoplastic lymphatics of lower extremity
  - Tortuous thoracic duct
  - Hypoplastic lymph nodes

GASTROINTESTINAL LYMPHOMA

Distinct subgroup of lymphoma that primarily arises in lymphoid tissue of the bowel rather than in lymph nodes.

GI lymphoma in otherwise healthy patients:
- Gastric lymphoma arising from mucosa-associated lymphoid tissue (MALT)
- Usually low-grade malignancy
- Represent 20% of malignant small bowel tumors; usual age: 5th to 6th decade
- Imaging features
  - Mass, nodule, fold thickening (focal or diffuse) confined to GI tract in 50%
  - Adenopathy, 30%
  - Extraabdominal findings, 30%
- Large ulcerated mass presenting as endoenteric or exoenteric tumor (differential diagnosis: gastrointestinal stromal tumor, metastatic melanoma, jejunal diverticulitis with abscess, ectopic pancreas)
- Aneurysmal dilatation: localized dilated, thick-walled, noncontractile lumen due to mural tumor; Auerbach plexus neuropathy

GI lymphoma in HIV-positive or immunosuppressed patients:
- Usually aggressive NHL with rapid spread, poor response to chemotherapy, short survival
- Widespread extraintestinal involvement, 80%
- Imaging features

GI abnormalities: nodules, fold thickening, mass
  - Splenomegaly, 30%
  - Adenopathy, 30%
  - Ascites, 20%

GRAFT-VERSUS-HOST (GVH) REACTION

Donor lymphocytes react against organs (GI tract, skin, liver) of the recipient after bone marrow transplant. Pathology: granular necrosis of crypt epithelium.

Imaging Features

- Classic finding: small bowel loops, which are too narrow, and featureless margins (ribbon bowel)
- Luminal narrowing is due to edema of the bowel wall.
- Flattening of mucosal folds (edema)
- Prolonged coating of barium for days

SCLERODERMA

Scleroderma or progressive systemic sclerosis (PSS) is a systemic disease that involves primarily skin, joints, and the GI tract (esophagus > small bowel > colon > stomach). Age: 30 to 50 years; female > male.

Imaging Features

Small bowel
- Dilation of bowel loops with hypomotility is a key feature.
- Mucosal folds are tight and closer together (fibrosis): hidebound appearance.
- Pseudosacculations along antimesenteric border, may involve both small and large bowel.
- Segmentation, fragmentation, hypersecretion are absent.

Other
- Dilated dysmotile esophagus, esophagitis, incompetent LES, reflux, stricture
- Dilated duodenum and colon (pseudo-obstruction)
- Pneumatosis cystoids coli (steroid therapy)
- Pulmonary interstitial fibrosis
- Acroosteolysis
- Soft tissue calcification

WHIPPLE DISEASE

Rare multisystem disease, probably of bacterial origin. Structures primarily involved include SI joints, joint capsule, heart valves, CNS, and jejunum.

Clinical Findings

- Middle-aged men, US, Northern Europe
- Diarrhea, steatorrhea
- Immune defects

Imaging Features

- 1- to 2-mm diffuse micronodules in jejunum
- No dilatation or increased secretions
- Nodal masses in mesentery (echogenic by US); nodes have low CT density
- Sacroiliitis

ENTERIC FISTULAS

Fistulas of small bowel with adjacent structures can be seen with Crohn disease, colorectal cancer, after surgery, and in diverticular disease.

Types

- Enteroenteric: small bowel → small bowel
- Enterocolonic: small bowel → colon
- Enterocutaneous: small bowel → skin
- Enterovesical: small bowel → bladder
- Enterovaginal: small bowel → vagina

Radiographic Workup

- Fistulogram (enterocutaneous fistula): injection of water-soluble contrast material through small catheter inserted into fistula
- UGI and SBFT
- Barium enema

Therapy

- Total parenteral nutrition to achieve "bowel rest"
- Postoperative fistulas usually heal spontaneously with conservative measures.
- Fistulas in active Crohn disease usually require excision of diseased bowel.
- Cyclosporine and other immunosuppressants have been used to heal fistulas in Crohn disease; more recently monoclonal antibody (infliximab) has been used.

DRUG CHEMOTHERAPY-INDUCED ENTERITIS

- Chemotherapeutic agents can induce spontaneous gastrointestinal edema, necrosis, and even perforation.
- Most common in long-term immunosuppressive treatment to prevent homograft rejection or in those receiving long-term chemotherapy for leukemia or lymphoma
- CT findings can be seen in diseased or disease-free intestinal segments.
- Chemotherapy-induced enteropathy appears as nonspecific focal or diffuse bowel wall thickening with or without the target sign or as regional mesenteric vascular engorgement and haziness, more often in distal small bowel.
- ACE inhibitors may cause angioedema resulting in reversible wall thickening.

INFECTIOUS ENTERITIS

Cryptosporidiosis

Cryptosporidium species are protozoa that frequently cause enteritis in AIDS patients but rarely in immunocompetent patients. Diagnosis is made by examination of stool or duodenal aspirate.

COMMON RADIOGRAPHIC PRESENTATIONS

Infection	Common Radiographic Patterns
Parasites	
Hookworms *(Necator, Ancylostoma)*	TFN
Tapeworms	FD
Ascaris	FD, intestinal obstruction
Infectious (Fig. 3-28)	
Yersinia enterocolitica	TFN, ulcers, TI
TB	Stricture → obstruction, TI
Histoplasmosis	TFN
Salmonellosis	TFN, TI
Campylobacter	TFN, loss of haustration, TI
Common in AIDS	
Cytomegalovirus	TF in cecum, pancolitis
Tuberculosis	TF in cecum; adenopathy (low central attenuation), TI
MAI	TFN, adenopathy (homogeneous)
Cryptosporidiosis	TFN
Giardiasis	TFN, largely jejunal, jejunal spasm

FD, worm seen as filling defect in bowel; MAI, *Mycobacterium avium-intracellulare*; TF, thickened folds; TFN, thickened folds with nodularity; TI, terminal ileum commonly involved.

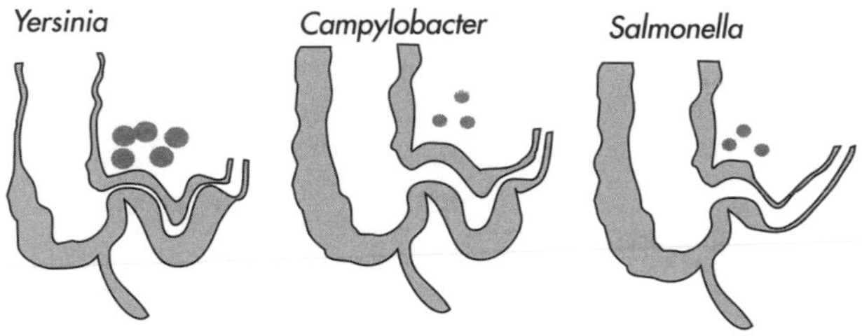

FIGURE 3-28

Imaging Features

- Thickened small bowel folds
- Dilatation of small bowel

INTESTINAL HELMINTHS

OVERVIEW

Organism (Treatment)	Route	Clinical Findings
Nematode (Mebendazole)		
*Ascaris lumbricoides**	Fecal-oral	Intestinal, biliary obstruction, PIE
Ancylostoma duodenale	Skin penetration	Iron-deficiency anemia, PIE
Necator americanus	Skin penetration	Iron-deficiency anemia, PIE
Strongyloides stercoralis	Skin penetration	Malabsorption, PIE
Nematode (Mebendazole)		
Trichuris trichiura	Fecal-oral	Rectal prolapse
Enterobius vermicularis	Fecal-oral	
Cestode (Praziquantel)		
Beef tapeworm (*Taenia saginata*)	Raw beef	
Pork tapeworm *(Taenia solium)*	Raw pork	Cysticercosis: CNS
Fish tapeworm	Raw fish	Vitamin B_{12} deficiency
Dwarf tapeworm	Fecal-oral	Diarrhea
Trematode (Praziquantel)		
Heterophyes heterophyes	Raw fish	Diarrhea
Metagonimus yokogawai	Raw fish	Diarrhea

*Worms in GI tract visible by barium studies.
CNS, central nervous system; PIE, pulmonary infiltrates with eosinophilia.

Ascariasis (Fig. 3-29)

Infection with *Ascaris lumbricoides* (roundworm, 15 to 35 cm long) is the most common parasitic infection worldwide.

Imaging Features

GI tract
- Jejunum > ileum, duodenum, stomach
- Worms visible on SBFT as longitudinal filling defects
- Enteric canal of worm is filled with barium
- Worms may cluster: "bolus of worm"
- Mechanical small bowel obstruction (SBO)
- Other complications: perforation, volvulus

Biliary tract
- Intermittent biliary obstruction
- Granulomatous stricture of bile duct (rare)
- Oriental cholangiohepatitis

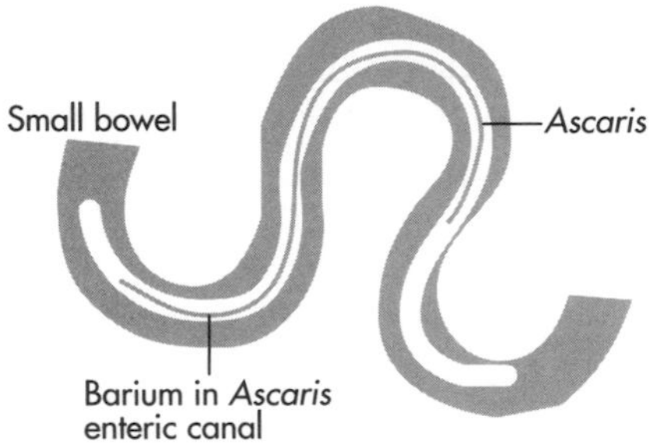

FIGURE 3-29

CARCINOID TUMORS

Carcinoid tumors arise from enterochromaffin cells.
Location:
GI tract, 85%
- Location: appendix, 50% > small bowel (33%), gastric, colon and rectum (2%); virtually never occur in esophagus

- 90% of small bowel carcinoids arise in distal ileum
- 30% of small bowel carcinoids are multiple; 40%-80% of GI tract carcinoids spread to mesentery

Bronchial tree, 15%
- 90% central, 10% peripheral

Other rare locations
- Thyroid
- Teratomas (ovarian, testicular)

Symptoms of GI carcinoids:
- Asymptomatic, 70%; obstruction, 20%; weight loss, 15%; palpable mass, 15%

CARCINOID SYNDROME

Ninety percent of patients with carcinoid syndrome have liver metastases. The tumor produces ACTH, histamine, bradykinin, kallikrein, serotonin (excreted as 5-HIAA in urine), causing:
- Recurrent diarrhea, 70%
- Right-sided endocardial fibroelastosis → tricuspid insufficiency, pulmonary valvular stenosis (left side of heart is spared because of metabolism by monoamine oxidase inhibitor in lung)
- Wheezing, bronchospasm, 15%
- Flushing of face and neck

Imaging Features
- Mass lesion in small bowel: filling defect
- Strong desmoplastic reaction causes angulation, kinking of bowel loops (tethered appearance), mesenteric venous congestion
- Mesenteric mass on CT with spokewheel pattern is virtually pathognomonic; the only other disease that causes this appearance is retractile mesenteritis (very rare).
- Stippled calcification in mesenteric mass
- Obstruction secondary to desmoplastic reaction
- Very vascular tumors (tumor blush at angiography, very hyperintense on T2-weighted images)
- Liver metastases (arterial phase indicated)

Complications
- Ischemia with mesenteric venous compromise
- Hemorrhage
- Malignant degeneration: gastric and appendiceal tumors rarely metastasize; small bowel tumors metastasize commonly.

RADIATION ENTERITIS

- Damage of small bowel mucosa and wall due to therapeutic radiation
- Highest to lowest tolerance: duodenum > jejunum, ileum > transverse colon, sigmoid colon > esophagus and rectum
- Tolerance dose (TD 5/5) is the total dose that produces radiation damage in 5% of patients within 5 years; TD 5/5 is 4500 cGy in small bowel and colon and 5000 cGy in rectum.
- Findings: mural thickening and luminal narrowing, usually in pelvic bowel loops, after treatment of gynecologic or urinary bladder cancers
- Long-term sequelae: narrowing or stenosis of affected segment; adhesions with angulation between adjacent loops; reduced or absent peristalsis

Colon

GENERAL

BARIUM ENEMA (BE)

Patient Preparation
- Clear liquid diet day before examination
- Magnesium citrate, 300 mL, afternoon before examination
- 50 mL castor oil evening before examination
- Cleansing enema morning of examination

Single-Contrast Technique
1. Insert tube with patient in lateral position.
2. Decide if need to inflate balloon for retention; if so, inflate under fluoroscopic control, being sure that balloon is in the rectum.
3. Fluoroscopy as the barium goes in.
4. Patient in supine position (as opposed to double-contrast study). Instill barium just beyond sigmoid colon. Take AP and two oblique spot films of sigmoid.
5. Try to follow head of column fluoroscopically.
6. Take spot views of both splenic flexure and hepatic flexure.
7. Spot cecum and terminal ileum. If a filling defect is encountered, palpate to see if it is sessile or floating.
8. Obtain overhead views and postevacuation films.

Double-Contrast Technique
1. Patient is in lateral position. Insert tube.
2. Patient supine: administer glucagon IV. Turn patient prone: this helps barium flow to the descending colon, decreases pooling in the rectum and sigmoid, and thereby is less uncomfortable. Instill barium beyond the splenic flexure. Stand patient up, bag to the floor, and let barium drain.
3. Place patient in horizontal prone position. Start slow inflation with air and rotate patient toward you into a supine position. Take spot views of the sigmoid in different obliquities (take spots

of any air-filled loop). When patient is supine, check to see if barium has already coated the ascending colon.
4. Stand patient up to facilitate coating of ascending colon. Drain as much barium as possible through rectal tube. Insufflate more air.
5. Spot views of splenic and hepatic flexure in upright position. Take spots in slightly different obliquities of both flexures.
6. Patient prone; put table down. Take spot views of the cecum and sigmoid.
7. Obtain overhead views:
   AP, PA
   Prone, cross-table lateral
   Decubitus
   Postevacuation films

Contraindications to BE

- Suspected colonic perforation (use water-soluble iodinated contrast)
- Patients at risk for intraperitoneal leakage (use Gastrografin):
  Severe colitis
  Toxic megacolon
  Recent deep biopsy
- If colonoscopy *needs* to follow enema; use water-soluble iodinated contrast
- Severe recent disease: myocardial infarction, cerebrovascular accident (CVA)

Complications of BE

- Perforation (incidence 1:5000), typically due to overinflation or traumatic insertion of balloon or fragile colonic walls
- Appearance of gas in portal venous system in patients with inflammatory bowel disease (no significant ill effects)
- Allergy to latex tips

Glucagon

Glucagon is a 29–amino acid peptide produced in A cells of the pancreas.

Physiologically, the main stimulus for glucagon release is hunger (hypoglycemia). Effects:

- Antagonist to insulin (increases blood glucose)
- Relaxation of smooth muscle cells
- Relaxation of gallbladder sphincter and sphincter of Oddi; increased bile flow

Glucagon is a useful adjunct (0.1 to 1 mg IV) to barium enema or whenever smooth muscle spasm is suspected producing "pseudostenotic lesion." Thus it can be used in evaluation of the esophagus, stomach, duodenum, small intestine, common bile duct, and colon. Contraindications include:

- Pheochromocytoma
- Insulinoma
- Glaucoma

CT COLONOGRAPHY (CTC)

- Replacing DCBE for detecting and screening of colonic neoplasms.
- Helically acquired axial images of the gas-distended colon are obtained during breath holding in both prone and supine positions.
- Images are combined into a detailed model of the colon subsequently viewed using either 2-D multiplanar reconstructions or primary 3-D endoluminal display.
- Standard examination does not require intravenous contrast and uses extremely low dose x-ray technique, typically 20% radiation of standard diagnostic CT, and approximately 10% less than double-contrast barium enema.
- Detection of large polyps (>10 mm) is comparable with optical colonoscopy (OC); detection of polyps 6 to 9 mm approximately equal to OC; detection of polyps <6 mm, OC is superior.
- Studies using latest techniques (primary 3-D visualization, fecal tagging) demonstrate sensitivity of 92% for polyps >10 mm; per patient specificity 96%
- Currently requires cathartic bowel preparation similar to that for fiberoptic colonoscopy

MR ENTEROGRAPHY (MRE)

- Performed to evaluate the small and large bowel in patients with inflammatory bowel disease
- MRE has the advantage of depicting extraluminal abnormalities, the ability to distinguish active from fibrotic strictures and better delineating fistulas. There is no ionizing radiation.
- Despite the advantages, there are some limitations, foremost the relatively long acquisition times. It may be difficult to identify early mucosal lesions.
- Optimal amount of oral contrast for MRE is approximately 1300 mL
- Types of oral contrast for MRE:
  - Positive: increased signal of bowel lumen on T1 and T2; solutions containing carbohydrate sugar alcohols (VoLumen) or gadolinium-based agents
  - Negative: decreased signal of bowel lumen on T1 and T2; iron oxide containing oral contrast (Gastromark)
- Typical patient preparation for MRE
  - Fasting for 6 hours before procedure
- Sequences for MRE
  - HASTE or SSFSE; insensitive to motion. Provides high contrast between lumen and bowel wall
  - High resolution ultrafast balanced GRE (FIESTA, True FISP). Insensitive to motion and provides uniform luminal opacification. Ideal for detection, mesenteric findings in patients with Crohn disease

- T2-weighted (fat saturated) or STIR. Ideal for detection of fistulas and for correlating inflammatory changes with gadolinium enhanced images.
- T1-weighted 3-D gradient echo sequence before and after gadolinium administration. Primarily used to assess bowel wall enhancement, extraluminal findings

POLYPS

A wide variety of colonic polyps exist. Nonneoplastic, hyperplastic polyps have been cited as the most frequent type for a long time.

OVERVIEW

	Single Polyp	Multiple Polyps
Neoplastic		
Epithelial	Tubular adenoma	Familial polyposis
	Tubulovillous adenoma	Gardner syndrome
	Villous adenoma	
	Turcot syndrome	
Nonepithelial	Carcinoid	
	Leiomyoma	
	Lipoma	
	Fibroma	
Nonneoplastic		
Hamartomas	Juvenile polyposis	Cronkhite-Canada syndrome
	Peutz-Jeghers syndrome	
Inflammatory	Benign lymphoid polyp	Juvenile polyp, benign lymphoid polyp
	Fibroid granulation polyp	Granulomatous colitis
Unclassified	Hyperplastic polyp	Hyperplastic polyposis

ADENOMATOUS POLYPS

Most common true colonic tumor (in up to 10% of the population by the 7th decade). Up to 50% of polyps are multiple.

Clinical Findings

- Asymptomatic
- Diarrhea
- Pain
- Hemorrhage

TYPES OF ADENOMATOUS POLYPS

	Tubular	Tubulovillous	Villous
Frequency	64%	27%	9%
Malignancy potential			
0.5-0.9 cm	0.3%	1%	2%
1-1.9 cm	4%	7%	6%
2.0-2.9 cm	7%	11%	17%

Location (Fig. 3-30)

- Rectum and sigmoid, 60%
- Descending colon, 15%
- Transverse colon, 15%
- Ascending colon, 10%

Differentiation of Benign and Malignant Polyps

- Histologic differentiation of polyps is invariably difficult radiographically, so the majority of lesions require endoscopic sampling.

BENIGN VERSUS MALIGNANT POLYPS

Feature	Benign	Malignant
Size*	<1 cm	>2 cm
Stalk	Present (pedunculated, thin)	Absent (sessile)
Contour	Smooth	Irregular, lobulated
Number	Single	Multiple
Underlying colonic wall	Smooth	Indented, retracted

*The larger the size of any polyp, the more likely it is malignant: <1 cm: 0.4%, 1 to 2 cm: 4%, >2 cm: >10%.

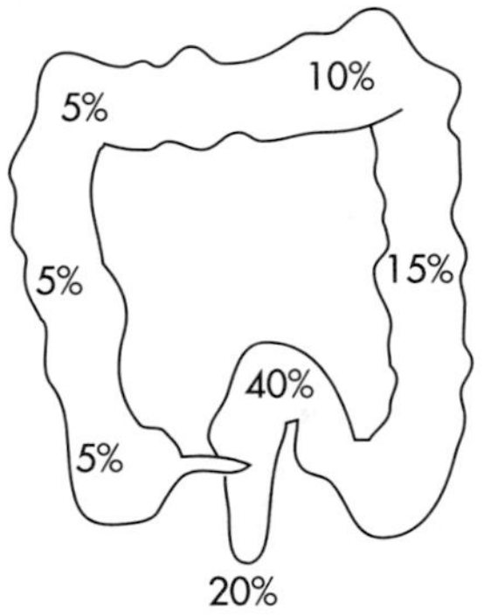

FIGURE 3-30

ADVANCED ADENOMA (Fig. 3-31)

- Polyp ≥1 cm, high-grade dysplasia
- Of all polyps <1 cm, the likelihood that a lesion is an advanced adenoma is 3% (the majority are hyperplastic and the rest are benign adenomas).

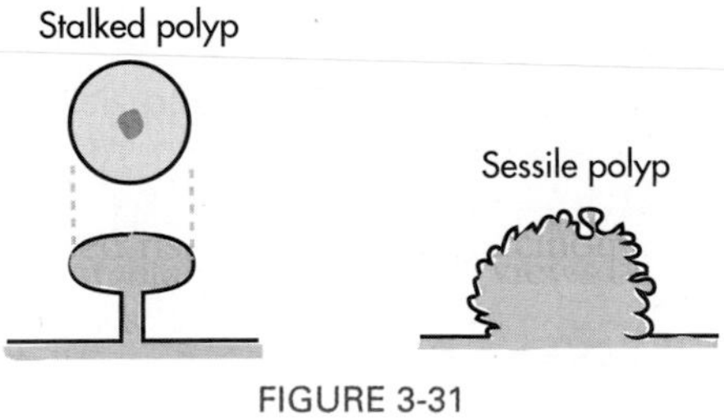

FIGURE 3-31

HYPERPLASTIC POLYPS

Focal proliferation of normal mucosa, hence not an adenoma. Hyperplastic polyps have no malignant potential. Hyperplastic polyps are due to excessive cellular proliferation in Lieberkühn's crypts. 75% of polyps occur distal to the splenic flexure, mostly in the rectosigmoid area.

Imaging Features

- Stalked polyp
- Sessile but <5 mm

POSTINFLAMMATORY POLYPS (PIPS)

Postinflammatory polyposis (pseudopolyposis, filiform polyps) represents a benign condition, not associated with cancer. PIPS occur most commonly in Crohn disease and ulcerative colitis due to regeneration of nonulcerated tissue.

Imaging Features

- Filiform polyps: thin, short, branching structures

DIFFERENTIATION OF TRUE POLYPS FROM PSEUDOPOLYPS

	Polyp	Pseudopolyp
Size	Uniform in size	Uniform in size
Form	Round, stalked, sessile	Y-shaped, filiform, irregular
Margins	Well delineated	Fuzzy (inflammation)
Colonic haustra	Preserved	Distorted (inflammation)

POLYPOSIS SYNDROMES

Familial Polyposis

- Most common intestinal polyposis syndrome (incidence 1:8000)
- Screening of family members of familial polyposis patients should start at puberty: malignant degeneration by 40 years (treatment: prophylactic total proctocolectomy)
- Usually >100 polyps
- Polyps may be sessile or stalked.
- Familial adenomatous polyposis syndrome (FAPS) is a common umbrella name under which Gardner and familial polyposis syndromes are included.

Gardner Syndrome

- Polyposis: colon 100%, duodenum 90%, other bowel segments <10%
- Hamartomas of stomach
- Soft tissue tumors: inclusion cysts, desmoids (30%), fibrosis
- Osteoma in calvarium, mandible, sinuses
- Entrapment of cranial nerves
- Malignant transformation in 100% if untreated
- Small bowel and pancreaticoduodenal malignancies
- Total colectomy recommended

Peutz-Jeghers Syndrome

- Second most common intestinal polyposis
- Autosomal dominant
- Hamartomas throughout GI tract except the esophagus
- Mucocutaneous pigmentations (buccal mucosa, palm, sole)
- Polyps have virtually no malignant potential.
- Slightly increased risk of stomach, duodenal, and ovarian cancer; benign neoplasm of testes, thyroid, and GU system

OVERVIEW

Type	Trait	Gastric	SB	Colon	Histology	GI Malignancy	Extraintestinal
Familial polyposis	AD	<5%	<5%	100%	Adenoma	100%	—
Gardner	AD	5%	5%	100%	Adenoma	100%	Osteoma, others*
Peutz-Jeghers	AD	25%	95%	30%	Hamartoma	Rare	Perioral pigmentation
Juvenile polyposis	AD	—	—	100%	Inflammatory	?	—
Turcot	AR	—	—	100%	Adenoma	100%	Glioma
Cronkhite-Canada	NH	100%	50%	100%	Inflammatory	None	Ectodermal changes
Cowden†	AD	—	—	—	Hamartoma	None	Oral papilloma‡
Ruvalcaba-Myhre†	AD	Yes	Yes	Yes	Hamartoma	None	Macrocephaly, penile macules, mental retardation, SC lipomas

*Soft tissue tumors, sarcomas, ampullary carcinoma, ovarian carcinoma.
†Extremely rare.
‡Gingival hyperplasia, breast cancer, thyroid cancer.
AD, autosomal dominant; AR, autosomal recessive; NH, nonhereditary; SB, small bowel; SC, subcutaneous.

Juvenile Polyposis
- Usually large polyps in rectum
- Usually single; 80% are located in the rectosigmoid.
- Present in children with bleeding, prolapse, or obstruction

Cowden Disease
- Multiple hamartoma syndrome
- Mucocutaneous pigmentations (buccal mucosa, palm, sole)
- Most common in rectosigmoid with lesions also present in esophagus
- Mucocutaneous lesions → facial papules, oral mucosal papillomatosis, acral keratoses, sclerotic fibromas
- Thyroid gland abnormalities: goiter, adenomas
- Breast cancer (ductal), bilateral in 30%
- Uterine and cervical carcinomas
- Transitional cell carcinoma of bladder and ureter

Lhermitte-Duclos Disease
- Gangliocytoma of cerebellar cortex

Turcot Syndrome
- Glioma polyposis syndrome
- Colonic adenomas with CNS gliomas and medulloblastomas

COLON CARCINOMA

GENERAL
Third most common cancer in both men and women. Risk factor: low-carbohydrate diet? Synchronous lesions, 5%; metachronous lesions, 3%.

CANCER RISK FACTORS
- Personal history of colorectal cancer or adenomatous polyps
- Personal history of chronic inflammatory bowel disease
- Strong family history of colorectal cancer or polyps (cancer or polyps in a first-degree relative younger than 60 or in two first-degree relatives of any age).

Note: A first-degree relative is defined as a parent, sibling, or child.

Family history of a hereditary colorectal cancer syndrome (familial adenomatous polyposis or hereditary nonpolyposis colon cancer)

Location
- Rectum, 35%
- Sigmoid, 25%
- Descending colon, 10%
- Ascending colon, 10%
- Transverse colon, 10%
- Cecum, 10%

Imaging Features (Fig. 3-32)
- Polypoid
- Ulcerative
- Annular constricting (apple core); <5 cm long
- Plaquelike (e.g., cloacogenic tumor at anorectal junction)
- Scirrhous carcinoma (rare): long (>5 cm) circumferential spread

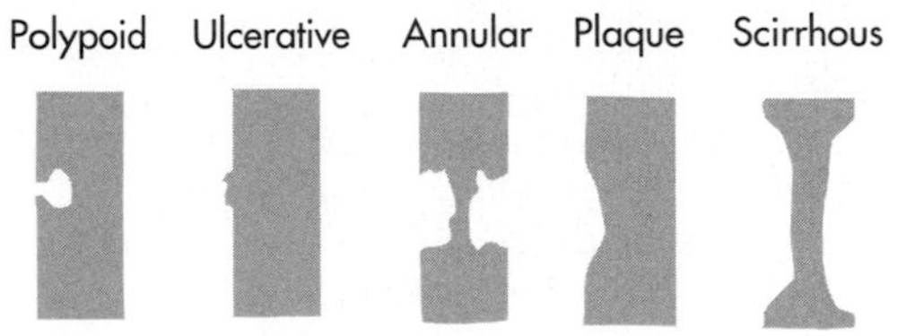

FIGURE 3-32

Complications
- Obstruction
- Intussusception (in polypoid lesions), rare
- Local perforation (simulates diverticulitis)
- Local tumor recurrence in 30%-50%
- Peritoneal spread

Staging (Fig. 3-33)
Dukes staging system
- Dukes A: limited to bowel wall, 15%
- Dukes B: extension into serosa or mesenteric fat, 35%
- Dukes C: lymph node metastases, 50%
- Dukes D: distant metastases: liver, 25%; hydronephrosis, 10%; peritoneal cavity, adrenal, 10%

TNM Classification
Tx: No description of the tumor's extent is possible.

Tis: The cancer is in the earliest stage. It has not grown beyond the mucosa (inner layer) of the colon or rectum. This stage is also known as carcinoma in situ or intramucosal carcinoma.

T1: Cancer has grown through the mucosa and extends into the submucosa.

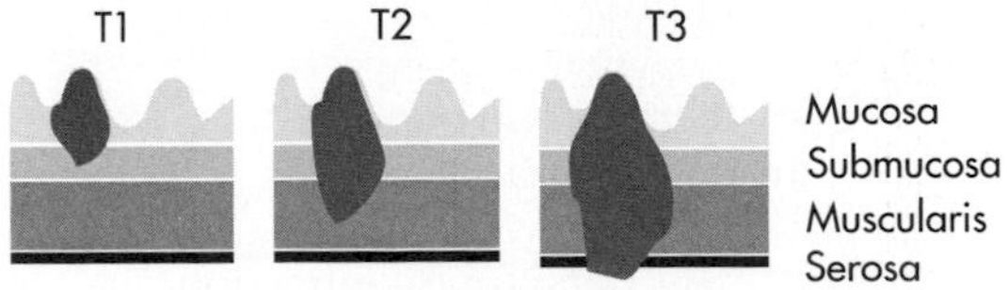

FIGURE 3-33

T2: Cancer has grown through the submucosa, and extends into the muscularis propria.
T3: Cancer has grown completely through the muscularis propria into the subserosa but not to any neighboring organs or tissues.
T4: Cancer has spread completely through the wall of the colon or rectum into nearby tissues or organs.
Nx: No description of lymph node involvement is possible because of incomplete information.
N0: No lymph node involvement.
N1: Cancer cells found in 1 to 3 nearby lymph nodes.
N2: Cancer cells found in 4 or more nearby lymph nodes.
Mx: No description of distant spread is possible because of incomplete information.
M0: No distant spread is seen.
M1: Distant spread is present.

Diagnostic Accuracy

Detection of lymph node metastases
- CT: 50%-70%
- MRI currently < CT

Detection of liver metastases
- Contrast-enhanced CT: 60%-70%
- MRI: 70%-80%

COLITIS

Etiology

Idiopathic inflammatory bowel disease
- Ulcerative colitis (UC)
- Crohn disease
- Behçet disease

Infectious colitis
Ischemic colitis
Iatrogenic
- Radiation
- Chemotherapy

Imaging Features

The imaging features of bowel inflammation (any etiology) depend mainly on the location of the process:

Mucosal inflammation
- Ulceration
  - Shallow: granularity of mucosa, aphthoid
  - Deeper: flasklike collections of barium: collar button
- Edema
  - Displacement of barium: translucent halo around central ulcer
- Spasm
  - Localized persistent contraction
  - Narrowing of bowel lumen

Submucosal inflammation
- Ulcers (deeper linear than in mucosal inflammation): cobblestone appearance
- Bowel wall thickening
  - CT: wall thickened (>3 mm with lumen distended)
  - Halo: fatty (chronic), gray (subacute or chronic), white (acute) with enhancement

Subserosal mesenteric inflammation
- Stranding in surrounding fat
- Inflammatory mass
- Fistula
- Creeping fat: excessive fat deposited around serosal surface (Crohn disease)

CROHN DISEASE (REGIONAL ENTERITIS) (Fig. 3-34)

Recurrent inflammatory condition of bowel due to altered immunity to intestinal flora. Lesions may occur in the entire GI tract but are most common in:
- Small bowel (especially terminal ileum), 80%
  - 30% only small bowel involved
  - 50% small bowel and colon involved
- Colon, 70%
  - 25% of patients with colonic disease have pancolitis (entire colon affected)
- Duodenum, 20%

Pathologic development of lesions: initial event → hyperplasia of lymphoid tissue in submucosa → lymphedema → aphthoid ulcerations → deeper ulcers → fistulas, abscesses → strictures

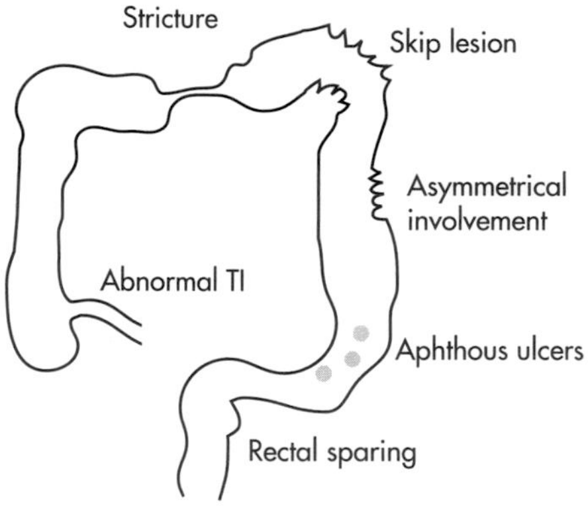

FIGURE 3-34

Imaging Features (Fig. 3-35)

Types of lesions
- Thickening of folds (edema)
- Nodular pattern (submucosal edema and inflammation)
- String sign: tubular narrowing of intestinal lumen (edema, spasm, scarring depending on chronicity)

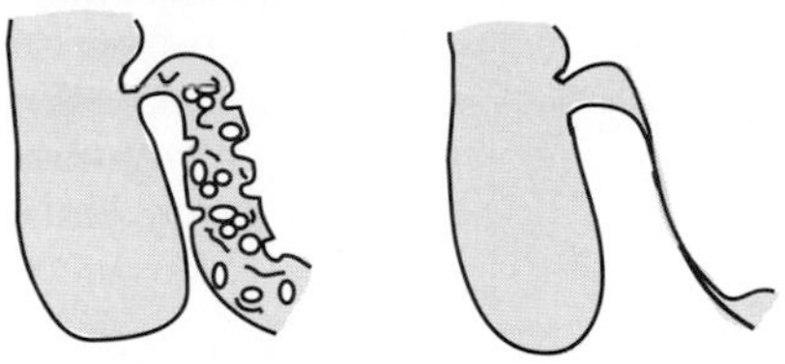

FIGURE 3-35

- Omega sign: asymmetric wall involvement results in contracture and C-shaped loop on small bowel series
- Ram's horn sign: loss of antral fornices with progressive narrowing from antrum to pylorus
- Ulcerations:
    - Aphthoid ulcers are early lesions and correspond to mucosal erosions (pinpoint ulcer in edematous mound up to 3mm in diameter and 2mm in depth).
    - Ulcers are irregularly scattered throughout GI tract and are interspersed with normal mucosa.
    - Ulcerations grow and fuse with each other in linear fashion and, with intervening edematous mucosa, produce an ulceronodular pattern ("cobblestone" appearance).
- Filiform polyposis: thin, elongated, branching mucosal lesions; represents proliferative sequelae of mucosa adjacent to denuded surface.
- Sinus tracts and fistulas originate in fissures or deep ulcers; characteristic of Crohn disease at advanced stages.
- Fatty thickening along mesenteric border (creeping fat) and paracolonic lymphadenopathy separate bowel loops.
- Fibrosis and scarring may result in:
    - Pseudodiverticula (fibrosis develops eccentrically)
    - Rigid, featureless bowel
    - Strictures and obstruction
    - Foreshortening of bowel

Spatial arrangement of lesions

- Transitional zones are typical; they occur between involved bowel loops and normal bowel.
- Skip lesions are typical: discontinuous involvement of bowel
- Lesions appear preferentially at mesenteric side of intestine.

Mural and Extramural Changes (CT Findings)

Primary intestinal findings

- Bowel wall thickening
    - Normally <3mm if well distended
    - Mean diameter in Crohn disease: 10mm
    - If >10mm, include pseudomembranous, ischemic, or CMV colitis in differential diagnosis.
- Circumferential submucosal low attenuation surrounded by higher outer attenuation: halo sign
- Inner and outer layers surrounding low-attenuation middle layer: target sign; middle layer of fat density; chronic, middle layer of water density

Peribowel inflammation ("dirty fat," "ground glass")

Mesentery

- Fat accumulates on serosal surfaces ("creeping fat")
- Inflamed mesentery fat (stranding, "misty")
- Adenopathy in small bowel mesentery common
- Comb sign: vasa recta stretched out along one wall of colon

Extraintestinal findings

- Gallstones
- Osseous complications (may cause pain)
    - Spondylitis
    - Sacroiliitis
    - Steroid complications: osteomyelitis, osteoporosis, avascular necrosis
- Renal stones, 7%

Complications (Fig. 3-36)

- Recurrence of disease after surgery (in contrast to UC, in which proctocolectomy is curative)
- Increased incidence of malignancies:
    - GI tract tumors
    - Lymphoma
- Toxic megacolon
- Fistulas
- Abscess formation

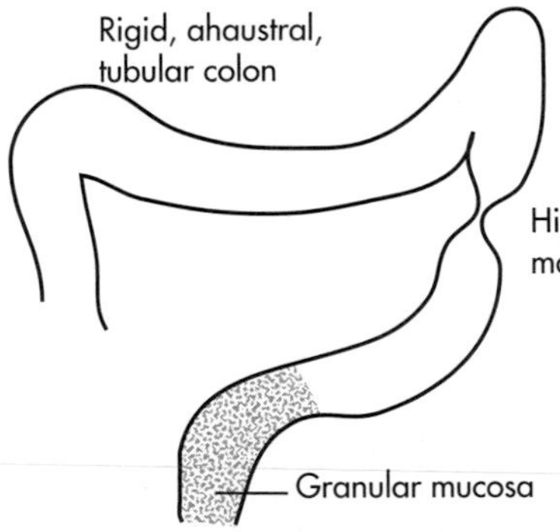

FIGURE 3-36

ULCERATIVE COLITIS (UC) (Figs. 3-37 and 3-38)

Unknown etiology. Clinical findings include diarrhea and rectal bleeding. Disease affects primarily mucosa (crypt abscesses) and typically starts in rectum.

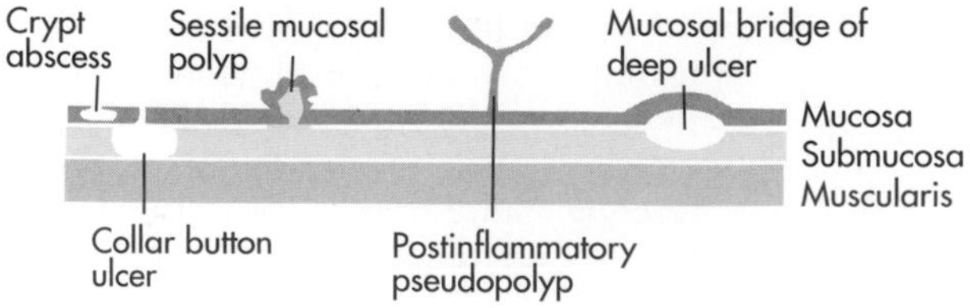

FIGURE 3-37

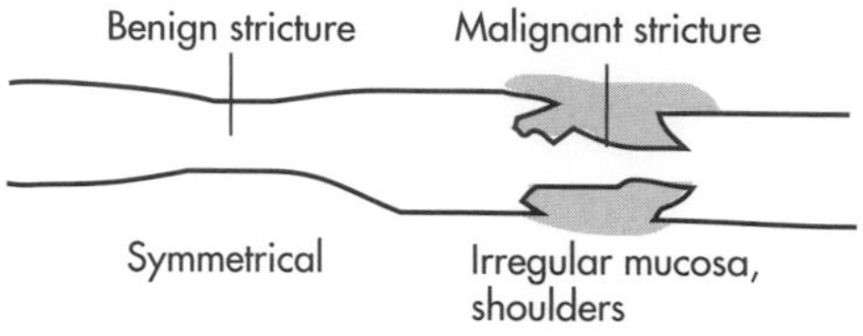

FIGURE 3-38

Associated Findings

- Joints, 25%: arthritis, arthralgia, ankylosing spondylitis
- Liver, 10%: sclerosing cholangitis, chronic active hepatitis, cholangiocarcinoma
- Skin: pyoderma gangrenosum, erythema nodosum
- Uveitis, episcleritis

Imaging Features

Ahaustral, foreshortened colon (lead pipe)
Granular mucosa, shallow confluent ulcerations
Polyps:
- Pseudopolyps
- Filiform polyps (regenerative mucosa, small thin, branching polyps)

Spread:
- Disease first and worst in rectum
- Continuous spread from distal to proximal colon
- Circumferential bowel involvement
- Backwash ileitis: only short segment of terminal ileum unlike Crohn disease, gaping ileocecal valve

Atypical imaging features:
- Atypical pattern of distribution: sparing of rectum (which may be healing), 5%
- Crohn-like findings: discontinuous disease in 5%-10% of patients

Mural and extramural changes (CT findings):
- Bowel wall thickening less than Crohn disease
- Distribution from rectum continuously proximal
- If pancolitis, terminal ileum may be affected for a very short length.
- Superimposed carcinoma: mass lesion or thick wall stricture
- Excessive fat surrounding rectosigmoid (creeping fat)
- Local lymph node enlargement; common in SB mesentery, infrequently the retroperitoneum

Complications

- Toxic megacolon: ahaustral transverse colon: >6 cm with pseudopolyps on KUB (can complicate most colitides)
- Strictures, obstruction: benign or malignant. Any stricture is suggestive of malignancy.
- Malignancy (5- to 30-fold higher risk than general population)
  - Annual incidence of 10% after the first decade
  - Multiple in 25% of cases
  - Often flat and scirrhous

SYNOPSIS

	Crohn Disease	Ulcerative Colitis
General Features		
Distribution	Skip lesions, entire GI tract	Confined to colon, distal terminal ileum
Symmetry	Eccentric	Concentric
Ulcers	Early: aphthoid ulcers (mucosa)	Superficial
	Late: deep ulcers (cobblestone)	
Fistula	Common	Rare
Pseudopolyps	Yes	20%
Toxic dilatation	Uncommon	Common
Strictures	Yes	Yes
Involvement		
Rectum	50%	95%
Anus	Perianal fistula and fissures	Normal
Terminal ileum	Narrowed, inflamed, fissured (cobblestone)	Dilated and wide open (backwash ileitis), gaping valve
Other		
Surgery	May exacerbate disease	Curative
Cancer risk	Uncommon	High
Recurrence	Common	Not after colectomy
Clinical Findings		
Diarrhea	++++	++++
Rectal bleeding	+++	++++
Pain	++++	+++
Weight loss	++	++
Fever	+++	+
Abdominal mass	++++	–
Malnutrition	+++	+

PERIANAL FISTULAS

Abnormal connection between epithelialized surface of the anal canal and skin.

Etiology:

- Primary; obstruction of anal gland, stasis, infection, fistula
- Secondary; iatrogenic (surgery), Crohn, infection, malignancy

Types

- Intersphincteric (common)
- Transsphincteric (common)
- Suprasphincteric
- Extrasphincteric (uncommon and seen in patients with multiple operations)

Imaging Features

- MRI is best technique for assessment
- Describe and classify type of fistula
- Distance of mucosal defect to perianal skin
- Secondary findings; abscesses, bowel wall abnormalities, reactive nodes

Treatment

- Fistulotomy
- Fistulectomy
- Sphincter saving fistulectomy
- Seton fistulotomy

BEHÇET DISEASE

Crohn mimic. HLA-B51 associated vasculitis.

Intestinal Manifestations

- Ulcers
- Strictures
- Fistulas

Extraintestinal Manifestations

- Oral, genital, skin ulcers
- Uveitis
- Aneurysms
- Arthritis

INFECTIOUS COLITIS

Some agents more commonly cause superficial lesions (similar to UC), and some are more likely to cause transmural inflammation (similar to Crohn disease). Infectious colitis is common in immunocompromised hosts.

ETIOLOGY OF INFECTIOUS COLITIS

Pathogen	Pattern	Comments
Campylobacter	SU, DU	Usually in distal colon
Shigella	SU	Most severe in rectosigmoid
Salmonella	SU, TI	Confined to colon
Gonococcus	SU	Rectum
Amebiasis	SU, DU	Diffuse but most severe in right colon (ameboma); small bowel rarely affected
Tuberculosis	DU	Loss of demarcation between cecum and terminal ileum (Stierlin sign); lymph nodes
Lymphogranuloma venereum	DU	Rectal strictures typical
Yersinia	DU	Typically terminal ileum, cecum
Strongyloides	SU	Duodenum, jejunum > colon
Trichuris trichiura (whipworm)		Rectal prolapse
Schistosomiasis		Hepatosplenomegaly
Chagas disease		Megacolon, megaesophagus

DU, deep ulcers (Crohn-Stierlin sign like); SU, superficial ulcers (UC-like); TI, more frequent terminal ileum affected.

CYTOMEGALOVIRUS (CMV) COLITIS

Occurs mainly in immunocompromised hosts.

Imaging Features

- Superficial (aphthoid) or deep ulcers
- Thick wall: >10 mm
- Localized distribution in cecum, terminal ileum, or universal colitis
- Radiographically may be indistinguishable from pseudomembranous colitis

TYPHLITIS (NEUTROPENIC COLITIS)

Acute necrotizing colitis involving the cecum, terminal ileum, and/or ascending colon in patients with leukemia undergoing therapy and/or immunosuppression. Incidence in autopsy series of young leukemia patients is 10%-25%. Unknown pathogenesis (leukemic bowel infiltration, intramural hemorrhage, necrosis, local ischemia). Indications for surgery include failed medical therapy, perforation, hemorrhage, pericecal abscess, and uncontrolled sepsis.

Clinical Findings

- RLQ pain, 50%
- Diarrhea, 40%
- Peritoneal signs in perforation

Imaging Features

- Marked thickening of cecum, terminal ileum, and/or ascending colon
- Pericecal fluid and soft tissue stranding more marked than in pseudomembranous colitis
- Complications: perforation, pericolonic abscess, pneumatosis

PSEUDOMEMBRANOUS COLITIS (PMC)

Colitis caused by colonic overgrowth of *Clostridium difficile* 1 to 6 weeks after administration of antibiotics (clindamycin, lincomycin > tetracycline, ampicillin; much less common causes: *Staphylococcus,* steroids, chemotherapeutic agents).

Clinical Findings

- Diarrhea
- Fever
- Pain
- Leukocytosis

Imaging Features (Fig. 3-39)

Plain films, abnormal in 40%
- Very thick haustral folds, thumbprinting, 40%
- Ileus, 40%

CT, abnormal in 60%
- Very thick (average 15 mm) colonic wall but preserved, thickened haustra (plaques, ulcers, edema)
- Contrast between thickened folds (accordion sign)
- Usually starts in rectum and progresses retrograde
- Largely left-sided disease; may be pancolitic
- Pericolonic fat changes, 35%
- Ascites, 35%

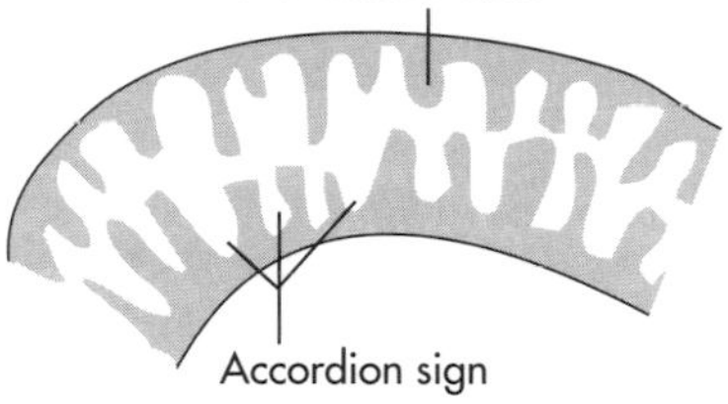

FIGURE 3-39

AMEBIASIS (Fig. 3-40)

Infection with *Entamoeba histolytica.* Common in Mexico, South America, Africa, and Asia. Clinical findings include diarrhea (bloody) and fever, but patient may be asymptomatic for long periods. Transmission is by direct person-to-person spread or contaminated water or food.

Imaging Features

- Colon
  - Cecum, right colon > transverse colon > rectosigmoid
  - Ulcers: initially punctate then confluent
  - Coned cecum
  - Stenosis from healing and fibrosis
  - Ameboma: hyperplastic granuloma (in 1% of cases)
  - Pericolic inflammation

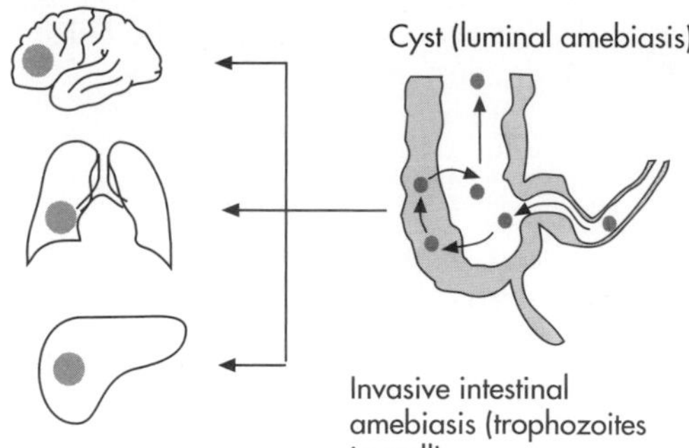

FIGURE 3-40

Other
- Fistula formation
- Intussusception due to ameboma (children)
- Liver abscess (very painful)
- Pleuropulmonary abscess
- Brain abscess
- Cutaneous extension (perianal region)

INTESTINAL TUBERCULOSIS (TB)

Types

- Primary intestinal TB
  - *Mycobacterium avium intracellulare* (AIDS)
  - *M. bovis* (cow's milk)
- Hematogenous spread from pulmonary TB
  - Location: cecum > colon > jejunum > stomach

Imaging Features

- Narrowed terminal ileum (Stierlin sign)
- Marked bowel wall thickening, short segments
- Ulcers, fissures, fistulas, stricture
- Marked hypertrophy: ileocecal valve (Fleischner's sign)
- Local adenopathy, may show low central density

COLITIS CYSTICA PROFUNDA

Benign look-alike disease characterized by the presence of submucosal, fluid-filled cysts. The disease is most commonly localized to the rectum (85%). Cysts can be up to 3 cm. Diagnosis is made histologically by exclusion of malignancy (cystic mucinous adenocarcinoma).

RECTAL LYMPHOGRANULOMA VENEREUM

Caused by *Chlamydia trachomatis.* Transmitted by sexual contact, usually in homosexual men. Major feature is bleeding. Purulent inflammation of inguinal lymph nodes occurs. Diagnosis is with Frei's intradermal test.

OTHER COLONIC DISEASES

DIVERTICULAR DISEASE (FIG. 3-41)

Colonic diverticula represent mucosal and submucosal outpouchings through the muscularis. Outpouchings occur mainly where vessels pierce the muscularis (i.e., between mesenteric and antimesenteric taenia). 95% of diverticula are located in sigmoid, in 20% the proximal colon also, never the rectum. Perforation causes diverticulitis. Clinical findings of pain, fever > bleeding.

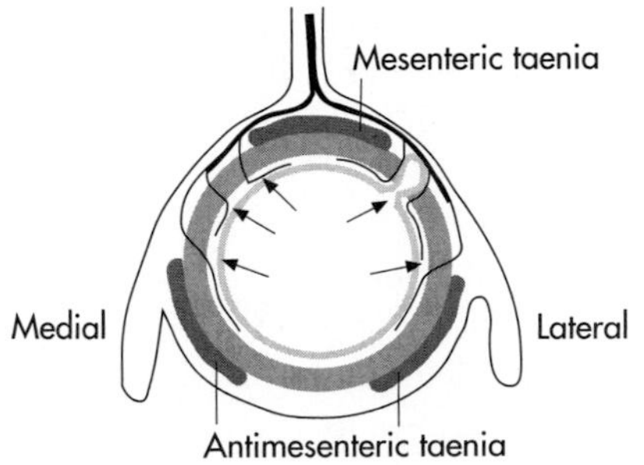

FIGURE 3-41

Diverticulosis

- Diverticula occur in two rows between taenia.
- Associated muscular hypertrophy

Diverticulitis (Fig. 3-42)

- Extravasation of barium from tip of diverticulum (microperforation), 20%
- Free intraperitoneal air: uncommon
- Intramural or paracolonic abscess
- Double tracking (intramural fistula): uncommon
- Fistula to bladder/uterus, 10%
- Muscular hypertrophy, 25%

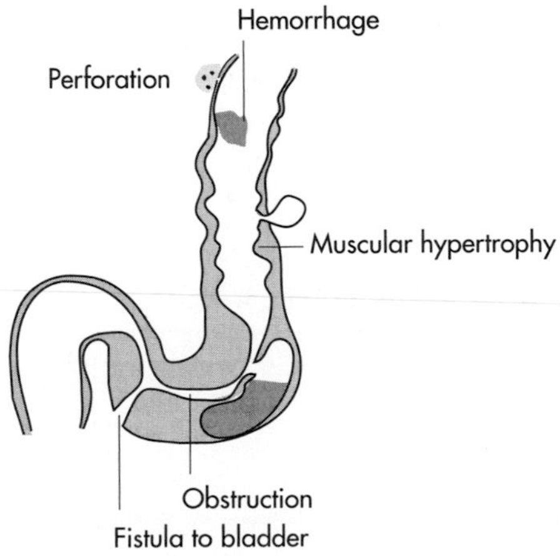

FIGURE 3-42

- Local penetration may lead to coexistent small bowel obstruction

Pearls

- Disease is common and worse in patients on steroids.
- Isolated giant sigmoidal diverticulum is a rare entity caused by ball-valve mechanism.
- Diverticulitis may be present without radiographically apparent diverticula.
- Underlying carcinoma may be obscured in patients >50 years of age, endoscopic evaluation indicated after resolution

GIANT SIGMOID DIVERTICULUM

Characteristic radiologic feature is a large balloon-shaped, gas-filled structure in lower abdomen located centrally in pelvis. Although it is rare, it is important to differentiate it from sigmoid and cecal volvulus.

Complications

- Diverticulitis
- Small bowel obstruction due to adhesions
- Perforation
- Volvulus of diverticulum

APPENDIX

The appendix is located about 3 cm below the ileocecal valve on the medial wall. Common abnormalities include:

Inflammation
- Appendicitis

Tumor
- Mucocele: abnormal accumulation of mucus, rupture leads to pseudomyxoma peritonei
- Cystadenoma, cystadenocarcinoma, adenocarcinoma
- Carcinoid (usually small tumor found incidentally at surgery)

APPENDICITIS (Fig. 3-43)

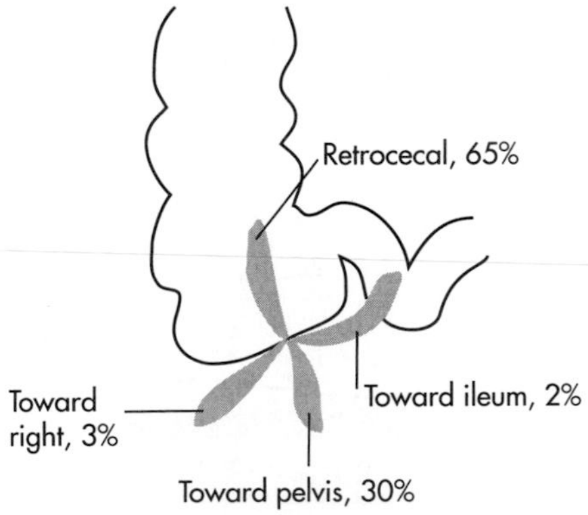

FIGURE 3-43

Appendicitis occurs secondary to obstruction of the appendiceal lumen/venous obstruction → ischemia → bacterial invasion → necrosis. Classic clinical signs are absent in one third of adults. Common causes of obstruction are:
- Appendicolith
- Lymphoid hypertrophy
- Tumor
- Intestinal worms (usually *Ascaris*)

Imaging Features (Figs. 3-44 and 3-45)

Plain film
- Calcified appendicolith, 10%
- Focal ileus
- Abscess

Barium enema
- Nonfilling of appendix; complete filling excludes appendicitis
- Mass effect on cecum, terminal ileum

CT
- Appendix thickness >6 mm
- Calcified appendicolith, 30%
- Stranding of fat (subtle important finding)
- Asymmetrical cecal wall thickening
- Only proximal filling and inflammation distally: tip appendicitis
- Lymph nodes in mesoappendix

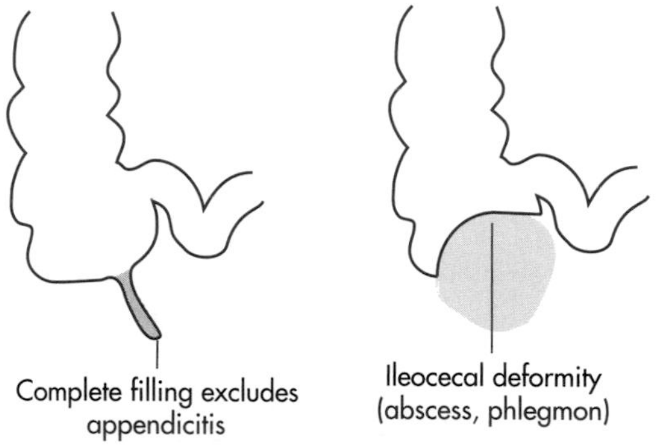

FIGURE 3-44

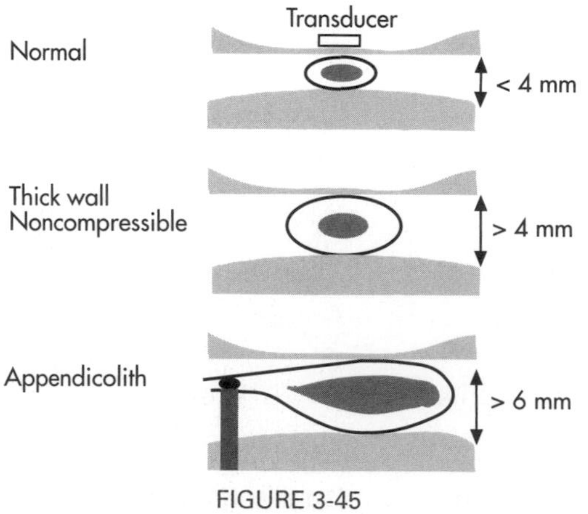

FIGURE 3-45

US
- Total appendiceal thickness >6 mm
- Noncompressible appendix
- >3-mm wall thickness
- Shadowing appendicolith

Choice of imaging study
- US (lower sensitivity than CT): children, pregnant women
- CT: all other patients, symptoms present >48 hours
- MRI during early pregnancy

MUCOCELE OF THE APPENDIX

Accumulation of mucus within abnormally distended appendix. Most cases are due to tumor (mucinous cystadenocarcinoma), whereas other cases are due to an obstructed orifice.

Imaging Features
- Nonfilling of appendix
- Smooth, rounded appendiceal mass
- Curvilinear calcification

EPIPLOIC APPENDAGITIS

Acute inflammation and infarction of epiploic appendages. Appendages are small adipose structures protruding from serosal surface of colon, seen along free taenia and taenia omentalis between cecum and sigmoid colon.
- Small oval pericolonic fatty nodule with hyperdense ring seen with surrounding inflammation
- Left lower quadrant more common than right lower quadrant
- Central area of increased attenuation indicative of thrombosed vein

ISCHEMIC BOWEL DISEASE

Basic underlying mechanism is hypoxemia that can be caused in small bowel by:
- Arterial occlusion (thrombotic, embolic, vasculitis), 40%
- Low flow states (reversible, nonocclusive), 50%
- Venous thrombosis, 10%

Ischemic bowel disease may occur in either superior mesenteric artery (SMA) or inferior mesenteric artery (IMA) distribution, or both.

CAUSES OF ISCHEMIC BOWEL DISEASE

	SMA	IMA	SMV
Occlusive	40%	5%	
Embolus			
Thrombosis			10%
Nonocclusive	50%	95%	
Hypoperfusion			

Imaging Features

SMA distribution

- Sick patients, hypotension, acidosis: high mortality
- Requires surgery, resection
- Plain film findings similar to SBO; may see "pink-prints" in SB wall
- Submucosal edema > pneumatosis > portal vein gas, 5%

IMA distribution

- Patients not very sick (mimics diverticulitis)
- Usually affects 1 to 3 feet of colon (splenic flexure to sigmoid)
- Rectum involved: 15%
- Invariably nonocclusive etiology
- Thumbprinting: hemorrhage and edema in wall
- Rarely pancolonic in distribution
- May also cause ulceration
- Conservative treatment: heals spontaneously; strictures rare
- CT: halo or target signs

VOLVULUS (Fig. 3-46)

Location: sigmoid > cecum > transverse colon. Predisposing factors: redundant loops of bowel, elongated mesentery, chronic colonic distention. Diagnosis is with barium enema study.

Sigmoid Volvulus

- Massively dilated sigmoid loop (inverted U) projects from pelvis to upper quadrant
- Proximal colonic dilatation is typical but not always present
- Typically occurs in elderly constipated patients

Imaging Features

- Massively dilated; devoid of haustra; U-shaped form
- Extends to upper abdomen

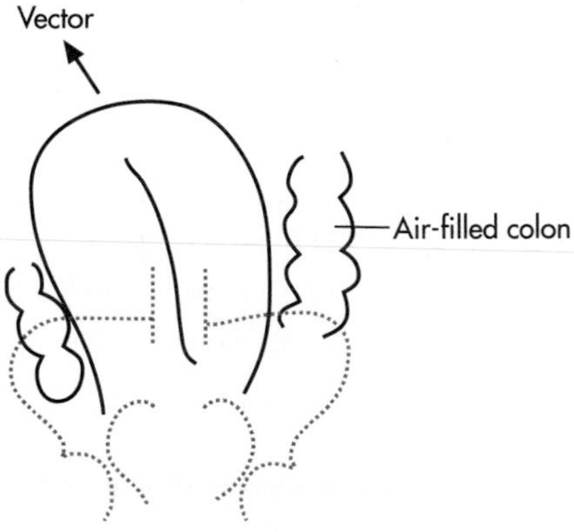

FIGURE 3-46

- Liver overlap sign: overlaps lower margin of liver
- Apex above T10
- Northern exposure sign: dilated twisted sigmoid colon projects above transverse colon
- Apex lies under left hemidiaphragm
- Inferior convergence into pelvis

Cecal Volvulus (Fig. 3-47)

- 35% of all cases of colonic volvulus
- Massively dilated cecum rotates toward midabdomen and points to left upper quadrant (LUQ); medially placed ileocecal valve produces soft tissue indentation with kidney or coffee bean appearance.
- Associated small bowel dilatation, decompressed distal colon
- Through foramen of Winslow: lesser sac hernia

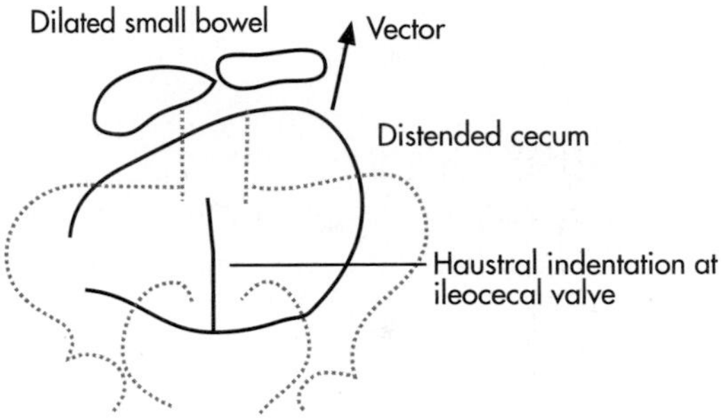

FIGURE 3-47

Cecal Bascule

- Mobile cecum is folded across the lower midabdomen horizontally.
- May mimic cecal volvulus but more likely located in pelvis and small bowel not dilated.

PSEUDO-OBSTRUCTION OF THE LARGE BOWEL (OGILVIE SYNDROME)

Dilatation of colon in elderly patients. Often history of cathartic abuse, anti-Parkinson medication, or metabolic abnormalities.

Imaging Features

- Dilated, ahaustral colon
- Often affects just proximal colon
- No mechanical obstruction
- Barium enema is diagnostic study of choice

TOXIC MEGACOLON (TMC)

Severe dilation of the transverse colon that occurs when inflammation spreads from the mucosa through other layers of the colon. The colon becomes aperistaltic and can perforate, carrying a 30% mortality rate. Anyone with UC or Crohn disease serious enough to

be at risk for toxic megacolon should be hospitalized and be closely monitored; many patients require surgery. Underlying causes include:
- UC (most common cause)
- Other colitides (uncommon): Crohn disease, pseudomembranous colitis, ischemic, infectious (CMV, amebiasis)

Imaging Features
- Dilated (>6 cm), transverse colon
- Ahaustral irregular colonic contour; may show intraluminal soft tissue masses (pseudopolyps)
- BE contraindicated; proceed to proctoscopy; gravity maneuvers (patient in prone, decubitus position) for plain film assessment
- Diameter of transverse colon should reduce as successful treatment proceeds

Liver

GENERAL

LIVER ANATOMY (Fig. 3-48)

The liver is anatomically subdivided into 8 segments, landmarked by hepatic and portal veins. Nomenclature:

Europe (liver divided into segments by hepatic veins)

Left liver: segments 2, 3, 4

Right liver: segments 5, 6, 7, 8

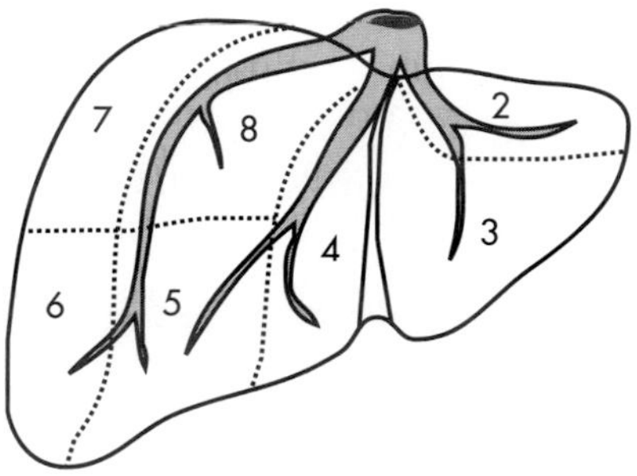

FIGURE 3-48

United States (liver divided by main lobar fissure 5, gallbladder fossa)

Left lobe: segments 2, 3

Right lobe: segments 4, 5, 6, 7, 8

Three hepatic ligaments are important because of their marker function (ligaments appear very hyperechoic relative to liver) in US.

HEPATIC LIGAMENTS

Ligaments and Spaces (Fig. 3-49, A-C)

US Doppler Waveforms (Fig. 3-50)

Hepatic veins
- Triphasic flow pattern
- Arterial contraction (right ventricle)

Portal vein
- Low-velocity (10 to 20 cm/sec) flow pattern
- Respiratory variation present
- Pulsation in portal vein flow is seen in tricuspid regurgitation, low body mass index

Hepatic artery
- Low impedance
- Arterial flow pattern
- Same flow direction as portal vein

Types of Contrast-Enhanced CT Techniques (CECT)

Liver is 8 to 10 HU higher than spleen on noncontrast CT.
- Hepatic artery contributes 25% of blood flow to liver
- Portal vein contributes 75% of blood flow to liver
- Most tumors have only arterial blood supply.

Dynamic Bolus CT (Portal Venous Phase Imaging for Hypovascular Lesions)
- 120 to 150 mL at 2 mL/sec
- 40-second delay for conventional CT
- 80-second delay for helical CT

Dynamic Bolus CT (Arterial Phase Imaging for Hypervascular Lesions)
- 20-second delay at 3 to 5 mL/sec

OVERVIEW

Ligament	Location	Landmark
Falciform ligament	Extends from umbilicus to diaphragm	Divides medial and lateral segments of left lobe
Ligamentum teres (round ligament = obliterated umbilical vein)	Hyperechoic structure in left lobe	Gastroesophageal junction
Main lobar fissure (major fissure, interlobar fissure, oblique ligament)	Extends from GB to porta hepatis	Divides right and left hepatic lobes (United States)
Fissure of ligamentum venosum	Between caudate lobe and lateral segment of left lobe	Contains hepatogastric ligament

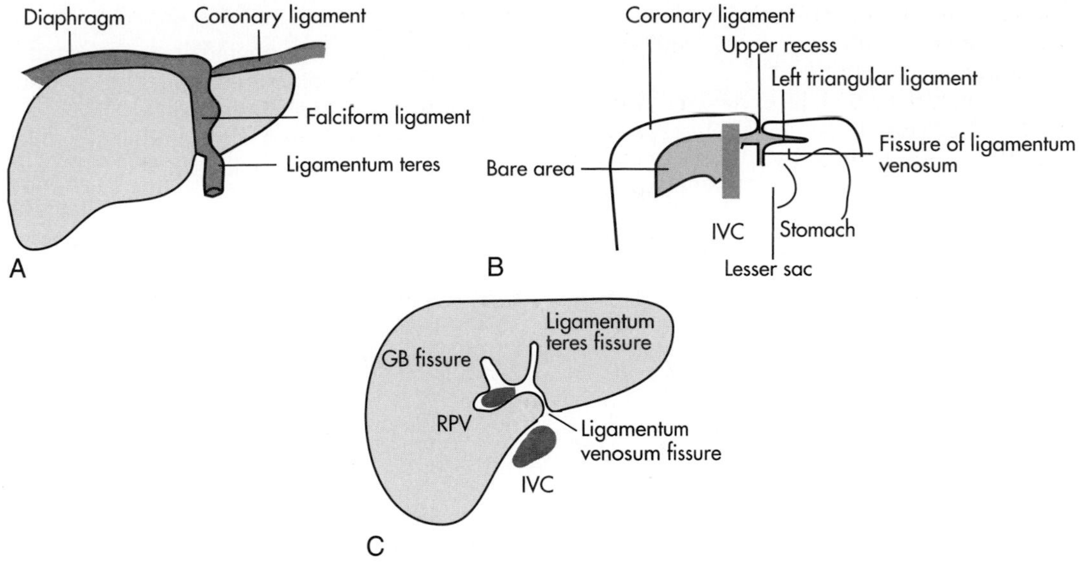

FIGURE 3-49

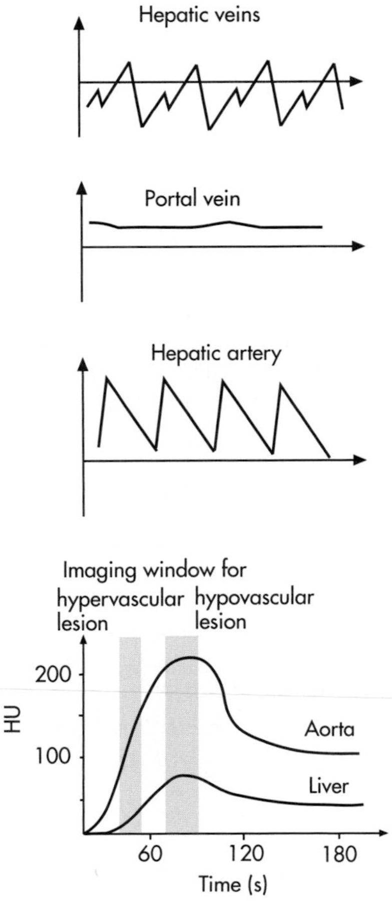

FIGURE 3-50

- Transient hyperattenuation of liver may be present (predominant arterial supply, decreased portal supply)
- Then 80-second delay as in portal venous phase

Delayed Equilibrium CT

- 10 to 20 minutes after contrast administration
- Retention of contrast may be observed in cholangiocarcinoma, fibrous tumors, or scars

Delayed High-Dose CT (Fig. 3-51)

Now rarely used.

- 60 g of iodine total
- 1%-2% of contrast material is excreted through liver
- 4 to 6 hours after injection, liver parenchyma is 20 HU increased.

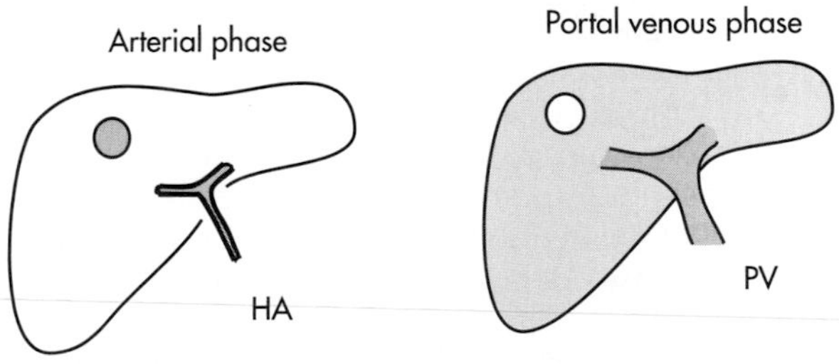

FIGURE 3-51

LIVER MRI

Specific sequences and parameters vary by field strength and vendors. Generic liver MRI protocol:

- SSFSE or fast gradient echo scout images
- Axial T1-weighted gradient echo in and out of phase images
- Axial fat saturated T2-weighted dual TE images; TE of 60 and 120 msec
- Axial DWI through liver
- Axial 3-D gradient echo T1-weighted images
- Axial 3-D gradient echo T1-weighted images after gadolinium administration (in arterial, portal venous, and in equilibrium phase)

MR ELASTOGRAPHY

New MR technique to noninvasively quantify the stiffness of the liver (or other organs).

A mechanical driver is placed adjacent to the liver to generate shear waves within the abdomen at a predetermined frequency (40-120 Hz).

MR images are then acquired with a gradient echo sequence as the waves propagate through the liver. The velocity and wavelength of the waves propagating depend on the stiffness of the tissue (velocity and wavelength increase with greater tissue stiffness). This technique can be used to assess liver fibrosis.

DIFFUSE LIVER DISEASE

HEPATITIS

Causes

Viral hepatitis
- Hepatitis A, B, non-A non-B, delta
- Other viruses: cytomegalovirus, Epstein-Barr, herpes simplex, rubella, yellow fever

Chemical hepatitis
- Alcohol
- Drugs: INH, halothane, chlorpromazine, phenytoin, methyldopa, acetaminophen
- Toxins such as CCl_4

Imaging Features

US
- GB wall thickening may occur.
- Increased echogenicity of portal triads in acute hepatitis (DDx: cholangitis), decreased echogenicity in chronic hepatitis
- Echogenicity: patterns are difficult to evaluate, and there exists considerable interobserver variability; only fatty liver substantially increases echogenicity of the liver.

MRI
- Increases in T1 and T2 relaxation times of liver
- High signal bands paralleling portal vessels (periportal edema) on T2W

CIRRHOSIS

Cirrhosis is defined as hepatic fibrosis with the formation of nodules that lack a central vein.

Types

- Chronic sclerosing cirrhosis: minimal regenerative activity of hepatocytes, little nodule formation, liver is hard and small.
- Nodular cirrhosis: regenerative activity with presence of many small nodules; initially the liver may be enlarged.

Causes

- Alcoholic (most common, Laënnec cirrhosis)
- Hepatitis B
- Biliary cirrhosis
- Hemochromatosis
- Heart failure, constrictive pericarditis
- Rare causes
  - Wilson disease
  - α_1-Antitrypsin deficiency
  - Drug induced

Imaging Features

Liver US features
- Small liver, increased echogenicity, coarse, heterogeneous
- Nodular surface
- Regenerating nodules: hypoechoic
- Simple cysts and hemangiomas are rare in cirrhotic livers
- Unequal distribution of cirrhosis in different segments (sparing):
  - Left lobe appears larger than right lobe.
  - Lateral segment of left lobe (segments 2, 3) enlarges; medial segment (segments 4A, 4B) shrinks
  - The ratio of the width of the caudate lobe (segment 1) to the right hepatic lobe (segments 5 and 6 or 7 and 8) is >0.6.

Portal hypertension (hepatic wedge pressure >10 mm Hg)
- Collaterals: left gastric, paraesophageal, mesenteric, retroperitoneal veins, splenorenal
- Splenomegaly
- Ascites

Complications

- Hepatocellular carcinoma (HCC) occurs in 10% of patients with cirrhosis; hemangiomas are much less common: 2%. In cirrhotic livers, HCC is best detected by helical CT or dynamic contrast MRI during arterial phase; delayed CT or noncontrast MRI has much lower sensitivity in lesion detection.
- Esophageal varices with bleeding

FATTY LIVER

Causes

- Obesity (most common cause)
- Alcohol
- Hyperalimentation

- Debilitation
- Chemotherapy
- Hepatitis
- Steroids, Cushing syndrome

Imaging Features

General

- Uniform decrease in density compared with vessels
- Focal fatty infiltration is usually geographic (straight borders) in distribution but may occasionally have all features of a tumor; areas of fatty liver are interspersed with normal liver.
- Focal fatty "mass" also occurs, most commonly adjacent to falciform ligament, usually anterolateral edge of medial segment
- Lack of mass effect: vessel distribution and architecture are preserved in areas of fat.
- Rapid change with time: fat appearance or resolution may be as fast as 6 days.
- Common areas of fatty sparing:
  Segment 1 (periportal region)
  Segment 4 (medial segment of left lobe)

US

- Visual criteria (most commonly used)
  Renal cortex appears more hypointense relative to liver than normal. Intrahepatic vessel borders become indistinct or cannot be visualized. Nonvisualization of diaphragm (because of increased beam attenuation)
- Quantitative
  Method uses backscatter amplitude measurements

CT

- The physiologic attenuation of liver parenchyma on unenhanced CT varies between 55 to 65 HU; normal liver is 10 HU denser than spleen; each milligram of triglyceride per gram of liver decreases density by 1.6 HU
- Fatty areas are hypodense (less dense than spleen) while normal liver appears relatively hyperdense.
- Hepatic and portal veins appear dense relative to decreased parenchymal density.
- Common focal fatty deposit: segment 4, anteriorly near fissure for falciform ligament

MRI

- Use fat saturation techniques to verify the presence of fat.

FOCAL CONFLUENT FIBROSIS

CT Findings

- Wedge-shaped area of low attenuation on noncontrast CT; T1 hypointense and T2 hyperintense on MRI
- Retraction of overlying liver capsule (90%)
- Total lobal or segmental involvement may be seen.
- Located in medial segment of left lobe and/or anterior segment of right lobe
- May show delayed persistent enhancement

GLYCOGEN STORAGE DISEASE

Enzyme deficiency results in accumulation of polysaccharides in liver and other organs.

GLYCOGEN STORAGE DISEASE

Type of Disease	Enzyme Deficiency	Organ Involvement
von Gierke	Glucose-6-phosphatase	Liver, kidneys, intestine
Pompe	Lysosomal glucosidase	All organs
Forbes, Cori	Debrancher enzyme	Liver, muscle, heart
Andersen	Brancher enzyme	Generalized amylopectin
McArdle	Muscle phosphorylase	Muscle
Hers	Liver phosphorylase	Liver
Tarui	Phosphofructokinase	Muscle

Imaging Features

Primary liver findings

- Hepatomegaly
- US: increased echogenicity (looks like fatty liver)
- CT: increased density (55 to 90 HU)

Other organs

- Nephromegaly

Hepatic complications

- Hepatic adenoma
- Hepatocellular carcinoma (uncommon)

GAUCHER DISEASE

Glucocerebrosidase deficiency leads to accumulation of ceramide in cells of the RES.

Clinical Findings

- Liver: hepatosplenomegaly, impaired liver function, hemachromatosis
- Bone marrow: anemia, leukopenia, thrombocytopenia, bone pain

Imaging Features

Liver

- Hepatomegaly

Spleen

- Splenomegaly (marked)
- Focal lesions (infarcts) typically have low density (CT) and are hyperechoic (US).

Musculoskeletal

- Erlenmeyer flask deformity of femur
- Generalized osteopenia
- Multiple lytic bone lesions
- Aseptic necrosis of femoral head

HEMACHROMATOSIS

Iron overload. Clinical finding is bronze diabetes: cirrhosis, diabetes mellitus, and hyperpigmentation.

TYPES

	Primary Hemochromatosis	Secondary Hemochromatosis
Genetics	Hereditary, autosomal recessive	Nongenetic cause of iron accumulation
Mechanism	Defect in intestinal mucosa, increased iron absorption	Multiple transfusions in bleeders
	Iron excess in parenchymal cells, most likely in liver, pancreas, myocardium, pituitary gland, thyroid, and synovium	Iron deposited in phagocytic cells in spleen and liver (Kupffer cells)
Clinical	Leads to cellular damage, organ dysfunction, and malignancy	Less toxic

Imaging Features

US
- Hyperechoic liver

CT
- Dense liver (>75 HU), much denser than spleen
- Intrahepatic vessels stand out as low-density structures.

MRI
- Liver, pancreas and myocardium markedly hypointense on T2-weighted and T1-weighted T2* gradient echo sequence in primary hemachromatosis, with sparing of spleen and bone marrow.
- In secondary hemochromatosis, there is decreased signal intensity of liver, spleen, and bone marrow with sparing of pancreas.
- Amount of iron can by quantified using gradient echo sequences with T2* weighting and progressively longer echo times. Free web sites allow calculation of estimated hepatic iron concentration (http://www.radio.univ-rennes1.fr/Sources/EN/Hemo.html)
- Iron deposition and decrease in signal intensity in the kidneys are only seen in intravascular hemolysis caused by mechanical stress in patients with heart valves, in patients with paroxysmal nocturnal hemoglobinuria, or in the hemolytic crisis of sickle cell disease.

Complication

- HCC in primary hemochromatosis

INFECTIONS

PYOGENIC ABSCESS

Pathogens: *Escherichia coli*, aerobic streptococci, anaerobes

Causes

- Ascending cholangitis
- Trauma, surgery
- Pylephlebitis

Imaging Features

- CT: hypodense mass or masses with peripheral enhancement, no fill-in
- Double-target sign: wall enhancement with surrounding hypodense zone (edema) 30% contain gas
- Percutaneous abscess drainage: any abscess can be drained percutaneously, particularly:
  - Deep abscesses
  - No response to treatment
  - Nonsurgical candidates

AMEBIC ABSCESS

Pathogen: *Entamoeba histolytica*

Imaging Features

- Abscesses do not contain gas unless secondarily superinfected.
- Irregular, shaggy borders
- Internal septations, 30%
- Multiple abscesses, 25%

Treatment

- Conservative: metronidazole
- Abscess drainage indicated if:
  - No response to treatment
  - Nonsurgical candidates

ECHINOCOCCUS (HYDATID DISEASE)

Humans are intermediate hosts of the dog tapeworm (*Taenia echinococcus*). The embryos penetrate the human intestinal mucosa and disseminate to liver and lungs > spleen, kidneys, bone, CNS. The disease is most prevalent in countries where dogs are used to herd livestock (e.g., Greece, Argentina, New Zealand). Two forms include:

- *Echinococcus granulosus* (hosts: dog, cattle): more common, few large cysts
- *E. multilocularis* (*alveolaris;* host: rodents): less common, more invasive

Most patients acquire disease in childhood. Initially, cysts are 5mm and then enlarge at a rate of 1cm/yr until they become symptomatic.

Imaging Features (Fig. 3-52)

E. granulosus
- Well-delineated cysts (multilocular > unilocular)
- Size of cysts usually very large

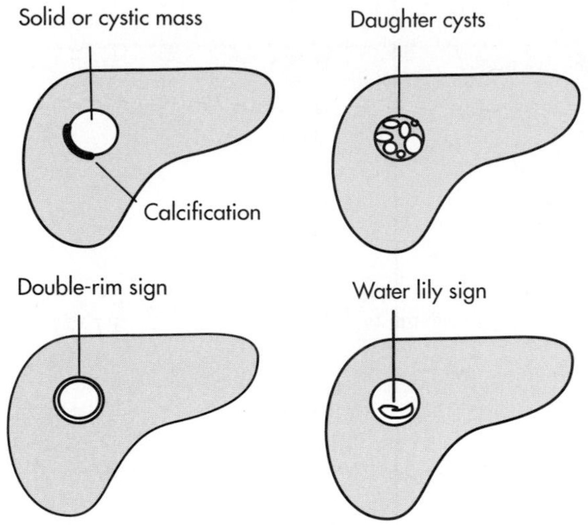

FIGURE 3-52

- Daughter cysts within larger cysts (multiseptated cyst) pathognomonic
- Rimlike cyst calcification, 30%
- Double-rim sign: pericyst, endocyst
- Water lily sign
- Enhancement of cyst wall

E. multilocularis
- Poorly marginated, multiple hypodense liver lesions
- Lesions infiltrative (chronic granulomatous reaction with necrosis, cavitation)
- Calcifications punctate and dystrophic, not rimlike

Classification of Cysts

Type I: Pure fluid collection, unilocular, well-defined cyst—amenable to percutaneous therapy

Type II: Partial/complete detachment of membrane floating in cyst—amenable to percutaneous therapy

Type III: Multiseptated or multilocular—amenable to percutaneous therapy

Type IV: Heterogeneous cystic mass—not amenable to percutaneous therapy

Type V: Calcified wall—not amenable to percutaneous therapy

Complications

- Rupture into peritoneal, pleural, pericardial cavity
- Obstructive jaundice due to external compression or intrinsic obstruction of biliary tree, biliary fistula
- Superinfection (bacterial) requiring prolonged drainage
- Anaphylaxis, shock, disseminated intravascular coagulation (DIC) <1%

Percutaneous Drainage

Surgical evacuation is procedure of choice. Percutaneous drainage is indicated in poor surgical candidates.

- <6 cm: aspiration with 19-gauge needle
- >6 cm: catheter placement 6 Fr for 1 day
  - Inject 15%-20% hypertonic NaCl (one-third cyst volume) or alcohol (one-half cyst volume) for 20 minutes with patient rotating during that period. Followed by catheter to gravity drainage.
- Prophylactic albendazole 20 mg/kg q12h PO for 1 week
- Anesthesia standby in case of hypersensitivity reaction
- Prophylactic 200 mg hydrocortisone IV before procedure
- Complications
  - Anaphylaxis, shock, DIC <1%
  - Biliary fistula
  - Superinfection (bacterial) requiring longer drainage
- Fluid analysis is positive for hydatid fragments in only 70%.

PELIOSIS HEPATIS

- Rare benign disorder associated with steroid medication, sprue, diabetes, vasculitis, hematologic disorders
- Bacillary peliosis hepatis is caused by *Bartonella* species in HIV-positive patients.
- Multiple spherical lesions with centrifugal or centripetal enhancement
- On angiography, lesions seen as multiple nodular vascular lesions on late arterial phase

TUMORS

TYPES OF HEPATIC TUMORS

OVERVIEW

Origin	Benign	Malignant
Hepatocellular	Adenoma	HCC
	Focal nodular hyperplasia	Fibrolamellar HCC
	Regenerating nodule	Hepatoblastoma
Cholangiocellular	Biliary cystadenoma	Cholangiocarcinoma
	Bile duct adenoma	Cystadenocarcinoma
Mesenchymal	Hemangioma	Angiosarcoma (Thorotrast)
	Fibroma, lipoma, others	Primary lymphoma (AIDS)
Heterotopic tissue	Adrenal	Metastases
	Pancreatic	

Whereas US is commonly used for the differentiation of solid and cystic masses, diagnostic modalities for further differentiation of solid tumors (>1 cm) are usually assigned to MR or CECT (MR is preferable). Two criteria are used for lesion characterization: signal intensity and morphologic features. Ultimately,

LESION CHARACTERIZATION BY MODALITY*

	Cyst	Hemangioma	FNH	Adenoma	HCC	Metastasis
Age	All ages	All ages	20-40	20-40	50-70	40-70
Sex	M = F	F > M	F >> M	F >> M	M > F	M = F
AFP	NI	NI	NI	NI	High	NI
Scar	No	In giant	Common	Occasional	Occasional	No
Calcification	Occasional	Yes	No	No	Rare	Rare
Rupture	Yes (rare)	Yes (rare)	No	Yes	Yes	No
US	Anechoic	Hyperechoic	Variable	Variable	Variable	Variable
CT	Hypodense	Enhancement †	Scar	Arterial enhancement	Capsule	Variable
	No enhancement	Early peripheral	Arterial phase		Arterial enhancement	
MRI	CSF intensity	CSF intensity	Liver intensity‡	Liver intensity	Liver intensity	Spleen
Angiography	Avascular	Hypervascular	Hypervascular	Hypervascular	Hypervascular	Variable
Scintigraphy§	Cold	Uptake	Uptake	Uptake	Cold	Cold

*Most frequent diagnostic pattern.
†Nodular peripheral with centripetal fill-in.
‡Arterial enhancement, with delayed enhancing central scar.
§Labeled RBC scan.
NI, not indicated.

the majority of lesions other than hemangiomas are sampled. It is difficult to characterize lesions <1 cm. Hyperechoic lesions with a hypoechoic halo are malignant until proved otherwise.

LESION CHARACTERIZATION BY MRI

Signal Intensity	
T1 hyperintense tumors	HCC
	Dysplastic nodule
	Dysplastic nodule
	Hemorrhagic tumors
	Melanoma
	Lesions in hemachromatosis livers
	Thrombosed portal vein
T2 hypointense tumors	Regenerating nodules
T2 lightbulb sign (lesion has CSF intensity)	Hemangioma
	Cysts
	Cystic metastases
	Cystadenocarcinoma
Other Morphologic Features	
Scars	Focal nodular hyperplasia
	Adenoma
	Hemangioma
Capsule	HCC
	Adenoma

HEMANGIOMA

Frequency: 4%-7% of population. 80% in females. Hemangiomas may enlarge, particularly during pregnancy or estrogen administration. Two types:

- Typical hemangioma (common): small, asymptomatic, discovered incidentally
- Giant hemangioma (>5 cm, uncommon), may be:
  - Symptomatic (hemorrhage, thrombosis)
  - Kasabach-Merritt syndrome: sequestration of thrombocytes in hemangioma causes thrombocytopenia (rare)

Imaging Features

US
- Hyperechoic lesions, 80%
- Hypoechoic lesions, which may have hyperechoic rim, 10%; especially in fatty liver
- Giant hemangiomas are heterogeneous.
- Anechoic peripheral vessels may be demonstrated by color Doppler US.
- Posterior acoustic enhancement is common (even in hypoechoic lesions).

CT
- Hypodense, well-circumscribed lesion on precontrast scan
- Globular or nodular intense peripheral enhancement during dynamic bolus phase, most characteristic findings on good bolus
- Fill-in occurs within minutes after administration of contrast (longer for giant hemangiomas) but also occurs often in metastases.

MRI
- Hyperintense (similar to CSF) on heavily T2W sequences (lightbulb sign)
- Postgadolinium peripheral nodular enhancement with centripetal fill-in
- Imaging modality of choice

Nuclear imaging (SPECT with ^{99m}Tc-labeled RBCs)
- Decreased activity on early dynamic images

- Increased activity on delayed (1 to 2 hours) blood pool images
- Only useful if lesion is >3 cm (limited spatial resolution)

FOCAL NODULAR HYPERPLASIA (FNH)

Rare hepatic neoplasm, most common in young women (75%). Composed of hepatocytes, Kupffer cells, and bile ducts. Association with oral contraceptives is questionable. Conservative management; no malignant transformation. 20% are multiple.

Imaging Features

General

- Mass lesion, usually difficult to detect because it has similar density, intensity, echogenicity as surrounding liver (normal hepatocytes, Kupffer cells, bile ducts)
- Central fibrous scar is common.
- 70% have normal or increased ^{99m}Tc sulfur colloid uptake; 30% have decreased uptake.

US

- Isoechoic
- May have central vascularity with spokewheel pattern on color Doppler

MRI

- Lesion isointense to liver; central scar hyperintense on T2W image.
- Arterial enhancement
- Delayed enhancement of central scar
- One-hour delayed enhancement after administration of Gd-BOPTA
- Angiography: hypervascular lesion

ADENOMA

Composed of hepatocytes; no bile ducts or Kupffer cells (cold on ^{99m}Tc sulfur colloid scan). Less common than FNH. Associated with oral contraceptives and glycogen storage disease (especially von Gierke disease). May resolve completely after discontinuation of hormone therapy. Liver adenomatosis appears to be a distinct entity. Although the adenomas in liver adenomatosis are histologically similar to other adenomas, they are not steroid dependent but are multiple, progressive, symptomatic, and more likely to lead to impaired liver function, hemorrhage, and perhaps malignant degeneration.

Complications

- Hemorrhage
- Infarction
- Malignant degeneration

Imaging Features

- Usually solitary, encapsulated. Patients with glycogen storage disease and liver adenomatosis may have dozens of adenomas detected at imaging and even more at close examination of resected specimens.
- CT: peripherally hypodense (lipid accumulation in hepatocytes). Because adenomas consist almost entirely of uniform hepatocytes and a variable number of Kupffer cells, it is not surprising that most of the adenomas are nearly isoattenuating relative to normal liver on unenhanced, portal venous phase, and delayed-phase images. In patients with fatty liver, adenomas are hyperattenuating at all phases of contrast enhancement and on unenhanced images as well.
- US features are nonspecific (may be isoechoic, hypoechoic, hyperechoic).
- MRI: Lesions may show fall in signal intensity on gradient echo out-of-phase images due to intralesional fat content. They are arterially enhanced with capsule seen on delayed images.
- Cold lesions by ^{99m}Tc sulfur colloid scan
- Angiography: varied appearance (hypervascular, hypovascular), no neovascularity pooling, or AV shunting

DIFFERENTIATING FEATURES OF FNH AND ADENOMA

Features	FNH	Adenoma
Sex preference	Female	Female
Hormone therapy	–/+	+++
Multiple	+++	++
Central scar	Yes	No
Internal hemorrhage	–/+	+++
Calcification	–/+	+
Arterial enhancement	Homogeneous	Inhomogeneous
Hepatobiliary liver contrast (Gd-BOPTA)	Uptake	No significant uptake
Reticuloendothelial liver contrast	Uptake	Uptake

Gd-BOFTA, gadolinium-benzyloxypropionic tetra-acetate

HEPATOCELLULAR CARCINOMA (HCC)

This is the most common primary visceral malignancy worldwide.

Incidence

- Asia, Japan, Africa: 5%-20%
- Western hemisphere: 0.2%-0.8%

Risk Factors

- Cirrhosis: 5% develop HCC
- Chronic hepatitis B: 10% develop HCC
- Hepatotoxins (aflatoxin, oral contraceptives, Thorotrast)
- Metabolic disease (galactosemia, glycogen storage disease) in pediatric patients

Imaging Features

General

- Three forms: solitary (25%), multiple (25%), diffuse (50%)
- Portal (35%) and hepatic vein (15%) invasion is common (rare in other malignancies).
- Metastases: lung > adrenal, lymph nodes > bone (10%-20% at autopsy, bone metastases may be painful)
- HCC typically occurs in abnormal livers (cirrhosis, hemochromatosis)

CT

- Hypodense mass lesion
- Lesion may appear hyperdense in fatty liver
- Enhancement: early arterial enhancement
  - Arterial supply, prominent AV shunting causes early enhancement, remains enhanced on PVP
  - Venous invasion, 50%
  - In cirrhotic livers, HCCs are best detected by helical CT or dynamic contrast MRI during arterial phase.
- Calcifications, 25%
  - More commonly seen in fibrolamellar HCC: 40% (better prognosis, younger patients, normal α-fetoprotein, central scar calcification)

US

- Most small HCCs are hypoechoic.
- Larger HCCs are heterogeneous.
- Fibrolamellar HCCs are hyperechoic.
- High-velocity Doppler pattern; feeding tumor vessels can be seen by color Doppler.

MRI

- T1W: hyperintense, 50% (because of fat in lesions); isointense, hypointense, 50%
- Hypointense capsule in 25%-40%
- T1-hyperintense and T2-hypointense lesion may represent a dysplastic nodule. Short-term follow-up MRI may be useful as there may be interval development of enhancement, capsule, and T2-hyperintensity suggesting progression to HCC.

Angiography

- Hypervascular
- AV shunting is typical.
- Dilated arterial supply

FIBROLAMELLAR HCC

- Malignant hepatocellular tumor with distinct clinical and pathologic differences from hepatocellular carcinoma
- Lobulated heterogeneous mass with a central scar in an otherwise normal liver
- Radiologic evidence of cirrhosis, vascular invasion, or multifocal disease—findings typical of hepatocellular carcinoma—uncommon
- Imaging features of fibrolamellar carcinoma overlap with those of other scar-producing lesions, including FNH, hepatocellular adenoma and HCC, hemangioma, metastases, and cholangiocarcinoma.
- The fibrous scar is usually hypointense on all MR sequences. This widely described imaging feature has been used to discriminate between fibrolamellar carcinoma and FNH. However, in rare cases, fibrolamellar carcinoma may demonstrate a hyperintense scar on T2W images, a finding that simulates the hyperintense scar characteristic of FNH.
- Dense heterogeneous enhancement in the arterial and portal phases. The scar usually does not enhance and is best visualized on delayed images.

METASTASES

30% of patients who die of malignancy have liver metastases. The liver is the most common site of metastatic disease from colorectal carcinoma: colon > stomach > pancreas > breast, lung. Up to 20% of patients die of liver metastases rather than the primary tumor.

Sensitivity for Lesion Detection

MR > CECT > noncontrast FDG PET-CT

Imaging Features

US

Echogenic metastases

- GI malignancy
- HCC
- Vascular metastases

Hypoechoic metastases

- Most metastases are hypovascular.
- Lymphoma
- Bull's eye pattern (hypoechoic halo around lesion)
  - Nonspecific sign but frequently seen in bronchogenic carcinoma
  - Hypoechoic rim represents compressed liver tissue and tumor fibrosis. Calcified metastases: hyperechoic with distal shadowing
- All mucinous metastases: colon > thyroid, ovary, kidney, stomach

Cystic metastases: necrotic leiomyosarcoma; mucinous metastases

CT

Best seen on portal venous phase images except for hypervascular lesions (arterial phase). Small lesions may fill in on delayed scans. Peripheral washout sign (when seen) is characteristic of metastases.

UNSUSPECTED HEPATIC LESIONS

Small lesions (<15 mm) of the liver are frequently detected during routine CT, MRI, and US studies of the abdomen ("incidentaloma"). In larger series, 70% of such lesions are benign and 30% are malignant. In the subset of patients with lesions <1 cm and no known primary lesion, virtually all lesions are benign. In the subset of patients with known malignant neoplasm, the percentage of malignant lesions is 50%.

ANGIOSARCOMA

- Rare malignancy
- Most common mesenchymal malignancy in liver in adults; tumor originates from endothelial cells.
- Risk factors: Thorotrast (10%), vinyl chloride, arsenic; hemochromatosis, neurofibromatosis
- Multilocular mass with disseminated appearance, cystic areas
- Can mimic hemangiomas on CT

EPITHELIOID HEMANGIOENDOTHELIOMA

- Female predominance
- Middle age
- Associated with OCs or vinyl chloride
- Predominant periphery of liver, intratumorous calcifications, changes of liver contour with capsular retraction and compensatory hypertrophy of normal liver, and invasion of portal and hepatic veins

ALCOHOL ABLATION OF LIVER TUMORS

Indication

HCC

- No extrahepatic spread
- ≤ 5 cm, single or multiple
- Child A or B cirrhosis

Metastases

- ≤ 5 cm, single lesion
- Vascular lesion (carcinoid, islet cell tumor)

Procedure

1. Localize hepatic lesion by US or CT.
2. Advance 20-gauge needle into tumor center, avoiding multiple perforations.
3. Slowly instill ethanol into tumor. We usually use 15 to 30 mL/lesion/setting.
4. Withdraw needle.
5. Lesions are typically treated at least three times or until no tumor is apparent.

Complications

- Major complications for which admission is necessary (10% by patient, 3% by procedure): bleeding, chest tube placement
- Minor complications (virtually all patients): pain, fever

Outcome

- Efficacy comparable to that of surgery for lesions
- The larger the lesion, the more difficult to treat.
- Metastases are more difficult to treat (alcohol diffuses less well, tumors have no capsule).

RADIOFREQUENCY ABLATION OF LIVER TUMORS

Alternating current at frequencies above 250 kHz is used to generate heat and destroy tumor tissue.

Indication

HCC

- Single tumor <5 cm, or as many as 3 nodules <3 cm each in the absence of vascular involvement or extrahepatic spread
- Liver cirrhosis in Child-Pugh class A or B

Metastases

- Four or fewer, 5 cm or smaller; ideal tumors for RF ablation are <3 cm, completely surrounded by hepatic parenchyma, 1 cm or more deep to liver capsule, and 2 cm or more away from large hepatic or portal veins.
- Palliation in patients with large liver tumors who have severe pain caused by capsular distention

Procedure

1. Conscious sedation
2. Localize hepatic lesion by US or CT.
3. Single or multiple electrodes used. The size of coagulated area can be increased by use of multiple electrodes or by using cluster probe (which may have up to 9 separate electrode tips).
4. Currently, three RF ablation systems are commercially available for clinical applications in the United States. One is the Radionics 200-Watt generator with internally cooled electrodes available as single needles or in a cluster array (Radionics, Burlington, MA). The length of the uninsulated electrically active tip ranges from 2 to 3 cm. The generator provides the option of automated pulsing of current. The other two systems provide umbrella-type electrodes placed via an introducer needle (RITA Medical Systems, Inc., Mountain View, CA; and Radiotherapeutics, Mountain View, CA). These latter two systems do not allow for internal cooling or pulsing of electrical current.
5. RF ablation can be performed using the following approaches: percutaneous, laparoscopy or laparotomy

Complications

More likely when tumor is superficial or close to hilar structures, there is prolonged ablation time, or several lesions are treated simultaneously

- Intraperitoneal hemorrhage, liver abscess, intestinal perforation
- Minor complications (virtually all patients): pain, fever

TRAUMA

The liver is the most common intraabdominal site of injury; however, one must inspect other organs (spleen, bowel) for coexistent trauma.

Types (Fig. 3-53)

- Subcapsular hematoma: hypodense or hyperdense lenticular fluid collection contained by the liver capsule; caused by blunt trauma
- Laceration: single or multiple stellate configurations usually of low density relative to enhanced parenchyma. Clots may appear high density; usually caused by penetrating or blunt trauma

Complications

- Perihepatic hemorrhage
- Intraperitoneal or extraperitoneal hemorrhage

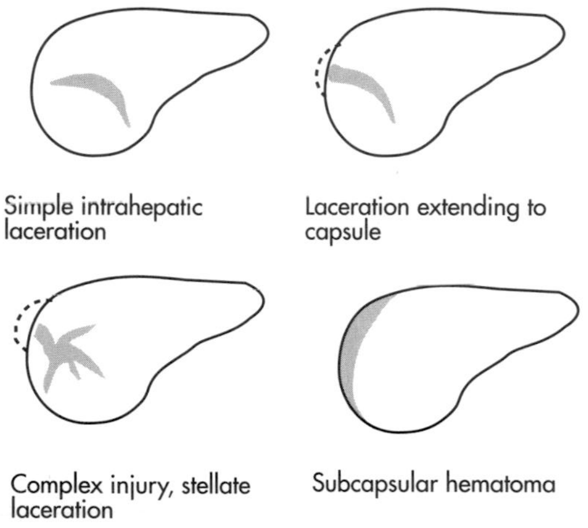

FIGURE 3-53

VASCULAR ABNORMALITIES

PORTAL HYPERTENSION

Criteria: hepatic wedge pressure >10 mm Hg

Causes

Presinusoidal

- Extrahepatic (obstruction of portal vein)
  - Thrombosis
  - Compression
- Intrahepatic (obstruction of portal venules)
  - Hepatic fibrosis: congenital, toxic (copper, polyvinyl chloride),
  - myelofibrosis, Wilson disease, sarcoid
  - Infection: malaria, schistosomiasis

Sinusoidal

- Cirrhosis (most common cause)
- Sclerosing cholangitis

Postsinusoidal

- Budd-Chiari syndrome
- Congestive heart failure

Imaging Features

- Portal vein diameter >13 mm
- US: reversal of flow in right portal flow with normal directional flow in the left portal vein feeding a recanalized umbilical vein
- Collaterals
  - Gastroesophageal varices via coronary vein, azygos
  - SMV collateral: mesenteric varices
  - Splenorenal varices
  - IMV collateral: hemorrhoids
  - Recanalization of umbilical vein: caput medusa
  - Unnamed retroperitoneal collaterals that communicate with phrenic, adrenal, and renal veins
- Splenomegaly
- Ascites
- Mural thickening of stomach, proximal colon: portal gastropathy/colopathy
- Portal biliopathy: Venous drainage of the CBD is handled by epicholedochal (Saint) and paracholedochal (Petren) venous plexi; dilatation of these veins due to extrahepatic portal venous obstruction can cause mural irregularities and compression of the biliary tree. Appears as irregular strictures of the extrahepatic and intrahepatic bile ducts, segmental dilated segments with beaded appearance, ectasia, and pruning of the intrahepatic bile ducts

ARTERIOPORTAL SHUNTING IN LIVER

Direct communications between branches of hepatic artery and portal vein. Appears as wedge-shaped areas of hyperattenuation on late arterial phase CT using fine collimation and contrast infusion rates of 3 to 5 mL/sec.

Types

Contribute arterial blood to the predominant portal venous blood supply of venous sinusoids.

- Transsinusoidal: These are most commonly seen in hepatic cirrhosis but may also occur due to focal infection or nodules of disease compromising portal circulation. When they are seen in cancer patients, attention should be paid to the apex of the lesion, where small metastases may be evolving.

- Transtumoral: Most common in the setting of HCC where a perinodular arteriolar plexus appears to cause a wedge of arterialized parenchyma. Both transsinusoidal and transtumor mechanisms contribute to this effect. This pattern is also seen after radiofrequency ablation.
- Transplexal: The walls of the large bile ducts carry a vascular plexus that communicates with hepatic artery and drains to both hepatic sinusoids and the portal vein. This type of shunting manifests from the perihilar level. They are encountered in cirrhosis, portal vein thrombosis, or occlusion and in the setting of lobar infection.

Arterioportal communication via vasa vasorum of portal vein
- Transvasal: Occurs commonly in conjunction with transplexal shunting and is commonly seen in portal vein occlusion or HCC.

BUDD-CHIARI SYNDROME (BCS)

Thrombosis of the main hepatic veins, branches of hepatic veins, or IVC; with possible extension to portal vein.

Clinical Findings

- Ascites
- Pain
- Hepatomegaly
- Splenomegaly

Causes

Idiopathic, 50%-75%

Secondary, 25%-50%
- Coagulation anomalies
  - Clotting disorders
  - Polycythemia
- Tumors: HCC, RCC
- Trauma
- Oral contraceptives, chemotherapy

Imaging Features

Veins
- Absent hepatic veins
- Flow in inferior vena cava (IVC) may be reversed, turbulent, diminished, or absent.
- Flow in portal vessels may be reversed or diminished.
- Intrahepatic collateral vessels
- Narrowing of the intrahepatic IVC

Liver parenchyma
- Hemorrhagic infarction appears hypoechoic by US.
- Caudate lobe is often spared (emissary veins drain directly into the IVC) and appears enlarged; small right lobe

CT
- Increased central (periportal) parenchymal enhancement
- Patchy peripheral enhancement: geographic zones of poorly opacified parenchyma interspersed with well-opacified zones

Pearls

- Hepatic venoocclusive disease, which causes progressive occlusion of small vessels, is clinically indistinguishable from BCS. Causes include:
  - Toxins from bush tea (Jamaica)
  - Chemotherapy
  - Bone marrow transplantation (GVH)

PORTAL VEIN THROMBOSIS

Causes

- Malignancy (HCC)
- Chronic pancreatitis
- Hepatitis
- Trauma
- Shunts
- Hypercoagulable states (pregnancy)

Imaging Features

US
- Echogenic thrombus in vein
- Portal vein enlargement
- Hepatofugal flow

CT
- Clot in portal vein with collaterals: gastroesophageal umbilical collateral vessels
- Cavernous transformation: numerous wormlike vessels at the porta hepatis reconstituting intrahepatic portal venous system
- Splenomegaly, ascites

Pearls

- Flow in hepatic artery and portal vein should always be in the same direction: hepatopetal flow.
- Opposite flow directions in portal vein and hepatic artery indicate hepatofugal flow.

HEPATIC ARTERY ANEURYSM

Decreasing order of frequency of abdominal aneurysms: aorta > iliac artery > splenic artery > hepatic artery. 10% of patients with hepatic artery aneurysm have sudden rupture. Hepatic pseudoaneurysm may occur secondary to pancreatitis.

TRANSPLANT

CRITERIA

Milan criteria are commonly used and have been adopted by the United Network of Organ Sharing. Identifies subgroup of patients with

primary or secondary liver malignancy who may benefit most from liver transplantation.
- Tumor size should be at least 2 cm.
- Maximum diameter of tumor is 5 cm if single, or no more than three liver tumors with maximum size of 3 cm.

COMPLICATIONS

- UGI bleeding (ulcer)
- Biliary: obstruction, leak, fistula, biloma, sludge
- Vascular complications
  - Hepatic artery thrombosis: most common serious vascular complication, more common in pediatric patients, usually necessitating retransplantation. US reveals no arterial flow within the liver. Pediatric patients may develop extensive collateralization to the liver. The waveforms of these collateral vessels are abnormal, showing parvus tardus waveform, RI of less than 0.5, and systolic acceleration time of greater than 0.1 second.
  - Hepatic artery thrombosis: usually occurs at the anastomotic site within 3 months of transplantation. Nonanastomotic stenosis may indicate rejection or hepatic necrosis.
  - Portal vein thrombosis: less frequent than hepatic artery thrombosis. US echogenic thrombus can be seen within the lumen of the vessel.
  - Hepatic vein thrombosis: quite rare because no surgical anastomosis is involved.
- Rejection, 40%

CT Features (after Transplantation)

- Atelectasis and pleural effusions are the most frequent CT features.
- Periportal increased attenuation (periportal collar) common (70%) and typical finding
- Ascites, 40%
- Splenomegaly
- Noninfected loculated intraperitoneal fluid collections
- Abscesses (hepatic, splenic, perihepatic, pancreatic)
- Hepatic infarction, 10%
- Hepatic hematoma
- Sludge (inspissated thick bile, 15%); may be extensive and cause "biliary casts"
- Splenic infarction
- Hepatic calcification
- Other
  - IVC thrombosis
  - Pseudoaneurysm of hepatic artery
  - Recurrent hepatic tumor

ERCP Findings (after Transplantation)

- Abnormal cholangiograms are seen in 80% of patients with hepatic artery stenosis (bile duct ischemia) but in only 30% of patients with patent hepatic artery. Abnormalities include:
  - Nonanastomotic strictures, 25% (up to 50% in hepatic artery stenosis)
  - Anastomotic strictures, 5%
  - Intraluminal filling defects (sludge, casts), 5%
  - Bile leaks, 5%

PASSIVE HEPATIC CONGESTION

- Congested liver in cardiac disease; stasis of blood in liver parenchyma due to impaired hepatic venous drainage
- Early enhancement of dilated IVC and hepatic veins on CT, due to contrast reflux from RA into IVC
- Heterogeneous reticulated mosaic parenchymal pattern of liver
- Periportal edema
- Enlarged liver and ascites

Cardiomegaly

HEPATIC SARCOIDOSIS (BOECK DISEASE)

Noncaseating granulomas are evident in multiple organs.
- Most common is nonspecific hepatosplenomegaly.
- Diffuse parenchymal heterogeneity or multinodular pattern with low attenuating nodules in liver and spleen that gradually become isodense after contrast
- Advanced disease may simulate cirrhosis.
- Nodules hypointense on T1W and T2W sequences
- Periportal adenopathy

HELLP SYNDROME

Hemolysis, elevated liver enzymes, low platelets.
- Variant of toxemia in primigravidas; rarely seen in multiparas
- Intrahepatic or subcapsular fluid collection (hematoma) on US or CT
- Liver infarction with small or large peripheral wedge-shaped hypoattenuating lesions

Biliary System

GENERAL

DUCTAL ANATOMY (Fig. 3-54)

Right hepatic duct (RHD)
- Right anterior superior (RAS) segment
- Right anterior inferior (RAI) segment
- Right posterior superior (RPS) segment
- Right posterior inferior (RPI) segment
- Caudate (C) segment

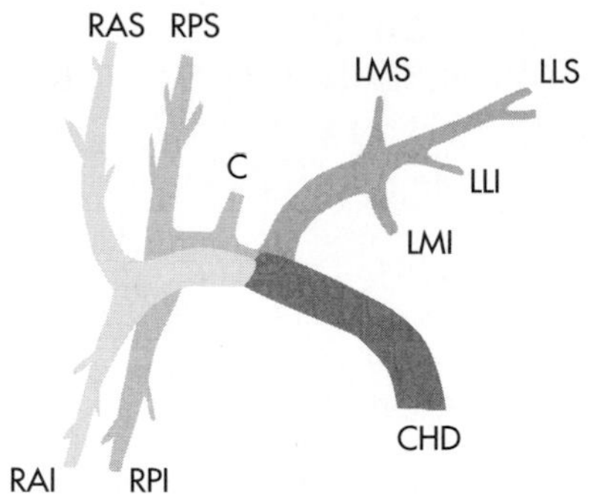

FIGURE 3-54

Left hepatic duct (LHD)
- Left medial superior (LMS) segment
- Left medial inferior (LMI) segment
- Left lateral superior (LLS) segment
- Left lateral inferior (LLI) segment

RHD and LHD form the common hepatic duct (CHD), which receives the cystic duct (CD) from the GB to form the common bile duct (CBD).

Variations of Intrahepatic Biliary Anatomy
- "Normal" anatomy as shown above, 60%
- Right posterior ducts drain directly into LHD, 20%
- Right posterior duct, right anterior duct, and LHD form CHD, 10%

Variations of Cystic Duct Insertion (Fig. 3-55)
- Normal insertion
- Low union
- Parallel course
- Anterior spiral course
- Posterior spiral course

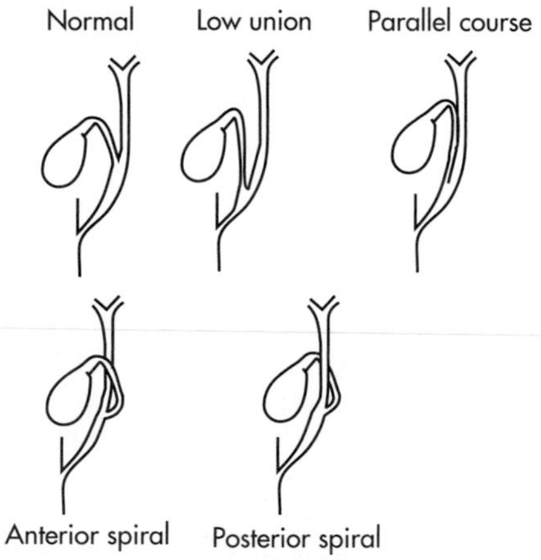

FIGURE 3-55

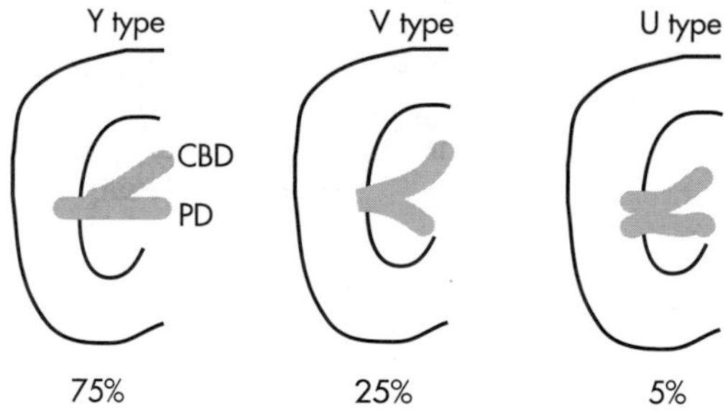

FIGURE 3-56

Variations of Papillary Insertion (Ducts within Papilla = Ampulla) (Fig. 3-56)

The CBD drains into the duodenum through the ampulla.

Variations of pancreatic duct (PD) and CBD insertion:
- Y type: CBD and PD combine before insertion into ampulla
- V type: CBD and PD insert jointly into ampulla
- U type: CBD and PD insert separately into ampulla

US Measurements of CHD (Fig. 3-57)

CHD measurements (inner wall to inner wall) are performed at the level of hepatic artery. Normal measurements:
- <7 mm in normal fasting patients <60 years; in 95% the CHD is <4 mm
- <10 mm in normal fasting patients age 60 to 100 years
- <11 mm in patients with:
  - Previous surgery
  - Previous CD obstruction
- Fatty meal challenge: if CHD enlarges more than 2 mm after fatty meal (Lipomul), it indicates obstruction.

Location of the hepatic artery relative to the CBD: (Fig. 3-58)

Most common (80%)
- Hepatic artery between CBD and portal vein

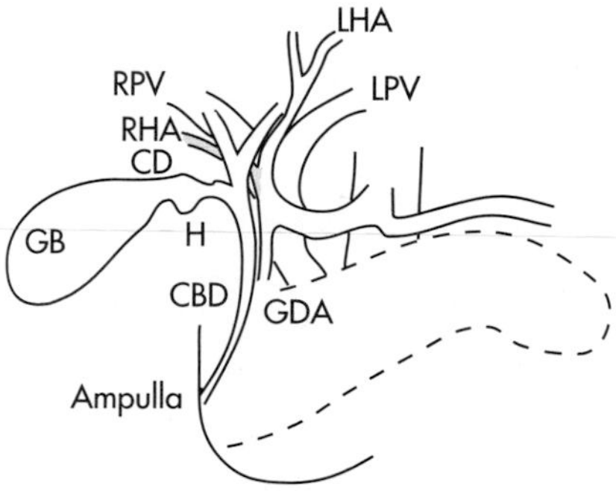

FIGURE 3-57

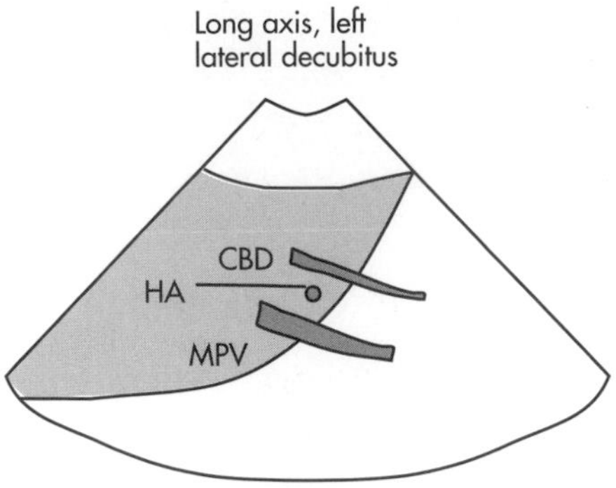

FIGURE 3-58

- Hepatic artery medial to main portal vein (MPV)
- CBD lateral to portal vein

Less common (20%)

- Hepatic artery anterior to CBD
- Hepatic artery posterior to portal vein

GALLBLADDER

US Measurements

- Wall ≤ 2 mm (distended GB)
- Maximum dimensions 5 x 10 cm

Variants

- Phrygian cap: fundal locule from septal-like invagination
- Junctional fold: fold between infundibulum and body; may be hyperechoic and cause posterior shadowing
- Agenesis of GB (rare); more common causes of nonvisualized GB
  - Previous cholecystectomy
  - Nonfasting
  - Chronic cholecystitis

ENDOSCOPIC RETROGRADE CHOLANGIOPANCREATOGRAPHY (ERCP)

Contrast-agent injection is performed through the endoscope after cannulation of papilla (Fig. 3-59) with CBD. Complications include:

- Pancreatitis, 5%
- Duodenal perforation
- Gastrointestinal bleeding

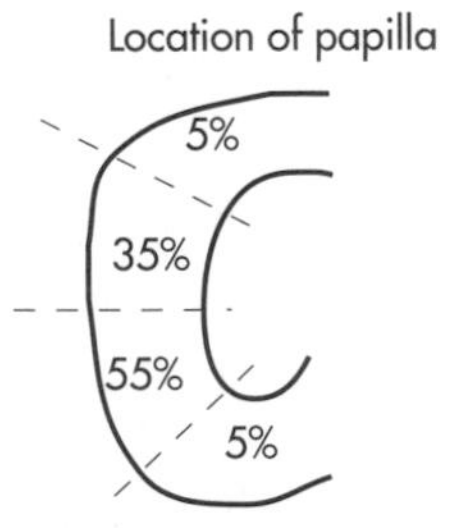

FIGURE 3-59

MAGNETIC RESONANCE CHOLANGIOPANCREATOGRAPHY (MRCP)

Fat-suppressed 2-D or 3-D heavily T2W sequences are obtained of the upper abdomen (e.g., fast spin-echo, spin-echo, echo-planar, gradient-echo). Bile appears hyperintense, and images of the entire biliary and pancreatic ductal system can be rendered by maximum signal intensity projection reconstruction. Common indications for MRCP usually include unsuccessful ERCP or a contraindication to ERCP and the presence of biliary enteric anastomoses (e.g., choledochojejunostomy, Billroth II anastomosis).

Advantages of MRCP over ERCP

MRCP (1) is noninvasive, (2) is cheaper, (3) uses no radiation, (4) requires no anesthesia, (5) is less operator dependent, (6) allows better visualization of ducts proximal to obstruction, and (7) when combined with conventional T1W and T2W sequences, allows detection of extraductal disease.

Disadvantages of MRCP

- Decreased spatial resolution, making MRCP less sensitive to abnormalities of the peripheral intrahepatic ducts (e.g., sclerosing cholangitis) and pancreatic ductal side branches (e.g., chronic pancreatitis)
- Imaging in the physiologic, nondistended state, which decreases the sensitivity to detect subtle ductal abnormalities
- Cannot perform therapeutic endoscopic or percutaneous intervention for obstructing bile duct lesions. Thus, in patients with high clinical suspicion for bile duct obstruction, ERCP should be the initial imaging modality to provide timely intervention (e.g., sphincterotomy, dilatation, stent placement, stone removal), if necessary.

Technique

MRCP is usually performed with heavily T2W sequences by using fast spin-echo or single-shot fast spin-echo pulse sequences and both a thick-collimation (single-section) and thin-collimation (multisection) technique with a torso phased-array coil. The coronal plane is used to provide a cholangiographic display, and the axial plane is used to evaluate the pancreatic duct and distal common bile duct. In addition, 3-D reconstruction by using a maximum-intensity projection (MIP) algorithm on the thin-collimation source images can be performed. The patients fast for 3 hours before the MRCP, thereby reducing unwanted signal from the intestine. Secretin (1 CU/kg IV) can be given to patients suspected of having pancreatic disease; this substance transiently distends the duct and allows better visualization of its morphologic features. Maximum dilatation occurs 2 minutes after secretin injection, and then the duct relaxes to baseline. Persistent dilatation implies papillary stenosis, and dilatation of side branches suggests chronic pancreatitis.

MRCP is comparable with ERCP in detection of obstruction, with a sensitivity, specificity, and accuracy of 91%, 100%, and 94%, respectively. It is 94% sensitive and 93% specific for detection of dilatation. MRCP may also allow more accurate assessment of ductal caliber in the physiologic state, unlike ERCP, with which ductal caliber may be overestimated because of injection pressure. MRCP is comparable with ERCP in detection of choledocholithiasis and superior to CT or US. Numerous studies have shown sensitivities of 81%-100% and specificities of 85%-100% for MRCP.

Pitfalls

Pitfalls include pseudo-filling defects, pseudodilatations, and nonvisualization of the ducts. Filling defects are usually due to stones, air, tumors, hemorrhage, or sludge. Infrequent causes of filling defects include susceptibility artifact from adjacent clips, metallic bile duct stents, folds, or flow voids.

BILIARY LITHIASIS

CHOLELITHIASIS

Gallstones occur in 10%-20% of the U.S. population. 30% are calcified. 30%-50% of patients are asymptomatic. Surgical removal is indicated in symptomatic and diabetic patients (high risk of acute cholecystitis).

Types

- Cholesterol stones are caused by precipitation of supersaturated bile (Western population, women > men, old age > young age).
- Pigment stones: precipitate of calcium bilirubinate (Asian population)
- Mixed stones (most common type)

Predisposing Factors

- Obesity
- Hemolytic anemia (pigment stones)
- Abnormal enterohepatic circulation of bile salts (Crohn disease, SB resection)
- Diabetes
- Cirrhosis
- Hyperparathyroidism

US Features

- Prominent posterior shadow (type I). Very small stones may not shadow: reposition the patient to heap up calculi.
- Mobility of stones; gravity-dependent movement; exception: stones impacted in neck or stones adherent to wall.
- Wall-echo-shadow (WES triad, double-arc sign) is seen if the GB is contracted (type II) and completely filled with stones; however, WES triad can also be seen with:
  - Porcelain GB (calcification of GB)
  - Emphysematous cholecystitis
- Highly reflective echo originating from the anterior surface of calculus

US SIGNS OF CHOLELITHIASIS

	Type I	Type II	Type III
US appearance	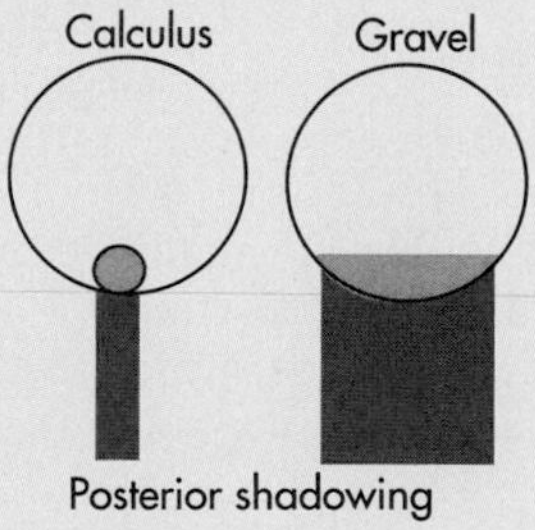	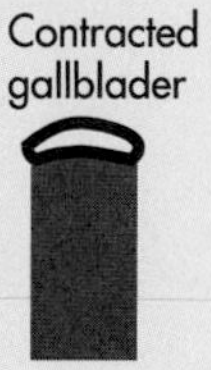	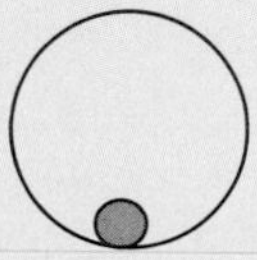
Sensitivity	Hyperechoic stone Posterior shadow Visible GB 100%	Hyperechoic stone Posterior shadow Nonvisible GB 90%-100%	Hyperechoic stone No posterior shadow Visible GB 50%-80%

Clean versus Dirty Shadows

The acoustic shadowing depends on:
- Size of stone (small stones may not shadow)
- Angle of beam
- Stone-beam focus distance
- Frequency of transducer

CLEAN VERSUS DIRTY SHADOWS

Clean Shadow	Dirty Shadow
Hypoechoic shadow with no echoes in it	Comet tail with echoes in shadow
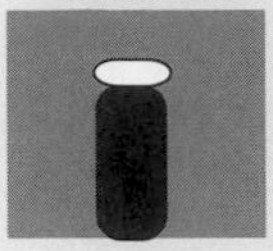	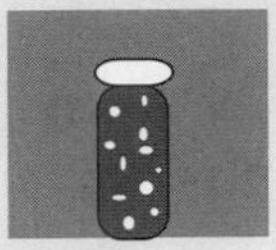
Rough surface	Smooth surface
Small radius of curvature	Large radius of curvature
Stones with calcification	Stones with high cholesterol content
	Bowel loops visualized rather than GB

CHOLEDOCHOLITHIASIS

Presence of stone or stones in the bile duct, typically associated with high-grade obstruction and jaundice. Diagnostic accuracy with US, 75%.

PAPILLARY STENOSIS

Sphincter of Oddi spasm; treat with papillotomy. Causes:

- Postcholecystectomy
- Stones
- Trauma
- AIDS cholangiopathy

SLUDGE

Sludge (echogenic bile) is a sonographic term that refers to layering particulate material (calcium bilirubinate and/or cholesterol crystals) within bile; no posterior shadowing. Causes include:
- Fasting (decreased CCK)
  - 10 days: 30% of patients have sludge
  - 6 weeks: 100% of patients have sludge
- Hyperalimentation (decreased CCK)
- Infection, obstruction

Implications

- Sludge is a common finding of stasis in the GB.
- Sludge is associated with infection/obstruction (cholecystitis) in 20% of ICU patients.
- Symptomatic patients (unexplained fever, RUQ pain, dilated GB with sludge) may benefit from percutaneous cholecystostomy.

MILK OF CALCIUM BILE

Concentration of intravesicular calcium salts in longstanding CD obstruction. Radiographically, GB contents appear dense.

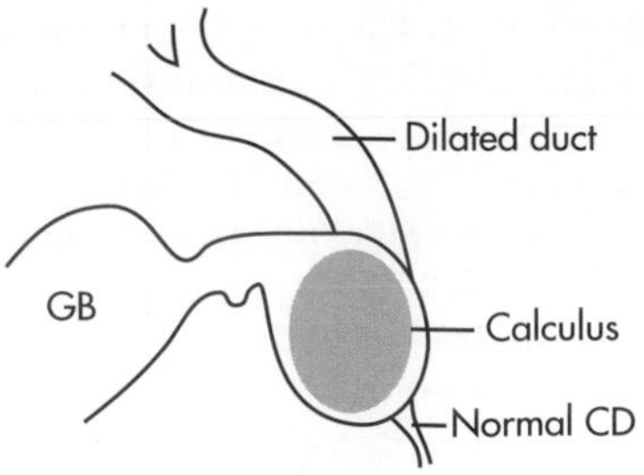

FIGURE 3-60

MIRIZZI SYNDROME (Fig. 3-60)

Impacted stone in the CD and surrounding inflammation causes compression and obstruction of CHD. The calculus may ultimately erode into the CHD or gut.

BILIARY-ENTERIC FISTULAS

Causes

- Chronic cholecystitis with erosion of a gallstone into the GI tract, 90%
- Penetration of posterior duodenal ulcer into CHD, 5%
- Tumor
- Trauma

Types

- Biliary-gastric
- Biliary-duodenal, 70% (most common; may cause gallstone ileus)
- Biliary-colonic
- Bouveret syndrome: obstruction of stomach or duodenum by stone
- Iatrogenic (ERCP, surgical): most common cause for biliary ductal gas

INFLAMMATION

ACUTE CHOLECYSTITIS (Fig. 3-61)

Causes

- Gallstone obstruction, 95%
- Acalculous cholecystitis, 5%

US Features

- Luminal distention >4 cm
- Wall thickening >5 mm (edema, congestion); thickening is usually worse on the hepatic side
- Gallstones; CD stones may be difficult to detect if they are not surrounded by bile.
- Positive Murphy's sign (sensitivity, 60%; specificity, 90%)
- Pericholecystic fluid

Complications

- Gangrenous cholecystitis: rupture of GB; mortality, 20% gangrene causes nerve death so that 65% of patients have a negative Murphy's sign.

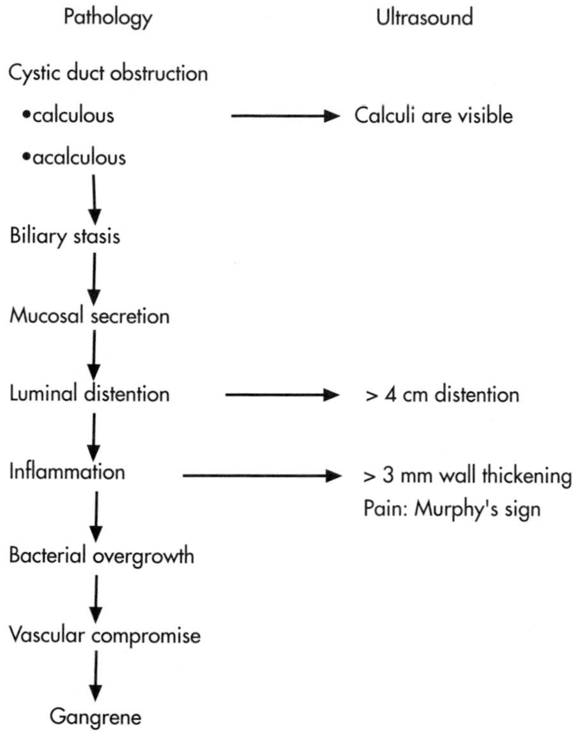

FIGURE 3-61

- Emphysematous cholecystitis, rare (40% occur in diabetics)
- Empyema

CHRONIC CHOLECYSTITIS

US Features

- GB wall thickening (fibrosis, chronic inflammation)
- Intramural epithelial crypts (Rokitansky-Aschoff sinuses)
- Gallstones, 95%
- Failure of GB to contract in response to CCK
- Porcelain GB: wall calcifications; increased risk of GB carcinoma

ACALCULOUS CHOLECYSTITIS (Fig. 3-62)

Clinical settings associated with acalculous cholecystitis:

- Trauma
- Burn patient
- Prolonged fasting (postoperative patients), hyperalimentation
- Diabetes
- AIDS
- Others: colitis, hepatic arterial chemotherapy, postpartum, vascular insufficiency

Imaging Features

US

- No calculi
- Sludge and debris
- Usually in critically ill patients
- Same findings as in calculous cholecystitis:
  - Sonographic Murphy's sign
  - GB wall thickening (>2 mm)
  - Pericholecystic fluid
  - May occur in absence of any of the above findings

HIDA scanning (see Chapter 12)

- Nonvisualization of GB

XANTHOGRANULOMATOUS CHOLECYSTITIS

Imaging Features

- Predominantly seen in women between the ages of 60 and 70 years. Patients present with signs and symptoms of cholecystitis: right upper quadrant pain, vomiting, leukocytosis, and a positive Murphy's sign.
- Gallstones
- Marked thickening of GB wall
- Inflammatory changes in contiguous hepatic parenchyma
- Difficult to differentiate from adenocarcinoma
- Complications are present in 30% of cases and include perforation, abscess formation, fistulous tracts to the duodenum or skin, and extension of the inflammatory process to the liver, colon, or surrounding soft tissues

AIDS (Fig. 3-63)

A variety of abdominal abnormalities are detected by US and/or CT in AIDS patients who are referred for abdominal pain, fever, and/or abnormal LFT:

- Hepatosplenomegaly, 30%
- Biliary abnormalities, 20%

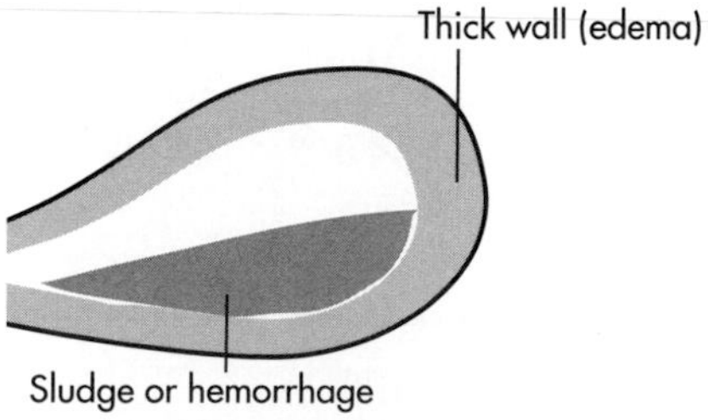

FIGURE 3-62

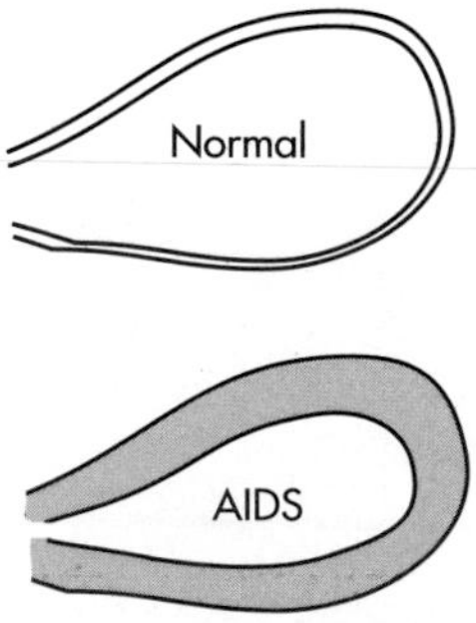

FIGURE 3-63

GB wall thickening, 7%
Cholelithiasis, 6%
Sludge, 4%
Biliary dilatation, 2%
- Lymphadenopathy, 20%
- Ascites, 15%

GB wall thickening is relatively common and may be marked, and its cause is often unknown. Only symptomatic patients should be treated for acalculous cholecystitis, which may be due to *Cryptosporidium* and/or cytomegalovirus.

ACUTE CHOLANGITIS

Infection of obstructed bile ducts. *E. coli* > *Klebsiella* > *Pseudomonas*.

Causes

- Choledocholithiasis (most common cause)
- Stricture from prior surgery
- Sclerosing cholangitis
- Infected drainage catheter
- Ampullary carcinoma

Imaging Features

- Dilatation of intrahepatic ducts; dilated CBD, 70%
- Pigment stones and sludge in intrahepatic bile ducts (pathognomonic)
- Biliary strictures, 20%
- Segmental hepatic atrophy, 30%
- Liver abscess, pancreatitis (less common complications)

RECURRENT PYOGENIC CHOLANGITIS (ORIENTAL CHOLANGIOHEPATITIS)

Endemic disease in Asia characterized by recurrent attacks of fever, jaundice, and abdominal pain. Cause: *Clonorchis sinensis* and *Ascaris* infections; however, at time of diagnosis these infections are typically absent. Bacterial superinfection. Very common in Asia. Young adults.

Imaging Features (Fig. 3-64)

Detection
- US is the primary screening modality of choice.
- CT is commonly used to assess the extent of disease.

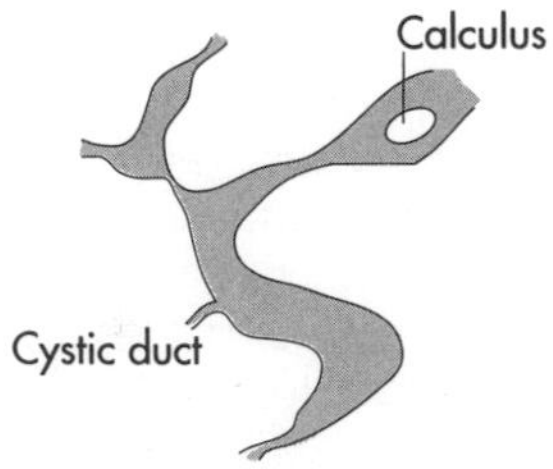

FIGURE 3-64

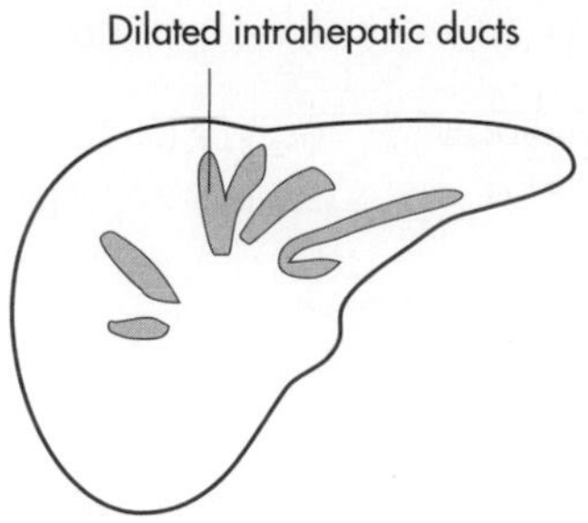

FIGURE 3-65

- Cholangiography (hepatic, ERCP or intraoperative) is mandatory to delineate intrahepatic biliary anatomy and to exclude high biliary strictures.

Morphologic features (Fig. 3-65)
- Biliary dilatation
  Extrahepatic biliary dilatation, 90%
  Intrahepatic biliary dilatation, 75%
  Left lobe and posterior right lobe most commonly affected
- Biliary strictures
- Intrahepatic calculi (hepatolithiasis)
  Contain calcium bilirubinate, cellular debris, and mucinous substance
  Typically hyperechoic and cast shadows
  Stones may not be sufficiently hyperdense to be detectable by CT.

Complications

- Intrahepatic abscess formation
- Hepatic atrophy due to portal vein occlusion
- Cholangiocarcinoma, 5%
- Pancreatic duct involvement, 20%.
- GB disease is present in only 20%.

SCLEROSING CHOLANGITIS (Fig. 3-66)

Chronic inflammatory process of intrahepatic (20%) and extrahepatic (80%) bile ducts that causes progressive narrowing. Chronic or intermittent obstructive jaundice is evident.

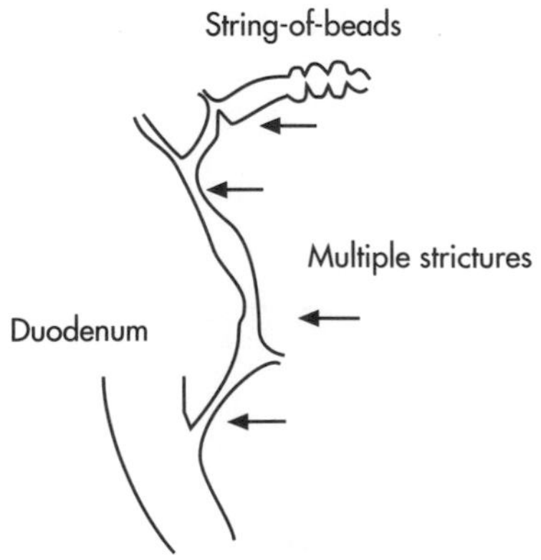

FIGURE 3-66

Types

Primary sclerosing cholangitis (idiopathic)
Secondary sclerosing cholangitis

- Inflammatory bowel disease (65%), usually ulcerative colitis
- Cirrhosis, chronic active hepatitis
- Retroperitoneal fibrosis
- Pancreatitis
- Some other rare diseases (e.g., Riedel thyroiditis, Peyronie disease)

Imaging Features

- Irregular dilatation, stenosis, beading of intrahepatic and extrahepatic bile ducts (seen best by cholangiogram): string-of-beads appearance
- Small "diverticula" of biliary tree are pathognomonic.
- Differential diagnosis:
  - Primary biliary cirrhosis (normal extrahepatic ducts)
  - AIDS cholangiopathy (may be associated with ampullary stenosis)
  - Sclerosing cholangiocarcinoma

Complications

- Cholangiocarcinoma, 10%
- Biliary cirrhosis
- Portal hypertension

HYPERPLASTIC CHOLECYSTOSES

Benign group of diseases with no neoplastic potential, uncertain clinical significance. Commonly seen in cholecystectomy specimen, less commonly identified by US or cholecystogram.

Adenomyomatosis

Most common form of hyperplastic cholesterolosis. There is marked hyperplasia of the GB wall. Epithelium herniates into the wall, forming Rokitansky-Aschoff sinuses. Findings may be focal (more common) or diffuse.

US Features

- Large Rokitansky-Aschoff sinuses (Fig. 3-67)
  - Hypoechoic sinuses if they contain bile
  - Hyperechoic sinuses if they contain sludge or calculi

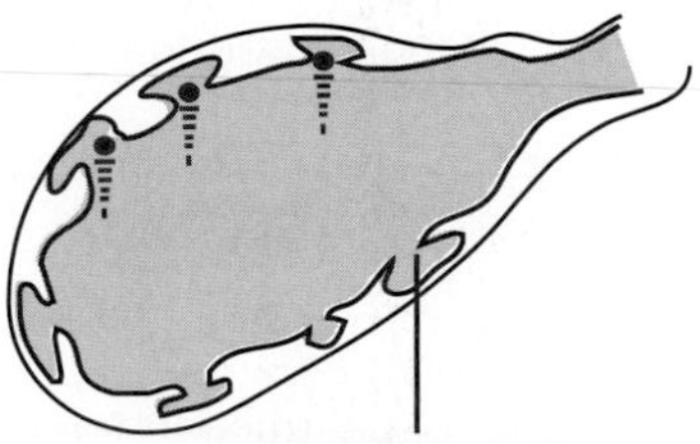

FIGURE 3-67

- High-amplitude foci in the wall (cholesterol crystals) that produce comet-tail artifacts (V-shaped, ring-down artifacts)
- Thickening of GB wall is common but nonspecific.
- Inflammation is not typical.
- Hypercontractility

CHOLESTEROLOSIS (STRAWBERRY GB)

Triglycerides and cholesterol are deposited in macrophages of GB wall. The cholesterol nodules stud the wall and give the GB the appearance of a strawberry.

US Features

- Lipid deposits (usually <1 mm) are echogenic.
- No shadowing
- Inflammation is not a prominent feature.
- Associated with multiple 0.5-mm polyps

GB ADENOMA

- Single or multiple (10%) 5 to 20 mm. 60% of the cases are associated with cholelithiasis. Found in 0.5% of cholecystectomy specimens (F > M) in normal population and to a higher degree in familial adenomatous polyposis and Peutz-Jeghers syndrome. Adenomas are usually asymptomatic and discovered incidentally during a radiologic evaluation of abdominal pain.
- Polyps >1 cm require a careful search for features associated with malignancy, such as thickening or nodularity of the GB wall; evidence of hepatic invasion, such as an indistinct margin between the liver and GB; biliary duct dilatation; and peripancreatic or hepatoduodenal ligament adenopathy.
- US: gallbladder adenomas are typically smoothly marginated. Intraluminal polypoid masses. Should raise concern for malignancy. The echo texture of adenomas is typically homogeneously hyperechoic; however, adenomas tend to be less echogenic and more heterogeneous as they increase in size. The additional finding of gallstones is common in patients with GB adenomas.
- CT: intraluminal soft tissue masses, isoattenuating or hypoattenuating relative to liver. They may be difficult to distinguish from noncalcified gallstones.

TUMORS

GB CARCINOMA

Biliary cancers (adenocarcinoma of the GB, cholangiocarcinoma) are the fifth most common GI malignancy

Associations

- Cholelithiasis in 90% (cholelithiasis per se is not carcinogenic)
- IBD (UC > Crohn disease)
- Porcelain GB, 15%
- Familial polyposis
- Chronic cholecystitis

Imaging Features

- Intraluminal soft tissue density (polypoid or fungating mass)
- Asymmetrically thickened GB wall
- Usually no biliary dilatation
- Cholelithiasis
- Direct invasion of liver
  - Direct extension, 50%
  - Distant liver metastases, 5%
- Gastrohepatic and hepatoduodenal ligaments
  - Ligamentous extension, 75%
  - Direct invasion into duodenum, 50%
  - Lymph node metastases, 70%
- Lymph nodes
  - Foramen of Winslow node
  - Superior and posterior pancreaticoduodenal nodes
  - Hepatic and celiac nodes
  - Peritoneal spread
  - Carcinomatosis, 50%
  - Intestinal obstruction, 25%

Cholangiocarcinoma

Adenocarcinoma of the biliary tree. Scirrhous type has worse prognosis than polypoid type. Jaundice, pruritus, and weight loss occur. Treatment is with pancreaticoduodenectomy (Whipple's procedure) or palliative procedures (stent placement, biliary bypass procedure).

Locations

- Hilar: originates from epithelium of main hepatic ducts or junction: Klatskin tumor
- Peripheral: originates from epithelium of intralobular ducts

Associations (Fig. 3-68)

- UC
- *Clonorchis* exposure in Asian population
- Caroli disease
- Benzene, toluene exposure

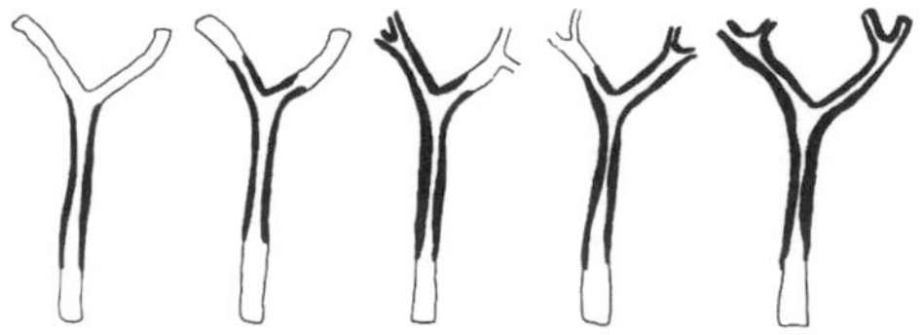

FIGURE 3-68

Imaging Features

- Dilated intrahepatic ducts with normal extrahepatic ducts
- Hilar lesions
  - Central obstruction
  - Lesions are usually infiltrative so that a mass is not usually apparent.
  - Encasement of portal veins causes irregular enhancement by CT.
- Peripheral lesions
  - May present as a focal mass or be diffusely infiltrative
  - Retain contrast materials on delayed scans
  - Occasionally invade veins
- ERCP patterns
  - Short annular constricting lesion, 75%
  - Long stricture, 10%
  - Intraluminal polypoid mass 5%

DIFFERENTIATION OF BILIARY STRICTURES

	MRCP or ERCP Findings	Risk Factors
Cholangiocarcinoma	Irregular biliary duct with abrupt luminal narrowing	Primary sclerosing cholangitis, ulcerative colitis, liver parasites, choledochal cysts
Benign stricture	Smoothly narrowed biliary duct, even with stricture	Recurrent cholangitis, surgical intervention
Primary sclerosing cholangitis	Multifocal intrahepatic strictures and dilatations	Ulcerative colitis
Autoimmune cholangitis	Smooth, thick wall, can have short or long stricture	May occur without autoimmune pancreatitis
Biliary stones	Round filling defects	Known biliary stone disease

Intrahepatic Cholangiocarcinoma

Adenocarcinoma arising from intrahepatic bile ducts. More common in Asia than in United States.

Imaging Features

- Biliary ductal dilatation distal to tumor
- Lesions have irregular borders with infiltrative margins
- Delayed peripheral to central enhancement due to fibrosis and hypovascularity
- Capsular retraction and vascular invasion

Biliary Cystadenoma

Biliary cystadenoma is an uncommon, multilocular cystic liver mass that originates in the bile duct and usually occurs in the right hepatic lobe. It typically occurs in women; many women complain of chronic abdominal pain. It may represent a congenital anomaly of the biliary anlage. Malignant transformation to cystadenocarcinoma occurs.

Imaging Features

- CT: lesions appear well defined and cystic. The wall and internal septations are often visible and help distinguish this lesion from a simple cyst. The cyst walls and any other soft tissue components typically enhance with contrast.
- MRI: variable appearance, depending on the protein content of the fluid and the presence of an intracystic soft tissue component.

BILE DUCT HAMARTOMA OR ADENOMA (VON MEYENBURG COMPLEX)

Benign tumor composed of disorganized bile ducts and ductules and fibrocollagenous stroma. The tumor is usually small (1 to 5 mm), although the nodules may coalesce into larger masses. Although bile duct hamartoma is benign, there have been reports of an association of cholangiocarcinoma with multiple bile duct hamartomas.

Imaging Features

- Nonspecific imaging appearance can simulate metastases or microabscesses; therefore, histologic diagnosis is required. Multiple bile duct hamartomas may simulate metastases or hepatic abscesses.
- CT: small, well-defined hypoattenuating or isoattenuating mass. Little if any enhancement is evident.
- MRI: usually hypointense on T1W images, isointense or slightly hyperintense on T2W images, and hypointense after administration of Gd-DTPA
- US: Hypoechoic lesions containing central echogenic focus with ring-down artifact due to cholesterol crystals

PERIBILIARY CYSTS

Found in cirrhosis, benign cystic lesions that encase but do not communicate with ducts. Related to peribiliary glands.

CYSTIC DISEASES

Cystic disease of the biliary tree can take several forms:

- Cyst in the main duct (choledochal cyst)
- Cysts in the main duct at the duodenal opening (choledochocele)
- Cysts in the small biliary branches within the liver (Caroli disease)
- Other cysts

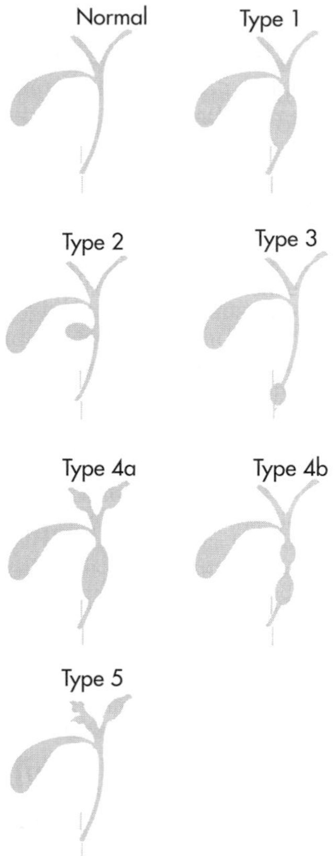

FIGURE 3-69

CHOLEDOCHAL CYST (Fig. 3-69)

Cystic dilatation of CBD (types 1, 2). Choledochal cysts are often lined with duodenal mucosa. They typically occur in children and young adults (congenital?). Most common in Asia (Japan), uncommon in United States. Because there is a 20-fold increased risk of bile duct malignancy, choledochal cysts are usually excised. Classic triad:

- Jaundice
- Abdominal pain (infection of bile)
- Palpable mass

CAROLI DISEASE SUBSET

Segmental cystic dilatation of intrahepatic (only) bile ducts (type 5, subset of choledochal cyst). Etiology unknown. Autosomal recessive. Sequence of events:

- Bile stasis predisposes to intrahepatic calculi.
- Secondary pyogenic cholangitis
- Intrahepatic abscesses
- Increased risk of cholangiocarcinoma

Associations

- Medullary sponge kidney, 80%
- Infantile polycystic kidney disease

Imaging Features

- Multiple cystic structures converging toward porta hepatis
- Beaded appearance of intrahepatic bile ducts
- Most of the cysts arranged in a branching pattern
- The "central dot sign" is a very specific sign of Caroli disease in which portal radicals are partially or completely surrounded by abnormally dilated and ectatic bile ducts on both sonography and CT.
- Sludge, calculi in dilated ducts

CHEMOTHERAPY CHOLANGITIS

- Iatrogenic cholangitis after intraarterial chemotherapy; ischemic cholangiopathy; in many cases, floxuridine has been used.
- Strictures of common hepatic duct, frequently involving biliary bifurcation.
- Sparing of distal common bile duct (disease hallmark)

INTERVENTION

LAPAROSCOPIC CHOLECYSTECTOMY

Technique

1. First, trocar is placed blindly in supraumbilical region (most common site of complications).
2. CO_2 is used to inflate the abdomen. Postoperatively, CO_2 is resorbed quickly, and persistent gas may indicate bowel perforation.
3. CD is dissected and clipped at both ends.
4. GB is removed via supraumbilical cannula.

Contraindications

- Acute cholecystitis, cholangitis
- Peritonitis, sepsis
- Pancreatitis
- Bowel distention
- Portal hypertension
- Morbid obesity

Complications (0.5%-5%)

- Biliary obstruction (clipping or thermal injury to CBD, postoperative fibrosis); usually requires percutaneous drainage
- Biliary leak causing peritonitis and/or biloma (cystic duct stump leak, injury to CBD, leak from small Luschka bile ducts draining directly into GB). Detection of bile leaks: HIDA scan, ERCP, transhepatic cholangiogram
- Other
  - Retained stones, stones dropped in peritoneal cavity (Morison's pouch)
  - Bowel perforation
  - Hemorrhage, infection

Bismuth Classification of Bile Duct Injury (Fig. 3-70)

Based on the level of traumatic injury in relation to the confluence of LHD and RHD.

- Type 1: injury >2 cm distal to confluence
- Type 2: injury <2 cm distal to confluence
- Type 3: injury immediately distal to confluence but with intact confluence
- Type 4: destroyed confluence

CHOLECYSTOSTOMY

Percutaneous cholecystostomy is often performed for acalculous cholecystitis in ICU patients with unexplained sepsis. In these patients, sonographic findings are not helpful in making the diagnosis of acute cholecystitis and a "trial" of cholecystostomy is often warranted (clinical response is typically seen in 60% of patients).

Indications

- Unexplained fever, suspected cholecystitis. Rationale for catheter placement is to decompress an inflamed GB.
- GB must be distended.
- GB wall may be thickened; GB may contain sludge.

Technique

1. Scan liver by US and choose appropriate entry site. Go through liver to minimize the occurrence of a bile leak.
2. Anesthetize skin.
3. Place 22-gauge spinal needle into GB under US guidance.
4. Place catheter into GB in tandem. Visualize catheter tip by US before deploying catheter.
5. Aspirate bile for culture. Connect catheter to collecting bag.

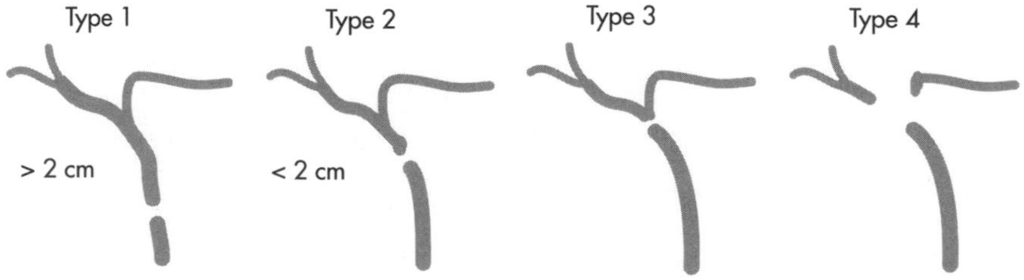

FIGURE 3-70

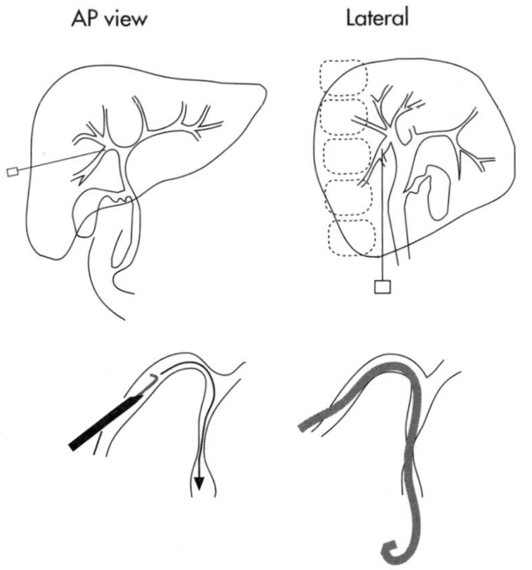

FIGURE 3-71

Management

- If there is no cholelithiasis, the catheter is usually left for ~3 weeks. At this point the catheter is clamped to make sure that there is adequate internal drainage. If the patient tolerates clamping, the catheter can be removed.
- If there is cholecystitis, the catheter is left in place until the patient is stable and can undergo a surgical cholecystectomy.
- Unlike patients with acalculous cholecystitis, patients with cholelithiasis have an irritant in the GB and thus a reason for inflammation to recur.

PERCUTANEOUS BILIARY PROCEDURES

Three types of percutaneous procedures are frequently performed:

- Transhepatic cholangiogram
- Biliary drainage
- Biliary stent placement

Transhepatic Cholangiogram

Indication: demonstration of biliary anatomy, first step before biliary drainage or stent placement. Steps in procedure:

1. Antibiotic coverage (particularly if biliary obstruction)
2. Using a lateral midaxillary approach, advance one-stick system into liver.
3. Attach extension tubing and syringe filled with contrast. Slowly inject contrast while retracting the needle under fluoroscopy. Repeat until opacification of bile ducts.

Biliary Drainage (Fig. 3-71)

Indication: biliary obstruction. Steps after transhepatic cholangiogram:

1. After cannulation of bile duct, advance a Nitinol guidewire (or the guidewire that comes with the one-stick access set) through the needle into the biliary system. Obtain as much purchase as possible. Remove needle.
2. Pass plastic catheter over guidewire. Exchange guidewire for a 0.038 metal wire or Terumo; pass guidewire into duodenum.
3. Dilate skin tract up to 12 Fr.
4. Place drainage catheter over guidewire (Cope, Ring catheters).
5. Perform catheter injection with contrast material to adjust placement of side holes.

Biliary Stent Placement

Indication: (malignant) biliary stricture; inability to place endoscopic stent. Steps:

1. Inject existing catheter to determine exact site of stricture.
2. Choose appropriate stent lengths.
3. Place ultrastiff guidewire; remove indwelling catheter.
4. Place 8-Fr peel-away sheath.
5. Deploy expandable stent (e.g., Wallstent).
6. Inject to confirm location. Leave safety catheter in. Remove guidewire.

Pancreas

GENERAL

PANCREATIC ANATOMY

Pancreatic Duct (Fig. 3-72)

- Duct of Wirsung enters into major papilla together with the CBD.
- Duct of Santorini empties into minor papilla.

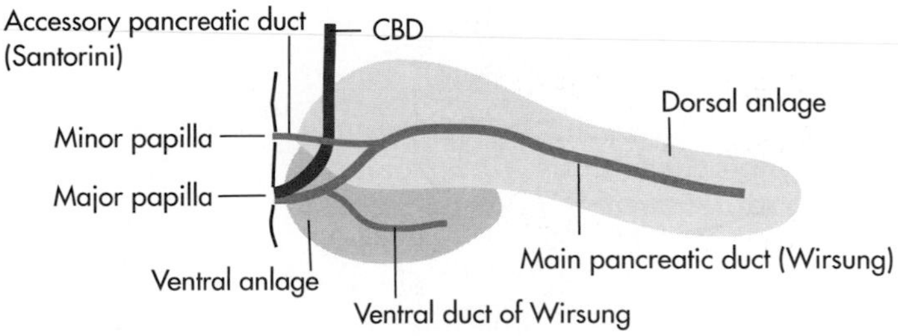

FIGURE 3-72

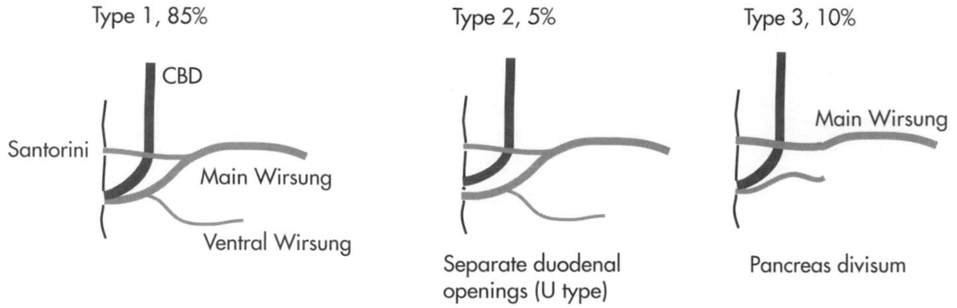

FIGURE 3-73

- Both pancreatic ducts communicate with each other near the neck of the pancreas, forming a single remaining duct that runs through the center of the body and tail of the pancreas.
- Upper size limit of main duct in young adults, 3 mm; elderly, 5 mm

Variations (Fig. 3-73)

- Type 1: normal anatomy, 85%
- Type 2: separate duodenal openings for pancreatic duct and CBD, 5%
- Type 3: pancreas divisum. Lack of fusion of dorsal and ventral pancreatic ducts. Occurs in 10% of population. Main pancreatic drainage is through the minor papilla. Up to 25% of patients with recurrent idiopathic pancreatitis have pancreas divisum. Pathophysiology of pancreatitis: orifice of duct of Santorini is relatively too small to handle secretions. ERCP: cannulization of the major papilla only allows visualization of the ventral duct.

Pancreas Dimensions (Fig. 3-74)

- Head, 2 cm
- Neck (anterior to portal vein), <1.0 cm
- Body and tail, 1 to 2 cm
- Cephalocaudate diameter, 3 to 4 cm

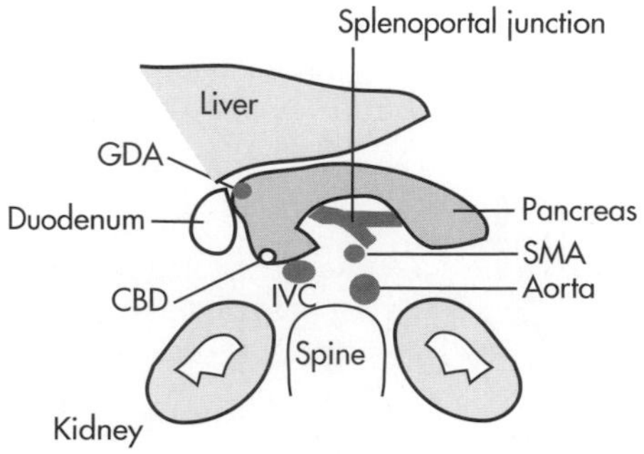

FIGURE 3-74

Fatty Infiltration (Fig. 3-75)

Fatty infiltration of the pancreas is common normal finding with increasing age.

- Fatty distribution is often uniform.
- Focal sparing around CBD is common.
- Lobulated external contour

Secretin Stimulation Test

Secretin (1 CU/kg) is given IV, and the pancreatic and CBD sizes are measured before and at 1, 5, 15, and 30 minutes. Secretin increases the volume and bicarbonate content of secreted pancreatic juice. Changes in duct diameter:

Normal volunteers
- Baseline duct size 1.9 mm (range: 1 to 3 mm)
- 70%-100% increase in duct size is normal.
- Return to baseline duct size within 30 minutes

Chronic pancreatitis
- No significant increase in pancreatic duct size

Functional ductal obstruction
- Pancreatic duct remains dilated 15 to 30 minutes after administration of secretin.

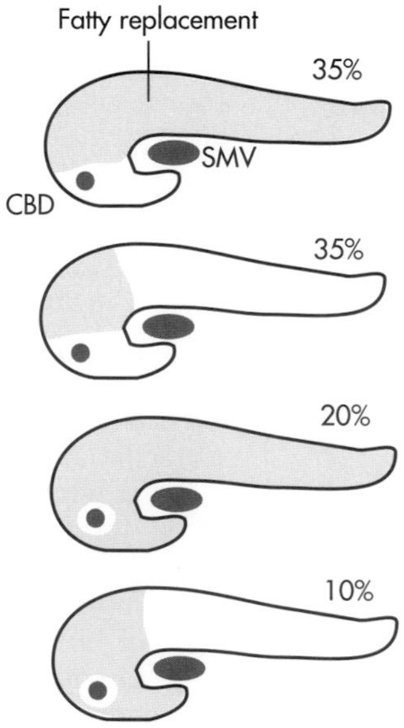

FIGURE 3-75

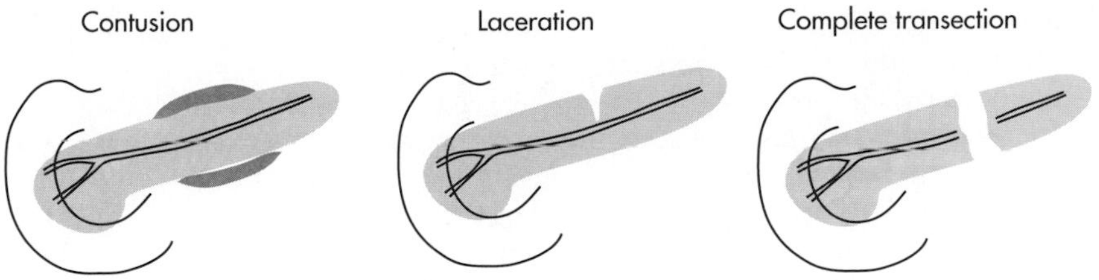

FIGURE 3-76

CONGENITAL ANOMALIES IN ADULTS

CYSTIC FIBROSIS

Pancreatic tissue largely nonexistent; often total fatty replacement is seen. End-stage disease: pancreatic insufficiency.

Imaging Features

US
- Increased echogenicity (fatty replacement)
- Small cysts are rarely visualized, although they are very common (1 to 3 mm).
- Large cysts (<5 cm) have been reported but are uncommon.

CT
- Pancreatic tissue totally missing; may see duct
- Small bowel may be dilated with "fecal appearing" contents
- Fibrosing colonopathy: wall thickening is the predominant proximal colon complication of enzyme replacement therapy

Annular Pancreas
- Results from abnormal migration of the ventral pancreas
- The pancreas surrounds and obstructs the duodenum.
- Appears as annular constriction of second portion of duodenum
- ERCP is the imaging study of choice; pancreatic duct encircles the duodenum.
- Increased incidence of pancreatitis and peptic ulcer disease

Ectopic Pancreatic Tissue
- Present in 1%-10% of population
- Sites
  - Stomach (antrum)
  - Duodenum
- Smooth, submucosal mass often with central umbilication (remnant of pancreatic duct)

PANCREATIC TRAUMA

Pancreatic injuries are due to either penetrating (stab, gunshot wounds) or blunt (motor vehicle accident) trauma.

Types of Injuries (Fig. 3-76)
- Simple superficial contusion with minimal parenchymal hemorrhage
- Deep laceration or perforation without duct injury
- Laceration with duct transection

Imaging Features

CT
- Fragmentation of gland
- Pancreatic hematoma
- Nonenhancing regions
- Peripancreatic stranding, exudate

Intraoperative pancreatography
- Should be performed to evaluate integrity of pancreatic duct (injury to the duct requires different surgery)

Delayed Complications
- Pancreatic fistula, 10%-20%
- Abscess, 10%-20%
- Pancreatitis
- Pseudocyst, 2%

PANCREATITIS

GENERAL

Classification

Acute pancreatitis
- Mild acute pancreatitis (interstitial edema)
- Severe acute pancreatitis (necrosis, fluid collections)
- Groove pancreatitis: inflammation localized to groove between duodenum and pancreatic head

Chronic pancreatitis

Causes

Common, 70%
- Alcoholic pancreatitis
- Cholelithiasis

Less common, 30%
- Postoperative, post-ERCP, abdominal trauma
- Hyperlipidemia, hypercalcemia
- Drugs: azathioprine, thiazides, sulfonamides
- Inflammation: PUD
- Hyperparathyroidism
- Pregnancy

Clinical Findings

Mild pancreatitis usually presents as pain, vomiting, and tenderness; progression to severe, acute pancreatitis is not common. Severe, acute pancreatitis is manifested by more dramatic symptoms and signs: shock, pulmonary insufficiency, renal failure, GI hemorrhage, metabolic abnormalities, flank ecchymosis (Grey Turner's sign), and/or periumbilical ecchymosis (Cullen's sign). The severity of acute pancreatitis can be assessed using Ranson (severe pancreatitis: >3 signs at onset) or APACHE II criteria (severe pancreatitis: >8 criteria during time of pancreatitis).

IMAGING OF ACUTE PANCREATITIS

CT Staging (Value of Predicting Clinical Outcome is in Dispute)

- Grade A: normal pancreatic appearance
- Grade B: focal or diffuse enlargement of pancreas
- Grade C: pancreatic abnormalities and peripancreatic inflammation
- Grade D: 1 peripancreatic fluid collection
- Grade E: >2 peripancreatic fluid collections and/or gas in or adjacent to the pancreas

Pearls

- By US, an inflamed pancreas appears hypoechoic relative to liver (reversal of normal pattern) because of edema.
- US is mainly used for investigation of gallstones and/or to follow the size of pseudocysts.
- Barium: colon cutoff sign

TERMINOLOGY AND COMPLICATIONS

Pancreatic Necrosis (Fig. 3-77)

- Diffuse parenchymal (>30% of pancreatic area) or focal areas (>3 cm) of nonviable parenchyma, peripancreatic fat necrosis, and fluid accumulation
- Accuracy of CECT for detection of pancreatic necrosis: 80%-90%

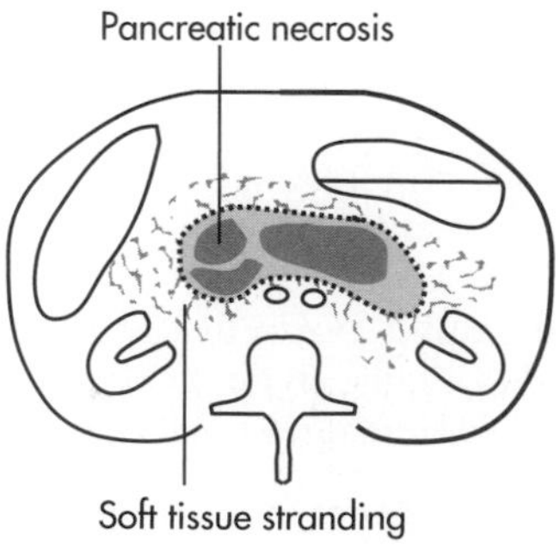

FIGURE 3-77

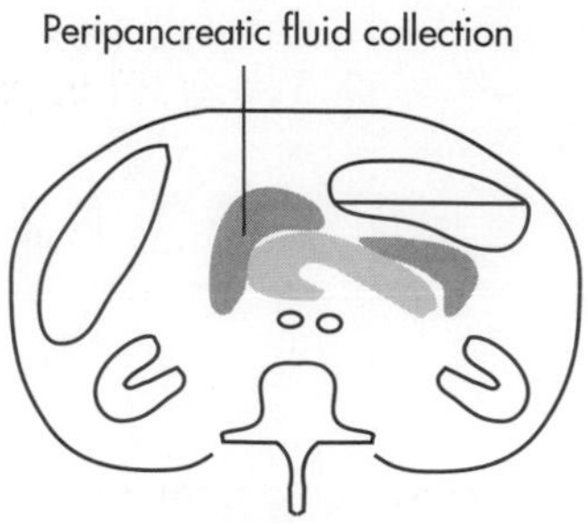

FIGURE 3-78

- Presence and extent of fluid associated with fat necrosis cannot be accurately determined by CT attenuation numbers.
- Prognosis: 30% necrosis = 8% mortality; 50% necrosis = 24% mortality; >90% necrosis = 50% mortality

Acute Fluid Collections (Formerly Called Phlegmon) (Fig. 3-78)

- Collections of enzyme-rich pancreatic fluid occur in 40% of patients.
- No fibrous capsule (in contradistinction to pseudocysts)
- Most common location is within and around the periphery of the pancreas. Fluid collections are not limited to the anatomic space in which they arise and may dissect into mediastinum, pararenal space, or organs (spleen, kidney, liver).
- Prognosis: 50% resolve spontaneously; the rest evolve into pseudocysts or are associated with other complications (infection, hemorrhage).
- Differentiation from pseudocyst difficult: test of time

Pseudocyst (Fig. 3-79)

- Encapsulated collection of pancreatic fluid, which is typically round or oval. The capsule is usually indistinguishable but may occasionally be identified. Caused by microperforation of the pancreatic duct; such a communication can be identified by ERCP in 50% of patients.

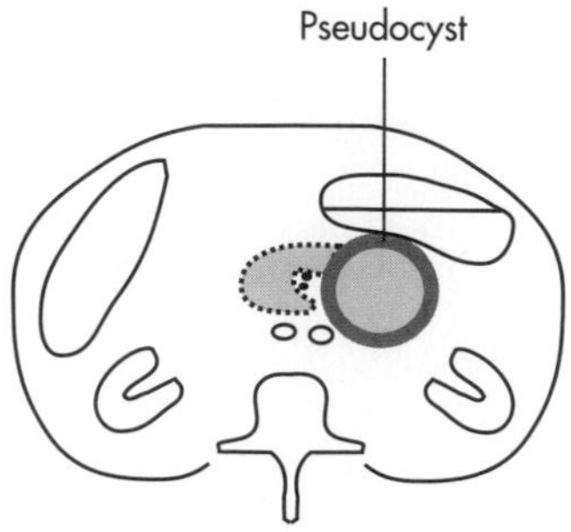

FIGURE 3-79

- Surgical definition of pseudocyst requires persistence at least 6 weeks from the onset of pancreatitis.
- Occurs in 40% of patients with acute pancreatitis and in 30% of patients with chronic pancreatitis
- Bacteria may be present but are often of no clinical significance; if pus is present, the lesion is termed a *pancreatic abscess*.
- Prognosis: 50% resolve spontaneously and are not clinically significant; 20% are stable and 30% cause complications such as:
  - Dissection into adjacent organs: liver, spleen, kidney, stomach
  - Hemorrhage (erosion into vessel, thrombosis, pseudoaneurysm)
  - Peritonitis: rupture into peritoneal cavity
  - Obstruction of duodenum, bile ducts (jaundice, cholangitis)
  - Infection

Pancreatic Abscess

- Intraabdominal fluid collection in or adjacent to the pancreas that contains pus. Effectively treated by percutaneous drainage
- Usually occurs >4 weeks after onset of acute pancreatitis
- UGI series: Mottled gas medial to C loop with duodenal narrowing

Infected Necrosis

- Necrotic pancreatic (and/or peripancreatic) tissue that can become infected; rarely specific signs of infection; precipitates surgical drainage if infected.
- Differentiation from pancreatic abscess is crucial for appropriate clinical treatment (see table below).

COMPARISON

Features	Pancreatic Abscess	Infected Necrosis
Location	In or adjacent to pancreas	In pancreas
Pancreas enhancement	Enhancement of periphery	Nonenhancement of necrotic pancreas
Gas	Very infrequent	Very infrequent
Time of appearance	>4 weeks after onset	Any time
Treatment	Percutaneous drainage	Surgical debridement
Prognosis	Better	Worse

Hemorrhage

- Usually occurs as a late consequence of vascular injury, commonly erosion into splenic or pancreaticoduodenal arteries
- May result from rupture of pseudoaneurysm

PERCUTANEOUS THERAPY

Needle Aspiration

- May be performed on any fluid collection, necrotic tissue, or hemorrhage to determine if infected
- Pseudocysts <5 cm should be monitored rather than aspirated because pseudocysts commonly resolve spontaneously; aspiration risks superinfection (in 10% of cases).

Percutaneous Drainage

- Fluid collections are amenable to drainage if there is clinical suspicion of infection: success rate is 70%.
- Pseudocysts >5 cm are good candidates for drainage; smaller pseudocysts should be monitored.
- Necrotic pancreatic tissue, soft tissue (peri)pancreatic collections, and hematomas are a contraindication to drainage; these entities usually require surgery.

CHRONIC PANCREATITIS (Fig. 3-80)

Progressive, irreversible destruction of pancreatic parenchyma by repeated episodes of mild or subclinical pancreatitis.

Causes

- Alcohol
- Hyperparathyroidism
- Hyperlipidemia
- Hereditary

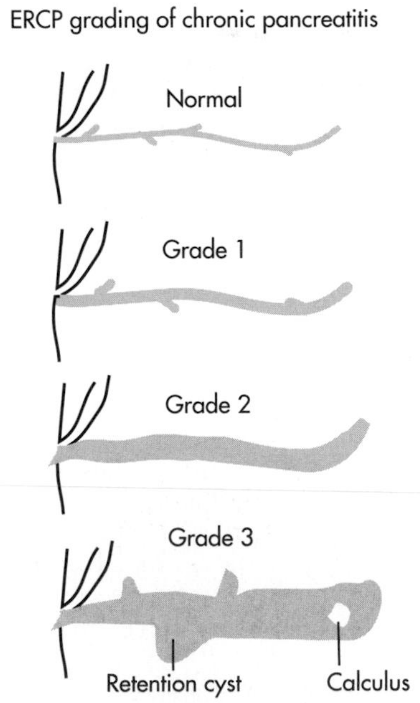

FIGURE 3-80

Imaging Features

Size
- Commonly small, uniformly atrophic pancreas
- Focal enlargement from normal or inflamed pancreas may be coexistent 40%

Tissue
- Fatty replacement
- Fibrosis
- Parenchymal calcifications, intraductal calculi

Irregular dilatation of pancreatic duct by ERCP: grade 1 to 3 (see Fig. 3-80); side branches may have clubbed appearance

Complications
- Pseudocysts, 30%
- Obstructed CBD, 10%
- Venous thrombosis (splenic, portal, mesenteric veins), 5%
- Increased incidence of carcinoma
- Malabsorption, steatorrhea, 50%

AUTOIMMUNE PANCREATITIS

A subset of patients with "chronic pancreatitis" have autoimmune pancreatitis (previously defined as idiopathic), for which no etiology has been identified to date. May occur alone or with other immune disorders; most patients have increased IgG and antinuclear antibody levels. Histologic diagnosis: dense lymphoplasmacytic infiltrate with scattered eosinophils. May be associated with autoimmune cholangitis. Treatment: steroids.

Imaging Features
- Ultrasound: focal hypoechoic, diffuse enlargement of gland; gland may be normal in appearance; CBD may be dilated.
- CT: often diffuse enlargement of pancreas, loss of normal surface indentations, tail retracted from splenic hilum, capsule-like rim enhancement around gland, peripancreatic adenopathy, no calcification, vascular encasement of CBD dilatation
- MRCP: diffuse irregular narrowing of pancreatic duct, proximal CBD dilated if disease localized to the head of the pancreas

GROOVE PANCREATITIS

Pancreatitis involving the pancreatic groove (potential space between head of pancreas, duodenum, and the CBD). Two forms:
- Segmental: involves pancreatic head with development of scar tissue in the groove
- Pure form: affects groove only sparing pancreatic head

Clinical manifestation related to duodenal and biliary obstruction; biliary strictures in 50%.

Factors related to development
- Peptic ulcer disease
- Gastric resection
- True duodenal wall cysts
- Pancreatic heterotopia
- Disturbance in flow of MPD

Imaging Features
- CT: Soft tissue in the pancreaticoduodenal groove with delayed enhancement; small cystic lesions along medial wall of duodenum
- MRI: Sheetlike mass in pancreaticoduodenal groove hypointense to pancreas on T1 and isointense to slightly hyperintense to pancreas on T2; delayed enhancement; cystic lesions in medial wall of duodenum seen in cystic dystrophy

HETEROTOPIC PANCREAS

Abnormally located pancreatic tissue with its own ductal system and no vascular neural or anatomic contact with the normal pancreas. Most common heterotopia in the GI system. Usually asymptomatic. Most common locations include:
- Duodenum 30%
- Stomach 25%; usually submucosal in location; prepyloric region along greater curvature in 90%
- Jejunum 15%
- Less common locations: Meckel's, ileum, GB, fallopian tubes, umbilicus, esophagus, spleen, mediastinum, and omentum

PANCREATITIS IN CYSTIC FIBROSIS

CF is autosomal recessive disease secondary to mutation of a gene encoding chloride channel; GI manifestations precede pulmonary manifestations with exocrine pancreatic insufficiency being most common (90%); CF is the most common cause of exocrine pancreatic insufficiency in young patients.

Imaging Features
- Fatty replacement with or without pancreatic glandular atrophy; most common CT finding
- Calcification, 7%
- Cyst formation; abnormalities in pancreatic duct (strictures, beading, dilatation, obstruction)
- Pancreatic cystosis: rare, entire pancreas replaced with multiple cysts of varying size

TROPICAL PANCREATITIS

Variant of chronic pancreatitis. Characterized by:
- Young age at onset; usually no alcohol abuse
- Associated with malnutrition
- Regional predisposition in tropical countries
- Rapidly progressive course with severe pancreatitis
- Presence of large intraductal calculi
- Increased risk of adenocarcinoma

Imaging Features

- Large pancreatic calculi within dilated pancreatic duct; up to 5 cm in size; may extend into side branches. In contrast, calculi in alcoholic-related chronic pancreatitis are small and speckled
- Parenchymal atrophy
- 15- to 25-fold increased risk of pancreatic adenocarcinoma

HEREDITARY PANCREATITIS

- Autosomal dominant disease involving mutation of the cationic trypsinogen gene
- Acute attacks begin in childhood
- Imaging features resemble those of tropical pancreatitis
- 50- to 70-fold increased risk of pancreatic adenocarcinoma

TYPES OF PANCREATIC TUMORS

Exocrine pancreatic tumor
- Pancreatic ductal adenocarcinoma (PDAC) represents 95% of all pancreatic cancers
- Cystic neoplasm (microcystic adenoma, macrocystic adenoma), 1%
- Intraductal papillary mucinous tumor (IPMT), 1%
- Rare tumors (acinar cell carcinoma, pleomorphic carcinoma, epithelial neoplasm)

Endocrine pancreatic tumor (islet cell neoplasm)
- Insulinoma
- Gastrinoma
- Nonfunctioning islet cell tumor

Other tumors
- Lymphoma
- Metastases
- Connective tissue tumors

ADENOCARCINOMA (PDAC)

Poor prognosis (1-year mean survival rate, 8%); 65% >60 years

Clinical Findings

- Jaundice
- Weight loss
- Courvoisier's sign (enlarged, nontender GB), 25%

Imaging Features (Fig. 3-81)

Mass effect
- 65% of tumors occur in head (5% curable), 35% in body and tail (incurable)
- Only part of pancreas is enlarged; global enlargement from associated pancreatitis is uncommon (15%).
- Compression of duodenum
- Enlargement may be subtle.

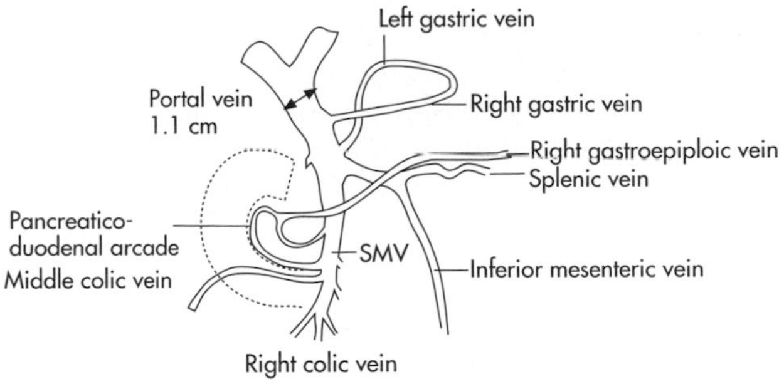

FIGURE 3-81

- Sensitivity: contrast-enhanced high-resolution CT > US
- Some small pancreatic tumors are better resolved by US than by CT because of texture changes.

Alterations of density (clue to diagnosis)
- On nonenhanced CT scans, tumors may appear subtly hypodense because of edema and necrosis.
- Tumor appears hypodense on bolus contrast-enhanced scans.
- Calcifications are very uncommon in contrast to cystic and islet cell tumors.

Ductal obstruction
- Pancreatic duct obstruction; pseudocysts are rare.
- Common bile duct obstruction with pancreatic duct obstruction (double duct sign: also seen with pancreatitis)
- Tumors in the uncinate process may not cause ductal obstruction.

Extrapancreatic extension
- Most commonly retropancreatic (obliteration of fat around celiac axis or SMA one sign of incurability)
- Porta hepatis extension
- Direct invasion of stomach, small bowel, etc.

Vascular involvement
- Arteries and veins are best evaluated by angiography or helical CT; rule out replaced right HA pre-Whipple
- Criteria for unresectability
  - SMA encased
  - Portal vein or proximal superior mesenteric vein (SMV) obstructed or largely encased
  - Tumors are still resectable if smaller branches are encased
  - Dilatation of smaller venous branches (>5 mm): an indirect sign of venous encasement

Metastases
- Liver (very common) > lymph nodes > peritoneal and serosal > lung

CYSTIC NEOPLASM

Mucin-producing cystic tumors should be considered when cystic lesions arise in the pancreas. Of all cystic pancreatic lesions, 10% are neoplastic, whereas the remainder represent benign lesions (simple cysts, VHL, pseudocysts).

Classification

- Mucin-producing tumors: malignant potential
  - Intraductal papillary mucinous tumor (IPMT)
  - Mucinous cystic neoplasm
- Serous cystadenoma: no malignant potential

OVERVIEW

Features	Serous Microcystic Adenoma (Benign)	Mucinous Cystic Neoplasm (Malignant Potential)
Number of cysts	>6	<6
Size of individual cysts	<20 mm	>20 mm
Calcification	40%: amorphous, starbursts	20%: rim calcification
Enhancement	Hypervascular	Hypovascular
Cyst content (aspiration)	Glycogen ++++	Mucin ++++
Other features	Central scar (15%)	Peripheral enhancement Spread: local, LN, liver
Demographics	Older patients (>60 years)	Younger patients (40-60 years)
Location	70% in head of pancreas	95% in body or tail of pancreas

DIFFERENTIATION OF CYSTIC LESIONS BY FLUID CONTENT

CYST ASPIRATION

Parameter	Pseudocyst	Serous Cystadenoma	Mucinous Cystadenoma	Mucinous Cystadeno-carcinoma
Cytology	Inflammatory	50% positive	Usually positive	Usually positive
CEA	Low	Low	High	High
CA 15-3	Low	Low	Low	High
Viscosity	Low	Low	High	High
Amylase	High	Low	Variable	Variable

INTRADUCTAL PAPILLARY MUCINOUS TUMOR (IPMT) OF PANCREAS

Rare pancreatic cystic neoplasms that arise from the epithelial lining of the pancreatic ducts and secrete thick mucin, which leads to ductal dilatation and obstruction. Synonyms: duct ectatic cystadenocarcinoma, intraductal papillary tumor, duct ectatic mucinous cystadenocarcinoma.

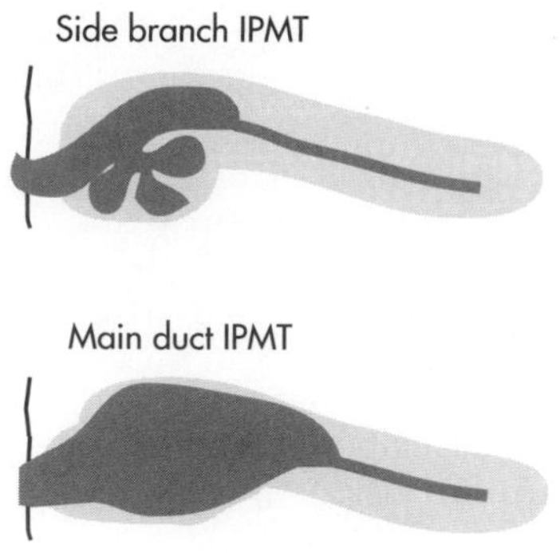

FIGURE 3-82

Types (Fig. 3-82)

- Side branch lesions
- Main duct lesions

Associations

- Adenocarcinoma, 25%
- Hyperplasia, 25%
- Dysplasia, 50%

Imaging Features

Location
- Head, uncinate, 55%
- Body, tail, 10%
- Diffuse, multifocal, 35%

Ductal abnormalities
- ERCP/MRCP: communicates with pancreatic duct, DDx: pseudocyst
- Combined main/side branch duct type, 70%
- Isolated side branch duct type, 30%
- Ductal dilatation, 97%
- "Masses of mucin"
- Clusters of small cysts from 1 to 2 cm in diameter

Signs of malignancy
- Size > 3 cm; if solitary and cyst < 3 cm, reexamine in 2 years
- Solid mass, mural nodule
- Main pancreatic duct >10 mm
- Intraluminal calcified content
- Diffuse or multifocal involvement
- Presence of diabetes

MUCINOUS CYSTIC NEOPLASMS (Fig. 3-83)

Large peripheral tumors surrounded by thick fibrous capsule. The cyst cavity is filled with mucinous material. Unlike IPMT, there is no connection to the pancreatic duct. Synonyms: mucinous macrocystic neoplasm, mucinous cystadenoma, mucinous cystadenocarcinoma, macrocystic adenoma.

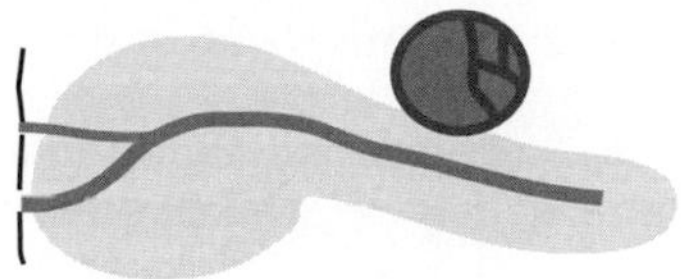

FIGURE 3-83

PANCREATOBLASTOMA

- Rare primary pancreatic neoplasm of childhood
- Usually affects patients between 1 and 8 years of age but has been reported in neonates and in adults
- A congenital form is associated with Beckwith-Wiedemann syndrome.
- Slow growing and usually large at presentation
- Large, well-defined, multilobulated masses with enhancing septa by CT; mixed echotexture seen on US.
- The tumors are soft and gelatinous and, if arising in pancreatic head, do not usually produce obstructive symptoms.

SOLID PSEUDOPAPILLARY NEOPLASM

- Synonyms: Frantz's tumor, solid and cystic acinar tumor, papillary epithelial neoplasm, solid and papillary epithelial neoplasm
- Large lesions of epithelial tissue that are slightly more common in body/tail. Well-demarcated, mixed solid and cystic hemorrhagic mass. Solid components with increased enhancement. May contain calcifications. Good prognosis after surgical resection.
- Women <50 years old

ACINAR CELL CARCINOMA

- Older men
- Less desmoplastic and often larger than pancreatic adenocarcinoma, may be encapsulated
- Invades rather than encases vessels
- Metastatic fat necrosis

ISLET CELL NEOPLASM

Islet cell tumors arise from multipotential stem cells: **a**mine **p**recursor **u**ptake and **d**ecarboxylation (APUD) system.

Classification

- Functional (85%): secretion of one or more hormones
- Nonfunctional

Insulinoma (Most Common Functional Tumor)

- Single, 70%; multiple, 10%; diffuse hyperplasia or extrapancreatic, 10%
- Malignant transformation, 10%
- 90% <2 cm
- Hypervascular, 70%
- Diagnostic accuracy: intraoperative US > pancreatic venous sampling > angiography > MRI > other
- Main symptoms: hypoglycemia

Gastrinoma (Second Most Common)

- Solitary, 25%; multiple, ectopic, in stomach, duodenum, etc.
- Gastrinoma triangle: formed by the cystic duct, 1st-3rd portions of duodenum, pancreatic head and neck
- 60% malignant transformation
- Mean tumor size: 35 mm
- Hypervascular, 70%
- Main symptoms: Zollinger-Ellison syndrome (diarrhea, PUD)

Nonfunctioning Islet Cell Tumors (Third Most Common)

- Most common in pancreatic head
- 80%-90% malignant transformation (5-year survival 45%)
- Usually large (>5 cm) and cause symptoms by exerting mass effect: jaundice, palpable
- Calcification, 20%
- Hypervascular at angiography
- Liver metastases enhance brightly on CT.
- Less aggressive than adenocarcinoma
- Better response to chemotherapy

Rare Islet Cell Tumors

- Less aggressive than adenocarcinoma
- Better response to chemotherapy
- VIPoma (vasoactive intestinal peptide)
  - WDHA syndrome (**w**atery **d**iarrhea, **h**ypokalemia, **a**chlorhydria)
  - 60% malignant transformation
- Somatostatinoma
  - Suppression of insulin, thyroid-stimulating hormone, growth hormone secretion (hyperglycemia)
  - 90% malignant transformation
- Glucagonoma
  - Diarrhea, diabetes, glossitis, necrolytic erythema migrans 80% malignant transformation

METASTASES

- Most hematogenous metastases are from RCC, lung cancer, breast cancer, or melanoma.
- Metastases from RCC are the most common metastases and can appear as hypervascular tumors, solitary or multiple.
- Direct invasion occurs most commonly from transverse colon (along mesocolon) or stomach.

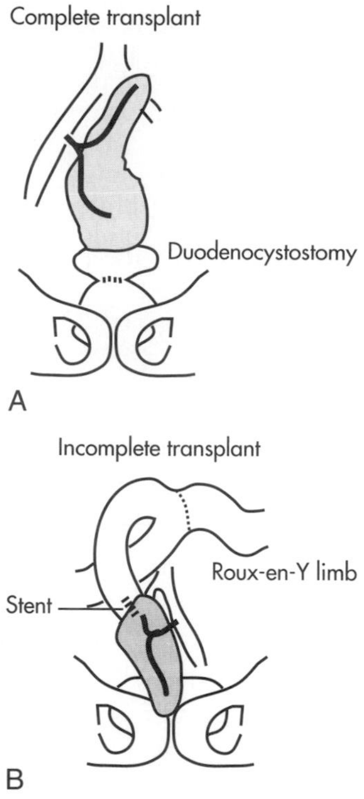

FIGURE 3-84

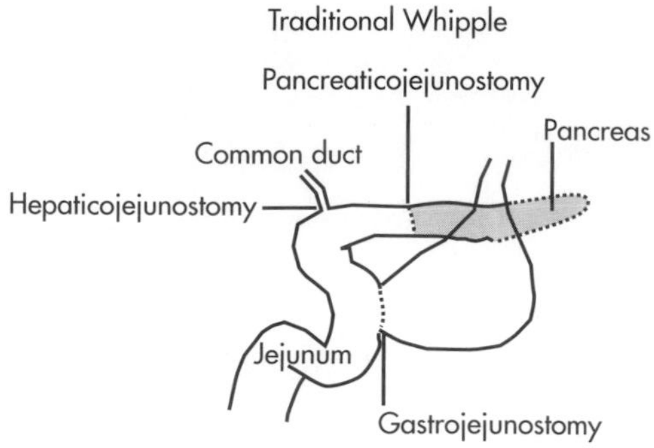

FIGURE 3-85

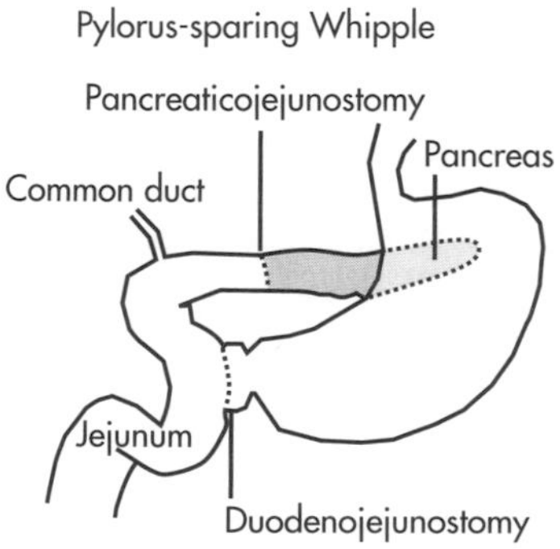

FIGURE 3-86

TRANSPLANT (Fig. 3-84)

Normal Imaging Features

- Pancreas is attached to bladder by duodenal interposition.
- Stent may be in place.

Complications

- Rejection, 35%
- Pancreatitis, 35%
- Peripancreatic abscess, 35%
- Peripancreatic hemorrhage, 35%
- Vascular thrombosis, 20%

WHIPPLE SURGERY (Fig. 3-85)

- The conventional standard Whipple procedure involves resection of the pancreatic head, duodenum, and gastric antrum. The GB is almost always removed. A jejunal loop is brought up to the right upper quadrant for gastrojejunal, choledochojejunal, or hepaticojejunal, and pancreatojejunal anastomosis.
- Some surgeons prefer to perform pancreatoduodenectomy to preserve the pylorus when possible (Fig. 3-86). In pylorus-preserving pancreatoduodenectomy, the stomach is left intact and the proximal duodenum is used for a duodenojejunal anastomosis.

Complications of Pancreatoduodenectomy

- *Delayed gastric emptying* is defined as the persistent need for a nasogastric tube for longer than 10 days and is seen in 11%-29% of patients.
- *Pancreatic fistula* is defined as surgical drain output of amylase-rich fluid greater than 5 mL/day at or beyond 7 to 10 days. Patients with the clinical diagnosis of pancreatic fistula usually undergo CT to assess for associated abscess formation, but approximately 80% of fistulas heal with conservative management. In 10%-15% of patients with pancreatic fistulas percutaneous drainage is required, and 5% of patients require repeat surgery.
- Wound infection
- Hemorrhage (can occur if replaced right hepatic artery is severed)
- Pancreatitis
- Abscess formation
- Biliary complications

Spleen

GENERAL

ANATOMIC VARIATIONS

Accessory Spleen (in 40% of Patients)

- Arises from failure of fusion
- Usually near hilum of spleen
- Usual size: <3 cm
- Usual shape: round

Lobulations (Very Common)

- Clefts cause lobulations
- Do not mistake clefts for splenic fractures.

Wandering Spleen

- Abnormal congenital development of the dorsal mesogastrium. Normally the posterior leaf of dorsal mesogastrium fuses with the parietal peritoneum anterior to the left kidney to form the lienorenal ligament, the most important stabilizer of splenic position. Failure of complete fusion of these structures allows for abnormal mobility of the spleen with a long splenic vascular pedicle. Because of the long pedicle, excessive intraperitoneal movement and torsion can occur. Laxity of suspensory ligaments allows spleen to move in abdomen.
- Confirm with ^{99m}TC sulfur colloid scan.

Polysplenia

- Multiple splenic nodules
- Left-sided liver
- Absence of gallbladder
- Cardiac anomalies
- Incomplete development of inferior vena cava

ASPLENIA

- Absence of spleen (exclude splenectomy)

CT APPEARANCE

- CT density of spleen is slightly less than that of liver.
- Inhomogeneous enhancement may normally occur early during contrast administration.

SPLENOMEGALY (Fig. 3-87)

Defined as splenic length >12 cm longest diameter on transverse image. The splenic index (multiply the 3 dimensions) is more accurate for determining splenic size. Normal: 120 to 480 cm^3. Most radiologists eyeball the size.

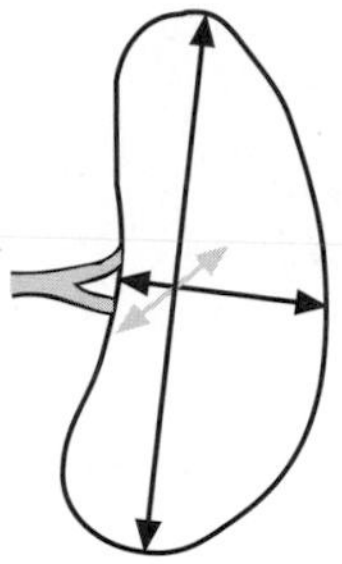

FIGURE 3-87

Common Causes

Tumor
- Leukemia
- Lymphoma

Infection
- AIDS related
- Infectious mononucleosis

Metabolic disorders
- Gaucher disease

Vascular
- Portal hypertension; may be associated with Gamma-Gandy bodies: benign siderotic nodules (hypointense by MRI).

TUMORS

CYSTS

- True cysts (epithelial lining): epidermoid
- False cysts (no lining): Trauma, infection, infarction

HAMARTOMA

Rare, benign tumors primarily composed of vascular elements. It can be asymptomatic, or anemia and thrombocytopenia may occur. May be hypodense or isodense; usually hyperechoic on US. Cystic and calcified elements may be present in large lesions.

HEMANGIOMA

Incidence: most common benign splenic tumor (14% of autopsy series).

Imaging Features

- Hyperechoic by US features (similar appearance as liver hemangioma)
- Well delineated, small
- Foci of calcification occur occasionally.

METASTASES

The most common malignancy of the spleen is lymphoma. Metastases are less common:
- Breast
- Lung
- Stomach
- Melanoma
- End-stage ovarian cancer

TRAUMA

INJURY

Mechanism

- Blunt trauma
- Penetrating trauma

Spectrum of Injuries

- Subcapsular hematoma (crescentic fluid collection)
- Intraparenchymal hematoma
- Laceration
- Fragmented spleen
- Delayed rupture (rare)

Imaging Features

- High-density (>30 HU in acute stage, i.e., <48 hours) blood in abdomen
- Blood clot is of high CT density and often located near source of bleeding: sentinel clot sign.
- Splenic contour abnormality
- Associated other trauma

SPLENOSIS

Autotransplantation of splenic fragments after trauma.

Location

- Mesentery, peritoneum, omentum
- Pleura
- Diaphragm

Imaging Features

- Small, enhancing implants
- Best imaged with ^{99m}RBC or ^{99m}Tc sulfur colloid
- Accumulation in most dependent portions: Morison's pouch, perihepatic space, paracolic gutter

VASCULAR

SPLENIC INFARCT

Common cause of focal filling defects on contrast-enhanced CT. Classically wedge shaped and peripheral but more commonly rounded, irregularly shaped, and random in distribution.

Causes

Cardiovascular
- Bacterial endocarditis, 50%
- Atheroma
- Valve vegetations
- Mitral stenosis

Tumor
- Lymphoproliferative
- Pancreas
- Inflammatory
- Pancreatitis

Other
- Sickle cell disease
- Polycythemia vera

AIDS

Splenic involvement is common in AIDS. CT has high sensitivity for detection (>90%) of splenic lesions and identification of associated findings in retroperitoneum, mesentery, and/or bowel.

Causes of Splenic Lesions

Tumor
- Kaposi sarcoma
- Lymphoma

Infectious
- *Mycobacterium tuberculosis:* low density, abnormal ileocecal region
- MAI: lymph nodes, jejunal wall thickening
- Fungus: *Candida, Aspergillus, Cryptococcus*
- Bacteria: *Staphylococcus, Streptococcus, Escherichia coli*
- Protozoa: *Pneumocystis carinii;* progressively enlarging lesions, calcification in spleen, liver, and lymph nodes

Peritoneum and Abdominal Wall

GENERAL

PERITONEAL SPACES (Figs. 3-88 and 3-89)

- Subphrenic (suprahepatic) space; divided by the falciform ligament into:
  - Right subphrenic space between diaphragm and liver
  - Left subphrenic space between diaphragm and spleen
- Morison's pouch is formed by:
  - Right subhepatic recess
  - Hepatorenal recess

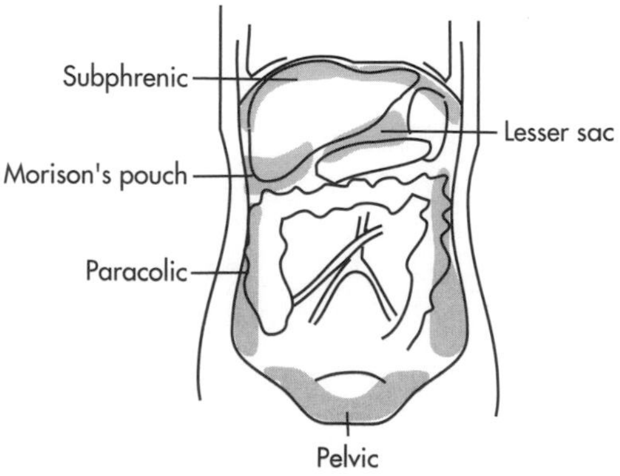

FIGURE 3-88

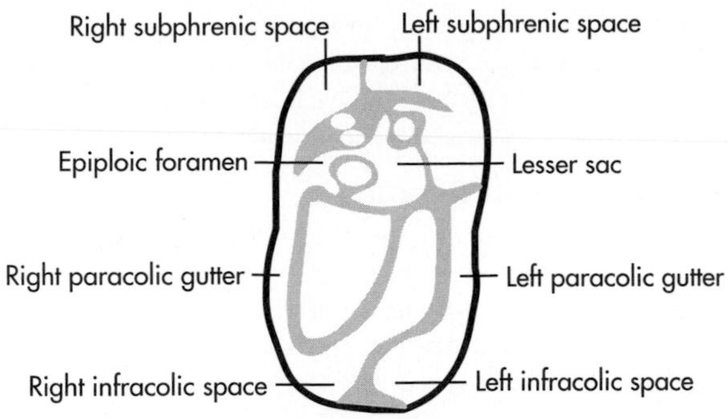

FIGURE 3-89

- Morison's pouch communicates with the lesser sac (via the epiploic foramen), the subphrenic space, and the right paracolic gutter. In supine position, Morison's pouch is the most dependent portion of the abdominal cavity and collects fluid (it is the most frequently infected space); the pelvic cul-de-sac is the other dependent space.
- Lesser sac (omental bursa): posterior to stomach and anterior to pancreas. Medial cephalad extent between lesser curvature and left hepatic lobe; roofed by gastrohepatic ligament. Access is by the epiploic foramen (Winslow).

PERITONEUM

ABSCESS DRAINAGE (Figs. 3-90 and 3-91)

Two techniques are frequently used to percutaneously treat abdominal and pelvic abscesses: trocar technique and Seldinger technique.

Trocar Technique

Commonly performed for large abscesses or collections with easy access.

1. Localize abscess by CT or US.
2. Anesthetize skin. Advance 20-gauge needle into abscess under imaging guidance. Obtain 2 to 5 mL of fluid for culture. Do not aspirate more because cavity will collapse.

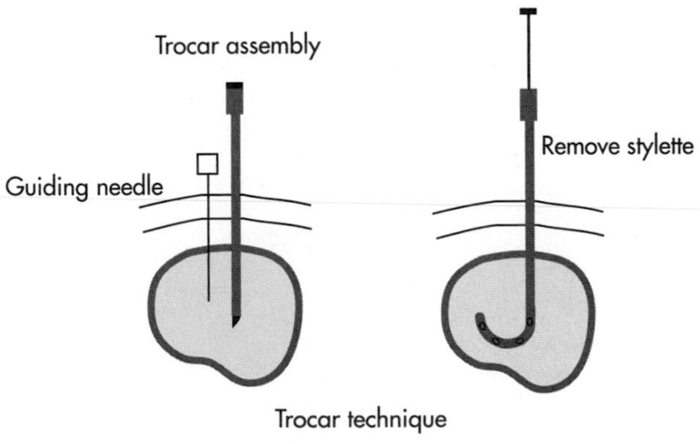

FIGURE 3-90

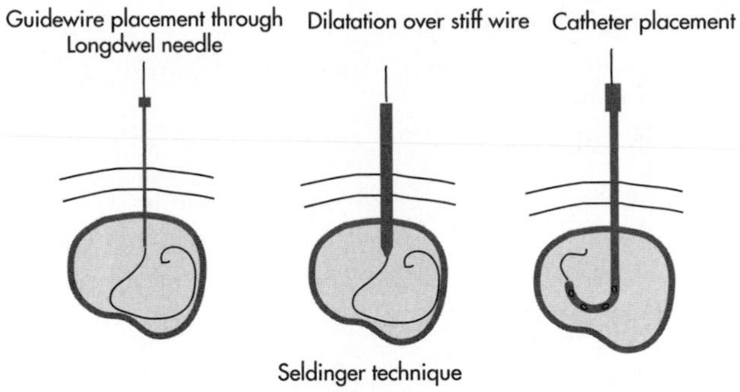

FIGURE 3-91

3. Make skin nick and perforate subcutaneous tissues.
4. Place 8- to 16-Fr abscess drainage catheter in tandem. Remove stylet.
5. Aspirate all fluid; wash cavity with saline.

Seldinger Technique

This is commonly performed for abscesses with difficult access or for necrotic tumors with hard rims.

1. Localize abscess.
2. Anesthetize skin. Localize abscess with 4-, 6-, or 8-inch Seldinger needle under imaging guidance.
3. Remove needle, leave outer plastic sheath. Pass guidewire (3-J) through plastic sheath into abscess cavity.
4. Dilate tract (8, 10, 12 Fr) over stiff guidewire.
5. Pass 8- to 16-Fr abscess drainage catheter over guidewire.
6. Remove stiffener and guidewire. Aspirate abscess.

PERITONEAL METASTASES (Fig. 3-92)

Most common origin: ovarian cancer, gastrointestinal cancer

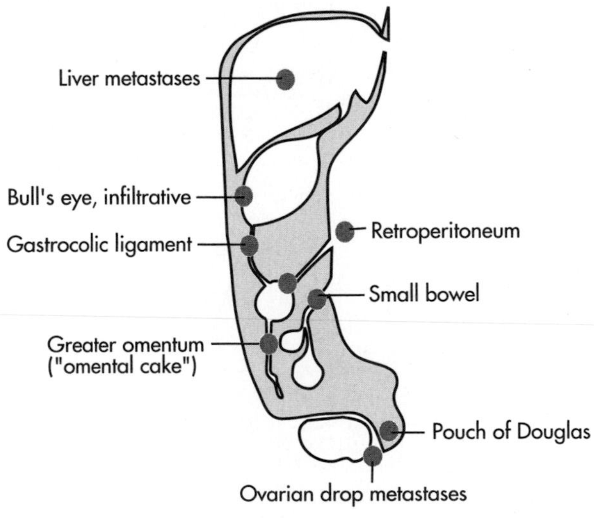

FIGURE 3-92

Imaging Features

- Greater omentum overlying small bowel: "omental cake"
- Masses on peritoneal surfaces (superior surface of sigmoid colon, pouch of Douglas, terminal ileum, Morison's pouch), gastrocolic ligament
- Malignant ascites (may enhance with Gd-DTPA due to increased permeability of peritoneum)

PERITONEAL INFECTION

- Often polymicrobial from bowel injury or perforation
- Gossypiboma: abscess involving retained sponge
- Tuberculous peritonitis may calcify
- Peritoneal nodularity in patients with IUD may be seen with actinomycosis

PSEUDOMYXOMA PERITONEI

Gelatinous substance accumulates in peritoneal cavity due to widespread mucinous cystadenocarcinoma (especially from the appendix or ovary, rarely from other sites).

Imaging Features

- Scalloped indentations of liver with or without calcification
- Thickening of peritoneal surfaces
- Septated "pseudo" ascites
- Thin-walled cystic masses

ABDOMINAL HERNIAS

Terminology (Fig. 3-93)

- Incarceration: a hernia that cannot be manually reduced
- Strangulation: occlusion of blood supply to the herniated bowel, leading to infarction. Findings include bowel wall thickening, hemorrhage, and pneumatosis, as well as venous engorgement and mesenteric edema.

Diaphragmatic Hernias

- Congenital diaphragmatic hernias (see also Chapter 11)
  Bochdalek hernia (posterior)
  Morgagni hernia (anterior)
- Traumatic hernia (left > right), may be masked by positive pressure ventilation

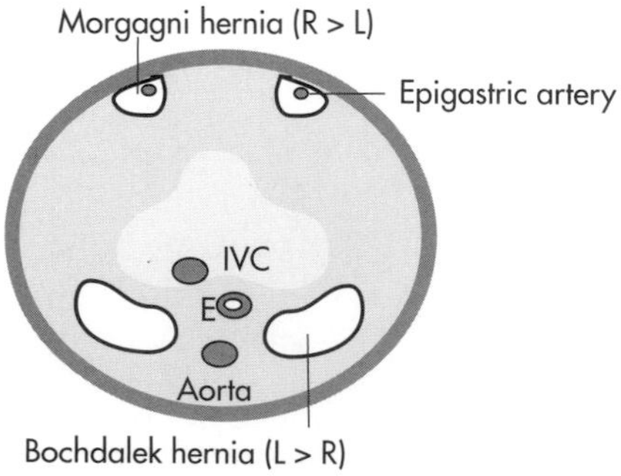

FIGURE 3-93

Abdominal Wall Hernias

- Spigelian hernias occur along lateral margin of rectus muscle through the hiatus semilunaris. Although these hernias protrude beyond the transverse abdominal and internal oblique muscles, they are contained within the external oblique muscle; thus, they may be difficult to detect on physical examination.
- Groin hernias
- Lumbar hernias occur through either superior (Grynfeltt) or inferior (Petit) lumbar triangle. The superior lumbar triangle is formed by the 12th rib, internal oblique, serratus posterior, and erector spinae muscles. The iliac crest, latissimus dorsi, and external oblique muscles form the inferior lumbar triangle. The inferior lumbar triangle is a site of laparoscopic nephrectomy ports.
- Richter hernia contains only a single side of a bowel loop may herniate but may still represent a clinically significant obstruction.

Internal Hernias (Rare)

- Paraduodenal hernia: L > R
- Small bowel grouped in saclike configuration
- Lesser sac hernia

GROIN HERNIAS (Fig. 3-94)

Types

Direct inguinal hernia

- Defect medial to inferior epigastric vessels, peritoneal sac protrudes through floor of inguinal canal
- Due to weakness in floor of inguinal canal

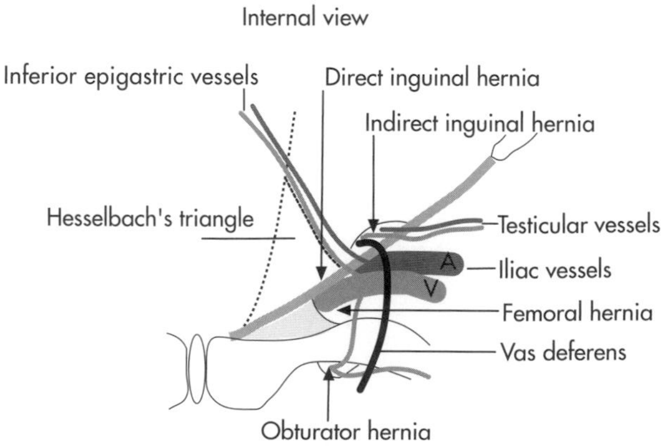

FIGURE 3-94

Indirect inguinal hernia
- Defect lateral to inferior epigastric vessels, peritoneal sac protrudes through internal inguinal canal
- Due to persistence of processus vaginalis

Femoral hernia
- Enlargement of femoral ring; peritoneal sac protrudes medial to femoral sheath.
- Women, due to increased intraabdominal pressure

Obturator canal hernia
- Occurs through the obturator foramen, between pectineus and obturator externus muscle;
- Has the highest mortality rate of all hernias
- Elderly women

MALIGNANT MESOTHELIOMA

Malignancy of mesothelial cells lining the peritoneum. Associated with asbestos.

Imaging Features
- Peritoneal soft tissue nodules, omental and mesenteric masses or nodules
- Ascites
- Bowel wall thickening
- Fixation of small bowel

ABDOMINAL WALL

ABDOMINAL WALL METASTASES

Origin: melanoma, skin tumors, neurofibromatosis, iatrogenic seeding, lymphoma (gastrostomy, biopsy)

Imaging Features
- Soft tumor mass in subcutaneous fat with or without focal bulging

ABDOMINAL WALL HEMATOMA

Causes
- Anticoagulant therapy
- Femoral catheterization
- Trauma

Imaging Features
- High-attenuation fluid collection: first several days with or without fluid-fluid level (hematocrit level). If there is no further bleeding, the high-density RBCs decompose to reduced-density fluid.
- Fluid-fluid level (hematocrit level)
- Usually confined to rectus muscle. About 2 cm below the umbilicus (arcuate line), the posterior portion of the rectus sheath disappears and fibers of all three lateral muscle groups (external oblique, internal oblique, and transversus abdominis) pass anterior to rectus muscle. This arrangement has imaging significance in that rectus sheath hematomas above the line are confined within the rectus sheath; inferior to the arcuate line, they are directly opposed to the transversalis fascia and can dissect across the midline or laterally into the flank.

MESENTERIC PANNICULITIS

Rare disorder characterized by chronic nonspecific inflammation involving the adipose tissue of the small bowel mesentery. When the predominant component is inflammatory or fatty, the disease is called *mesenteric panniculitis.* When fibrosis is the dominant component, the disease is called *retractile mesenteritis.* The latter is considered the final, more invasive stage of mesenteric panniculitis. The cause of this condition is unclear.

Imaging Features
- Well-circumscribed, inhomogeneous fatty small bowel mesentery displaying higher attenuation than normal retroperitoneal fat. The mass is usually directed toward the left abdomen, where it extends from mesenteric root to jejunum.
- Spiculated soft tissue mass: a carcinoid mesenteric mass look-alike

SCLEROSING PERITONITIS

Uncommon but important complication of chronic ambulatory peritoneal dialysis (CAPD). Incidence increases with duration of CAPD. Exact etiology is not known. Clinical onset is heralded by abdominal pain, anorexia, weight loss, and eventually partial or complete small bowel obstruction. Loss of ultrafiltration is common, as is bloody dialysis effluent.

Imaging Features
- Plain radiographs are normal early in disease. Later, curvilinear peritoneal calcification can be seen within the abdomen.
- Plain radiographs may also show centrally located, dilated loops of bowel with wall thickening, edema, and thumbprinting.
- CT shows peritoneal enhancement, thickening, calcification, as well as loculated intraperitoneal fluid collection. Adherent and dilated loops of bowel.
- Early diagnosis is essential, as cessation of CAPD and treatment with total parenteral nutrition, hemodialysis, immunosuppression, and/or renal transplantation may result in recovery.

MESENTERIC FIBROMATOSIS (DESMOID TUMOR)

Uncommon benign tumor but which is locally aggressive, infiltrates adjacent bowel wall and recurs following resection. There is an increased incidence in FAP and APC germline mutation. Associated with asbestos. Imaging: low attenuation on CT and high signal on T2 MR.

DESMOPLASTIC SMALL ROUND CELL TUMOR

Aggressive malignancy usually occurring in adolescents and young adults.

Imaging Features

- CT shows multiple peritoneal based soft tissue masses with necrosis and hemorrhage
- Hematogenous or serosal liver metastases can be present without detectable primary tumor.

Differential Diagnosis

ESOPHAGUS

DIVERTICULAR DISEASE (Fig. 3-95)

- Pharyngocele: usually lateral in hypopharynx
- Zenker's diverticulum (pulsion diverticulum)
- Traction diverticula; all layers involved: pulling usually by adhesions to mediastinal structures due to malignancy or TB; typically at level of bifurcation
- Pulsion: all layers, secondary to increased intraluminal pressure
- Pseudodiverticula: small outpouchings due to dilated mucus glands; associated with diabetes, alcoholism, candidiasis, obstruction, cancer
- Epiphrenic diverticulum
- Mimicking lesions:
  Paraesophageal hernia
  Esophageal perforation with contrast extravasation

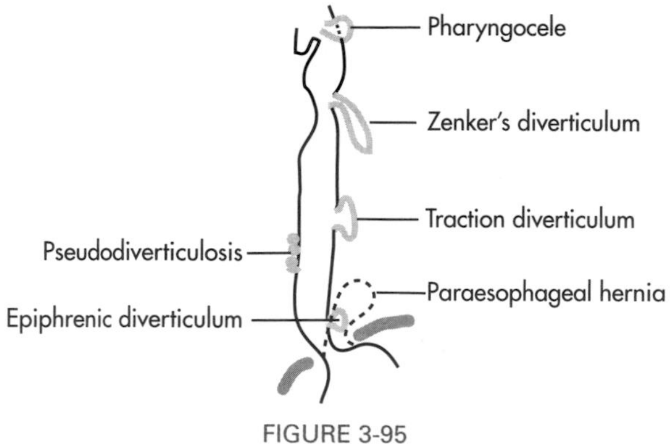

FIGURE 3-95

LUMINAL NARROWING (Fig. 3-96)

Webs
- Idiopathic
- Plummer-Vinson syndrome

Rings
- Congenital: vascular, muscular rings
- Schatzki's ring

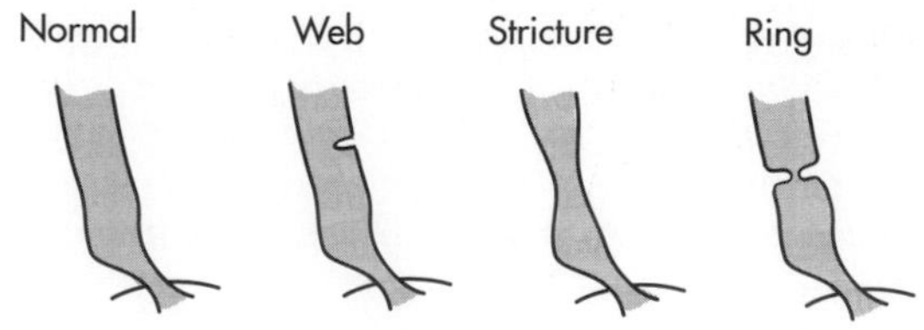

FIGURE 3-96

Stricture
- Skin lesions (epidermolysis, pemphigoid): proximal one third of esophagus
- Tumor
- Esophagitis (lye, Barrett's esophagus, infection, radiation, eosinophilic)
- Intubation
- Achalasia, scleroderma, Chagas disease

Extrinsic compression
- Vascular aortic arch, arch anomalies, aneurysm, left atrium
- Left bronchus
- Mediastinal tumors

MEGAESOPHAGUS (Fig. 3-97)

- Achalasia
- Scleroderma
- Dilatation secondary to distal narrowing
  Tumor
  Stricture
- Chagas disease
- Diabetic or alcoholic neuropathy
- Bulbar palsy

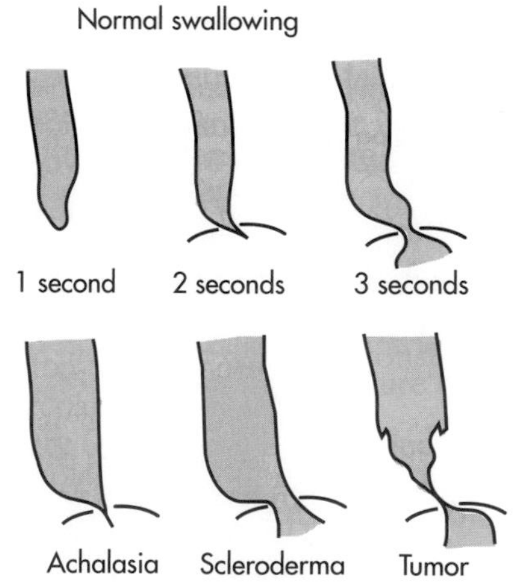

FIGURE 3-97

ESOPHAGEAL TEARS (CONTRAST EXTRAVASATION, FISTULA)

- Esophagitis
- Tumor
- Vomiting

Mallory-Weiss syndrome: only mucosa is disrupted (longitudinal, superficial tear), rarely visualized
Boerhaave syndrome: entire wall is ruptured (pneumomediastinum, extravasation of contrast)
- Tracheoesophageal fistulas (pediatric)
- Bronchopulmonary foregut malformation with communication to esophagus
  Bronchogenic cysts
  Extralobar sequestration (pediatric)
- Endoscopy

SOLITARY FILLING DEFECTS (MASS LESIONS)

Neoplasm
- Benign
  Leiomyoma, 50%
  Pedunculated fibrovascular polyp (especially upper esophagus), 25%
  Cysts, papilloma, fibroma, hemangioma
- Malignant
  Squamous cell carcinoma, 95%
  Adenocarcinoma, 5%
  Carcinosarcoma
  Lymphoma
  Metastases

Foreign bodies
Varices
- Uphill varices (portal hypertension), predominantly inferior location
- Downhill varices (superior vena cava obstruction), predominantly superior location

Extrinsic lesions (lymph nodes, engorged vessels, aneurysms, cysts)
Submucosal masses
- GIST
- Fibroma, neurofibroma, lipoma, hemangioma
- Duplication cyst
- Lymphoma

THICKENED FOLDS

- Early forms of esophagitis
- Neoplasm
  Lymphoma
  Varicoid carcinoma
- Varices

AIR-FLUID LEVEL

Hiatal hernia
Esophageal diverticulum
Any esophageal lesion caused by a motility disorder or a stricture
- Cancer
- Achalasia
- Scleroderma

STOMACH

APPROACH TO UGI STUDIES (Fig. 3-98)

GASTRITIS

- Erosive gastritis (corrosives, alcohol, stress, drugs)
- Granulomatous gastritis (Crohn disease, sarcoid, syphilis, TB, histoplasmosis)
- Eosinophilic gastritis (peripheral eosinophilia, 60%; hypoalbuminemia; hypogammaglobulinemia; hyperplastic polyps)
- Hypertrophic gastritis
  Ménétrier disease
  Zollinger-Ellison syndrome
  Idiopathic
- Recurrent gastric ulcer
  Zollinger-Ellison syndrome
  PUD
  Retained gastric antrum
  Drugs
- Miscellaneous
  Radiation (>4000 rad; gastritis occurs 6 months to 2 years after radiation)
  Ulcer
  Corrosives
  Rare causes of gastritis:
  - Pseudolymphoma
  - Suture line ulceration
  - Intraarterial chemotherapy

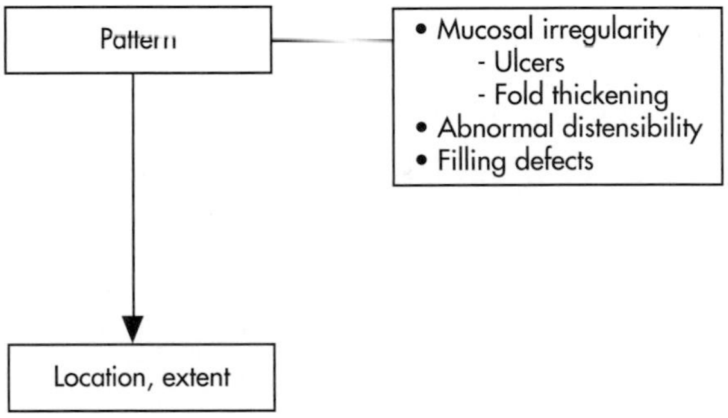

FIGURE 3-98

TARGET (BULL'S EYE) LESIONS (Fig. 3-99)

Ulcer surrounded by a radiolucent halo, multiple
Gastritis (aphthoid type, tiny ulcer)
- Erosive: NSAID, alcohol
- Granulomatous: Crohn disease
- Infections: candidiasis, herpes, syphilis, CMV

Submucosal metastases (large ulcer)
- Melanoma, Kaposi sarcoma >> all other metastases (breast, lung, pancreas)
- Lymphoma

Solitary, giant bull's eye (very large ulcer)
- Leiomyoma
- Sarcoma

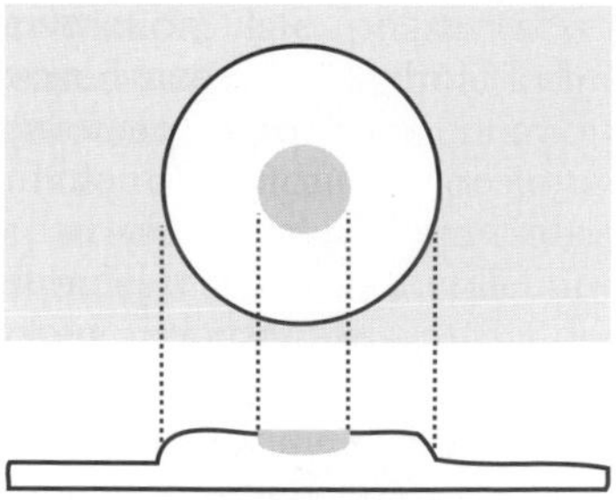

FIGURE 3-99

FILLING DEFECT (MASS LESION)

Any ingested material may cause a filling defect in the stomach; however, it should move from gastric wall with gravity. If it becomes very large, it may be confused with an immobile mass (bezoar); undigested vegetable material (phytobezoar); mass of matted hair (trichobezoar); mass of matted hair and undigested vegetable matter (trichophytobezoar). Fixed filling defects include.

Neoplasm
- Adenocarcinoma
- Lymphoma
- Leiomyosarcoma
- Metastases
- Kaposi sarcoma

Other
- Endometriosis
- Carcinoid
- Benign tumors: leiomyoma > lipoma, fibroma, schwannoma
- Polyps
- Varices
- Extramedullary hematopoiesis
- Ectopic pancreas

Extrinsic compression
- Spleen
- Pancreas
- Liver

SUBMUCOSAL LESIONS

- GIST
- Lipoma
- Ectopic pancreas
- Lymphoma

GIANT RUGAL FOLDS

Tumor
- Lymphoma

Inflammation
- Ménétrier disease
- Zollinger-Ellison syndrome
- Gastritis associated with pancreatitis
- Bile reflux gastritis
- Eosinophilic gastroenteritis

LINITIS PLASTICA

Linitis plastica (leather bottle stomach): marked thickening and irregularity of gastric wall (diffuse infiltration), rigidity, narrowing, and nondistensibility; peristalsis does not pass through linitis.

Tumor
- Scirrhous cancer (most common cause)
- Lymphoma
- Metastases (most common breast cancer)
- Pancreatic carcinoma (direct invasion)

Inflammation
- Erosive gastritis
- Radiation therapy

Infiltrative disease
- Sarcoid
- Amyloid (rare)
- Intramural gastric hematoma (rare)

Infection
- TB, syphilis

ANTRAL LESIONS (FIG. 3-100)

Tumor
- Adenocarcinoma
- Lymphoma
- Metastases

Inflammatory
- Crohn disease
- Peptic ulcer disease
- TB
- Sarcoid

Other (less extensive)
- Hypertrophic pyloric stenosis
- Pylorospasm
- Antral web

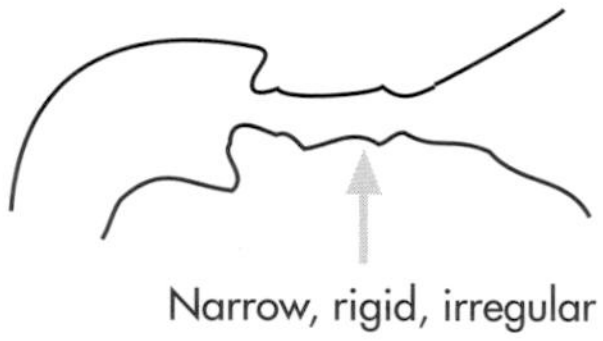

FIGURE 3-100

RAM'S HORN ANTRUM

Blunting of antral fornices with progressive tapering from antrum to pylorus
- Chronic PUD
- Scirrhous carcinoma
- Granulomatous disease (Crohn disease, TB, sarcoid, eosinophilic gastroenteritis)
- Caustic ingestion

FREE INTRAPERITONEAL AIR

- Surgery and laparoscopy and other radiologic interventions (most common cause)

- Perforated gastric or duodenal ulcer (second most common cause)
- Cecal perforation from colonic obstruction
- Pneumatosis coli
- Air through genital tract in females
- Perforated distal bowel (e.g., inflammatory bowel disease, diverticulitis, tumor) is usually associated with abscess and lesser amounts of free air

DUODENUM

FILLING DEFECTS

Neoplastic Filling Defects

Benign (often in first portion, asymptomatic)
- Adenoma (usually <1 cm)
- Leiomyoma
- Carcinoid
- Villous adenoma—near papilla, high malignant potential

Malignant (often distal to first portion, symptomatic)
- Adenocarcinoma at or distal to papilla (90% of malignant tumors)
- Metastases (direct invasion from stomach, pancreas, colon, kidney, etc., or hematogenous such as melanoma)
- Lymphoma

Other Filling Defects (Fig. 3-101)

Bulb
- Ectopic gastric mucosa
- Prolapsed antral mucosa
- Brunner gland hyperplasia
- Varices

Distal
- Benign lymphoid hyperplasia
- Ectopic pancreas
- Annular pancreas
- Papilla of Vater
- Tumor
- Edema with impacted or passed gallstone
- Choledochocele
- Duplication cyst
- Intraluminal diverticulum

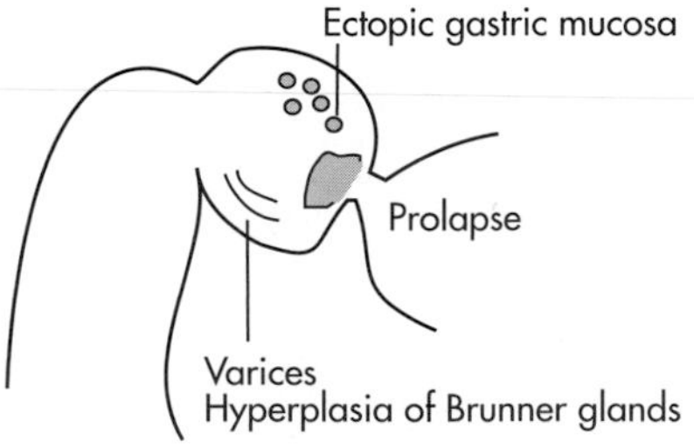

FIGURE 3-101

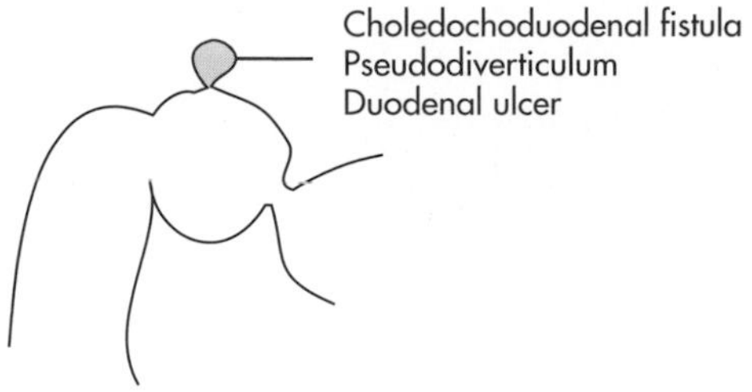

FIGURE 3-102

Malignancy of duodenal lesions depending on location
- Duodenal bulb: 90% are benign
- 2nd and 3rd portions: 50% are malignant
- 4th portion: 90% are malignant

LUMINAL OUTPOUCHINGS (Fig. 3-102)

Ulcer
- Ulcer with contained perforation
- Malignant ulcer (rarely primary)

Diverticulum
- Pseudodiverticulum: ulcer scarring
- Choledochoduodenal or cholecystoduodenal fistula
- True diverticulum medial, 2nd part duodenum

ULCER VERSUS DIVERTICULUM

Finding	Ulcer	Diverticulum*
Opposite incisura	Yes	No
Mucosal folds	Thickened, radiating	Normal
Spasm	Present	Absent
Symptoms	Yes	Unlikely

*Duodenal bulb: pseudodiverticulum; postbulbar duodenum; true diverticulum.

POSTBULBAR NARROWING (Fig. 3-103)

Neoplastic
- Adenocarcinoma
- Lymphoma
- Metastases (direct invasion from colon, kidney, pancreas, GB)
- GIST

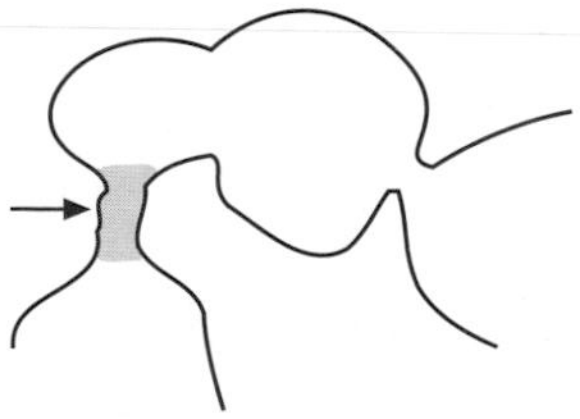

FIGURE 3-103

Inflammatory
- Intrinsic
  - Postbulbar ulcer
  - Duodenitis
  - Crohn disease
- Extrinsic
  - Pancreatitis

Other
- Annular pancreas
- Intramural diverticulum
- Duodenal duplication cyst
- Duodenal hematoma
- Aortic aneurysm (3rd portion)
- SMA syndrome (supine position causes partial obstruction of 3rd portion of duodenum by SMA), may be exacerbated by weight loss

DUODENAL FOLD THICKENING

- *H. pylori*
- Crohn disease
- Giardiasis
- Sprue
- Whipple disease
- Brunner gland hyperplasia
- Lymphoma
- Hematoma/trauma
- Pancreatitis

PAPILLARY ENLARGEMENT

- Normal variant
- Choledochocele
- Papillary edema
  - Pancreatitis
  - Acute duodenal ulcer
  - Impacted stone
- Ampullary tumor
  - Adenomatous polyp
  - Carcinoma

JEJUNUM AND ILEUM

DILATED GAS-FILLED BOWEL LOOPS (Fig. 3-104)

The following approach will ensure a correct determination of presence and level of obstruction in 80%.

Approach (Fig. 3-105, *A* and *B*)

1. Is there too much gas in dilated intestine (small bowel >3 cm, large bowel >6 cm)?
2. Where is the gas located (large or small bowel or both)?
3. Is the distribution of gas and/or fluid disproportionate between small and large bowel?
4. Is the cecum dilated?
5. Is there free peritoneal air (perforation)?

Small Bowel Obstruction (SBO)

Disproportionate distribution of gas is the key radiographic finding:
- Much more gas and fluid in small bowel compared to colon
- Much more gas in proximal small bowel compared to distal small bowel

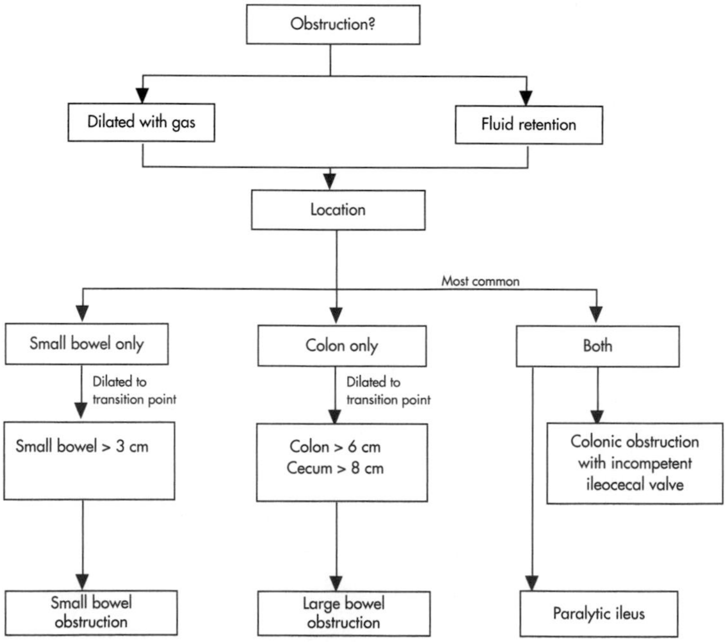

FIGURE 3-104

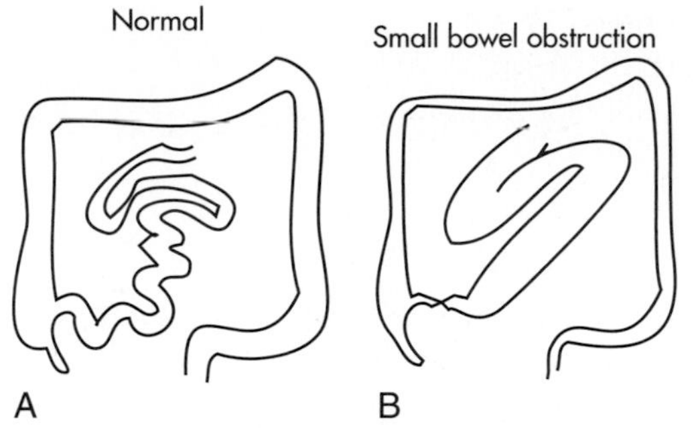

FIGURE 3-105

- Fluid retention parallels gas distribution: no fluid, no obstruction
- Closed loop obstruction: lumen occluded at 2 adjacent sites, obstructed loops distends with fluid; loop may twist; bowel may or may not be infarcted

Additional examinations in presumed acute SBO include:
- If very dilated or abundant fluid: CT (fluid acts as an intrinsic contrast material)
- If mild dilatation: CT with oral contrast or small bowel follow-through
- Enteroclysis: need to decompress bowel before study, best applied to nonacute situations

Colonic Obstruction (Fig. 3-106, A and B)

Cecal dilatation is the key radiographic finding:
- Cecum is invariably most dilated in colonic obstruction; however, it may also be very dilated in paralytic ileus (A > B).
- If the transverse colon is more dilated than the cecum (A < B), there is rarely an obstruction (exception: concomitant disease that intrinsically narrows the cecum, such as IBD).
- Fluid retention *not* necessarily seen in colonic obstruction

A useful initial screening procedure to rule out distal colonic obstruction is a prone KUB: if there is no obstruction, gas passes to the rectum. Barium enema is the definitive study. Do not perform UGI series in a patient with possible colonic obstruction (contraindicated because barium impacts in the colon).

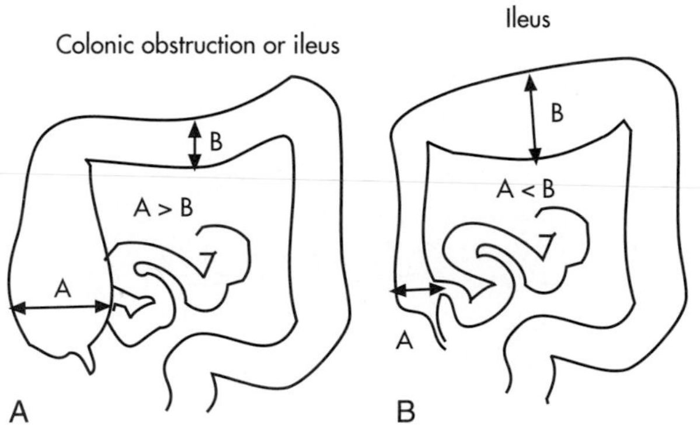

FIGURE 3-106

PARALYTIC (ADYNAMIC) ILEUS

Postoperative (most common)
Vascular
- IBD

Inflammatory (often localized ileus: sentinel loop)
- Pancreatitis
- Appendicitis
- Cholecystitis
- Diverticulitis
- Peritonitis

Metabolic
- Hypokalemia
- Hypocalcemia
- Hypomagnesemia

Medication
- Morphine, diphenoxylate (Lomotil)

MECHANICAL SBO

- Adhesions
- Hernias
- Tumors
- Gallstones
- Inflammation with strictures
- Gallstone ileus: pneumobilia, small bowel obstruction, stone within bowel lumen (e.g., may obstruct at ileocecal valve)

MALABSORPTION PATTERNS

Signs: dilution of barium (hypersecretion), flocculation of barium, moulage, segmentation of barium column, delay in transit.

Predominantly Thick/Irregular Folds

Mnemonic: "WAG CLEM:"
- **W**hipple disease
- **A**myloid
- **G**iardiasis (largely affects jejunum), graft-versus-host reaction, gammaglobulinopathy
- **C**ryptosporidiosis (largely affects jejunum)
- **L**ymphoma, lymphangiectasia, lactase deficiency
- **E**osinophilic gastroenteritis
- ***M****ycobacterium avium* complex, mastocytosis

Predominantly Thick/Straight Folds

- Ischemia
- Intramural hemorrhage
- Radiation
- Hypoproteinemia
- Venous congestion
- Cirrhosis

Predominantly Dilated Loops, Normal Folds

Mnemonic: "SOSO:"

- **S**prue is the single most important cause of true malabsorption.
- **O**bstruction or ileus
- **S**cleroderma
- **O**ther
  - Medication
    - **M**orphine
    - **L**omotil
    - **A**tropine
    - **P**ro-Banthine
  - Vagotomy

THICK FOLDS WITHOUT MALABSORPTION PATTERN (EDEMA, TUMOR HEMORRHAGE) (Fig. 3-107, *A* and *B*)

Criteria: folds >3 mm. By CT, the edema in small bowel wall may appear as ring or halo sign. Two types:

- Diffuse: uniformly thickened folds
- Focal: nodular thickening ("pinky printing"), analogous to "thumbprinting" in ischemic colitis, stack-of-coins appearance, picket fence appearance.

Causes

Submucosal edema
- Ischemia
- Enteritis
  - Infectious
  - Radiation
- Hypoproteinemia
- Graft-versus-host reaction

Submucosal tumor
- Lymphoma, leukemia
- Infiltrating carcinoid causing venous stasis

Submucosal hemorrhage
- Henoch-Schönlein disease
- Hemolytic-uremic syndrome
- Coagulopathies (e.g., hemophilia, vitamin K, anticoagulants)
- Thrombocytopenia, disseminated intravascular coagulation

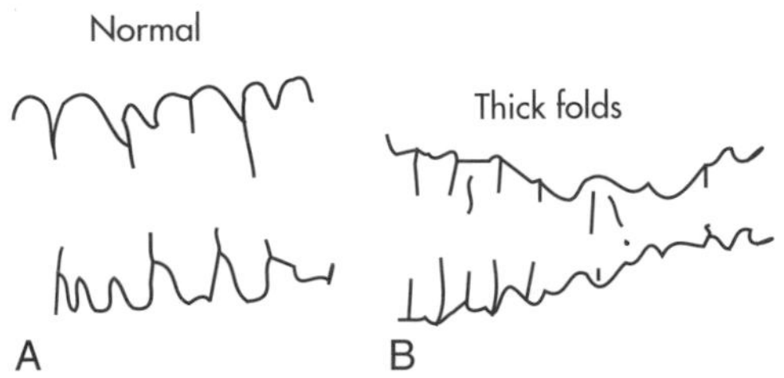

FIGURE 3-107

Nodules

- Mastocytosis
- Lymphoid hyperplasia
- Lymphoma
- Metastases
- Polyps
- Crohn disease

Small Bowel Stack of Coins Appearance

- Anticoagulation
- Vasculitis
- Trauma
- Ischemia
- Carcinoid

Small Bowel Luminal Narrowing

- Ischemia
- Vasculitis
- Hemorrhage
- Radiation
- Collagen vascular disease
- Inflammatory bowel disease
- Tumor
- Adhesions

CT Bowel Target Sign

- Ischemia
- Vasculitis
- Hemorrhage
- Inflammatory bowel disease
- Angioedema: ACEi, hereditary, allergic reaction
- Portal hypertension
- NSAIDs

Gracile Small Bowel

Tubular "toothpaste" appearance on small bowel series
- Graft-versus-host disease
- Cryptosporidium

SMALL BOWEL TUMORS

Benign tumors
- Adenoma (most common)
- Leiomyoma (second most common)
- Lipoma
- Hemangioma
- Neurogenic tumors (usually in neurofibromatosis)
- Other
  - Brunner gland hyperplasia
  - Heterotopic pancreatic tissue
  - Duplication cyst
  - Inverted Meckel's diverticulum

Malignant tumors
- Metastases
  - Melanoma
  - Kidney
  - Breast
  - Kaposi sarcoma

- Lymphoma, very variable appearance
- Carcinoid (most common primary; 50% are malignant and have metastases at time of diagnosis)
- GIST
- Sarcoma (sarcomatous degeneration of benign tumors: [e.g., leiomyosarcoma, lymphosarcoma]); usually large ulcerating tumors
- Adenocarcinoma (rare)

Polyposis syndromes

MESENTERIC BOWEL ISCHEMIA

Occlusive disease
- Emboli (atrial fibrillation, ventricular aneurysm)
- Arterial thrombosis (atherosclerosis)
- Venous thrombosis (portal hypertension, pancreatitis, tumor)

Nonocclusive disease (low flow)
- Hypotension
- Hypovolemia

SHORTENED TRANSIT TIME

- Anxiety
- Hyperthyroidism
- Medication
  - Metoclopramide
  - Neostigmine
  - Quinidine
  - Methacholine
- Partial SBO (paradoxical rapid propulsion to point of obstruction)

COLON

MASS LESIONS

Nonneoplastic polypoid abnormalities
- Normal lymphofollicular pattern
- Pneumatosis coli
- Colitis cystica profunda
- Amyloidosis
- Endometriosis
- Ischemic colitis

Polyps

Polyposis syndromes

Benign neoplasm
- Lipoma (common)
- Leiomyoma (rare)

Malignant neoplasm
- Adenocarcinoma
- Metastases
- Lymphoma

POLYPS

Hyperplastic polyps (90% of colonic polyps)
- Not true tumors
- No malignant potential

Adenomatous polyps (second most common type; 25% multiple)
- True tumors
- Malignant transformation
- Types
  - Tubular
  - Villous
  - Tubulovillous

Hamartomatous polyps (rare; Peutz-Jeghers syndrome)

ULCERS

Aphthoid Ulcers (Superficial)

- Crohn disease (in 50% of patients)
- Amebiasis
- Behçet syndrome
- CMV
- Herpes

Deep Ulcers

Inflammatory colitis
- Ulcerative colitis
- Crohn colitis
- Behçet syndrome

Infectious colitis
- Amebiasis
- TB
- *Salmonella*
- *Shigella*
- Histoplasmosis
- AIDS: *Candida,* herpes, CMV

Ischemic colitis

Radiation colitis

BOWEL WALL THICKENING (THUMBPRINTING)

Thumbprinting refers to luminal indentations the size of a thumb (due to edema, tumor, or hemorrhage). Morphology of accompanying haustral folds may be a clue to underlying diagnosis: preserved haustral folds: infection, ischemia; effaced haustral folds: tumor, IBD.

Edema
- Infectious colitis
  - Pseudomembranous colitis (*Clostridium difficile*) CMV colitis
  - *E. coli, Shigella, Salmonella,* amebiasis
  - Neutropenic colitis (typhlitis)
- IBD

Tumor
- Lymphoma, leukemia

Hemorrhage
- Ischemia
- Henoch-Schönlein disease, thrombocytopenia, DIC
- Coagulopathies (e.g., hemophilia, vitamin K, anticoagulants)

TUMOR-LIKE COLONIC DEFORMITY (Fig. 3-108, *A* and *B*)

Deformities may be symmetrical (circumferential, apple core) or asymmetrical.

Tumor
- Adenocarcinoma

Saddle shaped if asymmetrical

Apple core shaped if circumferential
- Metastases (common serosal implants: gastric, ovarian)

Inflammation
- Diverticulitis
- Focal inflammation
  - IBD: Crohn disease, UC
  - Infectious: ameboma, TB

Other
- Endometriosis
- Pelvic abscess
- Epiploic appendagitis

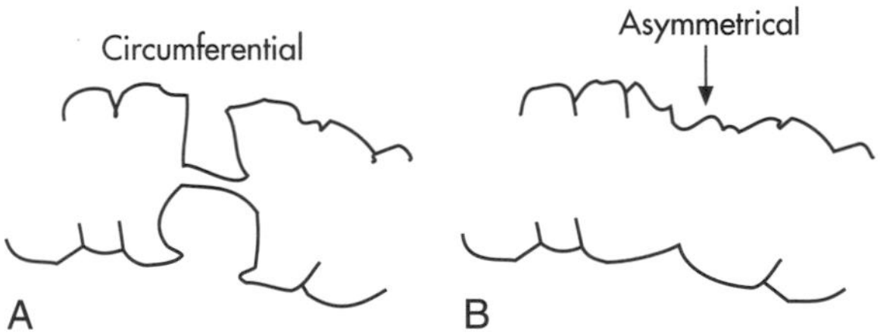

FIGURE 3-108

LONG (>10 CM) COLONIC NARROWING (Fig. 3-109)

- Scirrhous adenocarcinoma
- Lymphoma
- UC (with or without carcinoma)
- Crohn disease
- Ischemic stricture
- Radiation

AHAUSTRAL COLON

- Cathartic abuse (often right colon)
- UC, Crohn disease
- Amebiasis
- Aging (usually left colon)

COLONIC OBSTRUCTION

- Carcinoma, 65%
- Diverticulitis, 20%
- Volvulus, 5%
- Other
  - Impaction
  - Hernia

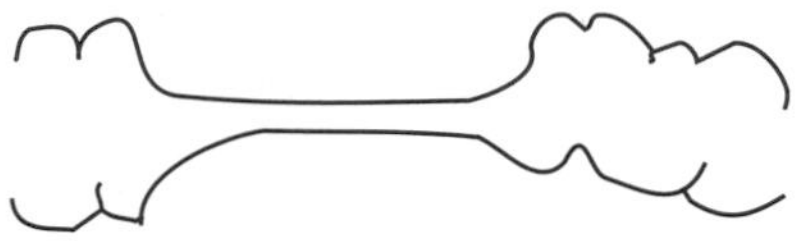
FIGURE 3-109

MEGACOLON

Descriptive term for abnormally distended transverse colon (>6 cm); most commonly used in conjunction with toxic megacolon.

Toxic megacolon (haustral deformity, pseudopolyps; risk of perforation; systemic signs)
- UC, Crohn disease
- Infectious: amebiasis, shigellosis, *Clostridium difficile*

Acute colonic distention (risk of perforation with cecum >9 cm)
- Obstructive: cancer
- Paralytic ileus
- Volvulus

Chronic megacolon (no or small risk of perforation)
- Cathartic colon (chronic laxative abuse)
- Colonic pseudoobstruction (Ogilvie syndrome, colonic ileus)
- Psychogenic
- Congenital (Hirschsprung disease)
- Chagas disease
- Neuromuscular disorders
  - Parkinsonism
  - Diabetes
  - Scleroderma
  - Amyloid
- Metabolic, drugs
  - Hypothyroidism
  - Electrolyte imbalances

ADULT INTUSSUSCEPTION (Fig. 3-110)

Ileoileal (40%) > ileocolic (15%) > other locations.

Idiopathic, 20%

Tumors, 35%
- Polyps, lipoma, 25%
- Malignant tumors (metastases, lymphoma, carcinoid), 10%

Other
- Meckel's diverticulum
- Adhesions
- Aberrant pancreas

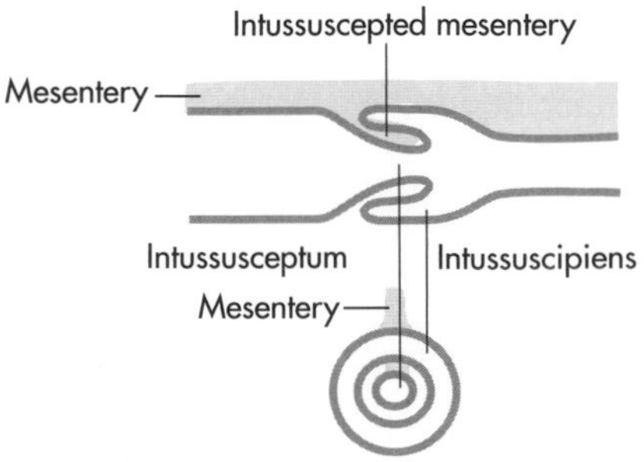

FIGURE 3-110

PNEUMATOSIS COLI

Pneumatosis cystoides (large, cystlike collection of air, few symptoms); associated with benign causes:
- COP
- Patients on ventilator
- Mucosal injury (rectal tube insertion, colonoscopy, surgery)
- Scleroderma
- Steroids
- Chemotherapy

Pneumatosis intestinalis (symptomatic); associated with serious causes:
- Infarcted bowel (tiny bubbles, linear gas collections)
- Necrotizing enterocolitis (neonates)
- Toxic megacolon
- Typhlitis

ILEOCECAL DEFORMITIES

Inflammation (coned cecum)
- Crohn disease: aphthous ulcers → linear fissures → nodules → cobblestone → stricture, spasm (string sign), fistula
- UC: valve is wide open (gaping), labia are atrophied, terminal ileum is dilated
- Amebiasis (predominantly affects cecum, not terminal ileum)
- TB: narrow cecum (Fleischner's sign), narrow Crohn's may produce same appearance, terminal ileum (Stierlin's sign)
- Typhlitis: inflammatory changes of cecum and/or ascending colon in neutropenic (immunosuppressed, leukemia, lymphoma) patients; caused by infection, bleeding, ischemia

Tumor
- Lymphoma
- Adenocarcinoma
- Carcinoid of ileum (desmoplastic response) or appendix
- Intussusception

PROCTITIS

- Condylomata acuminate (HPV)
- Lymphogranuloma venereum (chlamydia)
- Gonococcal proctitis
- UC, Crohn disease
- Herpes
- CMV

LIVER

LIVER MASSES

Solid masses
- Neoplasm
    - Benign: hemangioma
    - Malignant: primary, secondary
- Focal fatty liver (pseudotumor)
- Regenerating nodules in cirrhosis

Cystic masses
- Infectious
    - Echinococcosis
    - Amebiasis
    - Other abscesses (often complex and have debris)
- Benign masses
    - Simple liver cysts
    - Polycystic disease of the liver
    - von Meyenburg complexes
    - Peribiliary cysts
    - Biliary cystadenoma
    - Obstructed intrahepatic GB
    - Biloma
- Malignant masses
    - Cystadenocarcinoma
    - Cystic metastases: ovarian tumors
    - Necrotic tumors
    - Cholangiocarcinoma

ABNORMAL LIVER DENSITY (CT)

Increased Liver Density

- Hemachromatosis
- Glycogen storage disease

DIFFERENTIAL DIAGNOSIS OF COLITIS BY CT

	Wall Thickness (mm)	Submucosal Fat	SB Involvement	Left Colonic Involvement Only (o/o)	Ascites	Abscess
Crohn disease	>10	10%	60%	50	10%	35%
UC	<10	60%	5%	30	0%	0%
PMC	>10	5%	5%	30	50%	0%
Ischemic colitis	<10	0%	Uncommon	80	15%	0%
Infectious colitis	<10	0%	0%	0	50%	0%

- Wilson disease
- Drugs: amiodarone, cisplatin, gold
- Apparent increased density of liver parenchyma in patients with anemia (relative decreased blood density)

Decreased Liver Density

- Fatty liver (common)
    - Obesity, nutritional
    - Alcohol
    - Diabetes
    - Steroids
    - Chemotherapy

HYPERVASCULAR LIVER LESIONS

- Hemangioma
- Hemangioendothelioma, hemangiopericytoma, angiosarcoma (all rare), intrahepatic cholangiocarcinoma
- Metastases
    - Islet cell
    - Melanoma
    - Carcinoid
    - Renal cell cancer
    - Thyroid
    - Breast
    - Sarcoma

FAT-CONTAINING LIVER MASSES

- Hepatic adenoma
- HCC
- Metastases (liposarcoma, teratoma)
- Focal fatty infiltration
- Lipoma, AML

FOCAL LIVER LESIONS WITH CAPSULAR RETRACTION

- Metastases after treatment
- Cholangiocarcinoma
- Focal confluent fibrosis
- Primary sclerosing cholangitis
- Epithelioid hemangioendothelioma
- Hemangioma (rarely)

FOCAL LIVER LESIONS WITH CENTRAL SCAR

- FNH
- Fibrolamellar HCC
- Large cavernous hemangioma
- Cholangiocarcinoma
- Adenoma
- HCC (with central necrosis mimicking a scar)
- Metastases (with central necrosis mimicking a scar)

LIVER NODULES IN CIRRHOSIS

- Regenerative nodule: benign, proliferation of hepatocytes, precursor to dysplastic nodule and HCC. Regenerative nodules with hemosiderin are termed siderotic nodules. They are isointense on CT, hyperdense on noncontrast CT, and hypointense on T1 and T2.
- Dysplastic nodule: premalignant. Hyperintense on T1 and hypointense on T2. When malignancies develop they often appear as a nodule within a nodule, where the inner nodule has characteristic appearances (T1 hypointense, T2 hyperintense, arterial enhancement)
- HCC

HYPERECHOIC LIVER LESIONS

Round Lesions (Fig. 3-111)

- Hemangioma
- Hyperechoic metastases
    - Hypervascular metastases, sarcoma
    - Calcified metastases
- Primary liver tumors (contain fat)
    - HCC
    - Fibrolamellar HCC
- Focal fat, lipoma, angiomyolipoma (tuberous sclerosis)
- Gaucher disease

Linear Lesions

- Air in biliary tree
- Air in portal veins
- Biliary ascariasis

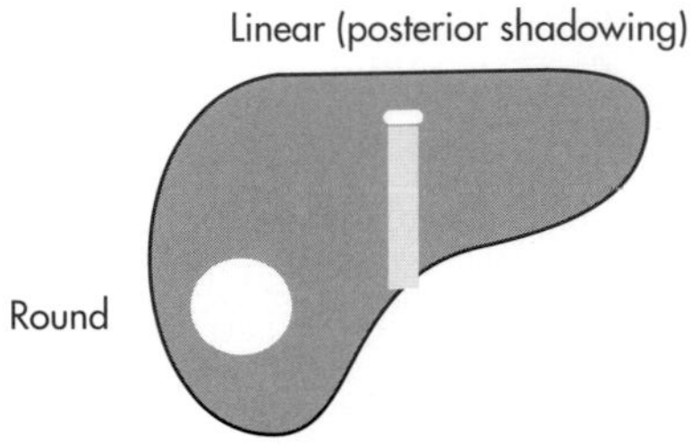

FIGURE 3-111

MULTIPLE HYPOECHOIC LIVER LESIONS

Tumor
- Metastases
- Lymphoma
- Multifocal HCC

Infection
- Multiple pyogenic abscesses
- Amebic abscesses
- *Echinococcus*
- Candidiasis
- Schistosomiasis

Other
- Regenerating nodules, cirrhosis
- Sarcoid
- Extramedullary hematopoiesis
- Hematomas
- Hemangioma

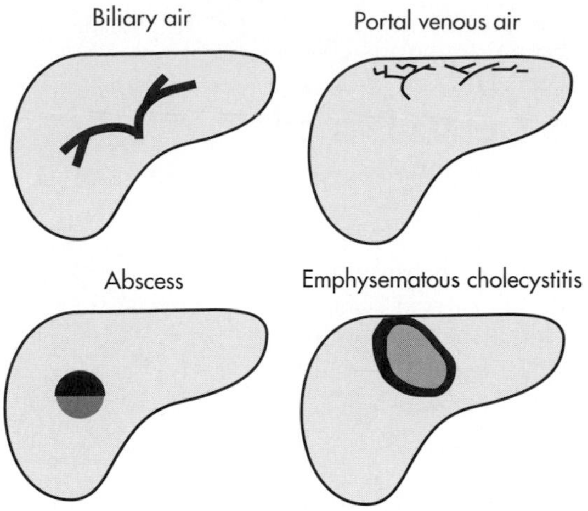

FIGURE 3-112

GAS IN LIVER (Fig. 3-112)

- Biliary gas (ERCP, surgery)
- Portal venous gas (bowel necrosis, diverticulitis); may produce short spikes on Doppler waveform
- Abscess
- Emphysematous cholecystitis

BILIARY SYSTEM

EXTRAHEPATIC BILIARY DILATATION (Fig. 3-113)

Levels of Obstruction

Intrapancreatic (most common)
- Pancreatic cancer
- Calculus
- Chronic pancreatitis

Suprapancreatic
- Primary biliary ductal carcinoma
- Metastatic lymph nodes

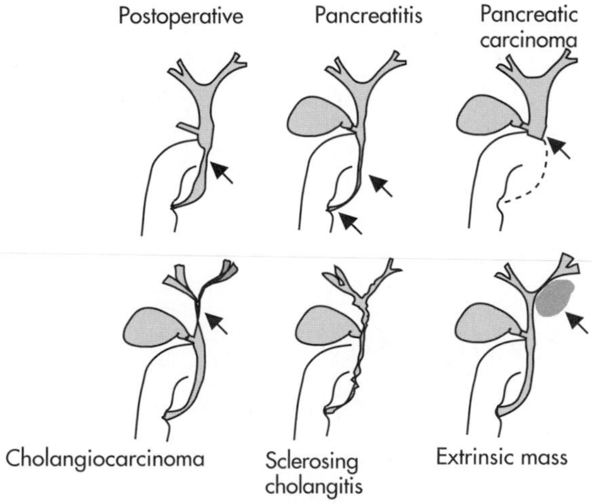

FIGURE 3-113

Portal
- Invasive GB carcinoma
- Surgical strictures
- Hepatoma
- Cholangiocarcinoma

Types of Obstruction

Tumor
- Abrupt termination of duct
- Mass adjacent to duct

Pancreatitis
- Smooth, long tapering

Lithiasis-related disease
- Calculus visible
- Meniscus sign (ERCP, CT), intrahepatic dilatation
- Mirizzi syndrome

Cholangitis
- Sclerosing cholangitis (50% have ulcerative colitis)
- AIDS cholangitis
- Intrahepatic biliary calculi (oriental cholangiohepatitis)

Caroli disease

Intrahepatic biliary neoplasm (rare)
- Cystadenoma
- Cystadenocarcinoma

Ultrasound Signs of Intrahepatic Dilatation (Fig. 3-114)

- Color Doppler flow is absent in dilated ducts.
- Acoustic enhancement behind dilated ducts; blood, in contrast, attenuates acoustic beam (high protein content).
- Double-duct sign: dilated biliary vessel accompanies portal veins.
- Caliber irregularity and tortuosity of dilated bile ducts; veins are always smooth and taper gradually.
- Spokewheel appearance at points of conversion of ducts

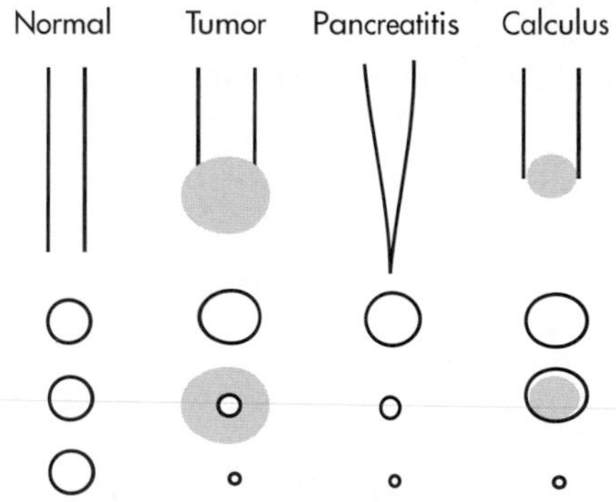

FIGURE 3-114

MULTIFOCAL DUCT NARROWING

- Primary sclerosing cholangitis
- AIDS cholangiopathy
- Metastases

- Chemotherapy
- Posttransplant ischemia

FILLING DEFECTS WITHIN BILIARY SYSTEM

- Calculi
- Clot
- Papillomas
- Cholangiocarcinoma
- Sludge balls

PERIPORTAL ENHANCEMENT

Thickened portal tracts with enhancement:
- Ascending cholangitis
- Schistosomiasis, TB, histoplasmosis
- Primary sclerosing cholangitis
- Primary biliary cirrhosis
- Sarcoidosis
- Cholangiocarcinoma

GALLBLADDER WALL THICKENING

GB wall thickening: >3 mm. Wall thickening typically appears as a hypoechoic region between two echogenic lines. When measuring wall thickening by US, a 5-MHz transducer should be used.

Diffuse (Concentric) Thickening (in order of decreasing frequency)

- Nonfasting GB (GB is usually <2 cm)
- Acute cholecystitis (50%-75% of patients have thickening)
- Chronic cholecystitis (<25% of patients have thickening)
- Portal venous hypertension (cystic vein dilatation causes edema)
- Hypoalbuminemia (must be <2.5 g/dL)
- Hepatitis
- AIDS (cryptosporidiosis, CMV, MAI)
- Vasculitis (e.g. lupus, HSP)
- Ascites
  - Benign ascites → GB wall thickening
  - Malignant ascites → no GB wall thickening

Focal (Eccentric) Thickening

- GB carcinoma (40% present with focal thickening; mass typically fills the GB)
- Metastases (melanoma >> gastric, pancreas)
- Benign tumors
  - Polyps (cholesterol, adenomatous)
  - Adenomyomatosis
- Tumefactive sludge adherent to GB wall
- AIDS

HYPERECHOIC FOCI IN GALLBLADDER WALL

- Calculus
- Polyp
- Cholesterol
- Emphysematous cholecystitis
- Porcelain GB

DENSE GALLBLADDER (CT)

- Hepatobiliary (vicarious) excretion of contrast material
- Calculi
- Milk of calcium bile
- Reflux of oral contrast agent after surgery
- Oral cholecystogram
- Hemorrhage (hematocrit effect)

PANCREAS

FOCAL PANCREATIC SIGNAL ABNORMALITY

Criteria: focal hypoechoic or hypodense pancreatic lesion
- Tumor
- Focal pancreatitis
- Adenopathy

PARADUODENAL PANCREATITIS

- Groove pancreatitis
- Cystic dystrophy of duodenum
- Paraduodenal wall cysts

CYSTIC PANCREATIC LESIONS

Differential Diagnosis by Features

(Figs. 3-115 and 3-116)

Unilocular
- Simple cyst (if multiple, consider VHL, CF, ADPKD)
- Pseudocyst postpancreatitis

Microcystic lesions
- Serous cystadenoma

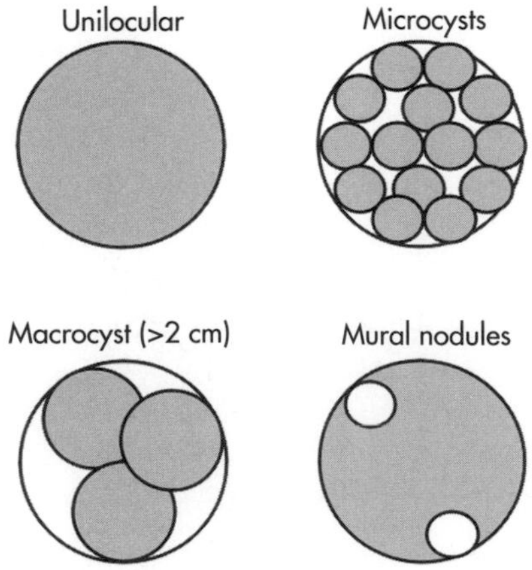

FIGURE 3-115

FIGURE 3-116

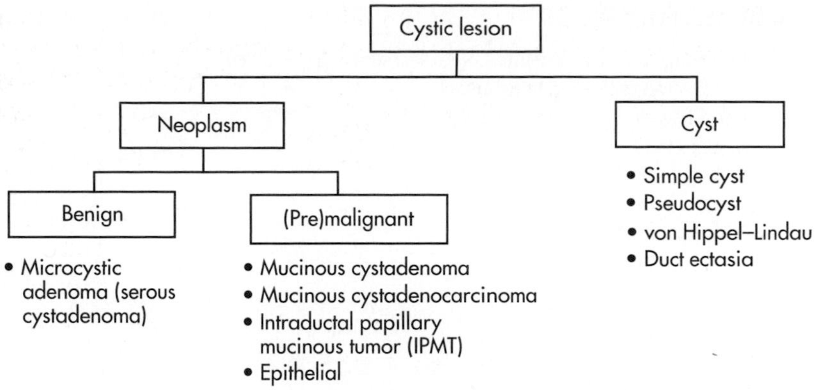

Macrocystic lesions
- Mucinous cystadenoma

Mural nodules
- Pancreatic adenocarcinoma

Differential Diagnosis by Incidence

Common cystic neoplasms
- Mucinous cystic neoplasm
- Serous cystadenoma
- Intraductal papillary mucinous tumor (IPMT)

Rare cystic neoplasms
- Solid pseudopapillary tumor
- Papillary cystic epithelial neoplasm
- Acinar cell cystadenocarcinoma
- Cystic teratoma
- Cystic choriocarcinoma
- Angiomatous neoplasms (lymphangioma, hemangioma)
- Paraganglioma

Solid tumors undergoing cystic change
- Cystic islet cell tumors
- Cystic necrosis of pancreatic adenocarcinoma

- Lymphoma
- Metastases (ovarian clear cell)
- Cystic teratoma
- Sarcoma

PANCREATIC CALCIFICATIONS

- Chronic pancreatitis
- Islet cell tumor
- Serous cystadenoma
- Mucinous cystic neoplasm
- SPEN
- Granulomatous disease (e.g., sarcoidosis, histoplasmosis)

FATTY REPLACEMENT OF PANCREAS

- CF
- Aging
- DM
- Obesity
- Steroids

HYPERECHOIC PANCREAS

The normal pancreas appears slightly hyperechoic relative to liver. Marked hyperechogenicity is seen in:
- Cystic fibrosis
- Pancreatic lipomatosis

SPLEEN

FOCAL SPLENIC LESIONS

Tumor
- Metastases (usually in end-stage disease); lymphoma, melanoma, ovary
- Hemangioma (common benign lesion)
- Lymphangioma
- Hamartoma
- Rare lesions: myxoma, chondroma, osteoma, hemangiosarcoma, fibrosarcoma

Infection (often calcified)
- Abscess
- Candidiasis (common in AIDS)
- TB, MAI
- Schistosomiasis (splenic nodules in 10%)
- *Pneumocystis jiroveci* (Frenkel 1999)

Other
- Infarcts
- Hematoma (trauma)
- Cysts: simple, hydatid
- Fatty nodules in Gaucher disease

Multiple hypodense lesions in spleen and liver
- Granulomatous disease (e.g., sarcoid)
- Lymphoma
- Metastases
- Candida
- TB, MAI

RIM-CALCIFIED CYSTIC LESIONS

- Echinococcus
- Traumatic cyst
- Metastases
- Intrasplenic aneurysm

CALCIFIED FOCI ON CT

- Healed granulomatous disease (e.g., sarcoid, TB, MAI, histoplasmosis)
- PCP
- Candida
- Treated lymphoma/mets

SPLENOMEGALY

Tumor
- Leukemia
- Lymphoma

Infection
- Infectious mononucleosis
- Histoplasmosis
- HIV

Metabolic disorders
- Gaucher disease
- Amyloid
- Hemochromatosis

Trauma

Vascular
- Portal hypertension
- Hematologic disorders (anemias, sickle cell, thalassemia, myelofibrosis, myelosclerosis)

PERITONEAL CAVITY

PERITONEAL FLUID COLLECTIONS

Water density
- Ascites
- Urinoma
- Biloma
- Seroma
- Lymphocele (after lymph node resection)
- Pancreatic pseudocyst
- Cerebrospinal fluid pseudocyst from VP shunt
- Duplication cyst
- Mesenteric cyst
- Ovarian cyst
- Lymphangioma

Complex (may be loculated, noncommunicating, heterogeneous signal intensity)
- Abscess
- Hematoma
- Pseudomyxoma peritonei
- Pancreatic necrosis

INTRAPERITONEAL CALCIFICATIONS

- Arterial calcification
- Appendicolith
- Mesenteric node
- Cholelithiasis
- Pancreatic calcification
- Porcelain GB
- Pseudomyxoma peritonei
- Renal/ureteral calculi
- Old hematoma, abscess
- Uterine leiomyoma
- Fetal skeletal part
- Pelvic phlebolith
- Teratoma
- Liver: echinococcal cyst

OTHER

AIDS

Common Gastrointestinal Manifestations by Cause

Infection
- CMV
- *Candida*
- Herpes
- *Cryptococcus*
- MAI

Tumor
- Kaposi sarcoma
- Lymphoma

Common Gastrointestinal Manifestations by Organ System

Esophagus
- Ulcers: *Candida*, CMV, herpes
- Sinus tracts: TB, actinomycosis

Proximal small bowel
- Ulcers: cryptococcosis
- Nodules: Kaposi sarcoma, MAI

Distal small bowel
- Enteritis: TB, MAI, CMV

Colon
- Colitis: CMV, pseudomembranous colitis
- Typhlitis

Biliary
- Strictures: CMV, cryptococcosis

LOW-DENSITY LYMPH NODES

- Infection: MAI, *Yersinia*
- Sprue/cavitary lymph node syndrome
- Metastases
- Necrotizing mesenteritis
- Whipple disease

ABDOMINAL TRAUMA

Injuries in decreasing order of frequency:
- Liver laceration (most common)
- Splenic laceration
- Renal trauma
- Bowel hematoma
- Pancreatic fracture
- Rare: GB injury, adrenal hemorrhage

ABDOMINAL COMPLICATIONS AFTER CARDIAC SURGERY

Incidence: 0.2%-2%. Most commonly, complications are related to ischemia (e.g., intraoperative hypotension, hemorrhage, vasculopathy, emboli, clotting abnormalities).

- GI hemorrhage, 50%
- Cholecystitis (emphysematous, acalculous, or calculus), 20%
- Pancreatitis, 10%
- Perforated peptic ulcer, 10%
- Mesenteric ischemia, 5%
- Perforated diverticular disease, 5%

Suggested Readings

Davis M, Houston J. *Fundamentals of Gastrointestinal Radiology.* Philadelphia: WB Saunders; 2002.

Eisenberg RL. *Gastrointestinal Radiology: A Pattern Approach.* 4th ed. Philadelphia: Lippincott Williams & Wilkins; 2003.

Federle MP, Jeffrey B, Desser T, et al. *Diagnostic Imaging: Abdomen.* 2nd ed. Amirsys: Salt Lake City; 2009.

Feldman M, Friedman L, Sleisenger M, eds. *Sleisenger and Fordtran's Gastrointestinal and Liver Disease.* 8th ed. Philadelphia: Saunders, an imprint of Elsevier; 2006.

Gedgaudas-McClees R. *Handbook of Gastrointestinal Imaging.* Vol 1. New York: Churchill Livingstone; 1987.

Ginsburg G, Kochman M. *Endoscopy and Gastrointestinal Radiology.* Vol 4. St. Louis: Mosby; 2004.

Gore RM, Levine MS. *Textbook of Gastrointestinal Radiology.* Vol 2. Philadelphia: WB Saunders; 2007.

Halligan S, Fenlon HM. *New Techniques in Gastrointestinal Imaging.* New York: Marcel Dekker; 2004.

Halpert RD, Goodman P. *Gastrointestinal Radiology: The Requisites.* 2nd ed. St. Louis: Mosby; 2006.

Jones B, Braver JM. *Essentials of Gastrointestinal Radiology.* Philadelphia: WB Saunders; 1982.

Laufer I, Levine M, Rubesin S. *Double Contrast Gastrointestinal Radiology.* 3rd ed. Philadelphia: WB Saunders; 1999.

Margulis AR, Burhenne HJ, eds. *Alimentary Tract Radiology.* 5th ed. St. Louis: Mosby; 1994.

Meyer MA. *Dynamic Radiology of the Abdomen: Normal and Pathologic Anatomy.* 5th ed. New York: Springer-Verlag; 2000.

Moss AA, Gamsu G, Genant HK. *Computed Tomography of the Body with Magnetic Resonance Imaging.* 2nd ed. Philadelphia: WB Saunders; 1992.

Rifkin M, Charbonneau J, Laing F. *Syllabus Special Course: Ultrasound.* Oak Brook, IL: Radiological Society of North America; 1991.

Rumack CM, Charboneau W, Wilson S. *Diagnostic Ultrasound.* St. Louis: Elsevier Science Health Science; 2004.

Taylor KJW. *Atlas of Ultrasonography.* 2nd ed New York: Elsevier Health; 1984.

Weissleder R, Stark DD. *MRI Atlas of the Abdomen.* London: Martin Dunitz; 1989.

CHAPTER 4

Genitourinary Imaging

CHAPTER OUTLINE

Kidneys

GENERAL

ANATOMY

The kidneys, renal pedicle, and adrenal glands are located in the perirenal space, which is bound by the anterior and posterior renal fascia (Gerota's fascia; for anatomy, see the section titled Retroperitoneum).

Renal Pedicle (Fig. 4-1)

- Renal artery
- Renal vein
- Collecting system and ureter
- Lymphatics

Collecting System

- Minor calyces: most kidneys have 10 to 14 minor calyces
- Major calyces
- Renal pelvis: may be completely within the renal sinus or partially "extrarenal"

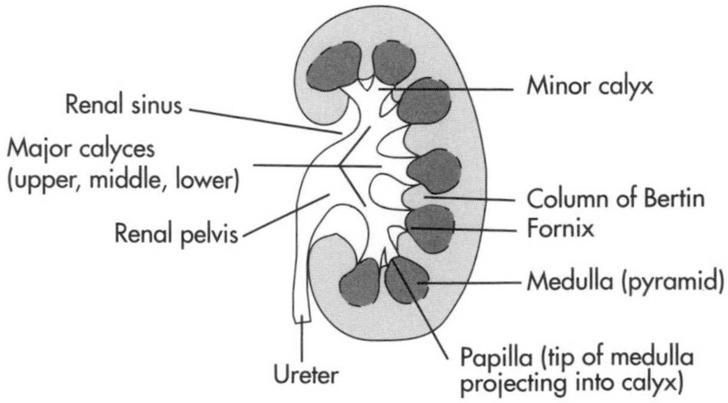

FIGURE 4-1

Orientation and Size of Kidneys

- Kidneys are 3 to 4 lumbar vertebral bodies in length, 12 to 14 cm long, and 5 to 7 cm wide.
- Intravenous pyelograms (IVPs) overestimate the true renal length because of magnification and renal engorgement from osmotic diuresis. Ultrasound (US) often underestimates the true renal length because of technical difficulties in imaging the entire kidney.
- Left and right kidney size should not vary more than 1 cm.
- Right kidney is 1 to 2 cm lower than the left kidney and slightly more lateral.
- Renal axis parallels axis of psoas muscles.

TECHNIQUES

BOLUS IVP

Today, IVPs are rarely used but are covered for historical purposes. The bolus administration ensures maximum concentration of contrast media in the kidney. Indication: healthy ambulatory patients (screening type urography [e.g., for urinary tract infection]), trauma.

Technique

1. Kidney, ureter, bladder (KUB)
2. Inject 100 mL of 30% contrast
3. 1-min and 5-min film of both kidneys
4. 10-min KUB and both obliques
5. Coned bladder view
6. Postvoid KUB

DRIP-INFUSION NEPHROTOMOGRAM

With drip infusion, the nephrogram persists longer, allowing more time for nephrotomography and special views, if necessary. Today, this is much less commonly performed than the bolus technique or computed tomography (CT). If calcifications are seen on the renal outlines, scout oblique films can be obtained to determine the exact location relative to the kidneys.

Technique

1. KUB and preliminary tomogram of kidneys (starting at 8 cm from back)
2. Drip infusion of 300 mL of Urovist 14% (or Conray-30) or 150 mL of Isovue 300 (or Omnipaque 300)
3. Obtain tomograms after 150 mL has been given. Usually 7 to 9 cuts are obtained.
4. Postinfusion KUB and both oblique views
5. Coned bladder view
6. Postvoid KUB

SUMMARY OF CONTRAST DOSE

	Body Weight	Dose of Contrast
Bolus Injection		
Children	5–25 kg	0.5 mL/kg
	25–50 kg	50 mL
Adult	>50 kg	100 mL (28-40 g iodine)
Infusion Technique		
Children	Contraindicated	
Adult	300 mL (33-45 g iodine)	

RETROGRADE PYELOGRAM

A catheter is placed in the distal ureter via cystoscopy and contrast is administered via the catheter by hand injection to opacify the collecting system (no parenchymal opacification). This technique is primarily used for PUL access and difficult nephrostomy placements.

PRETREATMENT PROTOCOL FOR IV IODINATED CONTRAST IN PATIENTS WITH PREVIOUS ALLERGIC REACTION

- Prednisone, 50 mg PO or IV, 13 hours, 7 hours, and 1 hour before contrast injection
- Diphenhydramine, 50 mg PO or IV, 30 to 60 minutes before contrast media injection

CT PROTOCOLS OF THE KIDNEY/URETERS

Hematuria Protocol

Single bolus CT technique

- Phase 1: Noncontrast CT of the abdomen and pelvis, including kidneys, ureters, and bladder
- Single bolus (100 to 150 mL, 300 to 320 mg of iodine/mL) of intravenous contrast material at 2-4 mL/sec
- Early images of kidney in nephrographic phase
- Excretory phase images (5 minutes following injection) through kidney, ureters, and bladder

Split bolus CT technique:

- Phase 1: Noncontrast CT of abdomen and pelvis. Immediately thereafter administer 30 mL of IV contrast and wait 5 to 10 minutes.
- Phase 2: Place patient back on scanner and inject 100 mL of contrast at 2 to 3 mL/sec, and scan patient prone from top of kidneys to pubic symphysis after 100 seconds.
- Phase 2 excretory phase (5 minutes) through the kidneys

Stone Protocol

- Noncontrast CT of the abdomen and pelvis using 5-mm collimation

Renal Mass Protocol

- Phase 1: noncontrast CT images of abdomen
- Phase 2: corticomedullary phase, 25-30 seconds after contrast injection, through kidneys
- Phase 3: nephrographic phase, 60-80 seconds after injection

PERCUTANEOUS NEPHROSTOMY (PCN)

Refers to percutaneous drainage of renal collecting system by catheter placement. Complications: 2%-4% (extravasation of contrast, bleeding)

Indications

- Hydronephrosis (acute, subacute obstruction)
- Pyonephrosis

Technique (Fig. 4-2)

1. Preprocedure workup:
   - Check bleeding status.
   - Antibiotic coverage: ampicillin, 1 g; gentamicin, 80 mg in patients with normal renal function and no contraindications
   - Review all films and determine on plain film where kidneys are located, especially in relation to colon, spleen, and pleural reflections.
   - US or IV contrast opacification of kidneys may be helpful in difficult approaches or nondilated collecting systems. IV contrast is less useful with severe obstruction because opacification may not occur or may be impractically delayed.
2. Local anesthesia, aiming for upper pole calyx with 20-gauge Chiba biopsy needle. Aspirate urine to check for position and for partial decompression of collecting system before contrast opacification.
3. Using a second needle/sheath system, aim for middle pole calyx. Skin insertion point is inferior and slightly lateral to calyx. When positive urine returns, advance 0.038-inch guidewire as far as possible. If wire coils in calyceal system, a Kumpe catheter may be useful for manipulation.
4. Dilate skin up to 12 Fr.

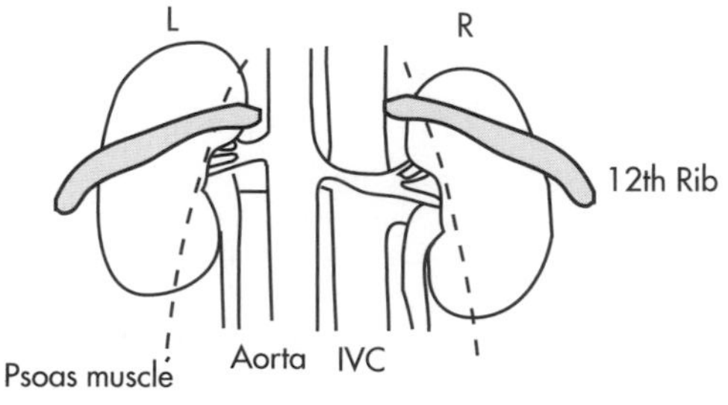

FIGURE 4-2

5. Pass 10-Fr PCN tube over guidewire. Remove stiffener and guidewire. Coil pigtail. Inject contrast to check position of catheter. Cut thread.
6. In the setting of infection, complete evaluation of the ureter via an antegrade injection is best deferred to a second visit.

CONGENITAL ANOMALIES

DUPLICATED COLLECTING SYSTEM

Bifid Renal Pelvis

One pelvis drains upper pole calyces; the other drains the middle and lower pole calyces. The two pelvises join proximally to the ureteropelvic junction (UPJ). Incidence: 10% of population. No complications.

Incomplete Ureteral Duplication

Duplications join distal to UPJ and proximal to bladder: Y-shaped ureters. No complications.

Complete Ureteral Duplication

See Chapter 11, Pediatric Imaging.

HORSESHOE KIDNEY

The two kidneys are connected across the midline by an isthmus. This is the most common fusion anomaly (other fusion anomalies: cross-fused ectopia, pancake kidney). The isthmus may contain parenchymal tissue with its own blood supply or consist of fibrous tissue.

Associations

- UPJ obstruction, 30%
- Ureteral duplication, 10%
- Genital anomalies
- Other anomalies: anorectal, cardiovascular, musculoskeletal anomalies

Complications

- Obstruction, infection, calculus formation in 30%
- Increased risk of renal malignancies, especially Wilms tumor
- Increased risk of traumatic injury

Imaging Features

- Abnormal axis of each kidney with lower calyx more medial than upper calyx
- Bilateral malrotation of renal pelvises in anterior position
- Isthmus lies anterior to aorta and inferior vena cava (IVC) but behind inferior mesenteric artery (IMA)

OTHER RENAL VARIANTS

- Persistent fetal lobation: scalloped appearance of renal outline; adjacent calyx is normal.
- Junctional parenchymal defect: fusion defect in upper pole of kidney that does not represent a

scar; echogenic linear defect extends from sinus; commonly seen in pediatric patients
- Septum of Bertin (upper pole 90%, bilateral 60%); associated with bifid renal pelvis
- Dromedary hump: parenchymal prominence in left kidney; results from compression of adjacent spleen
- Lobar dysmorphism: abnormally oriented lobe between upper and middle calyces; always points to posterior calyx, which is key to diagnosis on CT or IVP. By US this entity is indistinguishable from column of Bertin.
- Aberrant papilla: papilla indents infundibulum or pelvis rather than minor calyx
- Linear vascular impressions on renal pelvis and infundibula
- Ureteral spindle: dilatation of middle third of ureter at crossing of iliac vessels
- Sinus lipomatosis: large amount of fat in renal sinus
- Cross-fused ectopia; the ectopic kidney is inferior
- Nephroptosis (floating or wandering kidney): acquired condition with excessive descent of the kidney in erect position; differs from congenital pelvic kidney in that the paired renal arteries arise from their typical anatomic location.

CYSTIC DISEASE

CLASSIFICATION

Cortical cysts
- Simple cysts
- Complicated (complex) cysts

Localized cystic disease of the kidney
Medullary cystic disease
Polycystic renal disease
- Infantile polycystic disease
- Adult polycystic disease

Multicystic dysplastic kidney
Multilocular cystic nephroma
Cysts associated with systemic disease
- Tuberous sclerosis
- Von Hippel-Lindau disease

Miscellaneous cysts
- Hydatid
- Acquired cysts in uremia
- Extraparenchymal cysts
    - Parapelvic cysts
    - Perinephric cysts

SIMPLE CYSTS (Fig. 4-3)

Simple cysts (in >50% of population >50 years) probably arise from obstructed tubules or ducts. They do not, however, communicate with collecting system. Most commonly asymptomatic; rare findings include hematuria (from cyst rupture), HTN, cyst infection. Mass effect from large cysts may cause dull ache or discomfort.

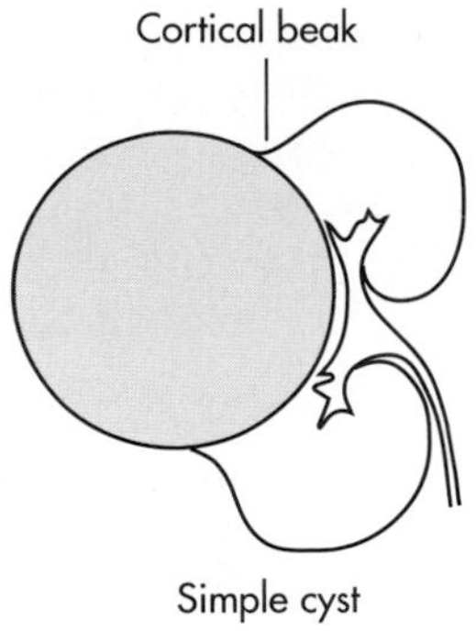

FIGURE 4-3

Imaging Features

IVP
- Lucent defect
- Cortical bulge
- Round indentations on collecting system
- "Beak sign" can be seen with large cysts.

US
- Anechoic
- Enhanced through-transmission
- Sharply marginated, smooth walls
- Very thin septations may occasionally be seen.

CT
- Smooth cyst wall
- Sharp demarcation from surrounding renal parenchyma
- Water density (<10-15 HU) that is homogeneous throughout lesion
- No significant enhancement after IV contrast administration (small increases of <5 HU, however, can be seen likely due to technical factors, not true enhancement)
- Cyst wall too thin to be seen by CT (with small cysts, volume-averaging may create the false appearance of a thick wall)

MRI
- Indications (rather than CT): renal insufficiency, solitary kidney, contrast allergy, patients with complex cystic renal masses needing multiple follow-up examinations
- End-expiration images are preferred because they are more reproducible in optimizing image coregistration and subtraction algorithms.
- Simple renal cysts are uniformly hypointense on T1W and hyperintense on T2W images with no perceptible enhancement after gadolinium. MRI can characterize extremely small renal cysts (>1 cm).

- Internal components of cystic masses and subtle enhancement are better appreciated by MRI than by CT.

Pearls

- True renal cysts should always be differentiated from hydronephrosis, calyceal diverticulum, and peripelvic cysts.
- Differentiate renal cyst from hypoechoic renal artery aneurysm using color Doppler US.
- Cysts that contain calcium, septations, and irregular margins (complicated cysts) need further workup.

COMPLICATED CYSTS

Complicated cysts are cysts that do not meet the criteria of simple cysts and thus require further workup.

Bosniak Classification

- Category 1: benign simple cyst.
  - Simple cysts contain low attenuation (0-20 HU) fluid and a hairline-thin smooth wall
  - Cysts do not contain septations, calcifications, or enhancing nodular soft tissue
- Category 2: minimally complicated cysts that are benign but have certain radiologic findings of concern.
  - This category includes septated (paper-thin septations) cystic, minimally calcified cysts, high-density cysts.
  - Fine calcification or a short segment of slightly thickened calcification may be present in the wall or septa.
  - Hyperattenuating cysts contain more fluid than water attenuation (i.e., >20 HU). In general, cysts that measure between 20 and 40 HU are proteinaceous cysts and will show findings of a simple cyst using US; those with attenuations over 40 to 50 HU are likely to be hemorrhagic cysts and will be complex under US. When a hyperattenuating renal mass is encountered on an unenhanced CT scan, the probability of the mass being benign is more than 99% as long as the attenuation is 70 HU or more and the mass is homogeneous.
- Category 2F (the "F" means to follow) lesions cannot be considered benign without some period of observation. These lesions are slightly more complicated (e.g., may contain multiple, hairline-thin septa that demonstrate perceived [not measurable] enhancement). There may be minimal smooth thickening of the wall or septa. They may contain thick irregular or nodular calcification. There are no enhancing soft tissue components. Hyperattenuating renal masses that exhibit all of the features of hyperattenuating cysts but are larger than 3 cm and are completely intrarenal are included also in this category. The recommended follow-up is to perform a CT or MR examination at 6 months, followed by yearly studies for a minimum of 5 years.
- Category 3: complicated cystic lesions that exhibit some radiologic features also are seen in malignancy.
  - This category includes multiloculated cystic nephroma, multiloculated cysts, complex septated cysts, chronically infected cysts, heavily calcified cysts, and cystic renal cell carcinoma (RCC).
  - Because these entities are difficult to separate radiologically, surgery is usually performed.
- Category 4 lesion: clearly malignant lesions with large cystic component.
  - Irregular margins, solid vascular elements.

CYST CATEGORIES (BOSNIAK)

Category (Bosniak)	US Features	Workup
Type 1: Simple cyst	Round, anechoic, thin wall, enhanced through-transmission	None
Type 2: Mildly complicated cyst	Thin septation, calcium in wall	CT or US follow-up
Type 3: Indeterminate lesion	Multiple septa, internal echoes, mural nodules	Partial nephrectomy, biopsy
	Thick septa	CT follow-up if surgery is high risk
Type 4: Clearly malignant	Solid mass component	Nephrectomy

Imaging Features

Septations

- Thin septa within cysts are usually benign.
- Thick or irregular septa require workup.

Calcifications

- Thin calcifications in cyst walls are usually benign.
- Milk of calcium: collection of small calcific granules in cyst fluid: usually benign

Thick wall

- These lesions usually require surgical exploration.

Increased CT density (>15 HU) of cyst content

- Vast majority of these lesions are benign.
- High density is usually due to hemorrhage, high protein content, and/or calcium.
- 50% appear as simple cysts using US.

The remainder of patients require a further imaging workup (to exclude soft tissue mass) or occasionally cyst puncture (analyze fluid, inject contrast).

CYST ASPIRATION

Indications for Cyst Aspiration

Diagnosis

- Complex, high-density cyst (type 2) ≥ 3 cm
- Evaluate fluid for character, as well as cytology.
- After aspiration, inject contrast ("cystogram") and obtain multiple projections so that all surfaces of the wall are smooth.

Therapy

- Most commonly performed for large cyst obstructing collecting system or causing dull, aching pain or, rarely, HTN (Page kidney)
- If the cyst is simple and the fluid is clear, yellow, and free-flowing, laboratory analysis is not necessary. Bloody or brownish fluid should be sent for cytology.

Cyst Ablation

If a symptomatic cyst recurs after aspiration, percutaneous ablation may be considered to avoid surgery.

1. Place 20-gauge needle into cyst and measure total volume aspirated. Some interventional radiologists prefer a small pigtail catheter.
2. Inject contrast to exclude communication with the collecting system, which would preclude alcohol ablation.
3. Inject absolute ethanol, 25% of the volume of cyst fluid aspirated.
4. Leave ethanol in place 15 to 20 minutes, turning the patient to different positions to maximize wall contact of alcohol with different surfaces.
5. Aspirate residual ethanol.

OTHER CYSTIC STRUCTURES

Milk of Calcium Cyst

- Not a true cyst but a calyceal diverticulum, which may be communicating or closed off
- Contains layering calcific granules (calcium carbonate)
- No pathologic consequence

Parapelvic Cyst

- Originates from renal parenchyma but expands into the renal sinus
- May cause compression of the collecting system

Peripelvic Cyst

- Originates from sinus structures, most likely lymphatic in origin
- May be indistinguishable from hydronephrosis on US, requiring an IVP or CT for definitive diagnosis
- Attenuated, stretched infundibula
- IVP differential diagnosis: renal sinus lipomatosis

Perinephric Cyst

- Located beneath the renal capsule
- Not true cysts; represent extravasated urine trapped beneath renal capsule (pseudocysts, uriniferous cysts, urinoma)

LOCALIZED CYSTIC DISEASE

Benign, acquired unilateral condition characterized by multiple cysts of varying size. Cysts, separated by normal renal parenchyma, may occupy the entire kidney or be more localized. Calcification of cyst walls may be present but the cyst wall has to be thin; it does not compromise renal function. No surgery necessary.

MEDULLARY CYSTIC DISEASE (MCD) (Fig. 4-4)

Spectrum of diseases characterized by tubulointerstitial fibrosis. Patients usually present with azotemia and anemia and subsequently progress to end-stage failure.

Types

- Familial nephronophthisis, 70%, autosomal recessive
  - Juvenile type, onset at age 3 to 5 years (most common); adult type
- Adult medullary cystic disease, 15%, autosomal dominant
- Renal-retinal dysplasia, 15%; recessive associated with retinitis pigmentosa

Imaging Features

- Small kidneys (as opposed to large kidneys in polycystic disease)
- Multiple small (<2 cm) cysts in medulla
- Cysts may be too small to resolve by imaging, but their multiplicity will result in increased medullary echogenicity and apparent widening of central sinus echoes.
- Cortex is thin and does not contain cysts.
- No calcifications

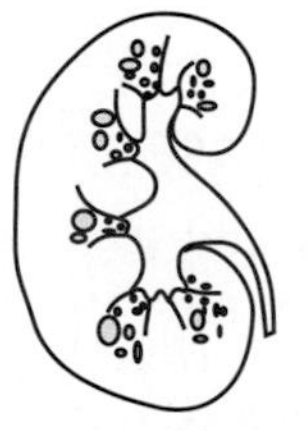

MCD

FIGURE 4-4

ADULT POLYCYSTIC KIDNEY DISEASE (APKD) (Fig. 4-5)

Cystic dilatation of collecting tubules, as well as nephrons (unlike MCD and infantile polycystic kidney disease in which only the collecting tubules are involved). Autosomal dominant trait (childhood type is autosomal recessive). Incidence: 0.1% (most common form of cystic kidney disease; accounts for 10% of patients on chronic dialysis). Slowly progressive renal failure. Symptoms usually begin in 3rd or 4th decade, but clinical onset is extremely variable, ranging from palpable cystic kidneys at birth to multiple cysts without symptoms in old age. Enlarged kidneys may be palpable. Treatment is with dialysis and transplant. No increased risk of malignancy.

Associated Findings

- Hepatic cysts, 70%
- Intracranial berry aneurysm, 20%
- Cysts in pancreas and spleen, <5%

Imaging Features

- Kidneys are enlarged and contain innumerable cysts, creating a bosselated surface.
- Calcification of cyst walls are common.
- Pressure deformities of calyces and infundibula
- IVP: "Swiss-cheese" nephrogram
- Cysts have variable signal characteristics.
  - CT: hypodense, hyperdense (hemorrhage, protein, calcium)
  - T1-weighted (T1W): some cysts contain clear, watery fluid (hypointense); others contain blood and protein (hyperintense); layering in some cysts is caused by cellular debris.
- Hepatic cysts

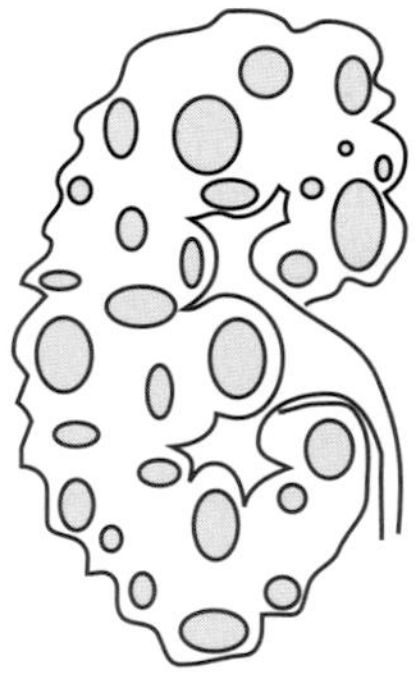

Polycystic kidney

FIGURE 4-5

UREMIC CYSTIC DISEASE (UCD)

40% of patients with end-stage renal disease develop renal cysts. Incidence increases with time on dialysis so that incidence of UCD is 90% in patients on dialysis for 5 years. Associated complications include:

- Incidence of malignancy is not as high as previously believed.
- Hemorrhage of cysts
- Cysts can regress after successful transplantation.

TUMORS

CLASSIFICATION

- Renal parenchymal tumors
  - Renal cell adenocarcinoma, 80%
  - Wilms tumor, 5%
  - Adenoma (thought to represent early RCC)
  - Oncocytoma
  - Nephroblastomatosis
  - Mesoblastic nephroma
- Mesenchymal tumors
  - Angiomyolipoma
  - Malignant fibrous histiocytoma
  - Hemangioma
  - Other rare tumors
- Renal pelvis tumors
  - Transitional cell carcinoma, <10%
  - Squamous cell carcinoma (SCC)
  - Other malignant tumors: undifferentiated adenocarcinoma tumors
  - Benign tumors: papilloma > angioma, fibroma, myoma, polyp
- Secondary tumors
  - Metastases
  - Lymphoma

RENAL CELL CARCINOMA (RCC)

Synonyms: renal adenocarcinoma, hypernephroma, clear cell carcinoma, malignant nephroma.

Clinical Findings

- Hematuria, 50%
- Flank pain, 40%
- Palpable mass, 35%
- Weight loss, 25%
- Paraneoplastic syndrome: hypertension (renin), erythrocytosis (erythropoietin), hypercalcemia (PTH), gynecomastia (gonadotropin), Cushing syndrome (ACTH)

Pathology

Clear cell type (65% of RCC). Cell origin: proximal tubule. Cytogenetic abnormalities: chromosome 3p deletions, mutations of von Hippel–Lindau (VHL) gene (tumor suppressor gene)

Papillary cell type (Chromophil) (15%). Cell origin: proximal tubule. Cytogenetic abnormalities: trisomies of chromosomes 3q, 7, 12, 16, 17, 20; loss of Y chromosome

Chromophobe cell type (10%). Cell origin: intercalated cell of cortical collecting duct. Cytogenetic abnormalities: monosomies of chromosomes 1, 2, 6, 10, 13, 17, and 21; –hypodiploidy

Oncocytoma (5%). Cell origin: Intercalated cell of cortical collecting duct. Cytogenetic abnormalities: loss of chromosomes 1 and Y

Unclassified cell type (5% of RCC). Sarcomas, collecting duct tumors, others

Risk Factors

- Tobacco use
- Long-term phenacetin use
- Von Hippel-Lindau disease (bilateral tumors)
- Chronic dialysis (>3 years)
- Family history

SUBTYPE OF RCC AND HEREDITARY ASSOCIATION

Clear cell RCC	Von Hippel–Lindau disease; tuberous sclerosis
Papillary RCC type 1	Hereditary papillary renal cell cancer
Papillary RCC type 2	Hereditary leiomyoma and renal cell carcinoma
Chromophobe and oncocytic neoplasms	Birt-Hodd-Dube
Medullary carcinoma	Sickle cell trait

Prognosis

5-year survival: stage 1, 2 = 50%, stage 3 = 35%, stage 4 = 15%

Tumors often have atypical behavior:
- Late recurrence of metastases: 10% recur 10 years after nephrectomy.
- Some patients survive for years with untreated tumor.
- Spontaneous regression of tumor has been reported but is very rare.

Imaging Features

Imaging findings
- Mass lesion: renal contour abnormality, calyceal displacement
- Large variability in signal characteristics on noncontrast CT and MRI depending on the degree of hemorrhage and necrosis
- Contrast enhancement is usually heterogeneous; strong contrast enhancement (>15 HU)
- Calcification, 10%
- Cystic areas (2%-5% are predominantly cystic)
- Filling defects (clots, tumor thrombus) in collecting system and renal veins
- US appearance
  - Hyperechoic: 70% of tumors >3 cm, 30% of tumors <3 cm
  - Hypoechoic

Angiography
- 95% of tumors are hypervascular.
  - Caliber irregularities of tumor vessels are typical (encasement).
  - Prominent AV shunting, venous lakes
- Angiography may be useful for detection in complicated and equivocal cases:
  - Small tumors
  - Underlying abnormal renal parenchyma
  - VHL disease
- Preoperative embolization with alcohol or Ivalon

MRI
- Venous invasion of tumor is better diagnosed by MRI.
- MRI allows scanning in alternate planes, which is beneficial for staging RCC.
- Using a 0.1-mmol/kg dose of Gd-chelate, the percent enhancement suggestive of RCC is 15%, obtained after 2 to 4 minutes of contrast administration (1.5T).
- DDX for enhancing renal lesions: RCC, oncocytoma, and angiomyolipoma. The likelihood of RCC increases with size and extension beyond kidney into Gerota's fascia.

Staging

- Stage I: tumor confined to kidney
- Stage II: extrarenal (may involve adrenal gland) but confined to Gerota's fascia
- Stage III: A: venous invasion (renal vein); B: lymph node metastases; C: both
- Stage IV: A: direct extension into adjacent organs through Gerota's fascia, B: metastases
  - Lungs, 55%
  - Liver, 25%
  - Bone, 20% (classic lesions are lytic, expansile)
  - Adrenal, 20%
  - Contralateral kidney, 10%
  - Other organs, <5%

Therapy

- Radical nephrectomy (entire contents of Gerota's fascia is removed)
- Chemotherapy
- Radiotherapy is used for palliation only.

RADIOFREQUENCY ABLATION OF RCC

Radiofrequency, cryoablation, and microwave ablation are noninvasive options for treating RCC. High-frequency alternating current is applied to a metallic applicator placed within the tumor. The surface area of the electrode is small, which results in a high current density at the electrode surface resulting in heat. When tissues reach temperatures greater than 50° C, they undergo necrosis.

Indications

- Comorbidities and contraindications to conventional or laparoscopic surgery
- Refusal of conventional surgery

- Compromised renal function; patients who have undergone a nephrectomy
- High risk of recurrence (e.g., von Hippel-Lindau disease)

Technical Factors

- Tumors >3 cm can be difficult to treat with current ablation technology. Larger tumors often require multiple overlapping ablations, which increase the risk of complications.
- Tumors >5 cm have a higher incidence of recurrence.
- Complete ablation of central tumors is difficult owing to heat sink effect of large vessels within the renal hilum. Also, ablating central tumors poses the risk of injury to the collecting system or ureter.
- Anterior location of tumors can lead to colonic injury.
- Tumors are ablated under general anesthesia or deep conscious sedation.
- CT is the preferred modality for renal tumor ablation because of high spatial resolution and its ability to image structures that need to be avoided. Ultrasound can also be used for superficial and peripheral exophytic lesions.

Complications

- Pain may last for several days to weeks.
- Postablation syndrome: fever, malaise, and body aches. Severity is related to volume of tissue ablated.
- Hemorrhage, often self-limited
- Injury to ureter, central collecting system, or adjacent organs

RENAL MASS BIOPSY CRITERIA

Most solid and complex cystic masses suspicious for primary renal malignancy are ultimately surgically removed. Established criteria for renal mass biopsy include:

Established

- Renal mass presenting in a patient with other primary malignancy to rule out metastasis
- Rule out focal pyelonephritis
- Comorbid disease increases risk for surgery (e.g., solitary kidney)
- Unresectable mass, confirmation of diagnosis before systemic therapy

Emerging

- Confirmation of diagnosis before percutaneous ablation
- Hyperdense homogeneously enhancing mass, which may be a lipid-poor AML
- Bosniak 3 lesion
- Multiple solid masses

LYMPHOMA

Incidence of renal involvement in lymphoma is 5% (non-Hodgkin lymphoma (NHL) > Hodgkin disease) at diagnosis and 30% at autopsy. Three patterns of involvement:

- Direct extension from retroperitoneal disease (common)
- Hematogenous dissemination (common)
- Primary renal lymphoma (i.e., no other organ involvement) is rare, because kidneys do not have primary lymphatic tissue.

Imaging Features

- Multiple lymphomatous masses (hypoechoic, hypodense), 50%
- Diffuse involvement of one or both kidneys
- Adenopathy

METASTASES

Incidence: 20% of cancer patients at autopsy. Common primary lesions are lung, breast, and colon cancer and melanoma.

ANGIOMYOLIPOMA (AML)

Hamartomas containing fat, smooth muscle, and blood vessels. Small lesions are not treated; large and symptomatic lesions are resected or embolized. Unlikely to bleed if <4 cm. Complication: tumors may spontaneously bleed because of their vascular elements.

Associations

- Tuberous sclerosis: 80% of patients with tuberous sclerosis have AML, typically multiple, bilateral lesions. However, <40% of patients with AML have tuberous sclerosis. In the absence of tuberous sclerosis, 5% of all AML patients will have multiple, bilateral AML.
- Lymphangiomyomatosis

Imaging Features

- Fat appears hypodense (CT), hyperechoic (US), and hyperintense (T1W). The presence of fat in a renal lesion is virtually diagnostic of AML. There have been only a few case reports of fat in RCC or in oncocytomas. 5% do not demonstrate fat on CT. *Caveat:* Be certain that fat associated with a large mass is not trapped in renal sinus or peripheral fat.
- Predominance of blood vessels
  - Strong contrast enhancement
  - T2W hyperintensity
- Predominance of muscle: signal intensity (SI) similar to that of RCC
- AMLs do not contain calcifications; if a lesion does contain calcification, consider other diagnosis, such as RCC.

- Angiography: tortuous, irregular, aneurysmally dilated vessels are seen in 3%. Presence depends on the amount of angiomatous tissue. Predominantly myxomatous AMLs may be hypovascular.

ADENOMA

Best described as adenocarcinoma with no metastatic potential. Usually detected at autopsy.

ONCOCYTOMA

These tumors arise from oncocytes (epithelial cell) of the proximal tubule. Although the majority of lesions are well differentiated and benign, these tumors need to be resected because of their malignant potential and the inability to differentiate from RCC preoperatively. Represent 5% of renal tumors.

Imaging Features

- Central stellate scar (CT) and spoke wheel appearance (angiography) are typical but not specific (also seen in adenocarcinoma).
- Well-defined, sharp borders
- Radiographically impossible to differentiate from RCC

Juxtaglomerular Tumor (Reninoma)

Secretion of renin causes HTN, hypernatremia, and hypokalemia (secondary aldosteronism). Most patients undergo angiography as part of the workup for hypertension. Tumors appear as small hypovascular masses. Rare.

RENAL PELVIS TUMORS

Most tumors arising from the renal pelvis are malignant with transitional cell cancer being the most common tumor. Papillomas are the most common benign tumor.

Inverted Papilloma

- No malignant potential
- 20% are associated with uroepithelial malignancies elsewhere, most commonly in bladder.

Transitional Cell Carcinoma (TCC)

- Tumors are often multifocal: 40%-80% of patients have bladder TCC. However, only 3% of patients with bladder TCC later develop upper tract TCC.
- Radiographic finding: irregular filling defect
- Obliteration of renal sinus fat and infiltration of renal parenchyma (faceless kidney)
- 60% recurrence on ipsilateral side
- 50% have lung metastases.
- Staging
  - Stage I: mucosal lamina propria involved
  - Stage II: into, but not beyond, muscular layer
  - Stage III: invasion of adjacent fat/renal parenchyma
  - Stage IV: metastases

Squamous Cell Carcinoma (SCC)

- Represent 5% of renal pelvis tumors and <1% of all renal tumors
- Frequently associated with leukoplakia or chronic irritation (nephrolithiasis, schistosomiasis)

Collecting Duct Carcinoma

- Uncommon yet distinct epithelial neoplasm of the kidney
- Aggressive malignancy derived from the renal medulla, possibly from the distal collecting ducts of Bellini
- Propensity for showing infiltrative growth, which differs from the typical expansible pattern of growth exhibited by most renal malignancies

Imaging Features

- By US, cortical renal cell carcinoma may be hypoechoic to normal renal parenchyma, isoechoic to renal parenchyma, hyperechoic to renal parenchyma, but hypoechoic to renal sinus fat, or isoechoic to renal sinus fat.
- By CT, the lesions are medullary in location and have an infiltrative appearance. The reniform contour of the kidney is maintained.
- By renal angiography, the tumors are usually hypovascular.
- By MR imaging, the tumors are hypointense on T2W images.

RENAL MASSES: WHAT THE UROLOGISTS WOULD LIKE TO KNOW

- Is the mass solid or cystic?
- Does it arise from parenchyma or collecting system?
- Size and exact location?
- Staging if malignant?
- Variant vascular or collecting system anatomy?

INDICATIONS FOR PARTIAL NEPHRECTOMY IN PATIENTS WITH RCC

- RCC in a solitary kidney
- Significant risk factors that predispose to the development of renal failure later in life (e.g., stone disease, chronic infection, vesicoureteric reflux)
- Solitary renal tumors <7 cm
- Tumors confined to kidney
- Location that will not require extensive collecting system or vascular reconstruction
- Elective indication

INFLAMMATION

URINARY TRACT INFECTION (UTI)

Most common pathogen is *Escherichia coli.* Less common organisms include other gram-negative bacteria: *Proteus, Klebsiella, Enterobacter, Pseudomonas,*

Neisseria, and *Trichomonas vaginalis*. "Sterile pyuria" refers to increased urinary white blood cell count (WBC) without being able to culture pathogens. Common causes of sterile pyuria:
- Tuberculosis (TB)
- Fungal infections
- Interstitial nephritis
- Glomerulonephritis

Risk Factors
- Urinary obstruction (e.g., benign prostatic hyperplasia, calculi)
- Vesicoureteral reflux
- Pregnancy (dilatation of ureters)
- Diabetes mellitus
- Immune deficiency
- Instrumentation

Complications
- Abscess formation
- Xanthogranulomatous pyelonephritis
- Emphysematous pyelonephritis
- Scarring and renal failure

ACUTE PYELONEPHRITIS

Acute bacterial infection of the kidney and urinary tract *(Proteus, Klebsiella, E. coli)*. Medical treatment is usually initiated without imaging studies. Role of imaging studies:

Define underlying pathology
- Obstruction
- Reflux
- Calculus

Rule out complications
- Abscess
- Emphysematous pyelonephritis
- Determine presence of chronic changes such as scarring

Common Underlying Conditions
- Diabetes mellitus
- Immunosuppression
- Obstruction

Types
- Focal type (lobar nephronia)
- Diffuse type: more severe and extensive

Imaging Features
Imaging studies (IVP, CT, US) are normal in 75%. In the remaining 25%, there are nonspecific findings:
- Renal enlargement (edema)
- Loss of the corticomedullary differentiation (edema)
- IVP findings:
  - Delay of contrast excretion
  - Narrowing of collecting system (edema)
  - Striated nephrogram
  - Ridging of uroepithelium
- Areas of decreased perfusion by contrast-enhanced CT
- Focal areas of hypodensity in lobar nephronia
- Complications: abscess, scarring

PYONEPHROSIS

Infected renal collecting system usually due to obstruction, calculi, 50% > tumor strictures > postoperative strictures. Penicillin and other antibiotics are sufficient in 35% of cases; remainder of patients require nephrectomy (depending on underlying cause).

Imaging Features
US
- Best study to differentiate pyonephrosis from uninfected hydronephrosis
- Echoes within collecting system
- Urine/debris levels
- Dense shadowing due to gas in collecting system
- Poor through-transmission

CT
- Best study to show cause and level of obstruction, as well as complications
- Dilated collecting system
- Allows detection of perinephric or renal abscess

Interventional procedures
- Aspiration for culture and sensitivity (definitive diagnostic study)
- Penicillin
- Formal antegrade pyelography should be deferred to a second visit so as not to cause sepsis.

RENAL ABSCESS

Usually caused by gram-negative bacteria, less commonly by *Staphylococcus* or fungus (candidiasis). Underlying disease: calculi, obstruction, diabetes, AIDS.

Imaging Features (Fig. 4-6)
- Well-delineated focal renal lesion
- Central necrosis (no enhancement with IV contrast)

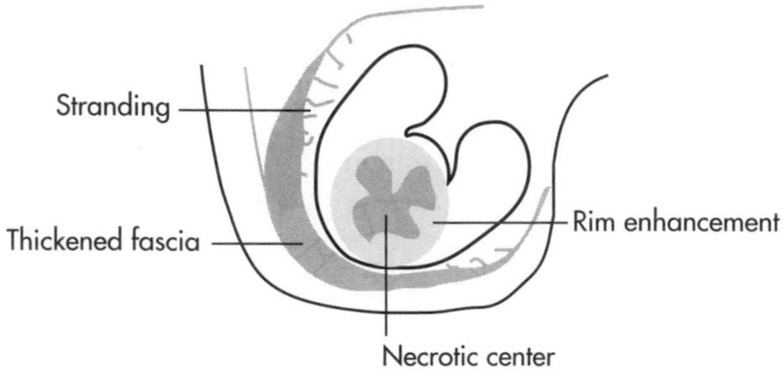

FIGURE 4-6

- Thickened, hyperemic abscess wall with contrast enhancement
- Perinephric inflammatory involvement:
  Thickening of Gerota's fascia
  Stranding of perirenal fat mass

Complications

- Retroperitoneal spread of abscess
- Renocolic fistula

PERINEPHRIC ABSCESS

Results most commonly from high-grade ureteral obstruction and infected kidney. Nonrenal causes include duodenal perforation, diverticular abscess, Crohn disease, infected pancreatic fluid collections, and spinal TB, which may spread and cause perirenal as well as psoas abscess. Treatment is with percutaneous drainage.

EMPHYSEMATOUS PYELONEPHRITIS

Most commonly caused by gram-negative bacteria in patients with diabetes mellitus; less commonly in nondiabetics with obstruction. Spectrum includes:

- Emphysematous pyelonephritis: gas in renal parenchyma and collecting system. Mortality: 60%-80%.
- Emphysematous pyelitis: gas in collecting system ("air pyelogram"). Mortality: 20%.

Imaging Features

- Gas in collecting system and/or renal parenchyma
- Gas may extend to Gerota's fascia (high mortality).

Treatment

- Nephrectomy
- In poor surgical candidates or in patients with focal disease, percutaneous drainage has been used as a temporizing or, occasionally, definitive therapy.

XANTHOGRANULOMATOUS PYELONEPHRITIS (XGP)

Chronic suppurative form of renal infection characterized by parenchymal destruction and replacement of parenchyma with lipid-laden macrophages. Diffuse form, 90%; focal form, 10%. 10% of patients have diabetes mellitus. Rare.

Imaging Features

- Large or staghorn calculus (thought to cause obstruction and inflammatory response), 75%; in the remaining 25% of patients, XGP is due to UPJ obstruction or ureteral tumors.
- Enlarged, nonexcreting kidney
- Multiple nonenhancing low attenuation masses (−10 to 30 HU): xanthomatous masses. The masses may extend beyond the kidney into the perinephric space. There may be a thin peripheral ring of enhancement.
- Fine calcifications may be present in xanthomatous masses.
- Thickened Gerota's fascia
- May be associated with psoas abscess

Replacement Lipomatosis

Also known as *replacement fibrolipomatosis,* replacement represents extreme form of renal sinus lipomatosis in which infection, long-term hydronephrosis, and calculi are associated with severe renal parenchymal atrophy. Calculi and inflammation are present in >70% of cases.

Imaging Features

- Enlarged renal outline, fatty lucent mass, and staghorn calculus
- IVP shows poorly or nonfunctioning kidney.
- On US, kidney is enlarged but has a preserved shape. Residual hypoechoic renal parenchymal rim is surrounded by hyperechoic areas of fatty proliferation in both renal hilum and perinephric space.
- CT is the imaging modality of choice to best demonstrate fatty characteristics.

Differential diagnoses for this condition include XGP, fat-containing tumors such as angiomyolipomas, lipoma, and liposarcoma. CT can aid in differentiating XGP because CT shows attenuation values of −5 to +15 HU in XGP, in contrast to replacement lipomatosis where the fatty tissues measure −100 HU. Fat-containing tumors usually produce a mass effect and show renal function, unlike replacement lipomatosis.

Tuberculosis

The genitourinary (GU) tract is the second most common site of tuberculous involvement after the lung. GU disease is typically due to hematogenous spread. Clinical findings include history of pulmonary TB, pyuria, hematuria, and dysuria.

Sites of Involvement

- Renal
- Ureteral
- Bladder
- Seminal vesicles, epididymis

Imaging Features of Renal Tuberculosis (Fig. 4-7)

Distribution

- Unilateral involvement is more common (70%) than bilateral (30%).

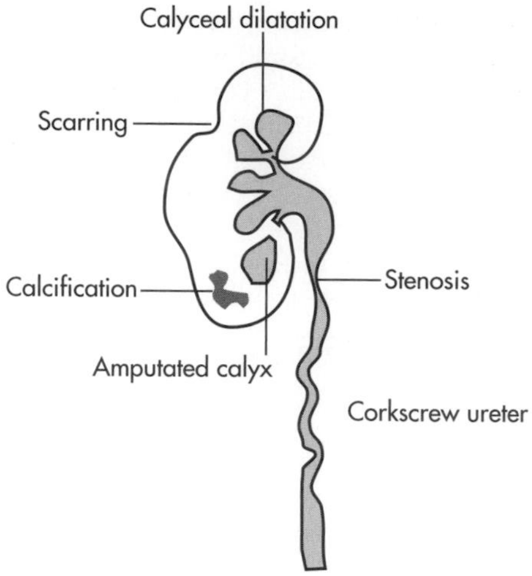

FIGURE 4-7

Size
- Early, kidneys are enlarged.
- Later, kidneys are small.
- Autonephrectomy (nonfunctioning kidney)

Parenchyma
- Parenchymal calcifications, 70%
- Calcification may take on multiple forms: curvilinear, mottled, or amorphous; "putty kidney" results when calcification has homogeneous, ground-glass appearance.
- Papillary necrosis; papillae may be irregular, necrotic, or sloughed.
- Tuberculoma
- Parenchymal scarring, 20%

Collecting system
- Mucosal irregularity
- Infundibular stenosis, hiked-up pelvis with narrowed pelvis pointing up
- Amputated calyx
- Corkscrew ureter: multiple infundibular and ureteral stenoses (hallmark finding)
- "Purse-string" stenosis of renal pelvis
- "Pipestem ureter" refers to a narrow, rigid, aperistaltic segment.
- Renal calculi, 10%

CANDIDIASIS

Most common renal fungal infections (coccidioidomycosis, cryptococcosis less common). Common in patients with diabetes mellitus.

Imaging Features

- Multiple medullary and cortical abscesses
- Papillary necrosis due to diffuse fungal infiltration
- Fungus balls in collecting system (mycetoma) cause filling defects on IVP; nonshadowing echogenic foci on US
- Hydronephrosis secondary to mycetoma
- Scalloping of ureters (submucosal edema)

RENAL MANIFESTATION OF AIDS

AIDS-related renal abnormalities are seen in most AIDS patients during the course of their illness. AIDS nephropathy refers to irreversible renal failure in 10% of patients and is seen in end-stage disease.

Imaging Features

- Increased cortical US echogenicity, 70%; (tubulointerstitial abnormalities)
- Renal enlargement without hydronephrosis, 40%
- Focal hypoechoic (US)/low attenuation (CT) lesions (infection, tumor), 30%

Other Renal Abnormalities

- Acute tubular necrosis (ATN)
- Interstitial nephritis
- Focal nephrocalcinosis
- Infection: Cytomegalovirus (CMV), aspergillus, toxoplasmosis, *Pneumocystis jiroveci* Frenkel 1999, histoplasmosis, *Mycobacterium avium-intracellulare* (MAI)
- Tumors: increased incidence of RCC, lymphoma, Kaposi sarcoma

Prostate Abnormalities

- Prostatitis: bacterial, fungal, viral
- Prostate abscess

Testicular Abnormalities

- Testicular atrophy: common
- Infection: bacterial, fungal, viral
- Tumors: germ cell tumors, lymphoma

NEPHROCALCINOSIS AND LITHIASIS

Renal calcifications can be located in renal parenchyma (nephrocalcinosis), in abnormal tissue (e.g., dystrophic calcification in cysts, tumors), or in the collecting system (e.g., nephrolithiasis, calculi).

CALCULI

Incidence: 5% of population; 20% at autopsy. Recurrence of stone disease, 50%. Symptoms in 50% of patients during first 5 years of stone presence. Predisposing conditions: calyceal diverticula, Crohn disease, some diversions, stents, renal tubular acidosis, hypercalcemia, and hypercalciuria. The radiographic density of a calculus depends mainly on its calcium content:

Calcium calculi (opaque), 75%
- Calcium oxalate
- Calcium phosphate

Struvite calculi (opaque), 15%
- Magnesium ammonium phosphate: "infection stones" (represent 70% of staghorn calculi,

remainder are cystine or uric acid calculi); struvite is usually mixed with calcium phosphate to create “triple phosphate” calculi.

Cystine calculi (less opaque)
- Cystinuria, 2%

Nonopaque calculi
- Uric acid (gout, treatment of myeloproliferative disorders), 10%
- Xanthine (rare)
- Mucoprotein matrix calculi in poorly functioning, infected urinary tracts; rare
- Protease inhibitor indinavir used in HIV treatment can result in radiolucent stones.

Imaging Features

Calculus (determine size, number, location)
- Radiopaque calculus, 90%
- Radiolucent calculi are best detected by IVP
- Renal calculi can be detected by US: hyperechoic focus (calculus), posterior shadowing; calculi 3 mm or less may not be detected.

CALCULUS VERSUS PHLEBOLITH

	Calculus	Phlebolith
Shape	Any shape 90% homogeneously opaque	Round, smooth Central lucency
Location	Along projected tract of ureter	In true pelvis (below distal ureter)

IVP
- Delayed and persistent nephrogram due to ureteral obstruction
- Column of opacified urine extends in ureter from renal pelvis to lodged calculus (diminished or absent peristalsis).
- Ureter distal to calculus is narrowed (edema, inflammation); may create false impression of stricture.
- Ureter proximal to calculus is minimally dilated and straightened: columnization; degree of dilatation has no relation to stone size.
- “Steinstrasse:” several calculi are bunched up along the ureter (common after lithotripsy).
- Halo appearance (edema) around distal ureter may resemble appearance of ureterocele (pseudoureterocele) or bladder carcinoma. Thickness of radiolucent halo of pseudoureterocele is typically >2 mm as opposed to ureterocele.

CT
- CT detects most calculi regardless of calcium content. The exceptions are matrix stones.
- Contiguous sections should be used to avoid gaps so as not to miss small stones; helical CT is very helpful in this regard.
- Dedicated CT protocol for stone search is performed; may need to follow with contrast-enhanced CT (CECT) to differentiate stone in ureter from phlebolith. Contrast-only CT may obscure a calcified ureteral calculus because it may blend in with high-density contrast material.
- Dual energy CT: Acquisition of CT data from two different energy spectra. Most urinary calculi, regardless of composition, appear as opaque densities by conventional CT. In dual energy CT, the differences in x-ray attenuation properties at high and low KvP allow more accurate renal stone differentiation between uric acid and calcium containing stones.

Location: three narrow sites in the ureter at which calculi often lodge
- UPJ: junction of renal pelvis and ureter proper
- At crossing of ureter with iliac vessels
- Ureterovesical junction (UVJ): insertion of ureters into bladder

Complications

- Forniceal rupture (pyelosinus backflow); inconsequential in isolation if urine is uninfected; chronic leak may result in periureteral/retroperitoneal fibrosis.
- Chronic calculous pyelonephritis
- XGP in the presence of staghorn calculus
- Squamous metaplasia (leukoplakia); more common in pyelocalyceal system and upper ureter than lower ureter or bladder. Cholesteatoma may result from desquamation of keratinized epithelium.
- SEC

Treatment Options

- Small renal calculi (<2.5 cm): extracorporeal lithotripsy
- Large renal calculi (>2.5 cm): percutaneous removal
- Upper ureteral calculi: extracorporeal lithotripsy
- Lower ureteral calculi: ureteroscopy

Extracorporeal Shock Wave Lithotripsy (ESWL)

- Best results with calcium oxalate and uric acid stones and calculi <2.5 cm. Larger calculi are better treated by percutaneous removal.
- Contraindications for ESWL include:
  - Patient not eligible for anesthesia
  - Severe bleeding
  - Pregnancy
  - Urinary tract infections
  - Nonfunctioning kidneys
  - Gross obesity
  - Small children
  - Tall patients (>200 cm)

- Distal obstruction
  - Calyceal neck stenosis
  - UPJ obstruction
  - Prostatic enlargement
  - Renal artery aneurysm
- Complications of ESWL
  - Intrarenal; subscapular and perinephric hematoma
  - Decrease in effective renal plasma flow

Indications for Percutaneous Nephrostomy

- Large stones requiring initial debulking (e.g., staghorn calculus)
- Calculi not responding to ESWL (e.g., cysteine stones)
- Body habitus precludes ESWL
- When patient has certain type of pacemaker
- Renal artery aneurysms
- Calculi >5 cm

CORTICAL NEPHROCALCINOSIS (Fig. 4-8)

Usually dystrophic calcification

Causes

- Chronic glomerulonephritis
- Cortical necrosis (due to ischemia)
  - Pregnancy
  - Shock
  - Infection
  - Toxins: methoxyflurane, ethylene glycol
- AIDS-related nephropathy
  - Glomerular sclerosis
  - Punctate calcifications MAI
- Uncommon causes
  - Rejected renal transplants
  - Chronic hypercalcemia
  - Oxalosis
  - Alport syndrome

Imaging Features

- Peripheral calcifications (medullary pyramids are spared)
- Tramline calcifications are classic: interface of necrotic cortex and viable subcapsular cortex
- Columns of Bertin may be calcified.
- US: hyperechoic cortex

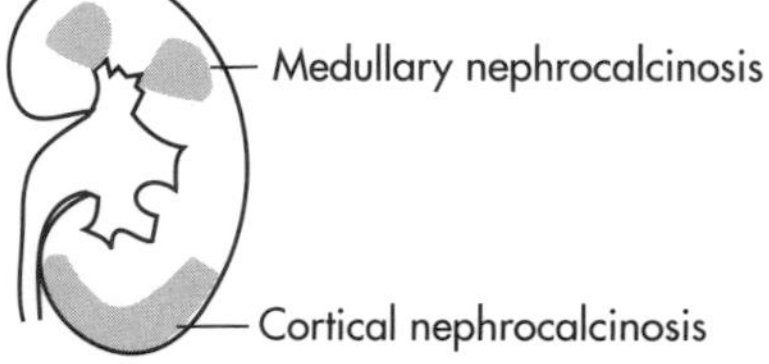

FIGURE 4-8

MEDULLARY NEPHROCALCINOSIS

Causes

- Hyperparathyroidism (hypercalciuria, hypercalcemia), 40%
- Renal tubular acidosis, 20%
- Medullary sponge kidney, 20%
- Papillary necrosis
- Lasix in infancy
- Other causes
  - Nephrotoxic drugs (amphotericin B)
  - Chronic pyelonephritis
  - Oxalosis may produce both medullary and cortical nephrocalcinosis

Imaging Features

- Bilateral, stippled calcification of medullary pyramids
- Calcifications may extend peripherally.
- US: hyperechoic medulla

PELVICALYCEAL SYSTEM (FIG. 4-9)

CONGENITAL MEGACALYCES

Congenital condition in which there are too many enlarged calyces (20 to 25; normal is 10 to 14). Associated with hypoplastic pyramids, resulting in polyclonal, faceted calyces rather than the blunting that is seen with obstruction. There is no obstruction, and the remainder of the collecting system is normal. Renal parenchyma and renal function are normal. Etiology is not known; there may be congenital underdevelopment of pyramids, "burnt-out" fetal obstruction or reflux or abnormal branching of collecting system. It is associated with megaureter.

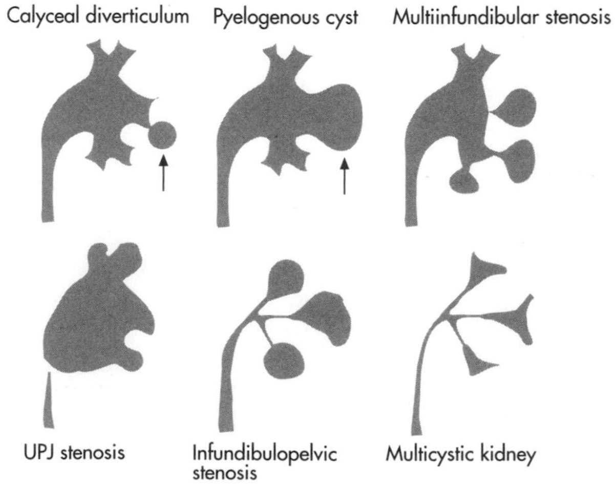

FIGURE 4-9

INFUNDIBULOPELVIC DYSGENESIS

Spectrum of diseases characterized by hypoplasia or aplasia of the upper collecting system:

- Calyceal diverticulum
- Pyelogenous cyst
- Multiinfundibular stenosis
- UPJ stenosis
- Infundibulopelvic stenosis
- Multicystic kidney

(PYELO)CALYCEAL DIVERTICULUM

Outpouching of calyx into corticomedullary region. May also arise from renal pelvis or an infundibulum. Usually asymptomatic, but patients may develop calculi.

- Type I: originates from minor calyx
- Type II: originates from infundibulum
- Type III: originates from renal pelvis

Imaging Features

- Cystic lesion connects through channel with collecting system.
- If the neck is not obstructed, diverticula opacify retrograde from the collecting system on delayed IVP films.
- May contain calculi or milk of calcium, 50%
- Fragmented calculi after ESWL may fail to pass because of a narrow neck. Percutaneous stone retrieval may be indicated.
- Cortical divot may overlie diverticulum

RENAL PAPILLARY NECROSIS (RPN)

RPN represents an ischemic coagulative necrosis involving variable amounts of pyramids and medullary papillae. RPN never extends to the renal cortex.

Causes

Ischemic necrosis
- Diabetes mellitus
- Chronic obstruction, calculus
- Sickle cell disease
- Analgesics

Necrosis due to infections
- TB
- Fungal

Imaging Features (Fig. 4-10)

Papillae
- Enlargement (early)
- Small collection of contrast medium extends outside the interpapillary line in partial necrosis.
- Contrast may extend into central portion of papilla in "medullary type" RPN.
- Eventually contrast curves around papilla from both fornices, resulting in "lobster-claw" deformity.

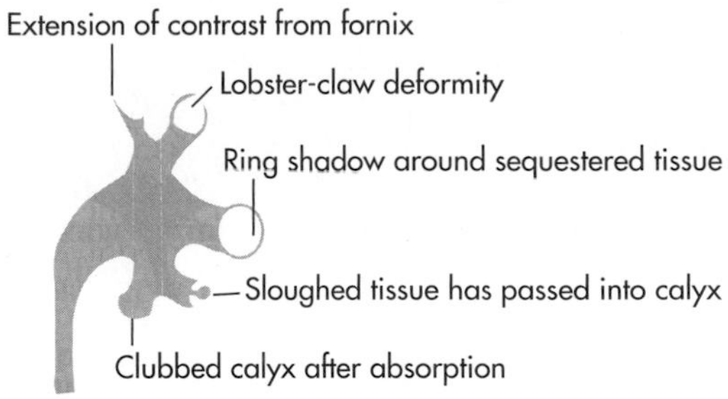

FIGURE 4-10

- Sequestered, sloughed papillae cause filling defects in collecting system: "ring sign."
- Tissue necrosis leads to blunted or clubbed calyces.

Multiple papillae affected in 85%. Rimlike calcification of necrotic papilla occurs.

MEDULLARY SPONGE KIDNEY (BENIGN RENAL TUBULAR ECTASIA; CACCHI-RICCI DISEASE) (Fig. 4-11)

Dysplastic dilatation of renal collecting tubules (ducts of Bellini). Cause: developmental. Usually detected in young adults (20 to 40 years) as an incidental finding. Usually there are no signs, but there can be urine stasis, UTI, calculi, and hematuria. In 10% progressive renal failure may develop. Relatively common (0.5% of IVP). May involve one or both kidneys or be confined to a single papilla.

Associations (Rare)

- Hemihypertrophy
- Associated with Beckwith-Wiedemann syndrome
- Congenital pyloric stenosis
- Ehlers-Danlos syndrome
- Other renal abnormalities: cortical renal cysts, horseshoe kidney, renal ectopia, APKD, RTA

Imaging Features

- Striated nephrogram (contrast in dilated collecting ducts), "brushlike" appearance
- Cystic tubular dilatation usually 1 to 3mm: occasionally larger, usually too small for CT resolution

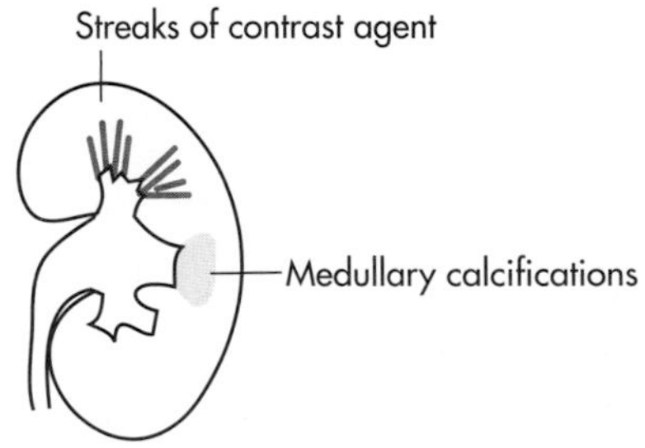

FIGURE 4-11

- Punctate calcifications in medullary distribution (located in dilated tubules), 50%
- Differentiate on IVP from "papillary blush," a normal variant, representing amorphous enhancement without tubular dilation, streaks, or globules; nephrocalcinosis; or pyramidal enlargement. Papillary blush is also an inconstant finding on successive IVPs.

OBSTRUCTION OF COLLECTING SYSTEM (Fig. 4-12)

Causes

- Calculi
- Tumor
- Previous surgery (ligation, edema, clot)

Imaging Features

IVP

Kidney

- Delayed nephrogram (peak enhancement at >30 minutes after IV injection, slow fading)
- Delayed renal (peak) density may be higher than in normal kidney.
- Faint radial striations of nephrogram
- Negative pyelogram: nephrogram with delayed pyelogram resulting in dilated unopacified calyces outlined by opacified parenchyma
- Dunbar's crescents (caliceal crescents): thin rings or crescents at interface with calyx and parenchyma resulting from contrast in dilated collecting ducts; disappear when collecting system is completely opacified
- Atrophy of renal parenchyma in chronic obstruction: "rim nephrogram" or "shell nephrogram"

Collecting system

- Blunting of forniceal angles
- Dilatation of ureter and pelvis; decreased or absent peristalsis
- Backflow

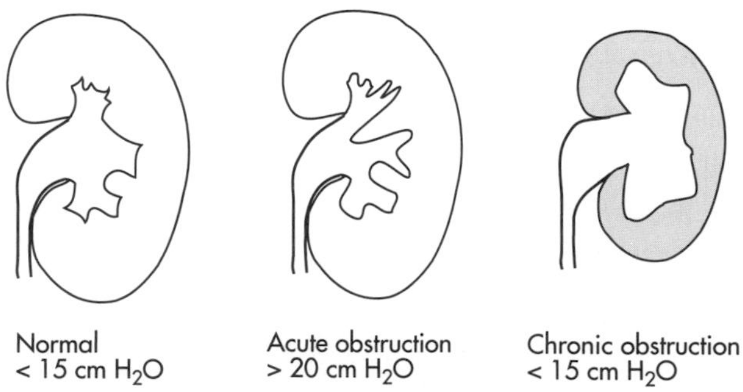

FIGURE 4-12

US

Sensitivity for detection of chronic obstruction: 90%

Sensitivity for detection of acute obstruction: 60%

Common causes of false-positive examinations:

- Extrarenal pelvis
- Peripelvic cyst
- Vessels: differentiate with color Doppler
- Vesicoureteral reflux, full bladder
- High urine flow (overhydration, furosemide)
- Corrected long-standing obstruction with residual dilatation
- Prune-belly syndrome

Common causes of false negative examinations:

- US performed early in disease before dilatation has occurred
- Distal obstruction

WHITAKER TEST

Pressure-flow study for determining ureteral obstruction or resistance in dilated, nonrefluxing upper urinary tracts. Useful test particularly in patients with surgically corrected obstruction having residual dilatation and/or symptoms. Because the test is invasive and time-consuming, it is usually reserved for cases with equivocal diuretic renograms.

1. Catheterize bladder and inject contrast to exclude refluxing megaureter.
2. Obtain percutaneous access to collecting system with 20-gauge needle.
3. Connect extension tubing, 3-way stopcock, and manometer to both antegrade needle and bladder catheter. The bases of both manometers have to be set at the same level as the tip of the antegrade needle.
4. Connect perfusion pump to antegrade needle and bladder catheter.
5. Obtain spot and overhead films during perfusion (intermittent fluoroscopic monitoring).
6. Pressures in collecting system and bladder are recorded during delivery of known flow rates (5, 10, 15 mL/min), and pressure differences are calculated.
7. Pressure difference of >15 mm is abnormal, and test should be terminated.

PYELORENAL BACKFLOW

Backflow of contrast material from collecting system into renal or perirenal spaces. Usually due to increased pressure in collecting system from retrograde pyelography or ureteral obstruction.

Types (Fig. 4-13)

- Pyelosinus backflow (forniceal rupture): extravasation along infundibula, renal pelvis, ureter

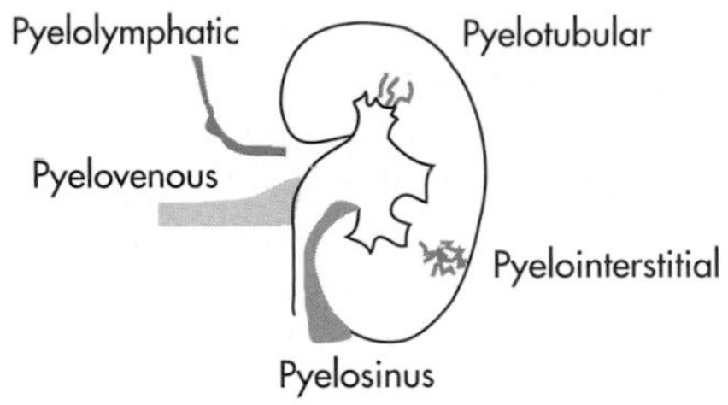

FIGURE 4-13

- Pyelotubular backflow (no rupture): backflow into terminal collecting ducts; thin streaks with fanlike radiation from the papillae
- Pyelointerstitial backflow: extravasation into parenchyma and subcapsular structures; more amorphous than pyelotubular backflow
- Pyelolymphatic backflow: dilated lymphatic vessels (may occasionally rupture): thin irregular bands extending from hilum or calyces
- Pyelovenous backflow: contrast in interlobar or arcuate veins; rarely seen because venous flow clears contrast material rapidly: renal vein extends superiorly from renal hilum.

TRAUMA

RENAL INJURY (Fig. 4-14)

Spectrum of renal injury in trauma:

Renal infarction
- Segmental branch
- Vascular pedicle avulsion

Hemorrhage (renal laceration, rupture)
- Intraparenchymal
- Extraparenchymal

Ruptured collecting system

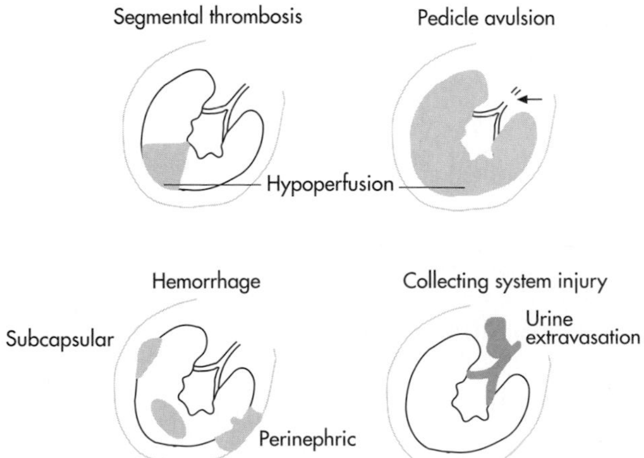

FIGURE 4-14

Mechanism
- Blunt trauma, 70%-80%
- Penetrating trauma, 20%-30%

Classification

Minor injuries (conservative treatment), 85%
- Hematomas
- Contusion (any injury that results in hematuria)
- Small lacerations
- Subsegmental renal infarcts

Moderate injuries, 10% (management controversial; 15%-50% will eventually require surgery)
- Urine leak
- Laceration communicating with collecting system

Major injuries (surgical treatment), 15%
- Multiple renal lacerations (rupture)
- Pedicle injury avulsion, thrombosis

Imaging Features

The optimum type of imaging study depends on stability of patient and symptoms (hematuria, blood at meatus, multiple bony fractures):
- CT is the study of choice.
- One-shot IVP: visualization of both kidneys excludes pedicle avulsion.
- Indications for angiography:
  - Nonvisualization of kidney on IVP in patient with abdominal trauma
  - Persistent hematuria in a patient with abdominal trauma
  - Hypotension or hypertension or persistent hematuria after an interventional urologic procedure

VASCULAR ABNORMALITIES

RENAL VEIN THROMBOSIS (RVT)

RVT may be caused by many conditions:
- Adults: tumor > renal disease > other causes (nephrotic syndrome, postpartum, hypercoagulable states)
- Infants: dehydration, shock, trauma, sepsis, sickle cell disease

Imaging Features

Renal vein
- Absence of flow (US, CT, MRI)
- Intraluminal thrombus
- Renal vein dilatation proximal to occlusion
- Renal venography: amputation of renal vein
- MRV or conventional venography: studies of choice

Kidneys
- Renal enlargement
- US: hypoechoic cortex (early edema); hyperechoic cortex after 10 days (fibrosis, cellular infiltrates) with preserved corticomedullary

differentiation; late phase (several weeks): decreased size, hyperechoic kidney with loss of corticomedullary differentiation
- IVP: little opacification, prolonged nephrogram, striated nephrogram (stasis in collecting tubules); intrarenal collecting system is stretched and compressed by edema
- CT may show low-attenuation thrombus in renal vein or simple renal enlargement with collaterals; prolongation of corticomedullary differentiation (CMD)
- Loss of CMD
- Scintigraphy (^{99m}Tc DTPA): absent or delayed renal perfusion and excretion, alternatively may be delayed and reveal a large kidney

Chronic thrombosis
- Small kidneys
- Collateral veins may cause pelvic and ureteral notches by extrinsic compression.

PAROXYSMAL NOCTURNAL HEMOGLOBINURIA

Rare acquired hemolytic disorder. The renal cortex appears hypointense on T2/T2* due to hemosiderin deposition.

RENAL INFARCTS (Fig. 4-15)

Renal infarcts may be focal and wedge shaped or larger, involving the anterior or posterior kidney or entire kidney. CECT or IVP may show thin, enhancing rim from capsular arteries.

Causes
- Trauma to renal vessels
- Embolism
  - Cardiac causes (e.g., atrial fibrillation, endocarditis)
  - Catheter
- Thrombosis
  - Arterial
  - Venous

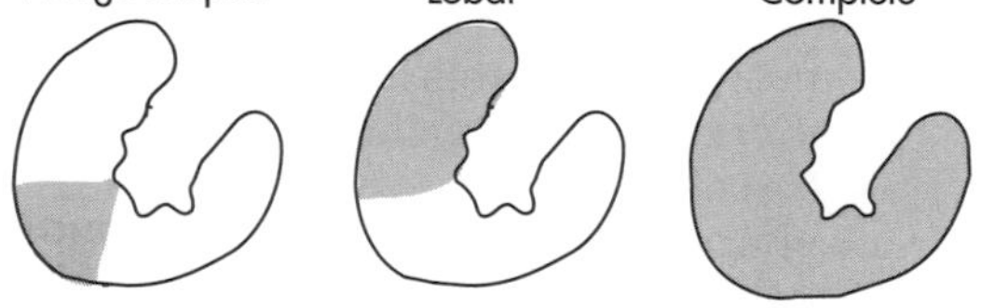

FIGURE 4-15

RENAL TRANSPLANT

DONOR EVALUATION

Transplant donor evaluation is most commonly done by CT or MRI and involves the following steps:
1. Location of kidneys. It is important that both kidneys are located in their normal retroperitoneal locations. Pelvic and horseshoe kidneys are associated with complex anomalous vascular and collecting systems, making them difficult to use for transplantation.
2. The presence of solid and complex cystic renal masses must be excluded. The contralateral kidney should be evaluated in the donor to exclude any neoplasm.
3. Number of renal arteries supplying the kidneys. Transplant surgeons prefer single arterial anastomosis in the recipient; the presence of multiple renal arteries increases the donor organ warm ischemia time and also increases the complexity of the operation.
   Left renal arteries that branch within 2 cm of the aorta are difficult to transplant because there is not a sufficient length of the main trunk for clamping and anastomosis in the recipient.
4. Accessory renal arteries to the lower pole of the kidneys must be identified. These arteries may supply the renal pelvis and proximal ureter; accidental injury to this vessel can predispose to ureteral ischemia and possible compromise of ureteral anastomosis.
5. Is aberrant renal venous anatomy present?
6. Are collecting system anomalies (duplication) present?

NORMAL RENAL TRANSPLANT

Morphology of normal transplanted kidney:
- Well-defined kidney, elliptical contour (i.e., not enlarged)
- CMD should be present but may not always be very well defined.
- Cortical echogenicity should be similar to liver echogenicity.
- The central echo complex should be well defined.

FUNCTIONAL EVALUATION OF TRANSPLANTED KIDNEY

- Normal perfusion and excretion by scintigraphy (MAG_3, DTPA)
- Resistive index ($P_{sys} - P_{diast}/P_{sys}$) should be <0.7 by Doppler US

COMMON TRANSPLANT COMPLICATIONS

- ATN
- Rejection
- Cyclosporine toxicity
- Arterial or venous occlusion
- Urinary leak
- Urinary obstruction

ACUTE TUBULAR NECROSIS (ATN)

Most common form of acute, reversible renal failure in transplant patients, usually seen within 24 hours. Other causes of ATN are:

Renal ischemia, 60%
- Surgery, transplant, other causes
- Pregnancy related

Nephrotoxins, 40%
- Radiographic contrast material, particularly in patients with diabetes
- Aminoglycosides
- Antineoplastic agents
- Hemoglobin, myoglobin
- Chemicals: organic solvents, $HgCl_2$

Imaging Features
- Smooth large kidneys
- Normal renal perfusion (MAG_3 angiography)
- Diminished or absent opacification after IV contrast administration
- Persistent dense nephrogram at late time points, 75%
- Variable US features:
  - Increased cortical echogenicity with normal corticomedullary junction
  - Increased echogenicity of pyramids

REJECTION
- Increased renal size, 90% (in chronic rejection, size is decreased)
- Thickened cortex may be hypoechoic or hyperechoic
- Large renal pyramids, edematous uroepithelium
- Indistinct corticomedullary junction
- Focal hypoechoic areas in cortex and/or medulla, 20%
- Increased cortical echogenicity, 15%
- Decrease or complete absence of central echo complex echogenicity
- Resistive index >0.7 by Doppler US; nonspecific

EVALUATION OF TRANSPLANT COMPLICATIONS (NUCLEAR SCANS, IVP)

Cause	Flow	Excretion
ATN	Normal	Reduced
Rejection	Reduced	Reduced
Vascular compromise	Reduced	Reduced

Pearls
- ATN is the only renal process with normal renal flow but reduced excretion.
- Hyperacute rejection has decreased flow but excretion on delayed images (opposite to ATN).
- Cyclosporine toxicity has similar pattern as ATN but occurs later in the posttransplant period.
- ATN rarely occurs beyond 1 month after transplant.
- Cyclosporine toxicity is uncommon within first month after transplant.
- MAG_3 results in better quality images in transplant patients with renal insufficiency compared with DTPA.

VASCULAR COMPLICATIONS
- Renal vein thrombosis: most occur in first 3 days after transplantation.
- Renal artery occlusion or stenosis. Anastomotic stenosis is treated with angioplasty with up to 87% success rate.
- Infarction
- Pseudoaneurysm of anastomosis: surgical treatment
- AV fistula: usually from renal biopsy; if symptomatic, embolization is performed.
- Ureterovesical anastomosis obstruction may result from edema, stricture, ischemia, rejection, extrinsic compression, or compromised position of kidney.

PERIRENAL FLUID COLLECTIONS
Perirenal fluid collections occur in 40% of transplants. The collections persist in 15%.

Causes
- Lymphocele: in 10%-20% of transplants at 1 to 4 months posttransplant. Usually inferomedial to kidney; linear septations are detectable in 80%. Most lymphoceles are inconsequential; if large and symptomatic or obstructing, percutaneous sclerosis with tetracycline or povidone-iodine may be tried.
- Abscess: develops within weeks; complex fluid collection; fever
- Urinoma: develops during 1st month; near UVJ; may be "cold" on nuclear medicine study if leak is not active at time of examination; may be associated with hydronephrosis
- Hematoma: hyperechoic by US; pain, hematocrit drop

Bladder and Urethra

URETER

ECTOPIC URETER
Ureter does not insert in the normal location in the trigone of the bladder (see also Chapter 11). Incidence: M:F = 1:6.

Clinical Findings
- UTI
- Obstruction
- Incontinence

Associations

- 80% have complete ureteral duplication.
- 30% have a ureterocele ("cobra head" appearance on IVP).

Insertion Sites

- Males: ureter inserts ectopically into the bladder > prostatic urethra > seminal vesicles, vas deferens, ejaculatory ducts.
- Females: ectopic ureter commonly empties into postsphincteric urethra, vagina, tubes, perineum.

RETROCAVAL URETER

Ureter passes behind inferior vena cava (IVC) and exits between aorta and IVC. Medial looping at L2-L3 level is seen on IVP. May result in ureteral narrowing and obstruction.

OVARIAN VEIN SYNDROME

Ureteral notching (vascular impression), dilatation, or obstruction as a result of ovarian vein thrombosis or varices. Usually associated with pregnancy. Normally the right gonadal vein crosses the ureter to drain into the IVC and the left gonadal vein drains into the left renal vein.

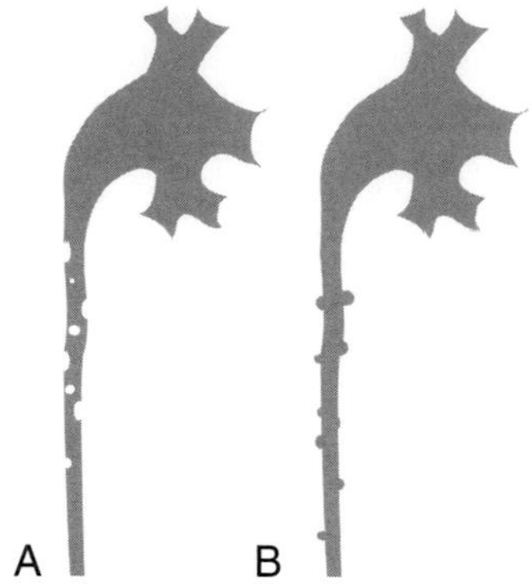

FIGURE 4-16

PYELOURETERITIS CYSTICA (Fig. 4-16, A)

Asymptomatic ureteral and/or pyelocalyceal cysts 2 to 4mm in diameter (may be up to 2cm), usually related to infection or calculi. Radiographically, there are small multiple intraluminal filling defects (cysts originate from degenerated uroepithelial cells). Most common in 6th decade, usually unilateral. May resolve with treatment of underlying infection or remain unchanged for months or years. Not a premalignant condition.

URETERAL PSEUDODIVERTICULOSIS (Fig. 4-16, B)

Outpouchings of 1 to 2mm produced by outward proliferation of epithelium into lamina propria. Associated with inflammation. 50% eventually develop a uroepithelial malignancy.

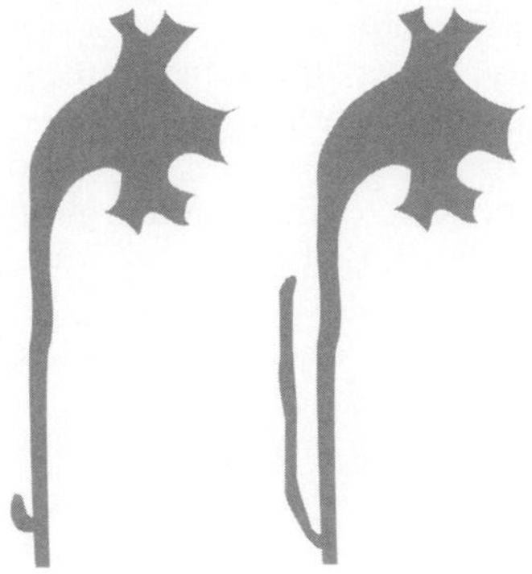

FIGURE 4-17

URETERAL DIVERTICULUM (Fig. 4-17)

Congenital blind-ending ureter. Probably due to aborted attempt at duplication.

MALACOPLAKIA

Rare inflammatory condition that most commonly affects the bladder. Yellow-brown subepithelial plaques consist of mononuclear histiocytes that contain Michaelis-Gutmann bodies. On IVP, multiple mural filling defects with flat or convex border are seen, giving a cobblestone appearance. Obstruction is a rare complication.

LEUKOPLAKIA

Ureteral involvement is less common than bladder and collecting system involvement.

URETERAL TUMORS

Types

Benign tumors
- Epithelial: inverted papilloma, polyp, adenoma
- Mesodermal: fibroma, hemangioma, myoma, lymphangioma
- Fibroepithelial polyp: mobile long intraluminal mass, ureteral intussusception

Malignant tumors
- Epithelial: transitional cell carcinoma, SCC, adenocarcinoma
- Mesodermal: sarcoma, angiosarcoma, carcinosarcoma

Prognosis

- 50% of patients will develop bladder cancer.
- 75% of tumors are unilateral.
- 5% of patients with bladder cancer will develop ureteral cancer.

Imaging Features

- Intraluminal filling defect
- Goblet sign: retrograde pyelogram demonstrates dilated ureteral segment distal to obstruction with filling defect and meniscus

- Bergman's coiled catheter sign: on retrograde pyelogram the catheter is typically coiled in dilated portion of ureter just distal to the lesion.

Sites of metastatic spread of primary ureteral neoplasm (at autopsy):
- Retroperitoneal lymph nodes, 75%
- Liver, 60%
- Lung, 60%
- Bone, 40%
- Gastrointestinal tract, 20%
- Peritoneum, 20%
- Other (<15%): adrenal glands, ovary, uterus

URETERAL DIVERSIONS

Ileal Loop (Fig. 4-18)

Ureter(s) drain into isolated ileal segment, which serves as an isoperistaltic conduit (not as a reservoir). May or may not have a surgical "intussusception" of conduit. 50% of patients have hydronephrosis immediately postoperatively; the hydronephrosis should resolve by 3 months. Common locations of strictures are at the ureteroileal anastomosis and where the left ureter enters the peritoneum.

Colon Conduit

Ureter(s) drain into isolated colon segment. Ureters are tunneled submucosally for antireflux.

Ureterosigmoidostomy

Distal ureter(s) drain into sigmoid colon; ureters are tunneled for antiperistalsis. Procedure is largely surpassed by ileal conduit nowadays because of complications (e.g., pyelonephritis, reflux, hyperchloremic acidosis, high risk of colon cancer).

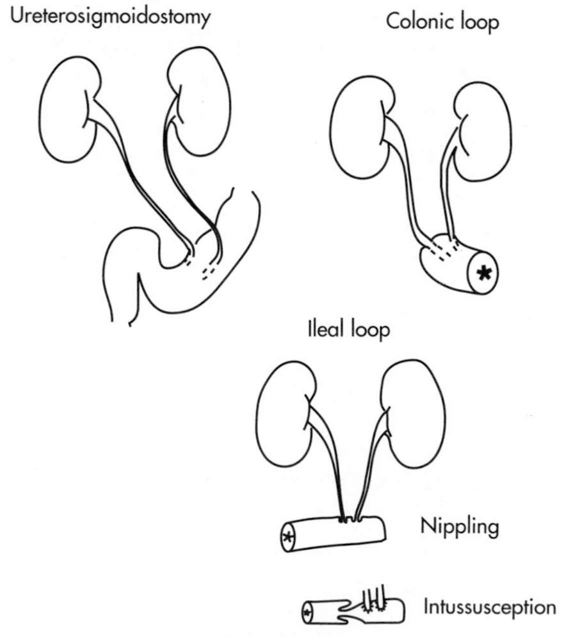

FIGURE 4-18

Loopogram

1. Insert 18- to 24-Fr Foley catheter with 5-mL balloon inflated in conduit.
2. Administer 30 to 50 mL of 30% water soluble contrast by gravity (<30 cm H_2O). Reflux in an ileal loop is a normal finding.
3. Search for drainage, stasis, stenosis, extravasation, calculi, or tumor.

BLADDER

CONGENITAL URACHAL ANOMALIES (Fig. 4-19)

Congenital urachal anomalies are twice as common in men as in women. There are four types:
- Patent urachus
- Umbilical-urachal sinus
- Vesicourachal diverticulum
- Urachal cyst

The majority of patients with urachal abnormalities (except those with a patent urachus) are asymptomatic. However, these patients may become symptomatic if these abnormalities are associated with infection.

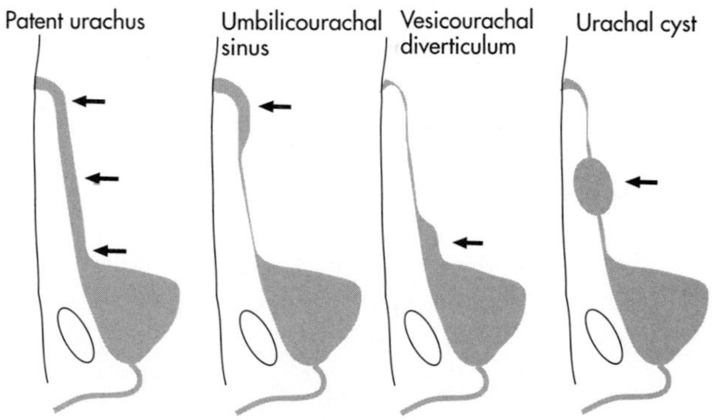

FIGURE 4-19

BACTERIAL CYSTITIS

Acute Cystitis

Pathogens: *E. coli* > *Staphylococcus* > *Streptococcus* > *Pseudomonas*

Predisposing Factors

- Instrumentation, trauma
- Bladder outlet obstruction, neurogenic bladder
- Calculus
- Cystitis
- Tumor

Imaging Features

- Mucosal thickening (cobblestone appearance)
- Reduced bladder capacity
- Stranding of perivesical fat

CHRONIC CYSTITIS

Repeated bacterial infections are usually due to such causes as reflux, diverticulum, or bladder outlet obstruction.

Imaging Features

- Cystitis cystica: serous fluid–filled cysts; multiple smooth round filling defects
- Cystitis glandularis: mucin-secreting glandular hypertrophy: multiple cystlike filling defects along mucosa
- Same findings as in acute cystitis

EMPHYSEMATOUS CYSTITIS

Infection (most commonly *E. coli)* that causes gas within the bladder and bladder wall. Conservative management unless there is coexisting emphysematous pyelonephritis. Predisposing diseases include:

- Diabetes mellitus (most common)
- Long-standing urinary obstruction (neurogenic bladder, diverticulum, outlet obstruction)

Imaging Features

- Gas in bladder wall
- Gas may enter the ureter
- Air-fluid level in bladder

TUBERCULOSIS

Chronic interstitial cystitis that usually ends in fibrosis. Typically coexists with renal TB.

Imaging Features

- Cystitis cystica or glandularis often coexists, causing filling defects in bladder.
- Small, contracted thick-walled bladder
- Mural calcification (less common)

SCHISTOSOMIASIS (BILHARZIOSIS)

Caused by *Schistosoma haematobium (S. japonicum* and *S. mansoni* affect GI tract). Infected humans excrete eggs in urinary tract; eggs become trapped in mucosa and cause a severe granulomatous reaction.

Imaging Features

- Extensive calcifications in bladder wall and ureter (hallmark)
- Inflammatory pseudopolyps: "bilharziomas"
- Ureteral strictures, fistulas
- SCC (suspect when previously identified calcifications have changed in appearance)

OTHER TYPES OF CYSTITIS

- Radiation cystitis occurs in 15% of patients receiving 6500 rad for pelvic malignancies.
- Cyclophosphamide treatment results in hemorrhagic cystitis in 40% of patients.
- Eosinophilic cystitis: severe allergic reactions
- Interstitial cystitis: most common in women; small, painful bladder

NEUROGENIC BLADDER

The detrusor muscle is innervated by S2-S4 parasympathetic nerves.

Types

- Spastic bladder: upper motor neuron defect
- Atonic bladder: lower motor neuron defect

BLADDER FISTULAS

Types and Common Causes

- Vesicovaginal fistula: surgery, catheters, cancer, radiation
- Vesicoenteric fistula: diverticular disease (most common cause), Crohn disease, cancer
- Vesicocutaneous fistula: trauma, surgery
- Vesicouterine fistula: cesarean section
- Vesicoureteral fistula: hysterectomy

LEUKOPLAKIA

Squamous metaplasia of transitional cell epithelium (keratinization). Associated with chronic infection (80%) and calculi (40%). Bladder > renal pelvis > ureter. Premalignant? Clinical findings include hematuria in 30% and passage of desquamated keratinized epithelial layers.

Imaging Features

- Mucosal thickening
- Filling defect

MALACOPLAKIA

Chronic inflammatory response to gram-negative infection. More prevalent in patients with diabetes mellitus. Michaelis-Guttman bodies in biopsy specimen are diagnostic.

Imaging Features

- Single or multiple filling defects
- Requires cystoscopy and biopsy to differentiate from TCC

BLADDER DIVERTICULUM

Types

Hutch diverticulum: congenital weakness of musculature near UVJ
- Usually associated with reflux

Acquired diverticulum in bladder outlet obstruction
- Usually multiple
- Not associated with reflux
- Complications
    - Infection
    - Calculi, 25%
    - Tumor, 3%

MALIGNANT BLADDER NEOPLASM

Clinical Finding

- Painless hematuria

Types and Underlying Causes

Transitional cell carcinoma, 90%
- Aniline dyes
- Phenacetin
- Pelvic radiation
- Tobacco
- Interstitial nephritis

SCC, 5%
- Calculi
- Chronic infection, leukoplakia
- Schistosomiasis

Adenocarcinoma, 2%
- Bladder exstrophy
- Urachal remnant
- Cystitis glandularis. 10% pass mucus in urine.

Imaging Features

Imaging findings
- Mass in bladder wall: US > contrast CT, MRI
- Obstructive uropathy due to involvement of ureteric orifices

Staging
- T1 = mucosal and submucosal tumors
- T2 = superficial muscle layer is involved
- T3a = deep muscular wall involved
- T3b = perivesicular fat involved
- T4 = other organs invaded
- N: The presence and distribution of malignant adenopathy affects the prognosis.

Treatment
- Nonmuscle invasive (only involvement of mucosa and lamina propria): typically resected endoscopically
- Muscle invasive (with extension into detrusor muscle or deeper): radical cystectomy and lymph node dissection

Urachal Carcinoma

Rare tumor (0.4% of bladder cancers, 40% of bladder adenocarcinomas) arising from urachus (fibrous band extending from bladder dome to umbilicus; remnant of allantois and cloaca). Tumors are usually located anterior and superior to dome of bladder in midline (90%). In contradistinction to bladder tumors, calcifications occur in 70%. 70% occur before the age of 20. Prognosis is poor. Histologically, this tumor is classified as:
- Adenocarcinoma, 90%
- SCC, TCC, sarcoma

BENIGN BLADDER TUMORS

- Primary leiomyoma (most common); ulcerated leiomyomas may cause hematuria.
- Hemangioma associated with cutaneous hemangiomas
- Neurofibromatosis
- Nephrogenic adenoma
- Endometriosis
- Pheochromocytoma

BLADDER CALCULI

Usually seen in patients with bladder outlet obstruction. Calculi usually form around a foreign body nidus (catheter, surgical clip). Calcium oxalate stones may have an irregular border (mulberry stones) or spiculated appearance (jack stones).

BLADDER OUTLET OBSTRUCTION

CAUSES

Adults	Children*
Benign prostatic hypertrophy	Posterior urethral valves (most common in males)
Bladder lesions	Ectopic ureterocele (most common in females)
Tumor	Bladder neck obstruction
Calculus	Urethral stricture
Ureterocele	Prune-belly syndrome
Urethral stricture	
Postoperative, traumatic	
Detrusor/sphincter dyssynergy	

* See Chapter 11, Pediatric Imaging.

Imaging Features (Fig. 4-20)

- Distended bladder with incomplete emptying (postvoid residual); best seen by US or IVP
- Increased bladder pressure causes formation of trabeculae and diverticula
- Enlarged prostate:
  - Rounded central filling defect at base of bladder
  - Hooking of ureters with massively enlarged prostate on IVP
- Upper urinary tract changes:
  - Reflux
  - Dilated ureter

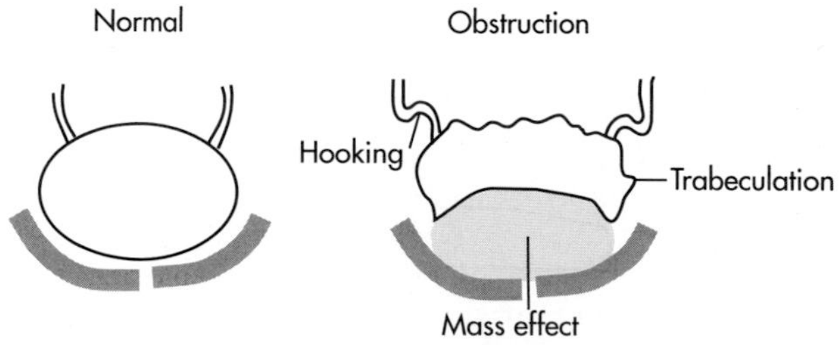

FIGURE 4-20

BLADDER INJURIES

Bladder injuries occur in 10% of patients with pelvic fractures; instrumentation and penetrating trauma are less common causes. There are two types of ruptures: extraperitoneal and intraperitoneal. The likelihood of rupture increases with degree of distention of the bladder at time of injury. Intraperitoneal rupture is treated surgically, whereas extraperitoneal rupture is treated conservatively with Foley catheter.

TYPES OF BLADDER RUPTURE

	Extraperitoneal, 45%	Intraperitoneal, 45%
Cause	Pelvic fractures (bone spicule), avulsion tear	Blunt trauma, stab wounds, invasive procedures
Location	Base of bladder, anterolateral	Dome of bladder (weakest point)
Imaging	Pear-shaped bladder	Contrast extravasation into paracolic gutters
	Fluid around bladder with displaced bowel loops	Urine ascites
	Paralytic ileus	

Classification of Bladder Injury

- Type 1: Bladder contusion
- Type 2: Intraperitoneal rupture
- Type 3: Interstitial bladder injury
- Type 4: Extraperitoneal rupture
- Type 4a: Simple extraperitoneal rupture
- Type 4b: Complex extraperitoneal rupture
- Type 5: Combined bladder injury

Radiographic Examinations in Suspected Bladder Injury

Retrograde urethrogram
- Should precede cystogram if there is suspicion of urethral injury such as blood at meatus, "high-riding" prostate, or inability to void

Cystogram
- 350 mL of 30% water-soluble contrast is administered.
- Obtain scout view, AP, both obliques, and postvoid films.
- 10% of ruptures will become evident on postvoid films.

CT cystogram
- Retrograde bladder distention is required before CT cystography.
- After Foley catheter insertion, adequate bladder distention is achieved by instilling at least 350 mL of a diluted mixture of contrast material under gravity control.
- Obtain contiguous 10-mm axial images from the dome of the diaphragm to the perineum, including the upper thighs.
- Obtain postdrainage images through the decompressed bladder.
- The normal CT cystogram will demonstrate a uniformly hyperattenuating, well-distended urinary bladder with thin walls. The adjacent fat planes will be distinct, with no evidence of extravasated contrast material.

CYSTOSTOMY

Indication

- Bladder outlet obstruction

Technique

1. Preprocedure workup:
   - Check bleeding status.
   - Antibiotic coverage: ampicillin, 1 g; gentamicin, 80 mg
   - Review all films and determine whether bowel loops lie anterior to bladder.
   - Place Foley catheter to distend bladder with contrast.
2. Local anesthesia with lidocaine (Xylocaine). Place long dwell needle into bladder and aspirate urine to check for position.
3. Advance stiff 0.038-inch guidewire and coil in bladder.
4. Dilate skin up to 16 Fr and then use a balloon catheter for further dilatation.
5. Place 16-Fr peel-away sheath. Pass 12-Fr Foley over guidewire. Remove guidewire. Inject contrast to check position of catheter.

MALE URETHRA

RETROGRADE URETHROGRAM (RUG) (Fig. 4-21)

- Posterior urethra = prostatic + membranous portions
- Anterior urethra = bulbous and penile portions
- Verumontanum: dorsal elevation in prostatic urethra that receives paired ejaculatory ducts and the utricle

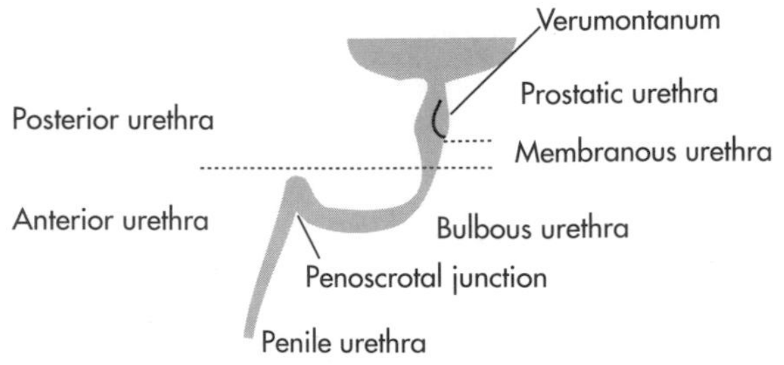

FIGURE 4-21

- Membranous urethra demarcates urogenital diaphragm; radiographically defined as the portion between the distal verumontanum and the cone of bulbous urethra
- Cowper glands in urogenital diaphragm; ducts empty into proximal bulbous urethra
- Littré glands in anterior urethra
- Utricle: müllerian duct remnant; blind-ending pouch in midline
- Fossa navicularis: 1-cm long dilatation of distal anterior urethra

URETHRAL INJURIES (Fig. 4-22)

Complications: strictures, impotence

Types

Complex trauma with pelvic fractures

- Type 1: urethra intact but narrowed, stretched by periurethral hematoma
- Type 2: rupture above urogenital diaphragm; extraperitoneal contrast, none in perineum; partial rupture: contrast seen in bladder; complete rupture: no contrast seen in bladder
- Type 3: rupture below urogenital diaphragm; contrast in extraperitoneal space and perineum

Soft tissue injury

- Straddle injury: injuries to penile or bulbous urethra

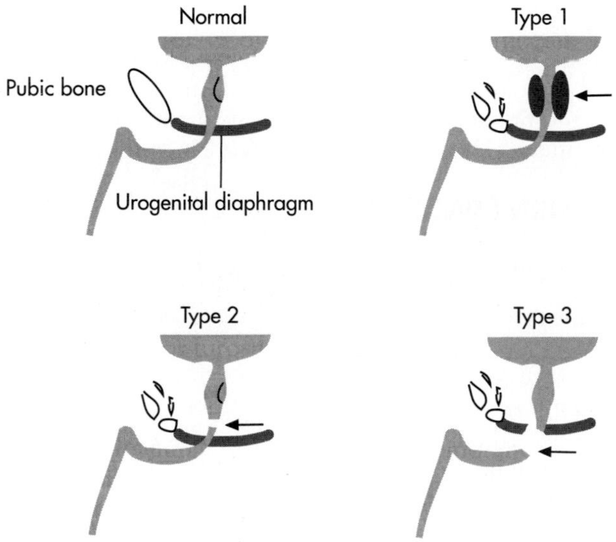

FIGURE 4-22

URETHRAL STRICTURES AND FILLING DEFECTS

Infection

- Gonococcal (most common, 40% of all strictures in United States), most common in bulbopenile urethra. Imaging Features: beaded appearance, retrograde filling glands of Littre
- TB: fistulas result in "watering can" perineum.
- Condylomata acuminata: HPV infection resulting in papillary filling defects on urethrogram

Trauma

- Instrumentation (e.g., transurethral resection of the prostate [TURP]): short, well-defined stricture in bulbomembranous urethra or penoscrotal junction
- Catheters: long, irregular, penoscrotal junction
- Injuries (straddle injury: bulbous urethra; pelvic fracture: prostatomembranous urethra)

Tumor (Rare)

- Polyps: inflammatory, transitional cell papilloma
- Malignant primaries: TCC, 15%; SCC, 80%; often associated with history of stricture
- Prostate cancer

FEMALE URETHRA

ANATOMY

- 2.5 to 4.0 cm long, ovoid or tubular
- Sphincter seen on US as a hypoechoic structure 1.0 to 1.3 cm in diameter
- Skene's glands, periurethral glands

INFECTION

- Usually seen in conjunction with cystitis
- Chronic irritation may result in polyps in the region of the bladder neck.
- Female urethral syndrome: chronic irritation on voiding. Radiographically, there is increased thickness of hypoechoic tissue by US; elevation of bladder on IVP

CARCINOMA

- Incidence in females 5 times that in males
- 90% in distal two thirds; 70% are SCC.
- TCC is usually posterior.

DIVERTICULA

- Female urethral diverticula usually acquired after infection, followed by obstruction of Skene's glands.
- If nonobstructed, 75% will be seen on postvoid IVP film, 90% on VCUG, remainder require double-balloon catheter positive-pressure urethrography.
- Calculi, 5%-10%
- Most common tumor is adenocarcinoma.

Retroperitoneum

GENERAL

Retromesenteric anterior interfascial space (RMS), retrorenal posterior interfascial space (RRS), anterior pararenal space (APS), anterior renal fascia (ARF), dorsal pleural sinus (DPS), lateroconal fascia (LCF), parietal peritoneum (PP), posterior pararenal space (PPS), perinephric space (PRS), posterior renal fascia (PRF), transversalis fascia (TF)

ANATOMIC TERMS (Figs. 4-23 and 4-24)

- *Interfascial plane:* Potential space between layers of renal, lateroconal, or transversalis fascia; result of fusion of embryonic mesentery
- *Anterior interfascial retromesenteric plane:* Potentially expansile plane between the anterior pararenal and perinephric spaces; continuous across the midline. It is an important potential route of contralateral spread of retroperitoneal collections.
- *Posterior interfascial retrorenal plane:* Potentially expansile plane between the perinephric space and posterior pararenal space; anterior pararenal, peritoneal, or intrafascial fluid may reside within the retrorenal space.
- *Lateroconal interfascial plane:* Potentially expansile plane between layers of lateroconal fascia; communicates with anterior and posterior interfascial planes at the fascial trifurcation.
- *Combined interfascial plane:* Potentially expansile plane formed by the inferior blending of the anterior renal, posterior renal, and lateroconal fasciae; continues into the pelvis, providing a route of disease spread from the abdominal retroperitoneum into the pelvis

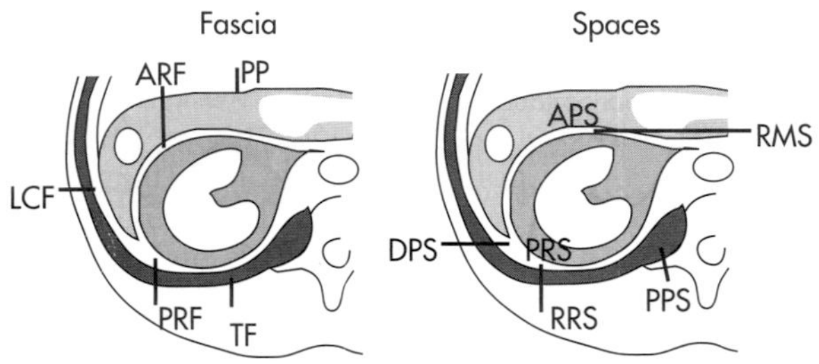

FIGURE 4-23

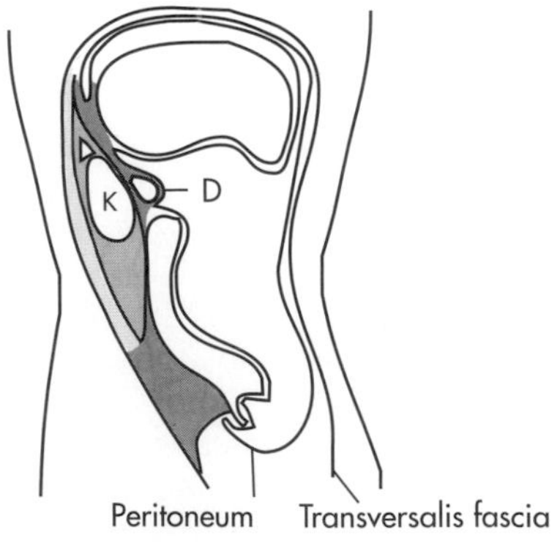

FIGURE 4-24

- *Fascial trifurcation:* Site at which the lateroconal fascia emerges from Gerota's fascia; anterior, posterior, and lateroconal interfascial planes communicate at the fascial trifurcation, usually located laterally to the kidney.
- *Anterior pararenal space:* between posterior peritoneum and anterior renal fascia; contains pancreas and bowel
- *Posterior pararenal space:* between posterior renal fascia and transversalis fascia; contains no organs. Fat continues laterally as properitoneal flank stripe.
- *Perirenal space:* between anterior and posterior renal fascia; contains kidney, adrenal gland, proximal collecting systems, renal vessels, and a variable amount of fat
- *Renal fascia* (Gerota's fascia) has an anterior and a posterior part. Renal and lateroconal fasciae are laminated planes composed of apposed layers of embryonic mesentery.
- *Lateroconal fascia* is formed by lateral fusion of anterior and posterior renal fascia.
- *Transversalis fascia*
- The *perinephric spaces* are closed medially.
- The *retromesenteric space* is continuous across midline.

PERINEPHRIC SPACE

The perinephric space contains a rich network of bridging septa, lymphatics, arteries, and veins. The perirenal lymphatics communicate with small lymph nodes at the renal hilum, and these, in turn, connect with periaortic and pericaval lymph nodes. This lymphatic network provides a potential route of spread for metastatic tumors into perinephric space.

BENIGN CONDITIONS

RETROPERITONEAL HEMATOMA

Causes

- Anticoagulation
- Trauma
- Iatrogenic
- Ruptured abdominal aortic aneurysm (particularly if >6 cm)
- Tumor: RCC, large angiomyolipoma

Imaging Features

- Dissection through retroperitoneal spaces
- Acute hemorrhage: 40 to 60 HU
- Hematocrit level

ABSCESS

Location and Causes

- Anterior pararenal space (>50%): pancreatitis
- Perirenal space: renal inflammatory disease
- Posterior pararenal space: osteomyelitis

RETROPERITONEAL AIR

Causes

- Trauma (perforation)
- ERCP
- Emphysematous pyelonephritis

RETROPERITONEAL FIBROSIS

Fibrotic retroperitoneal process that can lead to ureteral and vascular obstruction.

Causes

Idiopathic (Ormond disease), 70%

Benign

- Medication: methysergide, ergotamine, methyldopa
- Radiation, surgery
- Inflammation extending from other organs
- Retroperitoneal fluid: hematoma, urine

Malignant

- Desmoplastic reaction to tumors: HD > NHL > anaplastic carcinoma, metastases

Imaging Features

- Fibrotic tissue envelopes retroperitoneal structures.
- Fibrosis may enhance after contrast administration.
- Extrinsic compression of ureter
- Medial deviation of ureters
- Extrinsic compression of IVC, aorta, iliac vessels
- On T1W MRI, fibrous tissue appears hypointense. Active inflammation has an intermediate to hyperintense SI on T2W.
- Differential diagnosis: inflammatory aneurysm of the aorta; enhancing perianeurysmal soft tissue, which may obstruct ureters and IVC

PELVIC LIPOMATOSIS

Abnormal large amount of fatty tissue in pelvis compressing normal structures. Unrelated to obesity or race. May occur with IBD of rectum.

Imaging Features

- Elongation and narrowing of urinary bladder (pear shape)
- Elongation and narrowing of rectosigmoid
- Large amount of fat in pelvis

TUMORS

Retroperitoneal tumors may arise from muscle, fascia, connective tissue fat, vessels, nerves, or remnants of the embryonic urogenital ridge. 90% of retroperitoneal tumors are malignant and are usually very large (10 to 20 cm) at diagnosis.

Types

Mesodermal tumors

- Lipoma, liposarcoma
- Leiomyosarcoma
- Fibrosarcoma
- Malignant fibrous histiocytoma
- Lymphangiosarcoma
- Lymphoma

Neural tumors

- Neurofibroma, schwannoma
- Neuroblastoma
- Pheochromocytoma

Embryonic tumors

- Teratoma
- Primary germ cell tumor

LIPOSARCOMA

Fat-containing retroperitoneal tumors range in spectrum from lipomas (benign) to liposarcoma (malignant).

Imaging Features

- Nonhomogeneity with focal higher density structures (i.e., >−25 HU) is strong evidence of a liposarcoma.
- Tumors are classified histologically as lipogenic, myxoid, or pleomorphic. Myxoid and pleomorphic tumors are most common and may demonstrate little or no fat on CT.

LEIOMYOSARCOMA

Imaging Features

- Large mass
- Typically large areas of central necrosis
- Heterogeneous enhancement

Adrenal Glands

GENERAL

Arterial Supply

- Superior adrenal artery: branch of inferior phrenic artery
- Middle adrenal artery: branch of the aorta
- Inferior adrenal artery: branch of the renal artery

Venous Drainage

Each gland is drained by a single vein that enters into the:

- Inferior vena cava on the right
- Renal vein on the left

Physiology

Cortex divided into 3 zones:

- Zona glomerulosa (aldosterone)
- Zona fasciculata (ACTH dependent)

- Zona reticularis (Cortisol)

Medulla (epinephrine, norepinephrine)

Imaging Appearance

- Y configuration: each adrenal gland consists of an anteromedial ridge (body) and two posterior limbs best seen by CT/MR.
- Posterior limbs are close together superiorly but spread out interiorly (120°).
- Right adrenal lies adjacent to IVC throughout its extent.
- Left adrenal lies adjacent to splenic vessels at its cephalad margin.
- Size:
  - Limbs: 3 to 6 mm thick
  - Length of entire adrenal: 4 to 6 cm
  - Width of entire adrenal: <1 cm
  - Weight: 4 to 5 g/gland

MEDULLARY TUMORS

PHEOCHROMOCYTOMA

Pheochromocytoma is a subtype of a paraganglioma, a neuroendocrine tumor that arises from paraganglionic tissue. Rule of "10s": 10% of pheochromocytomas are extraadrenal, 10% are bilateral, and 10% are malignant. The most common location of an extraadrenal pheochromocytoma is the organ of Zuckerkandl (near aortic bifurcation).

Classification of Paraganglioma

Paraganglioma arising from adrenal medulla = pheochromocytoma

Aortosympathetic paraganglioma arising from the sympathetic chains and retroperitoneal ganglia = extraadrenal pheochromocytoma

Parasympathetic paragangliomas including chemodectomas (nonchromaffin paraganglioma)

- Glomus tympanicum
- Glomus jugulare
- Glomus vagale
- Carotid body tumor
- Others, not specified

Paraganglioma cells belong to the amine precursors uptake and decarboxylation (APUD) system. Cells may secrete catecholamines (epinephrine, dopamine, norepinephrine) or be nonfunctional.

Clinical Findings (Excess Catecholamines)

- Episodic (50%) or sustained (50%) hypertension, tachycardia, diaphoresis, headache (catecholamine-producing tumors); however, only 0.1% of hypertension is caused by pheochromocytomas.
- Elevated VMA in 24-hour urine in 50%
- Elevated serum catecholamines, urine metanephrines

Pharmacologic Testing

Diagnostic pharmacologic tests are potentially hazardous and may result in acute hypertension (stimulation tests) or hypotension (suppression tests). Careful monitoring is therefore necessary.

- Stimulators: glucagon, histamine, contrast material during arteriography
- Suppressors: clonidine, phentolamine.

Associations

- Multiple endocrine neoplasia in 5%; pheochromocytomas are usually bilateral and almost always intraadrenal.
- Neurofibromatosis (10% of patients have pheochromocytomas)
- Von Hippel-Lindau disease (10% of patients have pheochromocytomas)
- Familial pheochromocytosis (10% of all pheochromocytomas)

Imaging Features

Sensitivity for detection of functional tumors

- CT or MRI: 90%
- MIBG scintigraphy: 80%
- Octreotide scintigraphy

Appearance

- Adrenal mass
- Strong contrast enhancement (CT, angiography)
- Calcification
- MRI: very high SI ("light bulb") on T2W images. The SI is usually considerably higher when compared with adenomas or metastases.
- Percutaneous biopsy: method of choice for tissue diagnosis; biopsy of pheochromocytoma may precipitate acute hypertensive crisis, and pharmacologic prophylaxis is therefore indicated.
- Location: Adrenal, 85%; paraaortic, 8%; Zuckerkandl, 5%; urinary bladder, 1%

MULTIPLE ENDOCRINE NEOPLASIA (MEN) TYPE II

MEN type II (mucosal neuroma syndrome, multiple endocrine adenomatosis) is a rare autosomal dominant cancer syndrome. Clinically, MEN IIb is characterized by marfanoid habitus, coarse facial features with prognathism, and GI tract abnormalities (constipation, diarrhea, feeding difficulties).

Types

- MEN I: pituitary adenoma, parathyroid adenoma, pancreatic islet cell tumor
- MEN IIa: medullary thyroid carcinoma, pheochromocytoma, parathyroid adenoma
- MEN IIb: medullary thyroid carcinoma, pheochromocytoma, oral ganglioneuromas, other soft tissue tumors

CORTICAL TUMORS

APPROACH TO ADRENAL MASSES

Adrenal masses are best evaluated first by noncontrast CT according to the flow diagram on the right (Fig. 4-25). Points to remember:

- Enlarging masses are considered malignant until proved otherwise.
- Masses larger than 4 cm are also concerning for malignancy. In the absence of known primary malignancy, adrenal adenocarcinoma should be considered.
- Masses with attenuation averaging ≤ 10 HU are all considered adenomas.
- If the attenuation is more than 10 HU, the mass is considered indeterminate, and an enhanced and 15-minute delayed enhanced CT scan is obtained. An absolute percentage washout may be calculated as follows: APW = [(Enhanced – Delayed)/(Enhanced – Unenhanced)] x 100%. If the APW is >60%, the lesion is likely an adenoma. If an unenhanced study is unavailable, a relative percentage washout can be calculated as follows: RPW = [(Enhanced – Delayed)/(Enhanced)] x 100%. If the RPW >40%, the lesion is likely an adenoma.
- If the APW or RPW is less than about 60% or 40%, respectively, especially if the delayed attenuation value is more than 35 HU, the mass is considered indeterminate. If the patient has a new extraadrenal primary neoplasm with no other evidence of metastases, percutaneous adrenal biopsy is recommended to confirm adrenal metastasis. In a patient without cancer, surgery, follow-up CT, or adrenal scintigraphy with the use of radioiodinated norcholesterol (NP-59) is recommended, depending on the size of the mass and the other specific clinical features.
- Using 10 HU as a cutoff for diagnosis, the test has a sensitivity of 71% and a specificity of 98%.

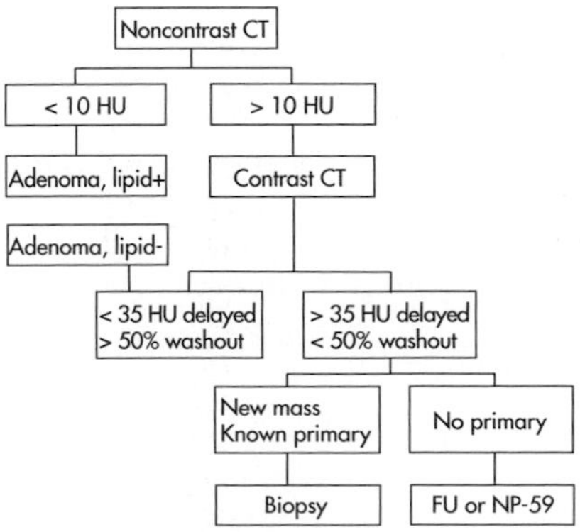

FIGURE 4-25

- 30% of adenomas have an attenuation value of more than 10 HU and are thus indistinguishable from other masses. 98% of homogeneous adrenal masses with a nonenhanced CT attenuation value of 10 HU or less will be benign (most will be adenomas).
- For the occasional adrenal mass that is detected by enhanced CT before the patient leaves the scanning table, a 15-minute delayed scan should be obtained and the above criteria applied.
- It is useful to refer to adenomas with nonenhanced CT attenuation values of 10 HU or less as lipid-rich and to refer to those with values of more than 10 HU as lipid-poor. The lipid-poor adenomas are an important subgroup because it is precisely these adenomas that cannot be characterized with nonenhanced CT densitometry.
- Although chemical shift MRI can be used to characterize lipid-rich adenomas with accuracy similar to that of nonenhanced CT, adenomas with only small amounts of lipid will not be detected.
- Chemical shift MRI may detect intracellular fat in adrenal adenomas, as manifested by a drop in lesion signal on out-of-phase images. Lesion signal intensity should be compared with that of spleen on both in-phase and out-of-phase images.
- Most adrenal cortical carcinomas are larger than 5 cm at presentation and often have demonstrable metastases. Typically, these tumors also have large amounts of necrosis, which would invalidate attempts to assess enhancement washout.
- An adrenal lesion demonstrating FDG uptake less than normal liver is likely an adenoma; although false-negative results on PET/CT may be seen with necrotic/hemorrhagic malignancy or BAC.

ADRENOCORTICAL CARCINOMA

50% of adrenocortical carcinomas are functioning (Cushing syndrome is the most common clinical manifestation). Prognosis is poor, because the tumor is usually large at time of diagnosis.

Imaging Features

- Mass usually >5 cm at time of diagnosis
- CT: heterogeneous enhancement because of areas of necrosis, hemorrhage; 50% have calcifications
- MRI: tumor appears hyperintense relative to liver T2W but is less hyperintense and usually much larger than pheochromocytoma.
- May extend into renal vein, IVC, or right atrium

ADRENAL METASTASES

Incidence: 25% at autopsy. Most common primary sites:

- Lung
  - Small cell carcinoma: 90% of adrenal masses detected by CT screening represent metastases
  - Non–small cell carcinoma: 60% of adrenal masses
- Breast
- Kidney
- Bowel
- Ovary
- Melanoma

Imaging Features (Fig. 4-26)

- Adrenal mass
- Bilateral masses
- Heterogeneous enhancement
- Indistinct, irregular margins
- SI of metastases by MRI is similar to that of spleen on T1W and T2W images. However, there is considerable overlap in SI between metastases and adenomas; the typical adenoma has an SI similar to that of adrenal tissue on T1W and T2W images.
- CT biopsy usually performed in equivocal cases

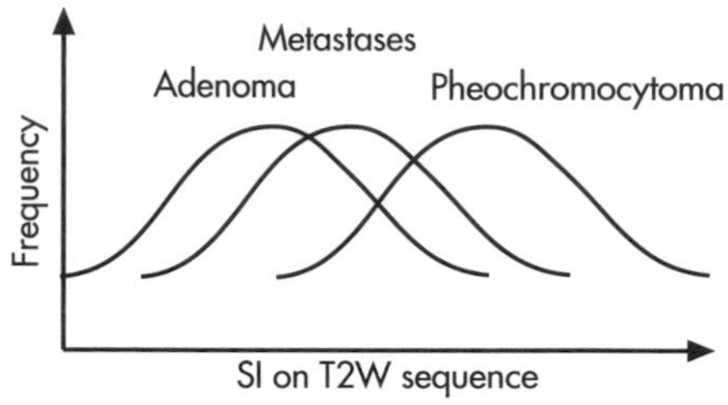

FIGURE 4-26

ADENOMA

Benign nonfunctioning adrenal adenomas are common (detected in 1%-3% of CT scans). Higher incidence in diabetes, hypertension, old age.

Imaging Features

CT

- Mass 1 to 5 cm
- <0 HU: diagnostic of adenoma (due to fat)
- 0 to 10 HU: diagnosis almost certain (follow-up or MRI)
- Calcification rare
- Slight enhancement with IV contrast

MRI

- Fat-suppression techniques are used to determine if a given lesion contains fat (e.g., in-phase/out-of-phase imaging, spin-echo fat-suppression imaging). If a lesion contains fat, it is considered an adenoma.

MYELOLIPOMA

Rare (250 cases reported up to 1994). Benign tumors are composed of adipose and hematopoietic tissue. Most common in the adrenal gland but extraadrenal tumors (retroperitoneum, pelvis, liver) have been reported. Usually very small and discovered incidentally at autopsy.

Imaging Features

- Area of obvious fat mass (low negative attenuation)
- May enhance with contrast administration
- Calcification, 20%
- US: hyperechoic mass superior to kidney

ADRENAL CYST

Rare lesion.

Classification

- Endothelial cyst (lymphangiectatic or angiomatous), 40%
- Pseudocyst (hemorrhage), 40%; may contain calcified rim
- Epithelial cyst, 10%
  - Cystic adenoma
  - Retention cyst
  - Cystic transformation of embryonal remnant
- Parasitic cysts (echinococcus), 5%

Imaging Features

- Mural calcification (15%), especially in pseudocysts and parasitic cysts
- Imaging findings of adrenal cyst are similar to those seen in cysts in other locations.

ADRENAL HEMORRHAGE

More common in neonates than adults.

Causes

- Hemorrhagic tumors
- Perinatal (common cause of calcification in later life)
- Severe trauma, traumatic hemorrhage, shock, postoperative, burn (traumatic hemorrhage is more common on the right)
- Anticoagulation, hemorrhagic diseases. Adrenal hemorrhage related to anticoagulation; usually occurs within the first month of treatment.
- Sepsis (disseminated intravascular coagulation, Waterhouse-Friderichsen syndrome)
- Adrenal venography (hemorrhage occurs in 10% of studies)
- Addison disease

Imaging Features

Acute hematoma

- High CT density (>40 HU)
- Enlarged adrenal gland

Old hematoma
- Liquefaction
- Fluid-fluid level
- May evolve into pseudocyst
- Typical MRI appearance of blood (see Chapter 6)

INFECTION

Most common causes are TB, histoplasmosis, blastomycosis, meningococcus, and echinococcus.
- TB may cause calcification and/or a soft tissue mass, which may have hypodense necrotic regions.
- Histoplasmosis usually preserves shape and may calcify.

FUNCTIONAL DISEASES

CUSHING SYNDROME

Excess steroid causes truncal obesity, HTN, hirsutism, cutaneous striae, and amenorrhea. Diagnostic studies: elevated plasma cortisol levels in 50%, elevated urinary 24-hour cortisol levels, abnormal dexamethasone suppression test (suppresses pituitary, not ectopic, ACTH production).

Causes

Adrenal hyperplasia, 70%
- Cushing disease (90% of adrenal hyperplasia): pituitary adenoma (ACTH hypersecretion). By imaging, 50% of patients will have normal adrenals and 50% will be diffusely enlarged. A small number will show macronodular enlargement.
- Ectopic ACTH (10% of adrenal hyperplasia): carcinoma of lung, ovary, pancreas
- Nonspecific hyperplasia is also associated with:
  - Acromegaly, 100%
  - Hyperthyroidism, 40%
  - Hypertension, 15%

Adenoma, 20%
Cortical carcinoma, 10%

HYPERALDOSTERONISM

Clinical Findings
- HTN
- Hypokalemia

Types

Primary (Conn disease)
- Adenoma, 75%
- Hyperplasia, 25%

Secondary (renal artery stenosis, reninoma)

Imaging Features
- Small tumors usually <2 cm
- Usually requires thin (1.5 to 3.0 mm) sections through the adrenal glands

ADRENAL INSUFFICIENCY

Clinical Finding
- Hyperpigmentation

Types

Primary (Addison disease; adrenal destruction)
- Autoimmune, idiopathic
- Infarction, hemorrhage
- Bilateral tumors: metastases
- Fungal

Secondary (hypopituitarism)

Imaging Features
- May be difficult to visualize small limbs
- Evidence of prior bilateral adrenal disease:
  - Metastases
  - TB
  - Hemorrhage

Male Pelvis

PROSTATE

NORMAL ANATOMY
- Peripheral gland: Peripheral zone and central zone
- Central gland: Transitional zone

US-GUIDED PROSTATE BIOPSY (Fig. 4-27)

Indications

Elevated prostate-specific antigen (PSA)

Technique
1. Obtain PSA, family history, and results of urologic examination.
2. Administer 3 days of oral antibiotics, 80 mg gentamicin IM immediately before biopsy.
3. Insert US probe with notch up (transverse view). Obtain the following views before biopsy (see lines in diagram):
   - Seminal vesicles midline
   - Prostate gland superior
   - Prostate gland midgland
   - Prostate gland apex
   - Obtain these views from the right and then the left gland rather than in midline.
4. Rotate notch 90° counterclockwise (sagittal view). Obtain the following views before biopsy (see lines in diagram):
   - Find urethra at apex (white lines of mucosa) and orient probe.

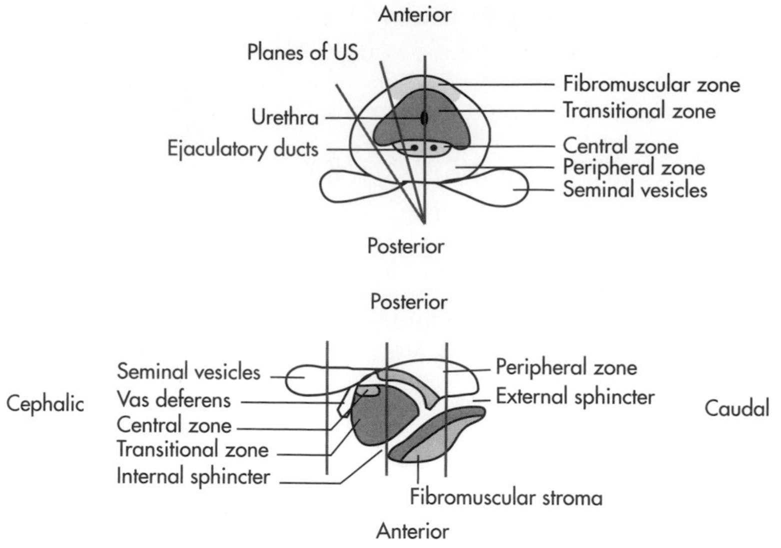

FIGURE 4-27

- Base views: midline, left, right
- Apex views: midline, left, right
- Measure volume of gland

5. Perform biopsy through guide. Line up right and left peripheral zones on transverse view. Usually multiple biopsies (6 to 8) are obtained. Use 18-gauge cutting needle (e.g., Biopty gun).

PROSTATE MRI (Fig. 4-28)

Indication

- Staging of known prostate cancer

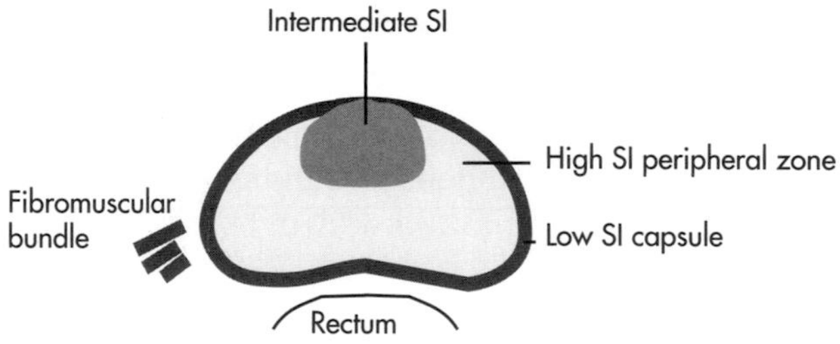

FIGURE 4-28

Technique

1. Glucagon, 1 mg IV
2. Endorectal surface coil
3. Fully inflate coil
4. Avoid rotation of coil
5. T1W imaging of pelvis/abdomen for adenopathy

BENIGN PROSTATIC HYPERPLASIA (BPH)

Imaging Features (Fig. 4-29)

IVP

- Bladder floor indentation
- Elevation of interureteric ridge, resulting in J-shaped ureters
- Bladder trabeculations, diverticula
- Postvoid residual urine

US

- Enlargement of central gland
- Hypoechoic or mixed echogenic nodules
- Calcifications within the central gland or surgical capsule
- Prostate volume >30 mL

CT

- Prostate extends above superior ramus of symphysis pubis

FIGURE 4-29

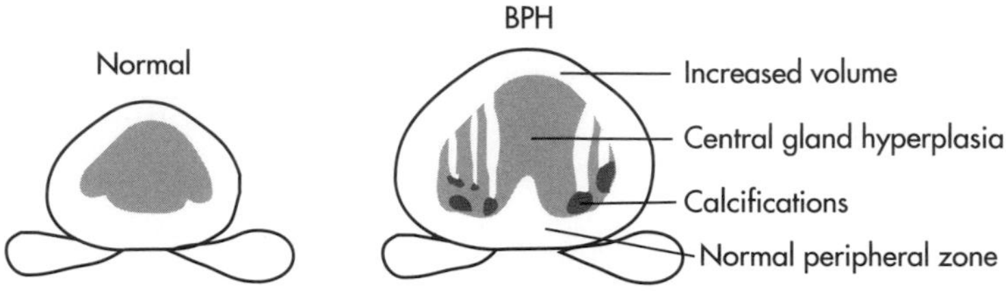

GRANULOMATOUS PROSTATITIS

Nodular form of chronic inflammation. The diagnosis is established by biopsy.
Relatively common.

Classification

- Nonspecific, idiopathic
- Infectious
  - Bacterial (TB, brucellosis)
  - Fungal
  - Parasitic
  - Viral
- Iatrogenic
  - BCG induced
  - Postsurgical, postradiation
- Systemic diseases
  - Allergic
  - Sarcoidosis
  - Autoimmune diseases

Imaging Features

US
- Hypoechoic nodules, 70%
- Diffuse hypoechoic peripheral zone, 30%

MRI
- Hypointense gland on T2W, 95%
- No enhancement with Gd-DTPA

PROSTATE CANCER

Represents 18% of all cancers in the United States (50,000 new cases a year). Second most common cause of cancer death in men in the United States; 30% are potentially curable at time of diagnosis. Incidence increases with age (uncommon before 50 years, median age 72 years). BPH does not predispose to cancer.

Screening (Controversial)

Prostate-specific antigen (PSA)
- Normal: 2 to 4U
- Cancer elevates PSA 10 times more than does BPH (per gram of tissue)
- Cancer: 1.8ng/mL PSA/gram of tissue (i.e., the higher, the more tumor)

Digital rectal exam
- Only 20% of palpable lesions are curable.
- False-negative rate of 25%-45%

US
- Most cancers are hypoechoic lesions in peripheral gland; however, only 20% of hypoechoic lesions are cancers.
- Isoechoic cancers, 40% (i.e., not detectable)

Origin

- Outer gland tumors (posterior and peripheral location), 70%

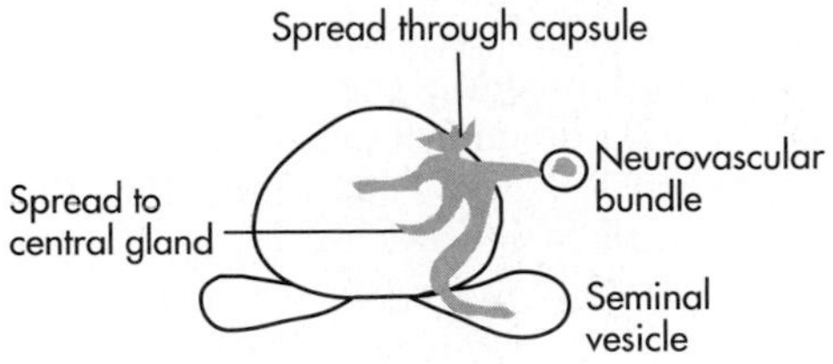

FIGURE 4-30

- Inner gland tumors (anterior and central location), 30%; inner gland tumors are not as rapidly invasive because of the presence of the surgical capsule and because there is no neurovascular bundle supply.

Imaging Features (Fig. 4-30)

US
- Sensitivity for detection of cancers is low with a specificity of approximately 60%; US is therefore mainly used to guide sextant biopsies.
- Appearance
  - Majority of tumors are hypoechoic.
  - Tumors may be hypervascular by Doppler US.
  - Suspect cancer if there are calcifications in the peripheral zone.
- Pattern of spread (Fig. 4-31)
  - Nodular
  - Nodular infiltrative
  - Infiltrative, spread along capsule, nonpalpable, nondetectable by US

CT
- Limited value in cancer detection and local staging; valuable for staging in abdomen

Bone scan
- Most commonly used technique to detect bone metastases
- Only 0.2% of patients with PSA <20 will have bone metastases in the absence of bone pain.

MRI
- On T2W images, prostate cancer usually demonstrates low SI in contrast to the high SI of the normal peripheral zone. Low SI in the peripheral zone, however, can also be seen in several benign conditions, such as hemorrhage, prostatitis, hyperplastic nodules, or posttreatment sequelae (e.g., as a result of irradiation or hormonal treatment).

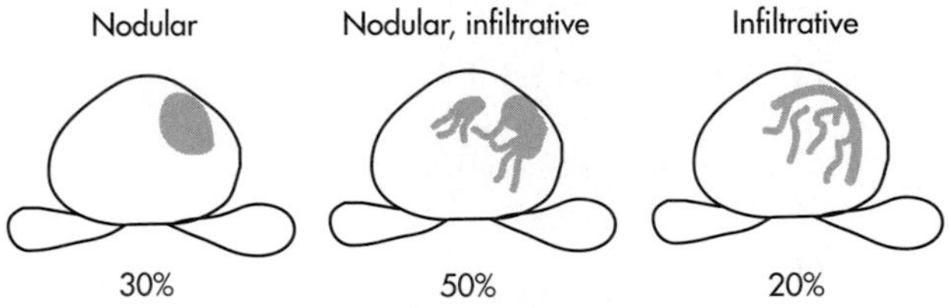

FIGURE 4-31

- Functional MRI techniques include diffusion weighted imaging (DWI), dynamic contrast enhanced imaging (DCE), and MR spectroscopy (MRS). DWI assesses the Brownian motion of free water in tissue. Normal prostate has high water diffusion rates, whereas tumors have restricted diffusion. These differences can be depicted on apparent diffusion coefficient (ADC) maps, which are obtained with multiple b-field gradient values. Prostate cancers are high in signal on raw high b-field DWI because of reduced diffusion and appear low in signal intensity on ADC maps.
- DCE-MRI depicts the vascularity and vascular permeability of tissue by following the time course of signal over time. The vasculature of tumor is heterogeneous, with highly permeable vessels that leak contrast material after injection. Tumor shows early, rapid enhancement and early washout out on DCE-MRI.
- 3-D proton MR spectroscopic metabolic mapping of the entire gland is possible with a resolution of 0.24 mL. Proton MR spectroscopy displays concentrations of citrate, creatine, and choline. Normal prostate tissue contains high levels of citrate (higher in the peripheral zone than in the central and transition zones). Glandular hyperplastic nodules, however, can demonstrate citrate levels as high as those observed in the peripheral zone. In the presence of prostate cancer, the citrate level is diminished or undetectable because of a conversion from citrate-producing to citrate-oxidating metabolism. The choline level is elevated owing to a high phospholipid cell membrane turnover in the proliferating malignant tissue. Hence, there is an increased choline-citrate ratio. Voxels are considered suspicious for cancer if the ratio of choline and creatine to citrate is at least 2 standard deviations (SDs) higher than the average ratio for the normal peripheral zone. Voxels are considered very suspicious for cancer if the ratio of choline and creatine to citrate is higher than 3 SDs above the average ratio.
- Extracapsular extension criteria on MR images
  - Neurovascular bundle asymmetry
  - Tumor envelopment of the neurovascular bundle
  - Angulated contour of the prostate gland
  - Irregular, spiculated margin
  - Obliteration of the rectoprostatic angle
- Seminal vesicle invasion criteria on MR images
  - Focal low SI of the seminal vesicle
  - Enlargement with a low-SI mass
  - Direct tumor extension from the base to the undersurface of the seminal vesicle
  - Expanded low-SI ejaculatory duct with low-SI seminal vesicle
- Pitfalls of MRI
  - Postbiopsy changes can mimic cancer.
  - BPH can extend into peripheral zone, simulating cancer.
  - Apical lesions are usually difficult to detect.
  - "Pseudolesions" are often present at gland base.
  - Image degradation by motion artifact
- MRI is a staging, not a screening, tool. It allows determination of the extension into seminal vesicles, bladder, and periprostatic fat.

OUTCOME BY MRI

MRI Findings	3-Year Recurrence
Tumor confined to gland	25%
Bulge of capsule	25%
Definitely stage C	100%

TNM staging

Tumor (T) stages are used to describe the stage of the cancer within the prostate itself.

- T1: No tumor can be felt upon DRE or seen with an imaging technique such as TRUS.
- T1a: The cancer is found incidentally during a transurethral resection of the prostate (TURP), a procedure used to reduce pressure on the urethra due to benign prostatic enlargement. Cancer is present in less than 5% of the tissue removed.
- T1b: Cancer is found after TURP and is present in more than 5% of the tissue removed.
- T1c: Cancer is found by needle biopsy that was done because of an elevated PSA.
- T2: Cancer can be felt upon DRE, but it is still confined to the prostate.
- T2a: Cancer is in one half or less of only one side (left or right) of the prostate.
- T2b: Cancer is in more than half of only one side (left or right) of the prostate.
- T2c: Cancer is in both sides of the prostate.
- T3: Cancer has begun to spread outside the prostate and may involve the seminal vesicles.
- T3a: Cancer extends outside the prostate but not to the seminal vesicles.
- T3b: Spread to the seminal vesicles
- T4: Spread to tissues next to the prostate such as the bladder's sphincter, the rectum, and/or the pelvic wall

Nodes (N) stages

- N0: No spread to the lymph nodes
- N1: One or more nearby lymph nodes involved

Metastases (M) stages

- M0: No spread beyond the regional nodes
- M1: Spread beyond the regional nodes
- M1a: Spread to distant lymph nodes outside of the pelvis
- M1b: Spread to the bones
- M1c: Spread to other organs such as lungs, liver, or brain (with or without bone disease)

The combined use of MRI and MR spectroscopy improves detection of tumors within the peripheral zone. It has also been shown to increase the specificity in the localization of prostate cancer in the peripheral zone. The ratio of choline and creatine to citrate in the lesion shows correlation with the Gleason grade, with the elevation of choline and reduction of citrate indicative of increased cancer aggressiveness. It has also been shown that metabolic and volumetric data obtained with MR spectroscopy correlate with the Gleason grade at pathologic examination. It has been recommended that the maximum ratio of choline and creatine to citrate combined with tumor volume at MR spectroscopy be used as an index to help predict tumor aggressiveness. Because Gleason grade is an important predictor of patient outcome, this finding provides a rationale for adding MRI and/or MR spectroscopy to the pretreatment evaluation of patients with prostate cancer.

Treatment Complications

- Urethral stricture
- Nervous injury (urinary incontinence, impotence)
- Cystitis, proctitis

SEMINAL VESICLE AND SPERMATIC CORD

SEMINAL VESICLE CYSTS

- Common, usually <3 cm
- Associated with ipsilateral renal agenesis
- Usually found incidentally in second or third decade
- Bilateral SV cysts seen in 40%-60% of ADPKD

SEMINAL VESICLE AGENESIS OR HYPOPLASIA

Unilateral SV Agenesis (Embryonic Insult Occurs Before 7th Week of Gestation)

- Associated with ipsilateral renal agenesis (80%)
- Other renal abnormalities (10%)
- Normal kidney (10%)

Bilateral SV Agenesis

- Mutations in cystic fibrosis transmembrane conductance regulator gene in 60%
- Associated with bilateral agenesis of VD
- Patients usually have normal kidneys

OTHER SEMINAL VESICLE (SV) DISEASE

- Abscess (usually due to prostatitis)
- Primary carcinoma (rare)
- Hypospermia due to strictures, reflux

TUMORS OF SEMINAL VESICLE AND VAS DEFERENS

Tumor Type	SV	VD
Benign	Cystadenoma, papillary adenoma, leiomyoma, teratoma, schwannoma, epithelial stromal tumor	Leiomyoma, fibroma
Malignant		
Common	Secondary neoplasm including bladder, prostate, or rectal cancer and lymphoma	Secondary neoplasm from prostate, bladder, or rectal cancer
Uncommon	Adenocarcinoma, leiomyosarcoma, rhabdomyosarcoma, angiosarcoma, müllerian adenosarcoma-like tumor, carcinoid, cystosarcoma phyllodes, seminoma	Sarcoma, inflammatory malignant fibrous histiocytoma, lymphoma
Nonneoplastic	Amyloidosis, hydatid cyst	Amyloidosis

SPERMATIC CORD

Spermatic cord contains the draining spermatic veins, the testicular artery, the vas deferens, and the draining lymphatics and nerves. Calcification of the vas deferens is associated with diabetes.

HEMATOSPERMIA

Seminal vesicle

- Congenial or acquired SV or ED cysts with or without stones
- Seminal vesiculitis
- Amyloidosis
- SV tumors (usually malignant)

Prostate

- Prostatic calculi
- Utricular or müllerian duct cysts (midline cysts)
- Prostatitis
- Amyloidosis
- BPH
- Biopsy
- TURP
- Irradiation

Urethra

- Urethritis or epididymal orchitis
- Urethral stricture or stent
- Urethral polyp

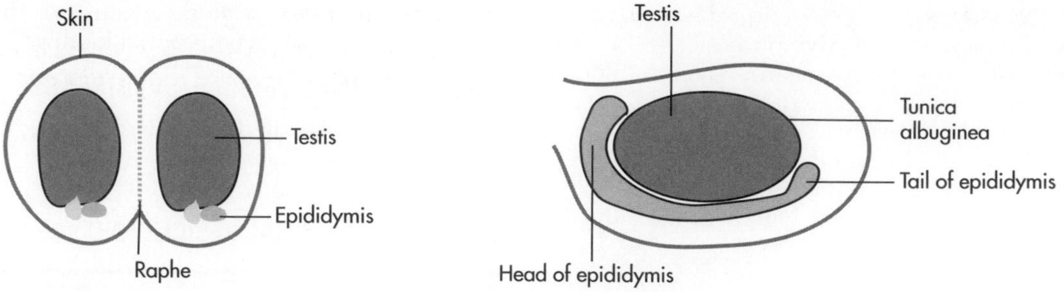

FIGURE 4-32

TESTIS AND EPIDIDYMIS

GENERAL (Fig. 4-32)

- Testes (5 × 3 × 3 cm) contain 250 pyramidal lobulations. There are 1 to 4 seminiferous tubules (30 to 70 cm long) per lobule, which converge into the rete testis. The rete testis communicates with the head of the epididymis via 10 to 15 efferent ductules.
- Epididymis contains 6 m of coiled tubules; the head is <10 mm in diameter and lies lateral to the superior pole of the testis; the body and tail are smaller (2 mm).
- Mediastinum testis: invagination of the tunica albuginea (fibrous capsule that envelops the testis)

Arterial Supply (Fig. 4-33)

- Main supply via testicular artery (from aorta)
- Cremasteric artery (via inferior epigastric)
- Differential artery (via inferior vesicle branch of internal iliac arteries; supplies the epididymis and vas deferens)

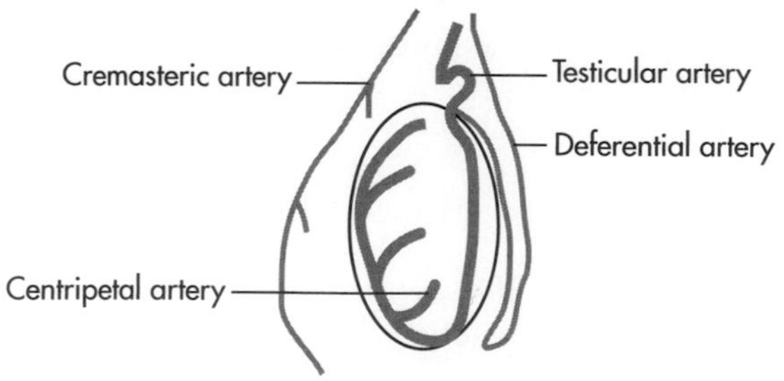

FIGURE 4-33

MRI EVALUATION OF TESTIS

- Surface coil
- Towel is placed under scrotum to raise testis between the thighs; second towel draped over scrotum and coil placed on towel; towels should be warm to prevent scrotal muscular contractions.
- Coronal T1W; axial, coronal, and sagittal T2W images acquired. Although not generally needed, gadolinium can be administered to characterize intermediate scrotal masses. T1W axial images of abdomen are done to search for adenopathy.
- Normal testis has homogeneous intermediate SI on T1W images and high SI on T2W images. The epididymis is isointense or slightly hypointense relative to testis on T1W and hypointense on T2W images.

CRYPTORCHIDISM

Undescended testes are present in 0.3% of adult men. 20% of these testes lie within the abdomen or pelvis. Unilateral maldescent in the adult is usually treated by surgical removal of the testes. Bilateral maldescent is treated with orchiopexy and biopsy (to exclude malignancy). Early orchiopexy reduces the risk of tumor later in life.

Complications

- Torsion
- Malignancy: 30-fold increased risk; the malignancy rate correlates with increasing distance of the testis from the scrotal sac.
- Testicular atrophy, resulting in infertility

TORSION

Types (Fig. 4-34)

Intravaginal torsion (common)

- Bell-clapper anomalous suspension: tunica vaginalis completely surrounds testis, epididymis, and spermatic cord so that they are freely suspended in scrotal sac.
- Testes twist within tunica vaginalis.
- 50%-80% are bilateral.

Extravaginal torsion (rare)

- Testis and its tunic twist at the external ring.
- Occurs in newborns

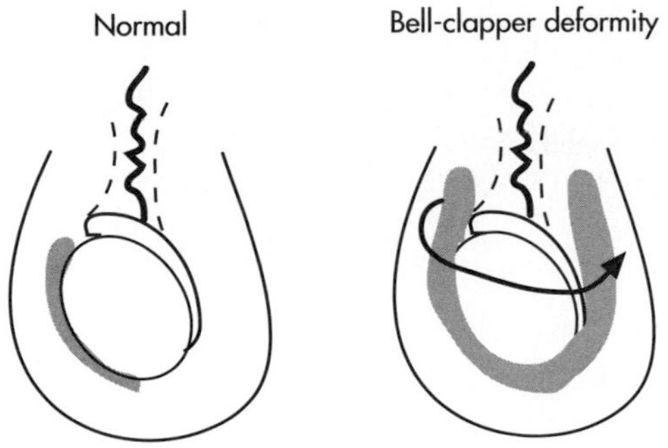

FIGURE 4-34

Imaging Features

Scintigraphy (see Chapter 12)

US

- Color Doppler
  - <4 hours: absent or decreased flow
  - Late: peritesticular inflammation: hypervascularity
- Gray-scale imaging
  - >4 hours: enlargement, heterogeneous echogenicity
  - Late: reactive hydrocele, atrophy

Treatment

- <4 hours: testes are usually salvageable
- >24 hours: testes are usually nonsalvageable (orchiectomy)
- Long-standing torsion: orchiectomy and contralateral orchiopexy

EPIDIDYMOORCHITIS (Fig. 4-35)

Results from retrograde spread of organism from bladder or prostate via the vas deferens. Common pathogens:

- Gonococcus
- Pyogenic *(E. coli, Pseudomonas)*
- Mumps
- TB

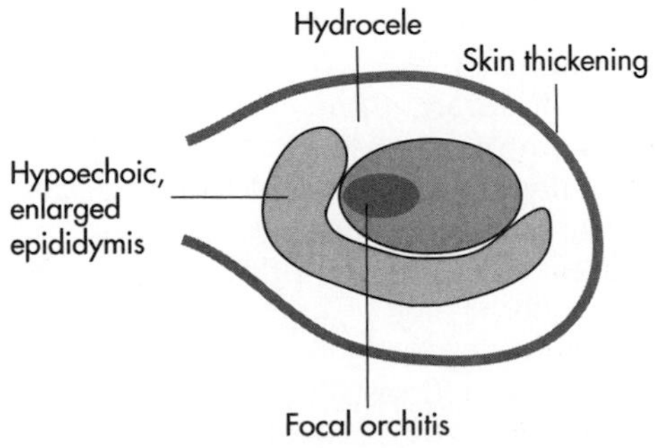

FIGURE 4-35

Imaging Features

- Epididymis and spermatic cord enlargement
- Decreased echogenicity of epididymis and cord
- Focal orchitis: peripheral hypoechoic region; all hypoechoic testicular lesions need to be followed by ultrasound until resolution; 10% of patients with testicular tumors present with orchitis.
- Reactive hydrocele or pyocele
- Thickening of the skin
- Calcification in chronic inflammation
- Color Doppler: hypervascularity in affected epididymis and/or testis

TESTICULAR ABSCESS

- Abscesses occur most commonly in patients with diabetes, genitourinary tuberculosis, or mumps. They are usually preceded or accompanied by epididymoorchitis.

US FEATURES

- Testicular enlargement
- Hypoechoic lesion
- Fluid-fluid level

VARICOCELE

Varicoceles represent dilated veins of the pampiniform plexus. They result from incompetent or absent valves in the spermatic vein. Varicoceles occur in 15% of adult males.

Clinical Findings

- Infertility
- Pain
- Scrotal enlargement

Location

- 90% of all varicoceles occur on the left side (drainage of left spermatic vein into the left renal vein at a right angle).
- 25% of varicoceles are bilateral.
- A solitary right-sided varicocele requires the exclusion of an underlying malignancy (tumor obstruction).

US Features (Fig. 4-36)

- Hypoechoic veins ("bag of worms")
- Veins >2 mm in diameter
- Dilated veins are easily compressed by transducer.
- Increase in venous size when patient is upright or performs Valsalva maneuver
- Color Doppler: flow is easily seen within varicocele and increases with Valsalva maneuver.

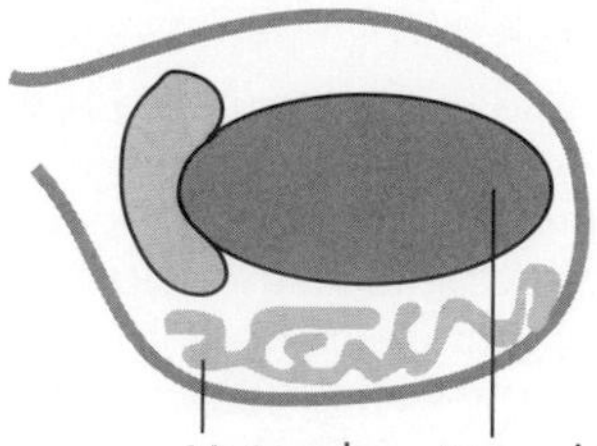

FIGURE 4-36

HYDROCELE

Simple fluid collection in scrotum. Most common cause of scrotal swelling.

Types

- Congenital: incomplete closure of processus vaginalis; spontaneous resolution by 18 months; associated with hernia
- Acquired:
  - Obstruction
  - Infection
  - Idiopathic

TRAUMA

Types (Fig. 4-37)

- Testicular contusion
- Testicular rupture: tear of tunica albuginea with extrusion of contents; requires emergency surgery to salvage testis and to prevent antibody formation against sperm
- Testicular fracture: fracture line (detectable in 30%) or loss of sharpness of tunica albuginea (70%)
- Hematoma: complex cystic mass ("Swiss cheese")
- Hematocele (blood-stained hydrocele)

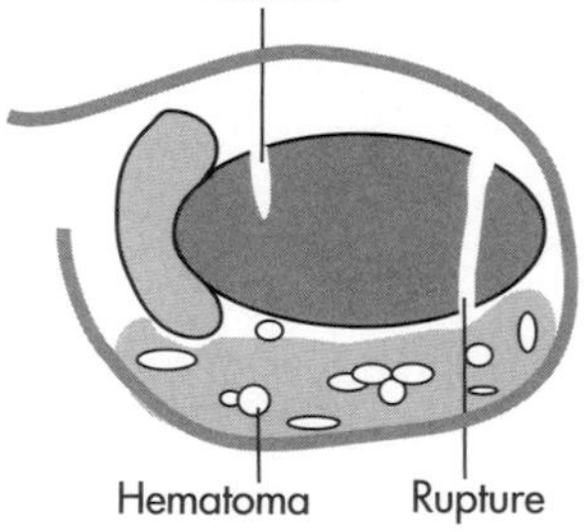

FIGURE 4-37

CYSTS

Causes: idiopathic, postinflammatory, posttraumatic

Types (Fig. 4-38)

- Epididymal cysts are very common; may be difficult to differentiate from spermatocele.

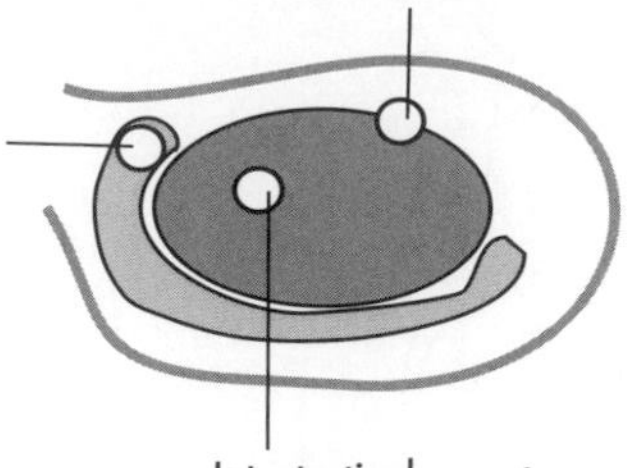

FIGURE 4-38

- Tunical cysts (mesothelial cysts) are common.
- Intratesticular cysts are uncommon (exclude malignancy).
- Rete testes dilatation is usually associated with epididymal cysts, older patients.

TESTICULAR MICROLITHIASIS

Multiple highly echogenic foci in testes. No known underlying disease. Associated with cryptorchidism, malignancy, Down and Klinefelter syndromes.

SCROTAL PEARL

Calcified loose body between membranes of tunica vaginalis. Solitary, echogenic focus with posterior shadowing. May represent a detached torsed appendix epididymis or appendix testis.

MALIGNANT TESTICULAR TUMORS

In the United States, there are 2500 new cases of testicular tumors per year. Testicular tumors are the most common malignancy in the age group 15 to 35 years. Tumor markers (AFP, HCG) aid in the early diagnosis and are important in follow-up.

Types

Germ cell tumors, 95%. Mnemonic: "SPECT:"

- Seminoma, 40%; extremely radiosensitive; good prognosis
- Embryonal carcinoma, 10%; more aggressive than seminoma
- Choriocarcinoma, 1%; very aggressive
- Teratoma, 10%
- Mixed tumors, 40%

Sex cord–stromal tumors

- Usually benign and endocrinologically active (e.g., Leydig cell tumor)

Metastases, 5%. Common primary lesions include:

- Prostate
- Kidney
- Lymphoma (most common testicular cancer in patients >60 years of age)
- Leukemia

Imaging Features

US

- High sensitivity (95%) for detection
- Tissue diagnosis is made by biopsy/removal of testis; only some tumors have more typical imaging features:
  - Seminoma: homogeneously hypoechoic
  - Embryonal cell carcinomas: cystic, heterogeneous, wild
  - Lymphoma: diffuse or multifocal testicular enlargement

Staging

- Retroperitoneal nodes (20% at presentation): CT > lymphangiography

Pearls

- Rule of thumb:
  - Intratesticular masses = malignant
  - Extratesticular masses = benign
- Seminoma presents later than other tumors (4th to 5th decade, may have two peak ages), most common in cryptorchidism
- Embryonal cancers (20%) are smaller and more aggressive than seminoma
- Choriocarcinomas (1%) are the most aggressive tumors
- Teratomas occur at younger age (10 to 20 years), good prognosis

BENIGN EPIDERMOID TUMOR

Represents 1% of all testicular tumors. Mean age: 20 to 40 years. US features include well-circumscribed hypoechoic lesions with echogenic capsule; may have "onion-skin" appearance; internal shadowing is due to calcifications.

PENIS

PEYRONIE DISEASE

Calcified plaques in the two corpora cavernosa.

Imaging Features

- Plaque usually located in periphery
- Hyperechoic, posterior shadowing of plaques
- Calcified plaques can also be seen by plain film.
- Septum between corpora may be thickened.

PENILE FRACTURE

Fracture of corpus cavernosa, with tear in tunica albuginea. May involve corpus spongiosum and urethra. Surgical emergency as contractures may result. Retrograde urethrogram is performed to assess for urethral injury.

- US: Tear of the tunica albuginea appears as a hypoechoic defect of the normally echogenic envelope surrounding the corpora.
- MRI: tear manifests as a high-signal defect in the normally T1- and T2-hypointense tunica albuginea, often with intracavernosal or extratunical hematoma.

VASCULAR IMPOTENCE

50% of cases of impotence are due to vascular causes:

- Arterial insufficiency, 15%-35%
- Venous insufficiency, 15%
- Coexistent insufficiency, 50%-70%

Imaging Features

US

1. Inject papaverine into corpora cavernosa.
2. Scan with Doppler while erection develops.
3. Measure peak velocities:
   - <25 cm/sec: severe arterial disease
   - 25 to 35 cm/sec: arterial disease
   - >35 cm/sec: normal

Arteriography

Cavernosography and cavernosometry for venous leaks

PENILE CANCER

Penile cancer is a relatively rare neoplasm in the developed world.

Etiology

- Presence of foreskin, which results in the accumulation of smegma. Therefore, the risk of this disease is three times higher in uncircumcised men than in circumcised men. Poor hygiene also contributes to the development of penile cancer through the accumulation of smegma and other irritants.
- The presence of phimosis has a strong association with penile cancer and is seen in 25% of cases of penile disease.
- Other risk factors include:
  - Chronic inflammatory conditions (e.g., balanoposthitis, lichen sclerosus et atrophicus), smoking, treatment with psoralens or ultraviolet A photochemotherapy, human papillomavirus 16, and human papillomavirus 18
  - The main prognostic factors for carcinoma of the penis are the degree of invasion by the primary tumor and the status of the draining lymph nodes.

Pathology

Primary neoplasms of the penis can be classified into the following histologic types: SCC, sarcoma, melanoma, basal cell carcinoma, and lymphoma. SCC accounts for more than 95% of all primary neoplasms of the penis. Sarcomas are uncommon penile neoplasms and include epithelioid sarcoma, Kaposi sarcoma, leiomyosarcoma, and rhabdomyosarcoma.

Secondary or metastatic tumors of the penis: in approximately 70% of cases, the primary tumor is located in the urogenital tract. Other primary cancers causing metastases to the penis include those of the colon, rectum, stomach, bronchus, and thyroid.

Imaging Features

- MRI is superior to CT in the evaluation of primary tumors.
- In general, T2W and gadolinium-enhanced T1W MRI sequences are the most useful in defining the local extent of a penile neoplasm.
- Primary penile cancers are most often solitary, ill-defined infiltrating tumors that are hypointense relative to the corpora on both T1W and T2W images.
- The tumors enhance on gadolinium-enhanced images, although to a lesser extent than the corpora cavernosa.
- Penile metastases typically manifest as multiple discrete masses in the corpora cavernosa and corpus spongiosum.

Female Pelvis

GENERAL

PELVIC US

Uterus

- Endometrium appears hyperechoic (specular reflection from endometrial cavity); a hypoechoic halo surrounding the endometrium represents hypovascular myometrium (subendometrial halo).

CYCLIC CHANGES OF ENDOMETRIUM

Stage	Endometrium	Appearance
Menstrual	<4 mm	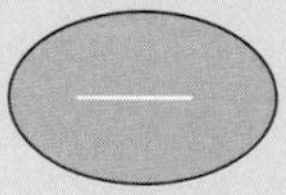
Proliferative	4-8 mm	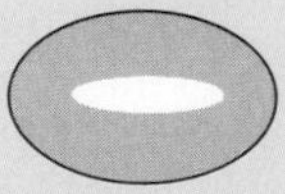
Secretory	7-14 mm	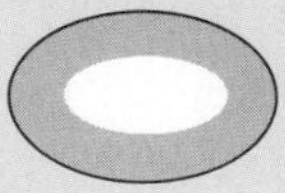

- Common age-related changes
  - Dilated peripheral uterine veins (hypoechoic)
  - Calcified arcuate arteries
- Version and flexion
  - Normal position, 80%: anteversion and anteflexion
  - Retroversion: entire uterus is tilted backward (uterus and cervix).
  - Retroflexion: only body and fundus are flexed posteriorly.
- Postmenopausal uterus (>2 years after the last menstrual period [LMP]; perimenopausal <2 years after LMP) may be difficult to see because of atrophy.
- Nabothian (retention) cysts of the cervix are common and usually insignificant.

Menstrual Cycle (Fig. 4-39)

Follicular (proliferative) phase

- Begins with day 1 of menses and continues until ovulation, usually on day 14 of a 28-day cycle
- Primordial follicles begin to grow under gonadotropin-releasing hormone/follicle-stimulating hormone (GnRH/FSH) stimulation (hypothalamic-pituitary axis); follicles may be visible sonographically as small cysts.
- Follicles secrete estrogen, which, through a negative feedback mechanism, causes a decrease in FSH; usually only one dominant follicle persists.
- Dominant follicle becomes visible by US at day 8 to 12; before ovulation, the dominant follicle undergoes rapid growth to reach a mean diameter of 20 to 24 mm by the time of ovulation.

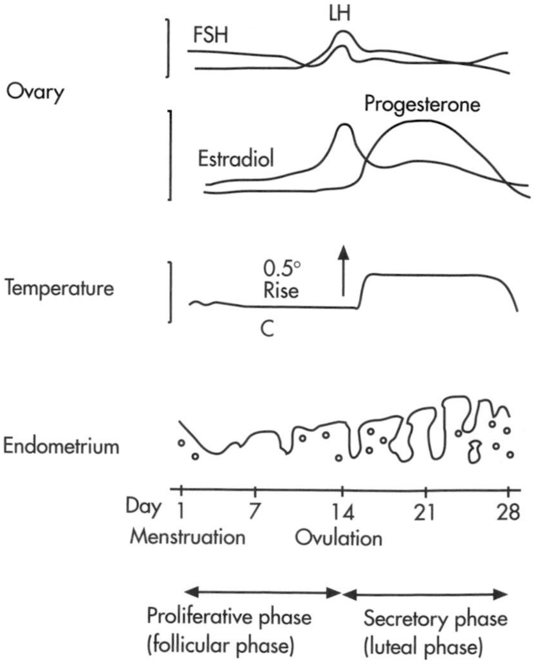

FIGURE 4-39

Ovulation

- Ovulation occurs as a result of a luteinizing hormone (LH) surge, which is induced by rising estrogen levels.
- US signs of impending ovulation (within 36 hours):
  - Decreased echogenicity around the follicle
  - Irregularity of the follicle wall (crenation)
  - A small echogenic core of tissue (cumulusoophorus) occasionally projects into the follicle.
- After ovulation there is sudden complete or partial collapse of the follicle; echoes appear within the cyst fluid.
- A small amount of free fluid may be noted in the cul-de-sac.

Secretory phase

- Granulosa cells (from the involuted follicle) form the corpus luteum, which synthesizes progesterone.
- Sonographically the corpus has a 2- to 3-mm thick echogenic rim and central cystic region that involutes over time unless fertilization occurs.
- Progesterone maintains the secretory endometrium, which is necessary for successful implantation.
- Thick hyperechoic appearance due to engorged glands
- Endometrial thickness is greatest during the secretory phase (7 to 14 mm).

Ovary

- Normal volume: multiply the three diameters and divide by 2; normal volume <18 cm^3 premenopausal, <8 cm postmenopausal
- Cyst (simple) size up to 4 cm can be normal during the menstrual cycle (mean cyst size is 2.5 cm).
- Structures that may simulate ovaries:
  - Iliac vessel in cross section
  - Bowel loops
  - Cervix containing multiple nabothian cysts
  - Lymph nodes
- Free fluid in the pelvis
  - Small amounts can be present during all phases of cycle (e.g., fluid from follicular rupture, estrogen-induced increased capillary permeability).
  - Large amounts of fluid are abnormal. Complex fluid with septations or nodularity is abnormal.

HYSTEROSALPINGOGRAM (HSG)

Indication: primarily used for infertility workup, as an anatomic study before in vitro fertilization (IVF), and occasionally for evaluation of congenital anomalies.

Technique

1. HSG should be performed only on days 6 to 12 after LMP (4-week cycle).
2. Insert 6-Fr Foley catheter into cervical canal using speculum and inflate balloon.
3. Inject 4 to 10 mL of 28% contrast agent (water-soluble) under fluoroscopy until contrast agent passes into peritoneal cavity. Normal tubal length, 12 to 14 cm.
4. In dilated fallopian tubes or contained peritubal adhesions, administer doxycycline (100 mg bid) for 10 days to prevent tuboovarian abscess. Patients with normal study do not require antibiotics.

Complications

- Pain
- Infection (<3%), usually in patients with hydrosalpinx and peritubal collections or adhesions
- Contrast allergy (venous or lymphatic intravasation); gadolinium can be used instead.
- Radiation: 100 to 600 mrad/ovary

Contraindications

- Active uterine bleeding/menses
- Active infection
- Pregnancy
- Uterine surgery within the last 3 days

PELVIC MRI

Indications: leiomyoma location, endometriosis, adenomyosis, congenital abnormalities, presurgical planning

Techniques (Fig. 4-40)

- T2W sequences are most useful for imaging of uterus.
- Obtain images in anatomic planes of uterus.
- Give glucagon to decrease bowel motility.
- Gd-enhanced, fast gradient-echo sequences for evaluation of malignancies; adnexal lesions
- Fat-saturation sequences to diagnose dermoids, endometriosis

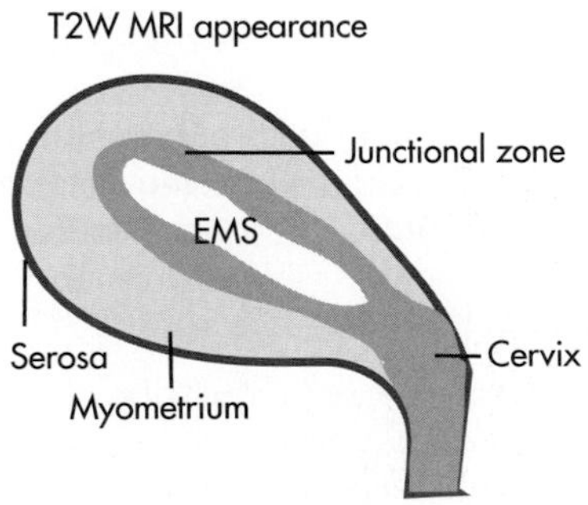

FIGURE 4-40

SI on T2W Sequences

- Endometrium, high SI
- Junctional zone (inner layer of compact myometrium), low SI
- Myometrium, intermediate SI
- Cervical stroma, low SI
- Serosal covering, low SI

TRANSVAGINAL DRAINAGE PROCEDURES

The transvaginal approach is an ideal route for drainage of pelvic collections because of the proximity of the vaginal fornices to most pelvic lesions. The transvaginal approach allows use of endoluminal US probe needle guides to permit extremely accurate and speedy needle or catheter placement.

Indications

- Gynecologic abscesses
- Nongynecologic pelvic abscesses
- Incomplete therapeutic transvaginal aspiration
- Biopsies

Complications

- Bleeding
- Bowel injury
- Inadequate catheter positioning
- Potential for superinfection of sterile fluid collections because of the semisterile route of access

UTERUS

UTERINE MALFORMATIONS (Fig. 4-41)

Incidence: 0.5%. Most often, duplication anomalies are discovered during pregnancy. Imaging modalities: US > MRI > HSG.

Types

Failure of fusion of the müllerian ducts: abnormal external contour
- Complete: uterus didelphys
- Partial: bicornuate uterus, arcuate uterus

Failure of resorption of the median septum: normal external contour
- Septate uterus: extends to uterine cervix
- Subseptate uterus: does not extend to uterine cervix

Arrested development of the müllerian ducts
- Bilateral (very rare): uterine aplasia
- Unilateral: uterus unicornis unicollis ± rudimentary horn

Complications

- Infertility and spontaneous abortions are common in septate uterus.
- Septate uterus: septum often consists of fibrous tissue rather than myometrium.

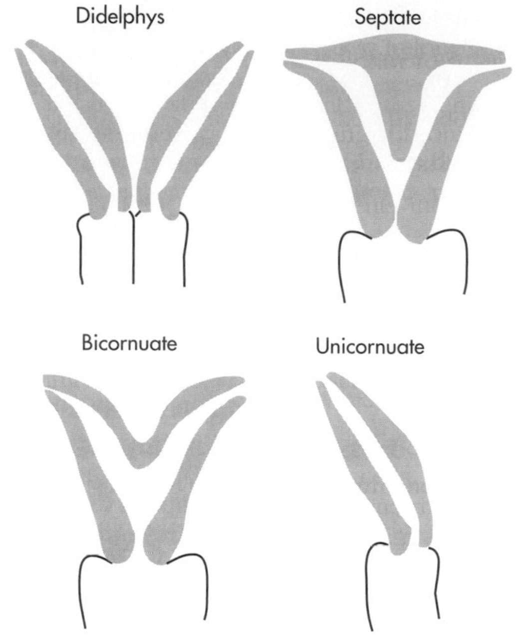

FIGURE 4-41

Highest incidence of reproductive failure (zygote cannot implant on fibrous tissue)
HSG: Intercornuate distance <4 cm, intercornual angle <75°
Treatment: hysteroscopic excision of septum
- Hydrometrocolpos: commonly seen in fusion anomalies
  - Uterine didelphys: one side may be obstructed by vaginal septum.
  - Rudimentary horn with no communication to uterine cavity
- Premature labor or uterine size cannot accommodate full-grown fetus.
- Malpresentation: distorted uterine anatomy

Associations

- Congenital GU anomalies are common, 50%.
  - Ipsilateral renal agenesis (most common)
  - Renal ectopia
- Mayer-Rokitansky-Küster-Hauser syndrome
  - Dysgenesis of müllerian ducts
  - Vaginal and/or uterine agenesis
  - Normal karyotype
  - Normal secondary sex characteristics
  - Renal anomalies
  - Normal ovaries; increased risk of endometriosis

IN UTERO DIETHYLSTILBESTROL (DES) EXPOSURE

- Uterine hypoplasia
- T-shaped uterus
- Increased risk of clear cell cancer of vagina

PELVIC INFLAMMATORY DISEASE (PID)

Spectrum of infectious diseases that present with pain, fever, discharge, and occasionally a pelvic mass.

Causes

Sexually transmitted diseases (most common)
- Gonorrhea
- *Chlamydia*
- Herpes

Pregnancy related
- Puerperal infection
- Abortion

Secondary PID
- Appendicitis
- Diverticulitis
- Actinomycosis in patients with IUD

US Features

- Endometrial fluid (nonspecific)
  Thick, irregular, and usually hypoechoic endometrium (must correlate with patient's age and cycle)
  Gas bubbles in endometrium are diagnostic.
- Hydrosalpinx or pyosalpinx: cystic and tubular adnexal mass
- Inflammatory pelvic mass lesion usually represents a tuboovarian abscess.
- Fibrosis and adhesions in end-stage disease

ASHERMAN SYNDROME

Uterine cavity synechiae that develop from trauma, DC, infection. HSG demonstrates irregular linear filling defects. May cause infertility.

PYOMETRA

Causes

- Malignancy
- Radiation
- Iatrogenic cervical stenosis

Imaging Features

- Endometrial canal filled with pus, blood
- Uterine enlargement

INTRAUTERINE DEVICE (IUD)

Complications

- Embedding
- Perforation
- 3-fold increased risk of PID (depends on IUD and string)
- Actinomycosis
- Associated pregnancy, spontaneous abortion

Radiographic Feature

- Hyperechoic (shadowing) structures in endometrial canal or myometrium if embedded

ADENOMYOSIS

Heterotopic endometrial glands and stroma are located within the myometrium ("internal endometriosis").

Clinical Findings

- Dysmenorrhea
- Bleeding
- Enlarged uterus
- Asymptomatic (5%-30%)

Imaging Features (Fig. 4-42)

MRI
- T2W MRI is study of choice.
- Focal or diffuse thickening of the junctional zone (>12 mm) is the key finding.
- High SI endometrial foci within junctional zone or myometrium
- Enlargement of uterus; globular shape

US
- US is nonspecific and less sensitive than MRI.
  Findings include heterogeneously increased echotexture, enlarged uterus, and myometrial cysts.

Hysterosalpingogram
- Outpouchings of contrast into wall

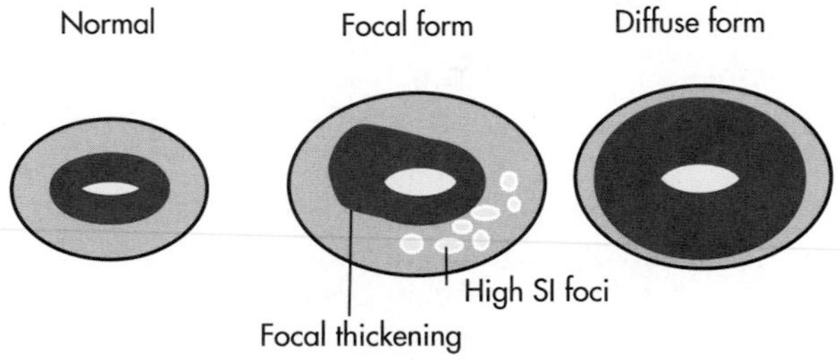

FIGURE 4-42

LEIOMYOMA (Fig. 4-43)

Uterine leiomyomas (fibroids) are the most common tumor of the uterus (in 25% of women >35 years). Fibroids arise from smooth muscle cells.

Clinical Findings

- Asymptomatic (most common)
- Uterine bleeding
- Pain
- Dysuria
- Infertility (especially if located in lower segment or cervix)
- Estrogen dependent
  May grow during pregnancy
  Regress after menopause

Location

- Intramural (myometrial): most common
- Submucosal: least common but most likely to produce symptoms

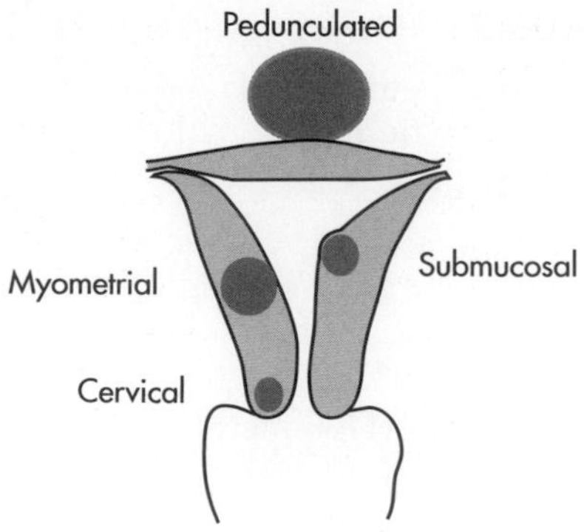

FIGURE 4-43

- Subserosal: frequently pedunculated
- Broad ligament: may simulate adnexal mass
- Cervical: uncommon

Complications

- Torsion if pedunculated
- Cervical fibroids may interfere with vaginal delivery and require cesarean section.
- Infertility
- Sarcomatous degeneration (very rare)

Imaging Features

US

- Fibroids are typically hypoechoic but may be heterogeneous:
  - Calcification, 25%
  - Degeneration: fatty (hyperechoic), cystic (hypoechoic)
  - Rarely may contain cystic center
- Deformation of uterine contour
- Often multiple
- Lipoleiomyomas appear uniformly echogenic.
- 20% of patients with fibroids have normal US.
- Transient muscular contraction (e.g., in abortion) may simulate the appearance of fibroid.

CT

- Differential enhancement relative to normal myometrium
- Same density as myometrium on noncontrast images
- Diagnosis is usually based on contour abnormalities of uterus.
- Coarse calcification may be present.

MRI

- Allows accurate anatomic localization of fibroids before planned surgery
- Simple fibroids are hypointense relative to uterus on T2W images.
- Atypical leiomyomas are hyperintense on T2W images, which may be due to mucoid degeneration or cystic degeneration.
- Isointense relative to uterus on T1W images

Extrauterine Leiomyomas

Arise from smooth muscle cells in blood vessels (inferior vena cava), spermatic cord, wolffian and müllerian duct remnants, bladder, stomach, and esophagus. Very rare.

Uterine Leiomyosarcomas

Typical presentation is as large masses with homogeneous SI. Suspect the diagnosis if a fibroid enlarges postmenopausally. Rare. Can have similar MR appearance as fibroid; look for areas of intermediate T2W SI that enhance or focal areas of arterial enhancement.

ENDOMETRIAL HYPERPLASIA

Caused by unopposed estrogen stimulation. Hyperplasia is a precursor to endometrial cancer. Clinical finding is bleeding.

Causes

- Estrogen-producing tumor
- Exogenous estrogen therapy (tamoxifen)
- Anovulation (any cause)
- Obesity
- Polycystic ovary (PCO)

Types

- Glandular-cystic (predominantly during reproductive years producing long menses and metrorrhagia). Hypoechoic spaces may be present within hyperechoic endometrium.
- Adenomatous (predominantly in menopause)

US Features

- Thick endometrial stripe
  - >4 mm postmenopausal
  - >8 mm postmenopausal, hormone-replacement or tamoxifen therapy
  - >14 mm premenopausal; difficult to assess sonographically in premenopausal patient, because there is overlap with normal

Tamoxifen

Antiestrogen (binds to 17β estrogen receptor) with weak estrogenic activity. Uses include:

- Breast cancer adjuvant therapy
- Improves lipid profile
- Osteoporosis

Tamoxifen is associated with increased incidence of:

- Endometrial hyperplasia
- Endometrial polyps
- Endometrial cancer
- Subendometrial cystic atrophy (anechoic areas in the subendometrial myometrium)

GARTNER'S DUCT CYST (Fig. 4-44)

Inclusion cyst of the mesonephric tubules (Gartner's duct). Located lateral to vagina. Represents one type of parovarian cysts.

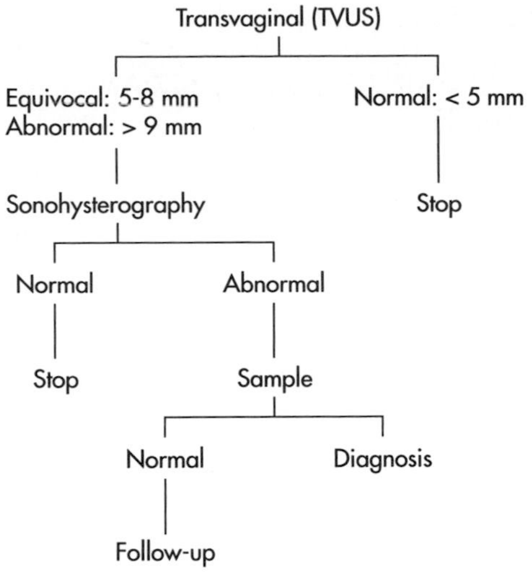

FIGURE 4-44

ENDOMETRIAL CARCINOMA

Adenocarcinoma. Risk factors (increased estrogen): nulliparity, failure of ovulation, obesity, late menopause.

Imaging Features

- Prominent, thick echogenic endometrium (usually cannot be differentiated from endometrial hyperplasia or polyps)
- Obstruction of internal os may result in:
  - Hydrometra
  - Pyometra
  - Hematometra
- Staging: (combined US and CT accuracy: 80%-90%)
  - Stages 1, 2: confined to uterus (tumor enhancement < myometrial enhancement)
  - Stages 3, 4: extrauterine
- MRI: variable appearance

CERVICAL CARCINOMA

Squamous cell carcinoma. Risk factors: condylomas, multiple sexual partners, sexually transmitted disease. Spread: local invasion of parametrium > lymph nodes > hematogenous spread.

Imaging Features

- Cervical stenosis with endometrial fluid collections (common)
- CT criteria for parametrial invasion (differentiates stage IIA from IIB, surgical vs. nonsurgical):
  - Irregular or poorly defined margins of lateral cervix
  - Prominent soft tissue stranding
  - Obliteration of periureteral fat plane
- Accuracy for detecting pelvic nodal metastases by CT: 65%
- MRI: tumor is high SI compared with hypointense cervical stroma:
  - FIGO stage 1B restricted to cervix; fully preserved hypointense rim of cervical stroma
  - Stage IIA invades upper two thirds of vagina; disruption of low SI vaginal wall
  - Stage IIB extends to parametrium; complete disruption of cervical stroma, irregularity or stranding within parametrial fat
- Staging
  - Stage IA: confined to cervix
  - Stage IB: may extend to uterus
  - Stage IIA: extension into upper vagina

CERVICAL CARCINOMA STAGING

	FIGO Staging	MRI Staging
0	Carcinoma in situ	Not visible
I	Confined to cervix	
	IA: Microscopic	
	IA-1: Stromal invasion <3 mm	No tumor visible
	IA-2: >3 mm, <5-mm invasion, <7-mm width	Small enhancing tumor may be seen
	IB: Clinically visible (>5 mm)	Tumor visible, intact stromal ring surrounding tumor
	IB-1: <4 cm	—
	IB-2: >4 cm	—
II	Extends beyond uterus but not to pelvic wall or lower one third of vagina	
	IIA: Vaginal extension, no parametrial invasion	Disruption of low-SI vaginal wall (upper two thirds)
	IIB: Parametrial invasion	Complete disruption of stromal ring with tumor extending into the parametrium
III	Extension to lower one third of vagina or pelvic wall invasion with hydronephrosis	
	IIIA: Extension to lower one third of vagina	Invasion of lower one third of vagina
	IIIB: Pelvic wall invasion with hydronephrosis	Extension to pelvic muscles or dilated ureter
IV	Located outside true pelvis	
	IVA: Bladder or rectal mucosa	Loss of low SI in bladder or rectal wall
	IVB: Distant metastasis	—

Stage IIB: parametrial involvement
Stage IIIA: extension into lower vagina
Stage IIIB: pelvic wall (hydronephrosis)
Stage IVA: spread to adjacent organs
Stage IVB: spread to distant organs

- Adenoma malignum: type of cervical carcinoma. Presents with water discharge; appears as cluster of Nabothian cysts but with enhancement, invasion, dissemination. Associated with Peutz-Jeghers syndrome and mucinous ovarian carcinoma. DDx: cystic endocervical hyperplasia.

FALLOPIAN TUBES

The normal fallopian tubes are not seen by TVUS (<4 mm). Visible fallopian tubes are always abnormal.

HYDROSALPINX (Fig. 4-45)

Causes

- PID
- Tumor
- Iatrogenic ligation
- Endometriosis

Imaging Features

- Convoluted cystic-appearing structure
- Echogenic wall
- Small polypoid excrescences along the wall
- Fluid-debris levels

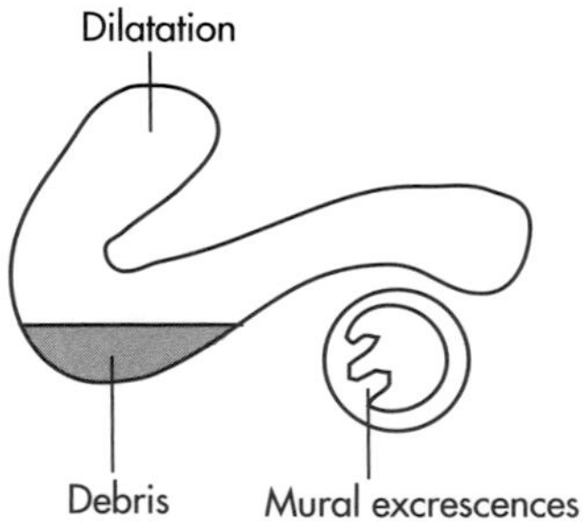

FIGURE 4-45

SALPINGITIS ISTHMICA NODOSA (SIN)

Diverticula-like invaginations of the epithelial lining herniating into myosalpinx. Unknown etiology. Frequently there is a history of prior PID. SIN indicates a 10-fold increase for ectopic pregnancy. DDx: TB.

OVARIES

CLASSIFICATION OF CYSTIC OVARIAN STRUCTURES

A small cystic ovarian structure should be considered normal (ovarian follicle) unless the patient is prepubertal, postmenopausal, or pregnant or the mean diameter is >25 mm (some authors use >20 mm). Types of cysts include:

Physiologic cysts (mean diameter <25 mm)
- Follicles
- Corpus luteum

Functional cysts (i.e., can produce hormones)
- Follicular cysts (estrogen), >25 mm
- Corpus luteum cysts (progesterone)
- Theca lutein cysts (gestational trophoblastic disease)
- Complications in functional cysts:
  - Hemorrhage
  - Enlargement
  - Rupture
  - Torsion

Other cysts
- Postmenopausal cysts (serous inclusion cysts)
- Polycystic ovaries
- Ovarian torsion
- Cystic tumors

FOLLICULAR CYSTS (Fig. 4-46)

When a mature follicle fails to involute, a follicular cyst (>2.5 cm in diameter) results.

Clinical Findings

- Asymptomatic (most common)
- Pain
- Hemorrhage
- Rupture

Imaging Features

- Usually anechoic, round, unilateral cyst ("simple cyst")
- If hemorrhage occurs, internal echoes are present.
- Size >25 mm at time of ovulation
- Usually resolve spontaneously (repeat US in 2 weeks [one-half cycle] or 6 weeks [one-and-one-half cycles] later)

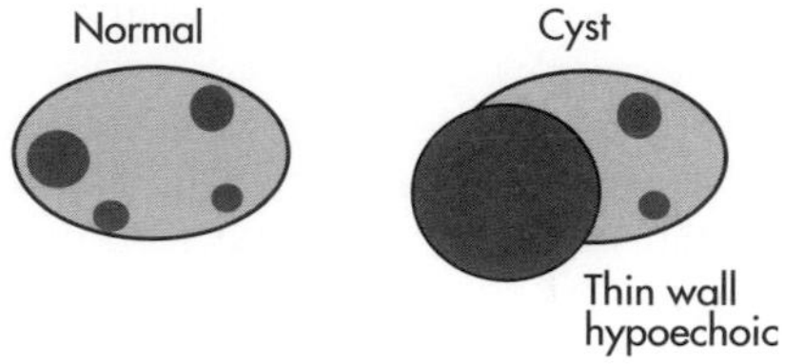

FIGURE 4-46

CORPUS LUTEUM CYST (CLC)

A corpus luteum cyst is a residual follicle after ovulation and normally involutes within 14 days. CLCs result from bleeding into or failed resorption of the corpus luteum. If an ovum is fertilized, the corpus luteum becomes the corpus luteum of pregnancy (maximum size at 8 to 10 weeks, resolves at 16 weeks).

Clinical Findings

- Pain
- More prone to hemorrhage and rupture

Imaging Features

- Unilateral, large lesions (5 to 10 cm)
- Hypoechoic with low-level echoes (hemorrhage)
- Usually resolve spontaneously
- Most common in first trimester of pregnancy

THECA LUTEIN CYSTS

These cysts develop in conditions with elevated β-HCG levels:

- Mole
- Choriocarcinoma
- Rh incompatibility (erythroblastosis fetalis)
- Twins
- Ovarian hyperstimulation syndrome

Imaging Features

- Largest of all ovarian cysts (may measure up to 20 cm)
- Usually bilateral and multilocular

PAROVARIAN CYSTS

Arise from embryonic remnants in the broad ligament. Relatively common (10% of all adnexal masses).

Imaging Features

- May undergo torsion and rupture
- Show no cyclic changes
- Specific diagnosis possible only if the ipsilateral ovary is demonstrated as separate structure

PERITONEAL INCLUSION CYSTS

These cysts represent nonneoplastic reactive mesothelial proliferations. Abnormal functioning ovaries and peritoneal adhesions are usually present. These cysts occur exclusively in premenopausal women with a history of previous abdominal surgery, trauma, PID, or endometriosis. Patients usually present with pelvic pain or mass.

Imaging Features

- Extraovarian location
- Spider web pattern (entrapped ovary): peritoneal adhesions extend to surface of ovary, distorting ovarian contour
- Oblong loculated collection, simulating hydrosalpinx or pyosalpinx
- Complex cystic appearance, simulating parovarian cyst
- Irregular thick septations accompanied by complex cystic mass, simulating ovarian neoplasm

OVARIAN REMNANT SYNDROME

Residual ovarian tissue after bilateral oophorectomy.

- Tissue left after surgery is hormonally stimulated.
- May result in functional hemorrhagic cysts
- Usually occurs after complicated pelvic surgeries

POSTMENOPAUSAL CYSTS

Postmenopausal cysts are not physiologic cysts, since there is not sufficient estrogen activity. Approach:

- TVUS should always be performed to determine that a cystic lesion is a simple, unilocular cyst. The incidence of malignancy in simple cysts <5 cm is low.
- Management:
  - <5 cm: US follow-up
  - >5 cm or change in size of smaller lesion: surgery
- Cysts that are not simple are considered neoplasms until proven otherwise.

POLYCYSTIC OVARIAN DISEASE (PCO, STEIN-LEVENTHAL SYNDROME)

PCO is a chronic anovulation syndrome presumably related to hypothalamic pituitary dysfunction. The diagnosis of PCO is made on the basis of clinical, biochemical, and sonographic findings; sonographic findings alone are nonspecific.

Clinical Findings

Triad of Stein-Leventhal syndrome

- Oligomenorrhea
- Hirsutism
- Obesity

Hormones

- Increased LH
- Increased LH/FSH ratio
- Increased androgens

Imaging Features (Fig. 4-47)

- Bilaterally enlarged ovaries with multiple small follicles, 50%

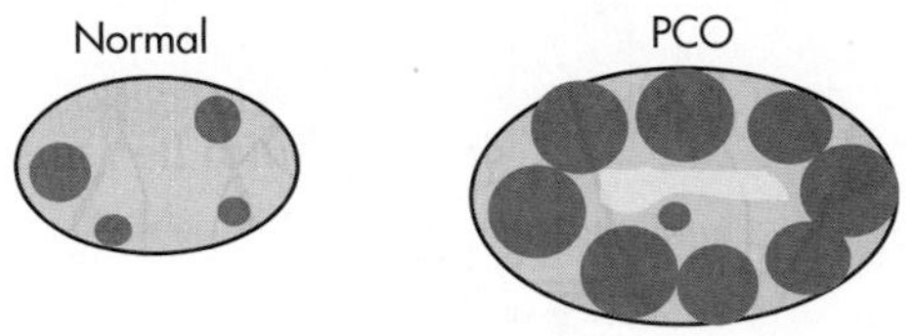

FIGURE 4-47

- Ovaries of similar size (key finding)
- >5 cysts, each of which is >5 mm
- Peripheral location of cysts
- Hyperechoic central stroma (fibrous tissue)
- Hypoechoic ovary without individual cysts, 25%
- Normal ovaries, 25%

ENDOMETRIOSIS

Ectopic endometrial tissue in ovary (endometrioma), fallopian tube, pelvis, colon, bladder, etc. Endometrial implants undergo cyclic changes, and hemorrhage occurs with subsequent local inflammation and adhesions.

MOST COMMON SITES FOR ENDOMETRIOTIC IMPLANTS AND ADHESIONS

Location	Implants (%)	Adhesions (%)
Ovaries	75	40
Anterior and posterior cul-de-sac	70	15
Posterior broad ligament	45	45
Uterosacral ligament	35	5
Uterus	10	5
Fallopian tubes	5	25
Sigmoid colon	5	10
Ureter	3	2
Small intestine	1	3

Types (Fig. 4-48)
- Diffuse peritoneal and ligamentous implants
- Endometrioma ("chocolate cyst")

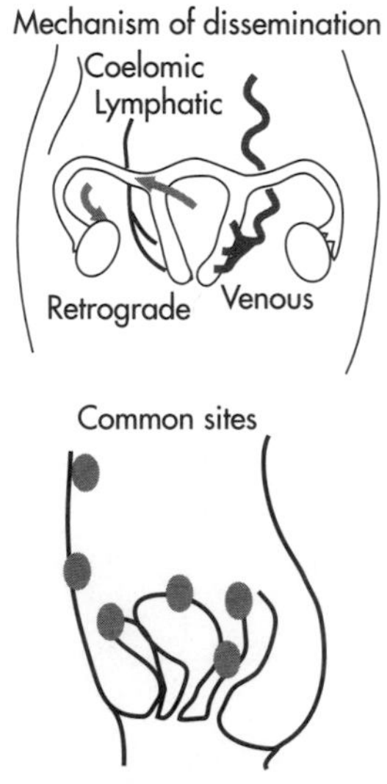

FIGURE 4-48

Imaging Features

Diffuse form
- Cannot be detected by US
- MRI may be useful.
- High SI on T1W and low SI on T2W (shading) are caused by the high iron content of endometrioma.

Endometrioma
- Cystic mass with low-level internal echoes
- May resemble a cystic neoplasm or hemorrhagic cyst

Uncommon manifestations
- Small bowel or colonic obstruction
- Bladder wall mass
- Anterior rectosigmoid abnormality
- Catamenial pneumothorax/hemothorax

OVARIAN TORSION

Often associated with neoplasm or cysts that act as lead points. Most common in children and adolescents. Extreme pain is usually the finding that makes one consider this diagnosis.

Imaging Features

- Enlarged ovary with multiple cortical follicles
- Color Doppler: absence of flow to affected ovary has been shown not to be diagnostic of ovarian torsion
- Fluid in cul-de-sac
- Nonspecific ovarian mass (common)
- CT: mass, inflammation, hydrosalpinx, hemoperitoneum, uterus deviated to side of torsion
- MRI: enlarged ovary with displaced follicles and low SI on T2W images due to interstitial hemorrhage. Peripheral enhancement may occur with gadolinium. Typical endometriomas and corpus luteum cysts do not have methemoglobin isolated to the rim and do not usually involve the entire ovary.

OVARIAN VEIN THROMBOSIS

Very rare cause of pulmonary thromboembolism. Right > left. Causes include:
- Infection (most common)
- Hypercoagulable states
- Delivery (especially cesarean section)

OVARIAN CANCER (Fig. 4-49)

Ovarian cancer (serous or mucinous cystadenocarcinoma) represents 25% of all gynecologic malignancies, with 20,000 new cases a year in the United States. Peak incidence is 6th decade. 65% of patients have distant metastases at time of diagnosis. Survival:
- Stage 1: 80%-90%
- Stage 2: 60%
- Stage 3-4: <20%

Types

OVARIAN NEOPLASIA

Type	Frequency	Example	US Pattern
Epithelial tumors (from surface epithelium that covers ovaries)	65%-75%	Serous or mucinous cystadenoma (carcinoma)	CCM
		Endometrioid carcinoma	CCM
		Clear cell carcinoma	CCM or SHM
		Brenner tumor	Small SHM
Germ cell tumors	15%	Dysgerminoma	SEM
		Embryonal cell cancer	CCM
		Choriocarcinoma	CCM
		Teratoma	Mixed (fat, cyst, calc)
		Yolk sac (endodermal sinus) tumor	SEM
Sex chord–stromal tumors	5%-10%	Granulosa cell tumor	CCM
		Sertoli-Leydig cell tumor	CCM
		Thecoma and fibroma	SHM
Metastatic tumors	10%	Primary uterine	
		Stomach, colon, breast	
		Lymphoma	

CCM, complex cystic mass; SEM, solid echogenic mass; SHM, solid hypoechoic mass.

BILATERAL OVARIAN TUMORS

	Serous Type	Mucinous Type
Benign cystadenoma	20% bilateral	5%bilateral
Malignant cystadenocarcinoma	50% bilateral	25% bilateral

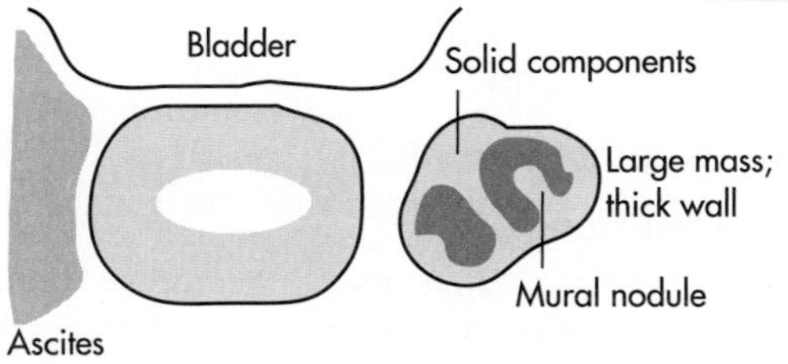

FIGURE 4-49

Risk Factors

- Family history
- Nulliparity
- High-fat diet, high-lactose diet

Screening

CA-125 serum markers
- Normal value is <35 U/mL.
- CA-125 is positive in 35% of patients with stage 1 ovarian cancer.
- CA-125 is positive in 80% of patients with advanced ovarian cancer.
- 85% of patients <50 years with elevated CA-125 have benign disease (PID, endometriosis, early pregnancy, and fibroids); that is, it is a useless screening test in patients under 50 years of age.
- More commonly elevated in patients with serous than mucinous tumors

Who should be screened:
- Patients with familial ovarian cancer; two types:
  - Hereditary ovarian cancer syndrome; autosomal dominant; 50% lifetime chance to get ovarian cancer → prophylactic oophorectomy
  - Familial history of ovarian cancer (first-degree relatives only); present in 7% of patients
- Screening of general population currently not recommended because of high-cost/low-benefit ratio (>$600,000 to detect one curable cancer)

Imaging Features

Adnexal mass
- Ovary
  - Premenopausal volume >18 cm^3 is abnormal
  - Postmenopausal volume >8 cm^3 is abnormal
- Findings suggestive of malignancy:
  - Thick, irregular walls
  - Septations >2 mm
  - Solid component
  - Size of cystic structure
    - <5 cm: 1% malignant
    - 5 to 10 cm: 6% malignant
    - >10 cm: 40% malignant
  - Ancillary features

Ascites
Hydronephrosis
Metastases to liver, peritoneal cavity, lymph nodes

Peritoneal cavity
- Implants in omentum (omental cake) and other peritoneal surfaces
- Pseudomyxoma peritonei represents intraperitoneal spread of mucin-secreting tumor that fills the peritoneal cavity with gelatinous material (sonographic appearance similar to ascites with low-level echoes).

Staging
- Stage 1: limited to ovary
- Stage 2: both ovaries involved ± ascites
- Stage 3: intraperitoneal metastases
- Stage 4: metastases outside peritoneal cavity

Tumor vascularity (Doppler) (Fig. 4-50)
- Need both criteria to diagnose malignancy:
  - High peak systolic velocity (>25 cm/sec)
  - Low-impedance diastolic flow
- Malignant tumors: resistive index (RI) <0.4, pulsatility index (PI) <1
- Tumor flow may be indistinguishable from normal luteal flow (repeat US within 14 days to differentiate)
- Problems:
  - Overlap in Doppler findings occurs between benign and malignant tumors.
  - Optimum cutoff value for malignant tumors has not been determined.

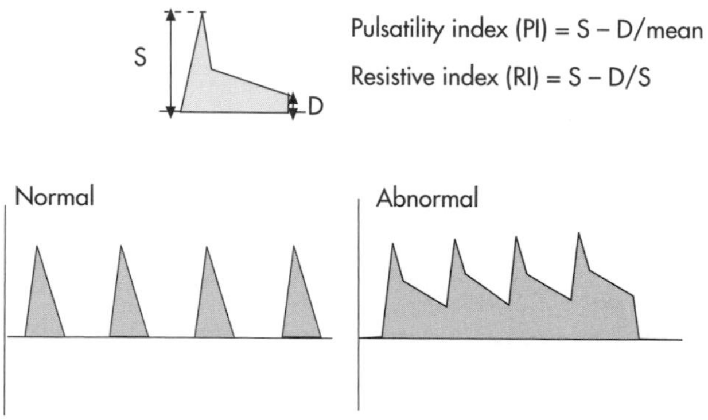

FIGURE 4-50

DERMOID, TERATOMA

GERM CELL TUMOR SPECTRUM

Tumor	Origin	Content
Teratoma	Ectoderm + mesoderm + endoderm	Any tissue element*
Dermoid	Ectoderm	Hair, teeth, sebaceous glands
Epidermoid	Only epidermis	Secretes watery fluid; not a true tumor (CNS)

*Fat (echogenic), pancreas, muscle, calcification, teeth, thyroid, etc.

Imaging Features of Dermoid

US
- Echogenic mass with acoustic shadowing
- May contain solid (isoechoic) and cystic (anechoic) components

CT
- Fatty mass with low HU
- Fat-fluid level
- Calcifications: tooth, rim calcification

MRI
- Protons from fat rotate near the Larmor frequency and are therefore very efficient T1-relaxation enhancers, which results in the high SI on T1W images seen with most ovarian dermoids and teratomas. Presence of fat within these masses is also the cause of chemical shift misregistration artifact in the frequency-encoding direction seen on SE images. The artifact occurs as a low SI boundary at the fat-water interface. Prefat and postfat saturation sequences may also help in identifying the fat.

Pearls
- Dermoids are common tumors in reproductive years.
- Bilateral, 10%.
- In the pelvis, dermoids have incorrectly been classified as cystic teratomas.
- Struma ovarii is a teratoma in which thyroid tissue predominates.
- Rokitansky nodule: raised protuberance, containing hair, bone, teeth

OTHER OVARIAN TUMORS

Dysgerminoma

5% of all ovarian neoplasms. These tumors are morphologically similar to seminomas in testes and germinomas in pineal glands. Highly radiosensitive. 5-year survival, 80%. Peak incidence <30 years.

Yolk Sac Tumors

Rare, highly malignant. Peak incidence <20 years. Increased α-fetoprotein (AFP) levels.

Endometrioid Tumor

Bilateral in 30%-50%. Histologically similar to endometrial cancer. 30% of patients have concomitant endometrial adenocarcinoma.

Clear Cell Carcinoma

Müllerian duct origin. 40% bilateral.

Brenner Tumor

Also know as transitional cell tumor. Rare and almost always benign. Usually discovered incidentally. Patients are typically asymptomatic. Solid fibrous tumors. Associated with cystadenomas or cystic teratoma in ipsilateral ovary in 30%. The high fibrous content accounts for the low SI on T2W images on MRI.

Granulosa Cell Tumors (Estrogen)

2% of ovarian neoplasms; low malignant potential, most common estrogen active tumor; 95% bilateral. Can have associated endometrial hyperplasia, polyps, or in 25% of cases endometrial carcinoma. The adult form (95% of tumors) manifests in postmenopausal women with irregular bleeding secondary to elevated estrogen levels. Juvenile form manifests in children or adolescents with pseudoprecocious puberty. May be solid or cystic on MR often with foci of T1 bright signal secondary to hemorrhagic cysts. Spongelike appearance on T2-weighted images is very specific.

Sertoli-Leydig Cell Tumors

Less than 0.5% of ovarian neoplasms. Majority are androgen secreting. Occurs in women younger than 30 years and is the most common ovarian neoplasm associated with virilization. Almost always unilateral. 15% are malignant.

Thecoma, Fibroma

Both tumors arise from ovarian stroma and typically occur in postmenopausal women:

- Thecoma: predominantly thecal cells; 1% of ovarian neoplasms
- Fibroma: predominantly fibrous tissue; 4% of ovarian neoplasms. Ascites and pleural effusions (Meigs syndrome) are present in 50% of patients with fibromas >5 cm. A widened endometrial stripe accompanied by an ovarian mass with low SI on T2W images can suggest a diagnosis of functional fibrothecoma with endometrial hyperplasia. The MR imaging appearance of fibroma and thecomas are similar; intermediate signal intensity on T1-weighted images and low signal intensity on T2-weighted images. Difficult to differentiate from pedunculated leiomyomas or Brenner tumors.

Krukenberg Tumor

Ovarian metastases result from stomach or colon primary tumor (signet ring cell types).

Meigs Syndrome

Pleural effusion and ascites from fibroma (original description) or other ovarian tumors and metastases (more recent use of terminology).

Pearls

- The approach to unilocular cysts depends on the age of the patient: in younger patients they are usually functional cysts, which may be hormonally active; in older women a cystic neoplasm is more common.
- A complex adnexal mass in a young woman usually represents a hemorrhagic cyst, endometrioma, tuboovarian abscess (TOA), or ectopic pregnancy; clinical setting helps to differentiate causes.
- Dermoids are the most common ovarian tumors in young women (<30 years). Tumors are often partially cystic and contain fat or calcium.

INFERTILITY

GENERAL

Affects 15% of couples. In most infertility programs, the current success rates of achieving a normal pregnancy are 10%-20%. The major causes (anatomic, functional) of infertility are:

Female (70%)

- Ovulatory dysfunction (hypothalamic-pituitary-ovarian axis), 25%
- Mechanical tubal problems, 25%
- Endometriosis, 40%
- Inadequate cervical mucus (poor estrogen response), 5%
- Luteal phase defects (poor progesterone response), 5%

Male (30%)

- Impotence
- Oligospermia, aspermia (many causes, including varicocele)
- Sperm dysfunction

Role of Ultrasound

- Monitor response to hormonal stimulation
- Percutaneous retrieval of mature oocytes
- Determine mechanical cause of infertility

Sonographic Signs During Menstrual Cycle

First part of cycle

- Early, several 5-mm cysts are seen; these cysts grow to 10 mm.
- Dominant follicle (>14 mm) can usually be identified from 8th to 12th day; follicles typically measure 18 to 28 mm.
- Follicles <15 mm usually do not develop to pregnancy.
- 5%-10% of patients have >2 dominant follicles.

Signs of impending (within 24 hours) ovulation (generally unreliable)

- Thickening and lack of distinction of follicular lining
- Thin hypoechoic layer surrounds follicle
- Folding in granulosa cell layer (crenation)

Signs of ovulation (generally reliable)

- Disappearance of follicle
- Collapsed follicle
- Follicle filled with low-level echoes
- Fluid in cul-de-sac

DRUG TREATMENT FOR OVULATION INDUCTION (Fig. 4-51)

Human Chorionic Gonadotropin

Used to induce ovulation once follicular development is complete. HCG has a biologic effect similar to LH but a longer blood half-life. Ovulation occurs 36 hours after administration of 10,000 IU (as opposed to 24 hours after LH).

Clomiphene Citrate (Clomid)

Nonsteroidal, synthetic weak estrogen agonist that binds to estrogen receptors in hypothalamus. Hypothalamus then releases GnRH, which produces FSH and LH. Requires an intact hypothalamic-pituitary-ovarian axis.

Pergonal

Used if clomiphene (Clomid) is not successful after 3 or 4 cycles. Pergonal contains human menopausal gonadotropins: 75% FSH and 25% LH. Used in conjunction with β-HCG to cause oocyte maturation and to trigger ovulation.

Leuprolide Acetate (Lupron)

GnRH analog used to shut off the hypothalamic-pituitary-gonadal axis. Used in conjunction with Pergonal to manage ovarian stimulation and ovulation.

Urofollitropin (Metrodin)

Pure FSH, an alternative/additive to Pergonal therapy. Originally used in patients with PCO and excess of LH.

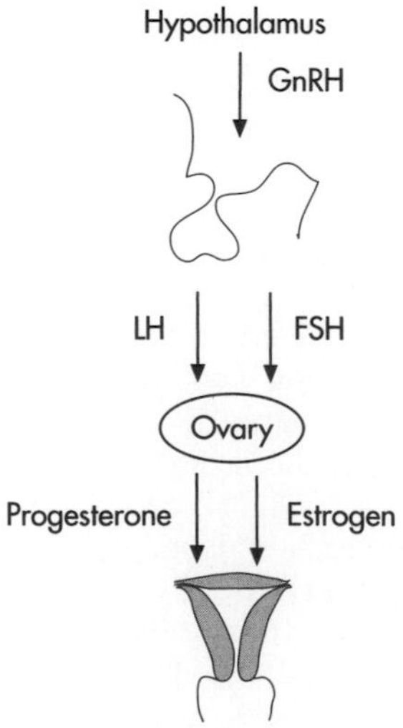

FIGURE 4-51

PROTOCOLS

Baseline US

- Use transabdominal ultrasound (TAS) and TVS.
- Perform on day 8.
- Exclude endometriosis, fibroids, parovarian cysts, hydrosalpinx, and unruptured cysts.

Subsequent Scans

- Performed daily with estrogen level determination (400 to 500 pg/mL per ovulatory follicle suggests oocyte maturity). US is useful to determine whether elevated estrogen levels are due to one large follicle or numerous small follicles.
- Growth rate of follicles is 1 to 2 mm/day.
- Measurement of follicular diameter (>18 mm) is used to time β-HCG administration.
- Determine endometrial thickness.

COMPLICATIONS OF HORMONAL TREATMENT

Ovarian Hyperstimulation

- Occurs in up to 40% of cycles
- May be due to fertility medications or pituitary adenoma (Brain MRI)
- Ovaries enlarge and contain multiple large lutein cysts; more commonly seen with Pergonal than with clomiphene therapy.
- Typically begins 3 to 10 days after β-HCG administration
- May last for 6 to 8 weeks
- Symptoms: lower abdominal pain, weight gain, ascites
- Complications: DIC; ascites, pericardial, pleural effusions, ectopic pregnancy, torsion, hemorrhage, DVT, PE, renal failure, hypotension, death

Multiple Pregnancies

Rate of multiple pregnancies is 25%.

OTHER

NORMAL PELVIC FLOOR ANATOMY

The female pelvic floor can be divided into three compartments, each supported by the endopelvic fascia and the levator ani muscle:

- Anterior containing the bladder and urethra
- Middle containing the vagina
- Posterior containing the rectum

The levator ani muscle complex consists of three muscle groups:

- Iliococcygeal muscle, which arises from the junction of the arcus tendineus fascia pelvis and the fascia of the internal obturator muscle

- Pubococcygeal muscle, which arises from the superior ramus of the pubis
- Puborectalis muscle, which arises from the superior and inferior pubic rami

In healthy women at rest, the levator ani muscles are in contraction, thereby keeping the rectum, vagina, and urethra elevated and closed by pressing them anteriorly toward the pubic symphysis. The components of the levator ani muscles are clearly seen on T2W MR images.

PELVIC FLOOR PROLAPSE

- Results from specific defects in the endopelvic fascia and may involve the urethra, bladder, vaginal vault, rectum, and small bowel (typically multiple)
- Patients present with pain, pressure, urinary and fecal incontinence, constipation, urinary retention, and defecatory dysfunction.
- Diagnosis is made primarily on the basis of findings at physical pelvic examination.
- Imaging is useful in patients in whom findings at physical examination are equivocal.
- Fluoroscopy, US, and MRI have been used for diagnosis, with MRI currently favored.

MRI Interpretation (Fig. 4-52)

- In healthy women, there is minimal movement of pelvic organs, even with maximal strain.
- Floor laxity: organ descent of 1 to 2 cm below the pubococcygeal line. Both H and M lines become elongated with Valsalva maneuver. $\Delta M > 1$ cm, $\Delta H > 1$ cm.
- Prolapse requiring surgical intervention: organ descent below the H line
- Enterocele: descent of small bowel >2 cm between vagina and rectum
- Anterior rectocele: anterior bulging of rectum
- Cystocele: bladder below H line

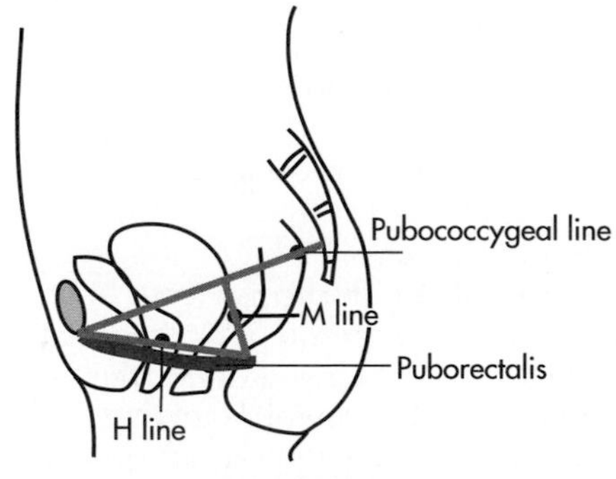

FIGURE 4-52

Differential Diagnosis

KIDNEYS

RENAL MASS LESIONS (Fig. 4-53)

Tumor
- Solid
- Cyst

Infection
- Lobar nephronia
- Abscess
- XGP

Congenital
- Duplicated collecting system
- Pseudotumors
  - Fetal lobulation
  - Dromedary hump
  - Column of Bertin
  - Suprahilar (less commonly infrahilar) "bump"
  - Lobar dysmorphism: doughnut sign on IVP or angiography

Trauma
- Hematoma

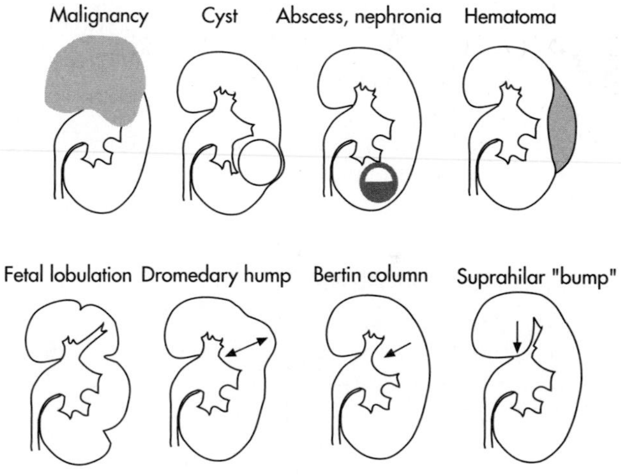

FIGURE 4-53

SOLID RENAL NEOPLASM

- RCC
- Wilms tumor
- Oncocytoma
- Adenoma
- Angiomyolipoma (fat density, hamartoma)
- Transitional cell carcinoma of the renal pelvis or calyces
- Metastases (multiple): lung, colon, melanoma, RCC
- Lymphoma

DIFFERENTIAL DIAGNOSIS OF RENAL MASSES BY LOCATION

Location	Intrarenal	<50% Protrusion	>50% Protrusion	In Collecting System
	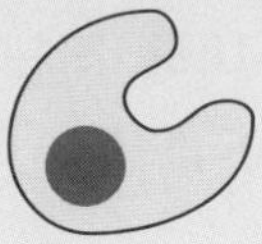	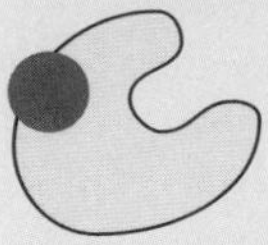	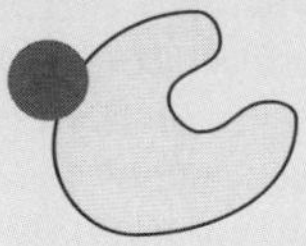	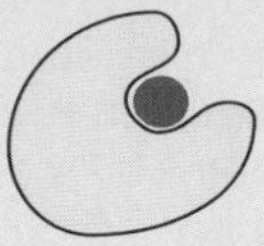
RCC	15%	15%	65%	5%
Metastases	55%	20%	25%	<5%
Renal TCC	80%	0%	0%	20%

CYSTIC RENAL MASSES

Tumors
- Cystic/necrotic RCC
- Multilocular RCC
- Cystic Wilms tumor

True cysts
- Cortical cysts
- Localized cystic disease
- Medullary cystic disease
- Adult polycystic kidney disease
- Cysts in systemic disease: VHL, tuberous sclerosis
- End-stage renal failure
- Infectious cysts

Other (use Doppler or color US for differentiation)
- Hydronephrosis/duplicated system
- Renal artery aneurysm
- Abscess

HYPERECHOIC RENAL MASS

- Angiomyolipoma
- RCC (the larger, the more likely to be hyperechoic)
- Milk of calcium cyst
- Nephritis
  - XGP
  - Emphysematous pyelonephritis
  - Focal nephritis
  - Candidiasis
- Hematoma
- Infarction
- Lesions that mimic true hyperechoic masses
  - Renal sinus fat
  - Duplicated collecting system

RENAL SINUS MASS

Tumors
- TCC
- RCC
- Lymphoma
- Bellini duct carcinoma

Other
- Renal artery aneurysm
- Renal sinus hemorrhage
- Complicated parapelvic cyst

WEDGE-SHAPED RENAL LESION

- Renal metastasis
- Infarction
- Lobar nephritis

MASSES IN THE PERINEPHRIC SPACE

- Renal cell carcinoma: perinephric pattern of spread is uncommon unless in bulky tumors
- Perinephric lymphoma: homogeneous, hypovascular, mildly enhancing, and associated with nonobstructive encasement of retroperitoneal vessels
- Posttransplantation lymphoproliferative disorder (PTD): lymphoma-like condition associated with Epstein-Barr virus infection; occurs in 2% of the recipients of solid-organ transplants. Often occurs in renal hilum; contrast enhancement is minimal.
- Retroperitoneal tumors (sarcomas, multiple myelomas, Castleman disease tumor) may involve the perinephric space by direct contiguous extension from retroperitoneum.
- Spontaneous (nontraumatic) perinephric hematomas arise from angiomyolipoma, renal cell carcinoma, polycystic kidney disease, and bleeding diathesis.
- Perinephric urinomas: obstructive forniceal rupture or trauma
- Perinephric abscess
- Renal lymphangiomatosis: rare benign malformation of the perinephric lymphatic system resulting in characteristic unilocular or multilocular thin-walled perinephric cysts
- Extramedullary hematopoiesis: seen in chronic anemia, blood dyscrasias such as leukemia, and

replacement of the normal bone marrow by tumor or bone overgrowth

- Retroperitoneal fibrosis: perinephric involvement rarely seen in isolation
- Rosai-Dorfman disease (sinus histiocytosis with massive lymphadenopathy): benign systemic histiocytic proliferative disorder; infiltrative hypodensity at the periphery of the kidney as a result of the accumulation of histiocytes with the imaging findings suggestive of a subcapsular rather than a perinephric process
- Erdheim-Chester disease (lipoid granulomatosis): progressive multisystem disorder characterized radiologically by bilateral symmetric medullary osteosclerosis with cortical thickening of long tubular bones, sparing the axial skeleton. Retroperitoneal and perinephric infiltration may occur.
- Renal cortical necrosis: destruction of the renal cortex with sparing of the renal medulla. In the acute setting, CT shows nonenhancement of the renal cortex, with the exception of a thin subcapsular rim, and normal medullary enhancement.
- Nephroblastomatosis: multiple well-defined round or ovoid foci in the periphery of the renal cortex
- Neurofibromatosis: may occasionally present as subcapsular masses

DIFFUSELY HYPERECHOIC KIDNEYS

- Inflammation
  - Glomerulonephritis
  - Glomerulosclerosis: HTN, DM
  - AIDS-related nephropathy
  - Interstitial nephritis: systemic lupus erythematosus (SLE), vasculitis
- Acute tubular necrosis
- Hemolytic uremic syndrome
- Multiple myeloma
- End-stage renal disease
- Medullary or cortical nephrocalcinosis
- Infantile polycystic kidney disease

RENAL CALCIFICATIONS

Tumors
- Cysts
- RCC

Infection
- Tuberculosis

"Metastatic" calcification
- Medullary nephrocalcinosis
- Cortical nephrocalcinosis

Collecting system
- Calculi

FAT IN KIDNEY

- Angiomyolipoma
- Lipoma
- Replacement lipomatosis

RENAL HEMORRHAGE

- Angiomyolipoma
- RCC
- Vasculitis (e.g., polyarteritis nodosa)
- Trauma

HYPOECHOIC PERIRENAL FAT

- Normal variant (in 10% of asymptomatic renal allografts)
- Perirenal hemorrhage (trauma, anticoagulants, adrenal hemorrhage)
- Cyst rupture
- SLE
- Polyarteritis nodosa

FILLING DEFECT IN COLLECTING SYSTEM (Fig. 4-54)

Tumor
- TCC
- Papilloma
- Leukoplakia, malacoplakia

Mobile filling defect
- Blood clot
- Sloughed papilla
- Calculus
- Fungus ball

Other
- Vascular impression, collateral vessels
- Artificial overlying bowel gas shadows mimicking filling defect

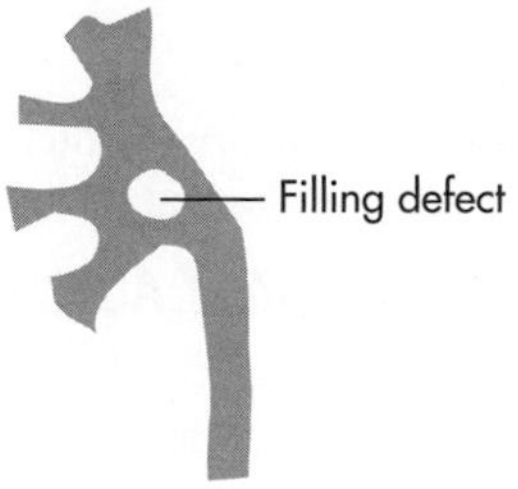

FIGURE 4-54

PAPILLARY NECROSIS (Fig. 4-55)

Mnemonic: "POSTCARD":
- **P**yelonephritis
- **O**bstruction (chronic)
- **S**ickle cell disease
- **T**B
- **C**irrhosis, ethanol
- **A**nalgesics: phenacetin
- **R**enal vein thrombosis
- **D**iabetes

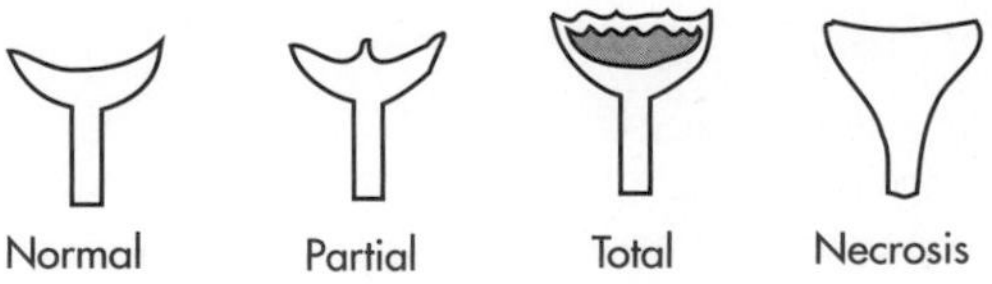

FIGURE 4-55

Unilateral:
- Pyelonephritis
- Obstruction
- TB
- Renal vein thrombosis

Bilateral:
- Sickle cell disease
- Cirrhosis, ethanol
- Diabetes

DELAYED (PERSISTENT) NEPHROGRAM (SAME DIFFERENTIAL DIAGNOSIS AS RENAL FAILURE)

Prerenal causes (15%)
- Renal artery stenosis
- Hypotension

Renal causes (70%)
- Acute glomerulonephritis
- Acute tubular necrosis: radiographic iodinated contrast agents, antibiotics, anesthesia, ischemia, transplants
- Acute cortical necrosis: pregnancy related, 70%; sepsis; dehydration
- Tubular precipitation: uric acid, hemolysis, myeloma
- Acute interstitial nephritis: antibiotics
- Papillary necrosis: analgesic, sickle cell, DM
- Renal vein thrombosis

Postrenal causes (15%)
- Obstruction: stone, stricture

Rule of thumb
- Symmetrical, bilateral: medical disease
- Asymmetrical, unilateral: surgical disease

EXTRACALYCEAL CONTRAST AGENT (Fig. 4-56)

Striations
- Medullary sponge kidney
- Early papillary necrosis

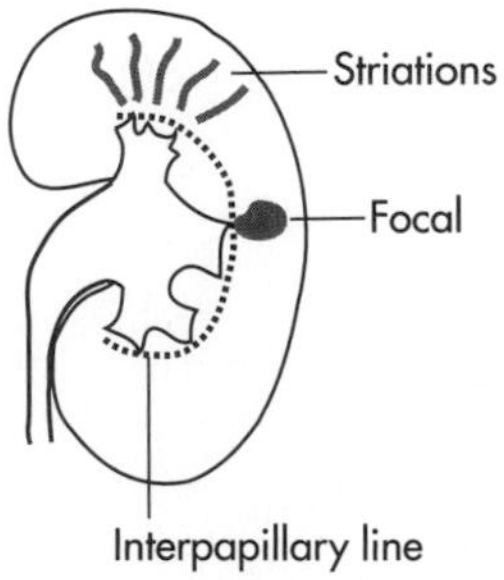

FIGURE 4-56

- Pyelosinus or pyelovenous backflow in obstruction
- Interstitial edema

Focal collections
- Late papillary necrosis
- Calyceal diverticulum
- Cavity from cyst rupture
- Abscess

DILATED CALYCES/COLLECTING SYSTEM (Fig. 4-57)

- Obstruction (calculi, tumor, acute, chronic)
- Papillary necrosis
- Congenital megacalyces
- Calyceal diverticulum
- Reflux

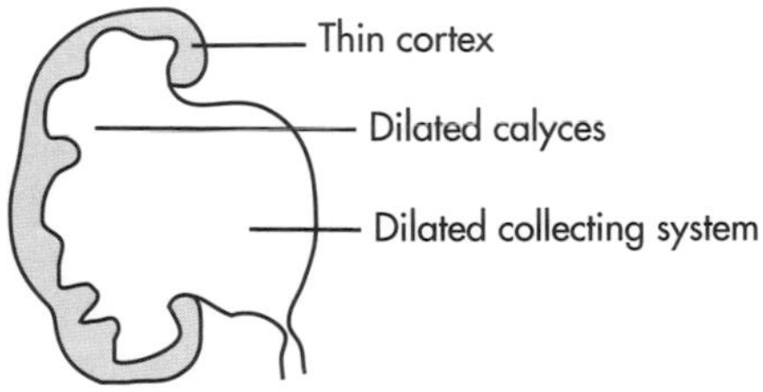

FIGURE 4-57

BILATERALLY ENLARGED KIDNEYS

Tumor
- Cystic disease (APCKD)
- Malignancy
  - Leukemia
  - Lymphoma
  - Multiple myeloma (protein deposition)

Inflammation (acute)
- Glomerulonephritis
- Interstitial nephritis
- Collagen vascular disease
- ATN

Metabolic
- Amyloid
- Diabetes mellitus
- Storage diseases, acromegaly

Vascular
- Bilateral renal vein thrombosis

BILATERALLY SMALL KIDNEYS

- Chronic inflammation: pyelonephritis, glomerulonephritis, interstitial nephritis
- Bilateral renal artery stenosis
- Reflux (chronic infection)

HYPERCALCEMIA

Mnemonic: "PAM SCHMIDT:"
- **P**arathyroid adenoma, hyperplasia
- **A**ddison disease

- **M**ilk alkali syndrome
- **S**arcoid
- **C**arcinomatosis
- **H**yperparathyroidism, secondary
- **M**yeloma
- **I**mmobilization
- **D** vitamin
- **T**hiazides

RENAL VEIN THROMBOSIS (RVT)

Acute thrombosis causes renal enlargement (congestion, hemorrhage). Chronic thrombosis results in small kidneys (infarction).

Causes

Tumor
- RCC (10% of patients have thrombosis)
- Other renal tumors (lymphoma, TCC, Wilms tumor)
- Adrenal tumors
- Gonadal tumors
- Pancreatic carcinoma
- Extraluminal compression of renal vein by retroperitoneal tumors

Renal disease (often with nephrotic syndrome)
- Membranous glomerulonephritis
- SLE
- Amyloidosis

Other
- Hypercoagulable states
- Extension of ovarian vein, IVC thrombosis
- Trauma, surgery
- Transplant rejection

URETER

DILATED URETER

Criteria: >8 mm, ureter visible in entire length, no peristaltic waves. Differentiation between mechanical obstruction and dilatation is possible by performing a Whitaker test or furosemide scintigraphy.

Obstruction
- Functional: primary megaureter
- Mechanical stenosis
    - Ureteral stricture
    - Bladder outlet obstruction
    - Urethral stricture

Reflux

Other
- Diuresis (e.g., furosemide, diabetes insipidus)

URETERAL STRICTURE

Wide differential (mnemonic: "TIC MTV"). Use IVP/retrograde pyelography to determine if there is a mass or a stricture and how long the narrowing is. CT/IVP (IVP reconstructed from CT) now combined.

- **T**umor
    - TCC
    - Metastases
    - Lymphadenopathy
- **I**nflammatory
    - TB (corkscrew appearance)
    - Schistosomiasis
    - Pelvic disease
        - Crohn disease
        - Pelvic inflammatory disease
- **C**ongenital
    - Ectopic ureterocele
    - Primary megaureter
    - Congenital stenosis
- **M**etabolic, drugs
    - Morphine
    - Methysergide: retroperitoneal fibrosis
- **T**rauma
    - Iatrogenic
    - Radiation
- **V**ascular
    - Aortic, iliac artery aneurysm
    - Ovarian vein syndrome
    - Lymphocele

MULTIPLE URETERAL FILLING DEFECTS (Fig. 4-58)

Wall
- Ureteritis cystica (more common in upper ureter)
- Allergic mucosal bullae
- Pseudodiverticulosis
- Vascular impressions (collateral veins in IVC obstruction)
- Multiple papillomas (more common in lower ureter)
- Melanoma metastases
- Suburothelial hemorrhage (less discrete than ureteritis cystica and associated with a coagulopathy)

Luminal
- Calculi (lucent, opaque)
- Blood clot

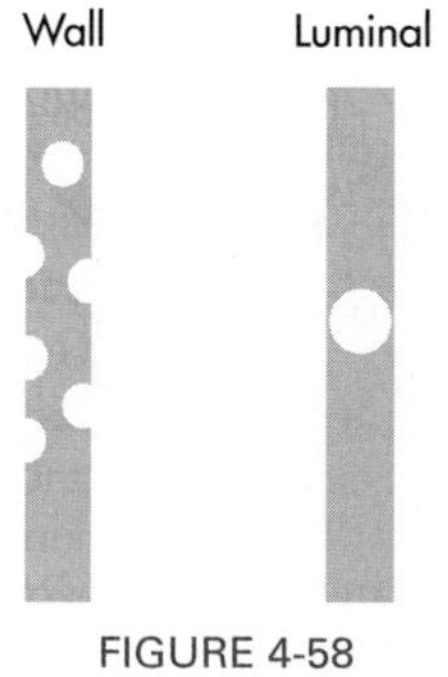

FIGURE 4-58

- Sloughed papillae
- Fungus ball
- Air bubbles

URETERAL DIVERTICULA (Fig. 4-59)

- Congenital
- Ureteritis cystica
- TB (also strictures)

DEVIATED URETERS

Normal ureters project over the transverse processes of the vertebral bodies.

Deviations occur laterally or medially.

Lateral Deviation

- Bulky retroperitoneal adenopathy
- Primary retroperitoneal tumors
- Aortic aneurysm
- Retroperitoneal fluid collection
- Malrotated kidney
- Ovarian/uterine masses

Medial Deviation

- Posterior bladder diverticulum (most common cause of distal medial deviation)
- Uterine fibroids
- Retroperitoneal fibrosis; associated with:
  - Aortic aneurysm: chronic leakage?
  - Methysergide/ergots
  - Idiopathic
  - Malignancy-related
- Postoperative (node dissection)
- Enlarged prostate (J-shaped ureter)
- Retrocaval ureter (only on right side)

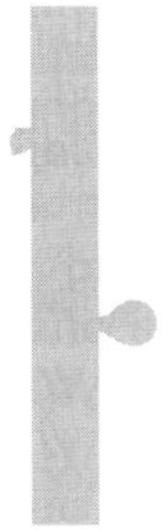

FIGURE 4-59

BLADDER

BLADDER WALL THICKENING (Fig. 4-60)

Criteria when distended: >5 mm, trabeculations, small bladder.

Tumor
- TCC
- Lymphoma

Inflammation
- Radiation cystitis
- Infectious cystitis
- Inflammatory bowel disease, appendicitis, focal diverticulitis

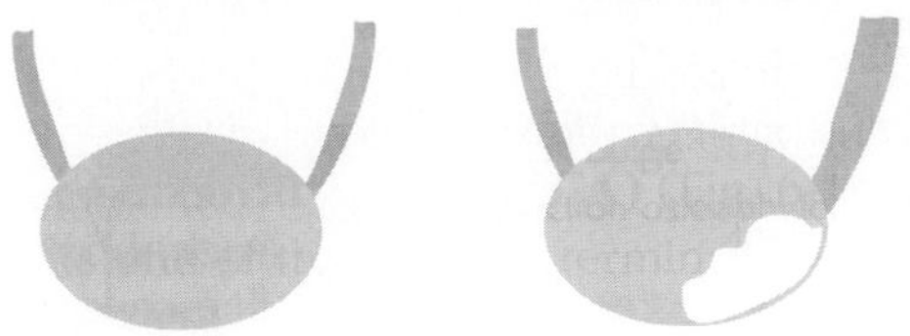

FIGURE 4-60

Outlet obstruction
- Benign prostatic hyperplasia
- Urethral stricture

Neurogenic

BLADDER FILLING DEFECT

Tumor
- Primary: TCC, SCC
- Metastases
- Endometriosis
- Polyps

Infection
- PID
- Parasitic infection: schistosomiasis
- Related to infection:
  - Leukoplakia, malacoplakia
  - Cystitis cystica, cystitis glandularis

Luminal
- Calculi
- Blood clot
- Foreign bodies
- BPH

BLADDER NEOPLASM

Primary
- TCC
- SCC
- Adenocarcinoma
- Pheochromocytoma from bladder wall paraganglia (10% are malignant)
- Rare tumors: rhabdomyosarcoma, leiomyosarcoma, primary lymphoma

Secondary
- Metastases
  - Hematogenous: melanoma > stomach > breast
  - Direct extension: prostate, uterus, colon
- Lymphoma

BLADDER CALCULI

- Chronic bacterial infection, 30%
- Chronic bladder catheterization (struvite stones)
- Bladder outlet obstruction, 70%
- Schistosomiasis
- Renal calculi (usually pass through urethra)

BLADDER WALL CALCIFICATION

Requires cystoscopy and biopsy
Mnemonic: "SCRITT:"

- **S**chistosomiasis
- **C**yclophosphamide (Cytoxan)
- **R**adiation
- **I**nterstitial cystitis
- **T**B
- **T**CC

AIR IN BLADDER

- Instrumentation, catheter
- Bladder fistula: diverticulitis, Crohn disease, colon carcinoma
- Emphysematous cystitis in patients with diabetes

TEARDROP BLADDER (Fig. 4-61)

Criteria: Pear-shaped or teardrop-shaped contrast-filled bladder:
circumferential extrinsic compression

Physiologic
- Normal variant
- Iliopsoas hypertrophy

Fluid
- Hematoma (usually from pelvic fracture)
- Abscess

Masses
- Pelvic lymphoma
- Pelvic lipomatosis (black males, hypertension)
- Retroperitoneal fibrosis

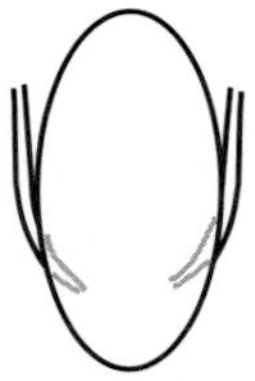

FIGURE 4-61

THE "FEMALE PROSTATE"

Criteria: Central filling defect at base of bladder in female patients

- Urethral diverticulum
- Urethral tumor
- Periurethritis
- Pubic bone lesion

ADRENAL GLANDS

ADRENAL MASSES

Tumor
- Adenoma, 50%
- Metastases, 30%
- Pheochromocytoma, 10%
- Lymphoma
- Neuroblastoma if <2 years
- Fatty lesions
  - Myelolipoma
  - Lipoma
- Cystic tumors
  - Simple cyst, 10%
  - Pseudocyst after previous hemorrhage

Other lesions
- Hemorrhage
- TB
- Wolman disease (acid cholesteryl ester hydrolase deficiency, very rare)

Cystic Masses

- Lymphangioma
- Hemangioma
- Epithelial cyst
- Adenoma, pheochromocytoma, metastasis
- Hemorrhage

Bilateral Masses

- Metastases
- Lymphoma
- Bilateral pheochromocytoma in:
  - MEN type II
  - VHL
  - Neurofibromatosis
- Granulomatous masses: TB, histoplasmosis

ADRENAL CALCIFICATIONS

- Tumor: neuroblastoma, pheochromocytoma
- Infection: TB, histoplasmosis, Waterhouse-Friderichsen syndrome
- Trauma: hemorrhage
- Congenital: Wolman disease

ADRENAL PSEUDOTUMORS

Criteria: soft tissue density in location of adrenal glands on plain films of abdomen

- Gastric fundus
- Accessory spleen
- Retroperitoneal varices
- Other lesions
  - Liver mass
  - Gallbladder mass
  - Renal mass

Adrenal pseudotumor by CT
- Gastric fundus or fundal diverticulum
- Varices
- Tortuous splenic artery
- Pancreatic tail
- Medial splenic lobulation

TESTES

SOLID TESTICULAR MASSES

Tumor
- Primary: germinal, 95%; nongerminal, 5%
- Metastases: prostate, kidney, leukemia, lymphoma

Infection
- Orchitis
- Abscess
- Granuloma

Trauma: fracture, rupture, hemorrhage, torsion

Other
- Atrophy
- Dilated rete testes

EXTRATESTICULAR ABNORMALITIES

- Epididymitis, diffuse or focal
- Spermatocele, epididymal cyst
- Hydrocele, hematocele, varicocele
- Tunical or mesothelial cyst
- Paratesticular hemorrhage, abscess
- Hernia
- Scrotal pearl
- Neoplasm (primary or metastatic)
  Benign: adenomatoid tumor, fibroma, leiomyoma
  Malignant: mesothelioma, sarcoma

EPIDIDYMAL MASS

- Focal epididymitis
- Adenomatoid tumor
- Embryonal rhabdomyosarcoma in children

PROSTATE

CYSTIC LESIONS (Fig. 4-62)

- Utricle cyst: Midline, intraprostatic, may communicate with posterior urethra and contain sperm, hypospadia
- Müllerian duct cyst: Midline, may rise above prostate, stones
- Cowper's duct cyst
- Ejaculatory duct cyst
- Prostatic retention cyst
- Seminal vesicle cyst
- Vas deferens cyst

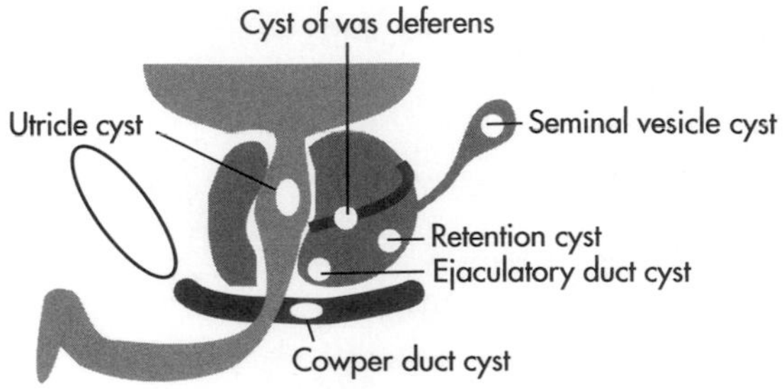

FIGURE 4-62

FEMALE PELVIS

APPROACH (Fig. 4-63)

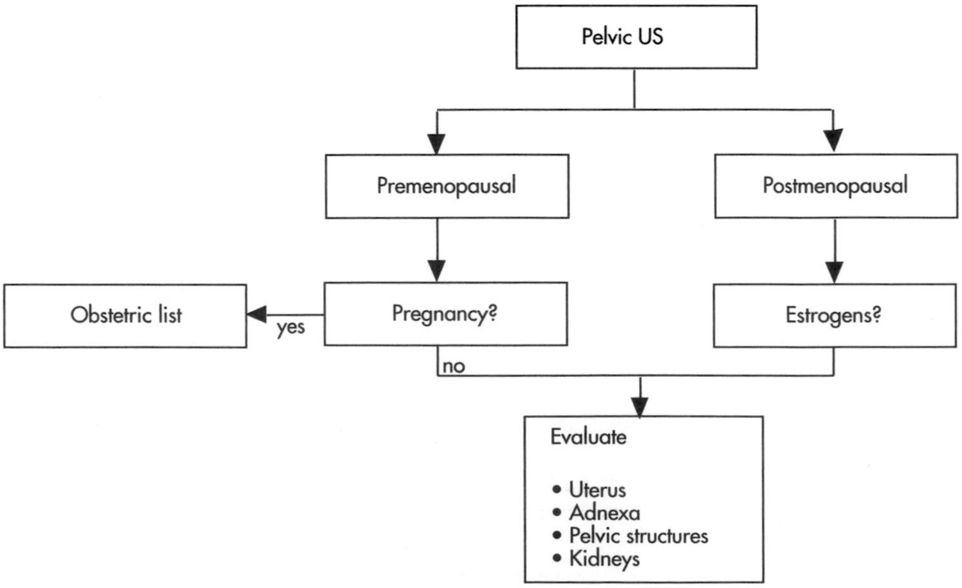

FIGURE 4-63

UTERUS

THICK HYPERECHOIC ENDOMETRIAL STRIPE (EMS) (Fig. 4-64)

Criteria: >4 mm in postmenopausal patients not taking hormone replacement therapy; >14 mm in premenopausal patients (varies with stage in cycle)

CAUSES OF THICK HYPERECHOIC ENDOMETRIAL STRIPE

Pregnancy Related	Postmenopausal
Normal early pregnancy	Hyperplasia
Ectopic	Tamoxifen, estrogen replacement
Incomplete abortion	Polyps
Molar pregnancy (cystic spaces can be missing early on)	Endometrial cancer

Pearls

- Endometrial cancer may be indistinguishable from other benign causes of thickened EMS; therefore, curettage is indicated in postmenopausal patient.
- A sonographically normal endometrium in a postmenopausal woman excludes significant pathology.
- Approach in postmenopausal patient:
  - EMS ≤ 4 mm: no further workup
  - EMS ≥ 4 mm (no hormone therapy): sonohysterogram to characterize; must sample endometrium.
  - EMS ≥ 8 mm (hormonal/tamoxifen therapy): sonohysterogram to characterize; stop hormones and obtain follow-up by US.

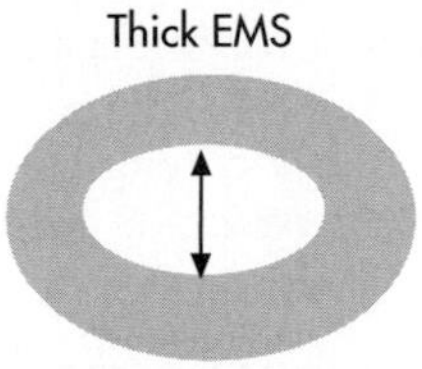

FIGURE 4-64

HYPOECHOIC STRUCTURES IN HYPERECHOIC ENDOMETRIUM (Fig. 4-65)

Premenopausal
- Molar pregnancy
- Retained placenta, abortus
- Degenerated placenta
- Degenerated fibroid

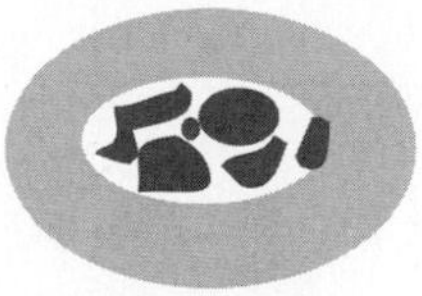

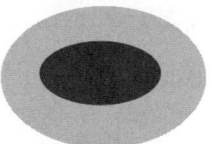

FIGURE 4-65

Postmenopausal
- Cystic glandular hyperplasia
- Endometrial polyps
- Endometrial carcinoma

FLUID IN UTERINE CAVITY (Fig. 4-66)

Acquired (cervical stenosis)
- Tumors: cervical cancer, endometrial cancer
- Inflammatory: endometritis, PID, radiation

Pregnancy related
- Early IUP
- Pseudogestational sac
- Blighted ovum

Congenital
- Imperforate hymen
- Vaginal septum
- Vaginal atresia
- Rudimentary uterine horn

FIGURE 4-66

UTERINE ENLARGEMENT OR DISTORTION

- Fibroids (most common cause)
- Adenomyosis
- Less common causes
  - Congenital uterine anomalies
  - Inflammation: PID, surgery
  - Endometriosis
  - Malignant tumors

UTERINE BLEEDING

- Endometrial hyperplasia or polyp (most common cause)
- Endometrial cancer
- Estrogen withdrawal
- Adenomyosis
- Submucosal fibroid
- Cervical cancer

UTERINE SIZE

Small Uterus

- Hypoplasia
- Nulliparity

- Synechiae
- DES exposure

Large Uterus

- Multiparity
- Pregnancy
- Molar pregnancy
- Neoplasm

PELVIC FLOOR CYSTIC MASSES

- Nabothian cyst: retention cyst of cervix
- Urethral diverticulum: usually posterolateral midurethra at level of pubic symphysis
- Skene's gland cyst/abscess: lateral to external urethral meatus
- Gartner's duct cyst: anterolateral upper third of vagina
- Bartholin cyst: Labia majora
- Hydrometrocolpos

SHADOWING STRUCTURES IN ENDOMETRIAL CAVITY (US)

- IUD
- Calcifications: fibroids, TB
- Pyometra (gas)

OVARIES AND ADNEXA

CYSTIC MASSES (Fig. 4-67)

Ovary

- Normal ovarian cysts (physiologic)
  - Follicle (mean diameter <25 mm); follicular cyst (mean diameter >25 mm)
  - Corpus luteum cyst
- Too many follicles: polycystic ovary, hyperstimulation syndrome
- Theca lutein cyst (with high levels of β-HCG)
- Cystic adnexal masses
  - Hemorrhagic cyst
  - Endometrioma ("chocolate cyst")
  - Ectopic pregnancy
  - Cystadenocarcinoma
  - TOA

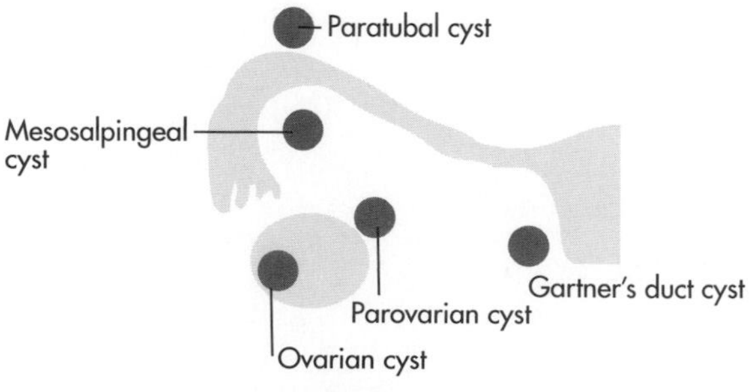

FIGURE 4-67

Tube

- Hydrosalpinx

Other

- Parovarian cyst
- Fluid in cul-de-sac
- Pelvic varices
- Lymphocele
- Bowel
- Pelvic abscess

COMPLEX PELVIC MASSES

Ovarian, parovarian (the "big 5")

- Ectopic pregnancy
- TOA
- Endometrioma, hemorrhagic cyst
- Ovarian torsion
- Tumor:
  - Benign: dermoid
  - Malignant: adenocarcinoma

Tubal

- Pyosalpinx

Uterine

- Pedunculated fibroid
- Extruded IUD
- Endometrial, cervical carcinoma (rare)

Other

- Pelvic abscess
- Appendicitis
- Diverticulitis
- Hematoma
- Pelvic kidneys
- Iliac aneurysm

Pearls

- US (gray scale or Doppler) cannot reliably distinguish benign from malignant ovarian tumors.
- MRI is useful to define etiology of solid, not cystic, masses.
- If a malignant lesion is suspected, scan the rest of the abdomen for metastases (liver, spleen, ascites).
- Always use Doppler imaging for cystic-appearing structures to exclude vascular origin (i.e., aneurysm).

MASSES WITH HOMOGENEOUS LOW-LEVEL ECHOES

- TOA
- Endometrioma
- Hemorrhagic cyst

SOLID OVARIAN MASS LESIONS

- Benign tumor: fibroma, thecoma, endometrioma, germ cell tumor
- Malignant ovarian tumors
- Metastasis

- Masses simulating ovarian tumor
  - Pedunculated fibroid
  - Lymphadenopathy

DILATED TUBES (HYDROSALPINX, PYOSALPINX, HEMATOSALPINX)

- Infection
- Tumor: endometrial or tubal carcinoma
- Endometriosis
- Iatrogenic ligation

TUBAL FILLING DEFECTS (HSG)

- Polyp
- Neoplasm
- Silicone implant
- Tubal pregnancy
- Air bubble from injection
- Asherman syndrome

TUBAL IRREGULARITY

- SIN
- Tubal diverticula
- Endometriosis
- Postoperative changes
- TB

PSEUDOKIDNEY SIGN (US)

Elliptical structure in pelvis or abdomen with an echogenic center (blood, prominent mucosa, infiltrated bowel wall) resembling the US appearance of a kidney.

- Inflammatory bowel disease
  - Crohn disease
  - Infectious colitis
- Tumor
- Intussusception
- Always exclude pelvic kidney.

Suggested Readings

Callen PW. *Ultrasonography in Obstetrics and Gynecology.* Philadelphia: Elsevier; 2008.

Dunnick NR, Sandler CM, Newhouse JH, et al. *Textbook of Uroradiology.* Philadelphia: Lippincott Williams & Wilkins; 2007.

Halpern EJ, Cochlin D, Goldberg B. *Imaging of the Prostate.* London: Taylor & Francis; 2002.

Pollack HM. *Clinical Urography: An Atlas and Textbook of Urological Imaging.* Philadelphia: WB Saunders; 2000.

Rumack CM, Charboneau W, Wilson S. *Diagnostic Ultrasound.* St. Louis: Elsevier Science; 2004.

Yoder IC. *Hysterosalpingography and Pelvic Ultrasound.* Baltimore: Lippincott Williams & Wilkins; 1988.

Zagoria RJ, Tung GJ. *Genitourinary Radiology: The Requisites.* St. Louis: Mosby; 2004.

CHAPTER 5

Musculoskeletal Imaging

CHAPTER OUTLINE

Trauma

GENERAL

FRACTURE

FRACTURE SYNOPSIS

Fracture	Finding
Spine	
Jefferson	Ring fracture of C1
Hangman's	Bilateral pedicle or pars fractures of C2
Teardrop (flexion)	Unstable flexion fracture
Clay-shoveler's	Avulsion fracture of spinous process lower cervical, high thoracic spine
Chance	Horizontal fracture through soft tissues and/or bone of thoracolumbar spine
Face	
Le Fort I	Floating palate
Le Fort II	Floating maxilla
Le Fort III	Floating face
Upper Extremity	
Hill-Sachs lesion (anterior dislocation)	Impaction fracture of posterolateral humeral head
Bankart lesion (anterior dislocation)	Fracture of anterior glenoid rim
Trough sign (posterior dislocation)	Linear impaction fracture of anterior humeral head
Reverse Bankart lesion (posterior dislocation)	Fracture of posterior glenoid rim
Monteggia fracture-dislocation	Ulnar fracture, proximal radial dislocation
Galeazzi fracture-dislocation	Radial fracture, distal radioulnar dislocation

FRACTURE SYNOPSIS—cont'd

Fracture	Finding
Essex-Lopresti	Radial head fracture and distal radioulnar subluxation
Colles	Distal radius fracture, dorsal angulation
Smith	Distal radius fracture, volar angulation
Barton	Intraarticular distal radial fracture/ dislocation
Bennett	Fracture-dislocation of base of first metacarpal
Rolando	Comminuted Bennett fracture
Boxer's	5th MCP shaft or neck fracture
Gamekeeper's thumb (skiers)	Ulnar collateral ligament injury of 1st MCP joint
Chauffeur's	Intraarticular fracture of radial styloid
Pelvis	
Duverney	Iliac wing fracture
Malgaigne	Sacroiliac (SI) joint or sacrum and both ipsilateral pubic rami
Bucket-handle	SI joint or sacrum and contralateral pubic rami
Straddle	Fracture of both obturator rings (all four pubic rami)
Lower Extremity	
Segond	Avulsion fracture of lateral tibial condyle; associated with anterior cruciate ligament (ACL) injury
Bumper	Intraarticular fracture of tibial condyle
Pilon	Intraarticular comminuted distal tibia fracture
Tillaux	Salter-Harris III of lateral distal tibia (due to later epiphyseal fusion)
Triplane	Salter III/IV fracture of distal tibia
Wagstaffe-Le Fort	Avulsion of the medial margin distal fibula
Dupuytren	Fracture of fibula above tibiofibular ligament
Maisonneuve	Proximal fibular fracture and disrupted ankle mortise or medial malleolar fracture
Lover's	Calcaneal fracture
Jones (dancer's)	Fracture of proximal 5th metatarsal shaft
Lisfranc	Tarsometatarsal fracture-dislocation
March	Stress fracture of metatarsal neck

Fracture Healing (Fig. 5-1)

Phases of healing:

Inflammatory phase
- Torn periosteum
- Blood clots in fracture line
- Inflammatory reaction

Reparative phase
- Granulation tissue replaces clot.
- Periosteum forms immature callus.
- Internal callus forms within granulation tissue.
- Cartilage forms around fracture.

Remodeling phase
- Woven bone in callus is replaced by compact bone (cortex) and cancellous bone (medullary cavity).

Terminology for Description of Fractures

Anatomic site of fracture
- In long bones, divide the shaft into thirds (e.g., fracture distal third of femur).
- Use anatomic landmarks for description (e.g., fracture near greater tuberosity).

Pattern of fracture
- Simple fracture: no fragments. Describe the direction of the fracture line:
  transverse, oblique, spiral, longitudinal
- Comminuted fracture (more than 2 fragments): T-, V-, Y-shaped patterns, butterfly fragments, segmental
- Complete or incomplete fractures

Apposition and alignment: defined in relation to distal fragments
- Displacement (e.g., medial, lateral, posterior, anterior)
- Angulation (e.g., medial, lateral, posterior, anterior)
- Rotation (internal, external)
- Overriding: overlap of fragments (bayonet apposition)
- Distracted: separated fragments

Adjacent joints
- Normal
- Dislocation
- Subluxation
- Intraarticular extension of fracture line

Specific Fractures

- Stress fractures:
  - Fatigue fracture: abnormal muscular stress applied to normal bone (e.g., march fracture)
  - Insufficiency fracture: normal muscular stress applied to abnormal bone (e.g., osteoporotic vertebral fracture)
- Pathologic fracture: fracture superimposed on underlying bone disease
- Intraarticular fracture: fracture line extends into joint
- Salter-Harris fracture: fractures involving growth plate
- Pseudofracture: fissurelike defects in osteomalacia (Looser's zones)
- Occult fracture: suspected but nonvisualized fracture on plain film; demonstrated by

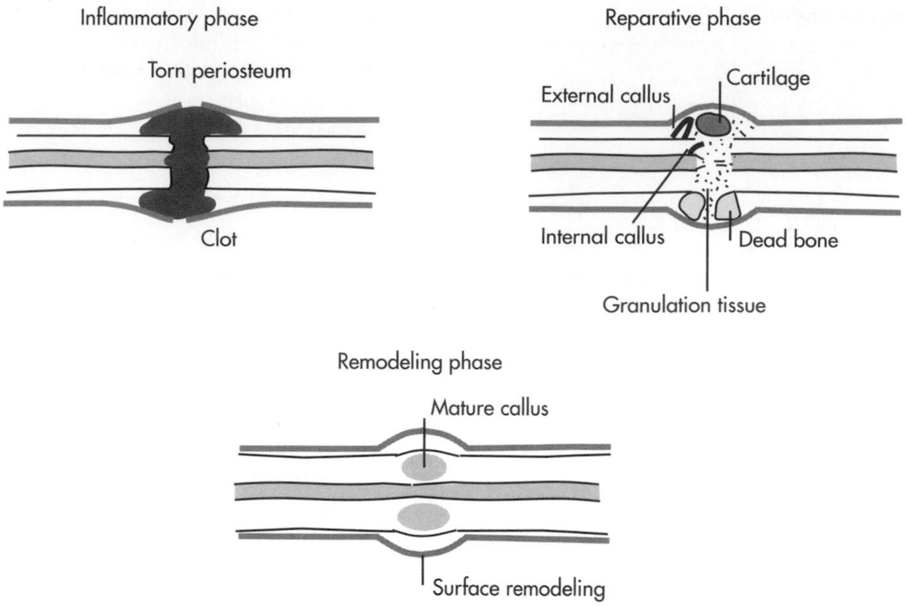

FIGURE 5-1

^{99m}Tc MDP scintigraphy or magnetic resonance imaging (MRI)
- Hairline fracture: nondisplaced fracture with minimal separation
- Avulsion fracture: fragment pulled away from bone at tendinous and ligament insertion (commonly at tuberosity)
- Apophyseal fracture: at growth centers such as ischial tuberosity and medial epicondyle; commonly avulsion fractures

RELEVANT ANATOMY (Fig. 5-2)

Long Bones

- Epiphysis
- Metaphysis
- Diaphysis

Types of Joints

Synovial joint (diarthrosis)
- Appendicular skeleton
- Facet joints of spine
- Atlantoaxial joints
- Lower two thirds of SI joints
- Acromioclavicular (AC) joint
- Uncovertebral joints

Cartilaginous joint (amphiarthrosis)
- Synchondroses
- Pubic symphysis
- Intervertebral disks

Fibrous joint (synarthrosis)
- Interosseous membranes
- Tibiofibular syndesmosis
- Sutures

Synovial Joint (Fig. 5-3)

In contradistinction to fibrous and cartilaginous joints, synovial joints allow wide ranges of motion and are classified according to axes of movement. The articular cartilage is hyaline. The most superficial layer has collagen fibrils parallel to the surface with microscopic pores to allow passage of electrolytes. This is also referred to as the *armor plate*. Deeper

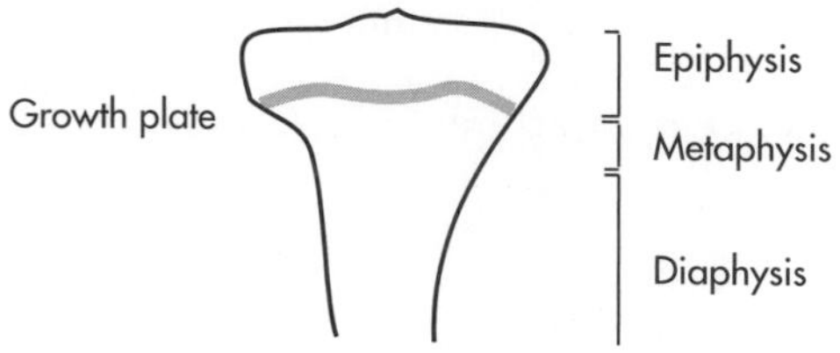

FIGURE 5-2

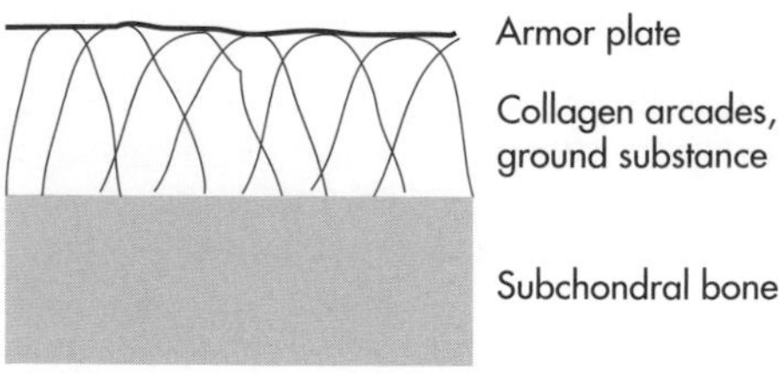

FIGURE 5-3

in the cartilage, collagen fibrils are arranged in arcades to give flexibility and allow for compression. Proteoglycans within the cartilage bind water to give a cushion effect.

FRACTURE COMPLICATIONS

Immediate
- Hemorrhage, shock
- Fat embolism
- Acute ischemia (5 P's: pulselessness, pain, pallor, paresthesia, paralysis)
- Spinal cord injury, epidural hematoma

Delayed
- Nonunion
- Osteoporosis due to disuse
- Secondary osteoarthritis
- Myositis ossificans
- Osteomyelitis
- Osteonecrosis
- Sudeck atrophy
- Volkmann ischemic contracture

ORTHOPEDIC PROCEDURES

Types of Repair

Reduction
- Closed: skin intact; may be performed in surgery under general anesthesia
- Open: requires exposing the fracture site in surgery

Fixation
- Internal: using fixation devices such as plates, screws, rods; a subsequent operation is usually necessary to remove hardware.
- External: cast or external fixator

Orthopedic Hardware

- Intramedullary rods: most of the intramedullary rods are hollow, closed nails; proximal and distal interlocking screws prevent rotation and shortening of bone fragments.
- Kirschner wires (K-wires): unthreaded segments of wires drilled into cancellous bone; if more than one wire is placed, rotational stability can be achieved; the protruding ends of the K-wire are bent to prevent injury; K-wires are most frequently used for:
  - Provisional fixation
  - Fixation of small fragments
  - Pediatric metaphyseal fractures
- Cerclage wires are used to contain bone fragments.
- Staples are commonly used for osteotomies.
- Plates
- Nails
- Screws

SPINE

CLASSIFICATION OF C-SPINE INJURIES

CLASSIFICATION

Type of Injury	Condition	Stability*
Flexion	Anterior subluxation	Stable†
	Unilateral facet dislocation	Stable
	Bilateral facet dislocation	Unstable
	Wedge compression fracture	Stable†
	Flexion teardrop fracture	Unstable
	Clay-shoveler's fracture	Stable
Extension	Posterior arch of C1 fracture	Stable
	Hangman's fracture	Unstable
	Laminar fracture	Stable
	Pillar fracture	Stable
	Extension teardrop fracture	Stable
	Hyperextension dislocation-fracture	Unstable
Compression	Jefferson fracture	Unstable
	Burst fracture	Stable
Complex	Odontoid fractures	Unstable
	Atlantooccipital disassociation	Unstable

*Stability is a function of ligamentous injury. Plain films in neutral position allow one to infer *instability* when certain fractures or dislocations are present. However, *stability* may not be inferred with 100% accuracy. The anterior subluxation injury in which films may appear within normal limits is an example. Clinical judgment is necessary to decide whether to do nothing, obtain flexion/extension films, or obtain an MRI.
†Possible delayed instability.

Biomechanics (Figs. 5-4 and 5-5)

Pearls

- 20% of spinal fractures are multiple.
- 5% of spinal fractures are at discontinuous levels.

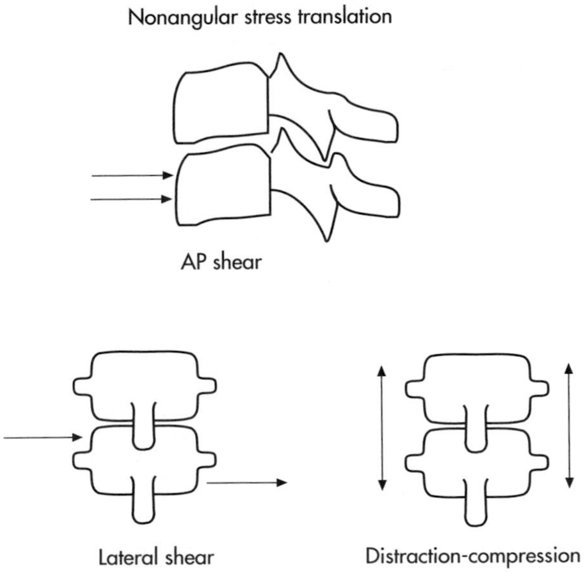

FIGURE 5-4

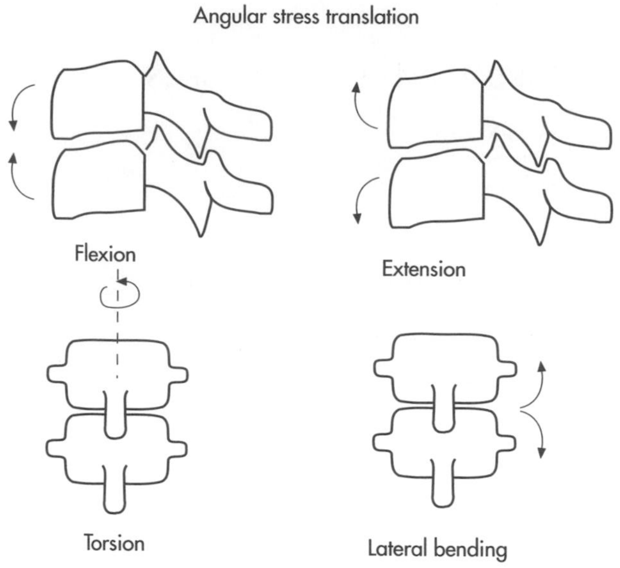

FIGURE 5-5

- Spinal cord injury occurs:
  At time of trauma, 85%
  As a late complication, 15%
- Cause of spinal fractures
  Motor vehicle accident (MVA), 50%
  Falls, 25%
  Sports related, 10%
- Most spinal fractures occur in upper (C1-C2) or lower (C5-C7) cervical spine and thoracolumbar (T10-L2) region.

APPROACH TO C-SPINE PLAIN FILM (Figs. 5-6 and 5-7)

1. Are all 7 cervical vertebrae well seen? If not, obtain additional views such as swimmer's view, computed tomography (CT), etc.

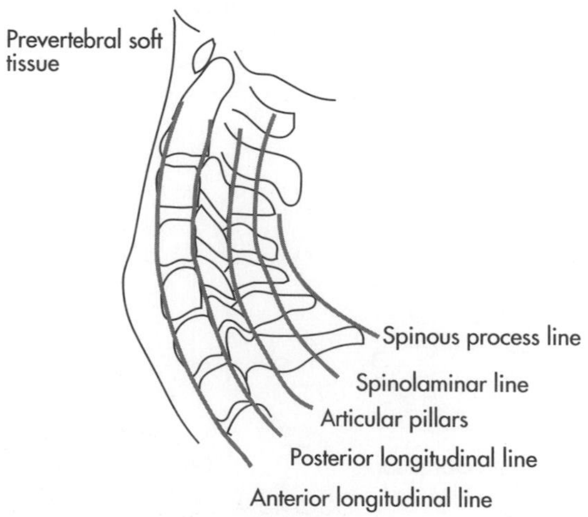

FIGURE 5-6

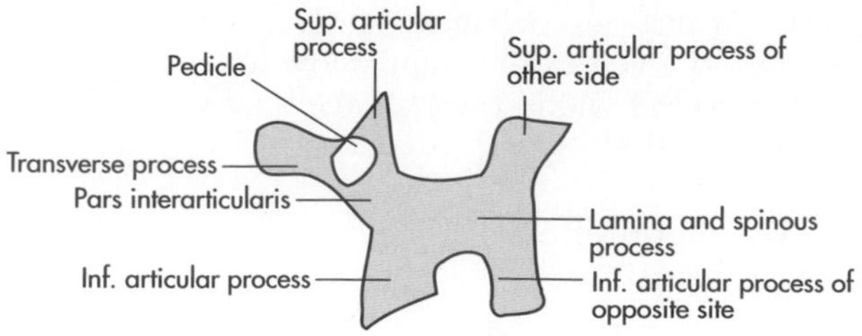

FIGURE 5-7

2. Is cervical lordosis maintained? If not, consider:
   - Positional
   - Spasm
   - Fracture/injury
3. Evaluate 5 parallel lines for stepoffs and/or discontinuity.
   - Prevertebral soft tissues
     C3-C4: 5 mm from vertebral body is normal (nonportable film)
     C4-C7: 20 mm from vertebral body is normal (not as reliable)
     Contour of soft tissues is as important as absolute measurements; a localized bulging anterior convex border usually indicates pathology.
   - Anterior longitudinal line
   - Posterior longitudinal line
   - Spinolaminar line
   - Posterior spinous process line
4. Inspect C1-C2 area.
   - Atlantodental distance
   - Adults: <3 mm is normal.
   - Children: <5 mm is normal.
   - Base of odontoid may not be calcified in children (subdental synchondrosis).
5. Inspect disk spaces.
   - Narrowing of disk spaces?
6. Transverse processes: C7 points downward, T1 points upward.

APPROACH TO CERVICAL SPINE INJURIES

1. Most suspected C-spine fractures are followed with thin-section CT with reformation for most accurate evaluation.
2. Patients with history/examination highly suggestive of cervical spine injury (high-speed accident) proceed directly to CT, followed by an out-of-collar lateral to clear cervical spine.
3. All individuals with signs/symptoms of cord injury require MRI.
4. It is also prudent to obtain CT in patients with unexplained prevertebral soft tissue swelling.

JEFFERSON FRACTURES (Fig. 5-8)

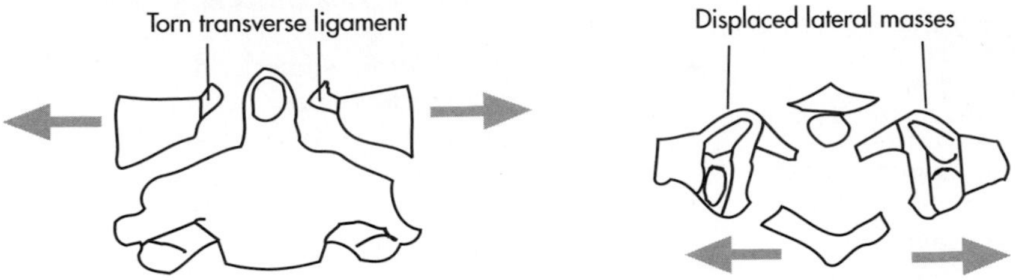

FIGURE 5-8

Compression force to C1 that usually results from blow to the vertex of the head (diving injury).

Consists of unilateral or bilateral fractures of both the anterior and posterior arches of Cl. Treatment is halo placement for 3 months.

Radiographic Features

- Key radiographic view: AP open-mouth
- Displacement of C1 lateral masses
  - <2 mm bilateral is always abnormal.
  - <1 to 2 mm or unilateral displacement can be due to head tilt/rotation.
- CT required for:
  - Defining full extent of fracture
  - Detecting fragments in spinal cord

FRACTURES OF THE ODONTOID PROCESS (DENS) (Fig. 5-9)

Various mechanisms: Anderson/D'Alonzo classification:

- Type I: fracture in the upper part of the odontoid (potentially unstable; rare fracture)
- Type II: fracture at base of the odontoid (unstable); highest rate of nonunion because fracture is above the accessory ligament and vascular supply
- Type III: fracture through base of odontoid into body of axis; best prognosis for healing because of larger surface area (unstable)

Radiographic Features

- Anterior tilt of odontoid on lateral view is highly suggestive of fracture.
- Plain film tomograms or CT with re-formations is helpful to delineate fracture line.
- Prevertebral soft tissue swelling (may be the only sign)
- Os odontoideum (type 1)
  - Congenital or posttraumatic
  - May be mechanically unstable

HANGMAN'S FRACTURE (Fig. 5-10)

Hyperextension and traction injury of C2.

Causes

- Hanging
- MVA (chin hits dashboard)

Radiographic Features

- Best demonstrated on lateral view
- Bilateral C2 pars (common) or pedicle (less common) fractures
- Anterior dislocation or subluxation of C2 vertebral body
- Avulsion of anterior inferior corner of C2 (ruptured anterior longitudinal ligament)
- Prevertebral soft tissue swelling

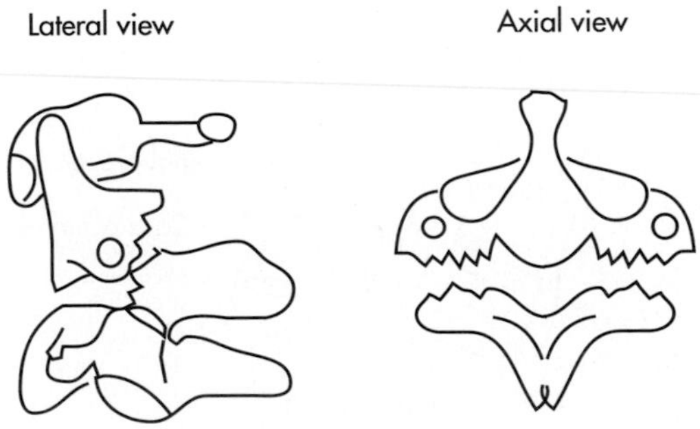

FIGURE 5-10

BURST (COMPRESSION) FRACTURE

Same mechanism as in Jefferson fracture but located at C3-C7. Injury to spinal cord (displacement of posterior fragments) is common. All patients require CT to evaluate

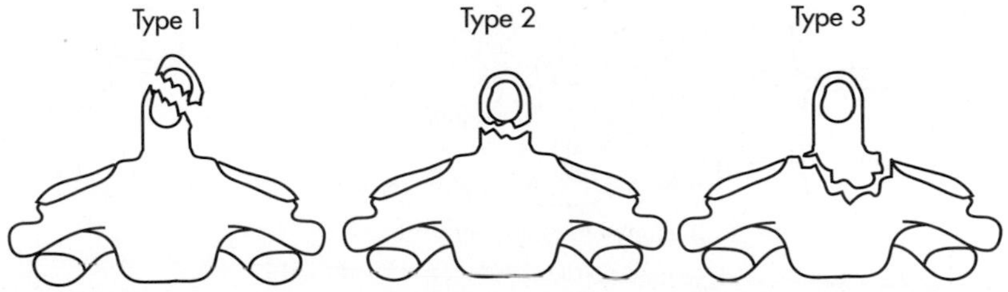

FIGURE 5-9

full extent of injury, to detect associated fractures, and to identify fragments in relation to spinal canal.

FLEXION TEARDROP FRACTURE (FLEXION FRACTURE-DISLOCATION)

The most severe C-spine injury. Results from severe flexion force and presents as clinical "acute anterior cord syndrome" (quadriplegia, loss of anterior column senses, retention of posterior column senses). Completely unstable.

Radiographic Features (Fig. 5-11)

- Teardrop fragment is major shear fragment from anteroinferior vertebral body.
- All ligaments are disrupted.
- Posterior subluxation of vertebral body
- Bilateral subluxated or dislocated facets
- Severe compromise of spinal canal secondary to subluxation of body and facets
- Not to be confused with:
  - Extension teardrop fracture (stable avulsive injury)
  - Burst fracture (stable comminuted fracture of centrum with variable neurologic involvement)

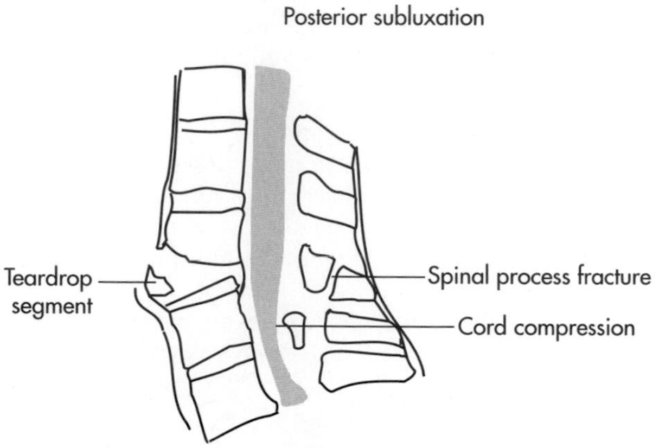

FIGURE 5-11

CLAY-SHOVELER'S FRACTURE (Fig. 5-12)

Oblique avulsive fracture of a lower spinous process, most commonly at C6-T1 levels (C7 > C6 > T1). Caused by powerful hyperflexion (shoveling).

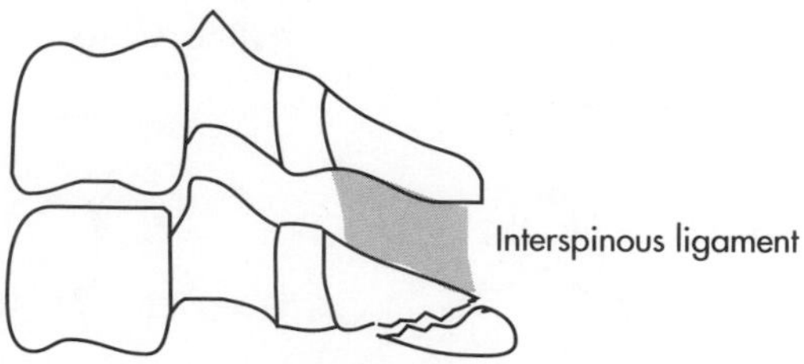

FIGURE 5-12

Radiographic Features

- Fracture through spinous process, best seen on lateral view
- If C6-C7 is not demonstrated on lateral view, obtain swimmer's view and/or CT.
- AP view: ghost sign (double-spinous process on C6-C7 caused by caudal displacement of the fractured tip of the spinous process)

WEDGE FRACTURE

Compression fracture resulting from flexion. Most fractures are stable.

Radiographic Features

- Loss of height of anterior vertebral body
- Buckled anterior cortex
- Anterosuperior fracture of vertebral body
- Differentiate from burst fracture
  - Lack of vertical fracture component
  - Posterior cortex intact

EXTENSION TEARDROP FRACTURE (Fig. 5-13)

Avulsion fracture of anteroinferior corner of the axis resulting from hyperextension.

Radiographic Features

- Teardrop fragment: avulsion by the anterior longitudinal ligament
- Vertical height of fragment ≥ horizontal width

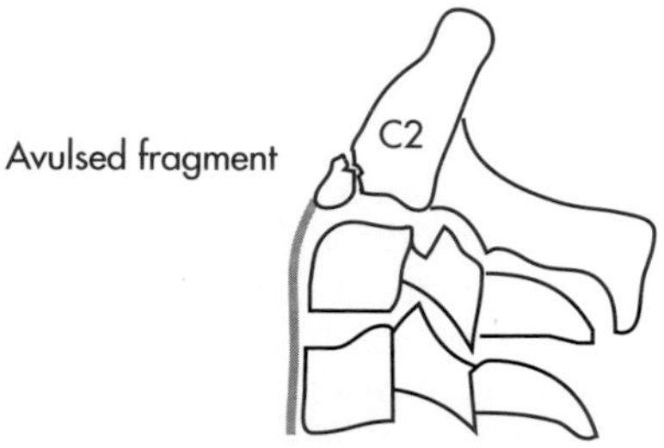

FIGURE 5-13

FACET DISLOCATION

Bilateral Facet Dislocation (Unstable) (Fig. 5-14)

Results from extreme flexion of head and neck without axial compression.

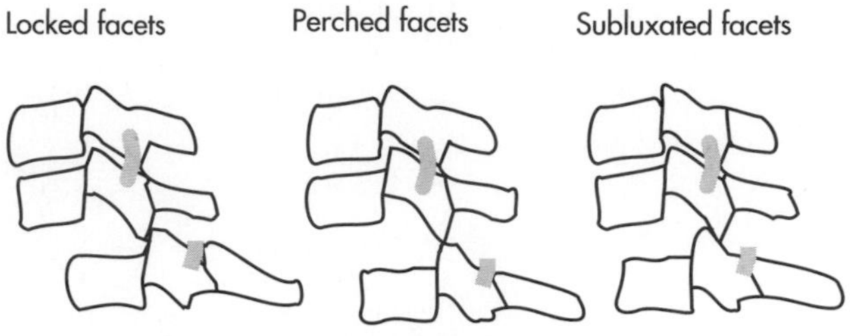

FIGURE 5-14

RADIOGRAPHIC FEATURES

- Complete anterior dislocation of the affected vertebral body by half or more of the vertebral body AP diameter
- Batwing or bowtie configuration of locked facets
- Disruption of posterior ligament complex, intervertebral disk, and anterior longitudinal ligament

Unilateral Facet Dislocation (Stable)

Results from simultaneous flexion and rotation.

RADIOGRAPHIC FEATURES

- Anterior dislocation of vertebral body less than half the AP diameter of the vertebral body
- Evidence of discordant rotation above and below involved level
- Disrupted "shingles-on-a-roof" on oblique view
- Facet within intervertebral foramen on oblique view
- Disrupted posterior ligament complex
- Best demonstrated on lateral and oblique views

ANTERIOR SUBLUXATION (HYPERFLEXION SPRAIN) (Fig. 5-15)

Anterior subluxation occurs when the posterior ligament complex is disrupted. Radiographic diagnosis can be difficult because muscle spasm may cause similar findings. Initially stable. Delayed instability occurs in 20%-50%.

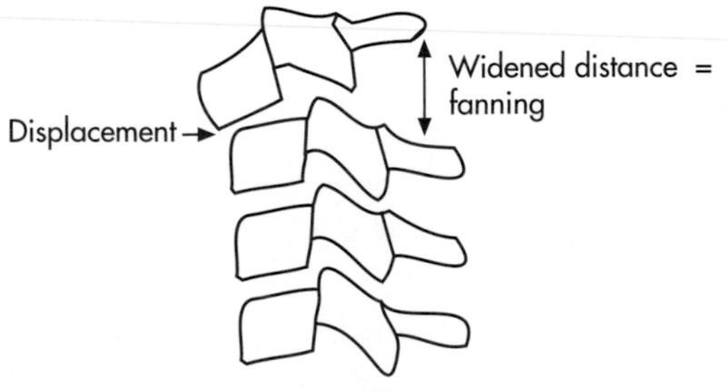

FIGURE 5-15

Radiographic Features

- Localized kyphotic angulation
- Widened interspinous/interlaminar distance (fanning)
- Posterior widening of disk space
- Subluxation at facet joints
- Anterior vertebral body may be displaced.
- In equivocal findings, voluntary flexion/extension views are helpful.

Hyperextension Fracture-Dislocation (Fig. 5-16)

Results from severe circular hyperextending force (e.g., impact on forehead). Characteristically results in anterior vertebral displacement, a finding more commonly seen in flexion injuries. Unstable.

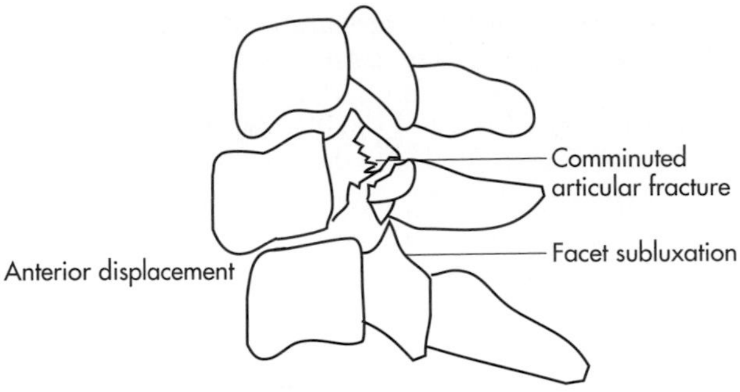

FIGURE 5-16

Radiographic Features

- Mild anterior vertebral displacement
- Comminuted articular mass fracture
- Contralateral facet subluxation
- Disrupted anterior longitudinal ligament and partial posterior ligamentous disruption

ATLANTOOCCIPITAL DISSOCIATION (Fig. 5-17)

Complex mechanism of injury. Complete dislocation is usually fatal.

Radiographic Features

- Prevertebral soft tissue swelling; a gap of more than 5 mm between the occipital condyles and the condylar surface of the atlas is highly suggestive of craniocervical injury.
- Wackenheim clivus line: a line drawn along the posterior aspect of the clivus toward the odontoid process. An abnormality is suspected when this line does not intersect or is tangential to the odontoid process.
- The traditional methods used to identify occipitoatlantal articulation injury included the power ratio and the "X" line of Lee. Each is dependent on identifying the opisthion and the spinolaminar line of C1. Anatomic variation and inconsistent visualization preclude consistent use of these methods.
- The current method uses the basion-axial interval (BAI) and is an easy and reliable method

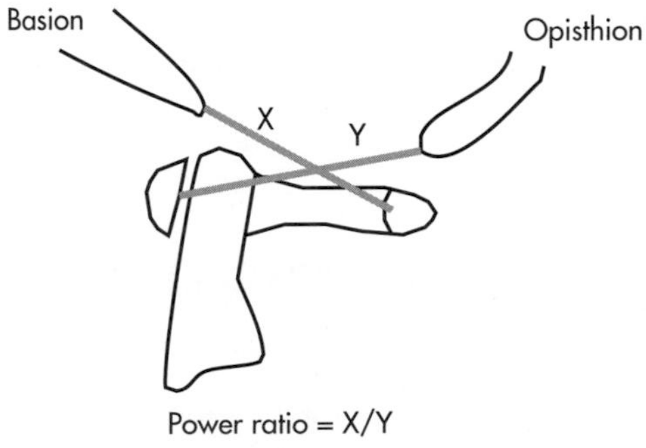

FIGURE 5-17

for assessing the occipitoatlantal relationship in patients of all ages. BAI is the distance between the basion and upward extension of the posterior axial line. Normally the BAI should not exceed 12 mm as determined on a lateral radiograph of the cervicocranium obtained at a target film distance of 1 meter.

- The vertical basion-dens distance should also be less than 12 mm.
- Anterior dissociation is more common.
- Posterior dissociation (subluxation) can be very subtle, especially if partial.

In atlantoaxial fixation (Fig. 5-18), the normal rotation of C1 on C2 cannot occur and the abnormal relationship between the atlas and the axis becomes fixed. Fielding and Hawkins have classified atlantoaxial rotatory subluxation into four categories:

- Type I, the most common type, demonstrates no displacement of C1.
- Type II demonstrates 3 to 5 mm of anterior displacement of C1 and is associated with abnormality of the transverse ligament.
- Type III demonstrates over 5 mm of anterior displacement of C1 on C2 and is associated with deficiency of the transverse and alar ligaments.
- Type IV, a rare entity, demonstrates C1 displacement posteriorly.

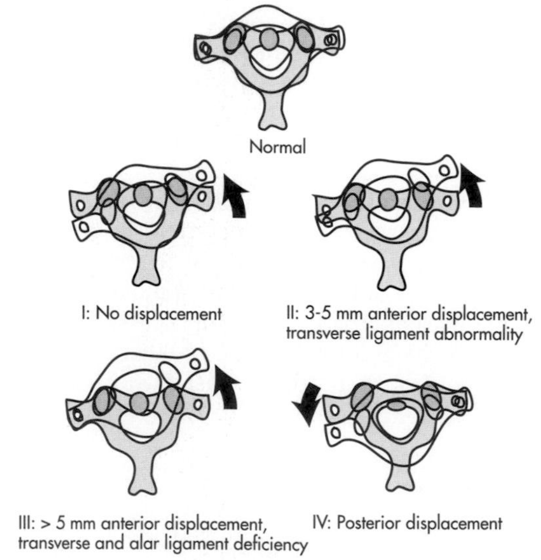

FIGURE 5-18

THORACIC AND LUMBAR FRACTURES

GENERAL

Most fractures occur at thoracolumbar junction (90% at T11-L4). All patients should have CT except for patients with:

- Stable compression fractures
- Isolated spinous or transverse process fractures
- Spondylolysis

Radiographic Features

- Widened interpedicular distance
- Paraspinal hematoma
- Unstable fractures:
  - Compression fracture >50%
  - Widened interlaminar space
  - Disrupted posterior elements

All fracture-dislocations

TYPES OF FRACTURES

Classified by mechanism or injury:

Compression or wedge fractures: anterior or lateral flexion
- Wedge-shaped deformity of vertebral body
- Decreased vertebral body height

Burst fracture: axial compression
- Comminution of vertebral body
- Bone fragments in spinal canal are common.

Chance fractures (lap seatbelt fracture, usually at L2 or L3 [Fig. 5-19]): distraction from anterior hyperflexion across a restraining lap seatbelt
- Horizontal splitting of vertebra
- Horizontal disruption of intervertebral disk
- Rupture of ligaments
- More than 50% of patients have associated small bowel and colon injuries (obtain abdominal CT).

Fracture-dislocations: combined shearing and flexion forces
- Spinal cord injury is common. Minor fractures
- Transverse process fractures
- Spinous process fractures
- Pars interarticularis fractures

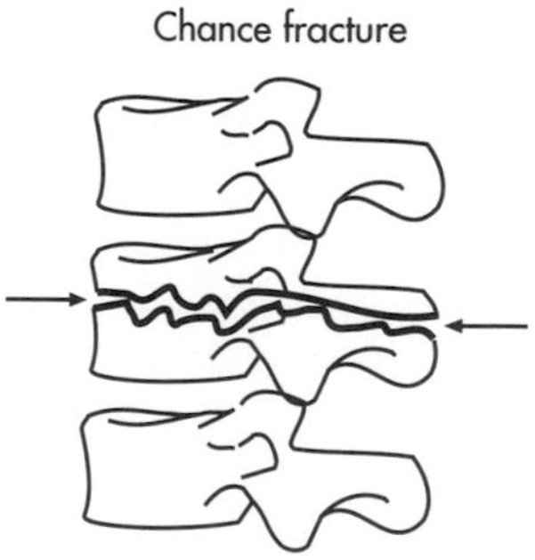

FIGURE 5-19

SPONDYLOLYSIS

Defect in the pars interarticularis (neck of the "Scottie dog"). Chronic stress fracture with nonunion. Typically in adolescents involved in sports. Most commonly at the L4 or L5 level.

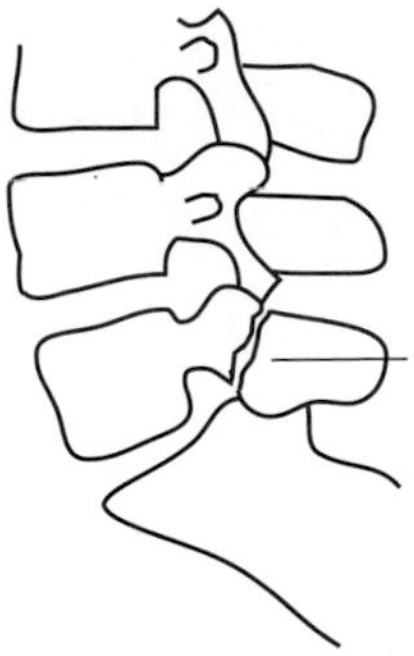

FIGURE 5-20

Radiographic Features (Fig. 5-20)

- Separation of pars interarticularis
- Spondylolisthesis common in bilateral spondylolysis
- If patient looks to right, the left pars is visualized by x-ray.
- Oblique view is usually diagnostic.
- CT or SPECT may be helpful in confirming diagnosis.

SPONDYLOLISTHESIS (Fig. 5-21)

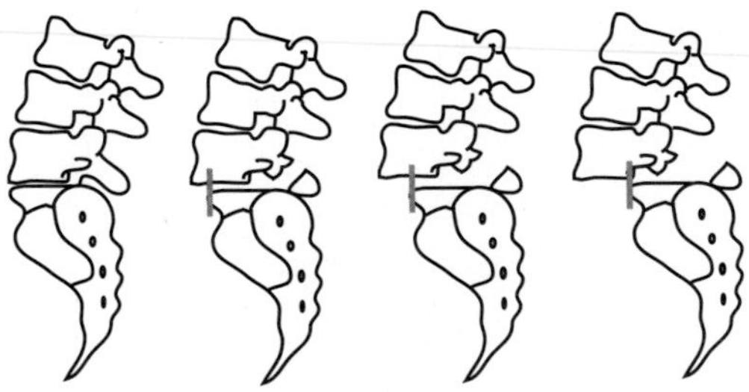

FIGURE 5-21

Ventral subluxation of a vertebral body due to bilateral pars defects.

- Four grades based on degree of anterior displacement
- 95% of spondylolisthesis occurs at L4-L5 and L5-S1.

PSEUDOSPONDYLOLISTHESIS (Fig. 5-22)

Secondary to degenerative disk disease and/or apophyseal degenerative joint disease. Use spinous process sign to differentiate from true spondylolisthesis. In true spondylolisthesis, the spinous process stepoff is above the level of vertebral slip; whereas in pseudospondylolisthesis, the stepoff is below the level of the slip.

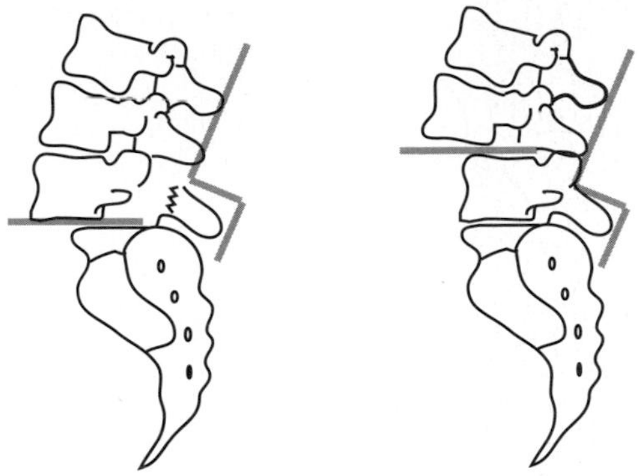

FIGURE 5-22

FACE

CLASSIFICATION OF FACIAL FRACTURES

General Category	Types	Need for CT
Orbital	Pure blow-out	Yes
	Impure blow-out	Yes
	Blow-in	Yes
Zygoma	Tripod fracture	Yes
	Isolated zygomatic arch	No
Nasal	Nondisplaced	No
	Comminuted	Variable
	Nasal-orbital-ethmoid	Yes
	Septal fracture/dislocation	Yes
Maxillary	Dentoalveolar	Yes
	Sagittal	Yes
	Le Fort fractures	Yes
Craniofacial (smash fractures)	Central craniofacial	Yes
	Lateral craniofacial	Yes
	Frontal sinus	Yes
Mandibular	Defined by site	Variable
	Flail mandible	Variable

APPROACH TO FACIAL FRACTURES (Fig. 5-23)

Facial radiographs are rarely obtained for facial fractures. Thin-section CT with re-formation is the preferred method of evaluation.

1. Incidence: nasal fractures > zygoma > other fractures
2. Facial series:
   - Waters view: three lines of the "elephant" should be traceable.
     - Maxillary sinuses
     - Orbital floor and rim
     - Nasal septum zygoma
   - Caldwell view
     - Orbital rim
     - Medial orbital wall
     - Sphenoid wings

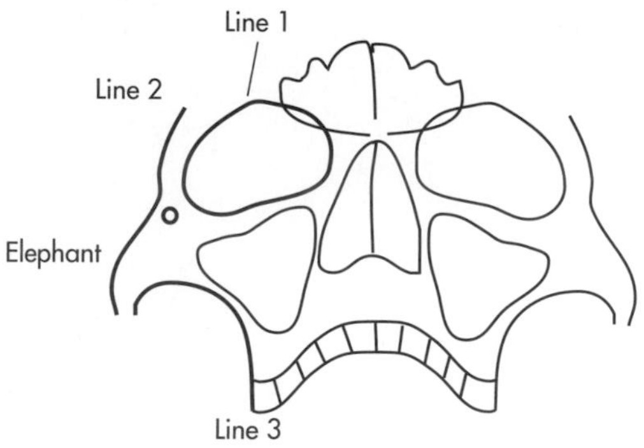

FIGURE 5-23

- Lateral view
  - Paranasal sinuses
  - Pterygoid plates
- Towne view
  - Mandible
- Base view (C-spine must be cleared first)
  - Zygoma
  - Mandible

3. Facial series is not adequate for nasal fractures:
   - Lateral (coned and soft tissue technique) views
   - Waters view
   - Occlusal view
4. Mandibular fractures require specific mandibular series:
   - Lateral, Towne, bilateral oblique views
5. Direct signs of fracture:
   - Cortical disruption, overlap, displacement
6. Indirect signs of fracture:
   - Asymmetry
   - Soft tissue swelling
   - Sinus abnormality (opacification, polypoid mass, air-fluid levels)
   - Orbital emphysema

ORBITAL FRACTURES

Pure Orbital Blow-out Fracture (Fig. 5-24)

Isolated fracture of the orbital floor or less commonly the medial wall; the orbital rim is intact. Mechanism: sudden increase in intraorbital pressure (e.g., baseball, fist).

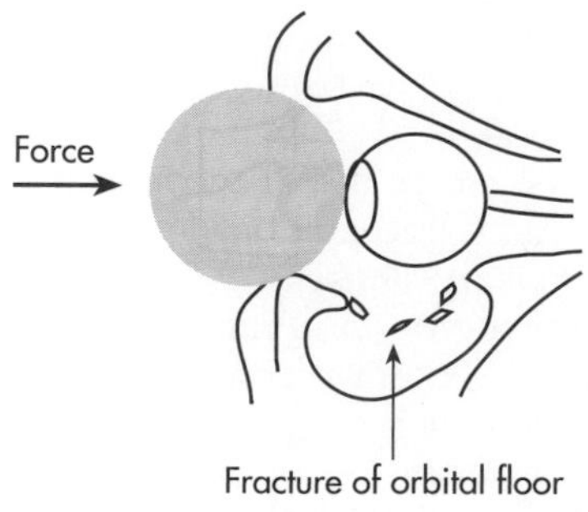

FIGURE 5-24

CLINICAL FINDINGS

- Diplopia on upward gaze (inferior rectus muscle entrapment)
- Enophthalmos (may be masked by edema)

RADIOGRAPHIC FEATURES (Figs. 5-25 and 5-26)

- Displacement of bone fragments into maxillary sinus (trap door sign)
- Opacification of maxillary sinus (hematoma)
- Orbital emphysema
- Caldwell and Waters views best demonstrate fractures.
- Using CT, evaluate for muscle entrapment and orbital content herniation.

Impure Orbital Blow-out Fracture

Associated with fracture of orbital rim and other facial fractures.

Orbital Blow-in Fracture

Impact to frontal bone causes blow-in of orbital roof. Associated with craniofacial fractures and frontal lobe contusion.

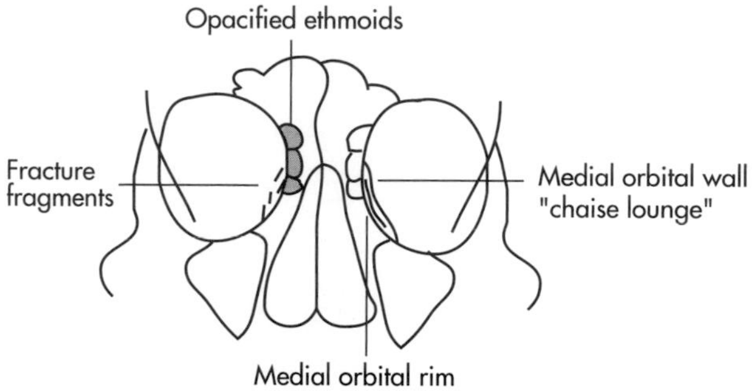

FIGURE 5-25

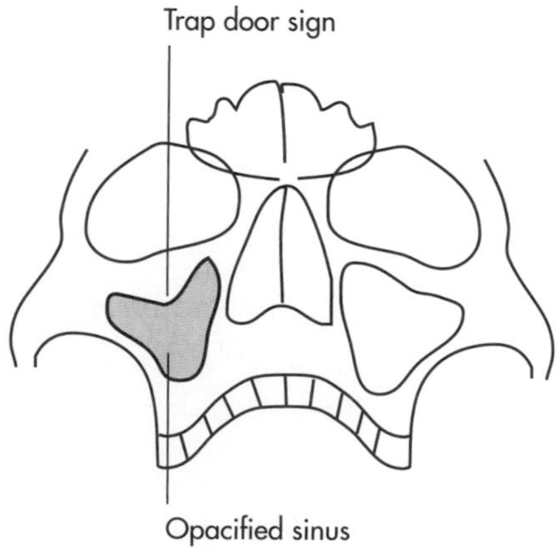

FIGURE 5-26

NASAL FRACTURES (Fig. 5-27)

Isolated nasal fractures are linear and transverse, result from a direct frontal impact, and usually occur in the lower one third of the nasal bone. More complex fractures result from lateral blows or more severe trauma and are often accompanied by other facial fractures.

Radiographic Features

- Most fractures are transverse and are depressed or displaced.
- Dislocation of septal cartilage is diagnosed by occlusal view or CT.
- Anterior nasal spine fracture is best evaluated by occlusal view.
- Do not mistake sutures and nasociliary grooves for fractures.

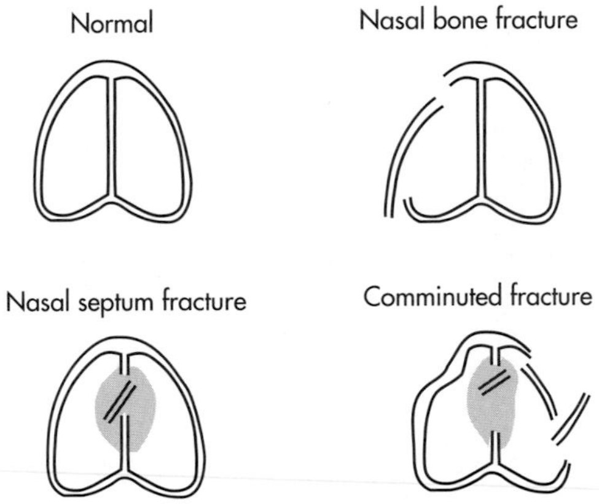

FIGURE 5-27

MANDIBULAR FRACTURES (Fig. 5-28)

The type of fracture depends on the site of impact. Most fractures are multiple and bilateral. The most common type of mandibular fracture is an ipsilateral fracture through the body of the mandible with a contralateral angle subcondylar fracture. Fractures typically occur in:

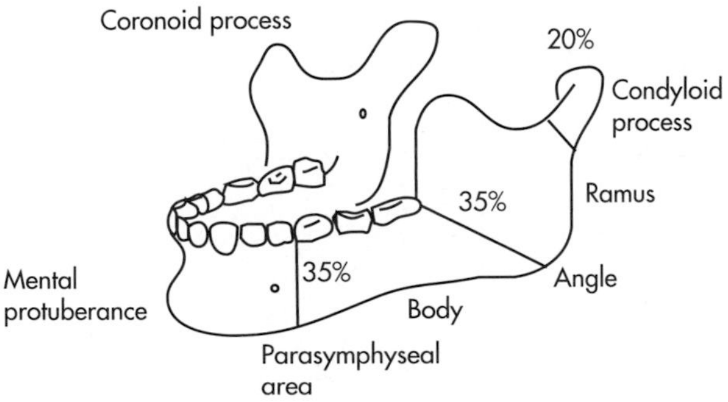

FIGURE 5-28

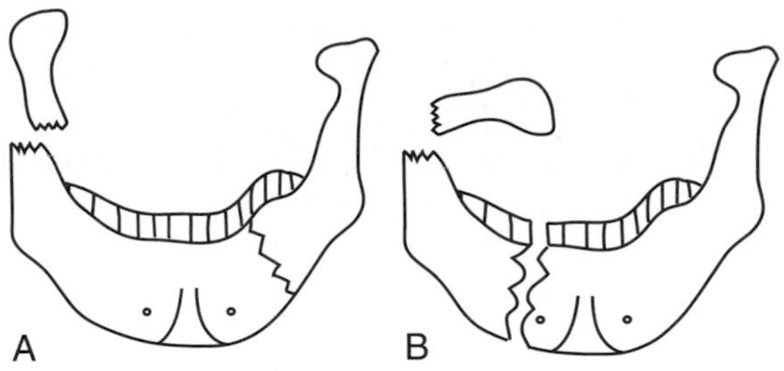

FIGURE 5-29

- Body (areas of weakness include mental or incisive foramen)
- Angle
- Subcondylar region (condylar neck)

Flail Mandible (Fig. 5-29, A and B)

Symphysis fracture with bilateral subcondylar, angle, or ramus fracture. Tongue may prolapse and obstruct airway.

ZYGOMA FRACTURES (Figs. 5-30 and 5-31)

Best view to demonstrate zygoma fracture is the base view to demonstrate the "jug handle."

Simple Arch Fractures

Simple fractures of the zygomatic arch are less common than complex fractures. Fracture lines occur most commonly:

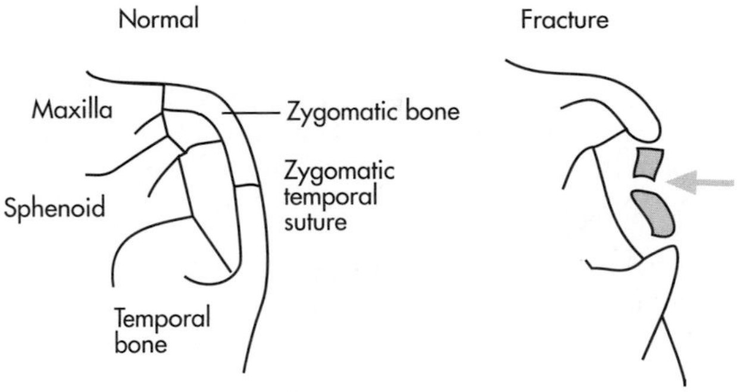

FIGURE 5-30

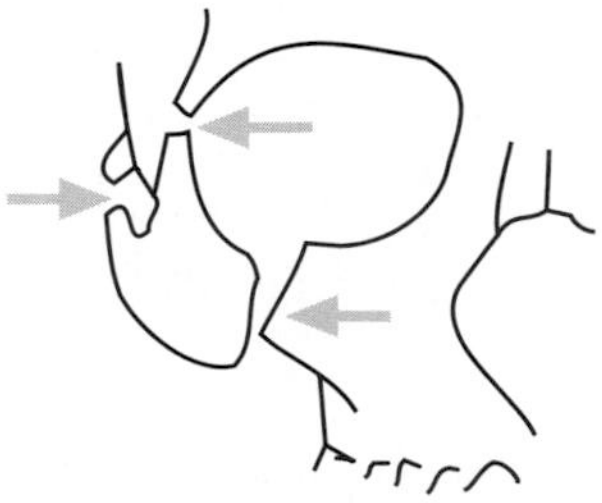

FIGURE 5-31

- Anteriorly at temporal process
- In midportion near zygomaticotemporal suture
- Posterior and anterior to condylar eminence

Complex Arch Fractures (Tripod Fracture)

- Diastasis of zygomaticofrontal suture
- Posterior zygomatic arch fracture
- Fracture of inferior orbital rim and lateral maxillary wall

MAXILLARY FRACTURES (Fig. 5-32)

Dentoalveolar Fracture

Fracture of the alveolar process of maxilla secondary to direct blow. May present clinically as loose teeth; managed as open fracture.

Sagittal Maxillary Fracture

Usually occurs with other injuries such as Le Fort fracture.

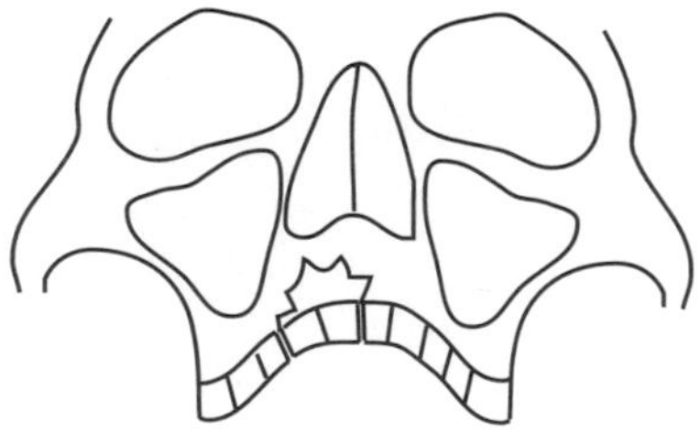

FIGURE 5-32

LE FORT FRACTURES (Figs. 5-33 and 5-34)

Fracture patterns that occur along lines of weakness in the face. Mechanism: severe force to face as would occur in motor vehicle accident. All Le Fort fractures involve the pterygoid plates of the sphenoid.

Le Fort Type I

This fracture produces a floating palate; fracture lines extend through:

- Nasal septum (vomer and septal cartilage)

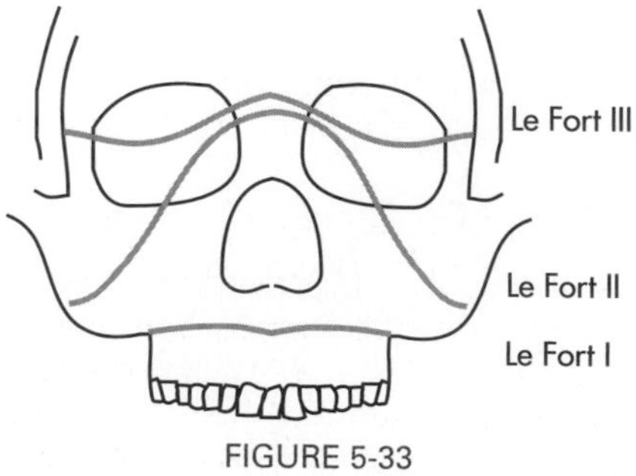

FIGURE 5-33

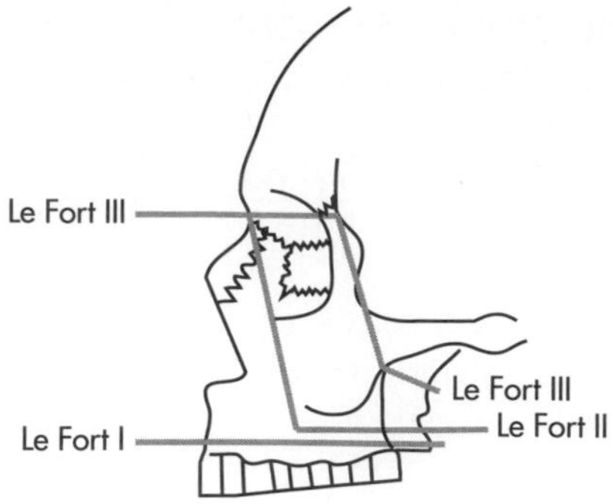

FIGURE 5-34

- Medial, anterior, lateral, posterior walls of maxillary sinus
- Pterygoid plates of sphenoid

Le Fort Type II

This fracture produces a floating maxilla; zygomatic arches are *not* included in this fracture; fracture line extends through:

- Nasal bone and nasal septum
- Frontal process of maxilla
- Medial orbital wall (ethmoid, lacrimal, palatine)
- Floor of orbit (inferior orbital fissure and canal)
- Infraorbital rim
- Anterior, lateral, posterior wall of maxillary sinus
- Pterygoid plates of sphenoid

Le Fort Type III

This fracture separates face from cranial vault and produces a floating face; the fracture line extends through:

- Nasal bone and septum
- Frontal process of maxilla
- Medial wall of orbit (lacrimal, ethmoid, palatine)
- Infraorbital fissure
- Lateral wall of orbit
- Zygomaticofrontal suture
- Zygomatic arch
- Pterygoid plates of sphenoid

SHOULDER

FRACTURE OF THE CLAVICLE (Fig. 5-35, A and B)

Common in children. Distal fragment is displaced inferior and medial. Sites of fracture include:

- Lateral third: 15%
- Middle third: 80%
- Medial third: 5%

Complications

- Laceration of vessels
- Nerve injuries
- Other associated fractures

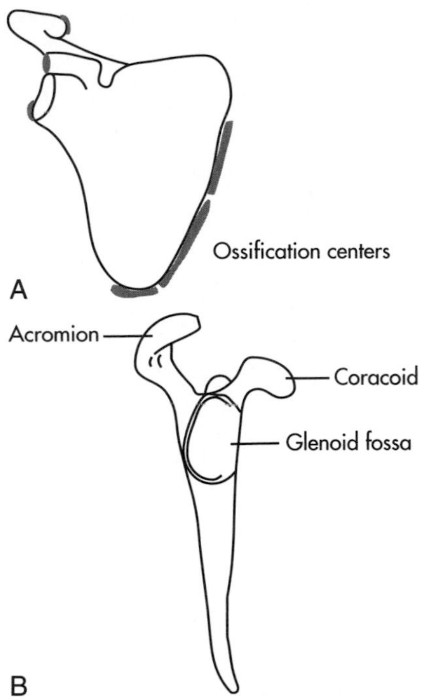

FIGURE 5-35

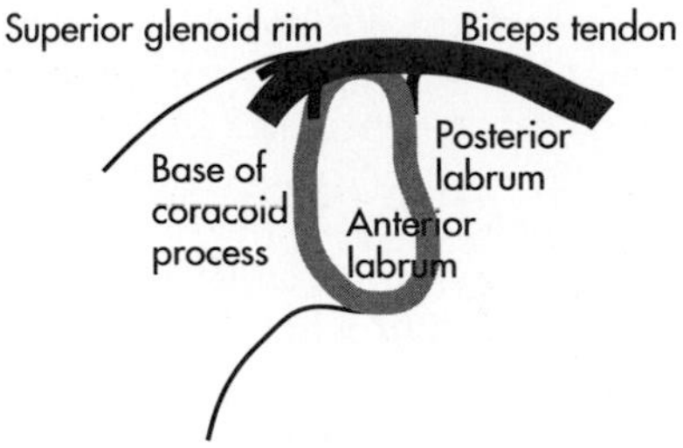

FIGURE 5-36

FRACTURE OF THE SCAPULA

Uncommon. Causes: motor vehicle accident, fall from height (direct impact injuries). Best radiographic view: transscapular view (Y-view), CT often helpful. Do not mistake ossification centers for fractures.

FRACTURE OF RIBS

- Fractures usually occur in lower 10 ribs.
- First and second rib fractures can occur after high energy trauma to chest and may be associated with severe mediastinal and vascular injury.
- Flail chest occurs when three or more ribs fracture and each rib fractures in two places (segmental fractures). Commonly associated with pulmonary contusion, laceration, pneumothorax, hemothorax, etc.

NORMAL MRI ANATOMY OF SHOULDER JOINT (Fig. 5-36)

- The glenoid labrum is a fibrocartilaginous structure that attaches to the glenoid rim and is about 4 mm wide. Anteriorly, the glenoid labrum blends with the anterior band of the inferior glenohumeral ligament. Superiorly, it blends with the biceps tendon and the superior glenohumeral ligament. It is usually rounded or triangular on cross-sectional images.
- The tendon of the long head of the biceps muscle attaches to the anterosuperior aspect of the glenoid rim. From its site of attachment, the biceps tendon courses laterally and exits the glenohumeral joint through the intertubercular groove where it is secured by the transverse ligament. In the adjacent diagram the biceps tendon attaches at the level of the superior labrum and glenoid. Note attachments to the (1) superior glenoid rim, (2) the posterior labrum, (3) the anterior labrum, and (4) the base of the coracoid process.
- The labral-bicipital complex is well visualized on transverse CT or MR arthrograms, as well as on coronal MR arthrograms and reconstructed images from coronal CT arthrograms.
- The glenohumeral ligaments play a role as shoulder stabilizers and consist of thickened bands of the joint capsule. The superior glenohumeral ligament is the most consistently identified capsular ligament. It can arise from the anterosuperior labrum, the attachment of the tendon of the long head of the biceps muscle, or the middle glenohumeral ligament.
- The middle glenohumeral ligament varies most in size and site of attachment to the glenoid. It typically has an oblique orientation from superomedial to inferolateral. It may attach to the superior portion of the anterior glenoid but more frequently attaches medially on the glenoid neck.
- The middle glenohumeral ligament may be absent or may appear thick and cordlike (e.g., Buford complex).
- The inferior glenohumeral ligament is an important stabilizer of the anterior shoulder joint and consists of the axillary pouch and anterior and posterior bands. The anterior band inserts along the inferior two thirds of the anterior glenoid labrum.

SHOULDER ULTRASOUND

Using a high-frequency linear transducer, US can be used to examine the rotator cuff, as well as biceps tendon, acromioclavicular joint, and bursae.

- Normal rotator cuff is hyperechoic and fibrillary (important to insonate perpendicular to tendon

plane to avoid anisotropy), is not compressible, and demonstrates an outer convex contour.
- Complete tear: nonvisualization of the tendon.
- Full-thickness tear: focal tendon defect/fluid; concave contour of bursal side of tendon; compressible tendon; cartilage interface sign (two parallel hyperechoic lines over humeral head)
- Partial-thickness tear: bursal side or articular side flattening with hypoechoic defect or heterogeneous echogenicity.
- Calcific hydroxyapatite deposits may manifest as dense or tiny calcifications with or without posterior acoustic shadowing. In calcific tendonitis, US may be used to guide fine needle aspiration and lavage.

DISLOCATIONS OF THE GLENOHUMERAL JOINT

Dislocation: separation of articular surface of glenoid fossa and humeral head that will not reduce spontaneously. Subluxation: transient incomplete separation that reduces spontaneously.

Anterior Dislocation (Fig. 5-37)

Most common type (95%) of dislocation. Usually due to indirect force from abduction, external rotation, and extension.

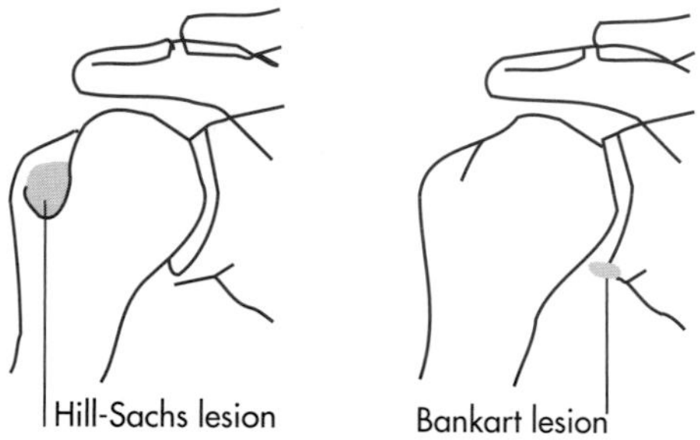

FIGURE 5-37

RADIOGRAPHIC FEATURES

- Humeral head lies inferior and medial to glenoid.
- Two lesions can occur as humeral head strikes the glenoid:
  Hill-Sachs lesion (posterosuperior and lateral) of humeral head (best seen on AP view with internal rotation) Bankart lesion (anteroinferior) of glenoid (may require CT)
- Bulbous distortion of the scapulohumeral arch (Moloney's arch)

Posterior Dislocation (Fig. 5-38)

Less common (5%); usually due to direct or indirect force. Associated with seizures or electrical shock.

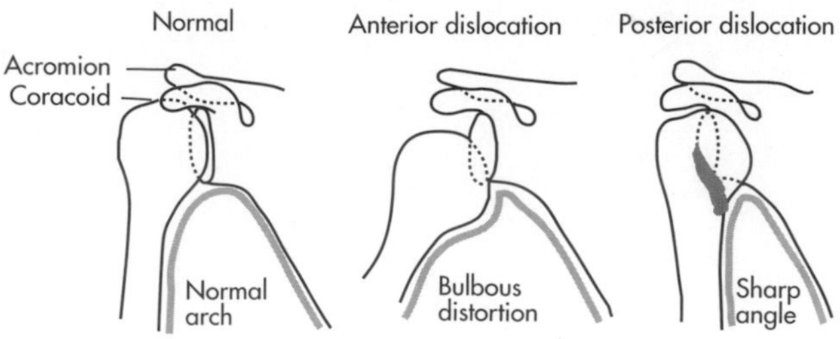

FIGURE 5-38

Radiographic Features

- Humeral head lies superior to glenoid.
- Trough sign: compression fracture of the anterior humeral surface, 15% (best seen on AP view with external rotation or axillary view)
- Sharp angle of the scapulohumeral arch (Moloney's arch)
- Posterior displacement is best seen on axillary view.
- 40° posterior oblique (Grashey view) may be needed: loss of glenohumeral space is diagnostic.
- Fixed in internal rotation

Inferior Dislocation

Also called *luxatio erecta:* the humeral head is located below the glenoid and the shaft of the humerus is fixed in extreme abduction. Complications of luxatio erecta include injuries to the brachial plexus and axillary artery.

PSEUDODISLOCATION OF GLENOHUMERAL JOINT

Inferior and lateral displacement of humeral head due to hemarthrosis that often occurs in fractures of humeral head or neck. Not a true inferior dislocation.

ROTATOR CUFF TEAR (Figs. 5-39 and 5-40)

The rotator cuff (inserts into anatomical neck and tuberosities of humerus) consists of four muscles. Mnemonic: "SITS":
- Supraspinatus
- Infraspinatus

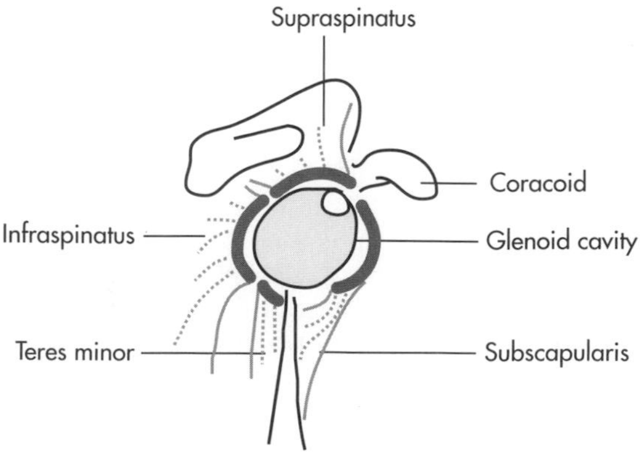

FIGURE 5-39

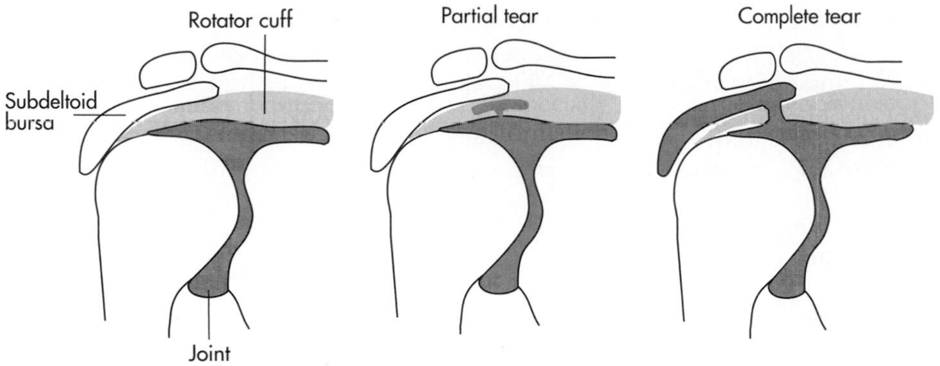

FIGURE 5-40

- Teres minor
- Subscapularis

Causes

- Degeneration
- Trauma
- Impingement

Radiographic Features

- Narrowing of acromiohumeral space to less than 6 mm (chronic rupture)
- Eroded inferior aspect of acromion (chronic rupture)
- Flattening and atrophy of the greater tuberosity of the humeral head
- Arthrogram
  - Opacification of subacromial-subdeltoid bursa
  - Contrast may leak into the cuff in partial tears
- MR arthrography is most accurate diagnostic study
  - Abnormal contrast/signal in supraspinatus tendon
  - Supraspinatus atrophy with tendon retraction
  - Accurate delineation of size/extent of tear possible
  - Allows evaluation of glenoid labrum

ANTERIOR-TO-POSTERIOR LESIONS OF THE SUPERIOR LABRUM (SLAP LESIONS)

- Type I: fraying or tear of the superior labrum
- Type II: detachment of the labral-bicipital complex from the superior glenoid
- Type III: bucket-handle tear of the superior labrum
- Type IV: bucket-handle tear with extension into the biceps tendon

MUSCLE ATROPHY

- Supraspinatus/infraspinatus: suprascapular nerve impingement in the suprascapular notch
- Parsonage-Turner syndrome: acute brachial neuritis. Early edema and thickening of supraspinatus and infraspinatus; later, atrophy.
- Infraspinatus: suprascapular nerve impingement after branch to supraspinatus in the spinoglenoid notch
- Teres minor (quadrilateral space syndrome): axillary nerve impingement in the quadrilateral space (bounded by teres minor superiorly, teres major inferiorly, humerus laterally, long head of triceps medially)

ADHESIVE CAPSULITIS (FROZEN SHOULDER)

Pain, stiffness, and limited range of motion from posttraumatic adhesive inflammation of the joint capsule.

Radiographic Features

- Decreased size of joint capsule
- Obliteration of axillary and subscapular recesses
- Disuse osteoporosis
- Arthrogram if persistent

ACROMIOCLAVICULAR SEPARATION (Fig. 5-41)

Most commonly results from athletic injury to AC joint

- Direct blow to AC joint (e.g., football)
- Severe arm traction
- Fall on hand or elbow with arm flexed 90°

FIGURE 5-41

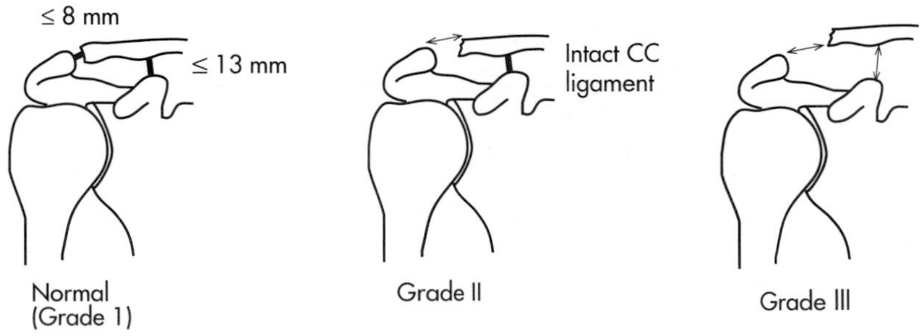

Radiographic Features

Technique
- AP view with 15° cephalad angulation is the preferred view for diagnosis.
- May need opposite shoulder for comparison
- May need stress views (10- to 20-lb weights)

Normal
- Acromioclavicular distance ≤8 mm
- Coracoclavicular distance ≤13 mm
- Inferior margin of clavicle lines up with inferior acromion.

AC joint injury
- Downward displacement of scapula/extremity
- Downward displacement and AC separation worsen with stress weights.
- AC widening = disrupted AC ligament
- Craniocaudad (CC) widening due to disrupted AC ligament

Six grade classifications (Rockwood):
- Grade I (mild sprain): normal radiograph
- Grade II (moderate sprain): increased AC distance; normal CC distance
- Grade III (severe sprain): increased AC and CC distance
- Grade IV: total dislocation; clavicle displaced superoposteriorly into the trapezius
- Grade V: total dislocation; clavicle displaced superiorly into neck
- Grade VI: total dislocation; clavicle displaced interiorly to subacromial or subcoracoid position

STERNOCLAVICULAR (SC) JOINT INJURY (Fig. 5-42)

Most injuries of the SC joint are dislocations resulting from a direct forceful impact. Although anterior dislocations are more common, posterior dislocations are more serious because the great vessels or trachea may be injured.

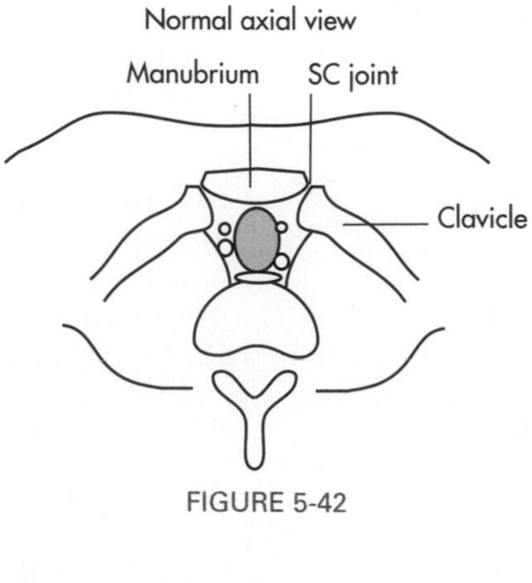

FIGURE 5-42

Radiographic Features

- Superior displacement of clavicle
- Many injuries occur as Salter fractures of medial clavicular epiphysis.
- CT is the examination of choice: thin section with coronal re-formation.
- Angled AP plain film (serendipity view) is not as helpful.

ARM

FRACTURES OF PROXIMAL HUMERUS

These fractures are common in osteoporotic elderly patients secondary to a fall on outstretched hand. 85% are nondisplaced; 4-segment Neer classification aids in treatment and prognosis.

4-Segment Neer Classification (Fig. 5-43)

Based on number and type of displaced segments. 4 segments: anatomic neck, surgical neck, greater tuberosity, lesser tuberosity. Displacement defined as (1) >1 cm separation of fragments or (2) >45° angulation.
- 1-part: no displacement (regardless of comminution); treated with sling
- 2-part: displacement of 1 segment; closed reduction
- 3-part: displacement of 2 segments, 1 tuberosity remains in continuity with the head; closed reduction
- 4-part: displacement of 3 segments; open reduction and internal fixation or humeral head replacement
- 2, 3, and 4-part fractures may have anterior or posterior dislocation.

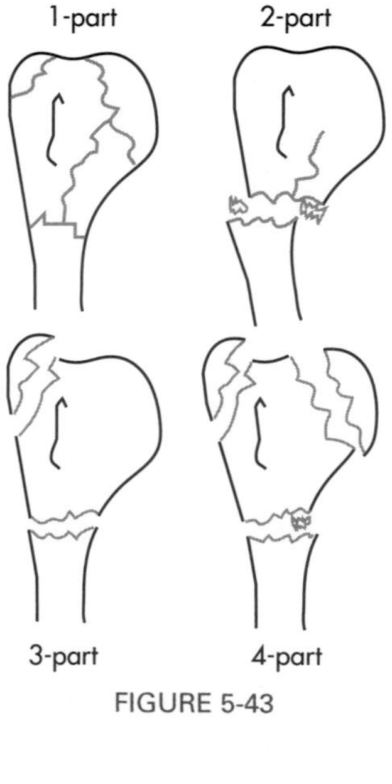

FIGURE 5-43

Radiographic Features

- Fracture lines according to Neer classification
- Pseudosubluxation: inferior displacement of humeral head due to hemarthrosis
- Subacromial fat-fluid level: lipohemarthrosis
- Transthoracic or transscapular views useful to accurately determine angulation

FRACTURES OF DISTAL HUMERUS (Figs. 5-44 and 5-45)

Classification

Supracondylar-extraarticular fracture (3 types)

- Type I: nondisplaced
- Type II: displaced with posterior cortical continuity
- Type III: totally displaced

Transcondylar-intraarticular fracture

Intercondylar (bicondylar)-intraarticular fracture (4 types)

- Type I: nondisplaced
- Type II: displaced
- Type III: displaced and rotated
- Type IV: displaced and rotated and comminuted

Complications

- Volkmann ischemic contracture (usually secondary to supracondylar fracture)
- Malunion (results in "cubitus varus" deformity)

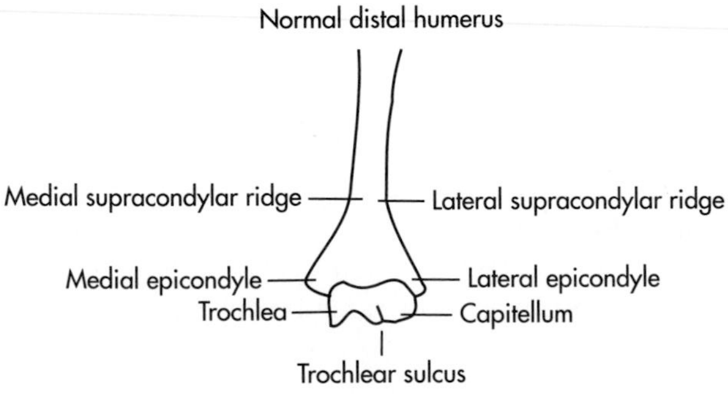

FIGURE 5-44

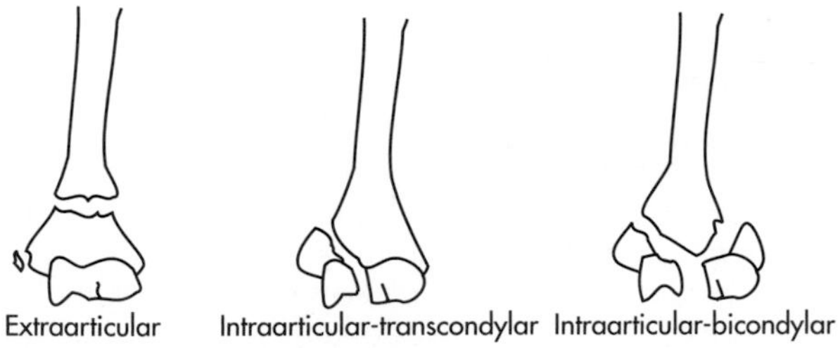

FIGURE 5-45

RADIAL HEAD FRACTURES

Common fracture that results from a fall on outstretched hand.

Treatment

- No displacement: splint, cast
- >3-mm displacement on lateral view: open reduction and internal fixation (ORIF)
- Comminuted: excision of radial head

Radiographic Features (Fig. 5-46)

- Positive fat pad sign
  - Anterior fat pad has the appearance of a sail (sail sign).
  - A positive posterior fat pad is a good indicator of a fracture that is not normally seen.
- Fracture line may be difficult to see on standard projections. If in doubt, obtain radial head view, oblique views, or tomograms.

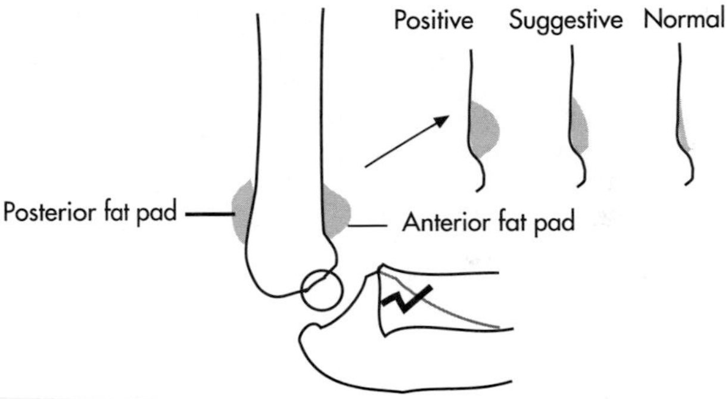

FIGURE 5-46

ULNAR FRACTURES

Isolated ulnar fractures are uncommon. Most fractures of the ulna also involve the radius (see below).

Olecranon Fracture

Result from direct fall on flexed elbow. Treated conservatively if nondisplaced. ORIF if displaced (by pull of triceps). Best view: lateral.

Coronoid Fracture

Usually in association with posterior elbow dislocations. Best view: radial head or oblique views.

ELBOW DISLOCATIONS

Different types of dislocations are defined by the relation of radius/ulna to distal humerus. Posterior dislocations of both the radius and ulna are the most common type (90%). Often associated with coronoid process or radial head fractures. Complication: myositis ossificans. Three types include:

- Ulna and radius dislocation (most common)
- Ulna dislocation only
- Radial dislocation only (rare in adults)

ULNAR COLLATERAL LIGAMENT TEAR

Baseball pitcher injury. Anterior band attaches to sublime tubercle of medial epicondyle and lies deep to common flexor tendon of elbow. Posterior band attaches to lateral aspect of ulna at supinator crest. MRI: T1 globular signal, increased T2 signal.

COMBINED RADIUS-ULNA FRACTURES AND DISLOCATIONS

Most (60%) forearm fractures involve both the radius and ulna.

Monteggia Fracture-Dislocation

Ulnar shaft fracture and radial head dislocation

Galeazzi Fracture-Dislocation

Distal radial shaft fracture and distal radioulnar dislocation

Essex-Lopresti Fracture-Dislocation

Comminuted radial head fracture and distal radioulnar subluxation/dislocation

COLLES FRACTURE (Fig. 5-47)

Mechanism of injury: fall on the outstretched hand with the forearm pronated in dorsiflexion. Most common injury to distal forearm, especially in osteoporotic females.

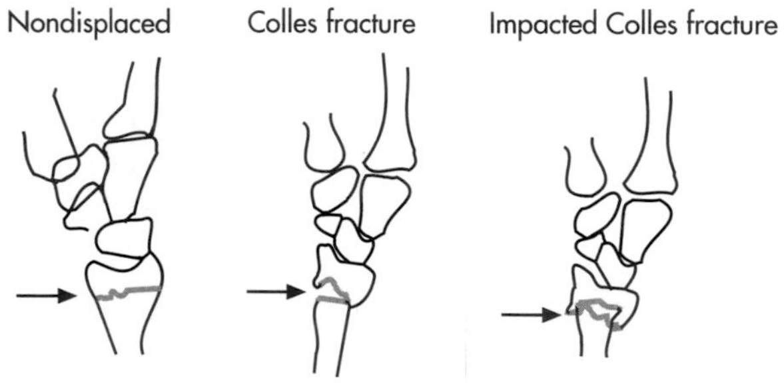

FIGURE 5-47

Radiographic Features

- Extraarticular fracture (in contradistinction to Barton fracture)
- Distal radius is dorsally displaced/angulated.
- Ulnar styloid fracture, 50%
- Foreshortening of radius
- Impaction

Complications

- Median, ulnar nerve injury
- Posttraumatic radiocarpal arthritis

OTHER RADIAL FRACTURES (Figs. 5-48 and 5-49)

Barton Fracture

Intraarticular fracture of the dorsal margin of the distal radius. The carpus usually follows the distal fragment. Unstable fracture requiring open reduction and internal fixation and/or external fixation.

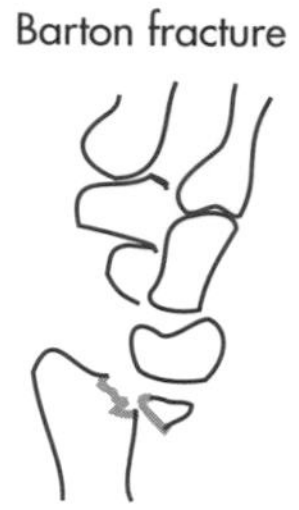

FIGURE 5-48

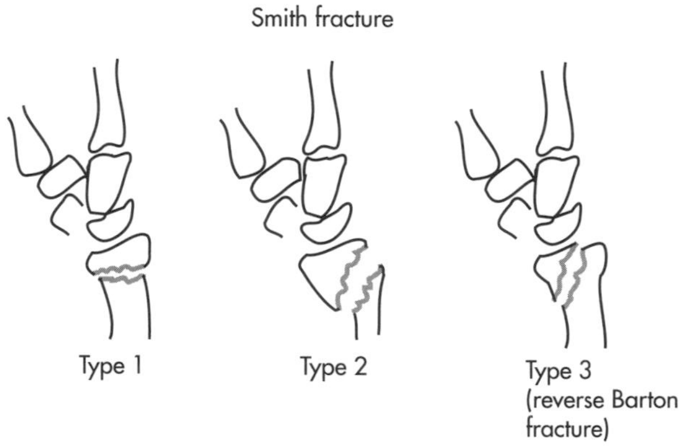

FIGURE 5-49

Smith Fracture

- Same as a Colles fracture except there is volar displacement and angulation of the distal fragment
- 3 types
  - Type 1: horizontal fracture line
  - Type 2: oblique fracture line
  - Type 3: intraarticular oblique fracture = reverse Barton fracture

Hutchinson Fracture (Fig. 5-50)

Intraarticular fracture of the radial styloid process. Also known as chauffeur's fracture.

CARPAL INSTABILITY

Most commonly due to ligamentous injury of the proximal carpal row (trauma or arthritis). Best diagnosed by stress fluoroscopy and/or plain film evaluation of the scapholunate and capitolunate relationships.

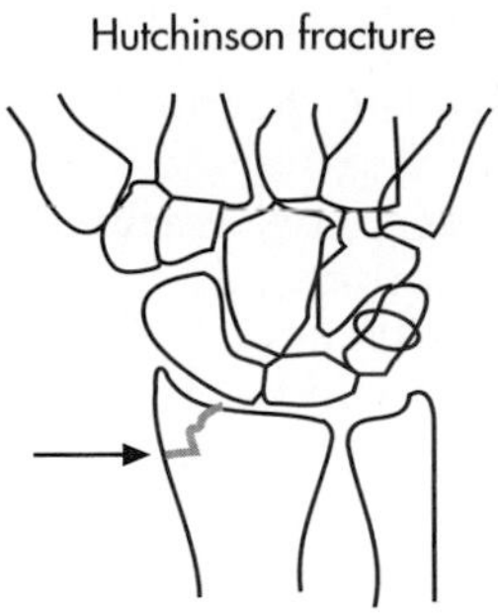

FIGURE 5-50

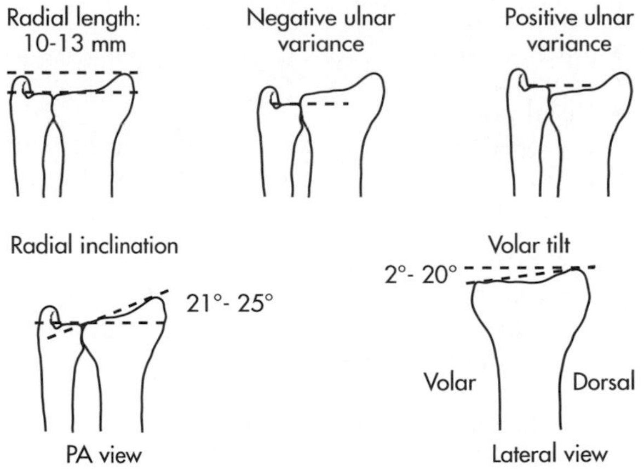

FIGURE 5-52

WRIST/HAND

WRIST ANATOMY (Fig. 5-51)

- Lunate
- Scaphoid
- Trapezium
- Trapezoid
- Capitate
- Hamate
- Triquetrum
- Pisiform

LINES OF ARTICULATIONS (Fig. 5-52)

Ulnar Variance

- Neutral ulnar variance (normal) 80% load by radius, 20% by ulna
- Negative ulnar variance (abnormal). Associated with Kienböck disease
- Positive ulnar variance (abnormal). Associated with:
  - Scapholunate instability
  - Ulnar impaction syndrome
  - Triangular fibrocartilage tear
  - Previous radial head excision
  - Aging

Standard radiographic assessment to quantify deformities associated with distal radius fractures should also consist of three radiographic measurements, which correlate with patient outcome:

- Radial length (radial height): on PA view, distance between line perpendicular to the long axis of the radius passing through the distal tip of the sigmoid notch at the distal ulnar articular surface of the radius and a second line at the distal tip of the radial styloid. This measurement is normally 10 to 13mm. A shortening of >3mm is usually symptomatic and leads to positive ulnar variance.
- Radial inclination (radial angle): on PA view, angle between line connecting the radial styloid tip and the ulnar aspect of the distal radius and a second line perpendicular to the longitudinal axis of the radius. The normal radial inclination ranges between 21° and 25°. Loss of radial inclination increases load across the lunate.
- Volar tilt of the distal radius (palmar tilt): on lateral view, the angle between a line along the distal radial articular surface and the line perpendicular to the longitudinal axis of the radius at the joint margin. The normal volar tilt averages 11° and has a range of 2° to 20°. DISI (see below) may result from an angle >25°.

SCAPHOID FRACTURE

Most common fracture of carpus. Mechanism: fall on outstretched hand in young adults.

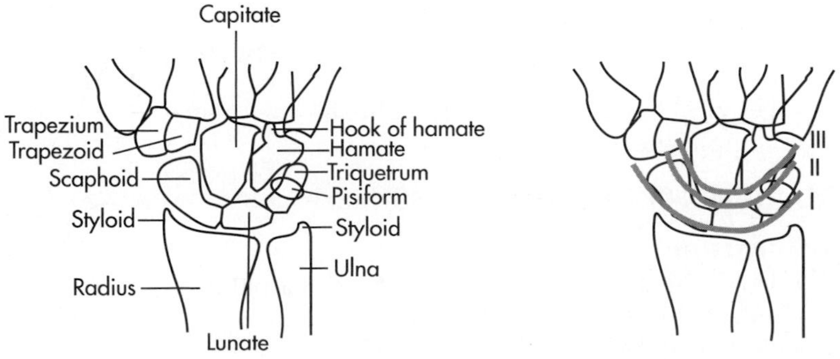

FIGURE 5-51

Locations:
- Waist, 70%
- Proximal pole, 20%
- Distal pole, 10%

Blood supply to the proximal pole enters at the waist; therefore, the proximal pole is at high risk for nonunion and osteonecrosis.

Radiographic Features

- Fracture may be difficult to detect on plain film.
- Scaphoid views (PA view in ulnar deviation) may be useful to demonstrate fracture.
- Loss of navicular fat stripe on PA view
- If a fracture is clinically suspected but not radiographically detected, use multidetector CT. In the absence of MDCT and high-quality re-formations, thin-section CT may be performed along the coronal and sagittal axis of the scaphoid:
  - Coronal position is obtained by placing the patient prone, with elbow flexed 90° and hand placed ulnar side down above the patient's head; images are acquired parallel to the dorsum of the wrist. Alternatively, with the palm side down, the hand and wrist are elevated 30° to 45° and images acquired parallel to the dorsal aspect of the scaphoid.
  - Long sagittal position can be obtained by placing wrist palm down with hand, wrist, and forearm at 45° angle to the long axis of the CT table. Anatomically, this alignment can be recognized by identifying the base of the thumb and the hard bone prominence on the middle portion of the distal radius (Lister tubercle).
- Bone scan: highly sensitive; increased uptake may represent fracture, and decreased uptake proximally may represent possible avascular necrosis (AVN). Does not offer anatomic detail or distinguish marrow edema/bone bruise from fracture.
- MRI: highly sensitive to fractures and allows imaging of planes along the long and short axes of the scaphoid
- Cast and repeat plain films in 1 week.

Prognosis

- Waist fracture: 90% heal eventually; 10% nonunion or proximal AVN
- Proximal fracture: high incidence of nonunion or AVN
- Distal fracture: usually heals without complications

FRACTURES OF OTHER CARPAL BONES

Triquetrum

- Dorsal avulsion at attachment of radiocarpal ligament (most common type of fracture)
- Best seen on lateral view

Hamate

- Hook of hamate fracture: diagnosis requires tomography, carpal tunnel view, or CT
- Other fractures are usually part of complex fracture-dislocations.

Kienböck disease (lunatomalacia)
- AVN of lunate secondary to (usually trivial) trauma
- Associated with ulnar minus variant
- Acute lunate fractures are rare.

WRIST DISLOCATIONS (Fig. 5-53)

The continuum of perilunate injuries ranges from disassociation to dislocation. Mechanism: backwards fall on extended hand. Each of the four successive stages progresses from radial to ulnar side and indicates increased carpal instability.

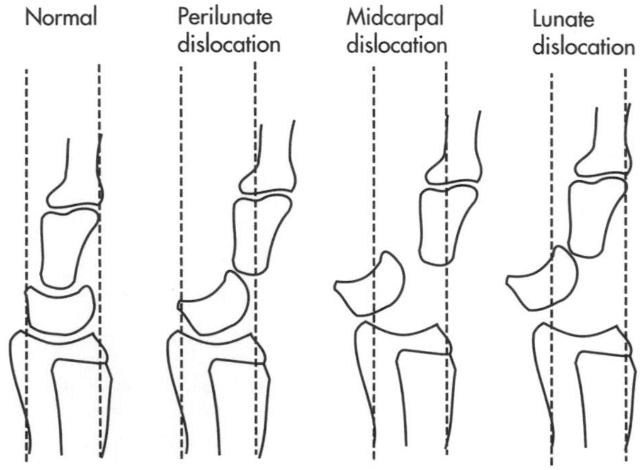

FIGURE 5-53

Scapholunate Dissociation (Stage 1)

- Rupture of scaphoid ligaments
- >3-mm gap between lunate and scaphoid (Terry-Thomas sign)
- Ring sign on PA view secondary to rotary subluxation of scaphoid

Perilunate Dislocation (Stage 2) (Fig. 5-54)

- Capitate dislocated dorsally
- Lunate maintains normal articulation with radius.

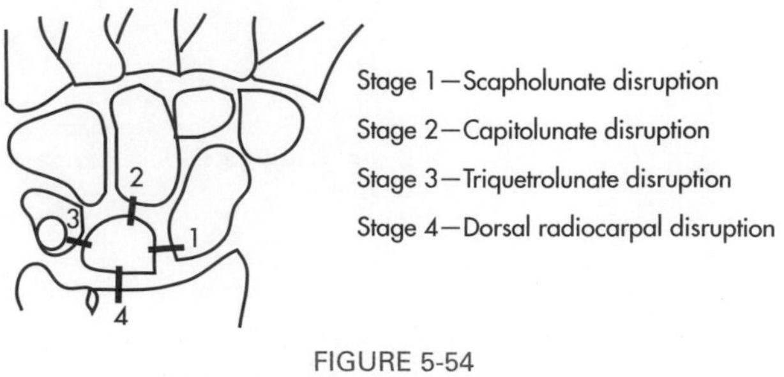

FIGURE 5-54

- May be accompanied by transscaphoid fracture, triquetrum fracture, capitate fracture, and radial styloid process fracture

Midcarpal Dislocation (Stage 3)

- Rupture of triquetral ligaments
- Capitate and carpus are dislocated dorsally.

Lunate Dislocation (Stage 4)

- Lunate dislocates volarly.
- Capitate appears aligned with the radius.

CARPAL INSTABILITY (Figs. 5-55 and 5-56)

Most commonly due to ligamentous injury of the proximal carpal row (trauma or arthritis). Best diagnosed by stress fluoroscopy and/or plain film evaluation of the scapholunate and capitolunate relationships.

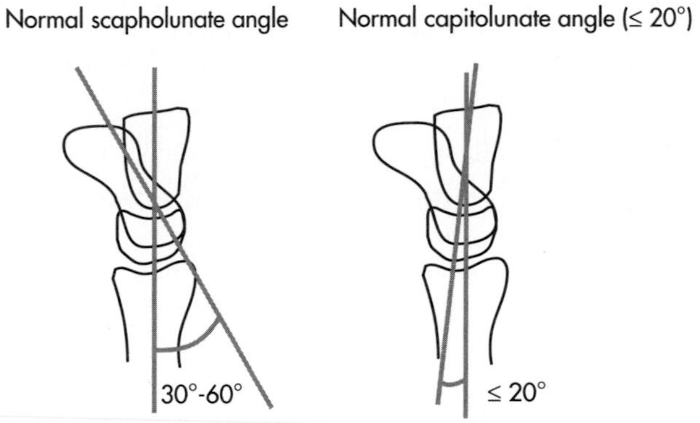

FIGURE 5-55

Scapholunate Dissociation

- Scapholunate angle >60°

Volar Intercalated Segment Instability (VISI)

- Increased capitolunate angle
- Volar tilt of lunate
- Scapholunate angle sometimes decreased
- Much less common than DISI

Dorsal Intercalated Segment Instability (DISI)

- Increased scapholunate and capitolunate angles
- Dorsal tilt of lunate

SCAPHOLUNATE ADVANCED COLLAPSE (SLAC)

Specific pattern of osteoarthritis (OA) associated with chronic scapholunate dissociation and chronic scaphoid nonunion. Calcium pyrophosphate dihydrate (CPPD) is the most common cause.

- Radial-scaphoid joint is initially involved, followed by degeneration in the unstable lunatocapitate joint as capitate subluxates dorsally on lunate.
- Radioscaphoid joint is first to be involved; capitolunate and STT joints follow.
- Capitate migrates proximally into space created by scapholunate dissociation.
- Radiolunate joint is spared.
- In end-stage SLAC, the midcarpal joint collapses under compression, and the lunate assumes an extended or dorsiflexed position DISI.

CT OF THE WRIST

Multidetector CT has revolutionalized evaluation of the wrist. Special patient positions are no longer necessary because high-quality reformatted images can be obtained along any plane from a multidetector CT dataset. However, for historical purposes, dedicated CT of the distal radius, ulna, and carpus can also be performed in several planes.

- CT in the transverse plane has been used to evaluate the distal radioulnar joint and the carpal bones or to further assess a longitudinal fracture. The coronal plane provides an image similar to the standard PA radiograph but will provide better soft tissue and bone detail than will a routine radiograph.

FIGURE 5-56

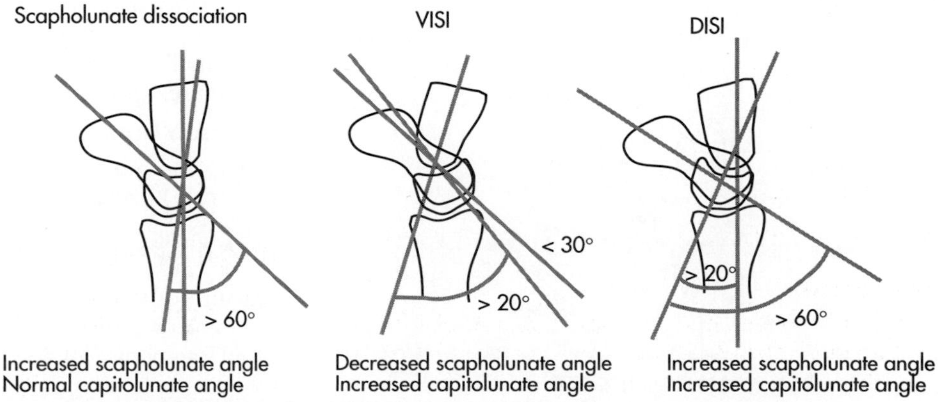

- Coronal CT also demonstrates the radiocarpal joint well.
- In general, 2-mm thick sections at 2-mm intervals will be satisfactory to show the anatomic detail of distal radius and ulnar fractures along articular surfaces.

When evaluating carpal bone fractures and displacements, it is sometimes of value to add 2-mm thick sections at 1-mm intervals in one plane for more anatomic detail, as for a scaphoid fracture.

EVALUATION OF DISTAL RADIAL FRACTURES (Fig. 5-57)

Fernandez and Jupiter, or mechanistic, classification system for distal radial fractures. This classification system closely mirrors prognosis. Fracture forces and comminution progressively increase from type I to type V:

- Type I: bending fractures; include metaphyseal Colles and Smith fractures. These are caused by tensile volar or dorsal loading, respectively, with subsequent comminution of the opposite cortex.
- Type II: shear fractures of the joint surface; includes volar and dorsal Barton injuries.
- Type III: compression fractures of the articular surface; includes die-punch fractures.
- Type IV: avulsion fractures and associated with radiocarpal fracture-dislocations; includes radial and ulnar styloid injuries.
- Type V: high-velocity injuries with comminution and often with bone loss; related to a complex interaction of multiple forces.

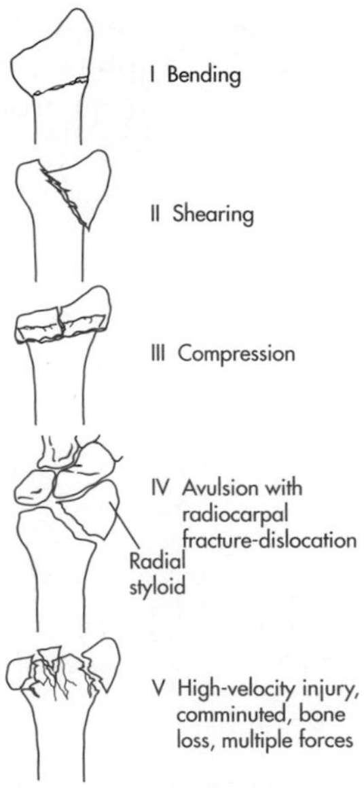

FIGURE 5-57

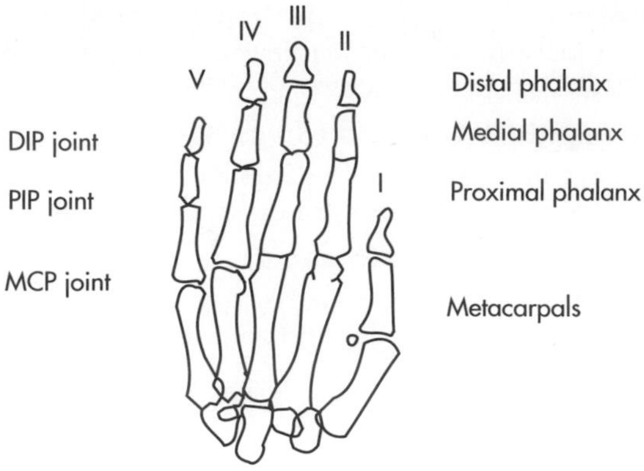

FIGURE 5-58

HAND ANATOMY (Fig. 5-58)

- Metacarpals
- Phalanges: distal, medial, proximal
- Joints: distal interphalangeal (DIP), proximal interphalangeal (PIP), MCP

FIRST METACARPAL FRACTURES (Fig. 5-59)

Bennett and Rolando fractures are intraarticular MCP fracture-dislocations of the thumb. These fractures must be distinguished from extraarticular fractures located distal to the carpometacarpal joint because the former may require open reduction.

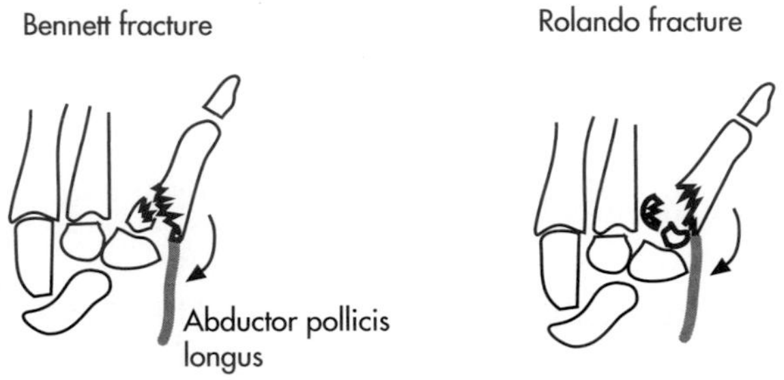

FIGURE 5-59

Bennett Fracture

- Dorsal and radial dislocation (force from abductor pollicis longus)
- Small fragment maintains articulation with trapezium.

Rolando Fracture

- Comminuted Bennett fracture; the fracture line may have a Y, V, or T configuration.

BOXER'S FRACTURE (Fig. 5-60)

Fracture of the MCP neck (most commonly 5th MCP) with volar angulation and often external rotation of the distal fragment. Simple fractures are reduced externally, whereas volar comminution usually requires ORIF.

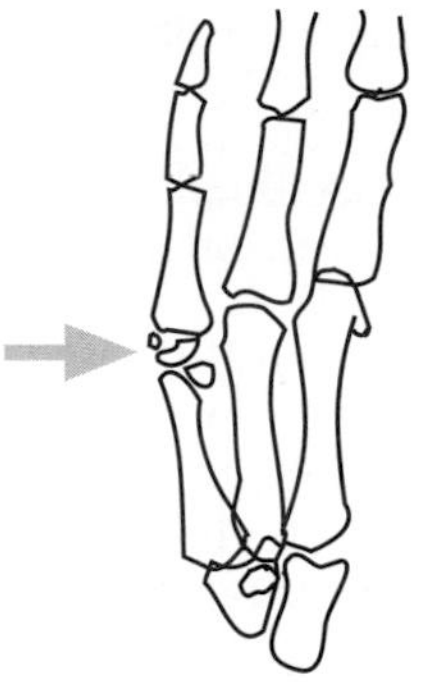

FIGURE 5-60

GAMEKEEPER'S THUMB (SKIER'S THUMB) (Fig. 5-61)

Results from disruption of ulnar collateral ligament. Often associated with a fracture of the base of the proximal phalanx. Common injury in downhill skiing (thumb gets hung up in ski pole). Stress views are required if no fracture is identified on routine plain films but is clinically suspected.

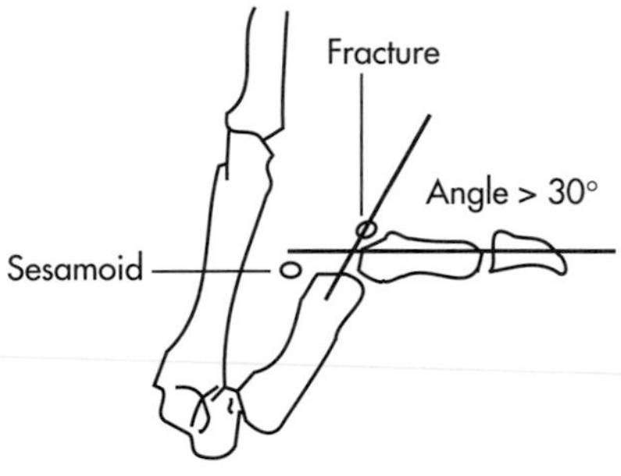

FIGURE 5-61

STENER'S LESION

Occurs in a subset of patients with gamekeeper's thumb, when the ulnar collateral ligament is completely torn and displaced superficial and proximal to the adductor pollicis aponeurosis, preventing the UCL from returning to its normal position. Detect with ultrasound or MR (yo-yo sign). Surgical lesion.

PHALANGEAL AVULSION INJURIES (Fig. 5-62)

Results from forceful pull at tendinous and ligamentous insertions.

Baseball (Mallet) Finger

- Avulsion of extensor mechanism
- DIP flexion with or without avulsion fragment

Boutonnière (Buttonhole) Finger

- Avulsion of middle extensor slip at base of middle phalanx
- PIP flexion and DIP extension with or without avulsion fragment

Avulsion of Flexor Digitorum Profundus

- Avulsion at volar distal phalanx
- DIP cannot be flexed.
- Fragment may retract to PIP joint.

Volar Plate Fracture

- Avulsion at base of middle phalanx
- PIP hyperextension

LOWER EXTREMITY

HIP ANATOMY (Figs. 5-63 and 5-64)

Acetabular lines and anatomy:

- Anterior column includes anterior aspect of the iliac wing, pelvic brim, superior pubic ramus, anterior wall of acetabulum, and teardrop. The column marker on plain radiographs are the iliopubic (iliopectineal line) and pelvic brim.
- Posterior column consists of posterior ilium, posterior wall of acetabulum, ischium, medial

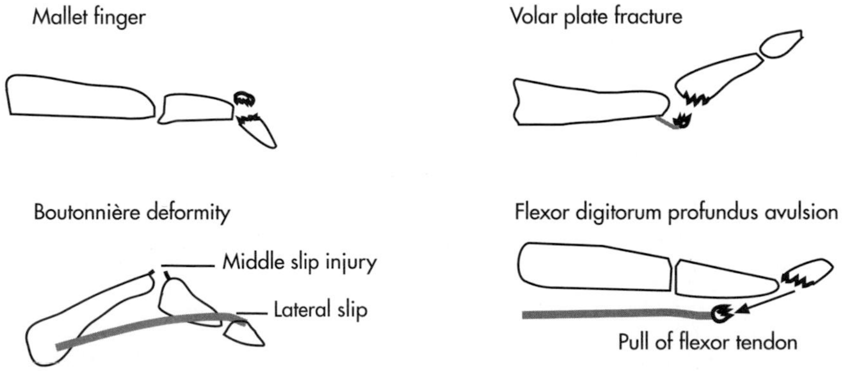

FIGURE 5-62

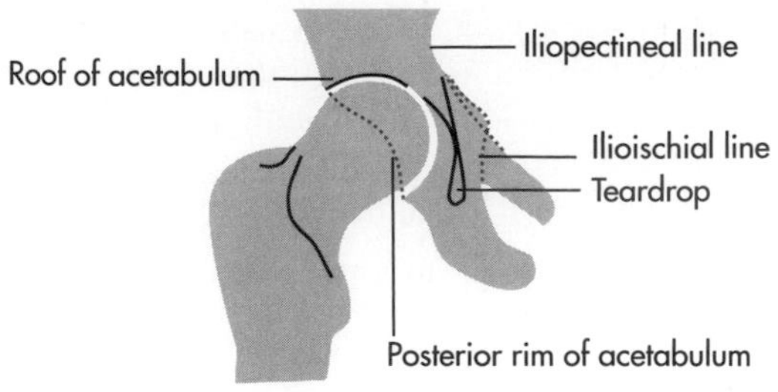

FIGURE 5-63

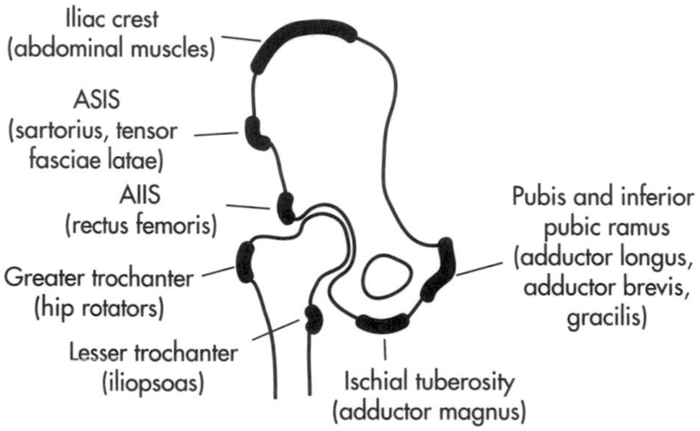

FIGURE 5-64

acetabular wall (quadrilateral plate). The marker on plain radiographs is the ilioischial line: posterior portion of quadrilateral plate of iliac bone.

- Teardrop: medial acetabular wall + acetabular notch + anterior portion of quadrilateral plate
- Roof of acetabulum
- Anterior rim of acetabulum
- Posterior rim of acetabulum

PELVIC FRACTURES (Fig. 5-65, A and B)

Classification

Stable fractures (single break of pelvic ring or peripheral fractures); more common

Avulsion fractures

- Anterior superior iliac spine: sartorius avulsion
- Anterior inferior iliac spine: rectus femoris avulsion
- Ischial tuberosity: hamstring avulsion
- Pubis: adductor avulsion

Other fractures

- Duverney fracture of iliac wing
- Sacral fractures
- Fracture of ischiopubic rami: unilateral or bilateral
- Wide-swept pelvis: external rotation (anterior compression) injury to one side and an internal rotation (lateral compression) injury to contralateral side

Unstable fractures (pelvic ring interrupted in two places); less common. Significant risks of pelvic organ injury and hemorrhage. All unstable fractures require CT before fixation for more accurate evaluation; the extent of posterior ring disruption is often underestimated by plain film.

- Malgaigne fracture: SI joint (or paraarticular fracture) and ipsilateral ischiopubic ramus fracture. Clinically evident by shortening of the lower extremity.
- Straddle: involves both obturator rings
- Bucket-handle: SI fracture and contralateral ischiopubic ramus fracture
- Dislocations
- Pelvic ring disruptions and arterial injury

  Sources of pelvic hemorrhage include arteries, veins, and osseous structures.

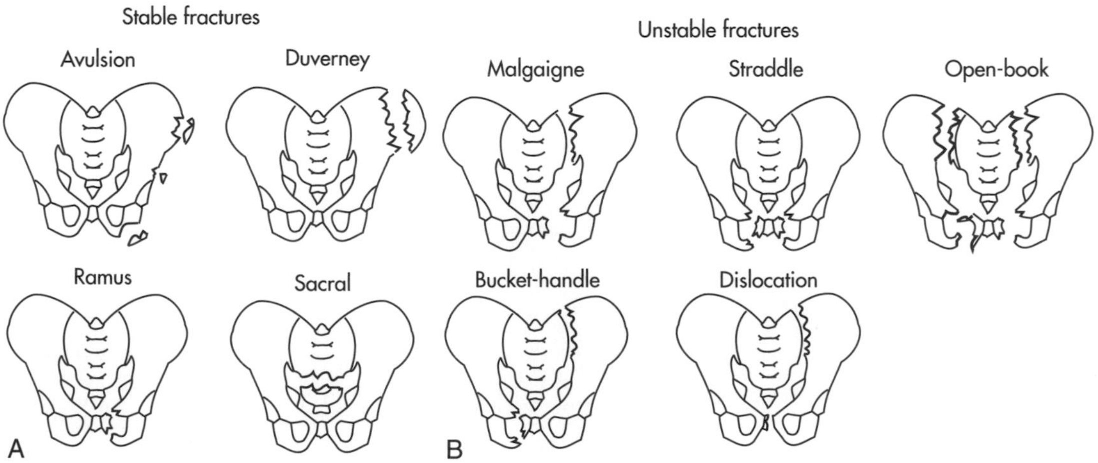

FIGURE 5-65

Arterial bleeding is usually from internal iliac artery branches. Frequency in descending order: gluteal, internal pudendal, lateral sacral, and obturator arteries.

High frequency of arterial hemorrhage in AP compression, vertical shear, crushed fracture of sacrum, and fractures extending into greater sciatic notch.

FRACTURE OF THE ACETABULUM (Fig. 5-66, A-C)

Classification (Letournel)

- Fracture of the anterior (iliopubic) column
- Fracture of the posterior (ilioischial) column
- Transverse fracture involving both columns
- Complex fracture: T-shaped, stellate

SACRAL FRACTURES (Fig. 5-66, D and E)

- Transverse fracture: direct trauma
- Vertical fracture: part of complex pelvic fracture
- Stress fractures: usually juxtaarticular and vertical
- One useful classification is the Denis classification:
  - Zone I: lateral to foramina—50% of cases; 6% with neurologic deficit
  - Zone II: transforaminal—34% of cases; 28% with neurologic deficit

Zone III: central canal involvement—8% of cases; 57% with neurologic deficit

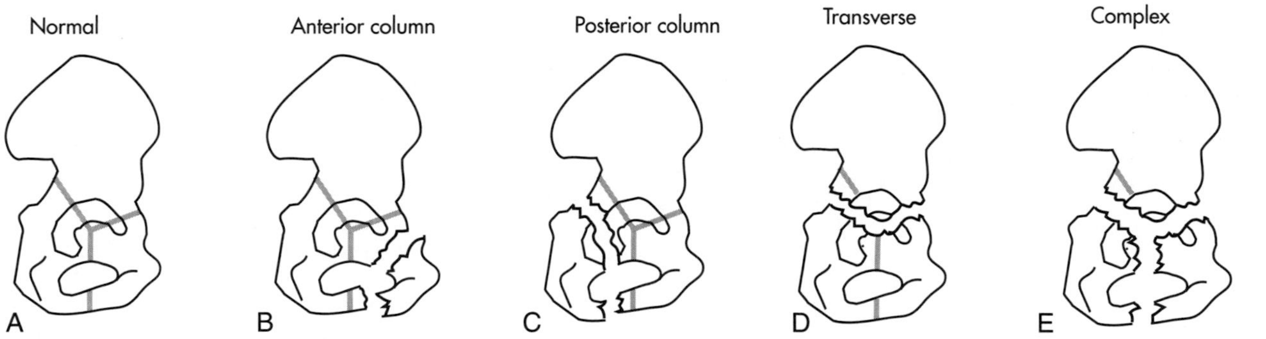

FIGURE 5-66

SOFT TISSUE INJURY (Fig. 5-67)

THIGH MUSCLES

	Origin	Insertion	Nerve
Flexors (Anterior)			
Iliopsoas	Vertebra/ilium	Lesser trochanter	Femoral, lumbar ventral rami
Rectus femoris	Anterior inferior iliac spine	Patellar ligament	Femoral
Vagh's group	Femur	Patellar ligament	Femoral
Sartorius	Anterior superior iliac spine	Medial tibial head	Femoral
Pectineus (adducts)	Iliopectineal line	Lesser trochanter	Femoral (obturator occasionally)
Extensors (Posterior)			
Adductors	Ischial tuberosity	Femur (adductor tubercle)	Obturator
Hamstrings			
Semitendinosus	Ischial tuberosity	Anteromedial tibial shaft	Tibial
Semimembranosus	Ischial tuberosity	Posteromedial tibial condyle	Tibial
Long head biceps	Ischial tuberosity	Fibular head	Tibial
Gluteus	Ilium, sacrum, ligaments	Femur (gluteal tuberosity)	Gluteal

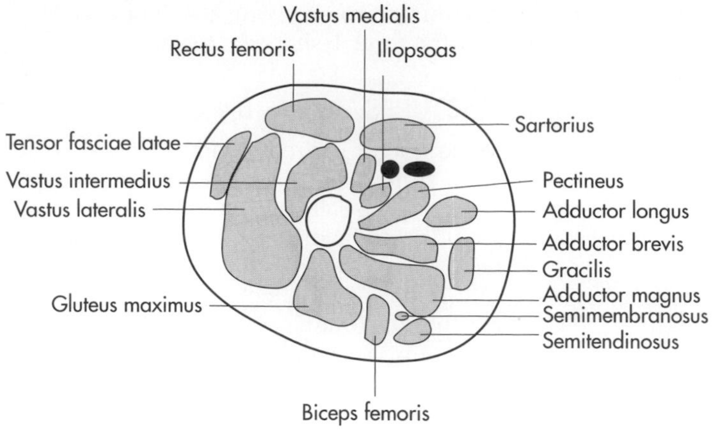

FIGURE 5-67

FRACTURES OF THE PROXIMAL FEMUR (Figs. 5-68 and 5-69)

Incidence: 200,000/year in the United States. Fracture incidence increases with age. In the old age group, mortality is nearly 20%.

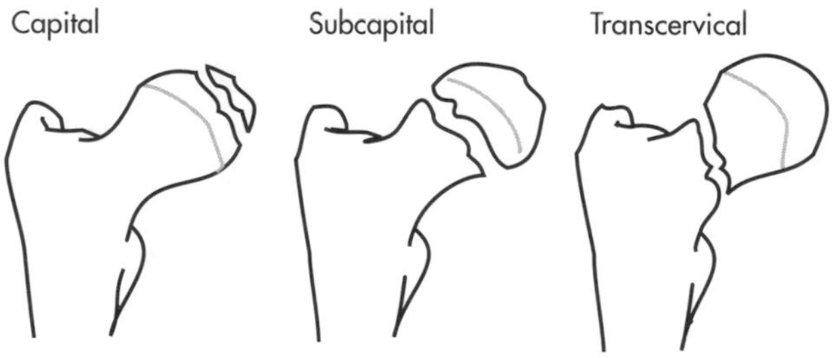

FIGURE 5-68

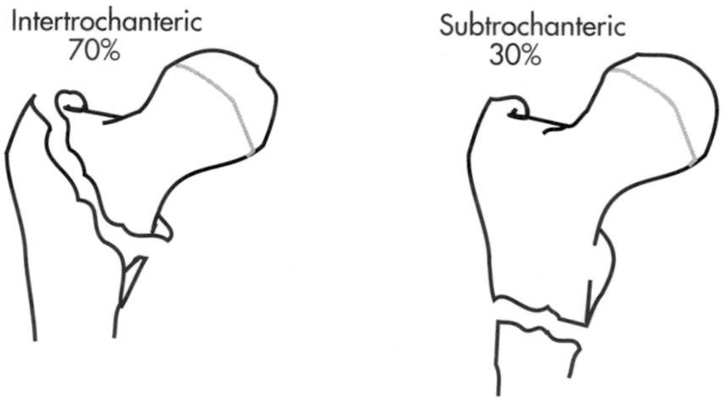

FIGURE 5-69

Classification

Intracapsular fracture involving femoral head or neck
- Capital: uncommon
- Subcapital: common
- Transcervical: uncommon
- Basicervical: uncommon

Extracapsular fracture involving the trochanters
- Intertrochanteric
- Subtrochanteric

FEMORAL NECK FRACTURES

Associated with postmenopausal osteoporosis. Patients often have distal radius and/or proximal humeral fractures.
- Garden classification: based on displacement of femoral head; this classification best predicts risk of AVN and nonunion (Fig. 5-70)
- MRI or bone scan helpful if plain films are equivocal

Treatment
- Bed rest: incomplete fractures
- Knowles pin
- Endoprosthesis if high risk of AVN or nonunion

Complications
- AVN (in 10%-30% of subcapital fractures) occurs secondary to disruption of femoral circumflex arteries.

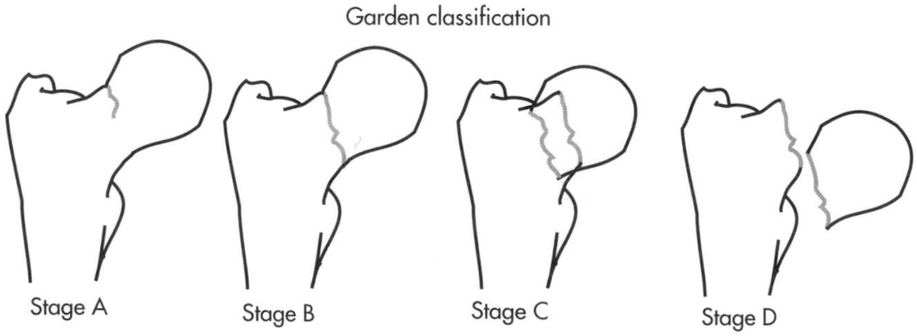

FIGURE 5-70

- Nonunion: obliquity of fracture influences prognosis (steep fractures have higher incidence of nonunion).

INTERTROCHANTERIC FEMORAL FRACTURES

Less common than subcapital fractures. Associated with senile osteoporosis.

- Simple classification: 2-, 3-, 4-, or multipart fracture, depending on number of fragments and involvement of trochanters
- Posteromedial comminution is common

Treatment

- Internal fixation with dynamic compression screw
- Valgus osteotomy

Complications

- AVN is rare.
- Coxa vara deformity from failure of internal fixation
- Penetration of femoral head hardware as fragments collapse
- Arthritis

DISLOCATION OF THE HIP JOINT

Classification (Fig. 5-71)

Posterior dislocation, 90%

- Femoral head lateral and superior to the acetabulum
- Posterior rim of acetabulum is usually fractured
- Sciatic nerve injury, 10%

Anterior dislocation, 10%

- Femoral head displaced into the obturator, pubic, or iliac region

Internal dislocation

- Always associated with acetabular fracture
- Femoral head protrudes into pelvic cavity

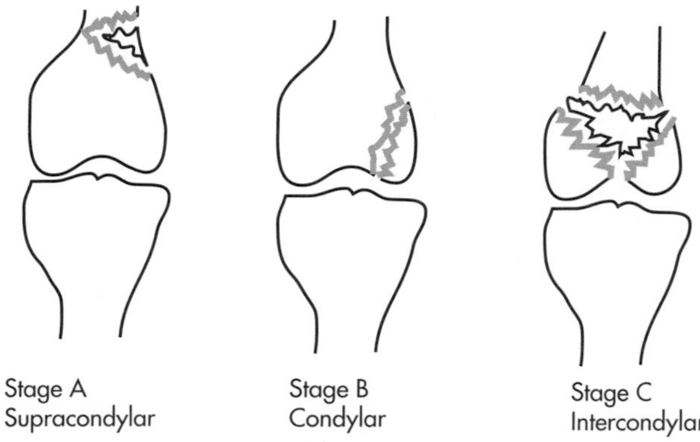

FIGURE 5-71

FRACTURE OF THE DISTAL FEMUR

Classification

Supracondylar

- Nondisplaced
- Displaced
- Impacted
- Comminute

Condylar Intercondylar

FRACTURE OF THE PROXIMAL TIBIA

Fender or bumper fracture: knee is struck by moving vehicle. Lateral (80%) plateau fracture is more common because most trauma results from valgus force; medial plateau fractures (10%); 10% combined medial and lateral fractures.

Classification (Müller) (Fig. 5-72)

- Type 1: split fracture of tibial condyle and proximal fibula (rare)
- Type 2: pure depression fracture of either plateau
- Type 3: combined types 1 and 2
- Type 4: comminuted fracture of both tibial condyles; lateral plateau is usually more severely damaged.

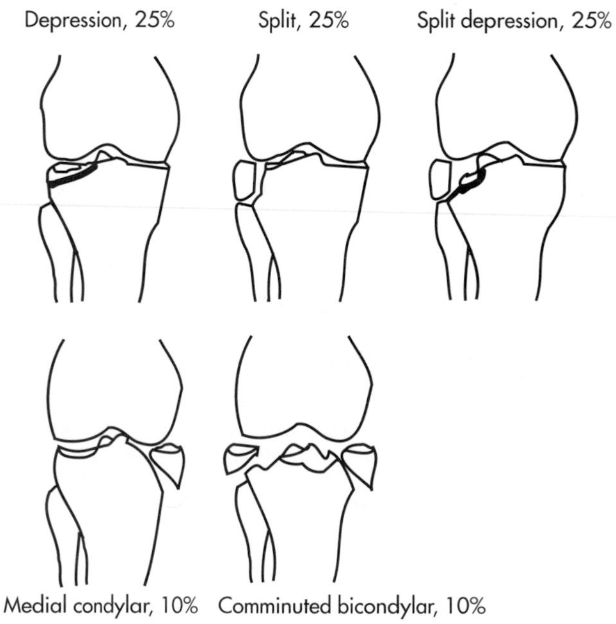

FIGURE 5-72

Radiographic Features

- Fractures of tibial plateau may not be obvious; plain films often underestimate the true extent of fractures; therefore, CT or tomography in AP and lateral projection is often necessary.
- Fat (marrow)-fluid (blood) interface sign (hemarthrosis) on cross-table lateral view
- Description of fractures:

Type of fracture: split, depression, etc.
Location: medial, lateral
Number of fragments
Displacement of fragments
Degree of depression

Complications

- Malunion (common)
- Secondary osteoarthritis (common)
- Concomitant ligament and meniscus injuries (i.e., medial collateral ligament [MCL])
- Peroneal nerve injury

TIBIAL STRESS FRACTURE

Classic runner's fracture is most commonly in proximal tibia.

- Zone of sclerosis with periosteal reaction
- Cortical thickening in posteromedial aspect of proximal tibia

FRACTURE OF THE PATELLA

Classification (Hohl and Larson):

- Vertical fracture
- Transverse (most common)
- Comminuted
- Avulsed

Differentiation of multipartite patella from fractured patella:

- Bipartite or multipartite patella is typically located at the superolateral margin of the patella.
- Individual bones of a bipartite or multipartite patella do not fit together as do the fragments of a patellar fracture.
- The edges of bipartite or multipartite patella are well corticated.

OSTEOCHONDRAL AND CHONDRAL FRACTURE

Shearing, rotary, and tangential impaction forces may result in acute fracture of cartilage (chondral fracture) or cartilage and bone (osteochondral fracture).

Radiographic Features

- Chondral fracture requires arthrography or MRI for visualization.
- Osteochondral fracture may be seen by plain film.

OSTEOCHONDRITIS DISSECANS (CHRONIC OSTEOCHONDRAL FRACTURE)

Painful, usually unilateral, disease in children and young adults. Results from chronic trauma: a segment of articular cartilage and subchondral bone becomes partially or totally separated. Locations: lateral aspect of medial femoral condyle (75%), medial aspect of medial femoral condyle (10%), lateral aspect of lateral condyle (15%), anterior femoral condyle.

Radiographic Features

- Earliest finding: joint effusion
- Radiolucent line separating osteochondral body from condyle (advanced stage)
- Normal ossification irregularity of posterior condyle may mimic osteochondritis dissecans.
- Best evaluated by MRI

PATELLAR DISLOCATION

The patella normally sits in the trochlear sulcus of the distal femur. The mechanism of dislocation is usually an internal rotation of the femur on a fixed foot. Almost always lateral with disruption of medial retinaculum. Medial facet of patella impacts on anterior lateral femoral condyle.

Radiographic Features

- Plain radiographs can be unremarkable except for joint effusion.
- MRI is the imaging modality of choice and shows:
  Hemarthrosis
  Disruption or sprain of medial retinaculum
  Lateral patellar tilt or subluxation
  Bone contusions in lateral femoral condyle anteriorly and in medial facet of patella
  Osteochondral injuries of patella
  Associated injuries to ligaments and menisci in 30%

PATELLAR TENDINITIS (JUMPER'S KNEE)

Overuse syndrome occurring in athletes involved in sports that require kicking, jumping, and running. These activities can place a tremendous stress on the patellofemoral joint, with eventual necrosis, fibrosis, and degeneration of patellar tendon leading to rupture.

- MRI is the imaging modality of choice.
- Enlarged proximal patellar tendon with areas of increased signal intensity on T1-weighted (T1W) and T2-weighted (T2W) images

MENISCAL INJURY (Fig. 5-73)

The most commonly injured meniscus is the medial one. The lateral meniscus is less commonly injured because it has greater mobility. Injuries to the lateral meniscus are associated with discoid meniscus.

Types

- Vertical (longitudinal) tears; most commonly from acute trauma
- Horizontal tears (cleavage tears) in older patients: degenerative
- Oblique tears
- Bucket-handle: may become displaced or detached. There are characteristic signs by MRI: double posterior cruciate ligament (PCL) sign

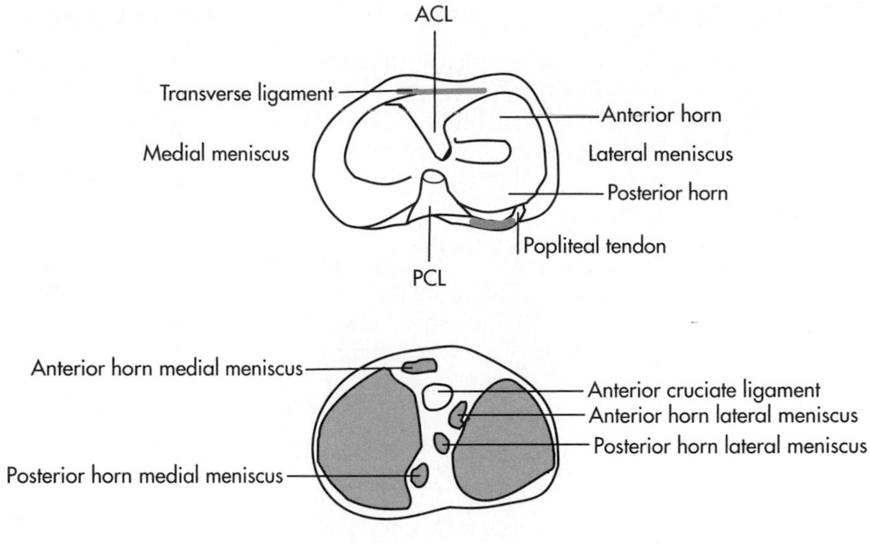

FIGURE 5-73

and flipped meniscus sign. The displaced fragment is typically seen within the intercondylar notch.

- Peripheral tear: meniscocapsular separation
- Truncated meniscus: resorbed or displaced fragment

MRI Grading of Tears (Fig. 5-74)

- Type 1: globular increased signal intensity, which does not communicate with articular surface. Pathology: mucinous, hyaline, or myxoid degeneration
- Type 2: linear increased signal intensity, which does not extend to articular surface. Pathology: collagen fragmentation with cleft formation
- Type 3: tapered apex of meniscus
- Type 4: blunted apex of meniscus
- Type 5: linear increased signal intensity, which extends to the articular surface. Pathology: tear
- Type 6: linear increased signal intensity, which extends to both articular surfaces
- Type 7: fragmented, comminuted meniscus

Pitfalls of Diagnosing Meniscal Tears by MRI (Fig. 5-75)

- Fibrillatory degeneration of the free concave edge of the meniscal surface is often missed by MRI because of volume averaging.
- Normal transverse ligament courses through Hoffa's fat pad and may be mistaken for an anterior horn tear. The ligament connects the anterior horns of medial and lateral menisci.
- Postmeniscectomy meniscus may have linear signal extending to articular surface as a result of intrameniscal signal.
- Pseudotears
  - Lateral aspect of posterior horn of lateral meniscus (popliteus tendon); medial lateral meniscus (ligament)

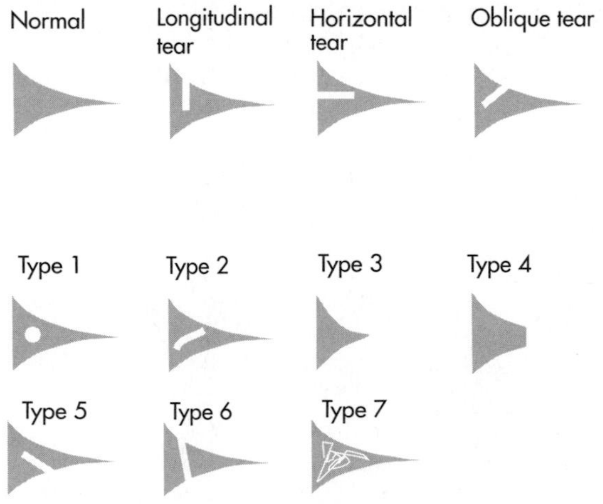

FIGURE 5-74

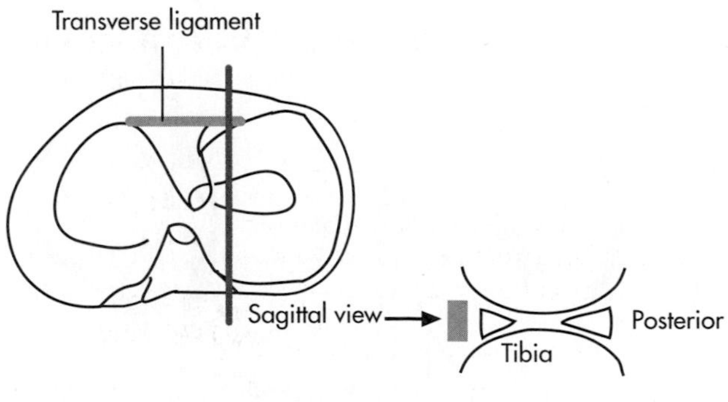

FIGURE 5-75

DISCOID MENISCUS

Morphologically enlarged meniscus (normal variant). Clinically presents as clicking of knee on flexion and extension. Diagnosed by MRI if three or more sagittal images show bridging between anterior and posterior horns. Prone to tears; almost always lateral.

MENISCAL CALCIFICATIONS

Common finding in many diseases (CPPD, hydroxyapatite, hyperparathyroidism, hemochromatosis, Wilson disease, gout, collagen vascular disease, idiopathic). Meniscal calcification is usually not detectable by MRI.

MENISCAL CYSTS

Formed by insinuation of joint fluid through a meniscal tear into adjacent tissues; therefore, meniscal cysts always occur with meniscal tears. Most common in lateral meniscus. Patient presents with knee pain and lateral joint swelling.

CRUCIATE LIGAMENT TEARS (Fig. 5-76)

The cruciate ligaments are intracapsular and extrasynovial. The anterior cruciate ligament (ACL) limits anterior translation of the tibia and hyperextension. The PCL limits anterior translation of the femur and hyperflexion. ACL tears are far more common than PCL tears and are often associated with other injuries.

Radiographic Features

- Plain films may show avulsion fragment of intercondylar eminence.
- MRI is the study of choice for diagnosing ligamentous injury.
- PCL is larger than ACL and better seen by MRI.
- MRI is useful for the assessment of complications after ACL reconstruction, including the Cyclops lesion (focal fibrotic nodule in the intercondylar notch

MRI SIGNS OF ACL INJURY

	Degree of Injury	Direct Signs	Indirect Signs
Mild sprain	Ligament edema	T2W hyperintensity	
Moderate sprain	Partial tear Some fibers intact	ACL edema/hemorrhage	Buckling of PCL ACL angulation Anterior tibial subluxation
Rupture	Complete tear	Wavy contour No ACL identified ACL discontinuity Edema/hemorrhagic mass	Lateral bone bruise MCL injury Medial meniscal injury
Chronic injury	Old mild/moderate sprains	Thickened ACL Thinned ACL Abnormal proton density signal No acute edema on T2W images	Anterior tibial subluxation

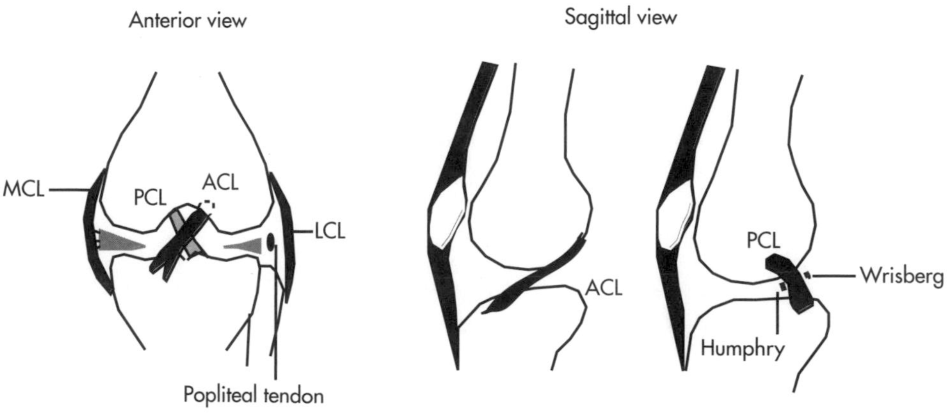

FIGURE 5-76

SEGOND FRACTURE (Fig. 5-77)

Small avulsion fracture involving the superolateral surface of the proximal tibia. Frequently associated with tears of lateral capsular ligament, ACL, and menisci. Segond fracture is in the midcoronal plane and must be differentiated from less common iliotibial band avulsion of Gerdy's tubercle seen more anteriorly on the tibia. MRI should be performed in all cases of Segond fracture to evaluate associated ligamentous injury.

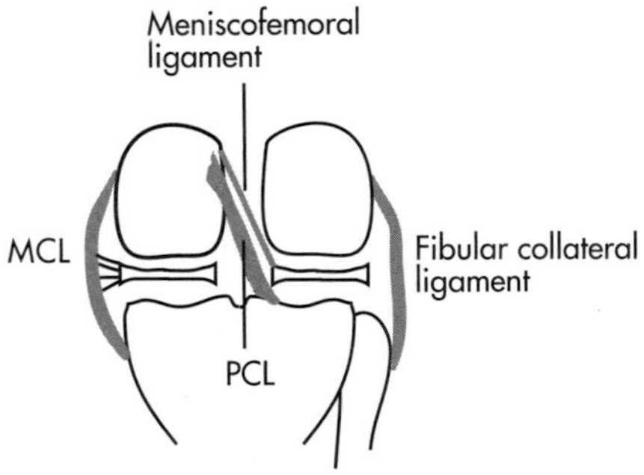

FIGURE 5-77

REVERSE SEGOND FRACTURE

Similar to Segond fracture but the fragment is located on the medial surface of the proximal tibia. Represents avulsion of the deep capsular component of the medial collateral ligament. Associated with tears of the posterior cruciate ligament (PCL), avulsions of the PCL from the posterior tibial plateau and tear of the medial meniscus. MRI should also be performed to evaluate associated injuries.

COLLATERAL LIGAMENTS

The medial collateral ligament (MCL) (injury common) is attached to the medial meniscus, so both are frequently injured together. The lateral collateral ligament (LCL) complex (injury less common) consists of the fibular collateral ligament, the biceps femoris tendon, and the iliotibial band.

Radiographic Features (Fig. 5-78)

- MRI criteria of injury are similar to those used for ACL and PCL tears
- O'Donoghue's triad (the "unhappy triad") results from valgus stress with rotation:
  - ACL tear
  - MCL injury
  - Medial meniscal tear (lateral compartment bone bruise)
- Pelligrini-Steida lesion: curvilinear calcification or ossification at site of femoral attachment of MCL indicates old MCL injury.

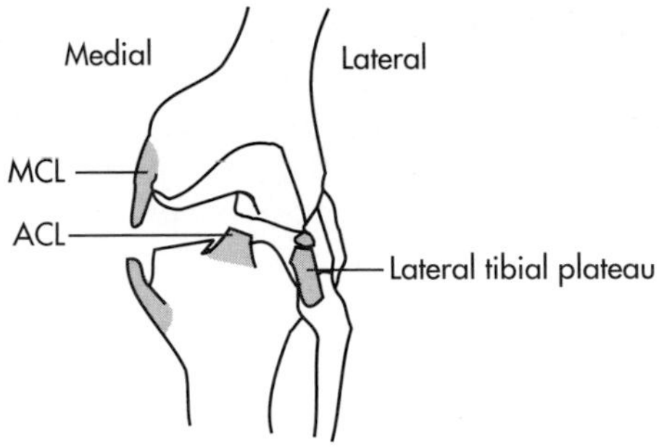

FIGURE 5-78

TENDON INJURY

Commonly occurs from acute trauma or overuse injury in athletes or degenerative tendinopathy in elderly.

Radiographic Features

Acute tendinitis
- Tendon enlargement
- Fluid in synovial sheath (in tenosynovitis)
- Abnormal MRI signal within tendon may indicate partial tear.

Chronic tendinitis
- Tendon thinning or thickening
- Intratendon signal does not increase on T2W images.

KNEE DISLOCATION

- Posterior, 75%
- Anterior, 50%
- Serious vascular injury to popliteal vessels occurs in 35% and to peroneal vessels in 25%.

ANKLE

ANKLE ANATOMY (Fig. 5-79)

ANKLE FRACTURES

Classification (Fig. 5-80)

Of the different classifications of injuries available, the Weber classification is the most useful. It uses the level of fibular fracture to determine the extent of injury to the tibiofibular ligament complex:

Weber A (below tibiofibular syndesmosis)
- Transverse fracture of lateral malleolus or rupture of LCL
- Oblique fracture of medial malleolus
- Tibiofibular ligament complex spared (stable)
- Results from supination-adduction (inversion)

Weber B (through tibiofibular syndesmosis)
- Oblique or spiral fracture of lateral malleolus near the joint
- Transverse fracture of medial malleolus or rupture of deltoid ligament

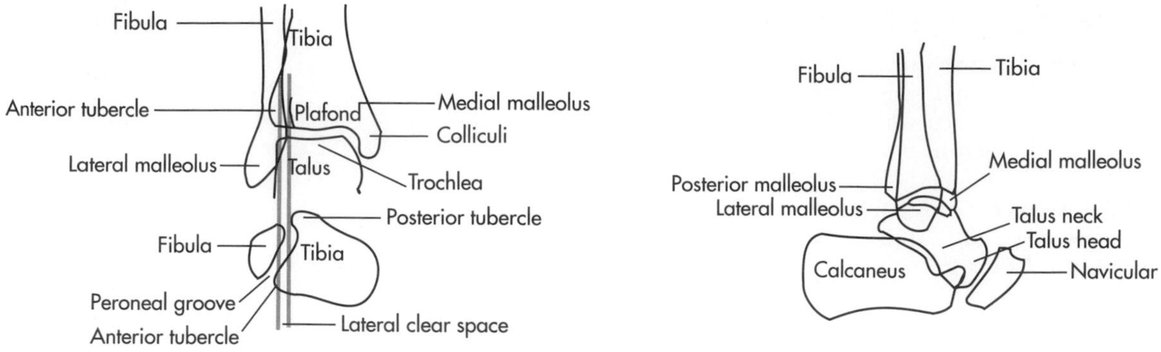

FIGURE 5-79

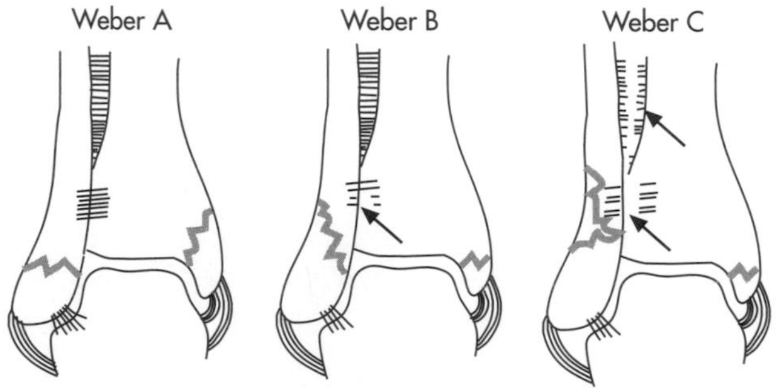

FIGURE 5-80

- Partial disruption of tibiofibular ligament complex
- Results from supination-lateral rotation or pronation-abduction

Weber C (above tibiofibular syndesmosis)

- Proximal fracture of fibula
- Transverse fracture of medial malleolus or rupture of deltoid ligament
- Rupture of tibiofibular ligament complex (lateral instability)
- Results from pronation-lateral rotation

Approach

1. Evaluate all three malleoli.
2. Assess ankle mortise stability (3- to 4-mm space over entire talus).
3. If an isolated medial malleolar injury is present, always look for proximal fibular fracture.
4. Obtain MRI or arthrography for accurate evaluation of ligaments.
5. Determine if the talar dome is intact.

TIBIAL FRACTURES

Pilon Fracture (Fig. 5-81)

Supramalleolar fractures of distal tibia that extend into tibial plafond. Usually associated with fractures of distal fibula and/or disruption of distal tibiofibular syndesmosis. Mechanism is usually due to vertical loading (e.g., in jumpers). Associated with intraarticular comminution. Complication: posttraumatic arthritis.

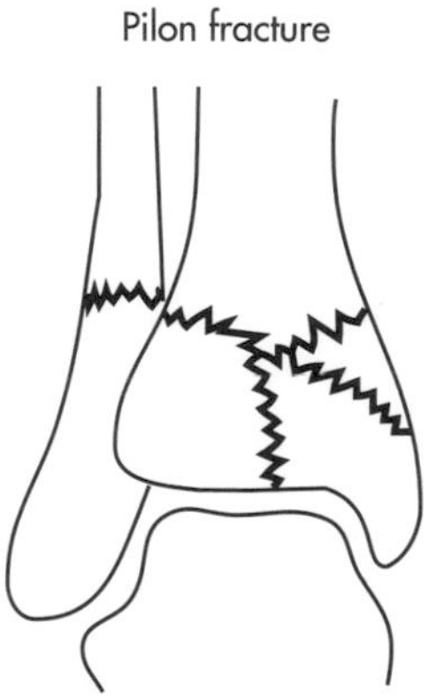

FIGURE 5-81

Tillaux Fracture (Fig. 5-82)

Avulsion of the lateral tibial margin. In children, the juvenile Tillaux fracture is a Salter-Harris type III because the medial growth plate fuses earlier.

Wagstaffe-Le Fort Fracture

Avulsion of the medial margin of the fibula at the attachment of the anterior tibiofibular ligament.

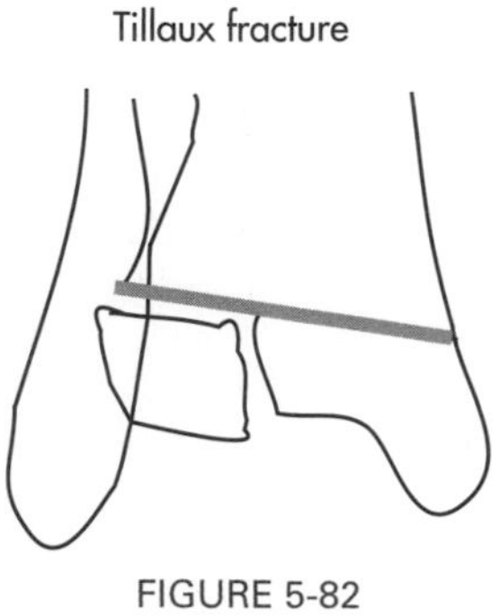

FIGURE 5-82

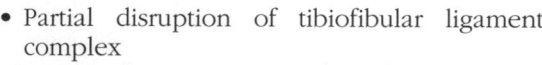

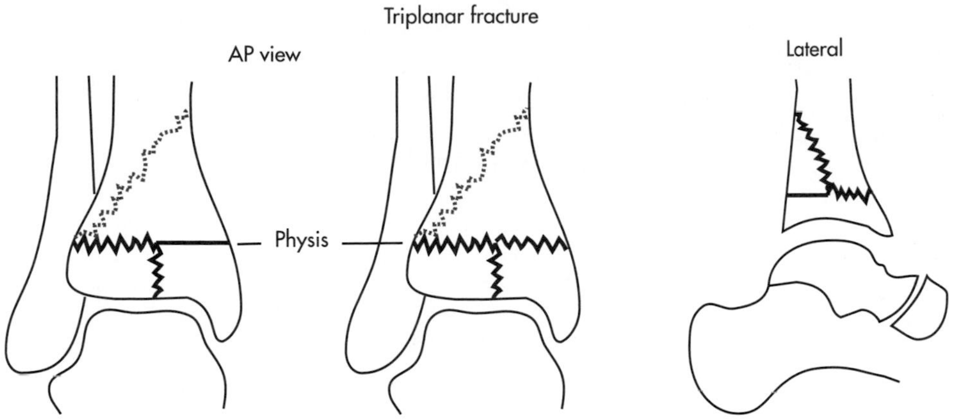

FIGURE 5-83

Triplanar Fracture (Fig. 5-83)

Childhood fracture with three fracture planes: vertical fracture of the epiphysis, horizontal fracture through the physis, and an oblique fracture through the metaphysis.

Tibial Insufficiency Fracture (Fig. 5-84)

Occurs in the distal tibia near plafond as opposed to tibial stress fractures, which occur in posterior proximal tibial diaphysis.

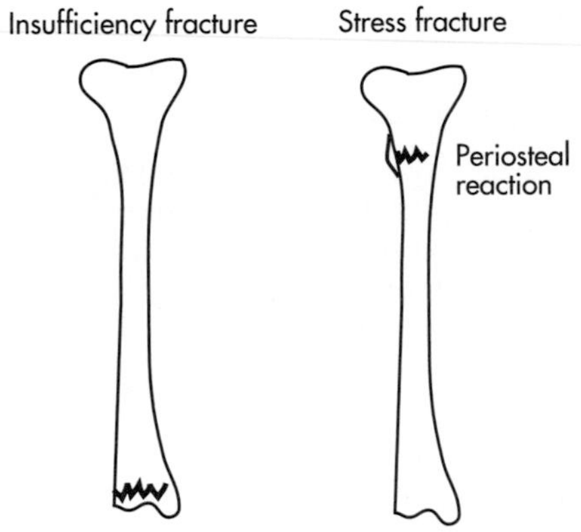

FIGURE 5-84

FIBULAR INJURY

Anatomy of Ligaments (Figs. 5-85 and 5-86)

Three groups of ligaments stabilize the ankle:

Medial collateral ligament (deltoid ligament, four parts)
- Anterior tibiotalar ligament
- Posterior tibiotalar ligament
- Tibiocalcaneal ligament
- Tibionavicular ligament

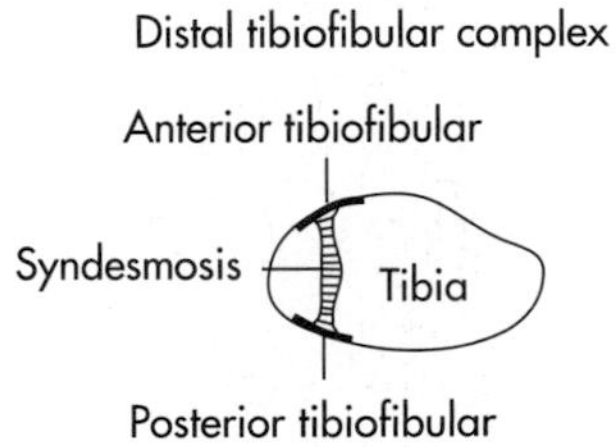

FIGURE 5-85

Lateral collateral ligament (three parts)
- Anterior talofibular ligament
- Posterior talofibular ligament
- Calcaneofibular ligament

Distal tibiofibular complex (most important for ankle stability)
- Anterior tibiofibular ligament
- Posterior tibiofibular ligament
- Tibiofibular syndesmosis

Tear of the Medial Collateral Ligament (Fig. 5-87)
- Plain film: soft tissue swelling
- Lateral subluxation of the talus
- Eversion stress views (5 to 10 mL of 1% lidocaine [Xylocaine] at site of maximum pain): >20° talar tilt is abnormal (angle between plafond and dome of talus on AP film)
- Arthrogram: leak of contrast beneath the medial malleolus

Tear of the Lateral Collateral Ligament
- Plain film: soft tissue swelling
- Medial subluxation of the talus
- Inversion stress views: <15° talar tilt is normal
- Arthrogram: leak of contrast beneath the lateral malleolus
- The anterior talofibular ligament is the most frequently injured ankle ligament.

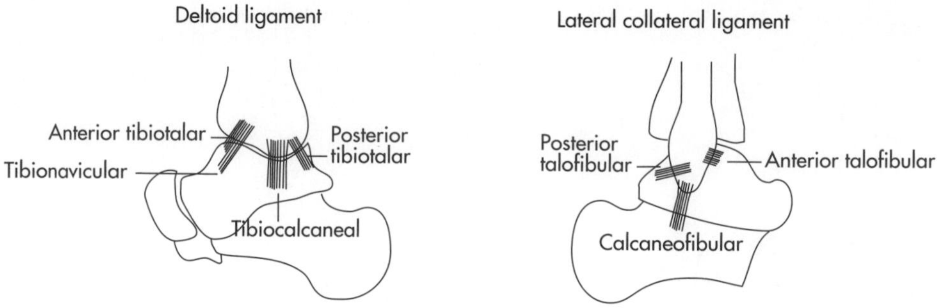

FIGURE 5-86

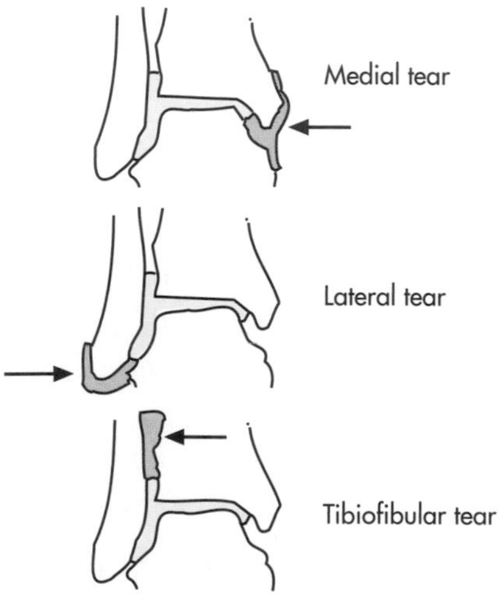

FIGURE 5-87

Tear of the Distal Anterior Tibiofibular Ligament

- Commonly associated with other ligament injuries
- Arthrogram: leak of contrast agent into the syndesmotic space

Maisonneuve Fracture

Spiral proximal fibular fracture associated with an ankle joint injury (named after a French surgeon). It is an important injury because it is easily overlooked clinically and occurs remote from the region covered by standard radiographs of the ankle. The presence of this fracture type implies a ligamentous ankle injury and disruption of the syndesmosis. It is categorized as Weber C.

FOOT

ANATOMY (Fig. 5-88)

CALCANEAL FRACTURES (Fig. 5-89)

Lover's Fracture

Results from axial load (e.g., fall from height)

Radiographic Features

- Decreased Boehler's angle (<20%); normal Boehler's angle does not exclude fracture.
- 75% are intraarticular (subtalar joint).
- 10% are bilateral.

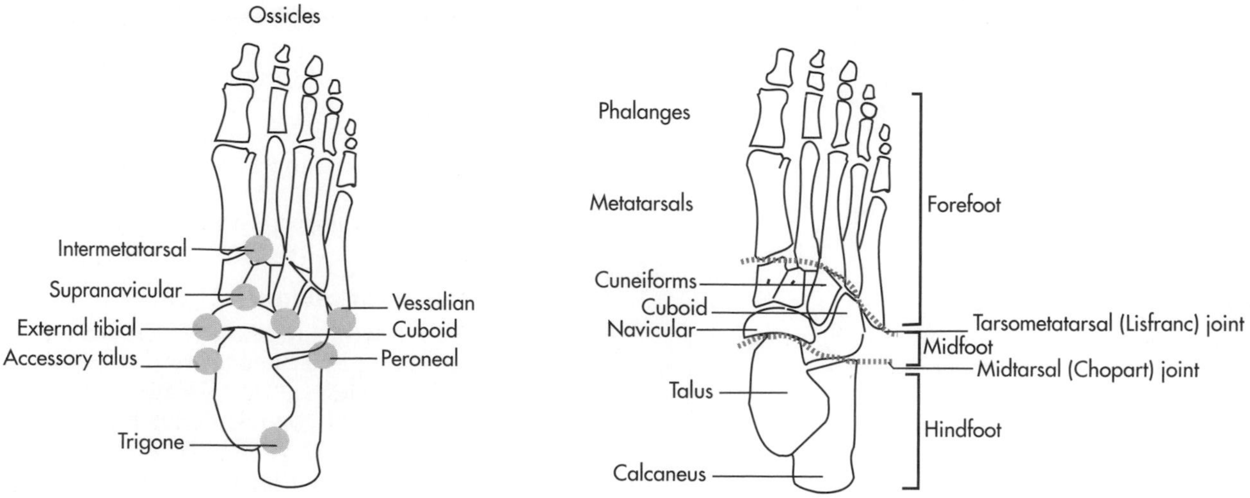

FIGURE 5-88

Normal Boehler's angle

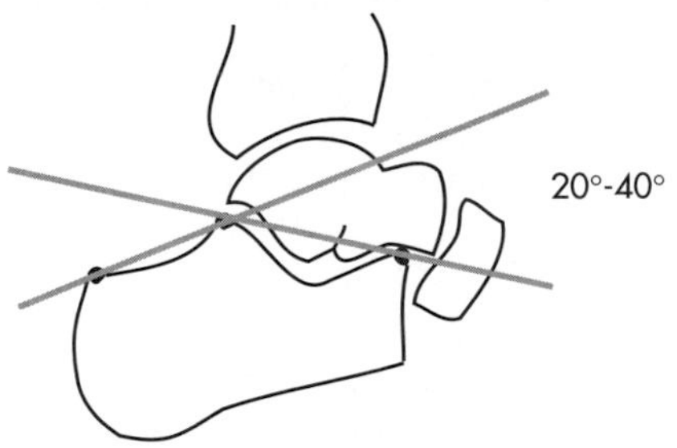

FIGURE 5-89

- Associated fractures:
  Thoracolumbar burst fracture (Don Juan fractures)
  Pilon fractures

Calcaneal Stress Fractures (Fig. 5-90)

Occurs in runners, diabetics, and elderly patients. Vertical linear appearance.

Achilles Tendon Tear

The Achilles tendon is formed by the confluence of the gastrocnemius and the soleus tendon. The critical zone, the site of most acute tears, is 2 to 6cm proximal to its calcaneal insertion site.

- Plain radiographs show marked soft tissue swelling behind the distal tibial and ankle with obliteration of the pre-Achilles fat pad.
- MRI in partial tears shows tendon enlargement and edema, intratendinous areas of increased signal intensity on T2W, and surrounding soft tissue edema.
- Incomplete tear; a tendinous gap is present and is filled with high signal blood and edema.

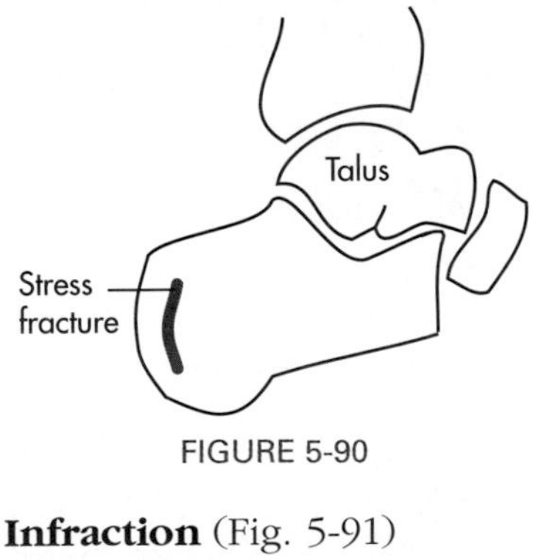

FIGURE 5-90

Freiberg Infraction (Fig. 5-91)

Osteochondrosis of metatarsal head secondary to repetitive trauma with flattening and sclerosis of head of second metatarsal leading to collapse of metatarsal head and fragmentation (late).

- Other metatarsals may also be involved.
- More common in females (3:1), ages 13-18
- Usually unilateral

Common fracture sites

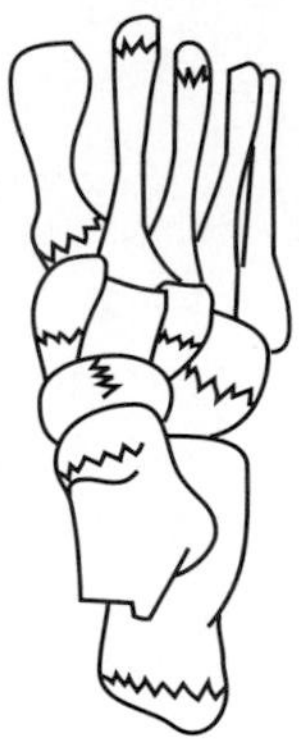

FIGURE 5-91

Talar Fractures

Articular cartilage covers 60% of talus; there are no muscle or tendon insertions. Ligamentous avulsions are most common. Other types:

- Talar neck fracture (aviator's astragalus). Complication: proximal AVN
- Osteochondral fractures of talar dome
- Osteochondritis dissecans of talar dome

Jones Fracture (Dancer's Fracture)

Fracture of proximal shaft of 5th metatarsal. Not due to peroneus brevis avulsion.

Located within 1.5cm from tuberosity. High rate of nonunion for which surgery may be indicated. Distinguished from avulsion fracture, which is more common, has a fracture line more perpendicular to the base, and usually does not require surgery.

Nutcracker Fracture of Cuboid

Cuboid fracture due to indirect compressive forces. Occurs when abduction of forefoot compresses cuboid between bases of fourth and fifth metatarsal distally and calcaneus proximally (like nut in a nutcracker).

LISFRANC FRACTURE-DISLOCATION (Fig. 5-92)

Named after Napoleon's surgeon, who described an amputation procedure at the tarsometatarsal joint. Dorsal dislocation of the tarsometatarsal joints. Most common dislocation of the foot. Usually a manifestation of a diabetic neuropathic joint (Charcot's joint). Two types: homolateral and divergent.

Radiographic Features

- Homolateral: lateral dislocation of metatarsals 1 to 5 or 2 to 5
- Divergent: lateral dislocation of metatarsals 2 to 5 and medial dislocation of first metatarsal
- Associated fractures of base of metatarsal and cuneiform bones
- May be very subtle at early stage

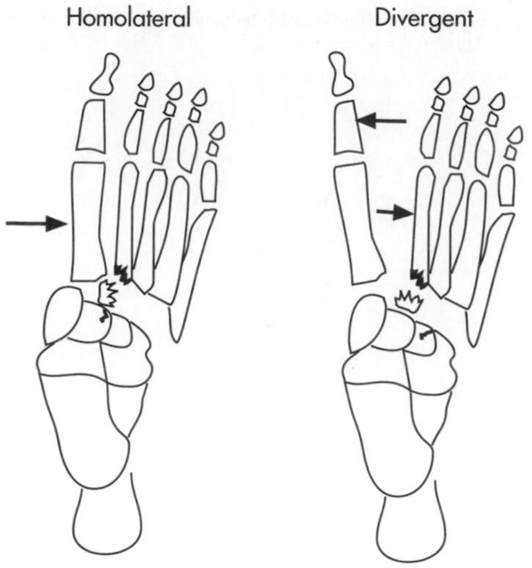

FIGURE 5-92

ORTHOPEDIC PROCEDURES

JOINT REPLACEMENT

Four types of materials are used:

- Polyethylene is used for concave articular surfaces (acetabulum, tibial plateau). Usually backed by metal to provide support. Polyethylene is radiolucent.
- Silastic is used for arthroplasty implants in foot and hands. Made radiopaque during production.
- Metal alloys; cobalt-chromium-molybdenum alloy; cobalt-chromium-tungsten alloy; titanium-aluminium-vanadium alloy
- Ultra high molecular weight polyethylene
- Methylmethacrylate is used as cement or is injected into the medullary space under high pressure. Made radiopaque during production.

Constrained prostheses have inherent stability (ball-in-socket); unconstrained prostheses rely on normal extraarticular structures to provide stability. The more constrained a prosthesis, the higher the likelihood of loosening. The less constrained a prosthesis, the more likely it will dislocate.

PROSTHETIC LOOSENING

Acute loosening is usually due to infection. Chronic loosening is due to mechanical factors; thus proper alignment is critical.

Radiographic Features

- Immediate postoperative plain films are usually obtained to document position and alignment and as baseline to demonstrate progression of loosening over time.
- Widening of the radiolucency at bone-cement or metal-bone interfaces to >2 mm indicates loosening.
- Migration of components
- Periosteal reaction
- Osteolysis is suggestive but not diagnostic of loosening.
- Cement fracture is a definite indicator of loosening.

Other Complications

- Polyethylene wear
- Dislocation of prosthesis
- Particle disease: lobulated areas of osteolysis around joint prosthesis due to macrophage-mediated reaction to particle debris (e.g., polyethylene, metal)
- Hematoma
- Heterotopic bone formation
  - Frequently seen after hip surgery for degenerative disease
  - Excessive bone formation interferes with motion
- Thrombophlebitis is frequent in the immediate postoperative course.
- Foreign body granulomatous reaction
- Leakage of acrylic cement
  - Intrapelvic leakage of cement (polymerization heat induced) leads to:
    - Vascular and neurologic damage
    - Necrosis
    - Genitourinary injury
  - To prevent accidental leaks, the following devices are used:
    - "Mexican hat" in acetabular drill holes
    - Wire mesh
- Infection. Imaging findings:
  - Extensive bone destruction
  - Air in soft tissue and /or joint
  - Extensive and aggressive periosteal reaction
  - Wide and irregular lucent zone
- Metal synovitis

HIP REPLACEMENT (Fig. 5-93)

Types of Prostheses

- Cemented (methylmethacrylate) Chamley or Chamley-Muller prostheses are usually implanted in older patients; occasionally the acetabular component may be fixed with screws while the femoral compartment is cemented.
- Sintered prosthesis (bone ingrowth into porous-coated prosthesis without cementing) is usually used for younger patients; loosening is difficult to assess other than by observing progressive motion of prosthesis.
- Modular prostheses are noncemented and consist of various components that optimize pressure distribution.

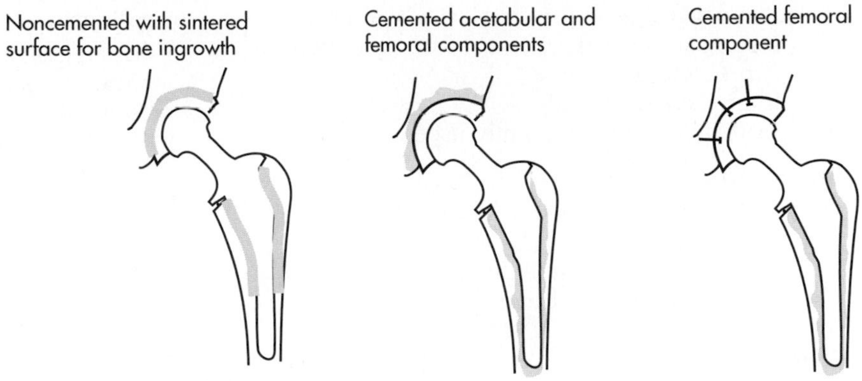

FIGURE 5-93

Types of Replacements (Fig. 5-94)

- Total: replacement of acetabulum and femoral head
- Partial hip replacement:
  - Bipolar (Bateman) prosthesis consists of cemented Miller femoral stem with a double acetabular (bipolar) compartment; for most of the movement, the femoral head articulates in the synthetic acetabulum; for extreme motion the synthetic acetabulum articulates with the real acetabulum; this prosthesis is used if the acetabulum is intact.
  - Simple (unipolar) prosthesis: there is only one acetabular compartment; may have accelerated acetabular wear.
- Infection cannot be excluded by radiographic studies. Joint aspiration is necessary.
- Cemented acetabular prostheses almost always fail.

KNEE REPLACEMENT (Fig. 5-95)

Types

- Nonconstrained prostheses: replacement of articular surface; relies on intact collateral and cruciate ligaments for stability
- Semiconstrained prosthesis: provides some stability to the knee through the design of components
- Tibial component most likely to loosen

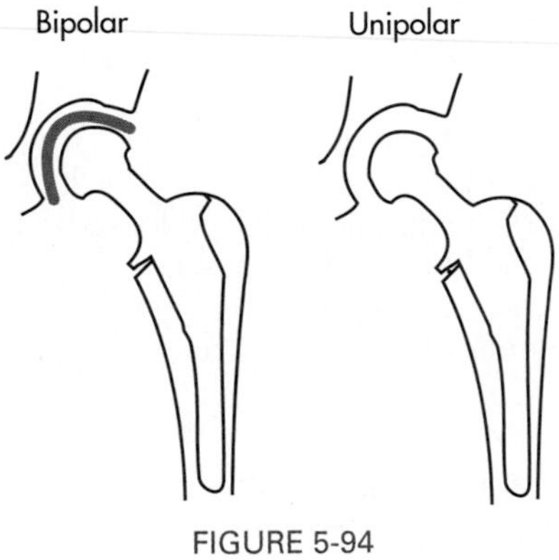

FIGURE 5-94

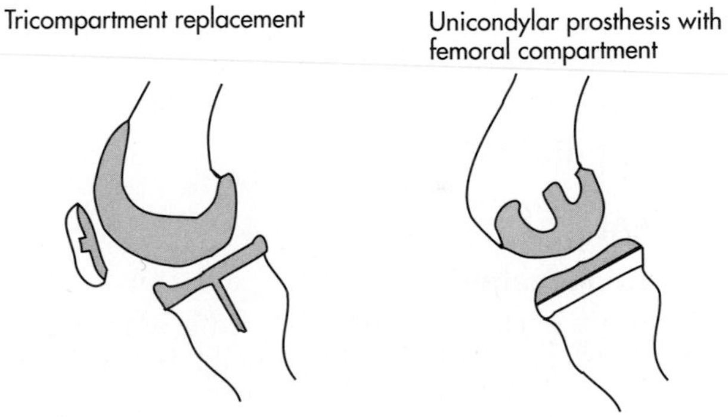

FIGURE 5-95

Pearls

- Many prostheses, even from different manufacturers, have a similar radiographic appearance.
- When a complication is suspected and plain films are unrevealing, a bone scan should be obtained.
- Bone scans are usually positive for 6 months after surgery; after 6 months, a negative scan is good evidence against loosening, infection, or fracture. Noncemented prosthesis can remain "hot" on bone scan for up to 2 years.
- Femoral components usually loosen earlier than acetabular components.

OTHER PROCEDURES

Arthrodesis

- Surgical fusion of a joint
- Achieved by removing articular cartilage, internal fixation, and fixing ends of articulating bones
- Common arthrodesis: spinal fusion, wrist fusion, and knee fusion

Osteotomy

- Surgical cut through the bone to correct alignment or length

Removal of bone for length discrepancy
Interposition of bone for lengthening procedures
Interposition of wedges
- Internal fixation is frequently used.

Bone Graft

- Used to stimulate bone growth and to provide mechanical stability
- Usually takes 1 year until the graft has been fully incorporated into the bone

SPINAL FUSION

Types

- Surgical fusion for fracture-dislocation, disk disease, spondylolisthesis, and scoliosis. Complications include:
  - Increased incidence of fracture/injury immediately above or below level of fusion
  - Pseudarthrosis
  - Spinal stenosis due to bony or ligamentous overgrowthv
  - Osteomyelitis, diskitis
- Congenital fusion (Klippel-Feil)
- Inflammatory arthritis: juvenile rheumatoid arthritis, ankylosing spondylitis, psoriatic arthritis
- Short-term stability depends on rods; long-term stability depends on bony fusion.
- Types of Harrington rods:
  - Distraction rods
  - Compression rods

ARTHROGRAPHY

GENERAL

General Principles

- Always obtain plain films before the arthrogram.
- All aspirated joint fluids should be sent for culture or other tests as indicated.
- Contrast agent is injected through long tubing.
- If the needle tip is intraarticular, the contrast should flow freely away from the needle tip.

Indications

- Ligamentous and tendinous tears
- Cartilage injuries
- Proliferative synovitis
- Masses and loose bodies
- Implant loosening

Contraindications

- Overlying skin infection
- Prior severe reaction to contrast media is a relative contraindication.

Complications

- Postarthrography pain is the most common complication (sterile chemical synovitis); begins 4 hours after procedure, peaks at 12 hours, and then subsides.
- Allergic reaction to contrast or lidocaine
- Infection
- Vasovagal reaction (may pretreat with atropine)

Preparation

Sterile preparation for arthrogram
- Determine puncture site fluoroscopically and mark skin.
- Scrub multiple times with povidone-iodine (Betadine) and then with alcohol.
- Drape and puncture.

Sterile preparation for hip aspiration/hip replacements
- Determine puncture site fluoroscopically and mark skin.
- Patient and radiologist are fully gowned.
- Drape fluoroscopy tower.
- Scrub multiple times with povidone-iodine (Betadine) and then with alcohol.
- Surgical draping

Anesthesia
- Lidocaine 1%, SC
- Lidocaine is bacteriostatic: do not use if aspirating joint (i.e., total hip replacement).

Type of Arthrogram

- Include epinephrine (1:1000) in contrast mixture to retard absorption (i.e., when subsequent CT is planned).
- Double-contrast arthrogram vs. single-contrast arthrogram
  - Single-contrast: noncalcified loose body (calcified loose body may be missed)
  - Double-contrast: cartilaginous injury (e.g., meniscus tear, labral tear)

PROTOCOL FOR ARTHROGRAPHY

Joint	Contrast Medium (mL)*	Epinephrine (mL)	Air (mL)	Comment
Shoulder	3	0.3	10	
Elbow	2+	For tomogram only	None	For loose body
Wrist	2+	None	None	
Hip	15	None	None	Single contrast
Knee	2	0.3	35	
Ankle	2	For tomogram only	None	

*30% lidocaine–1% +70% of Renografin-60 for single contrast, 1:1 mixture if followed by CT.

SHOULDER ARTHROGRAM (Fig. 5-96)

Patient Position

- Patient supine
- Arm externally rotated

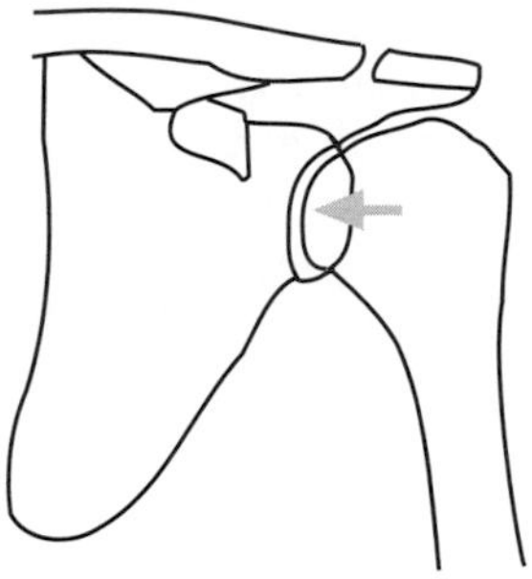

FIGURE 5-96

Procedure

- 21-gauge spinal needle
- Aim lateral to the joint space over the medial margin of the humeral head.
- Guide the needle medially off the humeral head and into the joint.
- Confirm the intraarticular location by injection of lidocaine. An alternative way to ensure intraarticular needle placement is to have contrast material in tubing and keep air in the needle.
  Intraarticular: free flow
  Extraarticular: air bounces back

Pearls

- Elevation of contralateral side may open joint space more.
- Most common problem is superficial needle placement.
- Connective tissue anterior to the joint may feel very dense.
- If needle is on humeral head in the correct position, it may be helpful to lessen the amount of external rotation (loosens the external capsule).

MR ARTHROGRAPHY OF THE SHOULDER

MR arthrography is performed by injecting 12 mL of a mixture of gadopentetate dimeglumine and saline (1:200 dilution) into the glenohumeral joint under fluoroscopic control. Coronal, transverse, and sagittal images are then obtained using T1W spin-echo sequences with or without fat saturation. The shoulder is placed in a neutral position or in slightly external rotation. Typical imaging parameters are as follows: section thickness, 2 to 3 mm; repetition time, 600 msec; echo time, <15 msec; field of view, 130 × 180; matrix size, 180 × 256; and number of signals acquired, 2.

HIP ARTHROGRAM (Fig. 5-97)

Injection Site

- Junction of femoral neck and head
- Puncture site is located 2 cm lateral to the femoral artery.

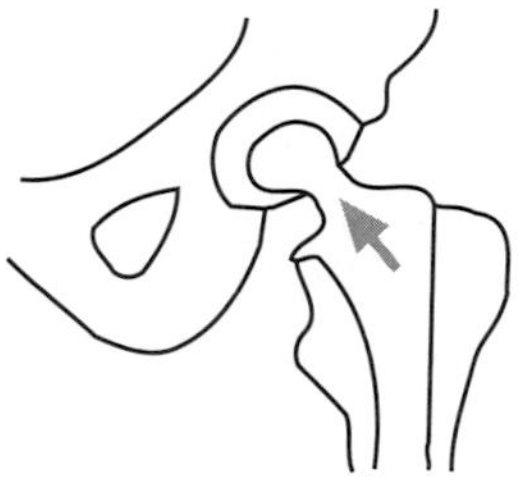

FIGURE 5-97

WRIST ARTHROGRAM (Fig. 5-98)

A complete arthrogram involves injection (25-gauge needle) of three separate compartments:

- Radiocarpal compartment (first injection); flexed wrist, localize midpoint of radioscaphoid space
- Midcarpal compartment (4-hour delay to allow resorption of contrast): inject space of Poirier
- Distal radioulnar joint

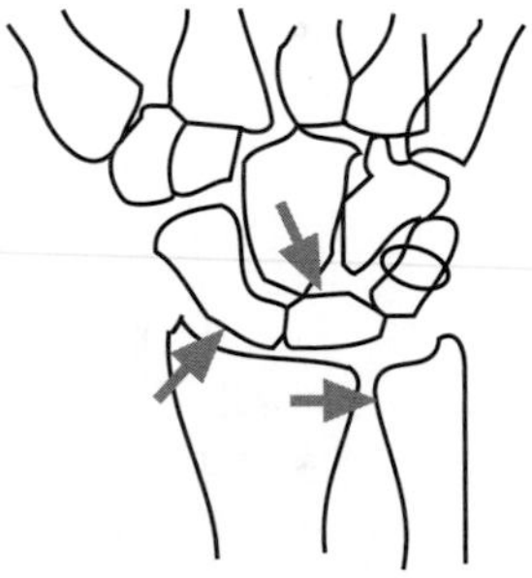

FIGURE 5-98

ANKLE ARTHROGRAM (Fig. 5-99)

- 25-gauge needle
- Mark midpoint tibiotalar joint and then turn the patient lateral.

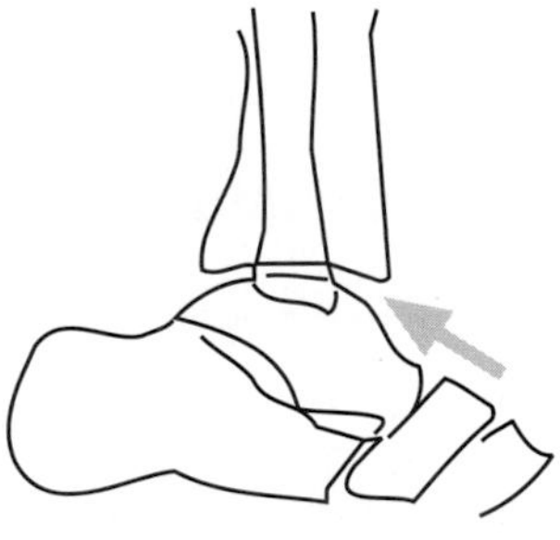

FIGURE 5-99

- Angle 25-gauge needle under the anterior tibial margin (start 1 cm caudal to the tibiotalar joint on the lateral view).
- Identify and avoid the dorsalis pedis artery.

BIOPSIES OF THE MUSCULOSKELETAL SYSTEM

INDICATIONS

- Primary or secondary bone tumors
- Osteitis
- Septic arthritis, diskitis

CONTRAINDICATIONS

- Bleeding diatheses
- Biopsies of inaccessible sites (odontoid process, anterior arch of C1)
- Soft tissue infection

TECHNIQUE

A CT scan is initially performed to localize the lesion. The entry point and the pathway are determined, avoiding nerve, vascular, and visceral structures. For peripheral long-bone biopsy, the approach has to be orthogonal to the cortex. This approach angle avoids slippage with the tip of the needle. The shortest path should be chosen. For flat bones such as scapula, ribs, sternum, and skull an oblique approach angle of 30° to 60° is used. For the pelvic girdle, a posterior approach is used avoiding the sacral canal and nerves. For vertebral body biopsy, different approach routes can be selected depending on vertebral level, the anterior route for cervical level, the transpedicular and intercostovertebral route for the thoracic level, and the posterolateral and transpedicular route for the lumbar level. For the neural posterior arch, a tangential approach is used to avoid damaging underlying neural structures.

COMPLICATIONS

- The major complication is septic osteitis. To avoid this complication, strict sterility during the intervention is mandatory.
- Hematoma
- Reflex sympathetic dystrophy
- Neural and vascular injuries
- Pneumothorax

PERCUTANEOUS PERIRADICULAR STEROID INJECTION

INDICATIONS

- Treatment of acute low back pain of diskogenic origin (without nerve paralysis) resistant to conventional medical therapy
- Postdiskectomy syndrome

TECHNIQUE

- Cervical level: The patient is placed supine with head slightly turned and in hyperextension.
- Lumbar level: The patient is placed prone. The entry point and pathway are determined by CT. After local anesthesia of the skin, a 22-gauge spinal needle is placed under CT guidance via a posterior approach near the painful nerve root.

In intracanalar infiltration, absence of cerebrospinal fluid (CSF) is verified by aspiration. Once the needle is in the epidural space, 1.5 mL of air is injected to confirm the extradural position of the needle tip. Then 2 to 3 mL of a long-acting steroid solution (cortivazol, 3.75 mg, is injected alone or mixed with 2 mL of 0.5% lidocaine). Using precise CT guidance, dural sac perforation is avoided. However, if the dura is perforated because of an adhesion of the dural sac to the ligamentum flavum or because of a mistaken maneuver, the needle must be pulled back slightly and checked for CSF leakage. If there is none, the corticosteroid is injected without anesthetic. During injection, the patient may experience a spontaneous recurrence of pain lasting a few seconds, brought on by dural stretch.

COMPLICATIONS

- Meningitis with neurologic damage (quadriplegia, multiple cranial nerve palsies, nystagmus) has been described after epidural or intrathecal injection of steroids if strict sterility is not respected. With precise CT monitoring, accidental intrathecal injection can be avoided.
- There is a risk of calcifications with use of triamcinolone hexacetonide as a long-acting steroid. This steroid is not recommended.
- At the cervical level, vertebral artery injury and intraarterial injection have been described. This can be avoided with precise CT guidance.

PERCUTANEOUS CEMENTOPLASTY

Percutaneous cementoplasty with acrylic cement (polymethylmethacrylate), also referred to as vertebral packing or vertebroplasty, is a procedure aimed at preventing vertebral body crushing and pain in patients with pathologic vertebral bodies.

INDICATIONS

- Symptomatic vertebral angioma
- Painful vertebral body tumor (particularly metastasis and myeloma), especially when there is a risk of compression fracture
- Severe, painful osteoporosis with loss of height or compression fracture of the vertebral body or both

CONTRAINDICATIONS

- Hemorrhagic diathesis
- Infection

- Lesions with epidural extension require careful injection to prevent epidural overflow and spinal cord compression by the cement.

COMPLICATIONS

- The major complication is a cement leak.
- Infection
- Patients experience temporary pain after the procedure but are usually free of symptoms within 24 hours. The postprocedural pain is usually proportional to the volume of cement injected. The majority of the patients have good packing of the vertebral body with more than 4 mL of acrylic cement injected.
- Allergic reactions, hypertension

Bone Tumors

GENERAL

APPROACH TO TUMORS (Fig. 5-100)

1. Determine aggressiveness (pattern of destruction and repair)
2. Tissue characterization by matrix (usually by CT)
3. Location of lesion
4. Age of patient

Some features have a higher diagnostic specificity than others. The most important ones are:
- Pattern of destruction (malignant versus benign)
- Pattern of matrix (to determine origin as osseous, cartilaginous, fibrous)

Pattern of Bone Destruction (Fig. 5-101)

Most important factor in determining the rate of growth or aggressiveness of the tumor. Cortical penetration is indicative of an aggressive lesion. Pattern types include:
Geographic lytic pattern

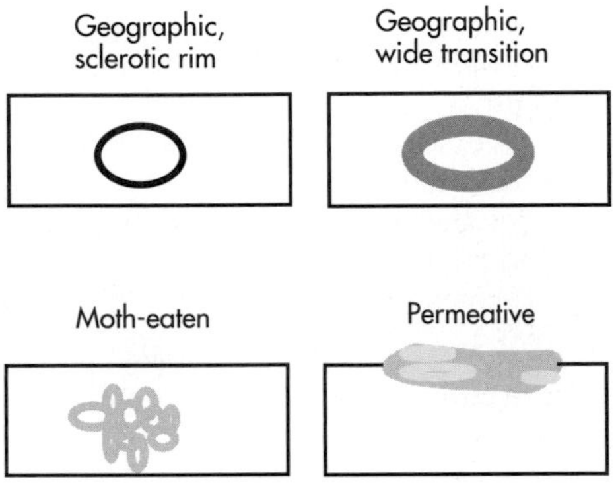

FIGURE 5-101

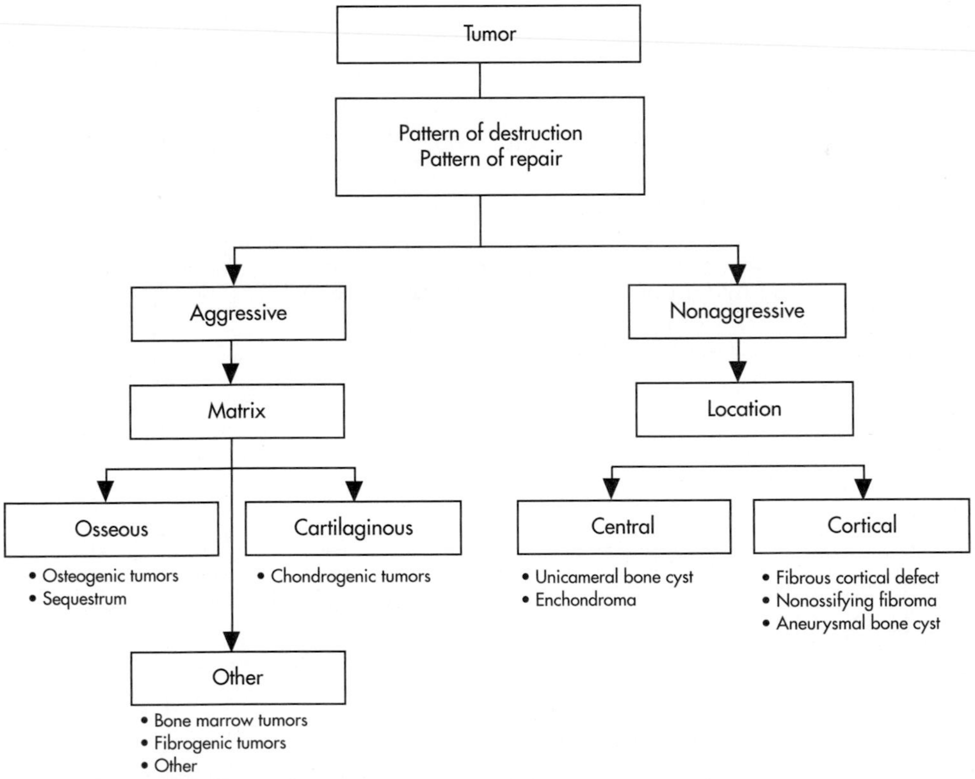

FIGURE 5-100

- Well-delineated, circumscribed hole in the bone
- Sclerotic rim indicates relatively slow growth.
- An ill-defined or wide transition zone indicates a moderately aggressive process.

Moth-eaten pattern
- Numerous small holes of varying size in cortical and trabecular bone
- Reflects aggressive behavior

Permeative pattern
- Numerous elongated holes along the cortex
- Occasionally, only a decrease in cortical bone density is visible.
- Reflects aggressive behavior

Radiographic Patterns of Lytic Bone Lesions

In order of increasing aggressiveness:
- Ia: Geographic lucency, well-defined sclerotic margin
- Ib: Geographic lucency, well-defined non-sclerotic margin
- Ic: Geographic lucency, ill-defined margin
- II: Moth-eaten
- III: Permeative

Pattern of Bone Repair (Fig. 5-102)

New bone (osteoblastic activity) is formed in response to destruction:

Periosteal response
- Buttressing (wavy periostitis; benign lesion)
  - Thick, single layer of periosteal reaction
  - Indicates slow growth or benignity
  - Nonspecific: hypertrophic pulmonary osteoarthropathy (HPO), atherosclerosis, benign tumors
- Aggressive patterns
  - Seen with rapidly progressive lesions such as malignancy or osteomyelitis
    - Lamination (onion-peel). Periosteum appears in layers.
    - Codman's triangle. Periosteum forms bone only at the margin of the tumor.
  - Spiculations
    - Sunburst pattern is seen in aggressive malignant lesions; spiculations commonly point to the center of the lesion.
    - Hair-on-end pattern is seen with lesions that invade the marrow cavity in long bones.

Endosteal response
- Thick rim of new bone indicates benign, slow growth (e.g., nonossifying fibroma [NOF], osteoma, Brodie abscess, fibrous dysplasia).
- Thin rim or no rim indicates a more active lesion.
- Mottled appearance
  - Results from bone intermingled with a permeative or moth-eaten pattern of destruction
  - Indicates invasiveness (malignant and nonmalignant causes)

Tissue Characterization

Tumor matrix refers to the neoplastic intercellular substance produced by tumor cells. CT is often required to adequately define the matrix. For example, an increased tumor density on plain film may be due to osteoid matrix or periosteal/endosteal response.

TUMOR MATRIX DEFINITION

Matrix	Benign	Malignant
Osteoid Matrix		
Does not always mineralize	Osteoid osteoma Osteoblastoma	Osteosarcoma
Mineralization is dense, homogeneous, cloudlike	Osteochondroma Bone island	
Chondroid Matrix		
Does not always calcify	Enchondroma	Chondrosarcoma
Calcifications in the form of arcs or circles	Osteochondroma (cap) Chondroblastoma Chondromyxoid fibroma	
Intermediate Matrix		
Diffuse uniform mineralization: ground glass	Fibrous dysplasia Osteoblastoma	Osteosarcoma
Cellular Matrix		
No calcification Radiolucent lesions	Fibrous tumors	Round cell tumors Fibrous tumors

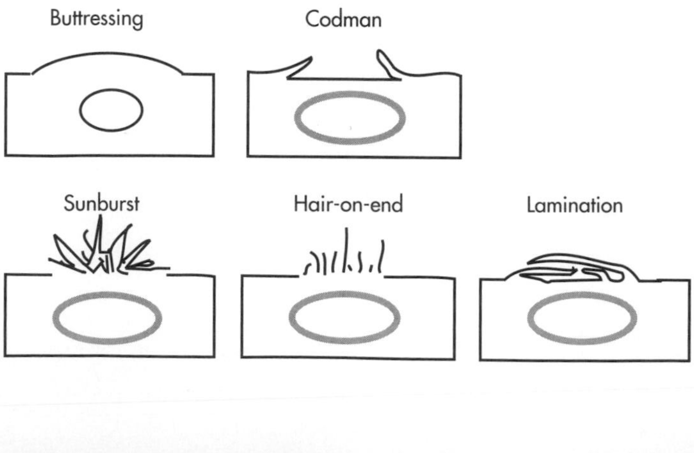

FIGURE 5-102

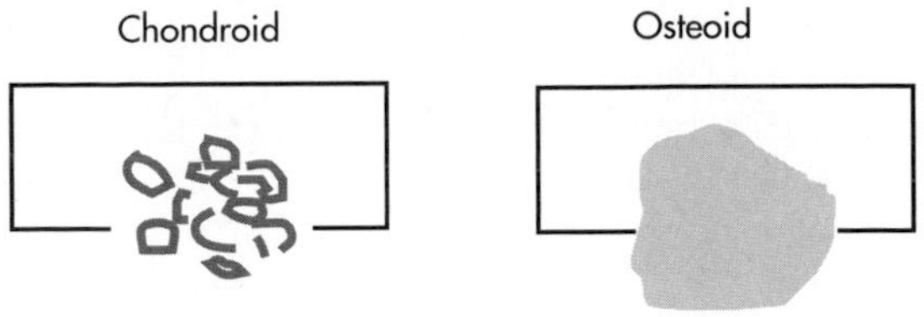

FIGURE 5-103

Pearls (Fig. 5-103)

- Mineralization of chondroid and osteoid matrix in tumors is often central (mature center, peripheral growth).
- Mineralization in benign lesions (e.g., bone infarcts, myositis ossificans) is often peripheral.

Location of a Lesion in the Skeleton

As a general rule, most primary tumors arise in areas of rapid growth (distal femur, proximal tibia, humerus), whereas metastases occur in well-vascularized red bone marrow (spine, iliac wings). The following tumors have a predilection for typical locations:

- Enchondromas: phalanges
- Osteosarcoma, giant cell tumor: around the knee
- Hemangioma: skull and spine
- Chondrosarcoma: innominate bone
- Chordoma: sacrum and clivus
- Adamantinoma: mid tibia

Location within Anatomic Regions

- Epiphysis: typical are cartilaginous and articular lesions such as chondroblastoma or eosinophilic granuloma (EG)
- Metaphysis: lesions of different causes (e.g., neoplastic, inflammatory, metabolic) have a predilection for the metaphysis (rich blood supply); therefore, this location alone is of limited differential diagnostic value.
- Epiphyseal/metaphyseal region: giant cell tumors
- Diaphysis: after the 4th decade of life, most solitary diaphyseal bone lesions involve the bone marrow.

Axial Location within a Bone (Fig. 5-104)

Refers to the position of the lesion with respect to the long axis of the bone.

- Central lesions (usually benign)
  - Enchondroma
  - Unicameral bone cysts
  - Eosinophilic granuloma (EG)
- Eccentric lesions
  - Aneurysmal bone cyst (ABC)
  - Osteosarcoma
  - NOF
  - Giant cell tumor (GCT)
  - Chondromyxoid fibroma
- Cortical lesions (most commonly benign)
  - Cortical defect
  - Cortical desmoid
  - Osteoid osteoma
  - Periosteal chondroma
- Parosteal lesions
  - All osseous, cartilaginous, and fibrous malignancies
  - Osteochondroma
  - Myositis ossificans (should be separate from bone)

INCIDENCE OF TUMORS BY LOCATION*

Tumor	Femur	Tibia	Foot	Humerus	Radius	Hand	Spine	Skull
Osteoid osteoma	30	25	10	5	1	10	5	1
Osteoblastoma	15	10	10	5	1	5	40	15
Osteosarcoma	40	15	1	15	<1	<1	2	5
Chondroma	10	3	5	5	2	55	1	1
Chondroblastoma	35	20	10	20	1	20	1	1
Chondrosarcoma	25	10	2	10	1	3	5	3
NOF	40	45	1	5	1	1	—	1
Fibrosarcoma	40	15	2	10	1	<1	5	5
GCT	35	30	2	5	10	5	5	1
Malignant fibrous histiocytoma	45	20	2	10	1	—	2	5
Hemangioma	5	3	5	3	1	2	25	35
Hemangiopericytoma	10	—	5	15	5	2	10	5
Neurofibroma	—	5	—	2	—	—	5	75
Chordoma	—	—	—	—	—	—	75	25
Simple cyst	30	5	1	55	1	1	—	—
ABC	15	15	10	10	3	5	15	5
Adamantinoma	3	80	1	5	1	1	—	—
Ewing tumor	40	30	3	10	2	1	5	1

*All numbers represent percentage of bone tumors in that location.

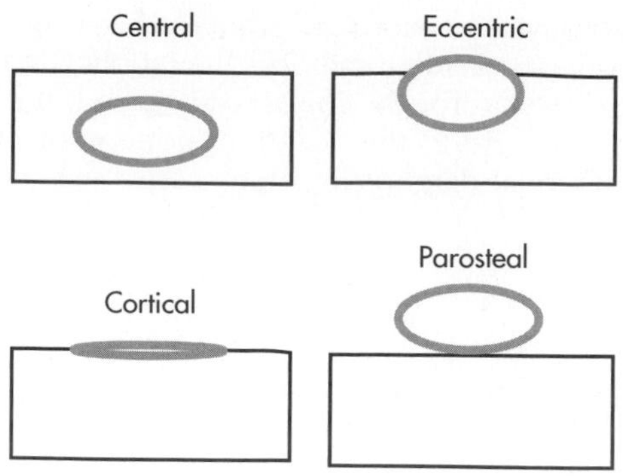

FIGURE 5-104

INCIDENCE

The numbers in the preceding table indicate the approximate percentage of tumors in that location.

BONE BIOPSIES

- Two general types of needles are used:
  - Needles to cut through cortical bone (trephine, Turkel, Ackerman)
  - Needles for predominantly soft tissue masses (Tru-Cut, spinal needle)
- Soft tissue biopsies are preferable over bone biopsies.
- The needle tip should hit the bone at a right angle, otherwise the needle tends to slide off the bone.
- Always biopsy the part of the lesion that will be resected. Likewise, the needle track should be within the surgical field (tumor seeding is rare but has been reported particularly with chondroid lesions and chordoma). Therefore, all biopsies require consultation of orthopedic surgeon regarding surgical approach.
- Complications: 1%-10%

BONE-FORMING TUMORS

OSTEOID OSTEOMA

The clinical hallmark of the lesion is pain (increased prostaglandins), especially at night, that is improved with aspirin. Age: 5 to 25 years. Treatment is with surgical excision, percutaneous thermal, or drill ablation. Preferred treatment currently is percutaneous radiofrequency ablation. Failure to remove entire lesion may lead to recurrence. Location: femur and tibia 55%, hands and feet 20%; 80% intracortical.

Radiographic Features

- Radiolucent nidus <2 cm in diameter (may contain bone matrix)
- Nidus surrounded by sclerosis; the sclerosis may obscure the detection of the nidus on plain films
- Lesion located on concave side in patients with painful scoliosis
- Synovitis may occur with periarticular or intracapsular lesions.
- Limb overgrowth in children
- CT is the study of choice for identifying number and location of nidus.
- Bone scan: hot spot
- Angiography: nidus has dense blush
- MRI: may have extensive reactive marrow edema

OSTEOBLASTOMA

Histologically similar to osteoid osteoma but radiographically distinct. Age: <30 years (80%). Treatment is with curettage. Two appearances:

- Expansile lytic
- Sclerotic >2 cm (giant osteoid osteoma)

DIFFERENTIATION OF OSTEOBLASTOMA FROM OSTEOID OSTEOMA

	Osteoblastoma	Osteoid Osteoma
Clinical	Rare	Common
	Rapidly increasing in size	Limited growth potential
	Pain inconsistent	Pain persistent (nocturnal)
Radiology	Expansile or >2 cm	<2 cm
	Variable sclerosis	Peripheral sclerosis

Location

- Spine (posterior elements): 40%
- Long bones of appendicular skeleton: 30%
- Hand and feet: 15%
- Skull and face: 15%

Radiographic Features

- Dense sclerotic bone reaction >2 cm
- Expansile, well-circumscribed lesion similar to ABC
- Variable central calcification and matrix
- Malignant, aggressive osteoblastoma may disrupt cortex and have a soft tissue component (may mimic an osteosarcoma).

OTHER BENIGN BONE-FORMING LESIONS

Bone Island (Enostosis)

Cortical type bone within cancellous bone. Islands may be 1 to 4 cm in size.

Homogeneously dense, well marginated. May be warm on bone scan.

Osteopoikilosis

Multiple epiphyseal enostoses.

Osteopathia striata

Linear longitudinal striations in metaphyses. Asymptomatic.

Osteoma

Localized masses of mature bone on the endosteal or periosteal surface of cortex, commonly in the skull or paranasal sinuses. Associated with Gardner syndrome.

OSTEOSARCOMA (OSA)

Second most frequent primary malignant bone tumor after multiple myeloma.

Incidence: <1000 new cases/year in United States. Age: 10 to 30 years. 5-year survival: parosteal 80% > periosteal 50% > conventional 20% > telangiectatic < 20%.

CLINICAL FINDINGS

- Pain
- Mass
- Fever

Types

Primary osseous OSA (95%)
- Conventional OSA
- Low-grade central OSA
- Telangiectatic OSA
- Small cell OSA
- Multicentric OSA

Juxtacortical OSA
- Parosteal OSA
- Periosteal OSA
- High-grade surface OSA

Secondary OSA
- Paget disease
- Prior radiation (3 to 50 years after radiation)
- Dedifferentiated chondrosarcoma

Location of Conventional OSA

- Tubular bones, 80%
  - Femur, 40% (75% of which occur around the knee)
  - Tibia, 15%
  - Humerus, 15%
- Other bones, 20%
  - Flat bones
  - Vertebral bodies

Radiographic Features

- Poorly defined, intramedullary, metaphyseal mass lesion that extends through the cortex
- Matrix:
  - Osteoid (osteoblastic OSA), 50%
  - Chondroid matrix (chondroblastic OSA), 25%
  - Spindle cell stroma (fibroblastic OSA), 25%
- Aggressive periosteal reaction: Codman's triangle, sunburst pattern
- Bone scan: increased uptake with activity extending beyond the true margins of the tumor (thought to be related to hyperemia)
- Skin lesions and metastases best detected by bone scan or MRI
- Pulmonary metastases best detected by high-resolution CT

Pearls

Role of imaging
- Presumptive diagnosis of OSA is made by plain film.
- CT useful for evaluation of matrix and of cortical penetration, and occasionally for biopsy
- MRI, bone scan, and chest CT are useful for staging.
- MRI may be better than CT for determining tumor margins.
- Detect metastasis (CXR)

Goals of cross-sectional imaging
- Determine extent of tumor within bone marrow and soft tissue
- Determine relationship to vessels and nerves
- Evaluate adjacent joints
- Detect skip lesions (MRI)
- Provide measurements needed for surgery

Telangiectatic OSA

Purely lytic lesion that lacks the highly aggressive appearance of a conventional OSA (tumor matrix, periosteal reaction) but is actually much more malignant and carries a worse prognosis.

Radiographic Features

- Large lytic lesion
- Cystic cavities filled with blood and/or necrosis
- May mimic ABC

Multicentric OSA

Synchronous osteoblastic OSA at multiple sites. Has a tendency to be metaphyseal and symmetrical. Occurs exclusively in children ages 5 to 10. Extremely poor prognosis.

Parosteal OSA

Low-grade OSA that occurs in an older age group (80% between 20 and 50 years).

Locations similar to those of conventional OSA.

Radiographic Features

- Posterior distal femur, 65%
- Attached to underlying cortex only at origin
- May wrap around bone
- Distinguishable from myositis ossificans by its zonal ossification; more mature ossification is located centrally but is located peripherally in myositis ossificans

Periosteal Osteosarcoma

Intermediate-grade OSA. Most commonly diaphyseal.

Radiographic Features

- No medullary involvement
- Cortical thickening or "saucerization"
- Entire tumor closely apposed to cortex

CARTILAGE-FORMING TUMORS

ENCHONDROMA

Benign cartilaginous neoplasm in the medullary cavity. Most enchondromas are asymptomatic but may present as pathologic fractures. Peak age is 10 to 30 years.

Location

- Tubular bones (hand, foot): 50%
- Femur, tibia, humerus

Radiographic Features

- Lytic lesion in bones of the hand or foot
- Chondroid calcifications: rings and arcs pattern ("O" and "C")
- Scalloped endosteum
- Expansion of cortex but no cortical breakthrough unless fractured
- No periosteal reaction or soft tissue mass

Pearls

- In the absence of a fracture, a painful enchondroma is considered malignant until proved otherwise.
- Malignant transformation occurs but is rare.
- Malignant transformation is more likely in central lesions.

ENCHONDROMATOSIS (OLLIER DISEASE)

Nonhereditary abnormality in which multiple enchondromas are present. Many lesions become stable at puberty. Risk of malignant transformation to chondrosarcoma is 25%.

Radiographic Features

- Multiple radiolucent expansile masses in hand and feet
- Hand and foot deformities
- Tendency for unilaterality

MAFFUCCI SYNDROME

Enchondromatosis and multiple soft tissue hemangiomas. Unilateral involvement of hands and feet. Malignant transformation is much more common than in Ollier disease.

OSTEOCHONDROMA (OSTEOCARTILAGINOUS EXOSTOSIS) (Fig. 5-105)

Cartilage-covered bony projection (exostosis) on the external surface of a bone. Most common benign bone lesion. Osteochondromas have their own growth plate and stop growing with skeletal maturity. Age: <20 years (adolescence) in 80% (10 to 35 years; male:female = 2:1). Symptoms are those of a slowly growing painless tumor. Treatment is with surgical resection if complications are present. Location: any bone with enchondral ossification but most commonly (85%): tibia, femur, humerus.

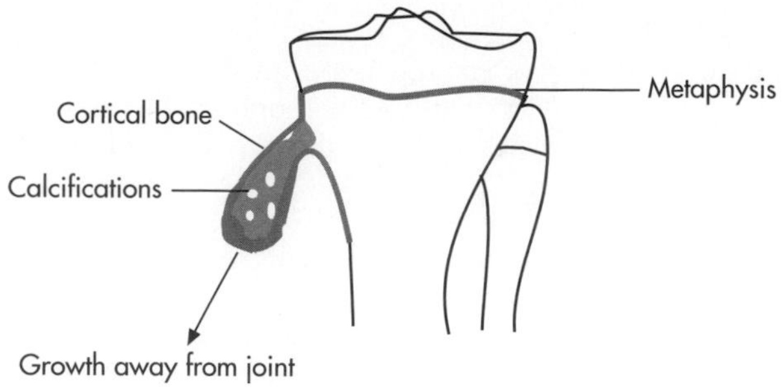

FIGURE 5-105

Radiographic Features

Two types:

- Pedunculated: slender pedicle directed away from growth plate
- Sessile (broad base)

Characteristic findings:

- Continuous with parent bone:
  - Uninterrupted cortex
  - Continuous medullary bone
- Calcification in the chondrous portion of cap; may be cauliflower-like
- Metaphyseal location (cartilaginous origin)
- Lesion grows away from joint
- MRI demonstrates cortical and medullary continuity between the osteochondroma and the parent bone as a distinctive feature.
- MRI is the best imaging modality for visualizing the effect of the lesion on surrounding structures and for evaluating the hyaline cartilage cap. Mineralized areas in the cartilage cap remain low signal intensity with all MRI pulse sequences, although as enchondral ossification proceeds, yellow marrow signal is ultimately apparent.

Complications

- Pressure on nerves and blood vessels
- Pressure on adjacent bone: deformation, fractures
- Overlying bursitis
- Malignant transformation (in <1%). Suspect if:
  - Pain in the absence of fracture, bursitis, or nerve compression
  - Growth of lesion after skeletal maturation
  - >1 cm of cartilaginous cap by CT, >2 cm by MRI
  - Dispersed calcifications in the cap
  - Enlargement of lesion
  - Increased uptake on bone scan (unreliable)

MULTIPLE OSTEOCARTILAGINOUS EXOSTOSES (MOCE)

- Hereditary autosomal dominant disease
- Knee, ankle, and shoulder are usually involved.
- Typically sessile and metaphyseal in location
- May simulate appearance of bone dysplasia

- Complications
  - Severe growth abnormalities
  - Malignant transformation rare but higher than in solitary osteochondromas (especially proximal lesions). Malignant transformation is usually into chondrosarcoma.

BIZARRE PAROSTEAL OSTEOCHONDROMATOUS PROLIFERATION (BPOP, NORA LESION) (Fig. 5-106)

Calcific masses attached to cortex without interruption of cortex. Unlike osteochondromas, BPOP does not have a cartilaginous cap. Involves small bones of the hands (volar) and feet, but may also involve skull, maxilla, and long bones. Can be confused with osteochondromas and malignancy.

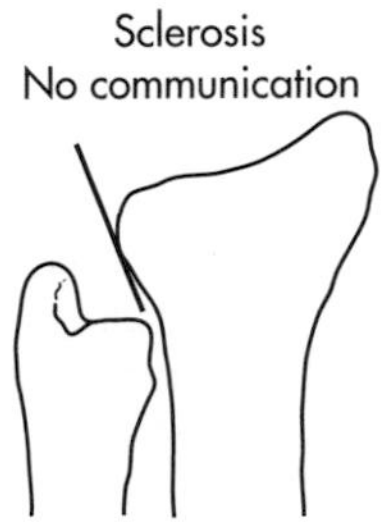

FIGURE 5-106

DYSPLASIA EPIPHYSEALIS HEMIMELICA (TREVOR DISEASE)

Intraarticular epiphyseal osteochondromas. Usually unilateral.

CHONDROBLASTOMA (CODMAN TUMOR)

Uncommon benign neoplasm that occurs almost exclusively in the epiphysis in immature skeleton. Lobulated geographic lucency eccentrically located along epiphysis. Location: around knee, proximal humerus. Treatment is with curettage.

CHONDROMYXOID FIBROMA

Uncommon benign neoplasm that consists mainly of fibrous tissue mixed with chondroid and myxoid tissue. Lesion typically appears lobulated, geographic and lytic; cartilaginous matrix is rarely seen. Location: 50% around knee, metaphysis. Treatment is with curettage.

CHONDROSARCOMA

Malignant cartilage-producing tumor. Mean age: 40 to 45 years. Most are low-grade asymptomatic tumors that are found incidentally. Location:

- 45% in long bones, especially the femur
- 25% innominate bone, ribs
- Most occur in the metaphysis but may extend to the epiphysis.

Radiographic Features

- Lytic mass that may or may not have chondroid matrix
- Medullary (central) chondrosarcomas arise within cancellous bone or the medullary cavity; may appear totally lytic.
- Exostotic (peripheral)) chondrosarcoma arises in the cartilage cap of a previously benign osteochondroma or exostoses; these tumors commonly have a chondroid matrix and an extraosseous soft tissue mass.
- Dedifferentiated chondrosarcoma is a high-grade tumor that frequently contains large areas of noncalcified tumor matrix.
- Degeneration to fibrosarcoma, MFH, or OSA in 10%

FIBROUS LESIONS

FIBROUS CORTICAL DEFECTS (FCD) AND NONOSSIFYING FIBROMA (NOF)

FCD and NOF are histologically identical (whorled bundles of connective tissue), cortically based lesions that differ only in the amount of medullary involvement. With time, lesions may sclerose and shrink.

DIFFERENTIAL DIAGNOSIS OF FCD AND NOF

Parameter	FCD	NOF
Age	4-7 years	10-20 years
Location	Cortex	Medullary involvement
Size	1-4 cm (small)	1-7 cm (large)
Clinical	Clinically silent	May cause pain, fracture
Treatment	None	Curettage if symptomatic

Radiographic Features (Fig. 5-107)

- Radiolucent cortical lesion with normal or sclerotic margins

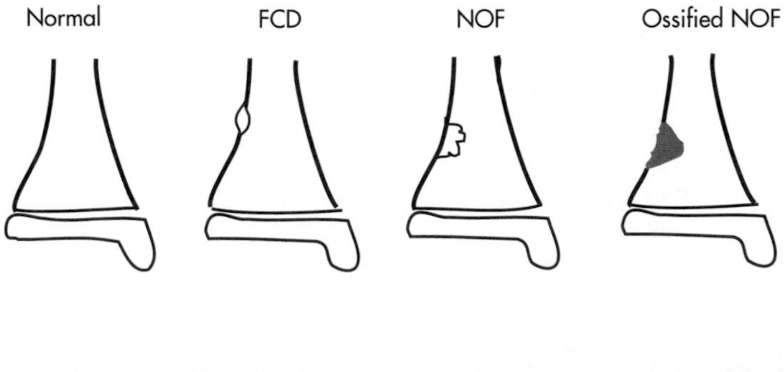

FIGURE 5-107

- Well-demarcated peripheral osseous shell
- Metaphyseal location: close to the growth plate, usually posteromedially
- Tibia and fibula are most commonly affected (90%).

Multiple NOF lesions: associated with neurofibromatosis and Jaffe-Campanacci syndrome (café-au-lait spots, hypogonadism, cryptorchism, mental retardation, and ocular and cardiovascular abnormalities)

FIBROUS DYSPLASIA (LICHTENSTEIN-JAFFE DISEASE)

Benign, developmental anomaly in which the medullary cavity is replaced with fibrous material, woven bone, and spindle cells. Age: 5 to 20 years. Fibrous dysplasia does not spread or proliferate; malignant transformation is rare (0.5%).

Associations

- Endocrine disorders
  - Hyperthyroidism
  - Hyperparathyroidism
  - McCune-Albright syndrome (precocious puberty)
- Soft tissue myxomas (Mazabraud syndrome)

Types

- Monostotic form, 85%
  - Femur (most common)
  - Tibia, ribs
  - Craniofacial
- Polyostotic form, 15% (peak age 8 years)
  - Femur, 90%
  - Tibia, 80%
  - Pelvis, 80%
  - Craniofacial

Radiographic Features

- Radiolucent expansile medullary lesions
- Degree of lucency depends on the amount of osteoid
- Typical ground-glass appearance is due to dysplastic microtrabeculae, which are not individually visible.
- Well-defined sclerotic margins, endosteal scalloping
- Bowing deformities: biomechanically insufficient bone (shepherd's crook deformity)
- Base-of-skull lesions tend to be sclerotic (in contrast to lucent lesions elsewhere).
- Frontal bossing, facial asymmetry
- Polyostotic form is often unilateral or monomelic.
- Bone scan: hot lesions

Variants (Fig. 5-108)

- Cherubism
  - Symmetrical involvement of mandible and maxilla
  - Familial inheritance

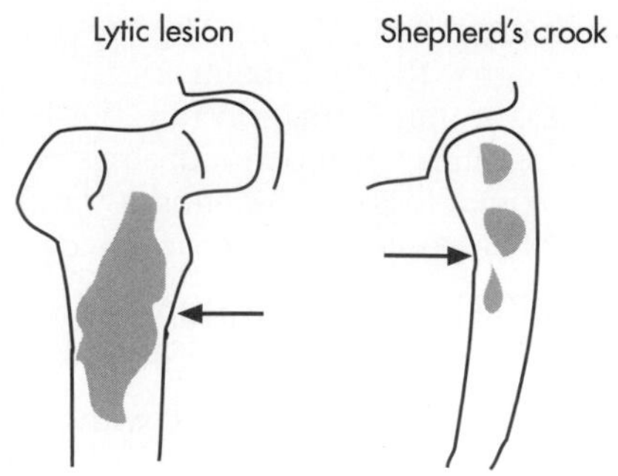

FIGURE 5-108

- McCune-Albright syndrome
  - Polyostotic unilateral fibrous dysplasia
  - Endocrine abnormalities (precocious puberty, hyperthyroidism)
  - Café-au-lait spots (coast of Maine)
  - Predominantly in girls
- Leontiasis ossea (craniofacial fibrous dysplasia)
  - Involvement of facial and frontal bones
  - Leonine facies (resembling a lion)
  - Cranial nerve palsies
- Fibrous dysplasia (pseudarthrosis of the tibia)
  - Young infants
  - Anterior tibial bowing
  - Pathologic fracture and subsequent pseudarthrosis

Complications

- Pathologic fractures
- Limb or growth deformity
- Sarcomatous transformation (very rare)

Pearls

- Fibrous dysplasia can mimic a variety of bone lesions.
- Pelvic involvement nearly always indicates polyostotic form; therefore, the ipsilateral femur is usually also involved.
- Painful fibrous dysplasia usually indicates the presence of a fracture.

OSSIFYING FIBROMA

Histologically and radiologically in the spectrum of fibrous dysplasia, osteofibrous dysplasia, and adamantinoma. Diagnosis is established by pathology. The former ossifying fibroma of the jaw is now classified as an ameloblastoma.

Radiographic Features

- Expansile cortical lesion of anterior tibial diaphysis
- Identical radiographic features to those of adamantinoma
- Occurs in younger age group than adamantinoma

DESMOPLASTIC FIBROMA (INTRAOSSEOUS DESMOID)

Histologically identical to soft tissue desmoid. Age: 50% occur in second decade. Location: metaphyses, pelvis, mandible.

Radiographic Features

- Expansile lytic lesion containing thick septations
- Difficult to distinguish from low-grade fibrosarcoma

MALIGNANT FIBROUS HISTIOCYTOMA (MFH)

Osseous MFH originates from histiocytes in the bone marrow. Although MFH is the most common soft tissue sarcoma in adults, osseous MFH is rare. Age: 40 to 60 years.

The tumor has a poor prognosis because of the high frequency of local recurrence (up to 80%) and hematogenous metastases to regional lymph nodes and distant sites (lungs > liver > brain, heart, kidney, adrenal glands, GI tract, bone). Osseous MFH may be:

- Primary
- Secondary
  - Paget disease
  - Dedifferentiation of a chondrosarcoma
  - Bone infarct
  - Postradiation

Location

- Bone MFH (rare): skeletal location of MFH is similar to that of osteosarcoma
- Soft tissues MFH: lower extremity > upper extremity > retroperitoneum
- Lung (extremely rare)

Radiographic Features

- Tumors have aggressive features: permeative or moth-eaten.
- Calcifications or sclerotic margins are rarely present.
- Periostitis is limited, unless a pathologic fracture is present.
- Density of tumor is similar to muscle (10 to 60 HU).
- Large soft tissue mass (common)

FIBROSARCOMA

Fibrosarcoma and malignant fibrous histiocytoma are clinically and radiographically indistinguishable.

LIPOSCLEROSING MYXOFIBROUS TUMOR (LSMFT)

Mnemonic: "**L**ucky **S**tripe **M**eans **F**ine **T**obacco:"

LSMFT of bone is a benign fibroosseous lesion that is characterized by a complex mixture of histologic elements, including lipoma, fibroxanthoma, myxoma, myxofibroma, fibrous dysplasia-like features, cyst formation, fat necrosis, ischemic ossification, and rarely cartilage. Despite its histologic complexity, LSMFT has a relatively characteristic radiologic appearance and skeletal distribution.

Radiographic Features

- Predilection for femur
- Geographic lesion with well-defined and sclerotic margins
- Mineralization within lesion is common.
- Unlike an intraosseous lipoma, LSMFT does not show macroscopic fat by CT or MRI as the fatty component is small and is admixed with more prominent myxofibrous and/or fibroosseous tissue.
- Prevalence of malignant transformation is between 10% and 16%.

BONE MARROW TUMORS

MARROW CONVERSION

Red to yellow marrow conversion generally progresses distal to proximal, starting at the epiphysis, then diaphysis, and metaphysis.

EOSINOPHILIC GRANULOMA (EG)

Langerhans cell histiocytosis is now the approved term for three diseases involving abnormal proliferation of histiocytes in organs of the reticuloendothelial system (RES):

- Letterer-Siwe: acute disseminated form, 10%
- Hand-Schüller-Christian: chronic disseminated form, 20%
- EG: only bone involvement, 70%

The radiologic manifestations of Langerhans cell histiocytosis may be skeletal or extraskeletal (involving any organ of the RES). Age: 1st to 3rd decade. Prognosis depends on degree of visceral involvement.

Radiographic Features

Appendicular, 20% (Fig. 5-109)

- Permeative, metadiaphyseal lytic lesion
- Cortical destruction may be present: pathologic fractures.

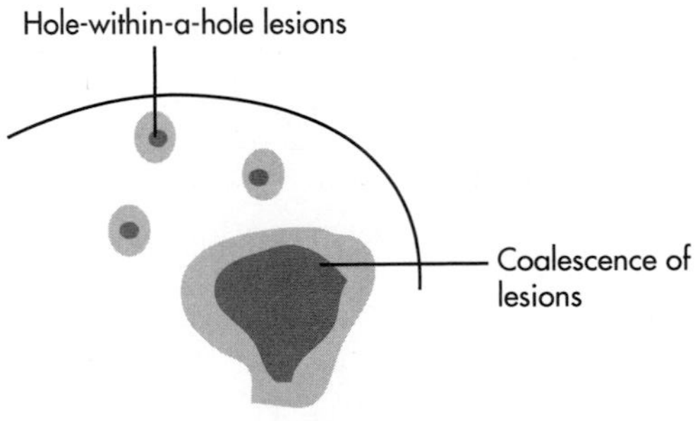

FIGURE 5-109

- Aggressive tumors may mimic osteomyelitis or Ewing sarcoma.
- Multifocal in 10%-20%

Skull, 50%
- Well-defined lytic lesions
- Beveled-edge appearance may produce hole-within-a-hole sign (outer table is more destroyed than inner table; button sequestrum); best seen by CT.
- Lesions may coalesce and form a geographic skull.
- In the healing phase, lesions may develop sclerotic borders.
- Floating tooth: lesion in alveolar portion of mandible

Spine and pelvis, 25%
- Vertebra plana: complete collapse of the vertebral body
- Vertebral lesions may produce scoliosis.

Extraskeletal Manifestation

Pulmonary involvement
- Alveolar disease (exudate of histiocytes)
- Interstitial pattern (upper lobe predominance)

CNS involvement
- Meningeal involvement
- Pituitary involvement

Other RES organ involvement
- Liver
- Spleen
- Lymph nodes

MULTIPLE MYELOMA

Most common primary bone tumor (12,000 new cases/year in the United States). Age: 95% > age 40. Composed of plasmacytes (produce IgG) with a distribution identical to that of red marrow:
- Vertebral bodies are destroyed before the pedicles are, as opposed to metastases in which pedicles are destroyed first.
- Axial skeleton is most commonly affected (skull, spine, ribs, pelvis).

Staging (Durie and Salmon Plus System) incorporates imaging findings
IA: Limited disease or plasmacytoma
IB: Mild diffuse disease with <5 focal lesions
IIA, IIB: Moderate diffuse disease, 5-20 focal lesions
IIIA, IIIB: Severe diffuse disease, >20 focal lesions

Clinical Findings

- IgA and/or IgG peak (monoclonal gammopathy) by electrophoresis
- Bence Jones proteins in urine (light-chain Ig subunit)
- Reversed albumin/globulin ratio
- Bone pain
- Anemia

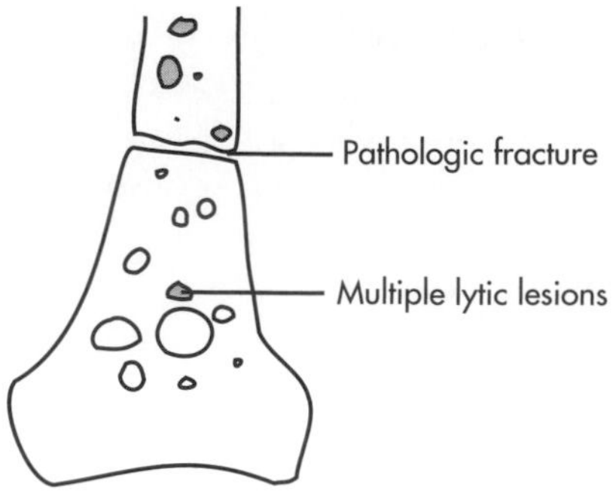

FIGURE 5-110

Types (Fig. 5-110)

- Multiple myeloma (multiple lesions)
  - Vertebra, 65%
  - Ribs, 45%
  - Skull, 40%
  - Shoulder, 40%
  - Pelvis, 30%
  - Long bones, 25%
- Solitary plasmacytoma. Common in vertebral body, pelvis, femur.

Radiographic Features

- Multiple myeloma has two common radiologic appearances:
  - Multiple, well-defined lytic lesions: punched-out lesions, 80%
  - Generalized osteopenia with vertebral compression fractures, 20%
- Plasmacytoma: tends to be large and expansile
- MRI: replacement of normal marrow (sensitive)
- Bone scan: normal scan, cold or hot lesions
- Skeletal survey: more sensitive than bone scan but still misses significant number of myeloma lesions
- Atypical findings (rare)
  - Myelomatosis
  - Sclerosing myeloma
  - Mixed lytic/blastic myeloma

DIFFERENTIATION OF MULTIPLE MYELOMA FROM METASTASES

Parameter	Multiple Myeloma	Metastases
Intervertebral disk	Yes	Rare
Mandible	Yes	Rare
Vertebral pedicles	No	Common
Large soft tissue mass	Yes	No
Bone scan	Cold, normal, hot	Hot, cold

Complications

- Pathologic fractures
- Amyloidosis, 10%
- Most plasmacytomas progress to multiple myeloma.

POEMS SYNDROME

Rare variant of sclerosing myeloma. Japanese predilection. Consists of:

- **P**olyneuropathy
- **O**rganomegaly
- **E**ndocrinopathy (gynecomastia, amenorrhea)
- **M** protein: sclerotic multiple myeloma
- **S**kin changes (hyperpigmentation)

EWING TUMOR

Relatively common malignant tumor derived from undifferentiated mesenchymal cells of the bone marrow or primitive neuroectodermal cells (small, round cell tumor).

Age: 5 to 15 years. Clinical finding is a mass; 35% of patients have fever, leukocytosis, elevated ESR, and thus the tumor clinically mimics infection. 5-year survival: 40%. Very rare in black population.

Location

- Diaphysis of lower extremity, 70%
- Flat bones (sacrum, innominate bone, scapula), 25%
- Vertebral body, 5%

Radiographic Features

- Aggressive tumor: permeative or moth-eaten osteolytic characteristics, cortical erosion, periostitis
- No tumor matrix
- Sclerotic reactive bone may be present.
- Extraosseous soft tissue mass is typical.
- Characteristically it is medullary in location but usually only the cortical changes are apparent on plain radiograph.
- Metastases (lung and bone): 30% at presentation

PRIMARY LYMPHOMA

Very rare; most osseous lymphomas are secondary. Primary osseous lymphoma is usually of the non-Hodgkin type.

Radiographic Features

- Permeative lytic lesion with similar appearance to other small, round cell tumors (e.g., Ewing's tumor)

METASTASES

GENERAL

BONE METASTASES

Adult Male	Adult Female	Children
Prostate, 60%	Breast, 70%	Neuroblastoma
Lung, 15%	Lung, 5%	Leukemia, lymphoma
Kidney, 5%	Kidney, 5%	Medulloblastoma
Other, 20%	Other, 20%	Sarcomas
		Wilms tumor

Spread of Metastases

- Hematogenous spread through arterial circulation to vascular red marrow; metastases are common around shoulders and hip joints due to residual red marrow.
- Hematogenous spread through retrograde venous flow (e.g., prostate)
- Direct extension (uncommon)
- Lymphangitic (rare)

Radiographic Features

The radiographic feature reflects the aggressiveness of the primary tumor. Pattern of destruction may be moth-eaten, geographic, or permeated. Metastases may be lytic, blastic, or mixed. Pathologic fractures are common.

Commonly lytic metastases

- Kidney
- Lung
- Thyroid
- Breast

Commonly sclerotic metastases

- Prostate
- Breast

Other sclerotic metastases (rare)

- Hodgkin lymphoma
- Carcinoid
- Medulloblastoma
- Neuroblastoma
- Transitional cell cancer (TCC)

SECONDARY LYMPHOMA

Skeletal abnormalities occur in 5%-50% of all lymphomas. The more immature the cell line, the greater the frequency of bone involvement.

Radiographic Features

- Usually aggressive tumors with no specific pathognomonic finding
- Suspect the diagnosis in lymphoma patients.
- Ivory vertebra is a manifestation of Hodgkin lymphoma.

OTHER BONE TUMORS

UNICAMERAL (SIMPLE) BONE CYST (UBC) (Fig. 5-111)

Common benign fluid-filled lesion of childhood of unknown cause. Age: 10 to 20 years. 50% of cysts present with pathologic fractures and pain. Most resolve with bone maturity.

Location

- Most common location: proximal metaphysis of the humerus or femur
- Long tubular bones, 90%
- Less common location: calcaneus, ilium (older patients)

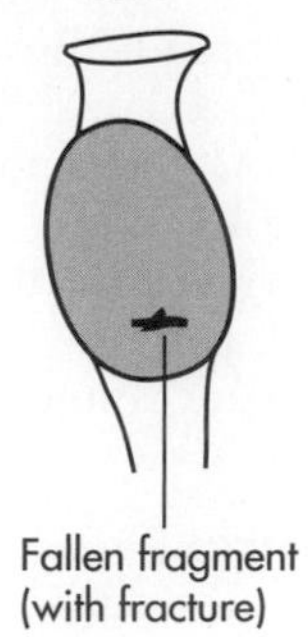

FIGURE 5-111

Radiographic Features

- Central (intramedullary) location; metadiaphyseal
- Tumor respects the physis
- Expansile lesion
- Fluid-filled cavities (fluid-fluid levels)
- Fallen fragment sign secondary to pathologic fracture is pathognomonic for UBC: fragment migrates to dependent portion of cyst.
- No periosteal reaction unless fractured

ANEURYSMAL BONE CYST (ABC) (Fig. 5-112)

Expansile nonneoplastic lesion containing thin-walled, blood-filled cystic cavities. Age: 5 to 20 years. Rapid progression (2 to 6 months) with acute pain. Two types:

- Primary nonneoplastic lesion, 70%
- Secondary lesion arising in preexisting bone tumors, 30% (chondroblastoma, fibrous dysplasia, GCT, osteoblastoma)

Location

- Posterior elements of spine
- Metaphysis of long tubular bones
- Pelvis

Radiographic Features

- Eccentric location (in contradistinction to UBC)
- Expansile
- Thin maintained cortex (best seen by CT) unlike in metastases (e.g., RCC) in which there is cortical breakthrough
- No periosteal reaction unless fractured
- Respects epiphyseal plate
- Large lesions may appear aggressive like lytic metastases.
- Fluid-fluid levels in cystic components

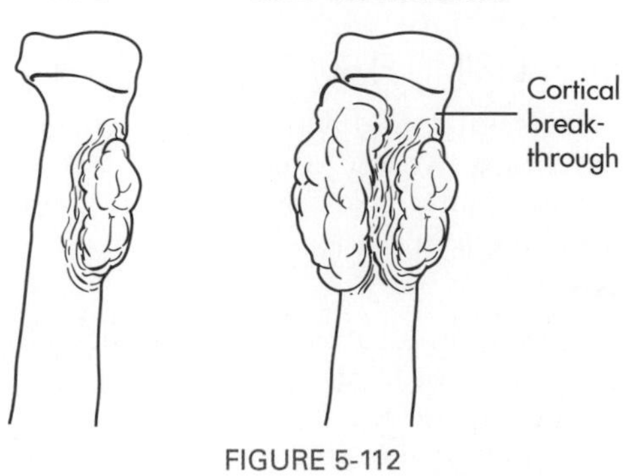

FIGURE 5-112

HEMOPHILIAC PSEUDOTUMOR

Incidence: 2% of hemophiliacs. Pathologically, pseudotumors represent hematomas with thick fibrous capsules caused by intraosseous, subperiosteal, or soft tissue hemorrhage. Painless expanding masses may cause pressure on adjacent organs. Pseudotumors destroy soft tissue, erode bone, and cause neurovascular compromise. Location: femur, pelvis, tibia.

Radiographic Features

- Large soft tissue mass with adjacent bone destruction
- Unresorbed hematoma increases in size over years.
- Calcifications common
- Periosteal elevation with new bone formation at the edge of the lesion
- Characteristic MRI appearance of hematoma (T1W):
  - Hypointense rim: fibrous tissue, hemosiderin deposition
  - Hyperintense center: paramagnetic breakdown products
- Fluid-blood levels may be present.

GIANT CELL TUMOR (FIG. 5-113)

Uncommon lesion thought to arise from osteoclasts. Typically occurs in epiphysis with metaphyseal extension. Age: after epiphyseal fusion. Location: 50% occur around knee. 10% are malignant (local spread, metastases).

Radiographic Features

- Lytic subarticular lesion
- Expansile
- Narrow transition; no sclerotic margin
- May erode into joint
- May be locally aggressive
- Pathologic fracture, 30%

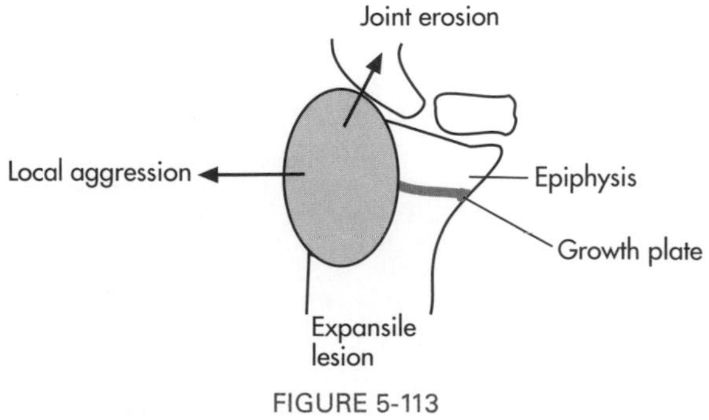

FIGURE 5-113

INTRAOSSEOUS HEMANGIOMA

Asymptomatic unless a complication occurs: pathologic fractures, rarely spinal cord compression (extension into epidural space, vertebral expansion, and hemorrhage). Location: vertebral body > skull > face. Middle age predilection.

Radiographic Features

- Corduroy appearance is pathognomonic: coarse, vertical trabecular pattern of vertebral body
- Radiolucent, slightly expansile intraosseous lesion in extraspinal sites

ADAMANTINOMA

Extremely rare locally aggressive tumor in the spectrum of osteofibrous dysplasia. Age: 20 to 50 years. Location: 90% in tibia.

Radiographic Features

- Sharply circumscribed lytic lesions with marginal sclerosis
- Occurs in middle one third of diaphysis and can be central or eccentric, multilocular, slightly expansile
- Satellite foci may occur in fibula.

CHORDOMA

Rare, slow growing, locally aggressive tumor arising from notochord remnants. The notochord represents the early fetal axial skeleton, which is later surrounded by cartilaginous matrix. As the cartilage ossifies, the notochord is extruded into the intervertebral regions, where it evolves into the nucleus pulposus of the intervertebral disk. Remnants of the notochord may occur at any position along the neural axis. Age: 30 to 70 years. Morbidity is secondary to extensive local invasion and recurrence. Distant metastases occur late in the disease. Treatment is with surgery and irradiation.

Location

- Sacrum, 50%
- Clivus tumors, 35%
- Vertebral bodies, 15%

Radiographic Features

- Nonspecific expansile lytic lesion
- Large soft tissue component
- Variable calcification

INTRAOSSEOUS LIPOMA

Asymptomatic lytic lesion. Location: proximal femur, fibula, calcaneus. May have central calcified nidus.

HEMANGIOENDOTHELIOMA

Low-grade malignant lesion of adolescents. Multifocal lytic lesions involving multiple bones of a single extremity, usually the hands or feet. Locally aggressive; rarely metastasize.

ANGIOSARCOMA

Highly malignant vascular tumor of adolescents/young adults. One third are multifocal. Commonly metastasize.

MASSIVE OSTEOLYSIS (GORHAM DISEASE)

Extensive cystic angiomatosis (hemangiomatous and lymphangiomatous) of bone in children and young adults. Idiopathic, but there frequently is a history of trauma. Location: shoulder and hip most common.

Radiographic Features

- Rapid dissolution of bone
- Spreads contiguously and crosses joints
- No host reaction or periostitis

GLOMUS TUMOR

Benign vascular tumor of the terminal phalanx, commonly subungual. Well-circumscribed, lytic, and painful. Clinical pain and terminal phalangeal location are characteristic.

MISCELLANEOUS LESIONS

MASTOCYTOSIS

Mast cell infiltration of skin, marrow, and other organs. Results in mixed lytic/sclerotic process (dense bones) with thickened trabecula; focal or diffuse. Organ involvement:

- Bone, 60%
  - Osteosclerosis, 20%
  - Osteoporosis, fractures (heparin-like effect), 30%
- GI, 35%
  - Peptic ulcers
  - Diffuse thickening of jejunal folds
  - Hepatomegaly, splenomegaly
  - Lymphadenopathy
  - Ascites
- Chest, 20%
  - Skin: urticaria pigmentosum
  - Fibrosis
  - Pulmonary nodules
- Other
  - Reaction to contrast medium
  - Associated malignancies, 30%: lymphoma, leukemia, adenocarcinoma

MYELOID METAPLASIA (MYELOFIBROSIS)

One of the myeloproliferative disorders in which neoplastic stem cells grow in multiple sites outside the marrow and the hematopoietic marrow is replaced by fibrosis. Only 50% demonstrate radiographic findings on plain films.

Radiographic Features

- Diffuse or patchy osteosclerosis
- Massive extramedullary hematopoiesis
    - Massive splenomegaly (100%)
    - Hepatomegaly

Paraspinal mass

PYKNODYSOSTOSIS (Fig. 5-114)

Autosomal recessive dysplasia

- Dwarfism
- Micrognathia
- Straight mandible
- Dense but fragile bones
- Acroosteolysis
- Wormian bones
- Underdeveloped paranasal sinuses and mastoid air cells

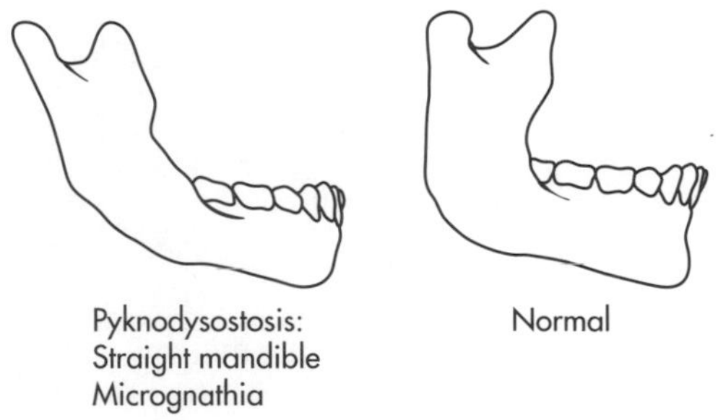

FIGURE 5-114

RADIATION-INDUCED CHANGES

Bone Growth

The major effect of radiation is on chondroblasts in epiphyses:

- Epiphyseal growth arrest (limb-length discrepancies)
- Slipped capital femoral epiphysis (damaged growth plate does not withstand shearing stress)
- Scoliosis (e.g., after radiation of Wilms tumor)
- Hemihypoplasia (i.e., iliac wing)

Osteonecrosis

Radiotoxicity to osteoblasts results in decreased matrix production. Pathologic fractures are not common. Radiation osteitis is most common in:

- Mandible, 30% (intraoral cancer)
- Clavicle, 20% (breast carcinoma)
- Humeral head, 14% (breast carcinoma)
- Ribs, 10% (breast carcinoma)
- Femur, 10%

Radiation-Induced Bone Tumors

- Enchondroma (exostosis) is the most common lesion.
- OSA, chondrosarcoma, and MFH are the most common malignant lesions.

SOFT TISSUE MASSES AND TUMORS

Nodular Fasciitis

Tender benign proliferation of fibroblasts and myofibroblasts that may be mistaken for sarcoma because of rapid growth. 20 to 40 years of age. Most commonly seen in the upper extremity (volar forearm).

Fibroma of the Tendon Sheath

Slow growing, painless, well-circumscribed lesion <3 cm in the extremities (upper 82%). Slow growing. 2:1 M:F ratio; 20 to 50 years.

Elastofibroma

Slow growing pseudotumor from chronic mechanical irritation, found frequently between the posterior chest wall and the inferomedial border of the scapula; >55 years old and more common in women.

Fibromatoses

Spectrum of fibrous soft tissue lesions that are infiltrative and prone to recurrence. Types: juvenile aponeurotic fibroma, infantile dermal fibromatosis, and aggressive fibromatosis (desmoid tumor).

Malignant Fibrous Histiocytoma

The most common soft tissue tumor in adults. Location: lower extremity is most common. Radiographic appearance is nonspecific (large mass); reactive pseudocapsule may be seen.

Liposarcoma

Second most common soft tissue tumor in adults. Location: buttocks, lower extremity, retroperitoneum. Fatty component is progressively replaced by soft tissue while degree of malignancy increases: variable reactive pseudocapsule.

Synovial Cell Sarcoma

Soft tissue sarcoma of questionable synovial origin. Age: 15 to 35 years. Location: most commonly around the knee. Approximately one third contain calcifications.

LIPOMA ARBORESCENS

Diffuse fatty infiltration of synovium of knee, usually monoarticular. May present with painless swelling. MRI demonstrates fat-signal frondlike projections of the synovium.

SYNOVIAL (OSTEO)CHONDROMATOSIS

Cartilaginous metaplasia of synovium. Ossified loose bodies, widened joint spaces, and erosions may be demonstrated on plain film. Cartilaginous loose bodies may be seen on MRI, which may be distinguished from PVNS by lack of low signal.

PIGMENTED VILLONODULAR SYNOVITIS (PVNS)

PVNS predominantly affects adults in their second to fourth decades. Two forms: diffuse (within the joint) and focal. PVNS can affect any joint, bursa, or tendon sheath; however, the knee is the most commonly involved (followed by hip, elbow, and ankle).

Radiographic Features

- Fibrohistiocytic proliferation of synovium manifests as noncalcified soft tissue masses on plain film that erodes into bone, creating large cystic cavities. Joint space narrowing can occur only late in its course.
- MRI characteristics diffuse low signal masses on T1W and T2W sequences lining the joint synovium. The masses represent synovial hypertrophy with diffuse hemosiderin deposits. Joint effusion occurs.
- The differential diagnosis for low signal intensity lesions on T1W and T2W in and around the joint includes PVNS, gout (the signal characteristics may be secondary to fibrous tissue, hemosiderin deposition, or calcification), amyloid (primary or secondary amyloidosis), fibrous lesions (fibromatosis, desmoid tumors included), and disorders causing hemosiderin deposition (hemophilia, synovial hemangioma, neuropathic osteoarthropathy). The deposition of hemosiderin from hemophilia is never as prominent as seen in PVNS.

Arthritis

GENERAL

APPROACH

Types of Arthritis (Fig. 5-115)

There are three types of arthritis (which often can be distinguished radiologically):

Degenerative joint disease

ABC APPROACH TO DIFFERENTIAL DIAGNOSIS OF ARTHRITIS

Parameter	Differential Diagnosis
Alignment	Subluxation, dislocation: common in RA and SLE
Bone	
Osteoporosis	Normal mineralization: all arthritides except RA
	Juxtaarticular osteopenia: any arthropathy; subtle findings have no differential diagnosis value
	Diffuse osteoporosis: only in RA
Erosions	Aggressive erosion (no sclerotic borders, no reparative bone): RA, psoriasis
	Nonaggressive erosion (fine sclerotic border): gout
	Location: inflammatory erosions occur at margins (mouse ear), erosions in erosive OA occur in the central portion of the joint (seagull)
Bone production	Periosteal new bone formation: psoriasis, Reiter syndrome (this is a feature that distinguishes RA from spondyloarthropathies due to tenosynovitis)
	Ankylosis (bony bridging of a joint): inflammatory arthropathies
	Overhanging edges of cortex: typical of gout (tophus)
	Subchondral bone (reparative bone beneath cortex): typical of OA
	Osteophytes (occur where adjacent cartilage has undergone degeneration and loss): typical of OA
Cartilage	
Joint space	Maintenance of joint space: any early arthropathy; only gout and PVNS maintain normal joint space in progressive disease
	Uniform narrowing: all arthritis except OA
	Eccentric narrowing: typical of OA
	Wide joint space: early inflammatory process
Distribution	
Monoarticular or polyarticular	Monarticular: infection, crystal deposition, or posttraumatic
Proximal/distal	Proximal joints: RA, CPPD, AS
	Distal joints: Reiter, psoriatic
	Symmetrical: RA, multicentric reticulohistiocytosis

ABC APPROACH TO DIFFERENTIAL DIAGNOSIS OF ARTHRITIS—cont'd

Parameter	Differential Diagnosis
SOFT TISSUES	
Swelling	Symmetrical around joint: seen in all inflammatory arthropathies but most commonly in RA asymmetrical: most commonly due to asymmetrical osteophytes rather than true soft tissue swelling; most common in OA
	Lumpy, bumpy soft tissue swelling: gout (tophus)
	Swelling of entire digit: psoriasis, Reiter (sausage digit)
Calcification	Soft tissue: gout (calcified tophus)
	Cartilage: CPPD
	Subcutaneous tissue: scleroderma (typical)

AS, ankylosing spondylitis; CPPD, calcium pyrophosphate dihydrate; OA, osteoarthritis; RA, rheumatoid arthritis.

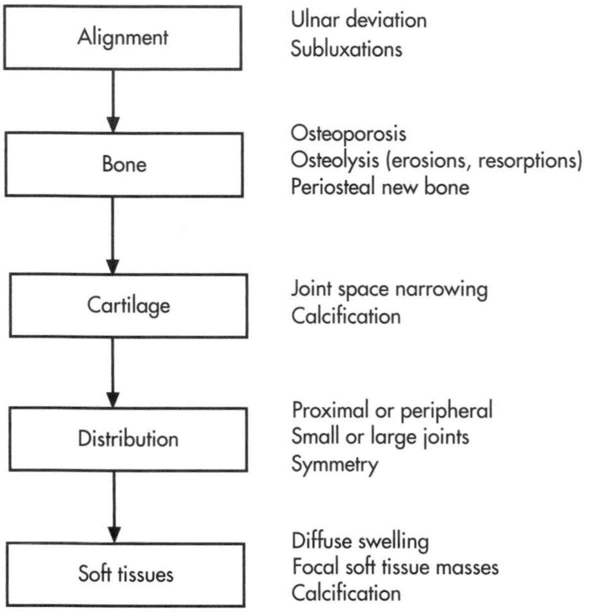

FIGURE 5-115

- Osteophytes
- Subchondral sclerosis
- Uneven loss of articular space

Inflammatory arthritis
- Erosions
- Periarticular osteoporosis common
- Soft tissue swelling
- Uniform loss of articular space

Metabolic arthritis
- Lumpy bumpy soft tissue swelling
- Marginated bony erosions with overhanging edges

DEGENERATIVE ARTHRITIS

GENERAL

Degenerative joint disease (DJD) = osteoarthritis (OA). Early changes include disruption of the armor plate of the articular cartilage. Subsequently, there is a progressive loss of macromolecular components from the ground substance, eventually exposing subchondral bone. Incidence: >40 million cases/year in the United States; 80% of population >50 years have radiologic evidence of OA. There are two types:

Primary OA
- No underlying local etiologic factors
- Abnormally high mechanical forces on normal joint
- Age related

Secondary OA
- Underlying etiologic factors: CPPD < trauma, inflammatory arthritis, hemochromatosis, acromegaly, congenital hip dysplasia, osteonecrosis, loose bodies
- Normal forces on abnormal joint

Clinical Findings

Characteristics of joint discomfort
- Aggravated by joint use; relieved by rest
- Morning stiffness <15 min

Joint examination
- Local tenderness
- Joint enlargement
- Crepitus
- Effusion
- Gross deformity
- Heberden's nodules
- Borchard's nodes

Joints most frequently involved: DIP, PIP, first carpometacarpal (CMC), hips, knees, spine, first metatarsal phalangeal (MTP)

Joints commonly spared: MCP, wrist, elbow, shoulder, ankles

No systemic manifestation

Synovial fluid
- High viscosity
- Normal mucin test
- Mild leukocytosis (<2000/mm^3)

Radiographic Features (Fig. 5-116)

Five hallmarks:
- Narrowing of joint space, usually asymmetrical
- Subchondral sclerosis

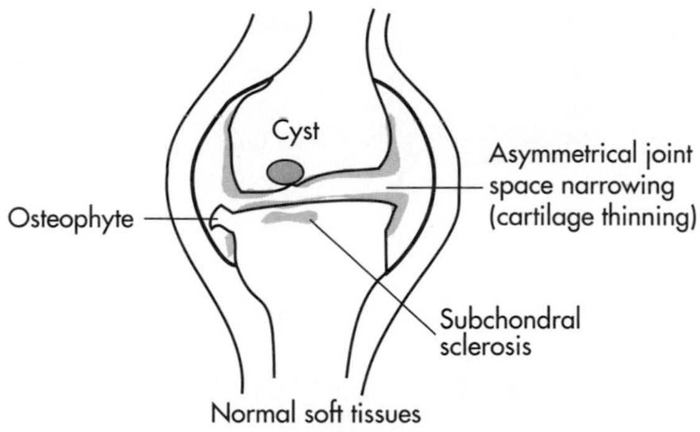

FIGURE 5-116

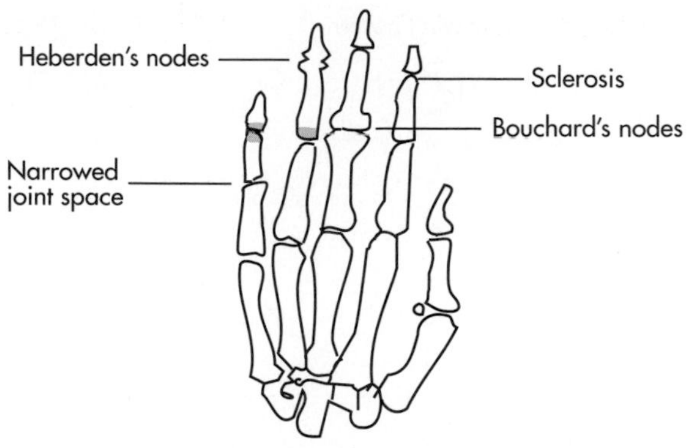

FIGURE 5-117

- Subchondral cysts (true cysts or pseudocysts)
- Osteophytes
- Lack of osteoporosis

Treatment Options

- Advanced OA: arthroplasty (e.g., total hip replacement [THR])
- Alternative surgical procedures:
  Osteotomy: sections of bone are excised to improve joint congruity and alignment, especially in young patients.
  Excision arthroplasty: excision of femoral neck; leads to extremity shortening and joint instability. Indications: (1) salvage operation for failed THR; (2) patients with limited weight-bearing activities.
  Arthrodesis: removal of articular cartilage with fusion of joint surfaces
- Antiinflammatory drugs: NSAIDs
- Experimental chondrocyte transplant

OSTEOARTHRITIS IN SPECIFIC LOCATIONS

Hip

- Joint space is narrowest superiorly at weight-bearing portion.
- Subchondral cyst formation (intrusion of synovium and synovial fluid into the altered bone); Egger's cysts: subchondral acetabular cysts
- Superolateral migration of the femoral head is common.
- Secondary OA of the hip is common and can be radiographically confusing.
- Postel's coxarthropathy: rapidly destructive OA of the hip joint that mimics Charcot's joint
- Protrusio acetabuli is uncommon.

Knee

- Medial femorotibial compartment is most commonly narrowed.
- Weight-bearing views are often helpful for assessment of joint space narrowing.
- Osteochondral bodies
- Patellar tooth sign (enthesopathy at the patellar attachment of the quadriceps tendon)
- Secondary OA occurs commonly after trauma and meniscectomy.

Hand (Fig. 5-117)

- Heberden's nodes in DIP
- Bouchard's nodes in PIP
- Asymmetrical peripheral involvement

Spine (Fig. 5-118)

- OA of the spine occurs in the apophyseal joints (diarthroses).
- Lower cervical and low lumbar spine are most commonly affected.
- Osteophytes may encroach on neural foramina (best seen on oblique views).
- Vacuum phenomenon: gas (N_2) in apophyseal joints is pathognomonic of the degenerative process.
- Degenerative spondylolisthesis (pseudospondylolisthesis)

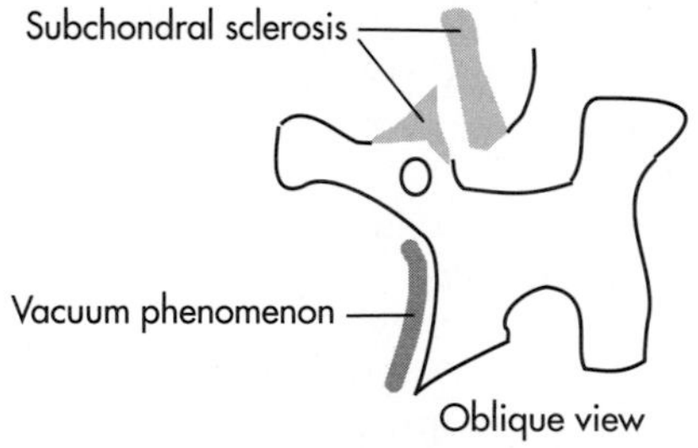

FIGURE 5-118

EROSIVE OSTEOARTHRITIS

OA with superimposed inflammatory, erosive changes. Characteristically affects middle-aged women.

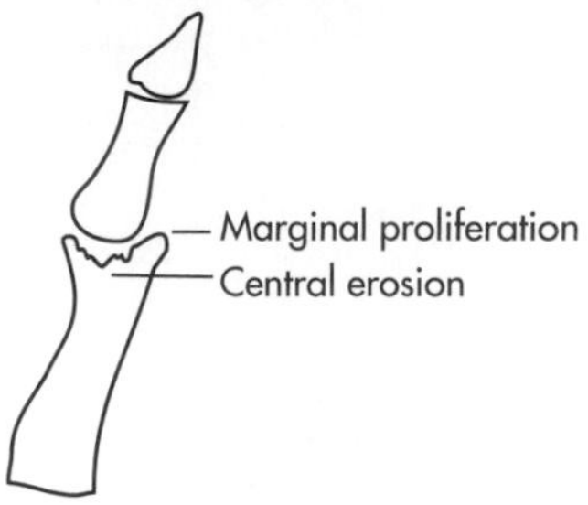

FIGURE 5-119

Radiographic Features (Fig. 5-119)
- Erosive and productive changes of DIP and PIP
- Gull-wing pattern: secondary to central erosions and marginal osteophytes
- Typical involvement of first CMC may help distinguish erosive OA from rheumatoid arthritis (RA), psoriatic arthritis, and adult Still disease.
- Interphalangeal fusion may occur.

DEGENERATIVE DISK DISEASE

Degenerative disk disease affects the intervertebral symphyses (amphiarthroses) and thus is not DJD (which affects diarthrodial joints). Degenerative disk disease and DJD often but not always occur together.

Radiographic Features
- MRI is imaging modality of choice for evaluating intervertebral disks.
- Disk signal abnormalities (loss of T2W bright signal) indicate degeneration.
- Decreased disk height
- Endplate changes
  - Modic I: dark TlW/bright T2W (vascular tissue ingrowth), enhances with contrast
  - Modic II: bright TlW/bright T2W (fatty change)
  - Modic III: dark TlW/dark T2W (sclerosis)
- Disk contour abnormalities
  - Bulges
  - Protrusions or extrusions (see Chapter 6)
- Plain film findings
  - Disk space narrowing
  - Vacuum phenomenon in disk space
  - Endplate osteophytes and sclerosis

SPONDYLOSIS DEFORMANS (Fig. 5-120)

Degenerative changes of the annulus fibrosis result in anterior and anterolateral disk herniations. Traction osteophytes may form secondarily and project several millimeters from the endplate. Disk spaces are usually well preserved.

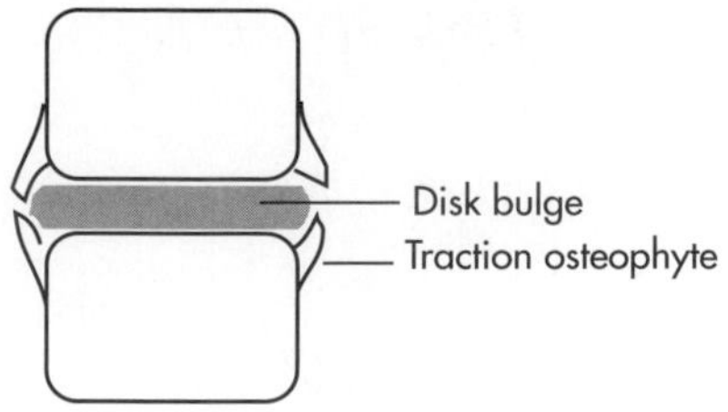

FIGURE 5-120

DIFFUSE IDIOPATHIC SKELETAL HYPEROSTOSIS (DISH, FORESTIER DISEASE)

Severe productive bone formation in the soft tissues around the spine, resulting in bulky flowing osteophytes. Most common site is thoracic spine. Unknown etiology. Clinical signs and symptoms are mild compared with radiographic appearance.

Radiographic Features
- Flowing osteophytes of at least four contiguous vertebral bodies
- Preserved disk height
- No sacroiliitis or facet ankylosis
- Calcification of ligaments and tendons
- Associated with hypertrophic DJD
- May be associated with ossification of the posterior longitudinal ligament
- If seen in a child, consider JRA

INFLAMMATORY ARTHRITIS

GENERAL

There are three types of inflammatory arthritis:
- Autoimmune arthritis
  - RA
  - Scleroderma
  - Systemic lupus erythematosus (SLE)
  - Dermatomyositis
- Seronegative spondyloarthropathies
  - Ankylosing spondylitis
  - Reiter syndrome
  - Psoriasis
  - Enteropathic arthropathies
- Erosive OA

ADULT RHEUMATOID ARTHRITIS

Epidemiology
- Female: male = 3:1
- Approximately 2 million people suffer from rheumatoid arthritis in the United States
- HLA-DW4 related

Diagnosis
- Classic RA: 7 criteria (from table below)
- Definite RA: 5 criteria
- Probable RA: 3 criteria

DIAGNOSTIC CRITERIA FOR RHEUMATOID ARTHRITIS

Criterion	Comment
Morning stiffness	Indicator of inflammation
Pain on motion	In at least one joint
Swelling of one joint	No bony growth (indicates DJD)
Swelling of another joint	
Symmetrical swelling	DIP Involvement excluded
Subcutaneous nodules	Exclude CPPD deposition disease
Typical radiologic changes	See below
Positive rheumatoid factor	>1: 64
Synovial fluid	Poor mucin clot formation
Typical synovial histopathology	
Histopathology of rheumatoid nodules	

Radiographic Features (Fig. 5-121)

Early changes
- Periarticular soft tissue swelling (edema, synovial congestion)
- Periarticular osteoporosis in symmetrical distribution (hallmark)
- Preferred sites of early involvement
  Hands: 2nd and 3rd MCP joints
  Feet: 4th and 5th MTP joints

Late changes
- Erosions (pannus formation, granulation tissue) first attack joint portions in which protective cartilage is absent (i.e., capsular insertion site).
- Erosions of the ulnar styloid and triquetrum are characteristic.
- Subchondral cyst formation results from synovial fluid, which is pressed into bone marrow through destroyed cartilage.
- Subluxations
- Carpal instability
- Fibrous ankylosis is a late finding.

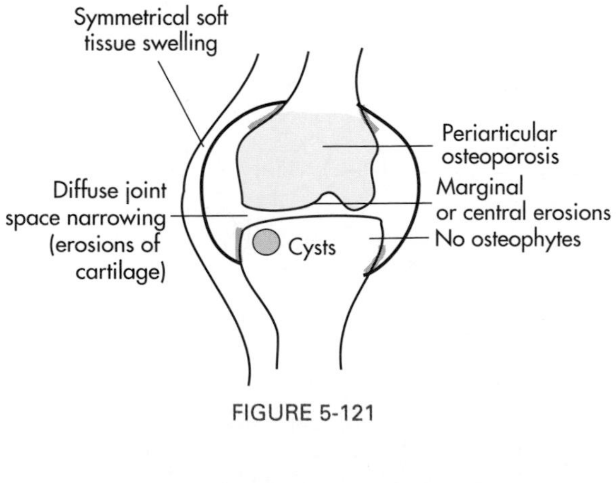

FIGURE 5-121

Extraarticular Manifestations of Rheumatoid Arthritis

Abdominal
- Secondary renal disease: glomerulonephritis, amyloid, drug toxicity
- Arteritis: infarction, claudication

Pulmonary
- Pleural effusion
- Interstitial fibrosis
- Pulmonary nodules
- Caplan syndrome: pneumoconiosis, rheumatoid lung nodules, RA
- Pneumonitis (very rare)

Cardiac
- Pericarditis and pericardial effusion, 30%
- Myocarditis

Felty syndrome
- RA
- Splenomegaly
- Neutropenia
- Thrombocytopenia

RHEUMATOID ARTHRITIS IN SPECIFIC LOCATIONS

Hand (Fig. 5-122)
- MCP ulnar deviation
- Boutonnière deformity: hyperextension of DIP, flexion of PIP
- Swan-neck deformity: hyperextension of PIP, flexion of DIP
- Hitchhiker's thumb
- Telescope fingers: shortening of phalanges due to dislocations
- Ulnar and radial styloid erosions are common.
- Wrist instability: ulnar translocation, scapholunate dissociation

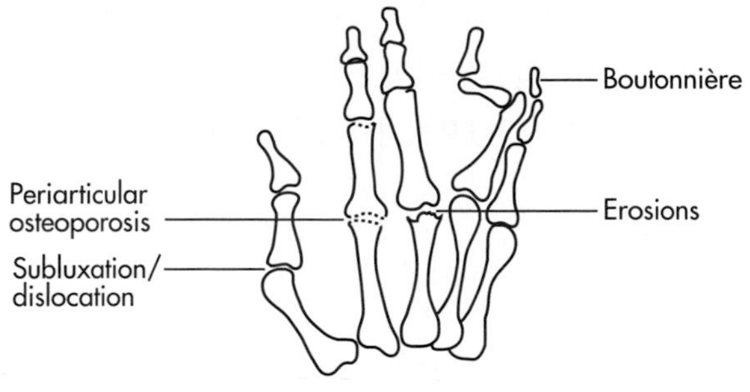

FIGURE 5-122

Shoulder (Fig. 5-123)
- Lysis of distal clavicle
- Rotator cuff tear
- Marginal erosions of humeral head

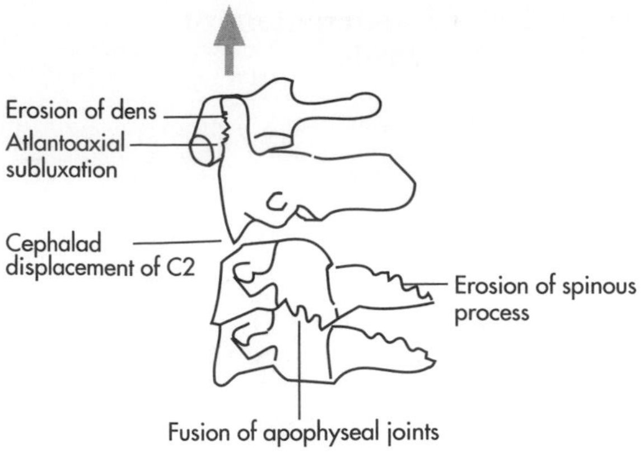

FIGURE 5-123

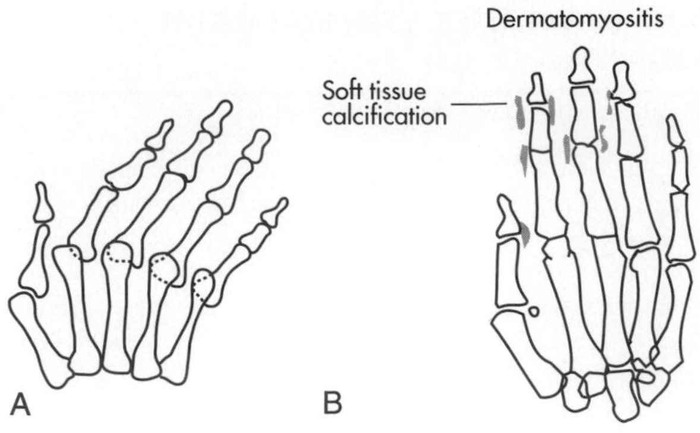

FIGURE 5-124A

Hip

- Concentric decrease in joint space
- Protrusio deformity
- Secondary OA is common

Spine

- Synovial joint erosions
  - Erosions in odontoid
  - Erosions in apophyseal joints
- Atlantoaxial subluxation and impaction
  - >3 mm separation between odontoid and C1 in lateral flexion
  - Due to laxity of transverse cruciate ligament and joint destruction

SCLERODERMA (SYSTEMIC SCLEROSIS)

Manifests as soft tissue abnormalities in addition to erosive arthritis.

Radiographic Features

- Soft tissue calcification
- Acroosteolysis: tuft resorption results from pressure of tight and atrophic skin
- Soft tissue atrophy
- Erosive changes of DIP and PIP

SYSTEMIC LUPUS ERYTHEMATOSUS (SLE) (Fig. 5-124A)

Nonerosive arthritis (in 90% of SLE) resulting from ligamentous laxity and joint deformity. Distribution is similar to that seen in RA.

Radiographic Features

- Prominent subluxations of MCP
- Usually bilateral and symmetrical
- No erosions
- Radiographically similar to Jaccoud arthropathy
- Soft tissue swelling may be the only indicator.

DERMATOMYOSITIS (Fig. 5-124B)

Widespread soft tissue calcification is the hallmark.

ANKYLOSING SPONDYLITIS (AS)

Seronegative spondyloarthropathy of the axial skeleton and proximal large joints. Clinical: males >> females. HLA-B27 in 95%. Insidious onset of back pain and stiffness. Onset: 20 years.

Radiographic Features (Fig. 5-125)

- SI joint is the initial site of involvement: bilateral, symmetrical
  - Erosions: early
  - Sclerosis: intermediate
  - Ankylosis: late
- Contiguous thoracolumbar involvement Vertebral body "squaring:" early osteitis
  - Syndesmophytes
  - Bamboo spine: late fusion and ligamentous ossification
  - Shiny corners: sclerosis at edges of endplates
  - Dagger sign, trolley track sign: one or three dense lines along spine due to ossification of interspinous and supraspinous ligaments.
- Anderson lesion and pseudarthrosis of ankylosed spine (fracture); may be seen in DISH
- Enthesopathy common
- Arthritis of proximal joints (hip > shoulder) in 50%
  - Erosions and osteophytes

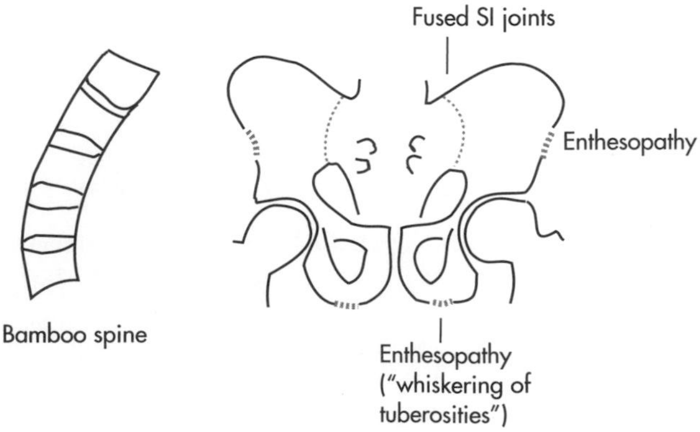

FIGURE 5-125

Associations

- Inflammatory bowel disease (IBD)
- Iritis
- Aortitis
- Pulmonary fibrosis of upper lobes

DIFFERENTIATION OF LUMBAR OSTEOPHYTES

Osteophytes

Extension of the vertebral endplates in the horizontal direction. Osteophytes are smaller in DJD and larger in psoriatic arthritis and Reiter syndrome (calcifications of periarticular soft tissues that become contiguous with the spine).

Syndesmophytes

Calcification of the outer portion of the annulus fibrosus such as in AS.

REITER SYNDROME (Figs. 5-126 through 5-128)

Seronegative spondyloarthropathy with lower extremity erosive joint disease. Clinical: males >> females. HLA-B27 in 80%. Follows either nongonococcal urethritis or bacillary dysentery *(Shigella, Yersinia, Salmonella)*.

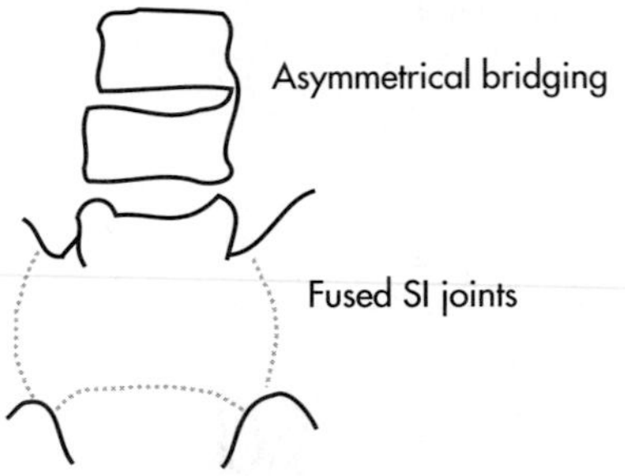

FIGURE 5-126

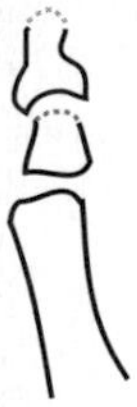

Pencil-in-cup deformity

FIGURE 5-127

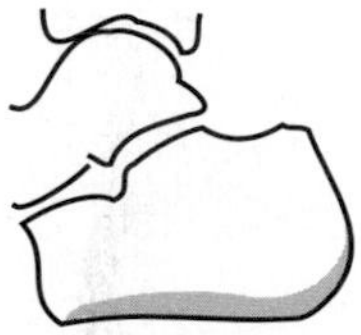

Heel enthesopathy
(periosteal new bone formation)

FIGURE 5-128

Clinical Findings

- Classic triad occurs in minority of patients:
  - Urethritis or cervicitis
  - Conjunctivitis
  - Arthritis
- Balanitis, keratoderma blennorrhagicum
- Back pain and heel pain are common.

Radiographic Features

- Predominant involvement of distal lower extremity
  - MTP > calcaneus > ankle > knee
- Earliest changes (erosive arthropathy) are often in feet:
  - MTP erosions
  - Retrocalcaneal bursitis
  - Enthesopathy and erosions at Achilles tendon and plantar aponeurosis insertion
- Bilateral sacroiliitis (less common than in AS), 30%
  - Asymmetrical: early
  - Symmetrical: late
- Bulky asymmetrical thoracolumbar osteophytes with skip segments. Spine involvement is similar to psoriatic arthritis.
- Periostitis is common.
- Hand involvement (pencil-in-cup deformity) may occur but is much less common than in psoriasis.

PSORIATIC ARTHRITIS

Seronegative spondyloarthropathy (inflammatory upper extremity polyarthritis) associated with psoriasis (10%-20% of patients with psoriasis will develop arthritis). In 90%, the skin changes precede the arthritis; 10% develop the arthritis first. HLA-B27 in 50%. Positive correlation between:

- Severity of skin lesions and joint disease
- Nail changes and DIP involvement

Types (Fig. 5-129)

- Asymmetrical oligoarthritis (most common type): DIP and PIP of hands
- Spondyloarthropathy of SI joints and spine, 50%
- Symmetrical polyarthritis that resembles RA
- Arthritis mutilans: marked hand deformity ("opera glass" hand)
- Classic polyarthritis with nail changes and variable DIP abnormalities

Radiographic Features

- Combination of productive and erosive changes (distinguishable feature from RA)
- Bone production
  - Mouse ears: bone production adjacent to erosions
  - Ivory phalanx: sclerosis of distal phalanx
- Erosions are aggressive.

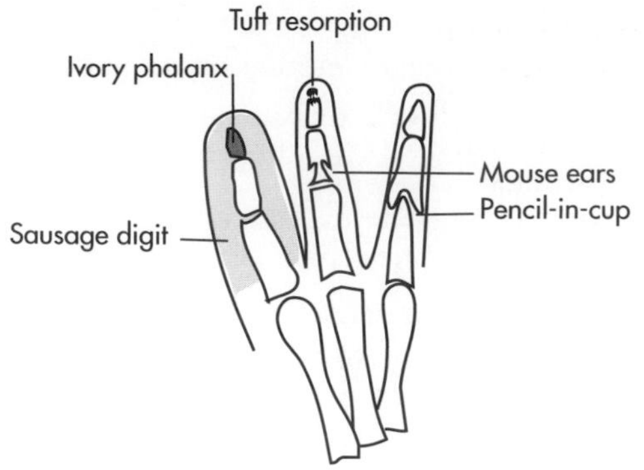

FIGURE 5-129

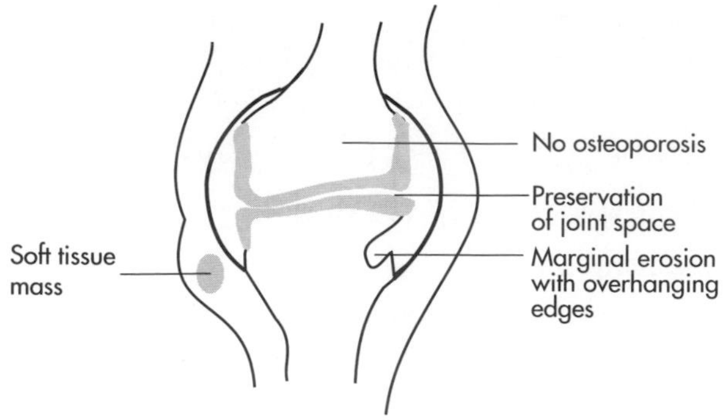

FIGURE 5-130

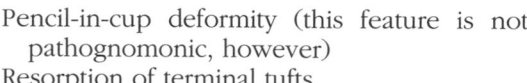

Pencil-in-cup deformity (this feature is not pathognomonic, however)
Resorption of terminal tufts

- Ankylosis (10%): most common in hands and feet
- Soft tissue swelling of entire digit: sausage digit
- Joint space loss is usually severe.
- Sacroiliitis is usually bilateral.
- Periostitis ("fluffy") is common.

Pearls

- SI and spine involvement of psoriatic arthritis is indistinguishable from Reiter's disease.
- Hand disease predominates in psoriasis; foot disease predominates in Reiter disease.
- Spine disease can be differentiated from AS by asymmetrical osteophytes and lack of syndesmophytes.
- SI involvement is more common and tends to be more symmetrical in AS.
- In one third of patients, the diagnosis of psoriatic arthritis cannot be made on the basis of radiographs.

ENTEROPATHIC ARTHROPATHIES

Patients with IBD or infection may develop arthritis indistinguishable from Reiter disease or AS. HLA-B27 is often positive. Underlying disease:

- Ulcerative colitis (10% have arthritis)
- Crohn disease
- Whipple disease
- *Salmonella, Shigella, Yersinia* enteritis infection

METABOLIC ARTHRITIS

GENERAL (Fig. 5-130)

Metabolic deposition diseases result in accumulation of crystals or other substances in cartilage and soft tissues. Depositions alter the mechanical properties of cartilage causing microfractures; crystals in the joint fluid elicit acute synovial inflammation. Ultimately, secondary arthritis develops.

Presentations

- Acute inflammatory arthritis
- Chronic destructive arthropathy

Types

Crystal deposition diseases
- Sodium urate: gout
- CPPD
- Basic calcium phosphate (e.g., calcium hydroxyapatite)

Other deposition diseases
- Hemochromatosis
- Wilson disease
- Alkaptonuria
- Amyloidosis
- Multicentric reticulohistiocytosis
- Xanthomatosis

Endocrine
- Acromegaly

GOUT (Fig. 5-131)

Heterogeneous group of entities characterized by recurrent attacks of arthritis secondary to deposition of sodium urate crystals in and around joints. Hyperuricemia not always present; 90% of patients are male.

Urate crystals are strongly birefringent under polarized microscopy.

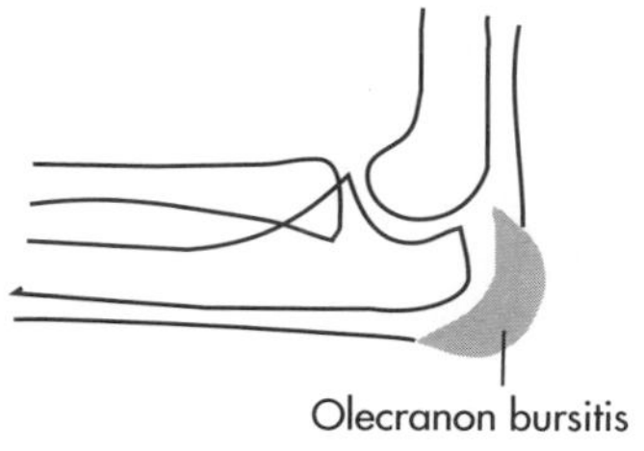

FIGURE 5-131

Causes

Uric acid overproduction, 10%
- Primary: enzyme defects in purine synthesis
- Secondary: increased turnover of nucleic acids
  - Myeloproliferative and lymphoproliferative diseases
  - Hemoglobinopathies, hemolytic anemias
  - Chemotherapy
  - Alcohol, drugs

Uric acid underexcretion, 90%
- Primary: reduced renal excretion of unknown cause
- Secondary
  - Chronic renal failure (any cause)
  - Diuretic therapy (thiazides)
  - Alcohol, drugs

Endocrine disorders (hyperparathyroidism or hypoparathyroidism)

Radiographic Features (Fig. 5-132)
- Lower extremity > upper extremity; small joints > large joints
- First MTP is most common site: podagra
- Marginal, paraarticular erosions: overhanging edge
- Erosions may have sclerotic borders.
- Joint space is preserved.
- Soft tissue and bursa deposition
  - Tophi: juxtaarticular, helix of ear
  - Bursitis: olecranon, prepatellar
- Erosions and tophi only seen in long-standing disease
- Tophi calcification, 50%
- Chondrocalcinosis

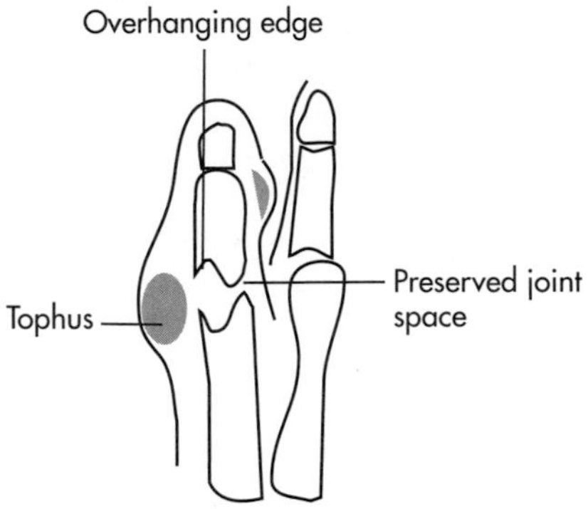

FIGURE 5-132

CALCIUM PYROPHOSPHATE DIHYDRATE DEPOSITION (CPPD) DISEASE

Intraarticular deposition of CPPD ($Ca_2P_2O_7 \cdot H_2O$) resulting in chondrocalcinosis and a pattern of DJD in atypical joints.

Terminology
- *Chondrocalcinosis:* calcification of hyaline cartilage and fibrocartilage, synovium, tendons, and ligaments. Chondrocalcinosis has many causes of which CPPD deposition is only one; not all patients with CPPD deposition have chondrocalcinosis.
- *CPPD deposition:* chondrocalcinosis secondary to CPPD. May or may not be associated with arthropathy.
- *CPPD arthropathy:* structural arthropathy secondary to CPPD
- *Pseudogout:* subset of patients with CPPD deposition disease who have a clinical presentation that resembles gout (i.e., acute intermittent attacks).

Radiographic Features (Fig. 5-133)
- Two main features:
  - Chondrocalcinosis
  - Arthropathy resembling OA
- Chondrocalcinosis present in:
  - Hyaline cartilage: linear calcification, especially in knee
  - Fibrocartilage: menisci, triangular fibrocartilage complex of wrist, glenoid and acetabular labra, symphysis pubis, intervertebral disks
- Synovial, capsular, ligament, and tendon calcification may occur but are not common.
- Arthropathy differs from OA in distribution: predominance of knee (patellofemoral predilection), radiocarpal joint, second and third MCP involvement
- Subchondral cysts are common and are distinctive.

Associations
- Primary hyperparathyroidism
- Gout
- Hemochromatosis

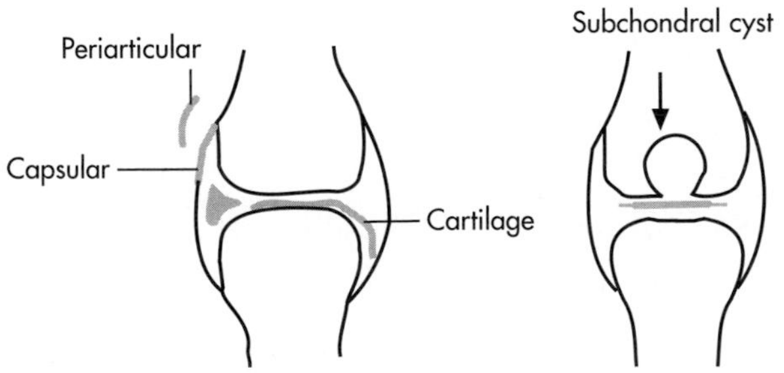

FIGURE 5-133

BASIC CALCIUM PHOSPHATE (BCP) DEPOSITION DISEASE

BCP (calcium hydroxyapatite) deposition is predominantly periarticular as opposed to intraarticular CPPD. The crystal deposition causes periarticular inflammation without structural joint abnormalities.

Radiographic Features

Periarticular calcifications occur primarily:

- Near insertions of supraspinatus tendon
- In flexor carpi ulnaris tendon near pisiform bone
- In Milwaukee shoulder: rotator cuff, subacromial subdeltoid bursa
- In hand: MCP, interphalangeal joints

HEMOCHROMATOSIS ARTHROPATHY

Develops in 50% of patients with hemochromatosis. Secondary to iron deposition and/or concomitant CPPD deposition. Arthropathy changes are similar to those seen in CPPD.

Radiographic Features

- Same distribution and productive changes as in CPPD
- Distinctive features:
    - Beaklike osteophytes on MCP heads (4th and 5th)
    - Generalized osteoporosis

WILSON DISEASE

Defect in the biliary excretion of copper results in accumulation of copper in basal ganglia, liver, joints, and other tissues. Autosomal recessive.

Radiographic Features

- Same distribution as CPPD
- Distinctive features:
    - Subchondral fragmentation
    - Generalized osteoporosis

INTRAARTICULAR HYDROXYAPATITE CRYSTAL DEPOSITION DISEASE: MILWAUKEE SHOULDER

Elderly women; shoulder pain and decreased mobility

Radiographic Features

- Amorphous calcification
- Glenohumeral joint narrowing
- Subchondral sclerosis
- Bone destruction
- Rotator cuff disruption
- Acromiohumeral abutment

ALKAPTONURIA (OCHRONOSIS)

Absence of homogentisic acid oxidase results in tissue accumulation of homogentisic acid. Homogentisic acid deposits in hyaline cartilage and fibrocartilage cause a brown-black pigmentation. Autosomal recessive.

Radiographic Features

- Dystrophic calcification: intervertebral disks are most commonly affected.
- Cartilage, tendons, ligaments
- Generalized osteoporosis
- OA of SI and large peripheral joints

AMYLOID ARTHROPATHY

10% of patients with amyloid have bone or joint involvement. Amyloid may cause a nodular synovitis with erosions, similar to that seen in RA.

Radiographic Features

- Bulky soft tissue nodules (i.e., shoulder pad sign)
- Well-marginated erosions
- Preserved joint space
- Wrists, elbows, shoulders, hips

MULTICENTRIC RETICULOHISTIOCYTOSIS

Systemic disease of unknown origin. Similar radiographic features as gout and RA. Red skin nodules.

Radiographic Features

- Nodular soft tissue swelling
- Sharply demarcated marginal erosions
- Mostly distal phalangeal joints
- Bilateral and symmetrical
- Absence of periarticular osteopenia

HEMOPHILIA

Arthropathy is secondary to repeated spontaneous hemarthroses, which occur in 90% of hemophiliacs. 70% are monoarticular (knee > elbow > ankle > hip > shoulder).

Radiographic Features

Acute episode

- Joint effusion (hemarthrosis)
- Periarticular osteoporosis

Chronic inflammation and synovial proliferation

- Epiphyseal overgrowth
- Subchondral cysts
- Secondary OA
- Distinct knee findings
    - Widened intercondylar notch
    - Squared patella
    - Similar radiographic appearance as JRA
- Distinct elbow findings
    - Enlarged radial head

Enlarged trochlear notch

TUMORAL CALCINOSIS

Rare, hereditary condition in which lobulated calcified painless masses are found along the extensor surfaces of large joints. No erosions. Amorphous, cystic, and multilobulated calcifications located in a periarticular distribution. CT may reveal cystic spaces with fluid-fluid levels (sedimentation sign). Treatment: Surgical excision with phosphate deprivation.

INFECTIOUS ARTHRITIS

GENERAL

Infectious arthritis usually results from hematogenous spread to synovium and subsequent spread into the joint. Direct spread of osteomyelitis into the joint is much less common. The diagnosis is made by joint aspiration.

Organism

- *Staphylococcus aureus* (most common)
- β-*Streptococcus* in infants
- *Haemophilus* in preschoolers
- Gram-negative organisms in diabetes mellitus, alcoholism
- Gonococcal arthritis in sexually active young patients (80% women)
- *Salmonella* is seen in sickle cell disease; however, the most common infection in patients with sickle cell disease is *Staphylococcus.*
- Tuberculosis (TB): granulomatous infection
- Fungal infections in immunocompromised patients
- Viral synovitis is transient and self-limited.
- *Borrelia burgdorferi:* Lyme arthritis

Radiographic Features

Plain film
- Joint effusion
- Juxtaarticular osteoporosis
- Destruction of subchondral bone on both sides of the joint

Bone scan
- Useful if underlying osteomyelitis is suspected

MRI
- Joint effusion
- Sensitive in detecting early cartilage damage

TUBERCULOUS ARTHRITIS

Radiographic Features

- Phemister triad
  - Cartilage destruction (occurs late)
  - Marginal erosions
  - Osteoporosis
- Kissing sequestra in bones adjacent to joints
- Location: hip, knee, tarsal joints, spine
- Spine: Pott disease (see Chapter 6)

DISK SPACE INFECTION

Usually there is primary hematogenous spread to vertebral body endplate and subsequent spread to intervertebral disk.

Radiographic Features

- Destruction of intervertebral disk space and endplates, process crosses the disk, unlike tumors (disk destruction occurs later compared with pyogenic infection)
- Paravertebral abscess
- MRI is most sensitive imaging modality.
- Vacuum phenomenon virtually rules out infection.

SPECTRUM OF OSTEOMYELITIS AND SEPTIC ARTHRITIS ON PLAIN FILM

Periosteal reaction
- Thin, linear periosteal reaction
- Thick periosteal reaction
- Laminated ("onion peel")
- Codman's triangle

Bone destruction
- Permeating bone lesion
- Punched-out bone
- Moth-eaten
- Geographic
- Aggressive osteolysis
- Well-defined osteolytic lesion with thick sclerotic border

Localized cortical thickening
Ground glass
Diffusely dense bones
Chronic sclerosing osteomyelitis: low level bone pain over long term; dense sclerosis without associated lucency and no short-term change over serial radiographs
Sequestrum
Septic arthritis
Disk space narrowing with endplate erosion
Diabetics: skin ulcer

NEUROPATHIC ARTHRITIS (CHARCOT JOINT)

Primary loss of sensation in a joint leads to arthropathy. Distribution helps determine etiology.

Causes

- Diabetes neuropathy: usually foot
- Tertiary syphilis (tabes dorsalis): usually knee
- Syringomyelia: usually shoulder
- Other
  - Myelomeningocele
  - Spinal cord injury
  - Congenital insensitivity to pain
  - Any inherited or acquired neuropathy

Radiographic Features

Common to all types
- Joint instability: subluxation or dislocation
- Prominent joint effusion
- Normal or increased bone density

Hypertrophic type, 20%
- Marked fragmentation of articular bone
- Much reactive bone

Atrophic type, 40%
- Bone resorption of articular portion

Combined type, 40%

Metabolic Bone Disease

GENERAL

Bone tissue consists of:
- Extracellular substance
  - Osteoid: collagen, mucopolysaccharide
  - Crystalline component: calcium phosphate, hydroxyapatite
- Cells
  - Osteoblasts
  - Osteoclasts

Bone is constantly absorbed and replaced with new bone. Disturbances in this equilibrium result in either too much bone (increased radiodensity, osteosclerosis) or too little bone (decreased density = osteopenia).

OSTEOPENIA

Osteopenia is a nonspecific radiographic finding that indicates increased radiolucency of bone. Bone density may be difficult to assess because of technical factors (kVp, mA) that influence the radiographic appearance.

Types
- Osteoporosis: decreased amount of normal bone
- Osteomalacia: decreased bone mineralization
- Marrow replacement: bone replaced by tumor, marrow hyperplasia, or metabolic products
- Hyperparathyroidism: increased bone resorption

OSTEOPOROSIS

Classification

Primary osteoporosis (most common): unassociated with an underlying illness
- Type I osteoporosis: postmenopausal
- Type II osteoporosis: senile
- Idiopathic juvenile osteoporosis

Secondary osteoporosis (less common)
- Endocrine disorders
  - Hypogonadism
  - Hyperthyroidism
  - Cushing disease
  - Acromegaly
- Nutritional
  - Malabsorption syndromes
  - Alcoholism
  - Scurvy
- Hereditary metabolic or collagen disorder
  - Osteogenesis imperfecta
  - Marfan syndrome
  - Ehlers-Danlos syndrome
  - Homocystinuria
  - Hypophosphatasia
  - Wilson disease
  - Alkaptonuria
  - Menkes syndrome
- Drugs
  - Heparin
  - Exogenous steroids

Radiographic Features (Fig. 5-134)
- Osteopenia: 30%-50% of bone has to be lost to be detectable by plain film
- Diminution of cortical thickness: width of both MCP cortices should be less than half the shaft diameter
- Decrease in number and thickness of trabeculae in bone
- Vertebral bodies show earliest changes: resorption of horizontal trabeculae
- Empty box vertebra: apparent increased density of vertebral endplates due to resorption of spongy bone
- Vertebral body compression fractures: wedge, biconcave codfish bodies, true compression
- Pathologic fractures
- Qualitative assessment: Singh index is based on trabecular pattern of proximal femur. Patterns:
  - Mild: loss of secondary trabeculae
  - Intermediate: loss of tensile trabeculae
  - Severe: loss of principal compressive trabeculae

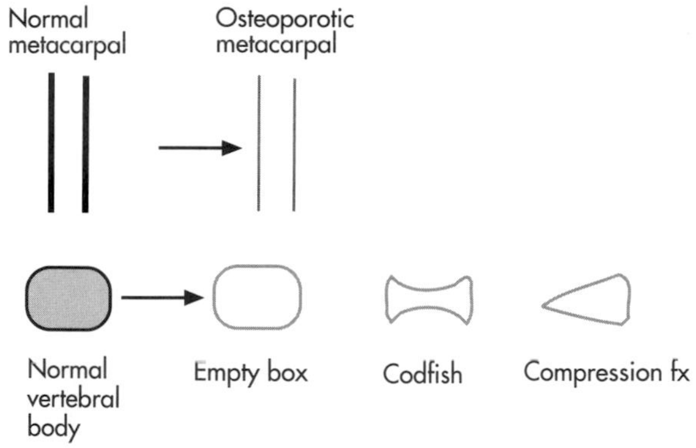

FIGURE 5-134

Quantitative Bone Densitometry (Fig. 5-135)

Predicts the risk for developing fractures. Three methods are available:
- Single-photon absorption
  - Measures cortical bone density of radial shaft
  - 2 to 3 mrem exposure
    - Precision: 1%-3%

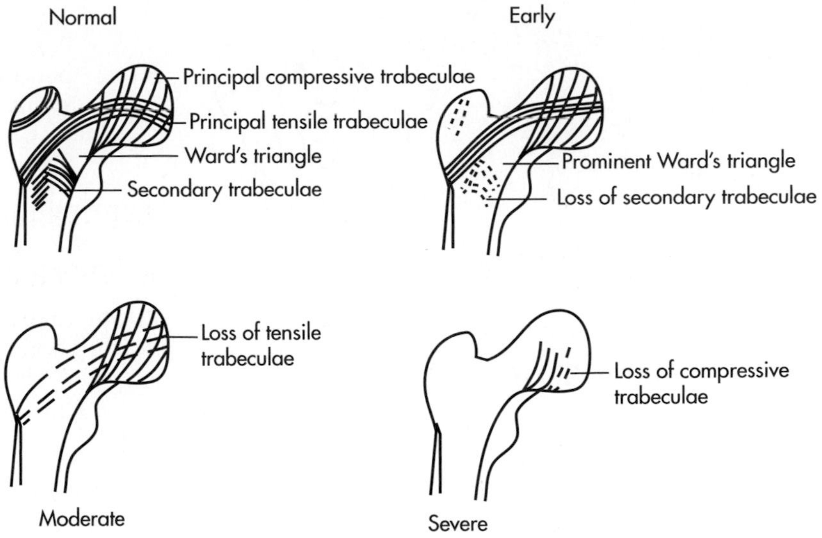

FIGURE 5-135

- Dual-photon absorption with radionuclide or dual-energy x-ray
  - Measures vertebral and hip bone density (cortical and trabecular)
  - 5 to 10 mrem exposure
  - Precision: 2%-4%
  - Cannot account for soft tissue contribution to x-ray absorption
- Quantitative CT with phantom
  - Measures vertebral body density (trabecular only) 300 to 500 mrem exposure
  - Most effective technique for evaluation of bone density

Indications for measurements:
- Initiation of estrogen replacement therapy or phosphonate therapy
- To establish diagnosis of osteoporosis
- To assess severity of osteoporosis
- To monitor treatment efficacy

TRANSIENT OSTEOPOROSIS OF HIP JOINT

- Transient osteoporosis, which can be related to or be a variant of AVN
- Radiographs generally show osteopenia, whereas bone scanning demonstrates activities within the femoral head region.
- MRI usually shows diffuse marrow edema with decreased signal on T1W scans and more intense signal on T2W scans.
- Dual-energy x-ray absorptiometry is a good method to quantitatively assess bone density and the fracture risk of the proximal femur.

OSTEOMALACIA

Abnormal mineralization of bone is termed *osteomalacia* in adults and *rickets* in children. In the past, the most common cause was deficient intake of vitamin D. Today, absorption abnormalities and renal disorders are more common causes:

Nutritional deficiency of:
- Vitamin D
- Calcium
- Phosphorus

Absorption abnormalities
- GI surgery
- Malabsorption
- Biliary disease

Renal
- Chronic renal failure
- Renal tubular acidosis
- Proximal tubular lesions
- Dialysis induced

Abnormal vitamin D metabolism
- Liver disease
- Hereditary metabolic disorders

Drugs
- Phenytoin (Dilantin)
- Phenobarbital

Radiographic Features

- Generalized osteopenia
- Looser's zones (Fig. 5-136) (pseudofractures): cortical stress fractures filled with poorly mineralized osteoid tissue.
- Milkman's syndrome: osteomalacia with many Looser's zones
- Typical location of Looser's zones (often symmetrical)
  - Axillary margin of scapula
  - Inner margin of femoral neck
  - Rib
  - Pubic, ischial rami
- Osteomalacia may be indistinguishable from osteoporosis; however, Looser's zones are a reliable differentiating feature.

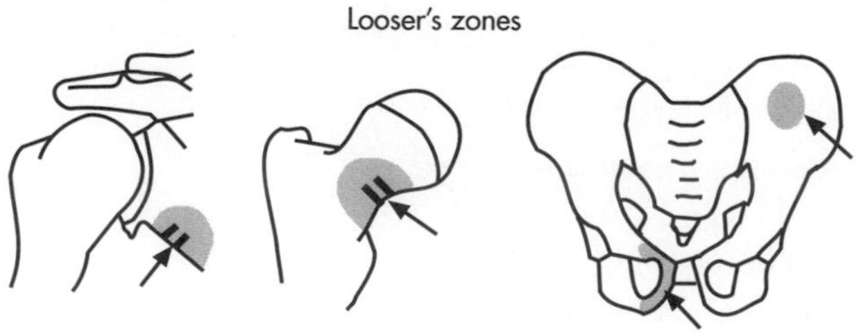

FIGURE 5-136

RENAL OSTEODYSTROPHY

Renal osteodystrophy is a general term that refers to a myriad of radiographic osseous changes in patients with renal failure. Radiographically, these changes are secondary to osteomalacia, secondary hyperparathyroidism, and aluminum intoxication.

Radiographic Features

Changes of osteomalacia
- Osteopenia and cortical thinning
- Looser's zones occur but are uncommon.

Changes of hyperparathyroidism
- Subperiosteal resorption (e.g., SI joint resorption)
- Rugger jersey spine
- Brown tumors
- Osteosclerosis
- Soft tissue calcification
- Chondrocalcinosis

SCURVY

Deficiency of vitamin C (ascorbic acid) impairs the ability of connective tissue to produce collagen. Never occurs before 6 months of age because maternal stores are transmitted to fetus. Findings are most evident at sites of rapid bone growth (long bones). Rare.

Radiographic Features (Fig. 5-137)

Children
- Generalized osteopenia
- Dense metaphyseal line (Frankel)
- Wimberger's sign: dense epiphyseal rim
- Corner sign: metaphyseal fractures (Pelkan spurs)
- Periosteal reaction (ossification) due to subperiosteal bleeding
- Hemarthrosis: bleeding into joint

Adults
- Osteopenia and pathologic fractures

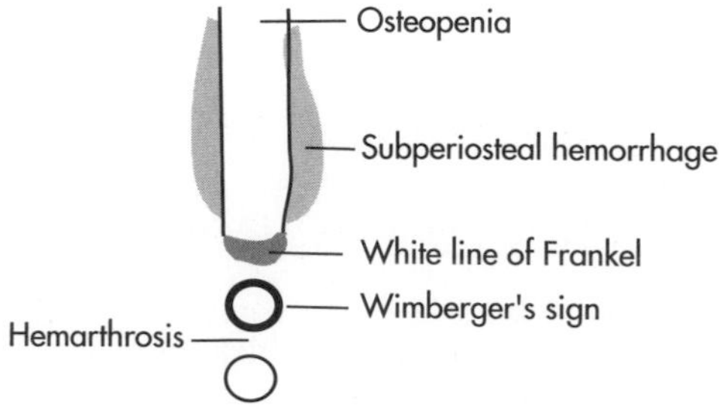

FIGURE 5-137

ENDOCRINE BONE DISEASE

HYPERPARATHYROIDISM (HPT)

Parathyroid hormone stimulates osteoclastic resorption of bone. HPT is usually detected by elevated serum levels of calcium during routine biochemical screening. Three types:
- Primary HPT:
  - Adenoma, 85% (single, 90%; multiple, 10%)
  - Hyperplasia, 12%
  - Parathyroid carcinoma, 1%-3%
- Secondary HPT: most often secondary to renal failure; rarely seen with ectopic parathyroid production by hormonally active tumor
- Tertiary HPT: results from autonomous glandular function after long-standing renal failure

Radiographic Features (Fig. 5-138)

- General osteopenia
- Bone resorption is virtually pathognomonic
  - Subperiosteal resorption
    - Radial aspect of middle phalanges (especially index and middle finger)
    - Phalangeal tufts
  - Trabecular resorption
    - Salt-and-pepper skull
  - Cortical resorption
    - Tunneling of MCP bones (nonspecific)
  - Subchondral resorption
    - Widened SI joint
    - Distal end of clavicle
    - Widened symphysis pubis
    - Can lead to articular disease
  - Subligamentous/subtendinous resorption
    - Inferior calcaneus
    - Trochanters, tuberosities
    - Anterior inferior iliac spine

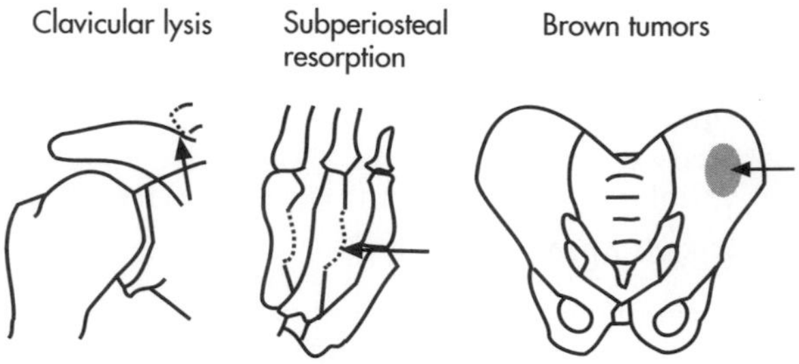

FIGURE 5-138

- Brown tumors (cystlike lesions) may be found anywhere in the skeleton but especially in the pelvis, jaw, and femur.
    - Loss of the lamina dura
    - Soft tissue calcification
    - Chondrocalcinosis
    - Complication: fractures

DIFFERENTIATION OF HYPERPARATHYROIDISM

Primary HPT	Secondary HPT
Brown tumors	Osteosclerosis
Chondrocalcinosis	Rugger jersey spine (renal osteodystrophy)
	Soft tissue and vascular calcification

THYROID ACROPACHY

Occurs 1 to 2 years after surgical thyroidectomy or radioablation for hyperthyroidism. Incidence: 5%.

Radiographic Features

- Thick periosteal reaction of phalanges and metacarpals
- Soft tissue swelling

ACROMEGALY (Fig. 5-139)

Elevated growth hormone (adenoma, hyperplasia) results in:

- Children (open growth plates): gigantism
- Adults (closed growth plates): acromegaly = gradual enlargement of hands and feet and exaggeration of facial features

Radiographic Features

The key feature is appositional bone growth: ends of bones, exostoses on toes, increase in size and number of sesamoid bones:

Hands
- Spade-shaped tufts due to overall enlargement
- Exostoses at tufts
- Widened joint spaces due to cartilage growth
- Secondary DJD

Feet
- Heel pad >25 mm (typical)
- Increased number of sesamoid bones

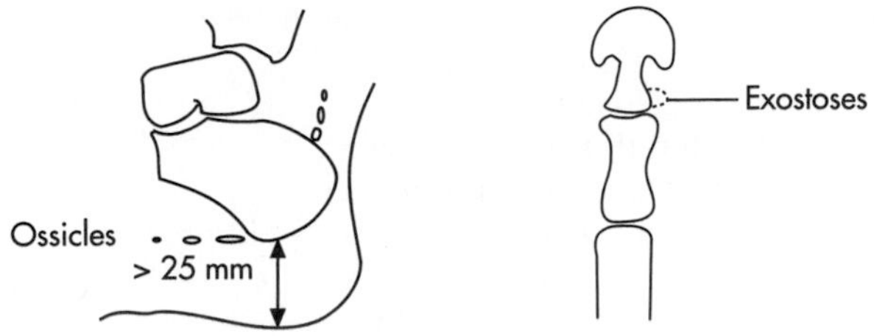

FIGURE 5-139

- Exaggerated bony tuberosities at tendon insertion sites
- Exostoses on 1st toe

Skull
- Thickening of skull bones and increased density
- Prognathism: protrusion of jaw
- Overgrowth of frontal sinuses (frontal bossing)
- Accentuation of orbital ridges
- Enlargement of nose and soft tissues
- Enlarged sella

Spine
- Posterior vertebral scalloping
- Lordosis

BONE MARROW DISEASE

CLASSIFICATION

Malignant infiltration
- Myeloma
- Leukemia/lymphoma
- Metastases (small cell tumors)

Secondary marrow hyperplasia
- Hemoglobinopathies
- Hemolytic anemias

Lysosomal storage diseases
- Gaucher disease
- Niemann-Pick disease: deficiency of sphingomyelinase; radiographically similar to Gaucher disease except that AVN and cystic bone lesions do not occur.

GAUCHER DISEASE

Deficiency of β-glucocerebrosidase leads to intracellular accumulation of glucosylceramide predominantly in cells of the RES. Autosomal recessive. Most common in Ashkenazi Jews.

Forms:
- Infantile form: lethal
- Adult form: more benign (see below)

Clinical Findings

- Liver: hepatosplenomegaly
- Spleen: focal lesions
- Bone marrow: pancytopenia, bone pain, characteristic foam cells

Radiographic Features (Fig. 5-140)

- Osteopenia
- Focal lytic lesions (expansile, cortical scalloping, no periosteal response), 50%
- Osteonecrosis, 50%; usually occurs combined as:
    - Medullary infarcts
    - Osteoarticular infarcts
- Modeling deformities (Erlenmeyer flask), 50%

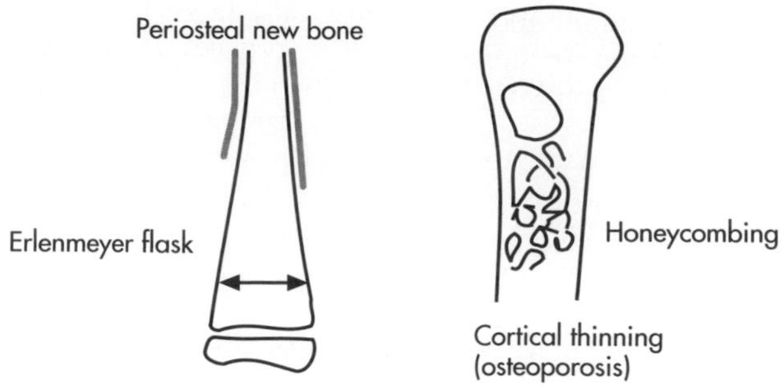

FIGURE 5-140

- Less common features
  - Periosteal response: bone-within-bone
  - H-shaped vertebra
  - Hair-on-end appearance of the skull

Complications

- OA
- Fractures, often multiple
- Increased risk for osteomyelitis

SICKLE CELL ANEMIA

Structural defect in hemoglobin (hemoglobin S; point mutation). Most hemoglobinopathies (over 250 are known) result in rigid hemoglobin and hemolysis.

Incidence: 1% of blacks. Diagnosis is confirmed by hemoglobin electrophoresis. Sickle cell disease (HbSS) has many bone findings, whereas sickle cell trait (HbAS) is only occasionally associated with bone infarcts. Hemoglobin sickle cell disease has the same bone findings but the spleen is enlarged.

Clinical Findings

- Hemolytic anemia, jaundice
- Skeletal pain (infarction, osteomyelitis)
- Abdominal pain
- High incidence of infections
- Chest pain: acute pulmonary crisis, infarcts

Radiographic Features (Fig. 5-141)

Hyperplasia of marrow
- Hair-on-end appearance of skull
- Pathologic fractures

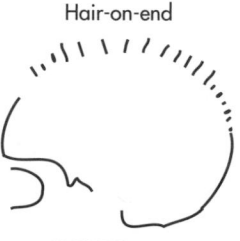

FIGURE 5-141

- Biconcave H-shaped vertebra
- Osteopenia

Vascular occlusion
- AVN occurs primarily in medullary space of long bones, hands, growing epiphyses
- Bone sclerosis from infarctions
- H-shaped vertebral bodies
- Involvement of growing epiphyses leads to growth disturbances
- Dactylitis (hand-foot syndrome): bone infarcts of hands and feet

Osteomyelitis
- High incidence: most caused by *Staphylococcus*
- *Salmonella* infection more common than in general population
- Most commonly at diaphysis of long bones
- Osteomyelitis and infarction may be difficult to distinguish.

Other
- Small calcified fibrotic spleen due to autoinfarction
- Cholelithiasis
- Progressive renal failure
- Papillary necrosis
- Cardiomegaly: high output congestive heart failure (CHF)
- Pulmonary infarcts

THALASSEMIA (COOLEY ANEMIA)

Genetic disorder characterized by diminished synthesis of one of the globin chains. Thalassemias are classified according to the deficient chain:

- α-Thalassemia: α-chain abnormality, Asian population
- β-Thalassemia: β-chain abnormality
- β-Thalassemia major (Cooley's anemia, Mediterranean anemia): usually fatal in 1st decade, transfusion dependent; 1% of American blacks, 7% of Greeks
- β-Thalassemia minor: nontransfusion dependent

Radiographic Features

Hyperplasia of marrow is the dominant feature.
- Expands the marrow space: hair-on-end skull, boxlike digits
- Modeling deformities of bone: Erlenmeyer flask deformity
- Premature closure of growth plates
- Paravertebral masses due to extramedullary hematopoiesis

Vascular occlusion
- Scattered bone sclerosis
- H-shaped vertebral bodies
- AVN less common than in sickle cell disease

Other
- Cardiomegaly and CHF
- Secondary hemochromatosis
- Cholelithiasis

SKELETAL MANIFESTATIONS OF ANEMIAS

	Sickle Cell	Thalassemia
Skull	Hair-on-end appearance	Severe hair-on-end appearance
Spine	Fish vertebra	Less common than in sickle cell anemia
Other bones	Osteonecrosis	Erlenmeyer flask
	Osteomyelitis	Arthropathy (hemochromatosis, gout)
	Growth arrest (decreased flow)	Osteoporosis
Spleen	Small (autoinfarction)	Large (hepatosplenomegaly)
Kidney	Papillary necrosis	—
Abdomen	Cholelithiasis	Cholelithiasis
Other	Pulmonary crisis	Transfusional hemachromatosis
	Cardiomegaly	Fatal in first decade (homozygous)
		Extramedullary hematopoiesis
		Cardiomegaly

MYELOFIBROSIS

Myeloproliferative disease in which bone marrow is replaced by fibrotic tissue.

Clinical Findings

- Splenomegaly (extramedullary hematopoiesis)
- Anemia (replacement of bone marrow)
- Changes in WBC, cell counts

Radiographic Features

Plain film
- Dense bones, 50%
- Paraspinal masses and splenomegaly (marrow production sites)

Bone scan
- Increased uptake
- Superscan

PAGET DISEASE (OSTEITIS DEFORMANS) (Fig. 5-142)

Chronic progressive disease of osteoblasts and osteoclasts resulting in abnormal bone remodeling. Probable viral etiology. Age: unusual <40 years. Usually polyostotic and asymmetrical: pelvis, 75% > femur > skull > tibia > vertebra > clavicle > humerus > ribs.

Stages

Active phase = lytic phase = “hot phase” (“hot phase” does not refer to bone scan)

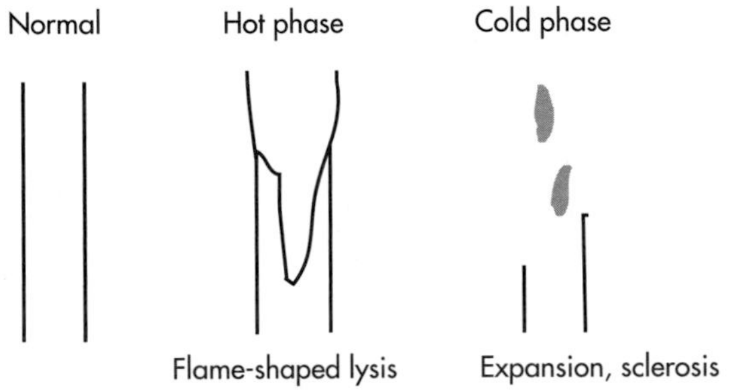

FIGURE 5-142

- Aggressive bone resorption: lytic lesions with sharp borders that destroy cortex and advance along the shaft (candle flame, blade of grass)
- Characteristically lesions start at one end of bone and slowly extend along the shaft.
- Bone marrow is replaced by fibrous tissue and disorganized, fragile trabecular.

Inactive phase = quiescent phase = “cold phase” (“cold phase” does not refer to bone scan)
- New bone formation and sclerosis: thickening of cortex and coarse trabeculations

Mixed pattern = lytic and sclerotic phases coexist
- Bowing of bones becomes a prominent feature.

Clinical Findings

- Often asymptomatic
- Painful, warm extremities
- Bowed long bones
- Neurologic disorders from nerve or spinal cord compression
- Enlarged hat size
- High-output CHF (increased perfusion of bone), increased metabolism
- Elevated serum alkaline phosphatase and urine hydroxyproline

Radiographic Features

Long bones
- Thickening of cortex and enlargement of bone
- Bowing of tibia and femur
- Lysis begins in subarticular location
- Candle flame: V-shaped lytic lesion advancing into diaphysis

Pelvis
- Thickening of iliopubic, ilioischial lines (early signs)
- Thickening of trabeculae
- Protrusio acetabuli

Skull
- Osteoporosis circumscripta: osteolytic phase, commonly seen in frontal bone
- Cotton-wool appearance: mixed lytic-sclerotic lesions
- Inner and outer table involved: diploic widening
- Basilar invagination with narrowing of foramen magnum: cord compression
- Neural foramen at base of skull may be narrowed: hearing loss, facial palsy, blindness

Spine
- Most common site of involvement
- Picture frame vertebral body: enlarged square vertebral body with peripheral thick trabeculae and inner lucency
- Ivory vertebra

Bone scan
- Extremely hot lesions in lytic phase
- Increased radiotracer uptake typically abuts one joint and extends distally
- Cold lesions if inactive (uncommon)

Complications

- Pathologic fractures
  - Vertebral compression fractures
  - Small horizontal cortical stress fractures in long bones (banana fracture, usually along convex border)
- Malignant degeneration <1% (osteosarcoma > MFH > chondrosarcoma)
- Giant cell tumors in skull and face, often multiple
- Secondary OA (increased stress on cartilage)
- Bone deformity (chronic stress insufficiency)
- High output

Pearls

- Bone scans are useful in determining the extent of the disease.
- Lesions in the lytic phase are very vascular: dense enhancement by CT.
- Always evaluate for sarcomatous degeneration.
- Treatment
  - Calcitonin (inhibits bone resorption)
  - Diphosphonate (inhibits demineralization)
  - Mithramycin (cytotoxin)

OSTEONECROSIS

Osteonecrosis (avascular necrosis, ischemic necrosis, aseptic necrosis) may be caused by two mechanisms:

- Interruption of arterial supply
- Intra/extraosseous venous insufficiency

The pathophysiology of all osteonecrosis is the same: ischemia → revascularization → repair → deformity → osteoarthrosis.

PATHOPHYSIOLOGY OF OSTEONECROSIS

Cause	Mechanism
Fractures (navicular bone, femoral neck)	Interruption of blood supply
Dislocation (talus, hip)	Ischemia (stretching of vessels)
Collagen vascular disease	Vasculitis
Sickle cell disease	Sludging of RBC
Gaucher disease	Infiltration of red marrow and vascular compromise
Caisson disease	Nitrogen embolization
Radiation	Direct cytotoxic effect
Pancreatitis, alcoholism	Fat embolization
Hormonal (steroids, Cushing disease)	Probable fat proliferation and vascular compromise
Idiopathic (Legg-Calvé-Perthes disease)	Unknown
Pregnancy	Unknown

Radiographic Features

Plain films

- Findings lag several months behind time of injury. These findings include areas of radiolucency, sclerosis, bone collapse, joint space narrowing, and, in the femoral head, a characteristic subchondral radiolucent crescent. Some of these represent late findings.
- Plain film staging system (Ficat)
  - Stage I: clinical symptoms of AVN but no radiographic findings
  - Stage II: osteoporosis, cystic areas and osteosclerosis
  - Stage III: translucent subcortical fracture line (crescent sign), flattening of femoral head
  - Stage IV: loss of bone contour with secondary osteoarthritis

MRI

- Most sensitive imaging modality: 95%-100% sensitivity
- Earliest sign is bone marrow edema (nonspecific)
- Early AVN: focal subchondral abnormalities (very specific)
  - Dark band on T1W/bright band on T2W
  - Double-line sign (T2W): bright inner band/dark outer band occurs later in disease process after the start of osseous repair
- Late AVN: fibrosis of subchondral bone
  - Dark on T1W and T2W images
  - Femoral head collapse
- Mitchell classification
  - Class A (early disease): signal intensity analogous to fat (high on T1W and intermediate on T2W)
  - Class B: signal intensity analogous to blood (high on T1W and T2W)
  - Class C: signal intensity analogous to fluid (low on T1W and high on T2W)
  - Class D (late disease): signal intensity analogous to fibrous tissue (low on T1W and T2W)
- MRI is helpful in planning treatment for AVN. Treatment options include core decompression, used in early disease, bone grafts, osteotomy, and electric stimulation.

Bone scanning

- Less sensitive than MRI

Complications

- Fragmentation
- Cartilage destruction with secondary DJD
- Intraarticular fragments
- Malignant degeneration (malignant fibrous histiocytoma [MFH], fibrosarcoma, chondrosarcoma)

KIENBÖCK DISEASE

Osteonecrosis of the lunate bone. Mean age: 20 to 30 years. Rare <15 years of age. Predilection for right wrist, males, heavy labor. High incidence of negative ulnar variance.

Radiographic Features

- Sclerotic lunate
- Occasionally a subchondral fracture is seen along the radial surface.
- Most patients develop arthritic changes.

SPONTANEOUS OSTEONECROSIS OF THE KNEE

Insufficiency fracture of the weight-bearing surface of the medial femoral condyle. Presents in elderly. Acute pain.

OSTEONECROSIS EPONYMS

Location	Name	Age	Frequency
Upper Extremities			
Humeral head	Haas	Adults	Rare
Humeral capitellum	Panner	Adolescents	Rare
Distal ulnar epiphysis	Burns	Children	Rare
Scaphoid	Preiser	Adolescents	+
Lunate	Kienböck	Adults	+
Metacarpal head	Dietrich	Adolescents	Rare
Entire carpus	Caffey	Children	Rare
Lower Extremities			
Femoral head	Legg-Calvé-Perthes	4-10	+++
Idiopathic coxa vara		6-16	++
Inferior patella	Sinding-Larsen-Johansson	8-12	+
Tibial tubercle	Osgood-Schlatter	10-16	++
Proximal medial tibial epiphysis	Blount	2-14	+
Talus	Diaz	Children	Rare
Distal tibia	Liffert-Arkin	Children	Rare
Calcaneal apophysis	Sever	5-15	Rare
Navicular	Köhler's bone	4-8	++
Middle cuneiform	Hicks	4-8	Rare
Metatarsal head	Frieberg	11-18	Rare
Fifth metatarsal base	Iselin	Adolescents	Rare
Trochanters	Mancl		Rare
Os tibiale externum	Haglund	Adults	Rare
Pelvis			
Ischiopubic synchondrosis	van Neck	Adolescents	Rare
Symphyseal synchondrosis	Pierson	Adolescents	Rare
Iliac crest	Buchman	Adolescents	Rare
Ischial tuberosity	Milch	Adolescents	Rare
Spine			
Vertebral body	Kümmell	4-8	Rare
Vertebral apophyses	Scheuermann	10-18	++

These osteonecroses are usually idiopathic in origin. If an osteonecrosis occurs as a complication of trauma (i.e., scaphoid) it is not called by its eponym but simply referred to as a posttraumatic AVN. Many of the eponyms are archaic, and some are questionable. For instance, some authors believe that Kümmell disease (manifests as vertebra plana and intervertebral vacuum phenomenon) may actually represent Langerhans cell histiocytosis.

Differential Diagnosis

FOCAL BONE LESIONS

FOCAL LESIONS

- Tumor
  - Metastases (common)
  - Primary (less common)
- Inflammation/infection/idiopathic
- Congenital
- Metabolic: brown tumors
- Trauma
  - Stress fracture
  - Insufficiency fracture
  - Pathologic fracture
- Vascular
  - Osteonecrosis

Infarct

BONE TUMORS

SYNOPSIS OF PRIMARY BONE TUMORS

Origin	Benign	Malignant
Osteogenic	Osteoma Osteoid osteoma Osteoblastoma	Osteosarcoma
Chondrogenic	Enchondroma Chondrosarcoma Osteochondroma Chondromyxoid fibroma	Chondroblastoma
Fibrogenic	Fibrous cortical defect Nonossifying fibroma Ossifying fibroma (Sisson) Desmoplastic fibroma Fibrous dysplasia	MFH Fibrosarcoma
Bone marrow	Eosinophilic granuloma	Ewing sarcoma Myeloma Lymphoma Leukemia
Other	Simple bone cyst Aneurysmal bone cyst Intraosseous ganglion Intraosseous lipoma Giant cell tumor Brown tumor Pseudotumor	Adamantinoma Chordoma Malignant giant cell tumor
Vascular	Hemangioma Lymphangioma Angiomatosis	Hemangioendothelioma Hemangio-pericytoma Angiosarcoma

Malignant Bone Tumors by Age

Up to age 10:
- Ewing sarcoma
- OSA
- Leukemia, lymphoma

Ages 11-20:
- OSA
- Ewing sarcoma
- Lymphoma, leukemia

Ages 21-30:
- OSA
- Lymphoma
- Ewing sarcoma
- MFH

Over age 30:
- Myeloma
- Metastases
- Lymphoma
- Chondrosarcoma
- MFH, fibrosarcoma
- OSA

BUBBLY LESIONS OF THE BONE (HELMS)

Mnemonic: "FEGNOMASHIC:"
- **F**ibrous dysplasia, fibrous cortical defect
- **E**nchondroma
- **G**CT
- **N**OF
- **O**steoblastoma
- **M**yeloma, metastases
- **A**neurysmal bone cyst (always eccentric)
- **S**imple unilocular bone cyst (always central)
- **H**yperparathyroidism (HPT), hemophilia
- **I**nfection
- **C**hondroblastoma

LYTIC EPIPHYSEAL LESIONS (Fig. 5-143)

Tumor
- GCT
- EG
- Chondroblastoma
- Metastases (rare)

Infection
- Osteomyelitis
- TB

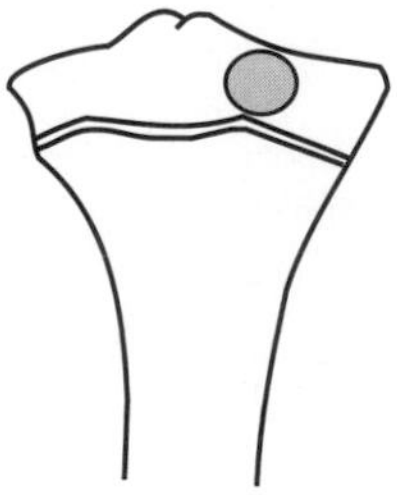

FIGURE 5-143

Subchondral cyst
- Arthropathy (CPPD, OA, RA, hemophilia)

Interosseous ganglion

SCLEROTIC METASTASES

- Prostate
- Breast
- Hodgkin lymphoma
- Other primary tumors
  - Carcinoid
  - Medulloblastoma
  - Bladder
- Lung

PERMEATIVE LESIONS IN CHILDREN

- Round cell tumors (see earlier)
- Infection
- EG
- OSA (rare)

PERMEATIVE LESIONS IN ADULTS

- Metastases
- Multiple myeloma
- Lymphoma, leukemia
- Fibrosarcoma

CORTICAL SAUCERIZATION

- Periosteal chondroma
- Surface chondrosarcoma
- Parosteal osteosarcoma

BONY SEQUESTRUM

Criterion: calcified nidus in a bone lesion
- Osteomyelitis
- EG (button sequestrum)
- Fibrosarcoma
- Osteoid osteoma (calcified nidus)

MALIGNANT TRANSFORMATION OF BONY LESIONS

- Fibrous dysplasia: fibrosarcoma, OSA, MFH
- Paget disease: OSA > chondrosarcoma, fibrosarcoma, MFH, lymphoma (rare)
- Osteomyelitis with draining sinus: squamous cell carcinoma (SCC)
- Radiation: OSA, chondrosarcoma, MFH
- Bone infarct: fibrosarcoma, MFH
- Ollier disease: chondrosarcoma
- Maffucci syndrome: chondrosarcoma
- Hereditary osteochondromatosis: chondrosarcoma

FOCAL SCLEROTIC LESION

Mnemonic: "TIC MTV:"
- Tumor
  - Benign
    - Osteoma
    - Osteoid osteoma, osteoblastoma

- Enchondroma
- Fibrous dysplasia
- Healing lesions: NOF, EG, brown tumor

Malignant
- Metastasis
- Sarcomas
- Lymphoma, leukemia

Any healing tumor (EG, brown tumor, treated metastases)

- **I**nfection
  - Osteomyelitis
    - Sequestration
    - Sclerosing osteomyelitis of Garré
- Congenital
  - Bone island
  - Melorheostosis
  - Fibrous dysplasia
- **M**etabolic
  - Paget disease
- **T**rauma
  - Stress fracture
  - Healing fracture
- **V**ascular
  - Osteonecrosis
  - Bone infarct

OSTEONECROSIS

Mnemonic: "ASEPTIC:"
- **A**nemias (hereditary)
- **S**teroids
- **E**thanol
- **P**ancreatitis, pregnancy
- **T**rauma
- **I**diopathic
- **C**aisson disease, collagen vascular diseases

JOINTS

DEGENERATIVE JOINT DISEASE (DJD)

Primary DJD, 90%

Secondary DJD, 10%
- Mechanical joint abnormality
  - Posttraumatic
  - Osteonecrosis
  - Injured menisci or ligaments
  - Bone dysplasias
  - Loose bodies
- Abnormal forces on a joint
  - Occupational
  - Postoperative
  - Bone dysplasias
- Abnormal cartilage within joint
  - Hemochromatosis
  - Acromegaly
  - Alkaptonuria
- Any inflammatory or metabolic arthritis

INFLAMMATORY ARTHRITIS

SYNOPSIS OF CLINICAL FEATURES

Feature	RA	AS	Psoriasis	Reiter Syndrome
Sex	Female	Male	Both	Young male
Peripheral distribution	Hand	Hip	Hand	Feet
Asymmetry	No	Yes	Yes	Yes
Sausage digits	No	No	Yes	Yes
Periosteal reaction	No	No	Yes	Yes
Sacroiliitis	No	Yes	Yes	Yes
Clinical	RF+	IBD	Nail, skin changes	Urethritis, conjunctivitis
HLA-B27	No	<90%	30%	80%

JACCOUD ARTHROPATHY

Ulnar and volar subluxation of metacarpals after streptococcal infection
- SLE
- Rheumatic fever
- Scleroderma

PERIARTICULAR OSTEOPENIA

- RA (also diffuse osteopenia)
- Scleroderma
- Hemophilia
- Osteomyelitis

SUBCHONDRAL CYSTS

Normal bone density
- DJD
- CPPD
- Seronegative spondyloarthropathies
- Gout
- Pigmented villonodular synovitis (PVNS)
- Synovial osteochondromatosis
- Neuropathic joint

Abnormal bone density
- Any of the above
- RA
- AVN

ACROOSTEOLYSIS (Fig. 5-144)

Mnemonic: "PINCH FO:"
- **P**soriasis
- **I**njury (thermal burn, frostbite)
- **N**europathy
  - Congenital insensitivity to pain
  - Diabetes mellitus
  - Leprosy
  - Myelomeningocele
- **C**ollagen vascular
  - Scleroderma
  - Raynaud disease

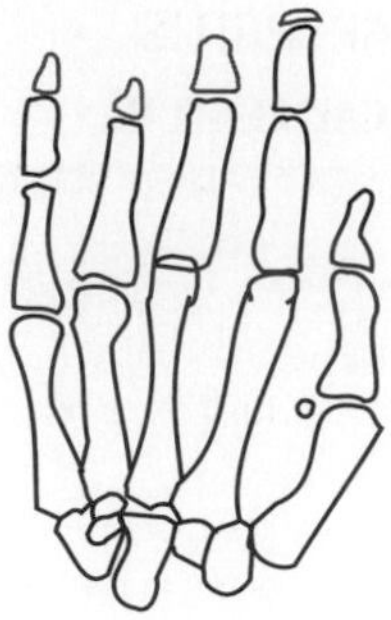

FIGURE 5-144

- **H**yperparathyroidism
- **F**amilial (Hadju-Cheney)
- **O**ther
    - Polyvinyl chloride (PVC) exposure (midportion)
    - Snake, scorpion venom, phenytoin, porphyria, epidermolysis bullosa

Transverse acroosteolysis
- Hyperparathyroidism
- Haju-Cheney
- PVC exposure

NEW BONE FORMATION IN ARTHRITIS

Periosteal new bone formation
- Psoriasis
- Reiter syndrome

Osteophytes
- OA
- CPPD

CALCIFICATIONS AND ARTHROPATHY (Fig. 5-145)

Periarticular
- Scleroderma (common)
- SLE (uncommon)

Articular
- CPPD
- Chondrocalcinosis (see later)

Joint space–related
- Neuropathic arthropathy
- Synovial osteochondromatosis
- Osteochondritis dissecans
- Osteochondral fracture

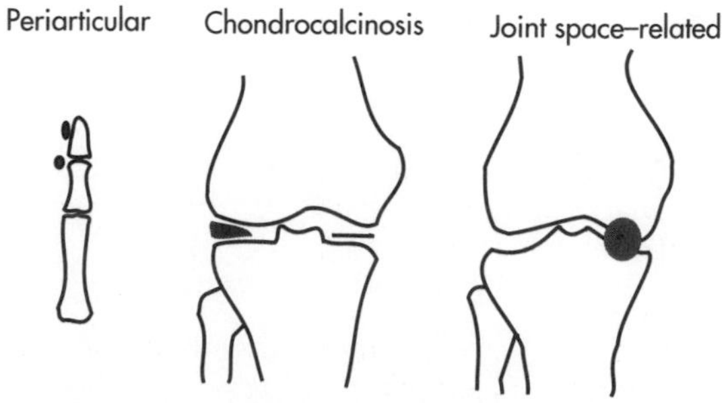

FIGURE 5-145

CHONDROCALCINOSIS

Mnemonic: "HOGWASH:"
- **H**yperparathyroidism
- **O**chronosis (alkaptonuria)
- **G**out
- **W**ilson disease
- **A**rthritides (any)
- (P)**s**eudogout: CPPD
- **H**emochromatosis

SOFT TISSUE SWELLING IN ARTHRITIS

Symmetrical bilateral swelling
- RA (most common)
- Any inflammatory arthritis

Asymmetrical swelling of one digit: sausage digit
- Psoriasis
- Reiter syndrome

Lumpy-bumpy soft tissue swelling
- Gout (tophus)
- Amyloidosis
- Multicentric reticulohistiocytosis
- Sarcoid

DIFFERENTIAL DIAGNOSIS OF ARTHRITIS BY DISTRIBUTION

Distal (distal and proximal interphalangeal joints)
- OA
- Psoriasis
- Reiter syndrome
- Multicentric reticulohistiocytosis

Proximal (MCP, carpus)
- RA
- CPPD
- Hemochromatosis
- Wilson disease

Ulnar styloid
- RA

MONOARTICULAR ARTHRITIS

Mnemonic: "CHRIST:"
- **C**rystal arthropathies
- **H**emophilia
- **R**A (atypical)
- **I**nfection (excluding Lyme disease and gonorrhea)
- **S**ynovial
    - PVNS
    - Synovial osteochondromatosis
- **T**rauma

Neuropathic Joint

Common
- Diabetes mellitus
- Spinal cord injury
- Myelomeningocele/syringomyelia
- Alcohol abuse

Uncommon
- Syphilis (tabes dorsalis)

- Congenital indifference to pain
- Neuropathies (e.g., Riley-Day)
- Amyloidosis

Clinical Syndromes Associated with Arthropathies

- Behçet disease: arthritis, orogenital ulcers, iritis, large artery, aneurysms, central nervous system (CNS) arteritis
- Reiter disease: arthritis, urethritis, conjunctivitis
- Still disease: juvenile RA (JRA), hepatosplenomegaly, lymphadenopathy
- Felty syndrome: RA, splenomegaly, neutropenia
- Jaccoud disease: arthritis after repeated episodes of rheumatic fever
- CREST syndrome: **c**alcinosis, **R**aynaud disease, **e**sophageal dysmotility, **s**clerodactyly, **t**elangiectasia
- Phemister triad (TB arthritis): osteoporosis, marginal erosions, slow cartilage destruction

Atlantoaxial Subluxation

- RA, JRA
- Seronegative spondyloarthropathies
- SLE
- Down syndrome
- Morquio syndrome
- Trauma

BONE DENSITY

DIFFUSE OSTEOSCLEROSIS (DENSE BONES)

Tumor
- Metastases
- Lymphoma/leukemia
- Myelofibrosis
- Mastocytosis (cutaneous flushing)

Congenital
- Osteopetrosis
- Pyknodysostosis
- Craniotubular dysplasias
- Sickle cell anemia
- Physiologic newborn

Metabolic
- Paget disease
- Renal osteodystrophy
- Fluorosis
- Hypervitaminosis A and D

Alternative mnemonic: "3MS PROOF:"
- **M**etastases
- **M**yelofibrosis
- **M**astocytosis
- **S**ickle cell anemia
- **P**yknodysostosis, Paget disease
- **R**enal osteodystrophy
- **O**steopetrosis
- **O**thers (dysplasias, hypothyroidism)
- **F**luorosis (heavy metal poisoning)

OSTEOPENIA

Localized osteopenia
- Disuse osteoporosis: pain, immobilization
- Arthritis
- Sudeck atrophy, reflex sympathetic dystrophy (periarticular)
- Paget disease (lytic phase)
- Transient osteoporosis
  - Transient osteoporosis of the hip
  - Regional migratory osteoporosis

Diffuse osteopenia
- Primary osteoporosis
- Secondary osteoporosis
  - Endocrine diseases
  - Nutritional deficiencies
  - Hereditary metabolic and collagen disorders
  - Medications
- Osteomalacia
  - Nutritional deficiencies
  - Abnormal vitamin D metabolism (inherited, acquired)
  - GI absorption disorders
  - Renal disease
  - Medications
- HPT
- Marrow replacement
  - Malignancy (e.g., myeloma)
  - Marrow hyperplasia (e.g., hemoglobinopathy)
  - Lysosomal storage diseases (e.g., Gaucher disease)

MULTIPLE SCLEROTIC LESIONS

Tumor
- Metastases
- Lymphoma/leukemia
- Osteomatosis (Gardner syndrome)
- Healing lesions
- Sclerotic myeloma (very rare)

Congenital
- Fibrous dysplasia
- Osteopoikilosis
- Tuberous sclerosis
- Mastocytosis

Metabolic
- Paget disease

Trauma
- Healing fractures

Vascular
- Bone infarcts

PERIOSTEUM

ASYMMETRICAL PERIOSTEAL REACTION

- Tumor
- Infection (osteomyelitis, soft tissue infection, congenital infection)
- Inflammation (psoriatic, Reiter disease, JRA)

- Trauma (fractures)
- Vascular (subperiosteal hemorrhage)

SYMMETRICAL PERIOSTEAL REACTION IN ADULTS

- Vascular insufficiency (venous > arterial)
- Hypertrophic pulmonary osteoarthropathy
- Pachydermoperiostosis
- Fluorosis
- Thyroid acropathy

HYPERTROPHIC PULMONARY OSTEOARTHROPATHY (HPO)

Causes

Intrathoracic tumor (removal of malignancy produces relief of HPO pain)
- Cancer: bronchogenic carcinoma, metastasis, lymphoma
- Pleura: benign fibrous tumor of the pleura, mesothelioma

Chronic pulmonary infection: bronchiectasis, abscess

Other entities that occasionally show periosteal bone formation but are more commonly associated with clubbing:
- GI: inflammatory bowel disease (ulcerative colitis, Crohn disease), celiac disease, cirrhosis
- Cardiac: cyanotic heart disease

Differential Diagnosis

- Vascular insufficiency
- Thyroid acropachy
- Pachydermoperiostitis
- Fluorosis
- Diaphyseal dysplasia (Englemen)
- Hypervitaminosis A

SKULL

SOLITARY LYTIC LESION

Tumors
- Metastases*
- Multiple myeloma*
- EG
- Epidermoid*
- Hemangioma*

Infections, inflammation
- Osteomyelitis (TB, syphilis especially)
- Sarcoidosis*

Congenital
- Fibrous dysplasia
- Encephalocele

Metabolic
- Paget disease*
- Hyperthyroidism

Trauma
- Leptomeningeal cyst

*Often present as multiple lesions.

DIFFUSE SKULL LESIONS

- Sickle cell anemia and thalassemia (hair-on-end appearance)
- HPT (salt-and-pepper skull)
- Paget disease (cotton-wool appearance)
- Fibrous dysplasia (predominantly outer table)
- Tuberous sclerosis (increased density of both tables)

MULTIPLE LYTIC LESIONS

Mnemonic: "POEMS:"
- **P**aget disease
- Parathyroid elevation (HPT)
- **O**steomyelitis
- **E**G
- **M**etastases
- Myeloma
- **S**arcoidosis

BASILAR INVAGINATION

Congenital
- Osteogenesis imperfecta
- Klippel-Feil syndrome
- Achondroplasia
- Chiari malformations
- Cleidocranial dysplasia

Acquired bone softening
- Paget disease
- HPT
- Osteomalacia, rickets
- Rheumatoid arthritis
- Marfan, Ehlers-Danlos
- Metastases

SPINE (Fig. 5-146)

VETEBRAL BODY

Abnormal density
- Picture frame:
  - Paget disease (cortex too prominent)
  - Osteoporosis (center too lucent)

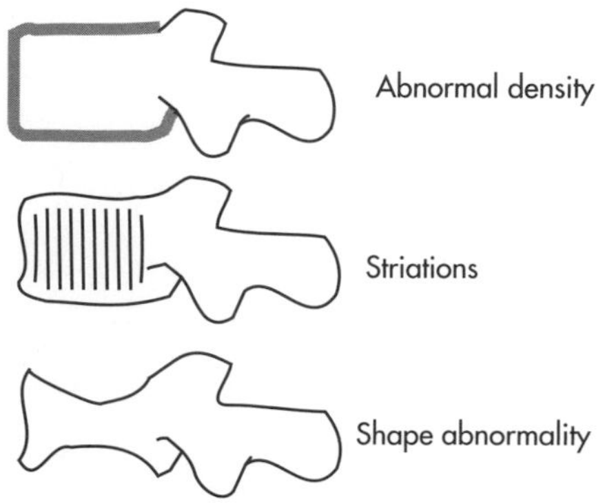

FIGURE 5-146

- Rugger jersey:
  - Renal osteodystrophy
- Ivory vertebral body
  - Metastases
  - Paget disease
  - Lymphoma
  - Infection
- Bone-in-bone:
  - Osteopetrosis

Striated vertebral body
- Multiple myeloma
- Hemangioma
- Osteoporosis
- Paget disease

Shape abnormalities
- Fish vertebra: sickle cell disease, thalassemias
- Squared vertebra: ankylosing spondylitis (AS), Paget disease, psoriasis, Reiter syndrome
- Vertebra plana; mnemonic: "PET SIT:"
  - **P**aget disease
  - **E**G (children)
  - **T**umor (hemangioma, metastases, myeloma, lymphoma)
  - **S**teroid
  - **I**nfection
  - **T**rauma

MRI: T1 marrow signal normally brighter than disk; marrow-replacing process if darker:
- Polycythemia vera
- Anemia
- Mastocytosis
- Myelofibrosis
- Leukemia
- Lymphoma
- Waldenström macroglobulinemia

SCLEROTIC PEDICLE

- Lymphoma
- Metastases
- Congenital absence
- Osteoblastoma, osteoid osteoma

VERTEBRAL OUTGROWTHS (Fig. 5-147)

Syndesmophytes
- AS

Flowing paraspinal ossification
- DISH

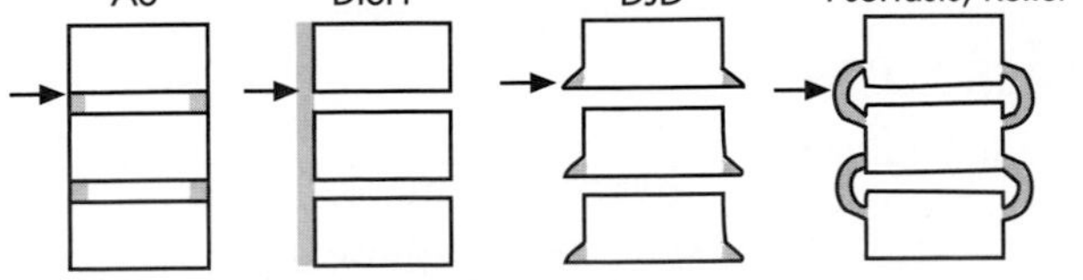

FIGURE 5-147

Small osteophytes
- Degenerative disease
- Spondylosis deformans

Large osteophytes
- Psoriasis (common)
- Reiter syndrome (uncommon)

POSTERIOR SPINAL FUSION

Congenital (Klippel-Feil syndrome)

Surgical fusion

Arthritides
- JRA (spinal fusion is more common than in RA)
- AS
- Psoriatic arthritis
- Reiter syndrome

Vertebral Body Lesion

- Metastases
- Myeloma
- Lymphoma
- EG
- GCT
- Hemangioma
- Sarcomas (rare)

POSTERIOR ELEMENT LESION

TYPES OF TUMORS

Anterior: Malignant	Posterior: Benign
Common	
Lymphoma	Osteoid osteoma
Myeloma	Osteoblastoma
Ewing sarcoma	ABC
Metastases	
Exceptions	
Hemangioma	
EG	
Giant cell tumor	

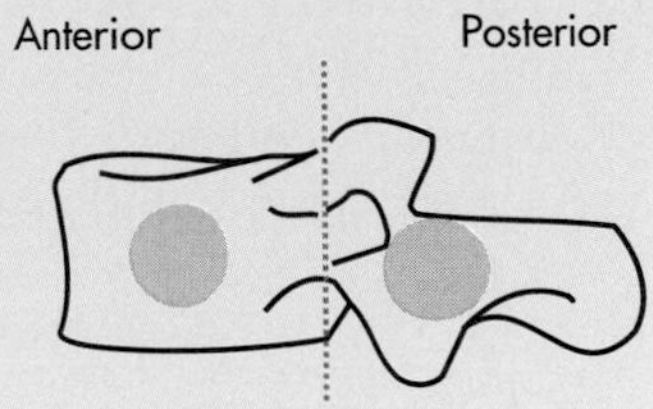

SOLITARY VERTEBRAL LESIONS

Mnemonic: "A HOG:"
- **A**BC
- **H**emangioma
- **O**steoblastoma/osteoid osteoma
- **G**iant cell tumor

POSTERIOR VERTEBRAL SCALLOPING

Increased intraspinal pressure
- Spinal canal tumors
- Syrinx

- Communicating hydrocephalus

Dural ectasia
- Neurofibromatosis
- Marfan syndrome
- Ehlers-Danlos syndrome

Congenital
- Achondroplasia
- Mucopolysaccharidoses (Morquio, Hunter, Hurler)
- Osteogenesis imperfecta (tarda)

Bone resorption
- Acromegaly

CALCIFIED DISKS

- DJD
- CPPD
- Ankylosing spondylitis
- JRA
- Hemochromatosis
- DISH
- Ochronosis/alkaptonuria

ANTERIOR VERTEBRAL SCALLOPING

- Aortic aneurysm
- Lymphadenopathy
- TB spondylitis
- Delayed motor development

ANTERIOR VERTEBRAL BODY BEAK (Fig. 5-148)

- Morquio syndrome (central beak)
- Hurler syndrome
- Achondroplasia
- Cretinism
- Down syndrome
- Neuromuscular disease

PLATYSPONDYLY

Diffuse
- Dwarf syndromes (thanatophoric, metatropic)
- Osteogenesis imperfecta

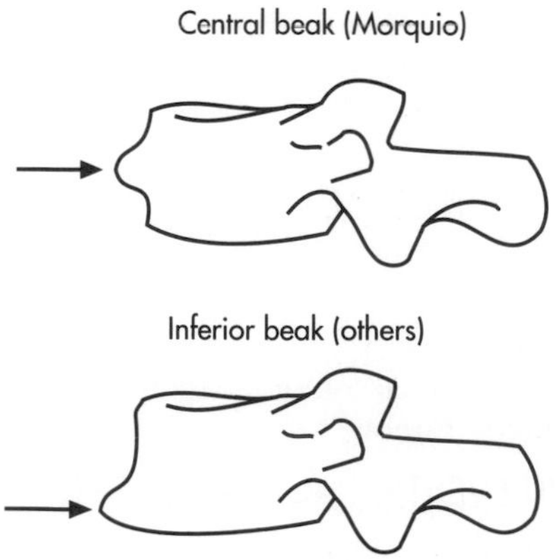

FIGURE 5-148

- Morquio syndrome
- Spondyloepiphyseal dysplasia

Solitary or multifocal
- Leukemia
- EG
- Metastasis/myeloma
- Sickle cell disease

SPINAL OSTEOMYELITIS VERSUS TUMOR

	Osteomyelitis	Tumor
Contiguity	Yes	No
Paraspinal soft tissue mass	Yes (abscess)	Less common
Disk space	Isocenter*	Not involved

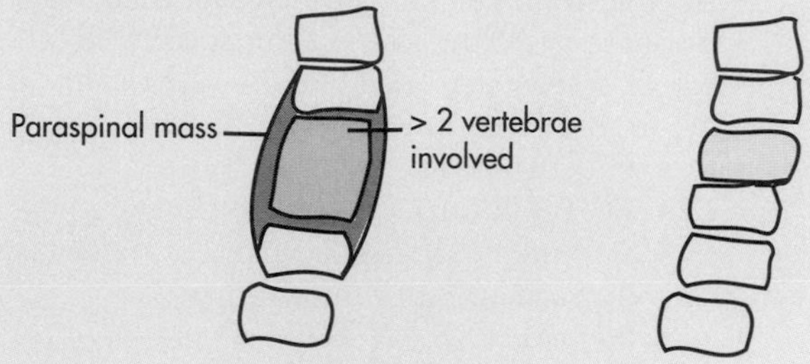

*Except for TB, which usually involves multiple levels but spares the disk.

PELVIS

PROTRUSIO ACETABULI (Fig. 5-149)

- Paget disease
- RA
- Osteomalacia, rickets
- Trauma
- Marfan syndrome
- AS
- Idiopathic

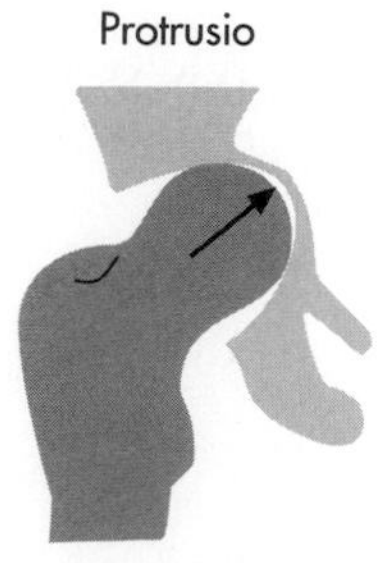

FIGURE 5-149

SACROILIITIS

Bilateral symmetrical
- AS
- Enteropathic spondyloarthropathy

- Psoriatic arthritis
- HPT
- DJD

Bilateral asymmetrical
- Reiter syndrome
- Psoriatic
- DJD

Unilateral
- Infection
- DJD
- Trauma
- RA

LYTIC LESIONS OF THE SACRUM

- Metastases
- Chordoma
- Plasmacytoma
- Chondrosarcoma
- GCT

LYTIC LESION OF ILIUM

- Fibrous dysplasia
- ABC
- Unicameral bone cyst (UBC)
- Hemophiliac pseudotumor
- Malignant lesions
  - Metastases
  - Plasmacytoma
  - Ewing sarcoma
  - Chondrosarcoma
  - Lymphoma

WIDENED PUBIC SYMPHYSIS

Congenital
- Bladder extrophy
- Epispadias
- Cleidocranial dysplasia
- Genitourinary or anorectal malformations

Bone resorption or destruction
- Pregnancy
- Osteitis pubis
- Infection
- Metastases
- HPT

LOWER EXTREMITY

ERLENMEYER FLASK DEFORMITY (Fig. 5-150)

Lack of modeling of tubular bones with flaring of the ends. Mnemonic: "CHONG:"
- **C**raniometaphyseal dysplasias
- **H**emoglobinopathies
  - Thalassemia
  - Sickle cell disease (often with AVN)
- **O**steopetrosis
- **N**iemann-Pick disease

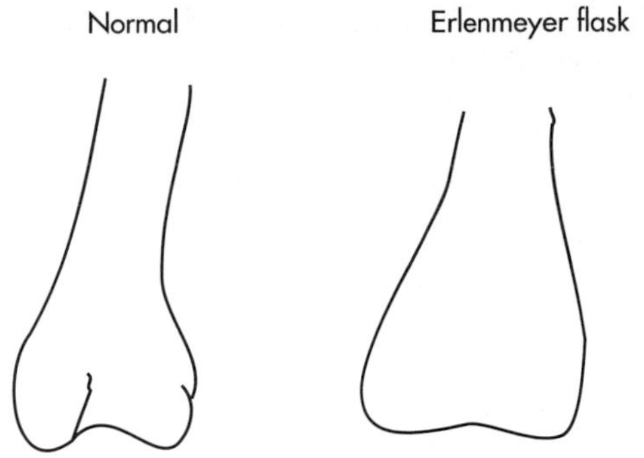

FIGURE 5-150

- **G**aucher disease (often with AVN)
- Other
  - Lead poisoning
  - Fibrous dysplasia
  - Osteochondromatosis
  - Enchondromatosis
  - Fibromatosis

GRACILE BONES (Fig. 5-151)

Overtubulation of the shaft with resulting prominent epiphyses. Mnemonic: "NIMROD:"
- **N**eurofibromatosis
- **I**mmobilization or paralysis
  - Poliomyelitis
  - Birth palsies
  - Congenital CNS lesions
- **M**uscular dystrophies
- **R**A (juvenile)
- **O**steogenesis imperfecta
- **D**ysplasias (e.g., Marfan syndrome, homocystinuria)

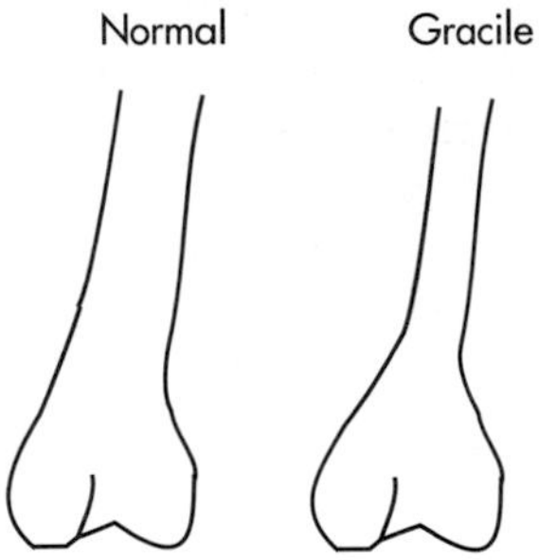

FIGURE 5-151

FEMORAL HEAD AVN

Mnemonic: "ASEPTIC LEG:"
- **A**lcoholism
- **S**ickle cell disease
- **E**xogenous steroids or RT
- **P**ancreatitis

- **T**rauma
  - Fracture/dislocation
  - Slipped capital femoral epiphysis
- Infection
- Caisson disease
- Legg-Calvé-Perthes
- Epiphyseal dysplasia
- Gaucher disease

MEDIAL TIBIAL SPUR (Fig. 5-152)

- Osteochondroma
- Blount disease
- Turner syndrome
- Posttraumatic lesion

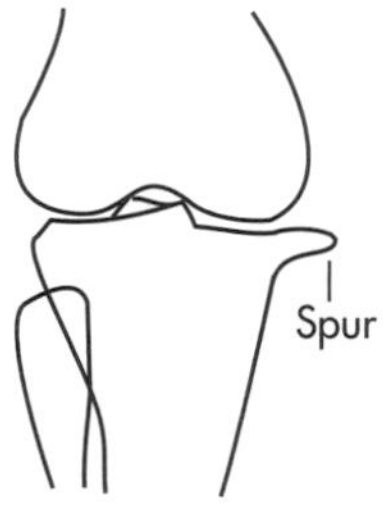

FIGURE 5-152

TIBIAL DIAPHYSEAL CORTICAL LESION

- Adamantinoma
- Osteofibrous dysplasia (ossifying fibroma)
- Fibrous dysplasia
- EG
- Metastases (adult)

HEEL PAD THICKENING

Criteria: thickness >25 mm. Mnemonic: "MAD COP:"

- **M**yxedema (hypothyroidism)
- **A**cromegaly
- **D**ilantin (phenytoin)
- **C**allus
- **O**besity
- **P**eripheral edema

WELL-CIRCUMSCRIBED LYTIC LESION IN CALCANEUS

- Lipoma
- Unicameral bone cyst
- Pseudotumor (hemophiliac)

PSEUDOARTHROSIS WITH BENT/BOWED BONES

Mnemonic: "ON OF:"

- **O**steogenesis imperfecta
- **N**F-1
- **O**steomalacia/rickets
- **F**ibrous dysplasia

DIGIT OVERGROWTH

- Macrodystrophia lipomatosa (fat, overgrowth in plantar nerve distribution)
- NF (multiple digits, bilateral)
- Proteus syndrome (multiple digits)
- Macrodactyly
- Hyperemia (Klippel-Trénaunay-Weber/hemangioma, JRA, infection)

WIDENED INTERCONDYLAR NOTCH

- Hemophilia
- JRA

UPPER EXTREMITY

LYTIC LESION OF THE FINGER

- Enchondroma
  - Solitary
  - Multiple (Ollier or Maffucci)
- Glomus tumor (close to nail, painful, enhances)
- Foreign body reaction
- Epidermoid inclusion cyst (history of trauma)
- Metastasis (lung, breast)
- Sarcoidosis
- Infection
- Erosive arthropathy
- Hemangioma

DIGITAL AMPUTATION

- Trauma
- Surgery
- Thermal injury
- Insensitivity to pain (DM, Lesch-Nyhan syndrome)
- Post meningococcemia (gangrene)

HOOKED OSTEOPHYTE (HAND)

- Hemochromatosis
- CPPD
- OA

ENLARGED EPIPHYSIS

- JCA
- Hemophilia
- Infection

SPADE TUFTS

- Acromegaly (ask for skull film to check pituitary)
- DISH
- Retinoid toxicity
- Reiter

EXPANDED MARROW (HAND)

- Thalassemia, sickle cell disease
- Fibrous dysplasia
- Gaucher disease
- Leukemia

ARACHNODACTYLY

- Marfan syndrome
- Homocystinuria (osteopenia)

ULNAR DEVIATION

- RA (erosions)
- SLE (no erosions)
- Jaccoud arthropathy (poststrep)

RADIAL HYPOPLASIA

- VACTERL complex (vertebral body anal, cardiovascular, tracheoesophageal, renal, limb anomalies)
- Fanconi anemia
- Holt-Oram syndrome
- Cornelia de Lange syndrome
- Thrombocytopenia–absent radius (TAR syndrome)

SHORT 4TH/5TH METACARPALS

- Pseudohypoparathyroidism
- Pseudopseudohypoparathyroidism
- Idiopathic
- Chromosomal anomalies (Turner, Klinefelter)
- Basal cell nevus syndrome
- Posttraumatic
- Postinfarct (sickle cell disease)

MADELUNG DEFORMITY (Fig. 5-153)

Premature fusion of ulnar aspect of radial epiphysis. Results in:

- Ulnar angulation of distal radius
- Decreased carpal angle
- Dorsal subluxation of ulna
- Unilateral or bilateral

Mnemonic: "HIT DOC:"

- **H**urler syndrome
- **I**nfection
- **T**rauma
- **D**yschondrosteosis (Leri-Weil syndrome)
- **O**steochondromatosis
- **C**hromosomal XO (Turner)

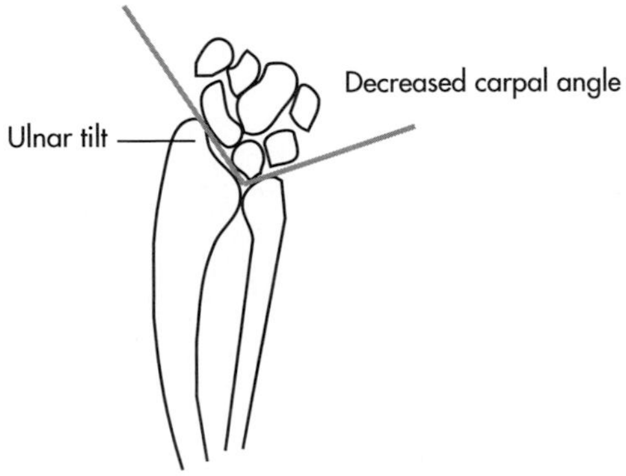

FIGURE 5-153

MISSING DISTAL CLAVICLE

- Erosion RA
- HPT
- Posttraumatic osteolysis
- Infection
- Metastases/myeloma
- Gorham disease
- Cleidocranial dysostosis
- Pyknodysostosis

HIGH-RIDING SHOULDER

- RA
- CPPD
- Rotator cuff tear

DISTAL CLAVICULAR EROSIONS

- RA
- HPT
- Trauma

SOFT TISSUES

SOFT TISSUE CALCIFICATION

Mnemonic: "TIC MTV:"

- **T**umor
  - Tumoral calcinosis
  - Synovial osteochondromatosis
  - Soft tissue tumor (sarcoma, hemangioma, lipoma)
- **I**nflammation/infection
  - Dermatomyositis
  - Scleroderma
  - Parasites
  - Leprosy
  - Pancreatitis (fat necrosis)
  - Myonecrosis
  - Bursitis/tendinitis
- **C**ongenital
  - Ehlers-Danlos syndrome
  - Myositis ossificans progressiva
- **M**etabolic
  - HPT (primary or secondary)
  - Metastatic calcification (any cause)
  - CPPD
  - Calcium hydroxyapatite deposition
- **T**rauma
  - Myositis ossificans
  - Burn injury
  - Hematoma
- **V**ascular calcification

SOFT TISSUE MASSES

Tumor

- Malignant fibrous histiocytoma
- Fatty tumors: lipoma, liposarcoma, fibromatoses

- Vascular tumors: hemangioma
- Nerve tumors: schwannoma, neurofibroma
- Metastasis
- Burns
- Hematoma
- Muscle: rhabdomyosarcoma, leiomyosarcoma

Other

- Myositis ossificans
- Abscess
- Hematoma
- Aneurysm

PSOAS ABSCESS

Mnemonic: "PASH:"

- **P**ott disease
- **A**ppendicitis
- **S**eptic arthritis
- **H**yperthyroidism

Suggested Readings

Berquist T. *MRI of the Musculoskeletal System*. Philadelphia: Lippincott Williams & Wilkins; 2005.

Bohndorf K, Pope TL, Imhof H. *Musculoskeletal Imaging: A Concise Multimodality Approach*. Stuttgart: Thieme; 2001.

Brower AC. *Arthritis in Black and White*. Philadelphia: WB Saunders; 1997.

Chew FS. *Musculoskeletal Imaging (The Core Curriculum)*. Philadelphia: Lippincott Williams & Wilkins; 2003.

Chew FS. *Skeletal Radiology: The Bare Bones*. Philadelphia: Lippincott Williams & Wilkins; 2005.

Greenspan A. *Orthopedic Radiology: A Practical Approach*. Philadelphia: Lippincott Williams & Wilkins; 2004.

Harris JH, Harris WH. *The Radiology of Emergency Medicine*. 4th ed; Philadelphia: Lippincott Williams & Wilkins; 2000.

Helms CA. *Fundamentals of Skeletal Radiology*. Philadelphia: WB Saunders; 2004.

Helms CA, Major NM, Anderson MW, et al. *Musculoskeletal MRI*. Philadelphia: WB Saunders; 2008.

Hodler J, von Schulthess GK, Zollikofer CL. *Musculoskeletal Diseases: Diagnostic Imaging and Interventional Techniques*. New York: Springer; 2005.

Manaster BJ, May DA, Disler DG. *Musculoskeletal Imaging: The Requisites*. St. Louis: Mosby; 2006.

Miller T, Schwitzer M. *Diagnostic Musculoskeletal Radiology*. New York: McGraw-Hill; 2004.

Resnick D. *Diagnosis of Bone and Joint Disorders*. 4th ed. Philadelphia: WB Saunders; 2002.

Resnick D, Kransdorf M. *Bone and Joint Imaging*. Philadelphia: WB Saunders; 2004.

Vahlensieck M, Genant HK, Reiser M. *MRI of the Musculoskeletal System*; Stuttgart: Thieme; 2000.

CHAPTER 6

Neurologic Imaging

CHAPTER OUTLINE

Imaging Anatomy

PARENCHYMAL ANATOMY

LOBAR ANATOMY (Fig. 6-1)

- Frontal lobe: anterior to central sulcus (Rolando)
- Parietal lobe: posterior to central sulcus
- Temporal lobe: inferior to lateral sulcus (Sylvius)
- Occipital lobe: posterior
- Limbic lobe
- Central (insular lobe)

BASAL GANGLIA (Fig. 6-2)

- Lentiform nucleus: putamen + globus pallidus
- Striatum: putamen + caudate nucleus
- Claustrum
- Caudate nucleus consists of:
  - Head (anterior)
  - Body
  - Tail (inferior)
- Subthalamic nucleus

THALAMUS (Fig. 6-3)

Contains over 25 separate nuclei and serves as a synaptic relay station. Organization:

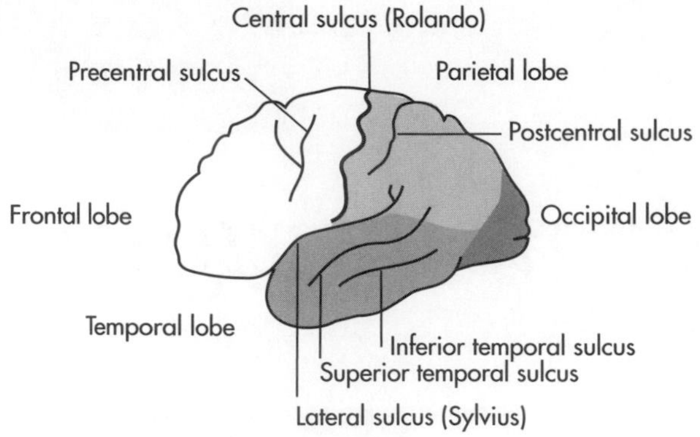

FIGURE 6-1

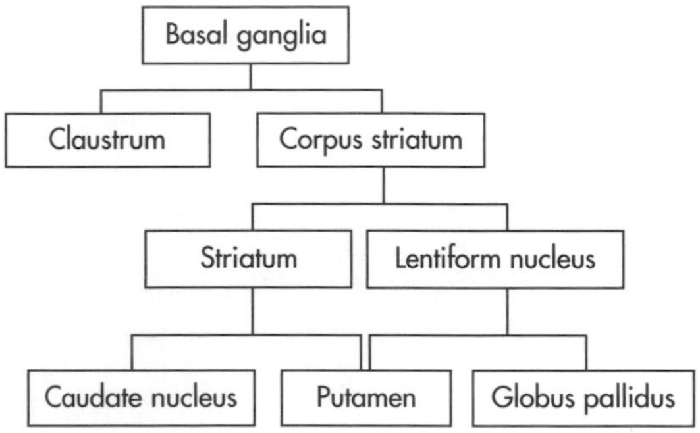

FIGURE 6-2

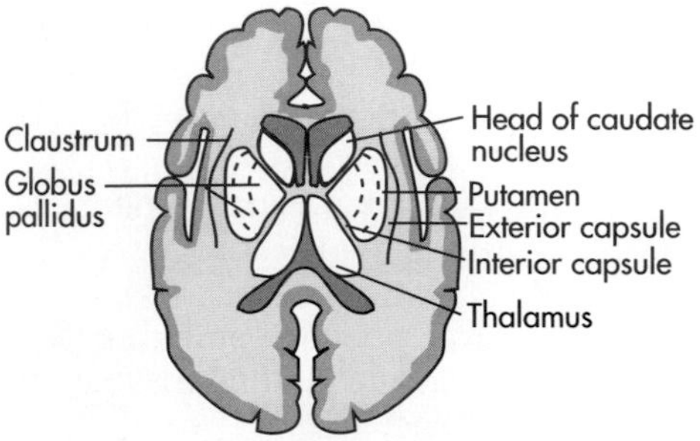

FIGURE 6-3

Thalamus
- Lateral nuclei
- Medial nuclei
- Anterior nuclei

Subthalamus
- Subthalamic nucleus
- Substantia nigra

Hypothalamus

CENTRAL SULCUS (CS) (Fig. 6-4)

1. Superior frontal sulcus/pre-CS sign (85% specific)
   - The posterior end of the superior frontal sulcus joins the pre-CS

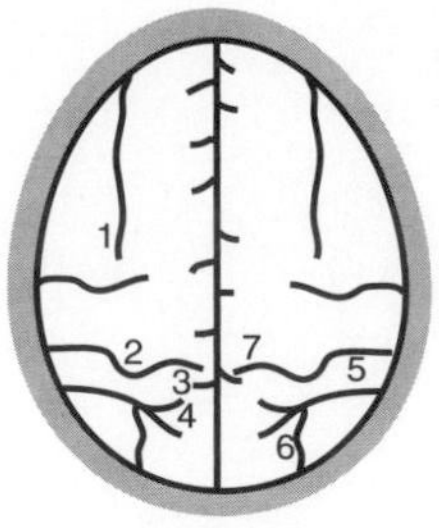

FIGURE 6-4

2. Sigmoidal hook sign (89%-98%)
   - Hooklike configuration of the central sulcus corresponding to the motor hand area
3. Pars bracket sign (96%)
   - Paired pars marginalis at or behind the CS
4. Bifid post-CS sign (85%)
5. Thin post-central gyrus sign (98%)
6. Intraparietal sulcus intersects the post-CS (99%)
7. Midline sulcus sign (70%)
   - Most prominent convexity sulcus that reaches the midline is the CS.

INFERIOR FRONTAL GYRUS ANATOMY (Fig. 6-5)

The inferior frontal lobe contains three subsections (forming an "M")
- Pars orbitalis (1)
- Pars triangularis (2)
- Pars opercularis (3)
- Pars triangularis and pars opercularis together form Broca's area
- Wernicke's area (4) — superior posterior temporal lobe

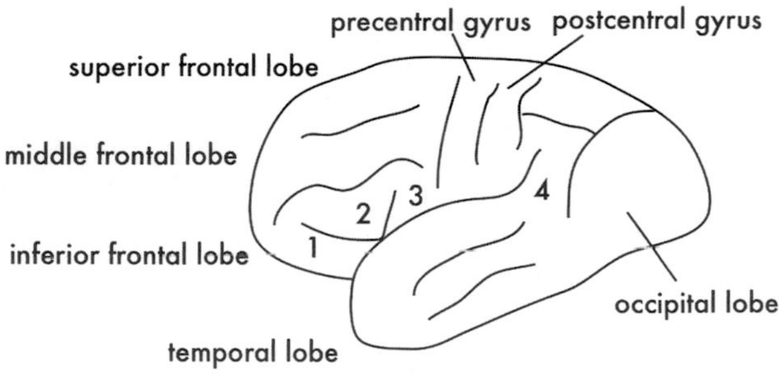

FIGURE 6-5

BRAIN MYELINIZATION (Fig. 6-6)

Neonatal and pediatric brains have different computed tomography (CT) and magnetic resonance imaging (MRI) appearances because of:
- Increased water content (changes best seen with T2-weighted [T2W] sequences)
- Decreased myelinization (changes best seen with T1-weighted [T1W] sequences)
- Low iron deposits

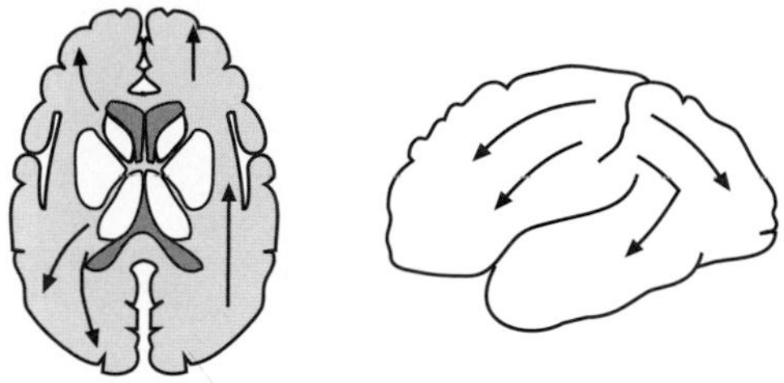

FIGURE 6-6

Brain maturation begins in the brainstem and progresses to the cerebellum and then to the cerebrum.

Characteristic MRI Appearance

Premature
- Smooth cortical surface, lacking cortical folding
- Gray-white matter (GWM) signal intensity reversal on T1W

Cortex is hyperintense.

Basal ganglia are hyperintense.

Neonate: myelinization of different structures depends on age

MRI DETECTION OF MYELIN BY REGION AND AGE

Region	T1W	T2W
Cerebellum	3 months	
Corpus callosum	5 months	7 months
Internal capsule		11 months
Frontal white matter		14 months
Adult pattern		18 months

VENTRICULAR SYSTEM

ANATOMY (Fig. 6-7)

Left and right lateral ventricles (1 and 2) connect to 3rd ventricle via a single T-shaped interventricular foramen (Monro). Anatomic aspects:
- Frontal horn
- Temporal (inferior) horn
- Occipital (posterior) horn
- Central part

Third ventricle connects to 4th ventricle via cerebral aqueduct of Sylvius. Anatomic aspects:
- Optic recess
- Infundibular recess
- Pineal recess
- Suprapineal recess
- Interthalamic adhesion (massa intermedia)

Fourth ventricle connects:
- Laterally to cerebrospinal fluid (CSF) via foramen of Luschka

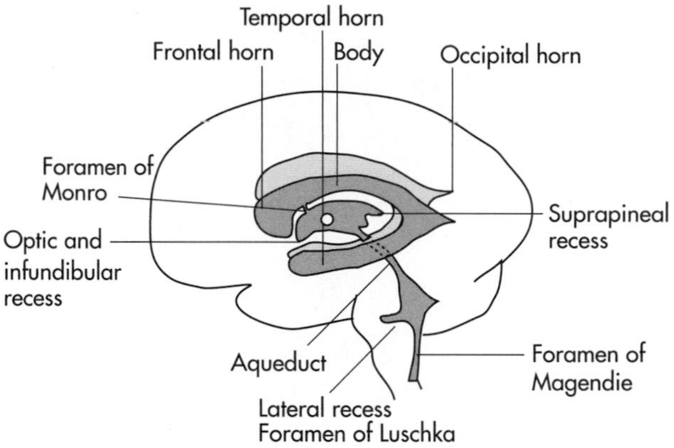

FIGURE 6-7

- Posteriorly to CSF via foramen of Magendie
- Inferiorly to central canal of spinal cord

CAVUM VARIANTS

Cavum Septum Pellucidum

- Separates frontal horns of lateral ventricles (anterior to foramen of Monro)
- 80% of term infants; 15% of adults
- May dilate; rare cause of obstructive hydrocephalus

Cavum Vergae

- Posterior continuation of cavum septum pellucidum; never exists without cavum septum pellucidum.

Cavum Velum Interpositum

- Extension of quadrigeminal plate cistern to foramen of Monro

PINEAL REGION ANATOMY (Fig. 6-8)

Location
- Posterior to 3rd ventricle
- Adjacent to thalamus

Normal pineal calcification
- 10% are calcified at 10 years of age.
- 50% are calcified at 20 years of age.
- Calcification should be approximately the size of the normal pineal gland
- Normal size of pineal calcification is <1 cm.

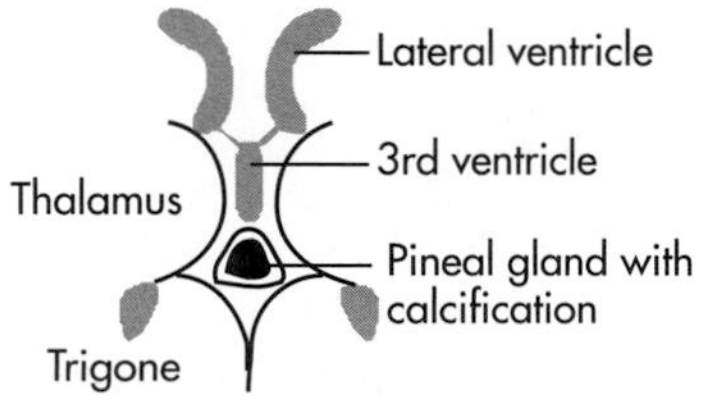

FIGURE 6-8

SELLA TURCICA

PITUITARY GLAND (Fig. 6-9, *A* and *B*)

COMPARTMENTS

Lobe	Origin	Hormones	MRI Features
Anterior (adenohypophysis)	Rathke's pouch*	PRL, ACTH, others	Intermediate signal
Intermediate	Rathke's pouch		Intermediate signal
Posterior (neurohypophysis)	Floor of 3rd ventricle	Oxytocin, vasopressin	Usually T1W hyperintense

*Rathke's pouch: roof of primitive oral cavity.
ACTH, adrenocorticotropic hormone; PRL, prolactin.

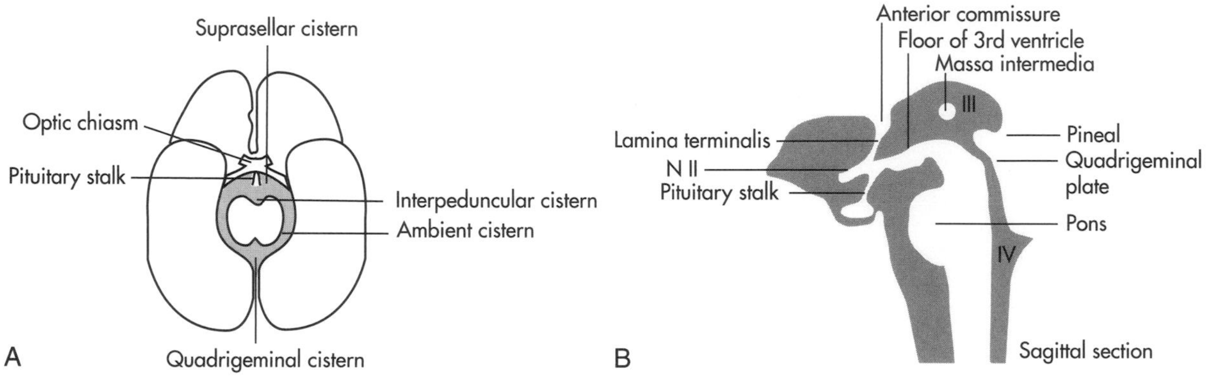

FIGURE 6-9

Normal height measurements (coronal MRI)
- 3 to 8mm in adults
- Up to 10mm during puberty; may be >10mm during pregnancy

Stalk
- 2 to 5mm in diameter
- Connects to hypothalamus
- Passes behind optic chiasm
- Enhances with contrast

Strong contrast enhancement of normal gland (no blood-brain barrier)

SUPRASELLAR CISTERN

Located above the diaphragma sella. Shape on axial sections:
- 5-pointed star shape (pontine level)
- 6-pointed star shape (midbrain level)

Contents of cistern:
- Circle of Willis
- Optic chiasm, optic tracts
- Cranial nerves (III, IV, V)
- Pituitary stalk

Cistern may herniate into sella: empty sella syndrome (usually asymptomatic with no consequence).

CAVERNOUS SINUS (Fig. 6-10)

Dura-enclosed venous channel containing:
- Internal carotid artery (ICA) and sympathetic plexus
- Cranial nerves: III, IV, V1, V2, VI

Connections of sinus:
- Ophthalmic veins
- Retinal veins
- Middle meningeal veins

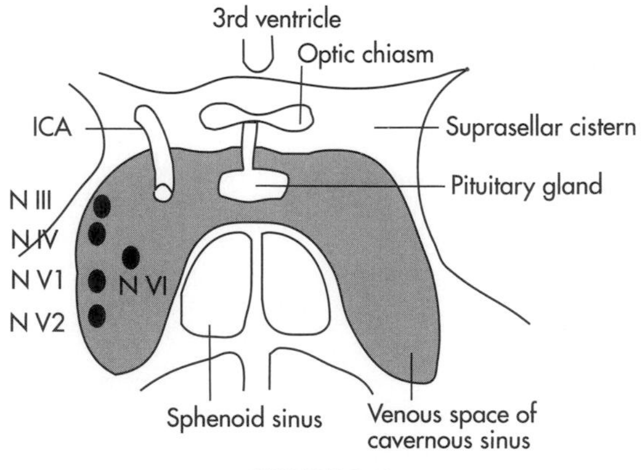

FIGURE 6-10

- Pterygoid vein
- Petrosal sinuses
- Sphenoparietal sinus

MECKEL'S CAVE (TRIGEMINAL CAVE)

Abuts the most posterior portion of the cavernous sinus (separate from cavernous sinus). Contains:
- Trigeminal nerve roots
- Trigeminal ganglion (gasserian ganglion)
- CSF

VASCULAR SYSTEM

EXTERNAL CAROTID ARTERY (ECA) (Fig. 6-11)

Eight main branches. Mnemonic: "SALFOPSM":
- **S**uperior thyroid artery
- **A**scending pharyngeal artery
- **L**ingual artery
- **F**acial artery
- **O**ccipital artery
- **P**osterior auricular artery
- **S**uperficial temporal artery
- **M**axillary artery

The major branches of the maxillary artery are:
- Middle meningeal artery through foramen spinosum
- Accessory middle meningeal artery through foramen ovale
- Descending palatine artery (greater palatine)
- Facial, sinus, and nasoorbital branches
- Sphenopalatine, infraorbital, posterior superior alveolar, artery of the vidian canal

Meningeal artery supply is from:
- ICA
  - Inferolateral trunk (ILT)
  - Meningohypophyseal trunk
  - Ophthalmic branches
- ECA
  - Middle meningeal artery
  - Accessory meningeal artery
  - Sphenopalatine artery

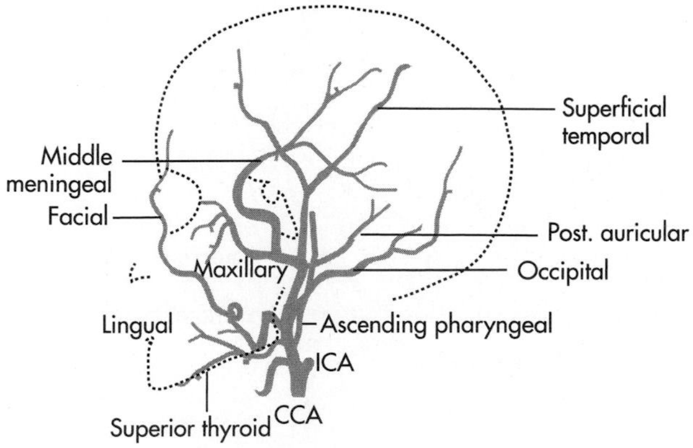

FIGURE 6-11

- Branches of ascending pharyngeal artery
- Branches of occipital artery

Vertebral artery
- Posterior meningeal artery

INTERNAL CAROTID ARTERY (ICA) (Fig. 6-12)

Four segments:
- Cervical segment
  - Usually no branches
- Petrous segment
  - Branches are rarely seen on angiograms.
  - Caroticotympanic artery
  - Vidian artery (inconstant)
- Cavernous segment
  - Meningohypophyseal trunk
  - ILT
- Supraclinoid segment (cavernous and supraclinoid segments = carotid siphon). Mnemonic: "SOPA":
  - **S**uperior hypophyseal artery (not routinely visualized)
  - **O**phthalmic artery
  - **P**osterior communicating artery (PCOM)
  - **A**nterior choroidal artery

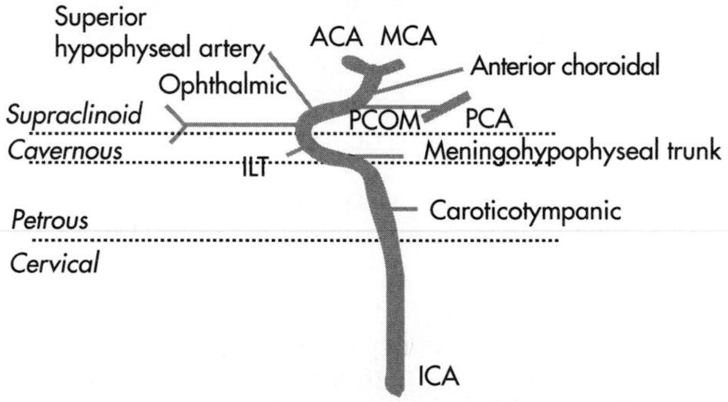

FIGURE 6-12

VERTEBROBASILAR SYSTEM (Fig. 6-13)

The vertebral arteries are the first branches of the subclavian arteries (95%). The left vertebral artery arises directly from the aortic arch (between left subclavian and common carotid) in 5%. The left artery is dominant in 50%; in 25% the vertebral arteries are codominant; in 25% the right artery is dominant. Vertebral arteries usually course through the C6-C1 vertebral foramina (but may start at C4) and then the foramen magnum.

Segments and Branches of Vertebral Arteries (Fig. 6-14)

Cervical segment (extradural)
- Muscular branches
- Spinal branches
- Posterior meningeal artery

Intracranial segment (intradural)

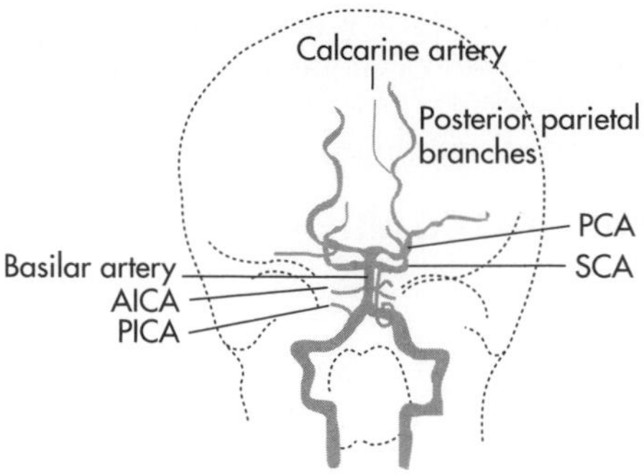

FIGURE 6-13

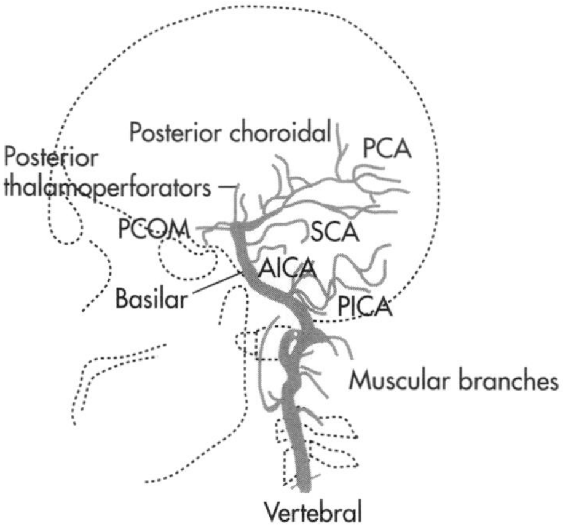

FIGURE 6-14

- Anterior spinal artery (ASA)
- Posterior inferior cerebellar artery (PICA)

Basilar artery

- Anterior inferior cerebellar artery (AICA)
- Superior cerebellar artery (SCA)
- Brainstem perforating arteries
- Posterior cerebral artery (PCA)

CIRCLE OF WILLIS (Fig. 6-15)

The circle is complete in 25% and incomplete in 75%. It consists of:

- Supraclinoid ICAs
- A1 segment of anterior cerebral arteries (ACAs)
- Anterior communicating arteries (ACOMs)
- PCOMs
- P1 segment of PCAs

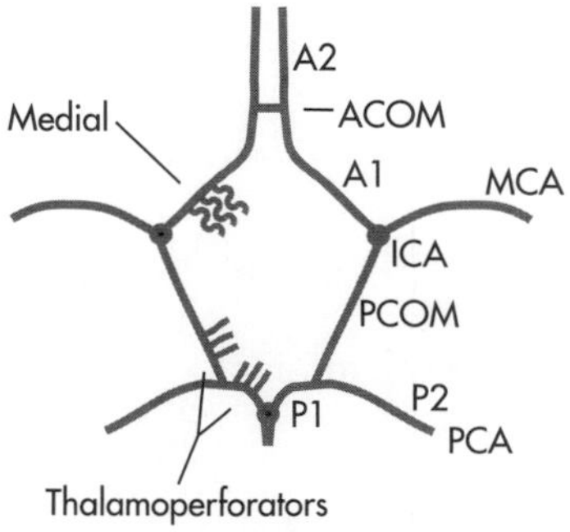

FIGURE 6-15

CEREBRAL ARTERIES

Anterior Cerebral Artery (ACA) (Fig. 6-16)

Represents one of the two ICA terminal branches

- A1 segment:
  - Origin to ACOM
  - Medial lenticulostriates
- A2 segment:
  - From ACOM
  - Recurrent artery of Heubner
  - Frontal branches
- Terminal bifurcation
  - Pericallosal artery
  - Callosomarginal artery

Middle Cerebral Artery (MCA) (Fig. 6-16)

Represents the larger of the two terminal ICA branches

- M1 segment:
  - Origin to MCA bifurcation
  - Lateral lenticulostriates
- M2 segment:
  - Insular branches
- M3 segment:
  - MCA branches beyond sylvian fissure

Posterior Cerebral Artery (PCA)

- P1 segment:
  - Origin to PCOM
  - Posterior thalamoperforators

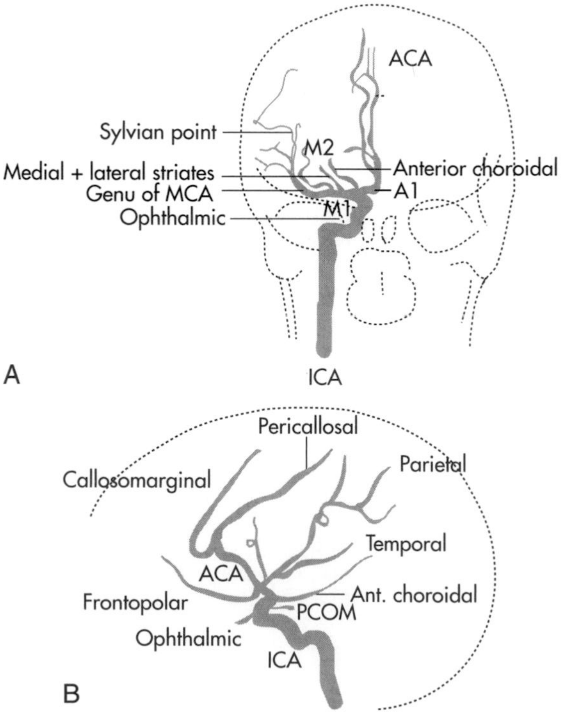

FIGURE 6-16

- P2 segment:
  - Distal to the PCOM
  - Thalamogeniculates
  - Posterior choroidal arteries
- Terminal cortical branches

NORMAL VARIANTS OF VASCULAR ANATOMY

Internal Carotid Artery (Fig. 6-17)

Mnemonic: "HOT Pepper:"

- **H**ypoglossal artery: ICA (C1-2) to basilar artery via hypoglossal canal
- **O**tic artery: petrous ICA to replace middle meningeal artery via middle ear (foramen spinosum may be absent)
- **T**rigeminal artery: cavernous ICA to basilar artery (most common), Neptune's trident sign on angiography
- **P**roatlantal intersegmental artery: cervical ICA to vertebrobasilar system

External Carotid Artery

- Middle meningeal artery arises from ophthalmic artery
- Variation in order of branching

Circle of Willis

- Hypoplasia of PCOM
- Hypoplasia or absence of A1 segment
- Fetal PCA (originates from ICA) with atretic P1
- Hypoplastic ACOM
- Infundibulum of PCOM: take-off of PCOM from ICA is from apex of a triangular- or funnel-shaped origin measuring <3mm; do not mistake for aneurysm

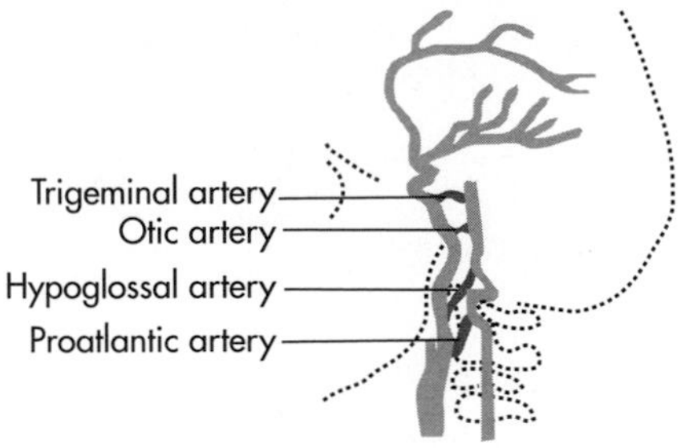

FIGURE 6-17

ANASTOMOSES BETWEEN ARTERIES

Between ICA and ECA via:

- Maxillary artery branches to ophthalmic artery
- Facial artery to ophthalmic artery
- Dural collaterals (occipital, ascending pharyngeal, middle meningeal)
- ECA → contralateral ECA → ICA

Between ECA and cerebral arteries

- ECA → middle meningeal artery → transdural → pial branches → ACA, MCA
- ECA → meningeal branches → vertebrobasilar artery

Between cerebral arteries

- Left ICA → ACOM → right ICA (circle of Willis)
- ICA → PCOM → basilar (circle of Willis)
- ICA → anterior choroidal → posterior choroidal → basilar
- Leptomeningeal anastomoses: ACA → MCA → PCA → ACA

Between ICA and posterior fossa (primitive embryonic connections; mnemonic: "HOT Pepper"; see earlier)

MENINGES AND VENOUS SINUSES (Fig. 6-18)

Meningeal Spaces

- Epidural space: potential space between dura mater (two layers) and bone
- Subdural space: space between dura and arachnoid
- Subarachnoid space: space between arachnoid and pia mater

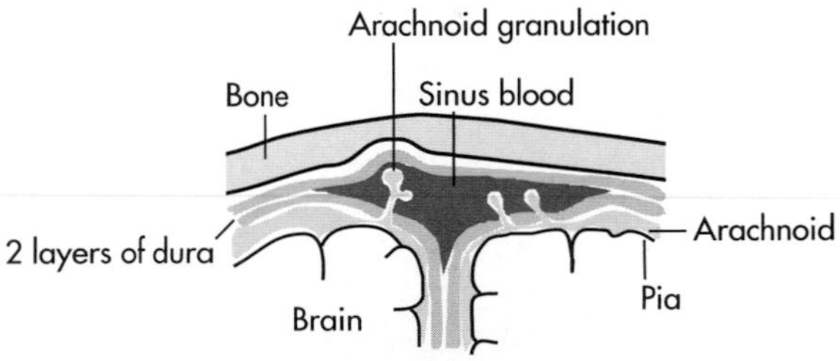

FIGURE 6-18

SINUSES (Fig. 6-19)

- Superior sagittal sinus: in root of falx
- Inferior sagittal sinus: in free edge of falx
- Straight sinus
- Great vein of Galen: drains into straight sinus

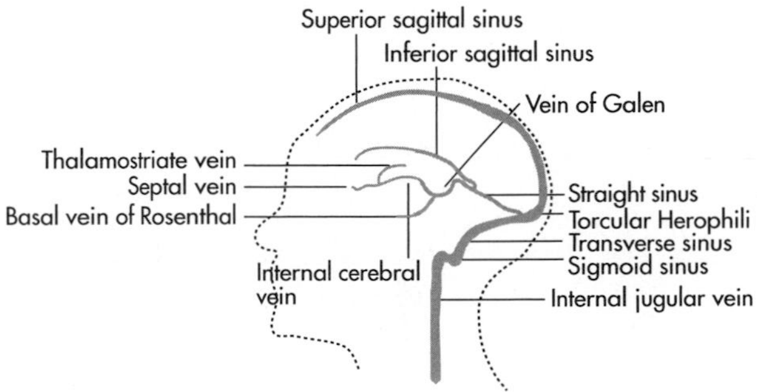

FIGURE 6-19

- Occipital sinus
- Confluence of sinuses (torcular Herophili)
- Left and right transverse sinus: drain from confluence
- Sigmoid sinus: drains into IJV
- Superior petrosal sinus: enters into transverse sinus
- Inferior petrosal sinus

VASCULAR TERRITORIES (Fig. 6-20)

ACA
- Hemispheric
- Callosal
- Medial lenticulostriate (Heubner)
  - Caudate head
  - Anterior limb of internal capsule
  - Septum pellucidum

MCA
- Hemispheric
- Lateral lenticulostriate
  - Lentiform nucleus
  - Caudate capsule
  - Internal capsule

PCA
- Hemispheric
- Callosal
- Thalamic and midbrain perforators
- Mesial inferior temporal lobe, occipital lobe

SCA
- Superior cerebellum

AICA
- Inferolateral pons
- Middle cerebellar peduncle
- Anterior cerebellum

PICA
- Medulla
- Posterior and inferior cerebellum

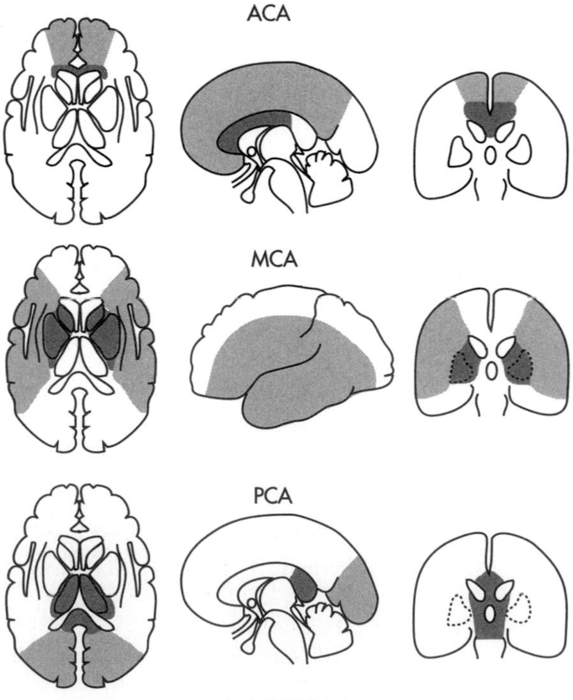

FIGURE 6-20

US OF CAROTID ARTERIES

B-Mode Imaging (Fig. 6-21)

Delineate CCA, ECA, ICA, bulb
- Vessel wall thickness
  - >1.0 mm is abnormal.
  - All focal plaques are abnormal.
- Plaque characterization
  - Determine extent and location
  - Plaque texture
    - Homogeneous (dense fibrous connective tissue)
    - Heterogeneous (intraplaque hemorrhage: echogenic center; unstable)
    - Calcified (stable)
  - Plaque surface
    - Irregular surface may represent ulceration
- Evaluation of stenosis
  - Measure visible stenosis in transverse and longitudinal planes. Use Doppler measurements for degree of stenosis
- Focal vs. segmental stenosis

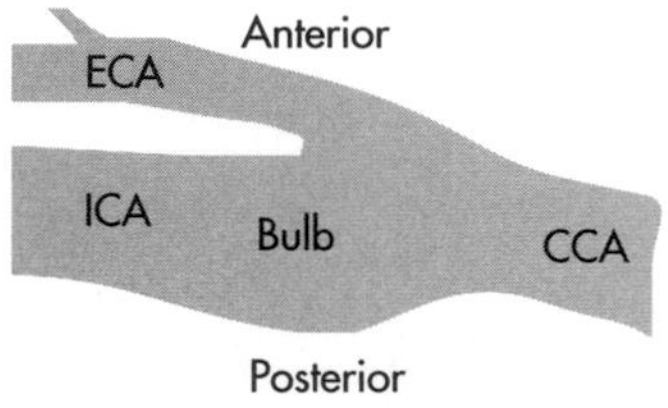

FIGURE 6-21

Doppler Imaging (Flow) (Fig. 6-22)

Doppler imaging displays velocity profile. Analysis of spectra:

1. Analysis of waveform
   - Components of curve
     - Peak diastolic flow
     - Peak systolic flow
     - Peak broadness
     - Flow direction
   - Shape of curves
     - High-resistance vessels (e.g., ECA)
     - Low-resistance vessels (e.g., ICA)
     - Intermediate-resistance vessels (e.g., CCA)

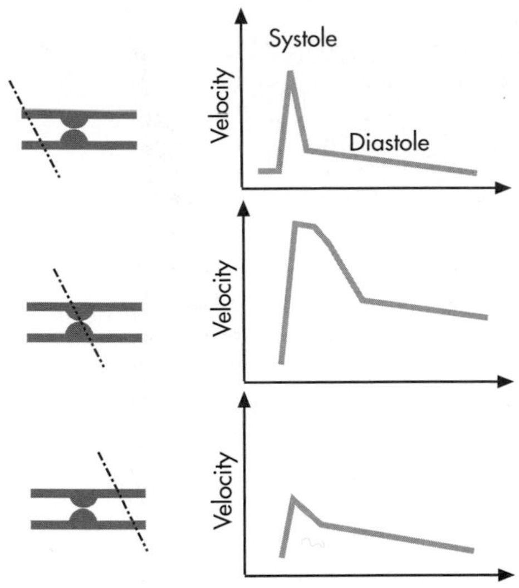

FIGURE 6-22

US DIFFERENTIATION BETWEEN ICA AND ECA

Parameter	ICA	ECA
Size	Large	Small
Location	Posterior and lateral	Anterior and medial
Branches	No	Yes
Temporal tap	No pulsation	Pulsation
Pulsatility	Not very pulsatile (low resistance)	Very pulsatile (high resistance)
Waveform	Low resistance Flow in systole and diastole	High resistance Flow in systole only

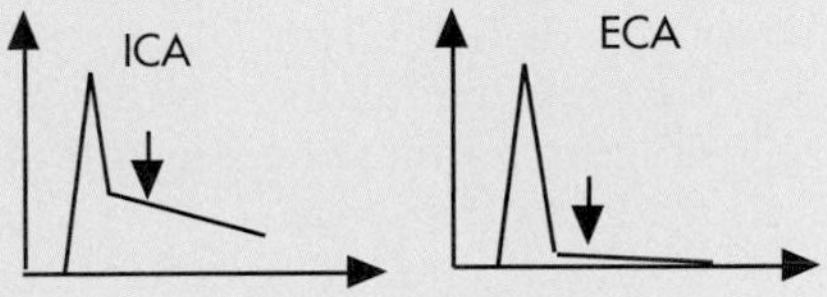

2. Spectral broadening (Fig. 6-23)
   When normal laminar blood flow is disturbed (by plaques and/or stenoses), blood has a wider range of velocities = spectral broadening.
   Two ways to detect spectral broadening:
   - The spectral window is obliterated.
   - Automated determination of bandwidth = spread of maximum and minimum velocities.
3. Peak velocities (Fig. 6-24)
   Flow velocities increase proportionally with the degree of a stenosis: flow of >250 cm/sec indicates a >70% stenosis.
   Carotid stent:
   50%-79% stenosis: >220 cm/sec and ICA/CCA ratio ≥ 2.7
   80%-99% stenosis: >340 cm/sec and ICA/CCA ratio ≥ 4.15

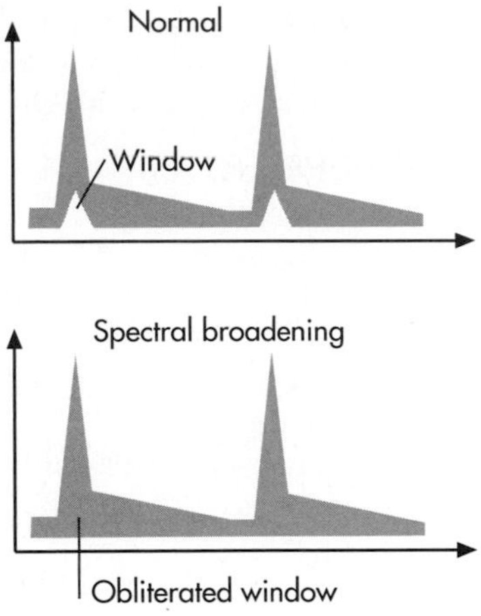

FIGURE 6-23

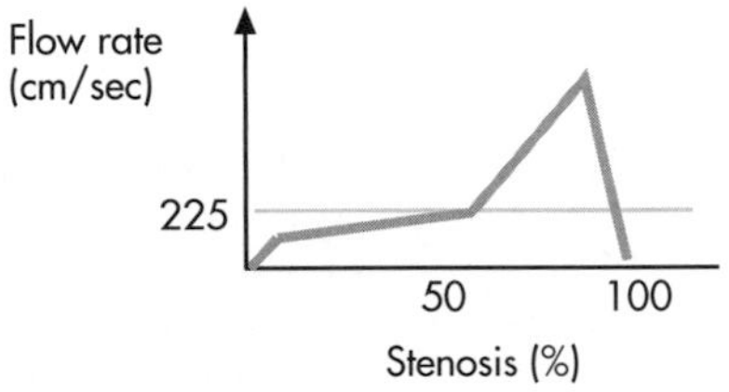

FIGURE 6-24

Color Doppler Ultrasound

Color Doppler imaging (CDI) displays real-time velocity information in stationary soft tissues. The color assignment is arbitrary but conventionally displayed in the following manner:

- Red: toward transducer
- Blue: away from transducer
- Green: high-velocity flow
- Color saturation indicates speed.
  Deep shades: slow flow
  Light shades: fast flow

Pearls

- Perform CDI only with optimal gain and flow sensitivity settings.
  Ideally the vessel lumen should be filled with color.
  Color should not spill over to stationary tissues.
- Frame rates vary as a function of the area selected for CDI: the larger the area, the slower the frame rate.
- Laminar flow is disrupted at bifurcations.
- Do not equate color saturation with velocity: green-tagged flow in a vessel may represent abnormally high flow or simply a region in the vessel where flow is directed at a more acute angle relative to the transducer.
- When color flow is not present in the expected vessel, increase pulse Doppler frequency, decrease filters, and apply Doppler imaging within the vessel to detect blood flow in slow

flow states such as pseudo-occlusion or no flow in an occluded vessel.
- The angle of insonation should be within 0° to 60°.

TRANSCRANIAL DOPPLER (TCD)

TCD measures the velocity of blood flow through the intracranial arteries. Commonly performed using the following windows:
Transtemporal — circle of Willis
Transorbital — carotid siphon and ophthalmic artery
Suboccipital or transforaminal — vertebral and basilar arteries

Indications
Vasospasm (esp. related to subarachnoid hemorrhage)
Stenosis/occlusion
Vasomotor reserve
Brain death
Monitoring of blood flow during surgery
Identification of feeder arteries in arteriovenous malformations

Criteria

	Velocity (cm/sec)	
Stenosis	**Anterior**	**Vertebrals and Basilar**
Mild	120-160	100-150
Mod	160-200	150-180
Severe	>200	>180

SPINE

SPINAL CANAL (Fig. 6-25)

Vertebral elements:
- Body
- Posterior elements
  Neural ring
- Posterior margin of vertebral body
- Pedicles

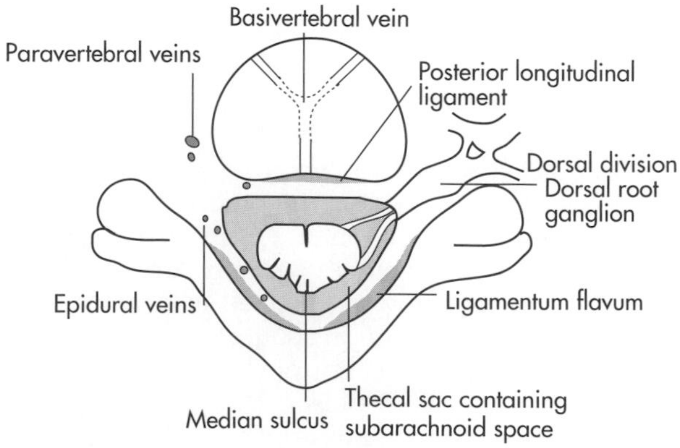

FIGURE 6-25

- Laminae
  Articular facets
  Transverse process

Recesses
- Subarticular recess
- Lateral recess

Disks
- Components:
  Nucleus pulposus (notochordal origin)
  Annulus fibrosus with peripheral Sharpey's fibers
- CT density (60 to 120 HU)
  Disk periphery is slightly denser than its center (Sharpey's fibers calcify).
  Disk is much denser than thecal sac (0 to 30 HU).
- MRI signal intensity
  T1W: hypointense relative to marrow
  PDW, T2W: hyperintense relative to marrow with hypointense intranuclear cleft

Ligaments
- Ligamentum flavum: attaches to lamina and facets
- Posterior longitudinal ligament: rarely seen by MRI except in herniations

Thecal sac
- Lined by dura and surrounded by epidural fat
- Normal AP diameter of thecal sac
  Cervical >7 mm
  Lumbar >10 mm
- MRI frequently shows CSF flow artifacts in thecal sac.

NEURAL STRUCTURES

Spinal cord
- AP diameter 7 mm
- Conus medullaris: 8 mm (tip at L1-L2)
- Filum terminale extends from L1 to S1.

Nerve roots (Fig. 6-26)
- Ventral root, dorsal root, dorsal root ganglion
- The dorsal and ventral nerve roots join in the spinal canal to form the spinal nerve. The nerve splits into ventral and dorsal rami a short distance after exiting the neural foramen.
  Below T1: spinal nerve courses under the pedicle for which it is named (e.g., L4 goes under L4 pedicle).

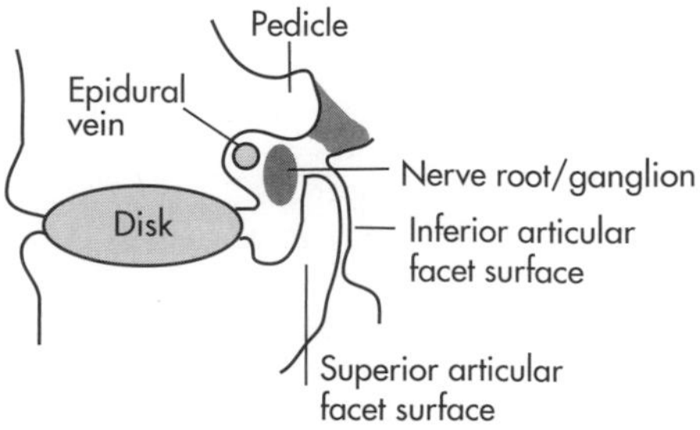

FIGURE 6-26

Above T1: spinal nerve courses above the pedicle for which it is named.

- Nerve roots lie in the superior portion of the intervertebral neural foramen.

Vascular Disease

INTRACRANIAL HEMORRHAGE (Fig. 6-27)

CT APPEARANCE OF INTRACRANIAL HEMORRHAGE

Acute hemorrhage (<3 days)
- Hyperdense (80 to 100 HU) relative to brain (40 to 50 HU)
- High density caused by protein-hemoglobin component (clot retraction)
- Acute hemorrhage is not hyperdense if the hematocrit is low (hemoglobin <8 g/dL).

Subacute hemorrhage (3 to 14 days)
- Hyperintense, isointense, or hypointense relative to brain
- Degradation of protein-hemoglobin product evolves from peripheral to central
- Peripheral enhancement may be present.

Chronic hemorrhage (>2 weeks)
- Hypodense

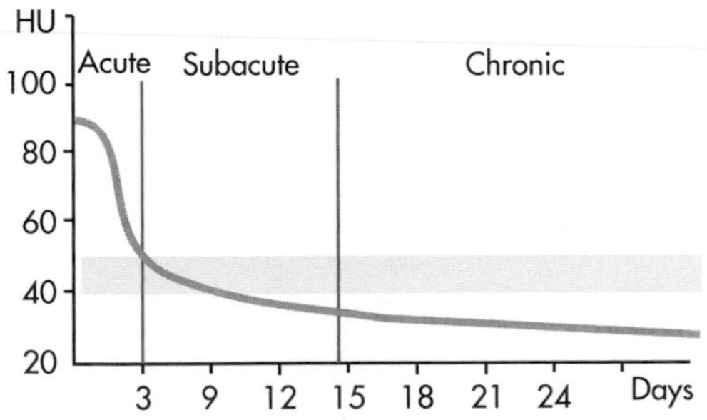

FIGURE 6-27

MRI APPEARANCE OF INTRACRANIAL HEMORRHAGE (Fig. 6-28)

Different iron-containing substances have different magnetic effects (diamagnetic, paramagnetic, superparamagnetic) on surrounding brain tissue. In the circulating form, hemoglobin (Hb) alternates between oxy-Hb and deoxy-Hb as O_2 is exchanged. To bind O_2, the iron (Fe) must be in the reduced Fe(II) (ferrous) state. When Hb is removed from the circulation, the metabolic pathways fail to reduce iron and Hb begins denaturation. The appearance of blood depends on the magnetic properties of blood products and compartmentalization.

Mnemonic: "I Be ID BD BaBy Doo Doo:"
- I = Isointense
- B = Bright
- D = Dark

Note: Gradient echo ("susceptibility") imaging exaggerates the T2W appearance of blood, and thus follows the same pattern as T2W (i.e., hypointense for acute, early subacute, and chronic hemorrhages).

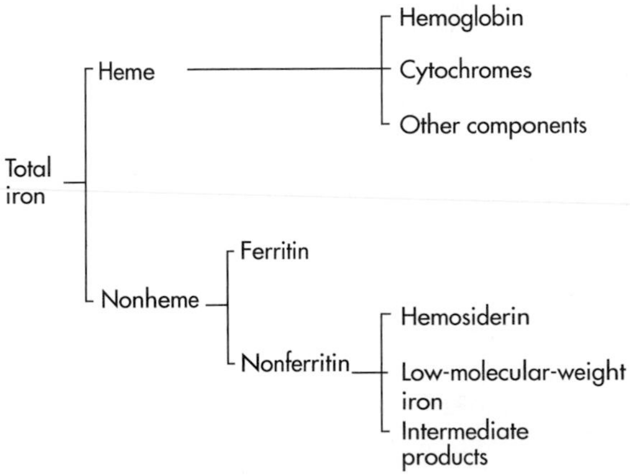

FIGURE 6-28

MRI APPEARANCE OF HEMORRHAGE

Stage	Biochemistry	Pathophysiology	Location	Magnetism	T1W/T2W (GRE) Appearance
Hyperacute (hr)	Oxy-Hb	Serum + RBCs	Intracellular	Diamagnetic	Isointense / Bright
Acute (1-2 days)	Deoxy-Hb	Deoxygenation	Intracellular	Paramagnetic	Isointense / Dark
Early subacute (2-7 days)	Met-Hb	Oxidation/ denaturation	Intracellular	Paramagnetic	Bright / Dark
Late subacute (1-4 wk)	Met-Hb	RBC lysis	Extracellular	Paramagnetic	Bright / Bright
Chronic	Hemosiderin Ferritin	Iron storage	Extracellular	Ferromagnetic	Dark / Dark rim

Isointense Bright Dark Dark rim

HYPERTENSIVE HEMORRHAGE

Occurs most commonly in areas of penetrating arteries that come off the MCA and/or basilar artery. Depending on size and location of hemorrhage, the mortality rate is high. Poor prognostic factors:

- Large size
- Brainstem location
- Intraventricular extension

Location

- Basal ganglia (putamen > thalamus), 80%
- Pons, 10%
- Deep gray matter, 5%
- Cerebellum, 5%

Imaging Features

- Typical location of hemorrhage (basal ganglia) in hypertensive patient
- Mass effect from hemorrhage and edema may cause herniation of brain.
- If the patient survives, the hemorrhage heals and leaves a residual cavity that is best demonstrated by MRI.

TUMOR HEMORRHAGE

Tumor-related intracranial hemorrhage may be due to coagulopathy (leukemia, anticoagulation) or spontaneous bleeding into a tumor. Most clinicians cite that the incidence of hemorrhage into tumors is 5%-10%. Tumors that commonly hemorrhage include:

- Pituitary adenoma
- Glioblastoma multiforme, anaplastic astrocytoma
- Oligodendroglioma
- Ependymoma
- Primitive neuroectodermal tumors (PNETs)
- Epidermoid
- Metastases

ANEURYSM

TYPES

Saccular aneurysm ("berry aneurysm"), 80%
- Developmental or degenerative aneurysm (most common)
- Traumatic aneurysm
- Infectious (mycotic) aneurysm, 3%
- Neoplastic (oncotic) aneurysm
- Flow-related aneurysm
- Vasculopathies (systemic lupus erythematosus [SLE], Takayasu's arteritis, fibromuscular dysplasia [FMD])

Fusiform aneurysm
Dissecting aneurysm

SACCULAR ANEURYSM

Berry-like outpouchings predominantly at arterial bifurcation points. Saccular aneurysm is a true aneurysm in which the sac consists of intima and adventitia. Etiology: degenerative vascular injury (previously thought to be congenital) > trauma, infection, tumor, vasculopathies. Present in approximately 2% of population; multiple in 20%; 25% are giant aneurysms (>25 mm). Increased incidence of aneurysm in:

- Adult dominant polycystic kidney disease (ADPKD)
- Aortic coarctation
- FMD
- Structural collagen disorders (Marfan syndrome, Ehlers-Danlos syndrome)
- Spontaneous dissections

Imaging Features (Fig. 6-29)

Interpretation of conventional angiography
- Number of aneurysms: multiple in 20%
- Location, 90% in anterior circulation
- Size
- Relation to parent vessel
- Presence and size of aneurysm neck

MRA
- Usually combined with conventional MRI
- Used to screen patients with risk factors (e.g., APKD)
- Low sensitivity for aneurysms <4 mm
- Need to verify presence of aneurysm by reviewing single-slice raw images

Complications

Rupture
- Subarachnoid hemorrhage
- Parenchymal hematoma
- Hydrocephalus

Vasospasm
- Occurs 4 to 5 days after rupture

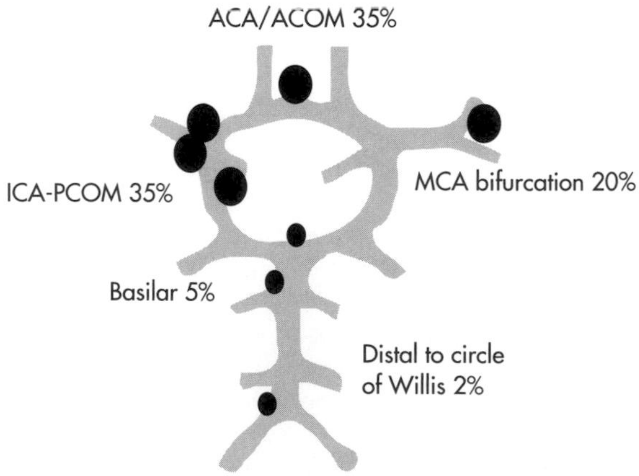

FIGURE 6-29

- Causes secondary infarctions
- Leading cause of death/morbidity from rupture

Mass effect
- Cranial nerve palsies
- Headache

Death, 30%

Rebleeding
- 50% rebleed within 6 months
- 50% mortality

In the presence of multiple aneurysms, one may identify the bleeding aneurysm using the following criteria:

- Location of subarachnoid hemorrhage (SAH) or hematoma adjacent to or around bleeding aneurysm
- Largest aneurysm is the one most likely to bleed
- Most irregular aneurysm is the one most likely to bleed
- Extravasation of contrast (rarely seen)
- Vasospasm adjacent to bleeding aneurysm

GIANT ANEURYSM

Aneurysm >25 mm in diameter

Clinical Findings

- Mass effect (cranial nerve palsies, retroorbital pain)
- Hemorrhage

Imaging Features

- Large mass lesion with internal blood degradation products
- Signet sign: eccentric vessel lumen with surrounding thrombus
- Curvilinear peripheral calcification
- Ring enhancement: fibrous outer wall enhances after complete thrombosis
- Mass effect on adjacent parenchyma
- Slow erosion of bone
  - Sloping of sellar floor
  - Undercutting of anterior clinoid
  - Enlarged superior orbital fissure

INFECTIOUS (MYCOTIC) ANEURYSM

Causes

- Bacterial endocarditis, intravenous drug abuse (IVDA), 80%
- Meningitis, 10%
- Septic thrombophlebitis, 10%

Imaging Features

- Aneurysm itself is rarely visualized by CT.
- Most often located peripherally and multiple (DDx: tumor emboli from atrial myxoma)
- Intense enhancement adjacent to vessel
- Conventional angiography is the imaging study of choice.

FUSIFORM (ATHEROSCLEROTIC) ANEURYSM

Elongated aneurysm caused by atherosclerotic disease. Most located in the vertebrobasilar system. Often associated with dolichoectasia (elongation and distention of the vertebrobasilar system).

Imaging Features

- Vertebrobasilar arteries are elongated, tortuous, and dilated.
- Tip of basilar artery may indent 3rd ventricle.
- Aneurysm may be thrombosed.
  - CT: hyperdense
  - T1W: hyperintense

Complications

- Brainstem infarction due to thrombosis
- Mass effect (cranial nerve palsies)

DISSECTING ANEURYSM

Following a dissection an intramural hematoma may organize and result in a saclike outpouching. Causes: trauma > vasculopathy (SLE, FMD) > spontaneous dissection.

Location: extracranial ICA > vertebral artery.

Imaging Features

- Elongated contrast collections extending beyond the vessel lumen
- MRA is a useful screening modality.
- CTA may be used for diagnosis and follow-up
- Angiography is sometimes required for imaging of vascular detail (dissection site).

SUBARACHNOID HEMORRHAGE (SAH)

Blood is present in the subarachnoid space and sometimes also within ventricles. Secondary vasospasm and brain infarction are the leading causes of death in SAH.

Causes

- Aneurysm (most common), 90%
- Trauma
- AVM
- Coagulopathy
- Extension of intraparenchymal hemorrhage (hypertension, tumor)
- Idiopathic, 5%
- Spinal AVM

Imaging Features (Fig. 6-30)

- CT is the first imaging study of choice.
- Hyperdense cerebrospinal fluid (CSF) usually in basal cisterns, sylvian fissure (due to aneurysm location), and subarachnoid space
- Hematocrit effect in intraventricular hemorrhage
- MRI less sensitive than CT early on (deoxy-Hb and brain are isointense)

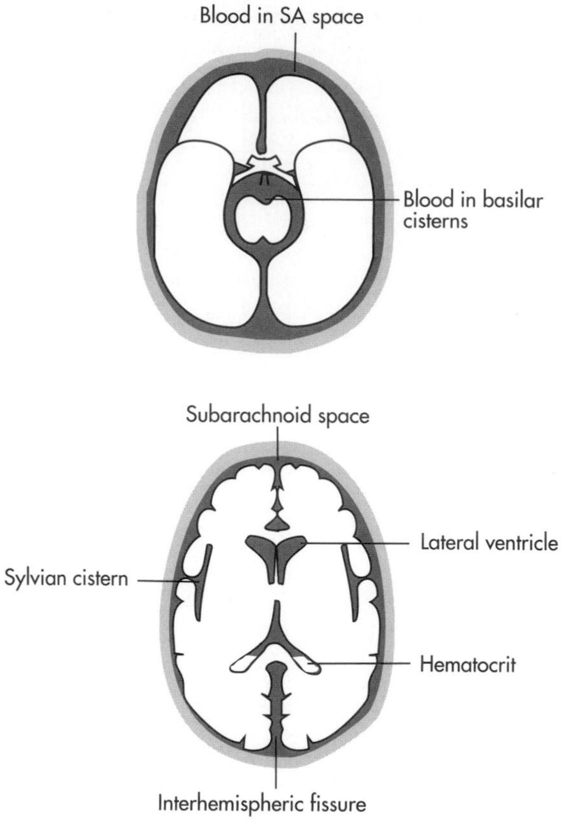

FIGURE 6-30

- MRI more sensitive than CT for detecting subacute (FLAIR bright)/chronic SAH (T2W/susceptibility dark)

Complications

- Hemorrhage-induced hydrocephalus is due to early ventricular obstruction and/or arachnoiditis.
- Vasospasm several days after SAH may lead to secondary infarctions.
- Leptomeningeal "superficial" siderosis (dark meninges on T2W): iron deposition in meninges secondary to chronic recurrent SAH. The location of siderosis corresponds to the extent of central myelin. Cranial nerves I, II, and VIII are preferentially affected because these have peripheral myelin envelope. Other cranial nerves have their transition points closer to the brainstem. If no etiology is identified, MRI of the spine should be performed to exclude a chronically bleeding spinal neoplasm such as an ependymoma or a paraganglioma.

VASCULAR MALFORMATION

TYPES OF VASCULAR MALFORMATIONS

There are four types of malformations:

- AVM
    - Parenchymal (pial) malformations
    - Dural AVM and fistula
    - Mixed pial/dural AVM
- Capillary telangiectasia
- Cavernous malformation
- Venous malformations
    - Venous anomaly
    - Vein of Galen malformation
    - Venous varix

ARTERIOVENOUS MALFORMATION (AVM)

Abnormal network of arteries and veins with no intervening capillary bed. 98% of AVM are solitary. Peak age is 20 to 40 years.

Types

- Parenchymal, 80% (ICA and vertebral artery supply; congenital lesions)
- Dural, 10% (ECA supply; mostly acquired lesions)
- Mixed, 10%

Imaging Features (Fig. 6-31)

- MRI is imaging study of choice for detection of AVM; arteriography is superior for characterization and treatment planning.
- Serpiginous high and low signal (depending on flow rates) within feeding and draining vessels best seen by MRI/MRA
- AVM *re*places but does not displace brain tissue (i.e., mass effect is uncommon) unless complicated by hemorrhage and edema.
- Edema occurs only if there is recent hemorrhage or venous thrombosis with infarction.
- Flow-related aneurysm, 10%
- Adjacent parenchymal atrophy is common as a result of vascular steal and ischemia.

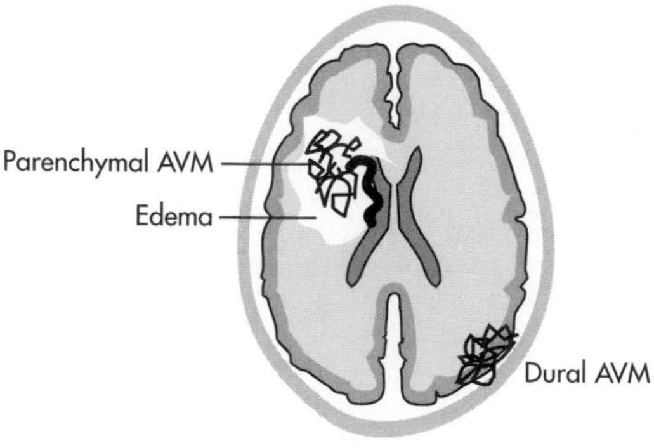

FIGURE 6-31

- Calcification, 25%
- Susceptibility artifacts on MRI if old hemorrhage is present.

Spetzler's Criteria

SPETZLER'S CRITERIA

	0	1	2	3
Eloquence	No	Yes	—	—
Draining vein	Superficial	Deep	—	—
Size	—	<3 cm	3-6 cm	<6 cm

- Higher score is associated with higher chance of hemorrhage
- Other factors associated with poorer prognosis/higher risk of hemorrhage:
  - Intranidal aneurysm
  - Aneurysm in the circle of Willis
  - Aneurysm in arterial feeder
  - Venous stasis

Complications

- Hemorrhage (parenchymal > SAH > intraventricular)
- Seizures
- Cumulative risk of hemorrhage is approximately 3% per year.

CAPILLARY TELANGIECTASIA

Nests of dilated capillaries with normal brain interspersed between dilated capillaries. Commonly coexist with cavernous malformation. Location: pons > cerebral cortex, spinal cord > other locations.

Imaging Features

- CT is often normal.
- MRI:
  - Foci of increased signal intensity on contrast-enhanced studies
  - T2W hypointense foci if hemorrhage has occurred
- Angiography is often normal but may show faint vascular stain.

CAVERNOUS MALFORMATION (Fig. 6-32)

Dilated endothelial cell-lined spaces with no normal brain within lesion. Usually detectable because cavernous malformation contains blood degradation products of different stages. Location: 80% supratentorial, 60%-80% multiple. All age groups.

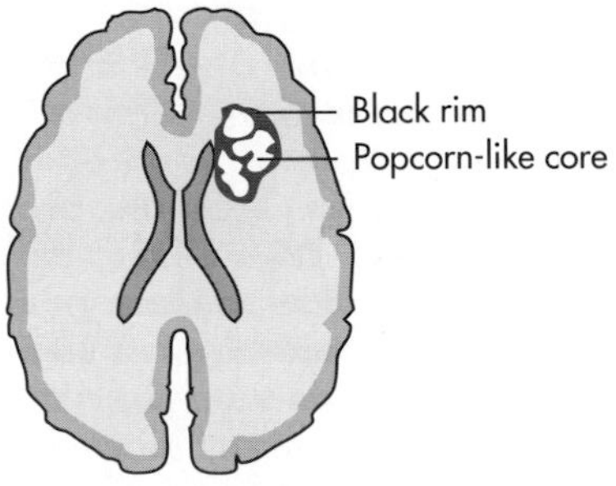

FIGURE 6-32

Clinical Findings

- Seizures
- Focal deficits
- Headache secondary to occult hemorrhage

Imaging Features (Fig. 6-33)

- MRI is the imaging study of choice.
- Complex signal intensities due to blood products of varying age
- "Popcorn" lesion: bright lobulated center with black (hemosiderin) rim
- Always obtain susceptibility sequences to detect coexistent smaller lesions.
- May be calcified
- Variable contrast enhancement
- Angiography is usually normal.

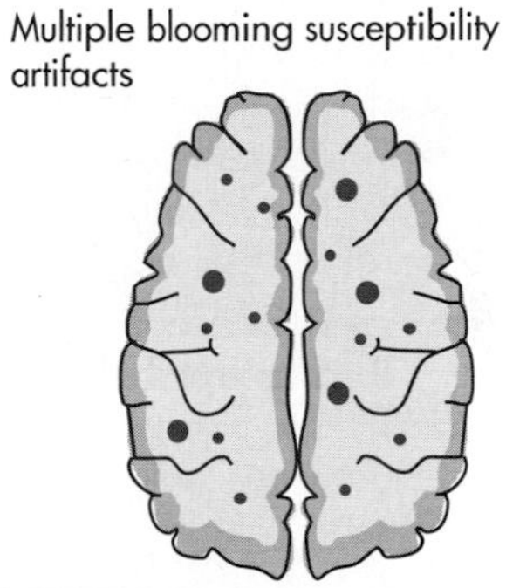

FIGURE 6-33

VENOUS ANOMALY (ANOMALOUS VEIN)

Multiple small veins converge into a large transcortical draining vein. Typically discovered incidentally. Venous angiomas per se do not hemorrhage but are associated with cavernous malformations (30%), which do bleed.

Imaging Features (Fig. 6-34)

Angiography
- Medusa head seen on venous phase (hallmark)
- Dilated medullary veins draining into a large transcortical vein

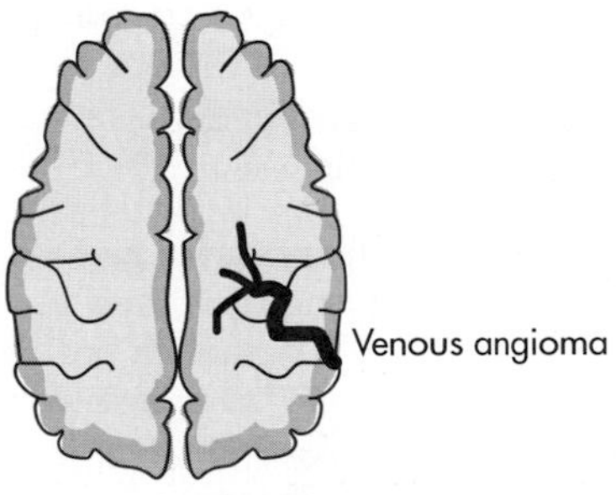

FIGURE 6-34

MRI
- Medusa head or large transcortical vein best seen on spin-echo images or after administration of gadolinium
- Location in deep cerebellar white matter or deep cerebral white matter
- Adjacent to the frontal horn (most common site)

Hemorrhage best detectable with MR susceptibility sequences, 10%.

VEIN OF GALEN AVM

Complex group of vascular anomalies that consist of a central AVM and resultant varix of the vein of Galen (incorrectly referred to as vein of Galen "aneurysm"). Two main types exist with the common feature of a dilated midline venous structure:

Vein of Galen AVM
- Primary malformation in development of vein of Galen
- AV shunts involving embryologic venous precursors (median vein of prosencephalon)
- Choroidal arteriovenous fistula with no nidus
- Absence of normal vein of Galen
- Median vein of prosencephalon does not drain normal brain tissue.
- Manifests as high-output congestive heart failure (CHF) in infants and hydrocephalus in older children

Vein of Galen varix
- Primary parenchymal AVM drains into vein of Galen, which secondarily enlarges.
- Thalamic AVM with nidus is usually the primary AVM.
- Uncommon in neonates
- Higher risk of hemorrhage than the vein of Galen AVM

Imaging Features

US
- First-choice imaging modality
- Sonolucent midline structure superior/posterior to 3rd ventricle
- Color Doppler ultrasound (US) to exclude arachnoid/developmental cyst

Angiography
- Used to determine type and therapy
- Endovascular embolization: therapy of choice

MRI
- Indicated to assess extent of brain damage that influences therapy

Chest radiography
- High-output CHF, large heart

STROKE

Stroke is a term that describes an acute episode of neurologic deficit. 80% of strokes are due to cerebral ischemia (embolic or thrombotic). Transient ischemic attacks (TIAs) are focal neurologic events that resolve within 24 hours; those that resolve after 24 hours are called *reversible ischemic neurologic deficits* (RINDs).

Causes

Cerebral infarction, 80%
- Atherosclerosis-related occlusion of vessels, 60%
- Cardiac emboli, 15%
- Other, 5%

Intracranial hemorrhage, 15%

Nontraumatic SAH, 5%

Venous occlusion, 1%

OVERVIEW OF COMMON CAUSES OF STROKE

Older Patient	Younger Patient	Child
Atherosclerosis	Emboli	Emboli from congenital heart disease
Cardiac emboli	Arterial dissections	Venous thrombosis
	Vasculopathy (FMD, vasculitis)	Blood dyscrasias (i.e., sickle cell disease)
	Drug abuse	

ATHEROSCLEROTIC DISEASE

Atherosclerosis represents the most common cause of cerebral ischemia/infarction. Carotid atherosclerosis causes embolic ischemia; intracranial atherosclerosis causes in-situ thrombotic or distal embolic ischemia. Location: ICA origin > distal basilar > carotid siphon, MCA.

Critical carotid stenosis is defined as a stenosis of >70% in luminal diameter. Patients with critical stenosis and symptoms have an increased risk of stroke and benefit from carotid endarterectomy. Patients with stenosis <70% or who are asymptomatic are usually treated medically.

Imaging Features

Gray-scale imaging (B-scan) of carotid arteries
- Evaluate plaque morphology/extent
- Determine severity of stenosis (residual lumen)
- Other features
  - Slim sign: collapse of ICA above stenosis
  - Collateral circulation

Doppler imaging of carotid arteries
- Severity of stenosis determined by measuring peak systolic velocity
  - 50%-70%: velocity 125 to 250 cm/sec
  - 70%-90%: velocity 250 to 400 cm/sec
  - >90%: velocity >400 cm/sec
- Stenoses >95% may result in decreased velocity (<25 cm/sec)
- 90% accuracy for >50% stenoses

- Other measures used for quantifying stenoses
  - End diastolic velocity (severe stenosis: >100 cm/sec)
  - ICA/CCA peak systolic velocity ratio (severe stenosis: >4)
  - ICA/CCA peak end-diastolic velocity ratio
- Innominate artery stenosis may cause right CCA/ICA parvus tardus
- CCA occlusion may result in reversal of flow in ECA

Color Doppler flow imaging of carotid arteries

- High-grade stenosis with minimal flow (string sign in angiography) is detected more reliably than with conventional Doppler US.

CT and MR angiography are used for confirmation of ultrasound diagnosis of carotid stenosis.

- On computed tomographic angiography (CTA), 1.0- to 1.5-mm residual lumen corresponds to 70%-90% stenosis.
- To determine complete occlusion versus a string sign (near but not complete occlusion), delayed images must be obtained immediately after the initial contrast images.
- At some institutions, carotid endarterectomy is performed on the basis of US and CTA/MRA if the results are concordant.
- Pitfalls of US and MRA in the diagnosis of carotid stenosis:
  - Near occlusions (may be overdiagnosed as occluded)
  - Postendarterectomy (complex flow, clip artifacts)
  - Ulcerated plaques (suboptimal detection)
  - Tandem lesions (easily missed)

Carotid arteriography (gold standard) is primarily used for:

- Discordant MRA/CTA and US results
- Postendarterectomy patient
- Accurate evaluation of tandem lesions and collateral circulation
- Evaluation of aortic arch and great vessels

CEREBRAL ISCHEMIA AND INFARCTION

Cerebral ischemia refers to a diminished blood supply to the brain. Infarction refers to brain damage, being the result of ischemia.

Causes

Large vessel occlusion, 50%

Small vessel occlusion (lacunar infarcts), 20%

Emboli

- Cardiac, 15%
  - Arrhythmia, atrial fibrillation
  - Endocarditis
  - Atrial myxoma
  - Myocardial infarction (anterior infarction)
  - Left ventricular aneurysm
- Noncardiac
  - Atherosclerosis
  - Fat, air embolism

Vasculitis

- SLE
- Polyarteritis nodosa

Other

- Hypoperfusion (borderzone or watershed infarcts)
- Vasospasm: ruptured aneurysm, SAH
- Hematologic abnormalities
  - Hypercoagulable states
  - Hb abnormalities (CO poisoning, sickle cell)
- Venous occlusion
- Moyamoya disease

Imaging Features

Angiographic signs of cerebral infarction

- Vessel occlusion, 50%
- Slow antegrade flow, delayed arterial emptying, 15%
- Collateral filling, 20%
- Nonperfused areas, 5%
- Vascular blush (luxury perfusion), 20%
- AV shunting, 10%
- Mass effect, 40%

Cross-sectional imaging

- CT is the first study of choice in acute stroke in order to:
  - Exclude intracranial hemorrhage
  - Exclude underlying mass/AVM
- Most CT examinations are normal in early stroke.
- Early CT signs of cerebral infarction include:
  - Loss of gray-white interfaces (insular ribbon sign)
  - Sulcal effacement
  - Hyperdense clot in artery on noncontrast CT (dense MCA sign)
- Edema (maximum edema occurs 3 to 5 days after infarction)
  - Cytotoxic edema develops within 6 hours (detectable by MRI).
  - Vasogenic edema develops later (first detectable by CT at 12 to 24 hours).
- Characteristic differences between distributions of infarcts
  - Embolic: periphery, wedge shaped
  - Hypoperfusion in watershed areas of ACA/MCA and MCA/PCA
  - Borderzone infarcts
  - Basal ganglia infarcts
  - Generalized cortical laminar necrosis
- Reperfusion hemorrhage is not uncommon after 48 hours.
  - MRI much more sensitive than CT in detection
  - Most hemorrhages are petechial or gyral.

CT AND MRI APPEARANCE OF INFARCTS

Factor	1st Day	1st Week	1st Month	>1 Month
Stage	Acute	Early subacute	Late subacute	Chronic
CT density*	Subtle decrease	Decrease	Hypodense	Hypodense
MRI	T2W: edema	T2W: edema	Varied	T1W dark, T2W bright
Mass effect	Mild	Maximum	Resolving	Encephalomalacia
Hemorrhage	No	Most likely here	Variable	MRI detectable
Enhancement	No	Yes; maximum at 2-3 weeks	Decreasing	No

*Due to cytotoxic and vasogenic edema.

- Mass effect in acute infarction
  - Sulcal effacement
  - Ventricular compression
- Subacute infarcts
  - Hemorrhagic component, 40%
  - Gyral or patchy contrast enhancement (1 to 3 weeks)
  - GWM edema
- Chronic infarcts
  - Focal tissue loss: atrophy, porencephaly, cavitation, focal ventricular dilatation
  - Wallerian degeneration: distal axonal breakdown along white-matter tracks

Pearls

- Cerebral infarcts cannot be excluded on the basis of a negative CT. MRI with diffusion-weighted imaging (DWI) and perfusion-weighted imaging (PWI) (see later discussion) should be performed immediately if an acute infarct is suspected.
- Contrast administration is reserved for clinical problem cases and should not be routinely given, particularly on the first examination.
- Luxury perfusion refers to hyperemia of an ischemic area. The increased blood flow is thought to be due to compensatory vasodilatation secondary to parenchymal lactic acidosis.
- Cerebral infarcts have a peripheral rim of viable but ischemic tissue (penumbra).
- Thrombotic and embolic infarcts occur in vascular distributions (i.e., MCA, ACA, PCA, etc.).
- MR perfusion/diffusion studies are imaging studies of choice in acute stroke.
  - DWI detects reduced diffusion coefficient in acute infarction, which is thought to reflect cytotoxic edema.
  - In patients with multiple T2W signal abnormalities from a variety of causes, DWI can identify those signal abnormalities that arise from acute infarction.
- 50% of patients with TIA have DWI abnormality.

DIFFUSION AND PERFUSION IMAGING IN STROKE

Standard diffusion protocol includes a DWI and an apparent diffusion coefficient (ADC) image. These are usually interpreted side by side. DWI: summation of diffusion and T2 effects, abnormalities appear as high signal. ADC: diffusion effects only; abnormalities appear as low signal.

Perfusion imaging is performed using the susceptibility effects of a rapid bolus injection of gadolinium administered intravenously. Rapid continuous scanning during this injection allows the signal changes associated with the gadolinium to be plotted over time for a selected brain volume. These time-signal plots can be processed to yield several possible parameters relating to cerebral perfusion.

Vascular parameters: mean transit time (MTT) is measured in seconds and is a measure of how long it takes blood to reach the particular region of the brain. Cerebral blood volume (CBV) is measured in relative units and correlates to the total volume of circulating blood in the voxel. Cerebral blood flow (CBF) is measured in relative units and correlates to the flow of blood in the voxel.

Interpretation

STROKE EVOLUTION ON MRI

Sequence	Hyperacute (<6 hr)	Acute (>6 hr)	Subacute (Days to Weeks)	Chronic
DWI	High	High	High (decrease with time)	Isointense to bright
ADC	Low	Low	Low to isointense	Isointense to bright
T2W/FLAIR	Isointense	Slightly bright to bright	Bright	Bright

- A typical infarct is DWI bright and ADC dark. Gliosis appears DWI bright due to T2 shine-through but is also bright on ADC.

- DWI is very sensitive for detecting disease (will pick up infarcts from about 30 minutes onward but is nonspecific and will also detect nonischemic disease).
- ADC is less sensitive than DWI, but dark signal is fairly specific for restricted diffusion, which usually means ischemia.
- Significance of a DWI-bright, ADC-dark lesion: this tissue will almost certainly go on to infarct and full necrosis. Rare instances of reversible lesions have been reported (venous thrombosis, seizures, hemiplegic migraine, hyperacute arterial thrombosis).
- EXP (exponential) is the map that "subtracts" the T2 effect. In equivocal cases, use EXP map as a problem solver (if it stays bright on the EXP map, then it is true restricted diffusion).
- MTT is highly sensitive for disturbances in perfusion but not good for prediction of later events. For example, an asymptomatic carotid occlusion would have a dramatically abnormal MTT, without the patient being distressed.
- CBV is a parameter that changes late in the ischemic cascade, and usually reduced CBV is also accompanied by restricted diffusion. Reduced CBV (and restricted diffusion) correlates well with tissue that goes on to infarction.
- CBF in the experimental setting can be used to predict the likelihood of brain tissue infarcting. In current clinical practice, a CBF abnormality exceeding the DWI abnormality (diffusion-perfusion mismatch) implies that there is brain at risk that has not infarcted yet. This brain at risk is the target of therapeutic interventions.

ROLE OF CT/CTA IN ACUTE STROKE

Important in early stages of stroke evaluation to facilitate thrombolytic therapy. CTA demonstrates the anatomic details of the neurovasculature from the great vessel origins at the aortic arch to their intracranial termination. Highly accurate in the identification of proximal large vessel circle of Willis occlusions and therefore in the rapid triage of patients to intraarterial (IA) or intravenous (IV) thrombolytic therapy.

Technique

- Noncontrast CT is performed initially to exclude hemorrhage; an absolute contraindication to thrombolytic therapy. Large parenchymal hypodensity (>⅓ of a vascular territory), typically indicating irreversible "core" of infarction, is a relative contraindication to thrombolysis.
- CTA/CTP imaging is performed on a multislice scanner, which enables acquisition of imaging data from entire vascular territories in <1 minute.
- The initial CT scan is performed at 140 kV, 170 mA, pitch = "high quality" (3 : 1), and a table speed of 7.5 mm/sec.
- Images are obtained from the skull base to the vertex. Slice thickness can be set at 2.5 mm, at 5 mm, or at both.
- Initial image review is in "real time," directly at the CT console. The use of narrow window-width settings, with a center level of about 30 HU (width of 5 to 30 HU), facilitates the detection of early, subtle, ischemic changes contiguous with normal parenchyma.
- Blood volume CTP is performed without repositioning the patient.
- Approximately 90 to 120 mL of nonionic, isoosmolar contrast is used for CTA from the skull base to the vertex, with a 25-second scan delay. A longer delay may be needed for patients with compromised cardiac function and atrial fibrillation.
- Initial scan parameters are as per the noncontrast CT scan described earlier. A second phase of scanning is performed immediately, with minimal possible delay, from the aortic arch to the skull base, with similar scan parameters except for an increase in the table speed to 15 mm/sec. Major advantages of first scanning the intracranial circulation include (1) obtaining the most important data first, which can be reviewed during subsequent acquisition; and (2) allowing time for clearance of dense IV contrast from the subclavian, axillary, and other veins at the thoracic inlet, reducing streak artifact.
- On a >16-slice scanner, CTA may be performed from the vertex to the aortic arch in one pass, with triggering of imaging when the contrast bolus reaches the arch ("smart prep"). This gets rid of the loss of contrast enhancement in the neck CTA usually seen with a two-stack protocol.

THERAPEUTIC OPTIONS

- To date, the only FDA-approved treatment for acute stroke is IV thrombolysis with recombinant tissue plasminogen activator (r-tPA), administered within 3 hours of stroke onset. If thrombolysis is applied beyond this time window, the increased probability of intracranial hemorrhage is considered unacceptable.
- The time window for treatment with IA agents is twice as long for the anterior circulation and indefinite for the posterior circulation (depending on risk-to-benefit ratios); however, IA thrombolysis—although of proven benefit in preliminary trials—has not yet received FDA approval. For thrombosis localized to the posterior circulation, the time

window for treatment may be extended beyond 6 hours due to the extreme consequences of loss of blood flow to the brainstem, despite the risk of hemorrhage.

- Advanced CTA/CTP imaging of acute stroke has the potential to not only help exclude patients at high risk for hemorrhage from thrombolysis but also identify those patients most likely to benefit from thrombolysis. Even without hemorrhage, treatment failure with thrombolytics is not uncommon.
- The choice between IA and IV thrombolysis depends on a variety of factors, including the time post ictus, the clinical status of the patient, and whether the clot is proximal (IA) or distal (IV). When typical findings of occlusive thrombus on CTA and decreased tissue enhancement on CTP are not present, the differential diagnoses include lacunar infarct, early small distal embolic infarct, transient ischemic attack, complex migraine headaches, and seizure.

LACUNAR INFARCTS

Lacunar infarcts account for 20% of all strokes. The term refers to the occlusion of penetrating cerebral arterioles, most often caused by arteriolar lipohyalinosis (hypertensive vasculopathy). Commonly affected are:

- Thalamoperforators (thalamus)
- Lenticulostriates (caudate, putamen, internal capsule)
- Brainstem perforator (pons)

Lacunar infarcts usually cause characteristic clinical syndromes: pure motor hemiparesis, pure hemisensory deficit, hemiparetic ataxia, or dysarthria-hand deficit.

Imaging Features

- MRI is the imaging study of choice.
- Small ovoid lesion (<1 cm): hyperintense on T2W and proton density–weighted (PDW) image.
- Location of lesions is very helpful in differential diagnosis:
  - Dilated perivascular or Virchow-Robin (VR) space
    - Can be large (giant VR space), can cause mass effect, and can have surrounding gliosis
    - More elongated appearance on coronal images

BASILAR ARTERY THROMBOEMBOLIC OCCLUSION

Risk Factors

- Atherosclerosis
- Cardiac arrhythmias
- Vertebral artery dissection
- Cocaine use
- Oral contraceptives

Top of Basilar Artery Syndrome

- Oculomotor dysfunction
- Third nerve and vertical gaze palsies
- Hemiataxia
- Altered consciousness

Imaging Features

- Unlike anterior circulation infarction, the duration of symptoms before treatment, age of patient, and neurologic a status at initiation of treatment do not predict the outcome of thrombolytic therapy.
- Basilar artery appears abnormally dense by CT.
- T2W hyperintensity is present in thalami, midbrain, pons, cerebellum, and occipital lobes.
- Absence of normal flow void in basilar artery and vertebral artery
- T1W with fat saturation may be useful to look for associated dissection.

CENTRAL NERVOUS SYSTEM (CNS) VASCULITIS

CNS vasculitis may be caused by a large variety of underlying diseases.

Differentiation may be possible by correlating systemic findings and clinical history, but a biopsy is often required for diagnosis.

Causes

Infectious vasculitis

- Bacterial, viral, fungal, tuberculosis (TB), syphilis
- HIV-related

Systemic vasculitis

- Polyarteritis nodosa
- Giant cell arteritis/temporal arteritis
- Takayasu's arteritis
- Kawasaki syndrome
- Behçet disease
- Collagen vascular diseases
- Serum sickness
- Allergic angiitis

Granulomatous vasculitis

- Sarcoidosis
- Wegener granulomatosis
- Granulomatous angiitis (primary and secondary)

Drug-related vasculitis

- Cocaine
- Amphetamines
- Ergots
- Heroin

Imaging Features

MRI

- Most MRI findings are nonspecific.
- T2W hyperintensities that progress rapidly are highly suggestive.
- Infarctions
- Hemorrhage

Angiography
- CTA may also show areas of focal narrowing, similar to catheter angiography.
- Catheter angiography is the more definitive imaging study, but findings are often also nonspecific.

Other imaging findings
- Vessel occlusions
- Stenoses
- Aneurysms

MOYAMOYA DISEASE

Idiopathic progressive vascular occlusive disease. Common in Japanese (moyamoya = puff of smoke). Most commonly there is occlusion of supraclinoid ICA and numerous meningeal, lenticulostriate, thalamoperforate collaterals; occasionally the posterior circulation is involved.

Imaging Features

- "Puff of smoke" on angiography: numerous collaterals supplying ACA and MCA
- Stenosis or occlusion of supraclinoid ICA
- MRI: multiple tiny flow voids on T2W images, which are collaterals; engorged collaterals may produce FLAIR bright sulci (Ivy sign)
- Similar radiographic findings can be seen in (mnemonic: "RAINS"):
  - **R**adiation vasculopathy
  - **A**therosclerosis
  - **I**diopathic (moyamoya)
  - **N**eurofibromatosis type I
  - **S**ickle cell disease

AMYLOID ANGIOPATHY

Amyloid deposition in walls of small vessels. Common in elderly normotensive patients.

Imaging Features

- Usually multiple areas of hemorrhage sparing the basal ganglia
- Foci of hemorrhage at corticomedullary junction
- MRI is the imaging study of choice (susceptibility sequences).

CADASIL

(Cerebral autosomal dominant arteriopathy with subcortical infarcts and leukoencephalopathy)

Hereditary stroke disorder, commonly presents with migraine headaches and TIA/strokes. Age: 40-50, though imaging feature may be detected earlier.

MRI Features

- Confluent T2 hyperintensities around periventricular white matter, pons, and basal ganglia.
- Predilection for the anterior temporal lobes.

VENOOCCLUSIVE DISEASE

Spectrum cerebral venous occlusion involving the following venous territories:
- Venous sinuses
- Cortical veins
- Deep cerebral veins (internal cerebral veins, basal vein of Rosenthal, vein of Galen)
- Unusual forms of venous stasis/occlusion (e.g., high-flow angiopathy associated with AVM)

VENOUS SINUS THROMBOSIS

Nonspecific clinical presentation. High mortality due to secondary infarction/hemorrhage.

Causes

- Pregnancy/puerperium
- Dehydration (particularly in children)
- Infection (mastoiditis, otitis, meningitis)
- Tumors with dural invasion
- L-Asparaginase treatment
- Any hypercoagulable state
- Trauma
- Oral contraceptives
- Blood dyscrasias and coagulopathies

Imaging Features (Fig. 6-35)

General
- CTV is the imaging method of choice, followed by MRV
- Location: superior sagittal sinus > transverse sinus > sigmoid sinus > cavernous sinus

Primary (sinus occlusion)
- Clot in sinus is hyperdense on noncontrast CT and hypodense on contrast-enhanced CT.
- Dural enhancement of sinus margin: delta sign
- MRI
  - Bright sinus on T1W and T2W (depending on stage)
  - Absence of flow void
- Pearl: If bilateral thalamic infarcts or infarcts do not conform to an arterial territory, suspect venous thrombosis.

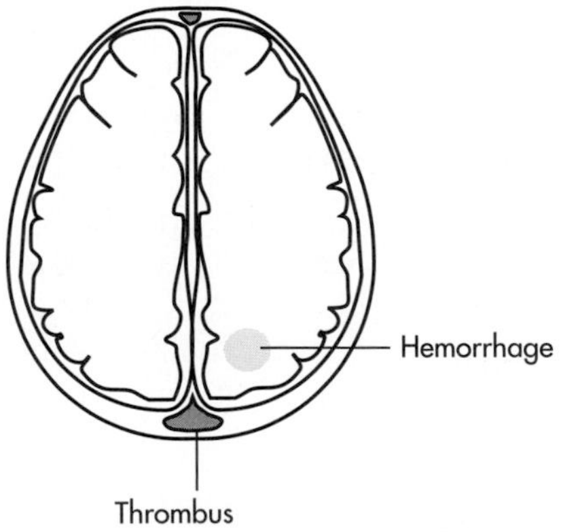

FIGURE 6-35

Secondary (effects of venous infarction)
- Subcortical infarctions, which may not follow arterial distribution
- Corticomedullary hemorrhage is common.

Trauma

GENERAL

CLASSIFICATION OF INJURY

Primary lesions (Fig. 6-36)
- Extraaxial hemorrhage
  - Subarachnoid hemorrhage
  - Subdural hematoma
  - Epidural hematoma
- Intraaxial lesions
  - Diffuse axonal injury
  - Cortical contusion
  - Deep cerebral gray matter injury
  - Brainstem injury
  - Intraventricular hemorrhage
- Fractures

Secondary lesions
- Brain herniations
- Traumatic ischemia
- Diffuse cerebral edema
- Hypoxic brain injury

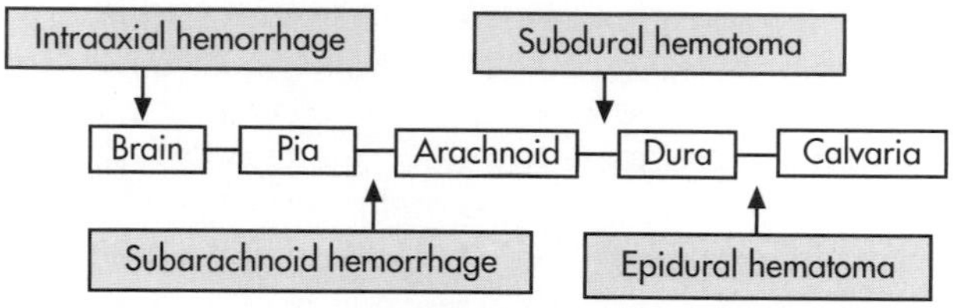

FIGURE 6-36

MECHANISM OF TRAUMATIC BRAIN INJURY (TBI)

Projectile (missile) injury
- Gunshot wounds
- Spear injury

Blunt injury (sudden deceleration or rotation)
- Automobile accident
- Fall from heights
- Direct blow

GLASGOW COMA SCALE

Minor head injury: score 13-15; moderate head injury: score 9-12; severe head injury: score ≤ 8.

Score

Eye opening
- Spontaneous = 4
- To sound = 3
- To pain = 2
- None = 1

Best motor response
- Obeys command = 6
- Localizes pain = 5
- Normal flexion = 4
- Abnormal flexion = 3
- Extension = 2
- None = 1

Best verbal response
- Oriented = 5
- Confused = 4
- Inappropriate words = 3
- Incomprehensible = 2
- None = 1

PRIMARY BRAIN INJURY

EPIDURAL HEMATOMA (EDH) (Fig. 6-37)

Types
- Arterial EDH, 90% (middle meningeal artery)
- Venous EDH, 10% (sinus laceration, meningeal vein)
  - Posterior fossa: transverse or sigmoid sinus laceration (common)
  - Parasagittal: tear of superior sagittal sinus

Large EDHs are neurosurgical emergencies. Small (<5 mm thick) EDHs adjacent to fractures are common and do not represent a clinical emergency. 95% of all EDHs are associated with fractures.

Imaging Features

Arterial EDH
- 95% are unilateral, temporoparietal
- Biconvex, lenticular shape
- Does not cross suture lines
- May cross dural reflections (falx tentorium), in contradistinction to subdural hematoma (SDH)
- Commonly associated with skull fractures
- Heterogeneity predicts rapid expansion of EDH, with areas of low density representing active bleeding.

Venous EDH
- More variable in shape (low-pressure bleed)
- Often requires delayed imaging because of delayed onset of bleed after trauma

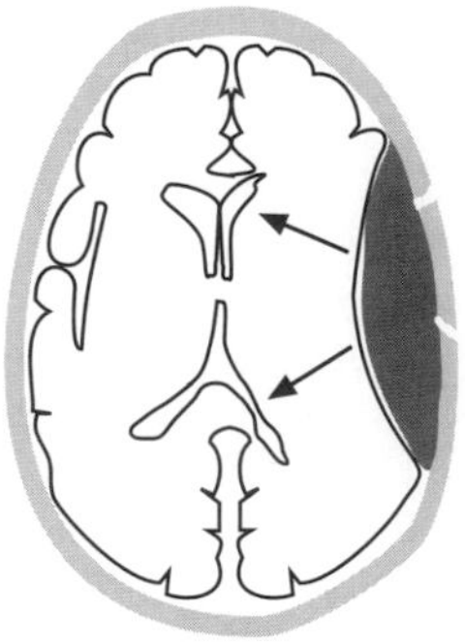

FIGURE 6-37

SUBDURAL HEMATOMA (SDH) (Fig. 6-38)

Caused by traumatic tear of bridging veins (rarely arteries). In contradistinction to EDH, there is no consistent relationship to the presence of skull fractures. Common in infants (child abuse; 80% are bilateral or interhemispheric) and elderly patients (20% are bilateral).

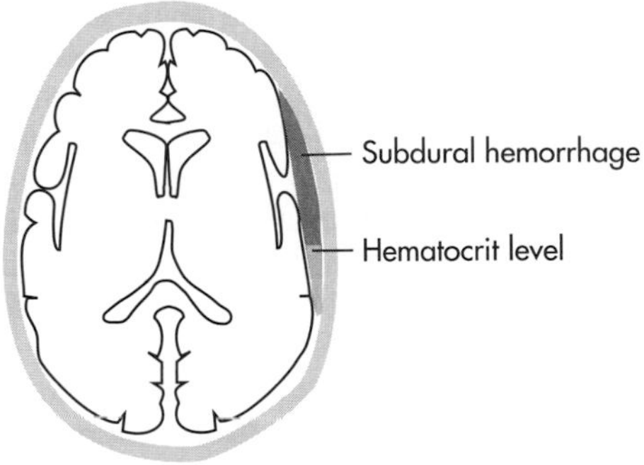

FIGURE 6-38

Imaging Features

Morphology of hematoma
- 95% supratentorial
- Crescentic shape along brain surface
- Crosses suture lines
- Does not cross dural reflections (falx, tentorium)
- MRI > CT particularly for:
  - Bilateral hematomas
  - Interhemispheric hematomas
  - Hematomas along tentorium
  - Subacute SDH

Other imaging findings
- Hematocrit level in subacute and early chronic hematomas
- Mass effect is present if SDH is large.

Acute SDH
- Hyperdense or mixed density

Subacute SDH (beyond 1 week)
- May be isointense and difficult to detect on CT
- Enhancing membrane and displaced cortical vessels (contrast administration is helpful)

Chronic SDH (beyond several weeks)
- Hypodense
- Mixed density with rebleeding
- Calcification, 1%

COMPARISON

	Epidural Hematoma	Subdural Hematoma
Incidence	In <5% of TBIs	In 10%-20% of TBIs
Cause	Fracture	Tear of cortical veins
Location	Between skull and dura	Between dura and arachnoid
Shape	Biconvex	Crescentic
CT	70% hyperintense, 30% isointense	Variable depending on age
T1W MRI	Isointense	

SUBDURAL HYGROMA

Accumulation of CSF in subdural space after traumatic arachnoid tear.

Imaging Features

- CSF density
- Does not extend into sulci
- Vessels cross through lesion.
- Main considerations in differential diagnosis:
  - Chronic SDH
  - Focal atrophy with widened subarachnoid space

DIFFUSE AXONAL INJURY (DAI)

DAI is due to axonal disruption from shearing forces of acceleration/deceleration. It is most commonly seen in severe head injury. Loss of consciousness occurs at time of injury.

Imaging Features (Fig. 6-39)

- Characteristic location of lesions:
  - Lobar gray matter (GM)/white matter (WM) junction
  - Corpus callosum
  - Dorsolateral brainstem
- Initial CT is often normal.
- Petechial hemorrhage develops later.
- Multifocal T2W bright lesions
- Susceptibility-sensitive gradient-echo sequences are most sensitive in detecting hemorrhagic shear injuries (acute or chronic) and can be helpful to document the extent of parenchymal injury (medicolegal implications) and to assess long-term prognosis (cognitive function) for patient and family.

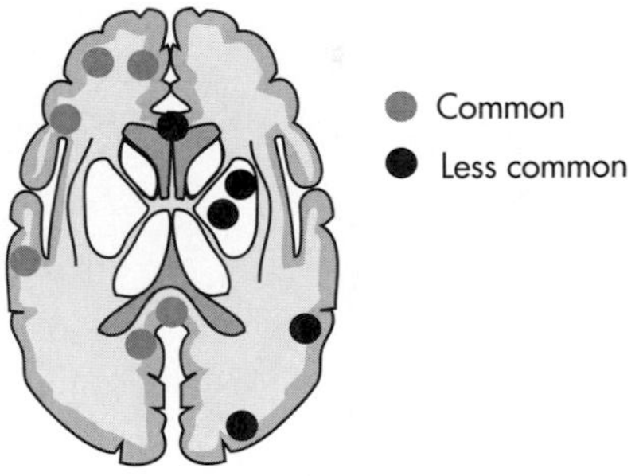

FIGURE 6-39

CORTICAL CONTUSION (Fig. 6-40)

Focal hemorrhage/edema in gyri secondary to brain impacting (or rotational forces) on bone or dura.

Imaging Features

- Characteristic location of lesions
  - Anterior temporal lobes, 50%
  - Inferior frontal lobes, 30%
  - Parasagittal hemisphere
  - Brainstem

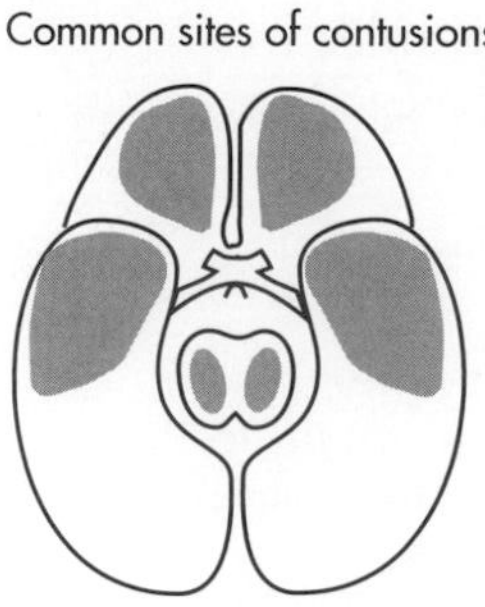

FIGURE 6-40

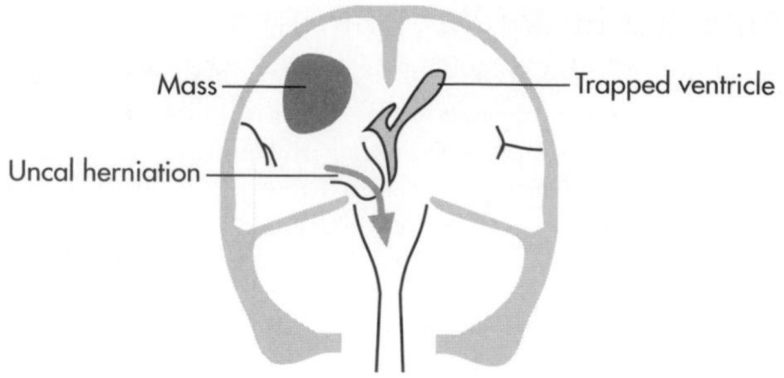

FIGURE 6-42

- Lesions evolve with time; delayed hemorrhage in 20%
- Initial CT is often normal; later on, low-density lesions with or without blood in them develop.
- Late: encephalomalacia

SECONDARY BRAIN INJURY

CEREBRAL HERNIATION (Fig. 6-41)

Mechanical displacement of brain secondary to mass effect. Herniation causes brain compression with neurologic dysfunction and vascular compromise (ischemia).

Types

- Subfalcine herniation
- Transtentorial (uncal) herniation
  - Descending
  - Ascending
- Tonsillar herniation

Imaging Features (Fig. 6-42)

Subfalcine herniation

- Cingulate gyrus slips under free margin of falx cerebri.
- Compression of ipsilateral ventricle
- Entrapment and enlargement of contralateral ventricle
- May result in ACA ischemia

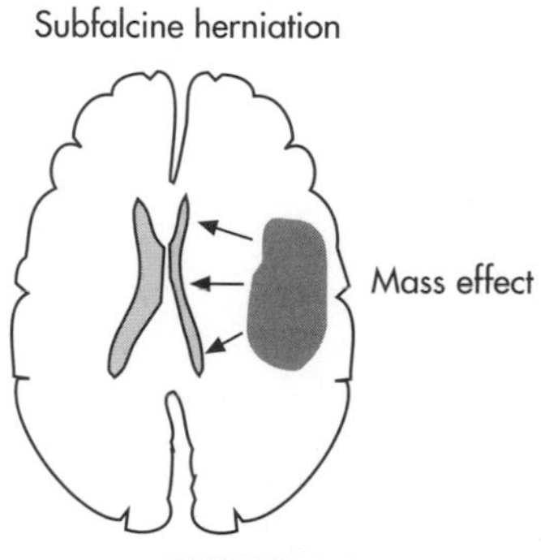

FIGURE 6-41

Descending transtentorial herniation (uncal) (Fig. 6-43)

- Uncus/parahippocampal gyrus displaced medially over tentorium
- Effacement of ipsilateral suprasellar cistern
- Enlargement of ipsilateral cerebellopontine angle (CPA) cistern
- Displaced midbrain impacts on contralateral tentorium.
  - Duret hemorrhage (anterior midbrain)
  - Kernohan's notch (mass effect on peduncle)
- PCA ischemia: occipital lobe, thalami, midbrain

Ascending transtentorial herniation

- Posterior fossa mass (i.e., hemorrhage) pushes cerebellum up through incisura.
- Loss of quadrigeminal cistern

Tonsillar herniation

- Cerebellar tonsils pushed inferiorly

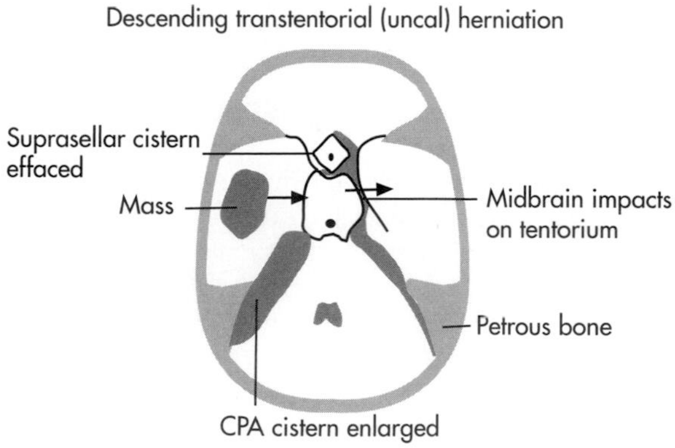

FIGURE 6-43

DIFFUSE CEREBRAL EDEMA

Massive brain swelling and intracranial hypertension secondary to dysfunction of cerebrovascular autoregulation and alterations of the blood-brain barrier. Underlying causes include ischemia and severe trauma. Ischemia may be primary (e.g., anoxic, drowning) or secondary to other brain injuries (e.g., large SDH) and may be followed by infarction. More common in children. High morbidity/mortality rates.

Imaging Features

- Findings develop 24 to 48 hours after injury.
- Effacement of sulci and basilar cisterns
  - Hint: the sulci near the vertex should always be present no matter how young the patient is, unless there is edema.
- Loss of perimesencephalic cisterns (hallmark)
- Loss of GM/WM interface (cerebral edema)
- White cerebellum sign: sparing of brainstem in comparison with hemispheres

ARTERIAL DISSECTION

Blood splits the media, creating a false lumen that dissects the arterial wall. Precise pathogenesis is unclear. Location: carotid artery (starts 2 cm distal to bulb and spares bulb) > ICA (petrous canal) > vertebral artery > others.

Underlying Causes

- Spontaneous or with minimal trauma (strain, sports)
- Trauma
- Hypertension
- Vasculopathy (FMD, Marfan syndrome)
- Migraine headache
- Drug abuse

Imaging Features

- CTA is preferred first study of choice—see intimal flap and caliber change
- MRI/MRA can also be performed.
  - T1W bright hematoma in vessel wall (sequence: T1W with fat saturation): must be interpreted in conjunction with MRA
  - MRA string sign
- Conventional angiography may establish the diagnosis and fully elucidate abnormal flow patterns.
- Long-segment fusiform narrowing of affected artery

Complications

- Thrombosis
- Emboli and infarction
- Intramural hemorrhage
- False aneurysm

CAROTID-CAVERNOUS SINUS FISTULA (CCF)

Abnormal connection between carotid artery and venous cavernous sinus. Ocular bruit.

Types

- Traumatic CCF (high flow)
- Spontaneous CCF
  - Rupture of aneurysm in its cavernous segment (less common; high flow)
  - Dural fistula (AVM) of the cavernous sinus (low flow); usually associated with venous thrombosis in older patients

Imaging Features

- Enlargement of ipsilateral cavernous sinus
- Enlargement of superior ophthalmic vein
- Proptosis
- Enlargement of extraocular muscles
- Angiographic embolization with detachable balloons (traumatic fistulas)

Neoplasm

GENERAL

CLASSIFICATION OF PRIMARY BRAIN TUMORS

Primary brain tumors constitute 70% of all intracranial mass lesions. The remaining 30% represent metastases.

- Gliomas (most common primary brain tumors)
  - Astrocytomas (most common glioma, 80%)
  - Oligodendroglioma, 5%-10%
  - Ependymoma
  - Choroid plexus tumors
- Meningeal and mesenchymal tumors
  - Meningioma, 20%
  - Hemangiopericytoma
  - Hemangioblastoma
- Neuronal and mixed glial/neuronal tumors
  - Ganglioglioma
  - Gangliocytoma
  - Dysembryoplastic neuroepithelial tumor (DNET)
  - Central neurocytoma
- Germ cell tumors
  - Germinoma
  - Teratoma
  - Mixed
- PNETs
  - Medulloblastoma
  - Retinoblastoma
  - Neuroblastoma
  - Pineoblastoma
  - Ependymoblastoma
- Pineal region tumors
- Pituitary tumors
- Nerve sheath tumor
  - Schwannoma
  - Neurofibroma
- Hematopoietic tumors
  - Lymphoma
  - Leukemia
- Tumor-like lesions
  - Hamartoma
  - Lipoma
  - Dermoid

Pearls

- Glial cells have high potential for abnormal growth. There are three types of glial cells: astrocytes (astrocytoma), oligodendrocytes (oligodendroglioma), and ependymal cells (ependymoma).
- Choroid plexus cells are modified ependymal cells, and tumors derived from them are therefore classified with gliomas.

LOCATION

The differentiation of intracerebral masses into intraaxial or extraaxial location is the first step in narrowing the differential diagnosis.

DETERMINING TUMOR LOCATION

Feature	Intraaxial Tumors	Extraaxial Tumors
Contiguity with bone or falx	Usually not	Yes
Bony changes	Usually not	Yes
CSF spaces, cisterns	Effaced	Often widened
Corticomedullary buckling	No	Yes
GM/WM junction	Destruction	Preservation
Vascular supply	Internal	External (dural branches)

FREQUENCY OF TUMORS (Fig. 6-44)

- Adults: metastases > hemangioblastoma > astrocytoma > lymphoma
- Children: astrocytoma > medulloblastoma > ependymoma

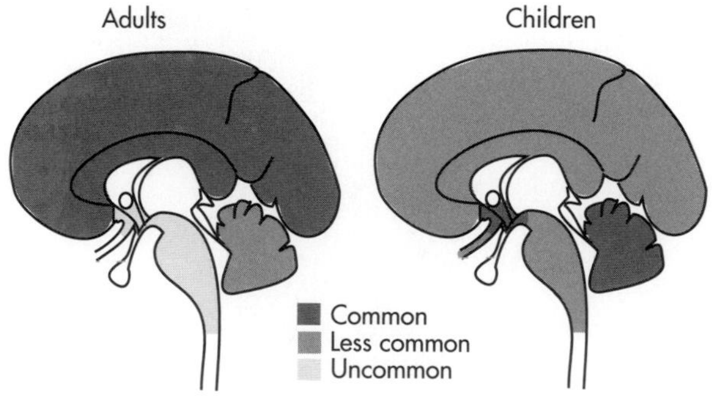

FIGURE 6-44

TUMOR EXTENT

Imaging modalities (see following table) are primarily used to diagnose the presence of a tumor. MR spectroscopy (see later discussion) and MR blood volume maps (high grade/hypervascular tumors — elevated blood volume) can differentiate with fairly good reliability between low-grade and high-grade tumors. This can be helpful in recognizing transformation of low-grade to high-grade tumor and in identifying high-grade components of otherwise lower-grade tumors to guide stereotactic biopsy. FDG-PET has no role in initial diagnosis, but may be useful for differentiating radiation necrosis. Once tumors are diagnosed, evaluation of tumor extension is important to:

- Determine site of stereotactic biopsy
- Plan surgical resection
- Plan radiation therapy

For many tumors, no imaging technique identifies their total extent. Gliomas often infiltrate the surrounding brain; microscopic tumor foci can be seen in areas that are totally normal on all MR sequences, including gadolinium-enhanced MRI.

TECHNIQUES FOR DETERMINING TUMOR EXTENT/ VIABILITY

	Determine True Extent of Tumor	Differentiate Viable versus Radiation Necrosis
Noncontrast CT	0	0
Contrast CT	++	0
T1W MRI	+	0
T2W MRI	+	0
Gd-DTPA MRI	+++	0
MRI blood volume/MRS	+	+
PET	+	++
MRI-guided biopsy	NA	+++

BRAIN EDEMA

TYPES OF BRAIN EDEMA

	Vasogenic	Cytotoxic
Cause	Tumor, trauma, hemorrhage,	Ischemia, infection
Mechanism	Blood-brain barrier defect	Na^+, K^+ pump defect
Substrate	Extracellular	Intracellular
Steroid response	Yes	No
Imaging	WM affected (cortical sparing)	GM and WM affected

On imaging it is difficult to identify between vasogenic and cytotoxic edema, and both can be present.

MASS EFFECT

Radiographic signs of mass effect:

- Sulcal effacement
- Ventricular compression
- Herniation
  - Subfalcine
  - Transtentorial (descending, ascending)
  - Tonsillar
- Hydrocephalus

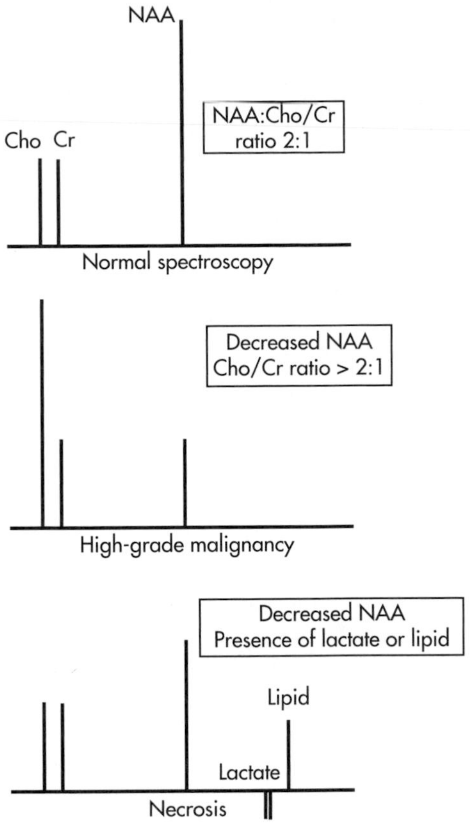

FIGURE 6-45

MR SPECTROSCOPY (Fig. 6-45)

- Useful metabolites
  Choline (Cho): 3.2 ppm
  - Cell turnover
  Creatine/phosphocreatine (Cr) ratio: 3.0 ppm
  N-acetyl aspartate (NAA): 2.0 ppm
  - Neuronal health
  Lipid: 1.25 ppm
  Lactate: usually an inverted doublet at 1.32 ppm
- Normal spectroscopy
  Cho/Cr ratio is near 1.
  NAA peak higher than either Cho or Cr (almost 2:1)
- Signs of high-grade malignancy
  High-grade neoplasm: Cho/Cr ratio > 2:1
  Decreased NAA peak: reflects neuronal loss
- Lactate or lipid peak: necrosis
  Often seen in posttreatment changes
- Sign suggesting metastasis over primary brain tumor: large lipid peak

GLIOMAS

ASTROCYTOMAS

Astrocytomas represent 80% of gliomas. Most tumors occur in cerebral hemispheres in adults. In children, posterior fossa and hypothalamus/optic chiasm are more common locations. The differentiation of types of astrocytoma is made histologically, not by imaging.

Classification

Fibrillary astrocytomas
- Astrocytoma, WHO grade I (AI)
- Astrocytoma, WHO grade II (AII)
- Anaplastic astrocytoma, WHO grade III (AA III)
- Glioblastoma multiforme, WHO grade IV (GBM IV)

Other astrocytomas
- Multicentric glioma (multiple lesions)
- Gliomatosis cerebri
- Juvenile pilocytic astrocytoma (in the cerebellum these lesions are typically cystic and have a mural nodule; tumors in the hypothalamus, optic chiasm, and optic nerves are usually solid and lobulated)
- Giant cell astrocytoma (in tuberous sclerosis): subependymal tumor growth along caudothalamic groove
- Xanthoastrocytoma
- Gliosarcoma

Associations

- Tuberous sclerosis
- Neurofibromatosis

OVERVIEW OF ASTROCYTOMAS

Parameter	Astrocytoma	Astrocytoma, Anaplastic	Glioblastoma Multiforme
Peak age	Younger patients	Middle-aged patients	50 years
Grade of malignancy	Low	High	High
Histology	Low-grade malignancy	Malignant	Very aggressive
Imaging features			
Multifocal	No	Occasionally	Occasionally
Enhancement (BBB)	±	++	+++
Edema*	Little or no	Abundant edema	Abundant edema
Calcification	Frequent	Less	Uncommon
Other			Hemorrhagic, necrotic

*The edema surrounding primary brain tumors tends to be less compared with metastatic tumors.

LOW-GRADE ASTROCYTOMA (AI, AII)

Represent 20% of all astrocytomas. Peak age: 20 to 40 years. Primary location is in the cerebral hemispheres.

Imaging Features

- Focal or diffuse mass lesions
- Calcification, 20%
- Hemorrhage and extensive edema are rare.
- Mild enhancement

ANAPLASTIC ASTROCYTOMA (AAIII)

Represent 30% of all astrocytomas. Peak age: 40 to 60 years. Primary location is in the cerebral hemispheres.

Imaging Features

- Heterogeneous mass
- Calcification uncommon
- Edema common
- Enhancement (reflects blood-brain barrier disruption [BBBD])

GLIOBLASTOMA MULTIFORME (GBM)

Most common primary brain tumor (represents 55% of astrocytomas). Age: >50 years. Primary location is in the hemispheres. Tumor may spread along the following routes:

- WM tracts
- Across midline via commissures (e.g., corpus callosum)
- Subependymal seeding of ventricles
- CSF seeding of subarachnoid space

Imaging Features

- Usually heterogeneous low-density mass (on CT)
- Strong contrast enhancement
- Hemorrhage, necrosis common
- Calcification is uncommon.
- Extensive vasogenic edema and mass effect
- Bihemispheric spread via corpus callosum or commissures (butterfly lesion)
- High-grade gliomas located peripherally can have a broad dural base and a dural tail, mimicking an extraaxial lesion.
- CSF seeding: leptomeningeal drop metastases

GLIOMATOSIS CEREBRI

Diffuse growth of glial neoplasm within brain. Usually there are no gross mass lesions but rather a diffuse infiltration of brain tissue by tumor cells. Age: 30 to 40 years. Rare. Poor prognosis (median survival <12 months). The MR appearances of gliomatosis may be similar to herpes encephalitis (T2 hyperintense), but the clinical presentations differ.

Imaging Features

- Gliomatosis predominantly causes expansion of WM but may also involve cortex.
- Usually nonenhancing lesions
- Late in disease, small foci of enhancement become visible.
- Leptomeningeal gliomatosis can mimic meningeal carcinomatosis or leptomeningeal spread of primary CNS tumors and cause marked enhancement.
- Important considerations in differential diagnosis for gliomatosis include:
    - Lymphomatosis cerebri
    - Multicentric glioma
    - Viral encephalitis
    - Vasculitis
    - Extensive active demyelinating disease such as acute disseminated encephalomyelitis (ADEM)

BRAINSTEM GLIOMA (Fig. 6-46)

Common pediatric posterior fossa tumor. Mean age: 10 years. 80% are anaplastic high grade; 20% are low grade and grow slowly. Locations: pons > midbrain > medulla.

Clinical Findings

- Cranial nerve VI and VII neuropathy
- Long tract signs
- Hydrocephalus

Imaging Features

- Enlargement of brainstem
- Posterior displacement of 4th ventricle (floor of the 4th ventricle should be in the middle of the Twining line: sella tuberculum—torcular)
- Encasement of basilar artery
- Cystic portions uncommon
- Hydrocephalus, 30%
- Enhancement occurs in 50% and is usually patchy and variable.
- Exophytic extension into basilar cisterns
- Focal tumors localized to the tectal plate are termed *tectal gliomas* and constitute a distinct

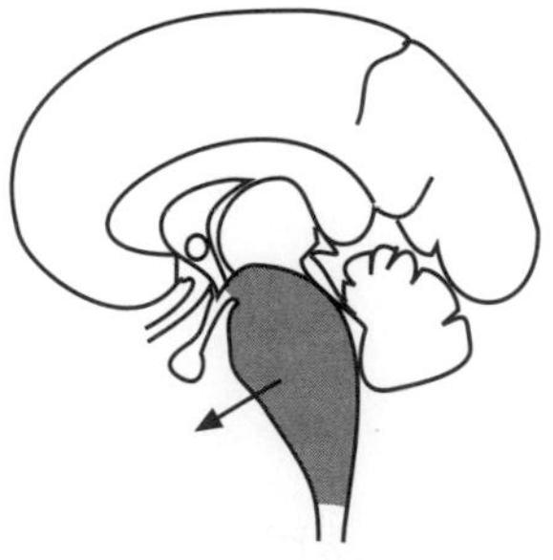

FIGURE 6-46

subset of brainstem gliomas. Because these tumors have good long-term prognosis and are located deep, they are usually followed without biopsy and with serial imaging to document stability. If a lesion extends beyond the tectum but is still confined to the midbrain, it is referred to as a *peritectal tumor* and carries a worse prognosis than that for purely tectal lesions. Peritectal tumors may be difficult to differentiate from pineal region tumors.

- Brainstem encephalitis may mimic a diffuse pontine glioma. Pontine gliomas have a worse prognosis when compared with tectal gliomas.

PILOCYTIC ASTROCYTOMA

Most common in children (represents 30% of pediatric gliomas); second most common pediatric brain tumor. Indolent and slow growing. Location: optic chiasm/hypothalamus > cerebellum > brainstem.

Imaging Features

- Cerebellar tumors are usually cystic and have intense mural enhancement.
- Calcification, 10%
- Optic chiasm/hypothalamic tumors are solid and enhance.
- Most in brainstem show little enhancement.

PLEOMORPHIC XANTHOASTROCYTOMA

Intraaxial mass in children and young adults, with predilection for temporal lobes Clinical: seizures, headaches

Imaging Features

- Cortically-based, often meningeal attachment
- Homogeneously enhancing
- May have cystic component

OLIGODENDROGLIOMA

Uncommon slow-growing glioma that usually presents as a large mass. Oligodendroglioma represents 5%-10% of primary brain tumors. Peak age: 30 to 50 years. "Pure" oligodendrogliomas are rare; usually tumors are "mixed" (astrocytoma/oligodendroglioma). The vast majority of tumors are located in cerebral hemispheres, the frontal lobe being the most common location. Intraventricular oligodendrogliomas are rare lesions. Many intraventricular lesions that were previously called oligodendrogliomas are now recognized as neurocytomas.

Imaging Features

- Commonly involve cortex
- Typically hypodense mass lesions
- Cysts are common.
- Large nodular, clumpy calcifications are typical, 80%
- Hemorrhage and necrosis are uncommon.
- Enhancement depends on degree of histologic differentiation.
- Pressure erosion of calvaria occurs occasionally.

EPENDYMAL TUMORS

The ependyma refers to a layer of ciliated cells lining the ventricular walls and the central canal. There are several histologic variants of ependymal tumors:

- Ependymoma (children)
- Subependymoma (older patients)
- Anaplastic ependymoma
- Myxopapillary ependymoma of filum terminale
- Ependymoblastoma (PNET)

EPENDYMOMA

Slow-growing tumor of ependymal lining cells, usually located in or adjacent to ventricles within the parenchyma:

- 4th ventricle (70%): more common in children
- Lateral ventricle or periventricular parenchymal (30%): more common in adults
  - Most common in children. Age: 1 to 5 years. Spinal ependymomas are associated with neurofibromatosis type 2 (NF2).

Imaging Features

- Growth pattern depends on location:
  - Supratentorial: tumors grow outside ventricle (i.e., resembles astrocytoma); remember to include ependymoma in the differential diagnosis of a supratentorial parenchymal mass lesion, particularly in a child.
  - Infratentorial: tumors grow inside 4th ventricle and extrude through foramen of Luschka into CPA and cisterna magna; this appearance is characteristic ("plastic ependymoma") and often helps to differentiate an ependymoma from a medulloblastoma.
- Hydrocephalus is virtually always present when in posterior fossa.
- Fine calcifications, 50%
- Cystic areas, 50%
- Hemorrhage

Differential Diagnosis for Supratentorial Ependymoma

- PNET: often peripheral and has more edema
- Malignant rhabdoid tumor: generally seen in infants and young children
- Glioblastoma multiforme: typically significant surrounding edema
- Anaplastic astrocytoma: may be indistinguishable but less likely to be in proximity of ventricular surface
- Metastatic disease: often multifocal with significant surrounding edema

SUBEPENDYMOMA

- Asymptomatic fourth ventricular tumor found in elderly males
- 66% arise in the fourth ventricle; 33% in lateral ventricles
- Unlike ependymomas, these tumors tend not to seed the subarachnoid space.
- Lesions often are multiple.

DIFFERENTIAL DIAGNOSIS OF LATERAL VENTRICULAR MASS

Location	Adult	Child
Atrium	Meningioma	CP papilloma
	Metastases	CP carcinoma
	CP xanthogranuloma	Ependymoma
Body	Subependymoma	Astrocytoma
	Oligodendroglioma	PNET
	Central neurocytoma	Teratoma
	Astrocytoma	CP papilloma
Foramen of Monro	Giant cell astrocytoma	Giant cell astrocytoma

CP, choroid plexus.

CHOROID PLEXUS PAPILLOMA/CARCINOMA

Rare tumors that arise from epithelium of choroid plexus. Peak age: <5 years (85%). 90% represent choroid plexus papillomas, 10% choroid plexus carcinomas. Typical locations include:

- Trigone of lateral ventricles (children)
- 4th ventricle and CPA (adults)
- Drop metastases to spinal canal

Imaging Features

- Intraventricular mass
- Ventricular dilatation due to CSF overproduction or obstruction
- Intense contrast enhancement
- Calcifications, 25%
- Supratentorial tumors are supplied by anterior and posterior choroidal arteries.
- Complications:
  - Hydrocephalus
  - Drop metastases to spinal dural space
- Papillomas and carcinomas are radiographically indistinguishable; both may invade brain and disseminate via CSF.

MENINGEAL AND MESENCHYMAL TUMORS

MENINGIOMA

Tumor originates from arachnoid cap cells. Age: 40 to 60 years. Three times more common in females. Represents 20% of all brain tumors. Meningiomas are uncommon in children and if present are commonly associated with NF2. 90% are supratentorial.

Classification

- Typical "benign" meningioma, 93%
- Atypical meningioma, 5%
- Anaplastic (malignant) meningioma, 1%-2%

Location

- Cerebral convexity along falx and lateral to it, 45%
- Sphenoid ridge, 20%
- Juxtasellar, 10%
- Olfactory groove, 10%
- Posterior fossa clivus, 10%
- Tentorium
- Uncommon locations:
  - Lateral ventricles (pediatric age group)
  - Optic nerve sheath (adult females)
- <1% of meningiomas may arise extradurally. These sites include intradiploic space, outer table of skull, skin, paranasal sinuses, parotid gland, and parapharyngeal space.

Imaging Features (Fig. 6-47)

CT signal intensity

- Hyperdense (75%) or isodense (25%) on noncontrast CT
- Strong, homogeneous enhancement, 90% (hallmark)
- Similar signal intensity as normal falx on enhanced and nonenhanced CT
- Calcifications, 20%
- Cystic areas, 15%

Morphology

- Round, unilobulated, sharp margin (most common)
- En plaque, pancake spread along dura (rare)
- Dural tail: extension of tumor or dural reaction along a dural surface
- Edema is absent in 40% because of the slow growth.

Bony abnormalities, 20% (Fig. 6-48)

- No changes (common)

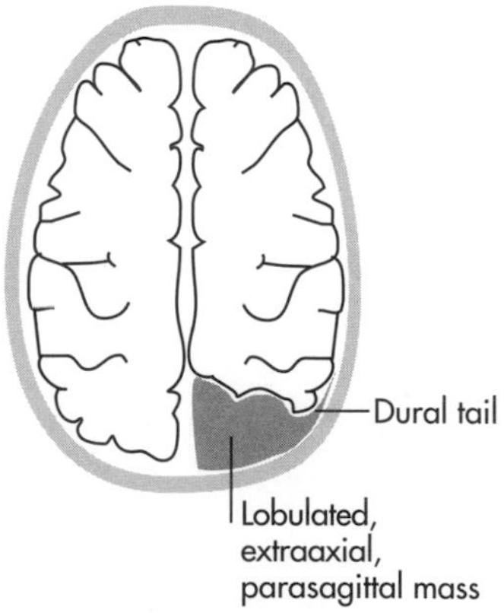

FIGURE 6-47

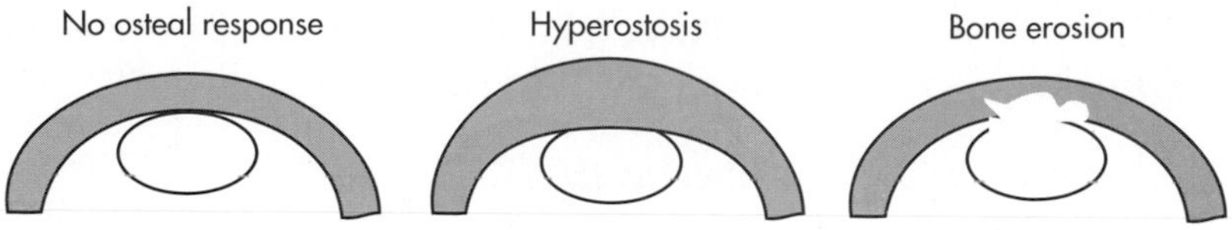

FIGURE 6-48

- Hyperostosis (common)
- Bone erosion (rare; if present may indicate malignant meningioma)
- Pneumosinus dilatans

MRI
- Tumors are typically isointense with GM.
- Strong gadolinium enhancement
- Best technique for detecting dural tail
- Dural tail (60%) is suggestive but not specific for meningioma.
- Increased vascular flow voids

Angiography (Fig. 6-49)
- Spokewheel appearance
- Dense venous filling
- Persistent tumor blush ("comes early and stays late")
- Well-demarcated margins
- Dural vascular supply

Atypical meningiomas (15% of all meningiomas)
- Necrosis causing nonhomogeneous enhancement, 15%
- Hemorrhage
- Peripheral low-density zones (trapped CSF in arachnoid cysts)

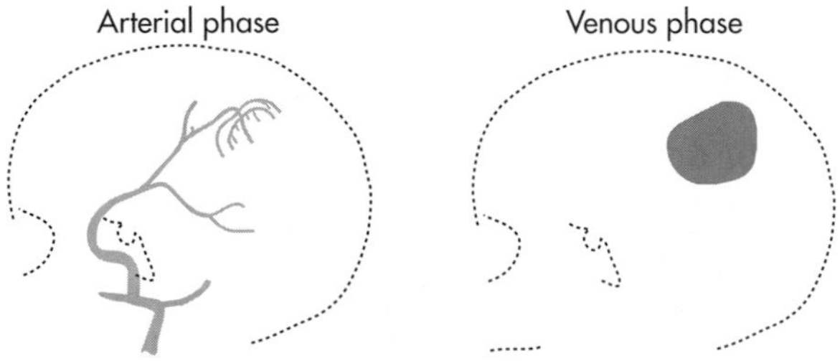

FIGURE 6-49

MALIGNANT MENINGIOMA

Presently there are no clear radiologic signs to predict malignancy in a meningioma other than:
- Rapid growth
- Extensive brain or bone invasion
- Bright on T2W imaging relative to brain (indicating meningothelial, angioblastic, hemangiopericytic elements as opposed to T2W hypointense benign meningiomas containing primarily calcified or fibrous elements)

Histologically, malignant meningiomas include the following cell types:
- Hemangiopericytoma
- Malignant fibrous histiocytoma (MFH)
- Papillary meningioma
- "Benign" metastasizing meningioma

HEMANGIOBLASTOMA

Hemangioblastomas are benign neoplasms of endothelial origin. Overall, hemangioblastomas are uncommon; however, they represent the most common primary cerebellar tumor in adult patients with VHL syndrome (hemangioblastomas occur in 35%-60% of VHL patients; the incidence of VHL syndrome in hemangioblastoma patients is 10%-20%). Multiple hemangioblastomas are pathognomonic for VHL syndrome: location: cerebellum > spinal cord (may be intramedullary or extramedullary) > medulla (area postrema).

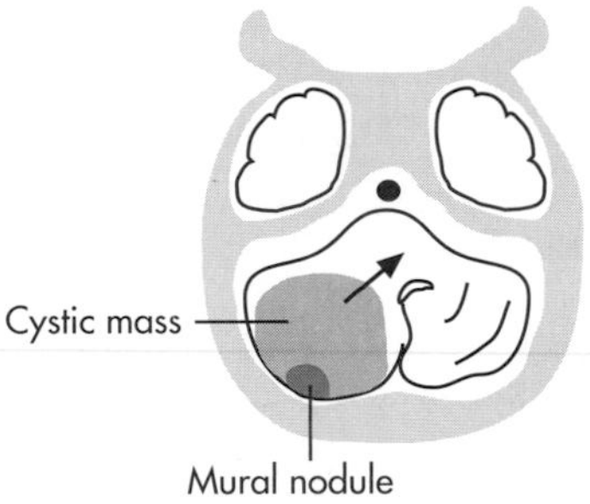

FIGURE 6-50

Cerebellar Hemangioblastoma, 80%

The tumor consists of a pial (mural) nodule with associated cysts. During surgery the nodule (not only the cystic contents) has to be removed entirely, otherwise tumor will recur. Angiography may be performed before surgery to demonstrate vascular supply. Three different appearances:
- Cystic lesion with an enhancing mural nodule, 75%. The cyst is generally not neoplastic and does not need to be resected unless there is evidence of tumor involvement (enhancement of cyst wall) (Fig. 6-50).
- Solid enhancing neoplasm, 10%
- Enhancing lesion with multiple cystic areas, 15%

Spinal Hemangioblastoma, 10%

Commonly located on posterior aspect of spinal cord. 70% are associated with syringomyelia or cystic component. Contrast-enhanced MRI optimizes visualization of the small mural nodule.

NEURONAL AND MIXED GLIAL/NEURONAL TUMORS

GANGLIOGLIOMA/GANGLIONEUROMA

Benign neoplasm of children/young adults with glial and neural elements. Low grade and slow growing.

- Clinical presentations: long-standing seizures
- Location: temporal > frontal > parietal
- Nonspecific cystic mass, often calcified, with variable enhancement.
  - May occasionally erode the inner table of the adjacent calvaria.
  - May metastasize throughout CSF pathways, with a pattern of multiple small subarachnoid cysts. In the cerebellum a ganglioglioma may mimic Lhermitte-Duclos disease.

DYSEMBRYOPLASTIC NEUROEPITHELIAL TUMOR (DNET)

Newly recognized tumor with distinctive histological features. Like ganglioglioma, DNET is strongly associated with epilepsy. Occurs in younger patients.

- A well-circumscribed, often mixed cystic and solid cortically based lesion in a patient with long-standing seizure should bring DNET to mind.
- FLAIR imaging is helpful in identifying small peripheral lesions that are similar to CSF signal intensity.
- Temporal lobe location is common (>60%), and the lesion often involves or lies close to mesial temporal structures; other locations include frontal lobe, followed by parietal and/or occipital lobes.

CENTRAL NEUROCYTOMA

Newly recognized tumor. Usually located in lateral ventricle, attached to ventricular wall. Calcification is common; mild to moderate enhancement. The tumor has feathery appearance on CT and MRI due to multiple cysts. It is usually attached to the septum pellucidum when arising from the lateral ventricle.

PRIMITIVE NEUROECTODERMAL TUMOR (PNET)

Undifferentiated aggressive tumors that arise from multipotent embryonic neuroepithelial cells. They are common in children. Can be seen in the sella/supersellar region — check for "trilateral retinoblastomas"

Types

- Medulloblastoma (infratentorial PNET)
- Primary cerebral neuroblastoma (supratentorial PNET)
- Retinoblastoma
- Pineoblastoma
- Ependymoblastoma

Common imaging features include intense contrast enhancement, dense cell packing, and aggressive growth.

MEDULLOBLASTOMA

PNET originating from roof of the 4th ventricle. Most common in childhood. Peak age: 2 to 8 years. Radiosensitive but metastasizes early via CSF. Associated with certain syndromes such as Gorlin syndrome (basal cell nevi, odontogenic keratocysts, falx calcification) or Turcot syndrome (colonic polyps and CNS malignancy).

Imaging Features (Fig. 6-51)

- Typically intense and homogeneous enhancement (hallmark)
- Cerebellar midline mass in 80%, lateral cerebellum 20%
- Dense cell packing (small cell tumor)
  - Hyperdense on noncontrast CT
  - May be intermediate signal intensity on T2W
- Hydrocephalus, 90%
- Rapid growth into cerebellar hemisphere, brainstem, and spine
- CSF seeding to spinal cord and meninges, 30%
- Systemic metastases can occur and appear as sclerotic lesions in bone. Metastases to abdominal cavity may occur via a ventriculoperitoneal (VP) shunt.
- Calcifications, 10%
- Atypical appearance and lateral cerebellar location are more common in older children.
- Strong enhancement

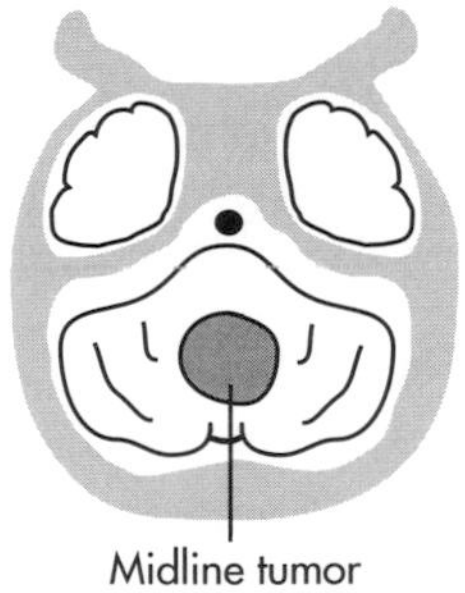

FIGURE 6-51

PRIMARY CEREBRAL NEUROBLASTOMA

Rare, malignant tumor. 80% in first decade.

Imaging Features

- Large supratentorial mass
- Necrosis, hemorrhage cyst formation common
- Variable enhancement (neovascularity)

DIFFERENTIATION OF CPA TUMORS

	Meningioma	Schwannoma	Epidermoid
Epicenter	Dural based	IAC	CPA
CT density	Hyperdense/isodense	Isodense	Hypodense
Calcification	Frequent	None	Occasional
Porus acusticus/IAC	Normal	Widened	Normal
T2W signal intensity relative GM	50% isodense	Hyperintense	Hyperintense
Enhancement	Dense	Dense	None

DYSPLASTIC GANGLIOCYTOMA OF CEREBELLUM (LHERMITTE DUCLOS)

Infiltrative masslike lesion, probably hamartomatous. FLAIR hyperintense with characteristic linear striations, no enhancement. Clinical: adults in 3rd decade, ataxia, Cowden syndrome.

NERVE SHEATH TUMORS

SCHWANNOMA (Fig. 6-52)

Benign tumor of Schwann cell origin. Almost all intracranial schwannomas are related to cranial nerves. 90% are solitary; multiple schwannomas are commonly associated with NF2. 90% of intracranial schwannomas are located in the CPA originating from cranial nerve VIII (acoustic neuroma). Locations include:

- CPA (CN VIII, most commonly from superior portion of vestibular nerve)
- Trigeminal nerve (CN V)
- Other intracranial sites (rare)
  - Intratemporal (CN VII)
  - Jugular foramen/bulb (CNs IX, X, XI)
- Spinal cord schwannoma
- Peripheral nerve schwannoma
- Intracerebral schwannoma (very rare)

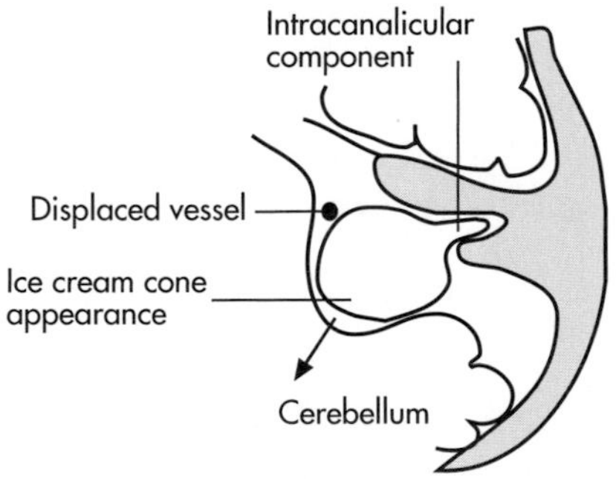

FIGURE 6-52

Imaging Features

Mass
- >2 mm difference between left and right IAC
- Erosion and flaring of IAC
- IAC >8 mm
- Extension into CPA (path of least resistance): ice cream cone appearance of extracanalicular portion

MRI/CT
- Isodense by CT
- MRI is more sensitive than CT.
- Dense enhancement: homogeneous if small; heterogeneous if large
- Gd-DTPA administration is necessary to detect small or intracanalicular tumors.
- May contain cystic degenerative areas
- Marginal arachnoid cysts
- Hyperintense on T2W

SUMMARY OF COMMON MASSES BY LOCATION

Location	Mass
Cisterna	Epidermoid cyst
	Dermoid cyst
	Lipoma
	Neuroenteric cyst
	Neuroepithelial cyst
Arteries	Aneurysm
	Ectasia
Skull base	Cholesterol granuloma
	Paraganglioma
	Apicitis
	Chordoma
	Chondroma
	Endolymphatic sac tumor
	Pituitary adenoma
Meninges	Meningioma
	Arachnoid cyst
	Metastases
Nerves	Cranial nerve V to XII schwannomas
Cerebellum	Glioma
Ventricle	Lymphoma
	Ependymoma
	Papilloma
	Hemangioblastoma
	Medulloblastoma
	DNET

Pearls

- Bilateral acoustic neuromas are pathognomonic for NF2.
- Although 90% of CPA schwannomas are of cranial nerve VIII origin, hearing loss is the most common presentation; hence, they are called *acoustic neuromas.*
- Meningiomas rarely extend into IAC but do not expand the IAC.

NEUROFIBROMA

Plexiform neurofibromas are unique to neurofibromatosis type 1 (NF1). They do not occur primarily in the cranial cavity but may extend into it from posterior ganglia or as an extension of peripheral tumors.

DIFFERENTIATION BETWEEN SCHWANNOMA AND NEUROFIBROMA

	Schwannoma	Neurofibroma
Origin	Schwann cells	Schwann cells and fibroblasts
Association	NF2	NF1
Incidence	Common	Uncommon
Location	CN VIII > other CN	Cutaneous and spinal nerves
Malignant degeneration	No	5%-10%
Growth	Focal	Infiltrating
Enhancement	+++	++/heterogeneous
T1W	70% hypointense, 30% isointense	Isointense with muscle
T2W	Hyperintense	Hyperintense

PINEAL REGION TUMORS (Fig. 6-53)

The pineal gland contributes to the circadian mechanism. Most pineal tumors occur in children and young adults. Patients may present with abnormal eye movement due to compression of the tectal plate (Parinaud syndrome: inability to gaze upward) or hydrocephalus from compression of cerebral aqueduct.

Germ cell tumors, >50%
- Germinoma (most common tumor): equivalent to seminoma in testes and dysgerminoma in ovary
- Teratoma
- Embryonal cell carcinoma
- Choriocarcinoma

Pineal cell tumors, 25%
- Pineocytoma (benign)
- Pinealoblastoma (highly malignant, PNET)

Glioma

Other tumors
- Meningioma
- Metastases
- Epidermoid/dermoid
- Arachnoid cyst
- Pineal cyst

TUMOR MARKERS

Tumor	HCG	AFP
Germinoma	–	–
Embryonal cell carcinoma	+	+
Choriocarcinoma	+	–
Yolk sac tumor	–	+

GERMINOMA

- Pineal region is most common location
- Males > females, age 10 to 30 years
- Sharply circumscribed enlargement of pineal gland
- Hyperdense on noncontrast CT/isodense on T2W (dense cell packing)
- Homogeneous intense enhancement
- Central calcification due to pineal engulfment (rare)
- May spread to ventricles and subarachnoid space via CSF
- In females, more commonly located in suprasellar location
- Sensitive to radiation therapy
- Germinomas located in the basal ganglia are often larger and more heterogeneous than those in pineal region.

TERATOMA

- Almost exclusively in male children
- Heterogeneous on CT and MRI
- Presence of fat and calcification is diagnostically helpful
- Little to no enhancement

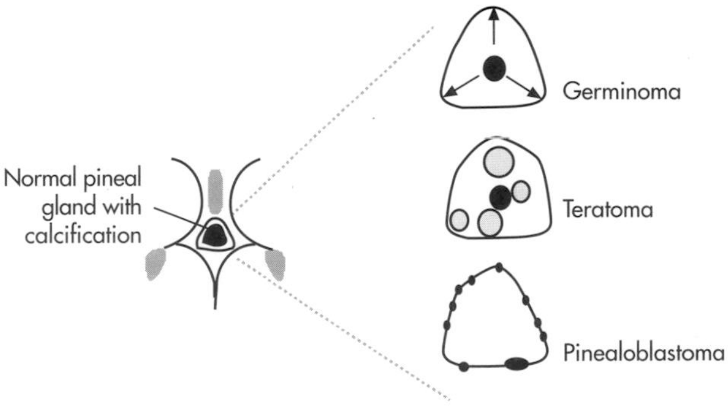

FIGURE 6-53

PINEALOBLASTOMA

- Highly malignant PNET
- In patients with trilateral retinoblastoma, pineoblastomas may develop in patients with familial and or bilateral retinoblastoma.
- "Exploded calcifications" along outside of mass

- Dense enhancement
- CSF dissemination

PINEOCYTOMA

- No male predilection
- Older age group, mean age 35 years
- Slow growing; dissemination is uncommon
- No helpful imaging features; cannot be distinguished by imaging features from a pineoblastoma

TUMOR-LIKE LESIONS

EPIDERMOID/DERMOID (Fig. 6-54)

Congenital tumor that arises from ectodermal elements in the neural tube before its closure. The concept of mesodermal elements within dermoids is probably incorrect; dermoids are of ectodermal origin.

SYNOPSIS

	Epidermoid	Dermoid
Content	Squamous epithelium, keratin, cholesterol	Also has dermal appendages (hair, sebaceous fat, sweat glands)
Location	Off midline	Midline
	CPA most common	Spinal canal most common
	Parasellar, middle fossa	Parasellar, posterior fossa
	Intraventricular, diploic space (rare)	
Rupture	Rare	Common (chemical meningitis)
Age	Mean 40 years	Younger adults
CT density	CSF density	May have fat
Calcification	Uncommon	Common
Enhancement	Occasional peripherally	None
MRI	CSF-like signal	Proteinaceous fluid
Other	5-10 times more common than dermoids	

DWI allows differentiation of epidermoid and arachnoid cysts. The ADC of an epidermoid cyst is significantly lower than that of an arachnoid cyst; therefore, epidermoid cysts have high-signal intensity on DWI, whereas arachnoid cysts, like CSF, have very low-signal intensity. Dermoid: may contain fat-fluid levels; rupture may produce headaches with scattered foci of fat in CSF spaces.

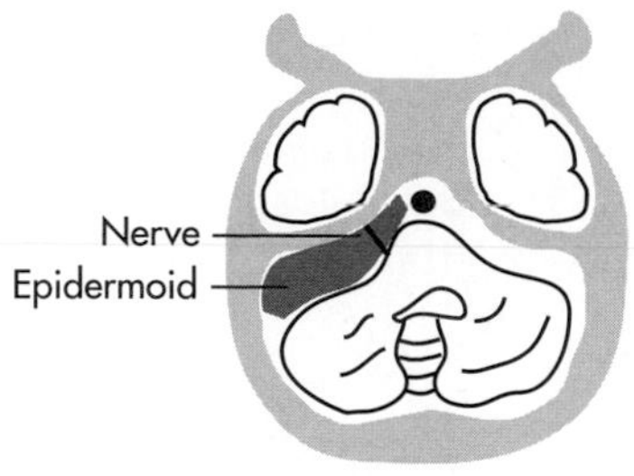

FIGURE 6-54

HYPOTHALAMIC (TUBER CINEREUM) HAMARTOMA

Mature, disorganized ectopic tissue. Two clinical presentations:

- Isosexual, precocious puberty
- Associated with Pallister-Hall syndrome—nonspecific facial anomalies, polydactyly imperforate anus, hypothalamic hamartoma
- No precocious puberty, gelastic seizures, intellectual impairment

Imaging Features

- CT: isodense, no enhancement (in contrast with hypothalamic gliomas)
- MRI T1W: similar signal intensity as GM, T2W: hyperintense
- The floor of the third ventricle should be smooth from infundibulum to mammillary bodies. Any nodularity should raise suspicion for a hamartoma in the right clinical setting.

LIPOMA

Asymptomatic nonneoplastic tissue (malformation, not a true tumor). 50% are associated with other brain malformations. Location: midline 90%; 50% are pericallosal.

Imaging Features

- Fat density on CT (-50 to -100 HU)
- Calcification
- Avascular, but callosal vessels may course through lesion
- MRI
    - Chemical shift artifact
    - Fat suppression sequences helpful
    - T1W and T2W hypointense relative to brain on conventional spin-echo sequences. On fast spin-echo sequences fat appears hyperintense.

HEMATOPOIETIC TUMORS

CENTRAL NERVOUS SYSTEM LYMPHOMA (Fig. 6-55)

Types

Primary lymphoma (1% of brain tumors), usually B-cell non-Hodgkin lymphoma (NHL); high incidence in immunocompromised hosts

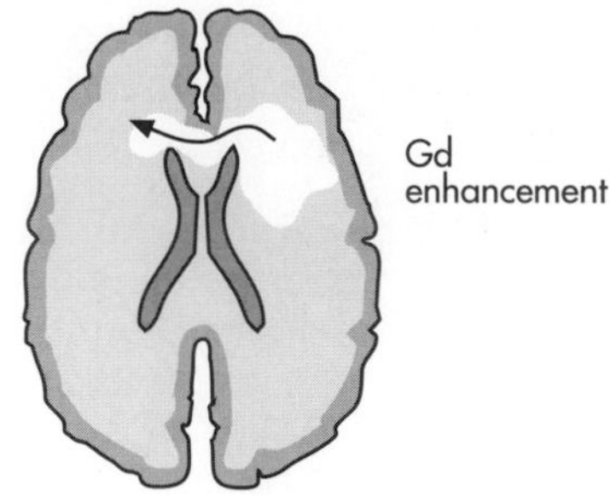

FIGURE 6-55

- Basal ganglia, 50%
- Periventricular deep WM
- Corpus callosum

Secondary lymphoma (15% in patients with systemic lymphoma)

- Leptomeningeal spread

Imaging Features

Growth patterns

- Solitary or multiple masses in deep GM and WM, predominantly periventricular
- Diffuse meningeal or paraventricular ependymal involvement
- Diffusely infiltrative (mimics WM disease or gliomatosis cerebri)
- Spread along VR perivascular spaces
- Intraspinal

Signal characteristics

- Intrinsic hyperdensity, on noncontrast CT, with less mass effect than the size of the lesion
- Primary CNS lymphoma (PCNSL) often involves the corpus callosum and mimics butterfly glioma.
- Location in deep gray nuclei with extension to ependymal surfaces
- PCNSL rarely involves spine, whereas secondary CNS involvement with systemic lymphoma commonly involves both brain (usually extraaxial) and spine.
- Isointense to GM on T2W (dense cell packing) or hyperintense
- Enhancement patterns
  - Dense homogeneous enhancement is most common.
  - Ringlike (central necrosis): more common in AIDS
  - Meningeal enhancement in secondary lymphoma
  - Fine feathery enhancement along VR spaces is typical.
- Calcification, hemorrhage, necrosis: multiple and large areas are typical in AIDS
- The tumor is very radiosensitive, and lesion may disappear after a short course of steroids. This may render the biopsy nondiagnostic.

AIDS-RELATED PRIMARY CNS LYMPHOMA

A solitary mass lesion in an AIDS patient is more often due to lymphoma than to infection. It may be difficult to distinguish PCNSL from toxoplasmosis in an AIDS patient with single- or multiple-enhancing lesions.

DIFFERENTIATION BETWEEN LYMPHOMA AND TOXOPLASMOSIS

	Lymphoma	Toxoplasmosis
Single lesion	+	±
Deep gray nuclear involvement	+	+
Hyperdense on noncontrast CT	++	±
Eccentric enhancing nodule	–	+
Callosal involvement	++	Rare
Ependymal spread	++	–
Subarachnoid spread	++	–
Thallium/FDG PET scanning	++	–
Spectroscopy	Elevated choline	Elevated lipid/lactate

METASTASES

Metastases account for 30% of intracerebral tumors. Location in order of frequency: junction GM and WM (most common) > deep parenchymal structures (common) > brainstem (uncommon). Metastases also occur in dura, leptomeninges, and calvaria. The most common primary lesions are:

- Bronchogenic carcinoma, 50%
- Breast, 20%
- Colon, rectum, 15%
- Kidney, 10%
- Melanoma, 10%

Imaging Features

- Gadolinium-enhanced MRI is the most sensitive imaging study. Triple dose Gd-DTPA or magnetization-transfer increases sensitivity of lesion detection.
- 80% of lesions are multiple.
- Most metastases are T2W bright and enhance.
- Some metastases may be T2W isointense/hypointense relative to:
  - Hemorrhage (e.g., renal cell carcinoma)
  - Mucin (e.g., gastrointestinal adenocarcinoma)
  - Dense cell packing (e.g., germ cell tumor)

- Vasogenic edema is common and greater than for primary tumors

Pearls

- Metastases and lymphoma are commonly multiple; gliomas are rarely multiple.
- A solitary enhancing brain tumor has a 50% chance of being a metastasis.
- Limbic encephalitis is a paraneoplastic syndrome associated with small cell lung cancer. MRI may demonstrate T2-hyperintensity in temporal lobes bilaterally; lesions which may enhance.

CARCINOMATOUS MENINGITIS

Leptomeningeal metastases are more common than dural metastases, although the two may coexist.

- Common primary neoplasms that cause carcinomatous meningitis include breast, lung, and skin (melanoma).
- MRI is more sensitive than CT for detection.
- Leptomeninges insinuate into cerebral sulci, which is a sign that helps distinguish a leptomeningeal process from a dural one.
- Subarachnoid tumor may be detected early by careful examination of cisternal segment of CN V and intracanalicular segment of CNs VII and VIII.

CYSTIC LESIONS

Various types of nonneoplastic, noninflammatory cysts are found intracranially:

- Arachnoid cyst
- Colloid cyst
- Rathke's cleft cyst
- Pineal cyst
- Neuroepithelial cyst
- Enterogenous cyst
- Intraparenchymal cyst

ARACHNOID CYST (LEPTOMENINGEAL CYST) (Fig. 6-56)

Not a true neoplasm; probably arises from duplication or splitting of the arachnoid membrane (meningeal maldevelopment). 75% occur in children. Location:

- Middle cranial fossa (most common), 40%
- Suprasellar, quadrigeminal cisterns, 10%
- Posterior fossa, 50%
- CPA
- Cisterna magna

Imaging Features

- Extraaxial mass with CSF density (CT) and intensity (MRI)
- Slow enlargement with compression of subjacent parenchyma
- No communication with ventricles
- Pressure erosion of calvaria

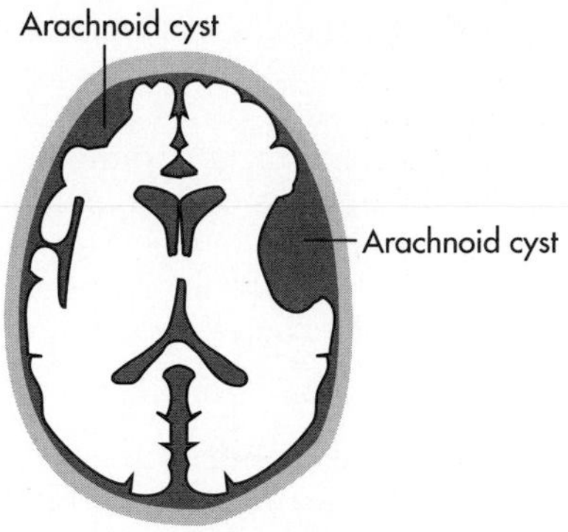

FIGURE 6-56

DIFFERENTIATION BETWEEN ARACHNOID CYST AND EPIDERMOID

	Arachnoid Cyst	Epidermoid
Signal intensity	Isointense to CSF on T1W Isointense to CSF on PDW Isointense to CSF on T2W	Mildly hyperintense to CSF Hyperintense to CSF on PDW Isointense to CSF on T2W
Enhancement	No	No
Margin of lesion	Smooth	Irregular
Effect on adjacent structures	Displaces	Engulfs, insinuates
Pulsation artifact	Present	Absent
DWI	Follows CSF	Restricted diffusion
FLAIR imaging	Suppresses like CSF	Hyperintense to CSF
Calcification	No	May occur

COLLOID CYST (Fig. 6-57)

Cyst arises in foramen of Monro region. Peak age: adults.

Clinical Findings

- Intermittent headaches and ataxia from intermittent obstructive hydrocephalus.

Imaging Features

- Typical location anterior to 3rd ventricle/foramen of Monro
- CT density: hyperdense 70%, hypodense (30%)

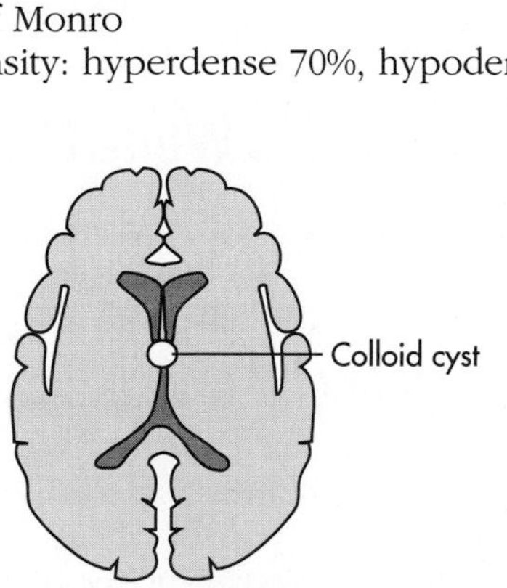

FIGURE 6-57

- MRI: variable signal intensity depending on paramagnetic content.
  - T1W hyperintense
  - T2W hypointense (most common)
- In differential diagnosis of lesions in foramen of Monro
- Subependymoma (less dense on noncontrast CT)
- Astrocytoma (isointense or hypointense on T1W)
- Lymphoma
- Meningioma
- Choroid plexus papilloma
- Tumefactive intraventricular hemorrhage
- Intraventricular neurocysticercosis

RATHKE'S CLEFT CYST

Cyst arises from embryologic remnant of Rathke's pouch (rostral outpouching during 4th week of embryogenesis; the precursor of anterior lobe and pars intermedia of pituitary gland).

Imaging Features

- Combined intrasellar and suprasellar location, 70%; purely intrasellar location, 20%
- Hypodense by CT, rim enhancement possible
- Hyperintense relative to brain on T1W imaging, variable signal intensity on T2W imaging

PINEAL CYST

- Distinguish from cystic pineocytoma or cystic astrocytoma by lack of growth, no solid component
- May be FLAIR hyperintense due to hemorrhage, protein
- May demonstrate peripheral enhancement or calcification

NEUROEPITHELIAL/NEUROGLIAL CYSTS

Can occur anywhere within the intraaxial CNS. More frequent in older age. Heterogeneous group of cysts comprising:

- Intraventricular ependymal cysts
- Choroid plexus cysts
- Choroid fissure cysts
- Brain parenchyma cysts

Degenerative and White Matter Disease

GENERAL

CLASSIFICATION OF DEGENERATIVE DISEASES

WM disease
- Demyelinating disease: acquired disease in which normal myelin is destroyed
- Dysmyelinating disease: hereditary inborn errors of myelin synthesis, maintenance, or degradation

GM disease
- Senile dementia, Alzheimer type (SDAT)
- Pick disease
- Vascular cortical dementia (multiinfarct dementia)
- Parkinson's disease
- Lysosomal storage diseases

Basal ganglia disorders
- Huntington disease
- Wilson disease
- Fahr disease
- Leigh disease

Toxic/infectious
- Creutzfeldt-Jakob
- Carbon monoxide
- Alchohol/Wernicke
- Seizure medication

DEGENERATION AND AGING

A variety of changes occur in the CNS with aging:

Diffuse cerebral atrophy
- Compensatory enlargement of ventricles, sulci, fissures, cisterns
- Loss of brain parenchyma

WM abnormalities
- Subcortical and central white matter abnormalities
- Periventricular WM abnormalities in 30% of older population. Causes include:
  - Microvascular disease (ischemic demyelination), gliosis, protein deposits, occasionally lacunar infarction
  - Periventricular and subcortical T2W bright signal abnormalities; no contrast enhancement, no mass effect
- VR spaces; état criblé: dilated perivascular spaces. Appearance:
  - Perivascular demyelination causes an increase in perivascular subarachnoid space (filled with CSF)
  - VR spaces always parallel CSF signal intensity (differentiate from WM lesions on PDW images)
  - Common locations: anterior perforated substance (most common), basal ganglia, centrum semiovale

Iron deposition in basal ganglia
- T2W hypointensity

WHITE MATTER DISEASE

CLASSIFICATION

Demyelinating disease
- Multiple sclerosis (MS)
- ADEM

- Toxin related
  - Central pontine myelinolysis
  - Paraneoplastic syndromes
  - Radiation therapy, chemotherapy
  - Alcoholism

Dysmyelinating diseases (leukodystrophies)

- Lysosomal enzyme disorders
- Peroxisomal disorders
- Mitochondrial disorders
- Amino acidopathies
- Idiopathic

MULTIPLE SCLEROSIS (MS)

Idiopathic demyelinating disease characterized by edematous perivascular inflammation (acute plaques) that progresses to astroglial proliferation and demyelination (chronic plaques). Thought to be an autoimmune process influenced by genetic and environmental factors. Mainly affects young white adults; slightly more common in females (60%). Clinical findings depend on anatomic location of lesions; monocular visual loss, gait difficulties, and sensory disturbances are most common. The diagnosis is based on a composite of clinical findings, laboratory data (evoked potentials, CSF oligoclonal bands) and imaging studies (McDonald's criteria). MRI allows the identification of dissemination in space and time. MRI also aids in monitoring treatment.

Imaging Features (Fig. 6-58)

MRI appearance of plaques

- Plaques are most commonly multiple. To support the diagnosis of MS at least three plaques of >5 mm should be present.
- Average size range: 0.5 to 3 cm
- Contrast enhancement may be homogeneous, ringlike, or patchy.
- Inactive plaques do not enhance.
- Bright signal intensity on T2W and PDW images
- Oblong, elliptical T2W bright structures at callososeptal interface
- Dawson's fingers: perivenular extension of elliptical structures into deep WM (sagittal T2/FLAIR useful)
- Tumefactive MS may mimic a brain tumor or infarct, but there is less mass effect than that seen with a tumor.

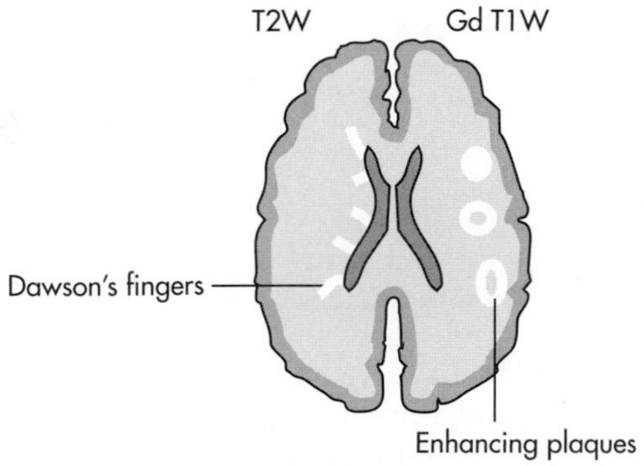

FIGURE 6-58

Distribution of plaques (Fig. 6-59)

- Supratentorial
  - Bilateral periventricular, 85%
  - Corpus callosum, 70%
  - Scattered in WM
  - GM (uncommon)
- Brainstem
- Cerebellum
- Spinal cord, 50%
- Optic nerve, chiasm
- Devic disease: plaques involving spinal cord and optic pathway, otherwise sparing brain

Other findings

- Cortical central atrophy, 20%-80%
- Atrophy of corpus callosum, 40%
- Hypointense thalamus and putamen on T2W (increased ferritin)
- Mass effect of very large plaques (>3 cm) may mimic tumors (uncommon)

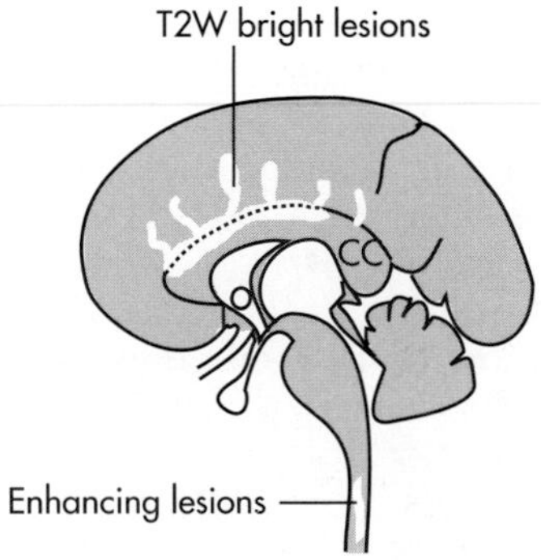

FIGURE 6-59

ACUTE DISSEMINATED ENCEPHALOMYELITIS (ADEM)

ADEM represents an immune response to a preceding viral illness or vaccination. Abrupt onset. More common in children. Indistinguishable from MS on imaging, although less likely to be periventricular. Also, thalamic involvement is rare in MS but not uncommon in ADEM. Involves corpus callosum. Monophasic in contradistinction to multiple sclerosis, which is polyphasic. Although it is a monophasic illness, not all lesions enhance at the same time because some lesions may be developing while others are resolving.

POSTERIOR REVERSIBLE ENCEPHALOPATHY SYNDROME (PRES)

High T2 signal abnormality in grey and subcortical white matter, often affecting posterior structures such as occipital and parietal lobes and brainstem. Enhancement variable. Posterior predilection may be due to relative sparse sympathetic innervation of the posterior circulation, with consequent poor autoregulatory function in context of blood pressure changes. Often reversible with treatment of inciting event; involvement of anterior structures does not preclude diagnosis. Clinical: headaches, visual disturbance, seizure, confusion.

Common Causes

- Hypertension
- Chemotherapy (e.g., cyclophosphamide)
- Eclampsia/pre-eclampsia
- Vasculitis

RADIATION/CHEMOTHERAPY-INDUCED CNS ABNORMALITIES

Common Causes

- Cyclosporine causes posterior confluent WM hyperintensity. Patients often present with blindness.
- Fluorouracil (5-FU), methotrexate (systemic)
- Intrathecal methotrexate
- Radiation and chemotherapy potentiate each other's toxic effects. Intrathecal methotrexate and whole brain radiation lead to progressive diffuse, deep WM T2W hyperintensity (disseminated necrotizing encephalopathy), potentially fatal

Two types of changes are observed:

Acute changes

- Occur during or immediately after course of radiation, resolve after therapy ends
- Changes usually represent mild edema, inflammation

Chronic changes

- Occurrence:
  - 6 to 8 months after nonfractionated therapy: proton beam, stereotactic therapy
  - 2 years after fractionated conventional radiation
- May be permanent
- Pathology: occlusion of small vessels, focal demyelination, proliferation of glial elements and mononuclear cells, atrophy
- Signal intensity changes: T2W bright, CT hypodense

CENTRAL PONTINE MYELINOLYSIS (CPM)

This disease entity is characterized by symmetrical, noninflammatory demyelination of the pons, the exact mechanism of which is unknown. Osmotic shifts due to rapid correction in patients with hyponatremia have been implicated. CPM is also seen in chronic alcoholics and malnourished patients and in patients undergoing orthotopic liver transplantation.

Imaging Features

- Diffuse central pontine hyperintensity on T2W images without mass effect or enhancement and with sparing of corticospinal tracts
- Extrapontine lesions are common in putamina and thalami.
- MRI may be negative initially on patient presentation, but lesions become apparent on follow-up scans.
- Differential diagnosis:
  - MS
  - ADEM
  - Ischemia/infarction
  - Infiltrating neoplasm

LEUKODYSTROPHIES

A heterogeneous group of diseases characterized by enzyme defects that result in abnormal myelin production and turnover. In some disorders (e.g., idiopathic group), the biochemical abnormality is unknown. Imaging findings are nonspecific in many instances and non-WM regions can be involved (e.g., basal ganglia, cortex, vessels).

General Categories

Lysosomal disorders

- Sphingolipidoses
- Mucolipidoses
- Mucopolysaccharidoses

Peroxisomal disorders

- Adrenoleukodystrophy
- Zellweger syndrome

Mitochondrial disorders

- MELAS syndrome (mitochondrial myopathy, encephalopathy, lactic acidosis, strokelike episodes)
- MERRF syndrome (myoclonic epilepsy with ragged red fibers)
- Leigh disease

Aminoacidopathies

- Phenylketonuria (PKU)
- Homocystinuria
- Others

Idiopathic

- Alexander disease
- Cockayne syndrome
- Pelizaeus-Merzbacher disease
- Canavan disease

Many entities have variable forms such as infantile, juvenile, and adult forms. Clinical manifestations overlap and include motor and intellectual deterioration, seizures, and progressive loss of function.

COMMON LEUKODYSTROPHIES

Name	Type	Deficiency	Comments
Metachromatic leukodystrophy	Lysosomal (AR)	Arylsulfatase A	Most common type
Krabbe disease	Lysosomal (AR)	Galactocerebroside β-Galactosidase	
Adrenoleukodystrophy	Peroxisomal (X-linked)	Acyl CoA synthetase	
Canavan disease	Cytosol (AR)	N-Acetylaspartylase	Spongy degeneration
Alexander disease	Unknown	Unknown	Sporadic
Pelizaeus-Merzbacher disease	Unknown	Proteolipid apoprotein	
Phenylketonuria	Amino acidopathy	Phenylalanine hydroxylase	Dietary treatment

Imaging Features

Macrocephaly
- Canavan disease
- Alexander disease

Frontal lobe predilection
- Alexander disease

Occipital lobe predilection
- Adrenoleukodystrophy

Contrast enhancement
- Adrenoleukodystrophy
- Alexander disease

Hyperdense basal ganglia
- Krabbe disease

Ischemic infarctions
- Mitochondrial disorders (MELAS, MERRF)
- Homocystinuria

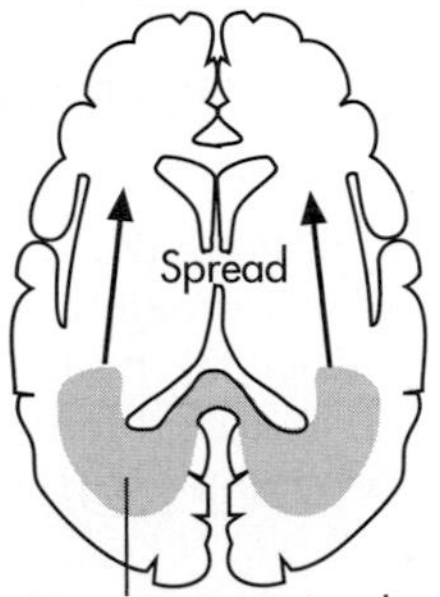

FIGURE 6-60

METACHROMATIC LEUKODYSTROPHY

Most common hereditary leukodystrophy; infantile form is most common. Age at presentation: <2 years in 80%. Death in childhood.

Imaging Features

- Most common abnormality: periventricular "butterfly" WM abnormalities
  - CT hypodense
  - T2W hyperintense
- Prominent feature: cerebellar WM involvement
- Other nonspecific findings that do not allow differentiation from other dysmyelinating diseases

ADRENOLEUKODYSTROPHY (ALD) (Fig. 6-60)

Defective fatty acid oxidation (X-linked recessive is the most common). Accumulation of long-chain fatty acids in GM and WM and adrenal cortex. Age group: preadolescent boys. CNS manifestations and adrenal insufficiency. Definitive diagnosis made by detecting long-chain fatty acids in cultured fibroblasts, RBCs, or plasma.

Imaging Features

Distribution
- Common (80%): disease starts in occipital regions and spreads anteriorly to involve frontal lobes and across corpus callosum
- Less common: disease starts in frontal lobes and spreads posteriorly
- Symmetrical

Signal intensities
- CT
  - Low attenuation (edema and gliosis)
  - Enhancement of leading edge (inflammation)
- MRI
  - T2W hyperintense with leading edge enhancement
  - Pontomedullary corticospinal tract involvement is a common finding in ALD and is unusual in other leukodystrophies.

End-stage: atrophy

GRAY MATTER DISEASE

DEMENTIA

Dementia occurs in 5% of population >65 years.

Types

- SDAT, 50%
- Multiinfarct dementia, 45%
- Less common causes (see following table)

DIFFERENTIAL DIAGNOSIS OF DEMENTIA

Disease	Atrophy	Characteristics	Imaging
SDAT	+	Temporal lobe, hippocampus	WM abnormalities not prominent
Multiinfarct dementia	+	Atrophy	Periventricular lacunae; cortical and subcortical infarction
NPH	-	Lacunae, basal ganglia	Communicating hydrocephalus
Binswanger*	+	Periventricular WM lesion	
Wernicke-Korsakoff†	+	Lacunae, basal ganglia, gyral and vermis atrophy	Medial thalamus T2W hyperintensity

*Subcortical arteriosclerotic encephalopathy.
†Clinically obvious (alcoholism, ataxia, ophthalmoparesis, thiamine deficiency).

SENILE DEMENTIA, ALZHEIMER TYPE (SDAT)

Most common degenerative brain disease and most common cortical dementia. Findings are nonspecific, so role of imaging is to exclude diseases that mimic SDAT: subdural hematoma, multiinfarct dementia, Binswanger disease, primary brain tumor, and normal pressure hydrocephalus (NPH).

Imaging Features

- No reliable CT or MR findings that allow specific diagnosis
- Diffuse enlargement of sulci and ventricles is most common imaging finding.
- Disproportionate atrophy of anterior temporal lobes, hippocampi, and sylvian fissures
- WM hyperintensities may occur but are not a prominent feature.
- Regional bilateral temporoparietal abnormalities:
  SPECT: decreased HMPAO perfusion
  PET: decreased perfusion/metabolism ($^{15}O_2$/^{18}FDG)
- Early: parietal temporal lobe hypometabolism
- Late: also involves frontal lobe
- Preservation of the sensorimotor strip

FRONTOTEMPORAL DYSPLASIA (PICK DISEASE) (Fig. 6-61)

Rare cortical dementia that commonly manifests before age 65 (presenile onset). Frontotemporal atrophy frontal horn enlargement, and parietooccipital sparing are typical imaging features.

- Differs from Alzheimer in less memory loss, more personality changes (irritability), loss of function, loss of interest, word finding difficulties

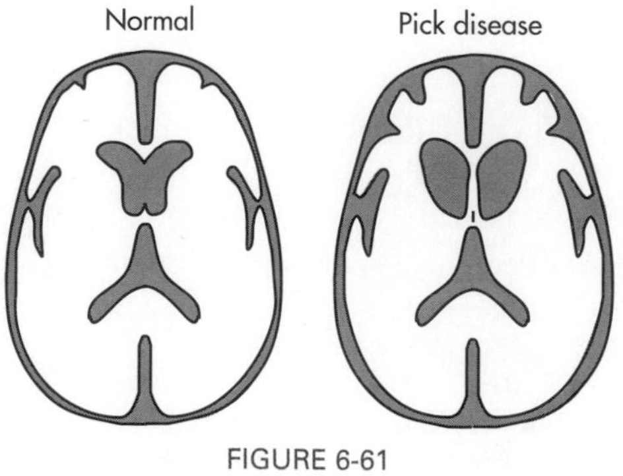

FIGURE 6-61

VASCULAR CORTICAL DEMENTIA

Ischemic dementia is the second most common form of dementia after SDAT.

Types

Multiinfarct dementia
- Cortical infarctions (territorial vascular infarctions)
- Enlarged sulci and ventricles
- Prominent T2W hyperintensities

Subcortical dementia (Binswanger disease)
- Periventricular hyperintensity (penetrating vessel ischemia)

- Hypertension is common.

PARKINSON DISEASE

Idiopathic extrapyramidal disease of the striatonigral system. Hallmark is loss of melanin-containing neurons in substantia nigra.

Clinical Findings

- Cogwheel rigidity
- Bradykinesia
- Tremor

Types

Parkinson disease
Secondary parkinsonism
- Neuroleptic drugs
- Trauma
- CO poisoning

Imaging Features

- MRI appearance is commonly normal.
- Decreased width of T2W dark compacta
- Iron-induced signal loss in basal ganglia best seen on T2W spin-echo and gradient-echo

images (black ganglia). Location of signal intensity change:
  Parkinson: globus pallidus
  Parkinson-plus: putamen
- Cerebral atrophy in chronic cases

PARKINSON PLUS SYNDROMES (PATIENTS WHO RESPOND POORLY TO ANTIPARKINSON MEDICATION) (Fig. 6-62)

Multisystem Atrophy (MSA)

Sporadic, progressive neurodegenerative disease of undetermined etiology, may have combinations of extrapyramidal, pyramidal, cerebellar, and autonomic dysfunction.

Types
- Striatonigral degeneration (SD)
- Shy-Drager syndrome (autonomic dysfunction)
- Olivopontocerebellar atrophy (OPCD)

Imaging features
- Volume loss of pons and cerebellum (SD and OPCD), olivary nucleus (OPCD)
- Slight T2 hyperintensity lateral margin of putamen (SD)
- Midbrain volume is preserved
- "Hot cross bun" sign in the pons on axial T2/FLAIR

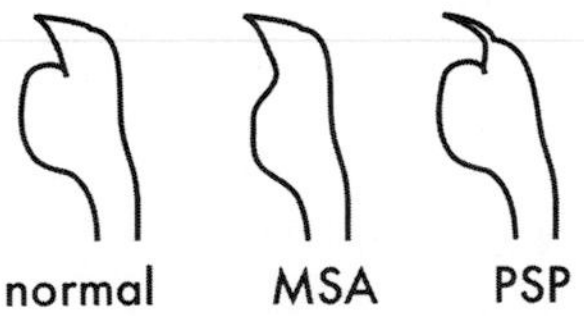

FIGURE 6-62

Progressive Supranuclear Palsy (PSP)

Progressive disease with vertical gaze abnormality, extrapyramidal and cognitive symptoms. ~60 years of age. Male:female 1.5:1.

Imaging Features
- Volume loss of the midbrain — Hummingbird sign
- Preservation of pons

AMYOTROPHIC LATERAL SCLEROSIS (ALS)

Progressive neurodegenerative illness. Unknown etiology but 5%-10% are familial cases.
- Abnormal high signal intensity in corticospinal tracts on PDW/FLAIR images, best seen at level of middle or lower internal capsule
- Low signal intensity within motor cortex

BASAL GANGLIA DISORDERS

BASAL GANGLIA CALCIFICATION

Basal ganglia calcification occurs in 1% of the general population. Unrelated to observed neurologic disturbances in many instances. Most patients with basal ganglia calcification have no symptoms. No data exist as to the amount of calcification that is pathologic.

Causes
- Idiopathic/physiologic aging (most common)
- Metabolic
  Hypoparathyroidism (common)
  Pseudohypoparathyroidism
  Pseudo-pseudohypoparathyroidism
  Hyperparathyroidism
- Infection (common)
  Toxoplasmosis
  HIV infection
- Toxin-related (uncommon)
  CO
  Lead poisoning
  Radiation/chemotherapy
- Ischemic/hypoxic injury
- Neurodegenerative diseases (rare)
  Fahr disease
  Mitochondrial disorders
  Cockayne disease
  Hallervorden-Spatz disease

HUNTINGTON CHOREA (Fig. 6-63)

Autosomal dominant inherited disease manifested by choreiform movements and dementia.

Imaging Features
- Caudate nucleus atrophy
- Boxcar appearance of frontal horns

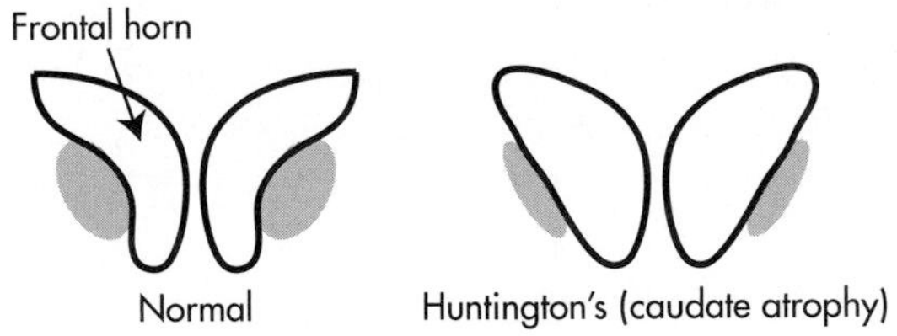

FIGURE 6-63

WILSON DISEASE

Caused by abnormality in the copper transport protein, ceruloplasmin. Autosomal recessive.

Imaging Features
- MRI appearance of the CNS may be normal.
- T2W hyperintense putamen and thalami
- Generalized atrophy
- Low-density basal ganglia on CT
- Hepatic cirrhosis

FAHR DISEASE

Historically, Fahr disease was a term applied to a large group of disorders characterized by basal ganglia calcification. It is now used to describe a small category of patients with basal ganglia calcification and symptoms of late-onset dementia with extrapyramidal motor dysfunction; autosomal dominant inheritance predominates. A more precise name is familial idiopathic striopallidodentate calcification. Calcification in the dentate nuclei and cerebral WM can also be present.

LEIGH DISEASE

Mitochondrial disorder of oxidative phosphorylation (pyruvate carboxylase deficiency thiamine pyrophosphate–ATP phosphoryl transferase–inhibiting substance, pyruvate decarboxylase deficiency, cytochrome oxidase deficiency). Suspect the diagnosis in children with lactic acidosis and abnormalities on MRI or CT of the basal ganglia.

Diagnosis

Suggestive:
- Elevated serum pyruvate/lactate levels
- Typical findings on CT

Definitive:
- Cultured skin fibroblast assay for mitochondrial enzyme deficiency
- Histology

Imaging Features
- Location: putamen > globus pallidus > caudate nucleus
- Symmetrical bilateral low-attenuation areas in basal ganglia on CT
- Lesions are T2W hyperintense.
- MRI is more sensitive than CT in lesion detection.

NEUROSARCOIDOSIS

Symptomatic CNS involvement is seen in <5% of cases. Serum or CSF angiotensin-converting enzyme level is elevated in 70%-80% of patients with pulmonary sarcoidosis.

Radiologic Features
- Plaquelike dural thickening on CT. These plaques are isointense on T1W and hypointense on T2W images.
- Homogeneous enhancement of involved dura and leptomeninges
- Can involve CSF spaces and parenchyma
- Typically small enhancing rim lesion with a peripheral enhancing nodule (scolex). Can be large and may obstruct CSF to cause hydrocephalus; can seed the entire neuraxis.
- Can cause significant edema in parenchymal lesions
- Calcifies as the cysts involute.
- Sarcoid is a great mimic; enhancing lesions may involve dura, leptomeninges, brain parenchyma, hypothalamic pituitary axis, and cranial nerves.

TOXIC/INFECTIOUS

CREUTZFELDT-JAKOB DISEASE (CJD)

Disease caused by prion, which may be acquired or familial. Classic CJD is more common in the elderly and causes progressive dementia over 4 to 5 months. A variant form of CJD (vCJD) has been reported in younger patients (20 to 30 years of age) with symptoms that are more insidious lasting over 1 year, with more psychiatric and behavioral symptoms.

Imaging Features
- Classical: DWI and FLAIR/T2: hyperintensity in caudate, putamen, and gray matter (may be asymmetric).
- Variant: DWI and FLAIR/T2 hyperintensity in the pulvinar (specific in the right clinical context).

CARBON MONOXIDE POISONING

Leading cause of death from poisoning in the United States. Early imaging findings demonstrate cerebral edema with or without petechial hemorrhages. Later typical findings of ischemic anoxia are present, showing restricted diffusion and T2/FLAIR hyperintensity in the global pallidus, cortex, hippocampus, and substantia nigra.

ALCOHOLIC AND WERNICKE ENCEPHALOPATHY

Most common cause of cerebellar volume loss. Poor nutrition from alcoholism causes damage to the brain stem and basal ganglia, resulting in ataxia and nystagmus (Wernicke). If severe amnesia and confabulation are present, then it is Korsakoff syndrome.

Imaging Features
- Alcoholism — generalized volume loss, most prominent in the cerebellum
- Marchiafava-Bignami — focal demyelination of splenium of corpus callosum
- Acute Wernicke

  Hyperintensity and enhancement
  - Periaqueductal gray
  - Mesial thalamus
  - Para-third ventricle
  - Mammillary body
- Chronic Wernicke
- Mammillary body volume loss (may also be seen in alcoholics without Wernicke)

SEIZURE MEDICATION

Long-term seizure medication use (e.g., dilantin, phenobarbital) can cause dilatation of cerebellar sulci and the fourth ventricle, and show hypometabolism of the cerebellum on FDG-PET. Dilantin can also cause thickening of the skull.

Hydrocephalus

GENERAL

CLASSIFICATION

Noncommunicating hydrocephalus
- Intraventricular, foraminal, or aqueductal obstruction

Communicating hydrocephalus
- Obstruction at level of pacchionian granulation (SAH, meningitis)
- Increased CSF production (rare): choroid plexus tumors
- NPH

APPROACH (Fig. 6-64)

SHUNT COMPLICATIONS

- Ventriculitis/meningitis
- Obstruction (increase in amount of hydrocephalus)
- Subdural hematomas or effusions
- Meningeal fibrosis

NONCOMMUNICATING HYDROCEPHALUS

Caused by obstruction of ventricles, foramina, or aqueduct. Ventricles are dilated proximal to the obstruction and normal in size distal to the obstruction.

Causes

Foramen of Monro obstruction
- 3rd ventricle tumors
  - Colloid cyst
  - Oligodendroglioma
  - Central neurocytoma
  - Giant cell astrocytoma in tuberous sclerosis
  - Ependymoma
  - Meningioma (rare)
- Suprasellar tumor

Aqueduct obstruction
- Congenital aqueduct stenosis
- Ventriculitis
- Intraventricular hemorrhage
- Tumors
  - Mesencephalic
  - Pineal, posterior 3rd ventricular region
  - Tectal glioma

4th ventricle obstruction
- Congenital: Dandy-Walker (DW) malformation
- Intraventricular hemorrhage
- Infection (cysticercosis)
- Subependymoma
- Exophytic brainstem glioma

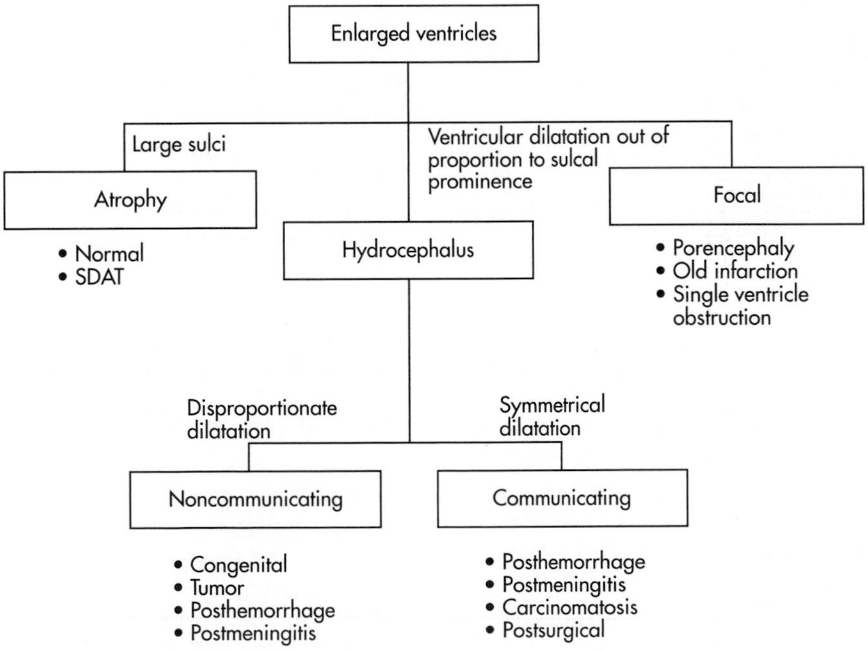

FIGURE 6-64

- Posterior fossa tumors: ependymoma, medulloblastoma, hemangioblastoma, metastasis, astrocytoma

Imaging Features

- Disproportionate dilatation of ventricles up to the point of obstruction
- Underlying abnormality causing the obstruction
- Ballooning of temporal horns ("Mickey Mouse ears") is a sensitive sign.
- Effacement of sulci due to mass effect
- Periventricular interstitial edema due to elevated intraventricular pressure and transependymal CSF flow T2W bright halo in noncompensated cases
- Absence of normal flow void in aqueduct by MRI
- Direct measurement of increased intracranial pressure via CSF puncture is sometimes performed for diagnostic purposes.

COMMUNICATING HYDROCEPHALUS

Results most commonly from extraventricular CSF pathway obstruction at the level of pacchionian granulations, basal cistern, or convexity.

Causes

- Meningitis
  - Infectious
  - Carcinomatous
- SAH and trauma
- Surgery
- Venous thrombosis

Imaging Features

- Following signs are the same as in noncommunicating hydrocephalus:
  - Ballooning of temporal horns
  - Effacement of sulci (mass effect)
  - Periventricular interstitial edema (T2W bright halo)
- Symmetrical dilatation of all ventricles
- The 4th ventricle is usually not very enlarged in convexity block hydrocephalus.

NORMAL PRESSURE HYDROCEPHALUS (NPH)

Form of communicating hydrocephalus in which there is no evidence of increased intracranial pressure. Clinical triad: gait incoordination, dementia, urinary incontinence. Clinical response to CSF tap is the gold standard for establishing the diagnosis.

Imaging Features

- No specific imaging findings
- Dilated ventricles
- Periventricular T2W bright halo (transependymal edema) is less common.
- Prominent cerebral aqueduct flow void

SPONTANEOUS INTRACRANIAL HYPOTENSION

The syndrome of intracranial hypotension results when CSF volume is lowered by leakage or by withdrawal of CSF in greater amounts than can be replenished by normal production. The syndrome is designated as spontaneous in absence of prior violation of the dura. Manifests as postural headache exacerbated by upright position. Diffuse dural enhancement seen in 100% of cases. Other findings that may not always be present include:

- Downward displacement of cerebellar tonsils and midbrain
- Flattening of pons against the dorsal clivus
- Draping of optic chiasm over the sella
- Distention of major dural venous sinuses
- Fast spin-echo T2W imaging of spine is performed to look for a spinal source of leak.
- An epidural blood patch may be an effective way to treat this condition. This procedure involves mixing a few milliliters of contrast with blood and using fluoroscopy to ensure instillation into the epidural space near suspected site of leak.

Infection

GENERAL

CLASSIFICATION BY INFECTIOUS AGENT

- Bacterial (purulent) infections
- Fungal infections
- Parasitic infections
- Viral infections

CLASSIFICATION BY LOCATION OF INFECTION

- Meningitis: pia or subarachnoid space and/or dura or arachnoid
- Empyema: epidural or subdural
- Cerebritis: intraparenchymal; early stage of abscess formation
- Intraparenchymal abscess
- Ventriculitis

BACTERIAL INFECTIONS

BACTERIAL MENINGITIS

Causes

- Neonates: Group B *Streptococcus, Escherichia coli, Listeria*
- Children: *Haemophilus, E. coli, Neisseria meningitidis*
- Adults: *S. pneumoniae, N. meningitidis*

Pathologically meningitis can be separated into:

- Leptomeningitis (most common): arachnoid and pia involved

- Pachymeningitis: dura and outer layer of arachnoid involved

Predisposing factors:
- Sinusitis
- Chronic pulmonary infection
- Tetralogy of Fallot
- Transposition of great vessels
- Other cyanotic heart disease

Imaging Features

Meningeal contrast enhancement
- Normal CT examination is initially most common finding.
- Convexity enhancement occurring later is a typical finding.
- Basilar meningeal enhancement alone is more common in granulomatous meningitis.

Cranial US in neonatal bacterial meningitis
- Subtle findings: abnormal parenchymal echogenicity
- Echogenic sulci, 40%
- Extraaxial fluid collections
- Ventricular dilatation
- Ventriculitis occurs in 70%-90% of cases of bacterial meningitis.
  - Normally thin ventricular wall thickens
  - Wall becomes hyperechoic
  - Debris in CSF

Complications

- Subdural effusion: common in infants and children
- Empyema
- Parenchymal extension: abscess and cerebritis
- Ventriculitis
- Hydrocephalus (communicating > noncommunicating)
- Venous infarctions secondary to venous thrombosis

TUBERCULOUS MENINGITIS

The most common CNS manifestation of TB followed by intraparenchymal tuberculoma. Spread is usually hematogenous from pulmonary TB. Basilar meningeal involvement by chronic granulomatous process leads to cranial nerve palsies.

Imaging Features

Basilar meningitis: indistinguishable from fungal, lymphoma, and sarcoid
- Intense contrast enhancement of basilar meninges (CT, MRI)
- Pituitary and parasellar involvement
- Pituitary or hypothalamic axis involvement
- T2W hypointense meninges
- Calcifications occur late in disease

Abscesses (tuberculoma)
- Rare unless immunocompromised or from endemic areas (Indian population)
- Usually solitary
- Nonspecific enhancing masslike lesions
- Cerebral hemispheres and basal ganglia
- Miliary form: multiple tiny intraparenchymal lesions

EMPYEMA

An empyema is an infected fluid collection in subdural (common) or epidural (uncommon) location. Empyemas are neurosurgical emergencies. Cause: sinusitis (most common), otitis, trauma, postcraniotomy.

Imaging Features

- Diffusion imaging is highly sensitive: lesions are DWI bright and ADC dark
- Subdural or epidural low-attenuation fluid collection with enhancement of adjacent brain
- Venous infarction → edema → mass effect → midline shift
- Thick, curvilinear enhancement of empyema
- Concomitant signs of sinusitis, otitis

BRAIN ABSCESS

Common Organism

- Children: *Staphylococcus* (especially after trauma), *Streptococcus*, pneumococcus
- Adults: mixed aerobic and anaerobic flora
- Immunosuppression: toxoplasmosis, cryptococcosis, candidiasis, aspergillosis, nocardiosis, mucormycosis (diabetes), TB, atypical mycobacteria

Mechanism

Hematogenous dissemination (most common)
- Intravenous drug abuse
- Sepsis

Direct extension
- Sinusitis
- Otitis, mastoiditis
- Open injury (penetrating trauma, surgery)

Idiopathic

Imaging Features

Diffusion imaging is highly sensitive to detect abscesses and empyemas.

Location
- Hematogenous seeding: multiple lesions at GM/WM junction
- Penetrating trauma or sinusitis: lesion around the entry site

Morphology
- Mass effect (abscessed cavity, edema)
- Ring or wall enhancement, 90%
- Restricted diffusion centrally
- Capsule forms in 7 to 14 days
  - Capsule is thinner on WM side because of lower perfusion to WM than to GM.

Because of the thinner capsule, daughter lesions (and intraventricular rupture) occur on the medial side.

Capsule is hypointense on T2W images.

Inner margin is often smooth.

Capsule formation may be delayed by steroid administration.

- Ventriculitis due to ventricular spread
  - Increased CSF density (elevated protein concentration)
  - Ependymal contrast enhancement
  - May cause ventricular septations and hydrocephalus
  - DWI bright
- Daughter lesions

FUNGAL INFECTIONS

Causes

Immunocompetent patients

- Coccidioidomycosis, histoplasmosis, blastomycosis

Immunocompromised patients (AIDS, chemotherapy, steroids, transplant recipients)

- Nocardiosis, aspergillosis, candidiasis, cryptococcosis, mucormycosis

Imaging Features

Basilar meningitis

- Intense contrast enhancement of basilar meninges (similar to TB)

Abscesses

- Early: granuloma
- Late: abscess with ring enhancement and central necrosis

Helpful features:

- Aspergillosis
  - Hemorrhagic infarcts from vascular invasion
  - Often coexistent sinus disease that has extended to CNS
  - T2W isointense/hypointense masslike lesions
- Mucormycosis: indistinguishable from aspergillosis
- Coccidioidomycosis: indistinguishable from TB
- Cryptococcosis: cystic lesions (gelatinous pseudocysts secondary to spread into VR spaces) in basal ganglia. Consider this diagnosis in an HIV-positive patient with communicating hydrocephalus. "Lacunar infarct"–like appearance in an HIV-positive patient may be secondary to cryptococcal gelatinous pseudocysts.

PARASITIC INFECTIONS

NEUROCYSTICERCOSIS (Fig. 6-65)

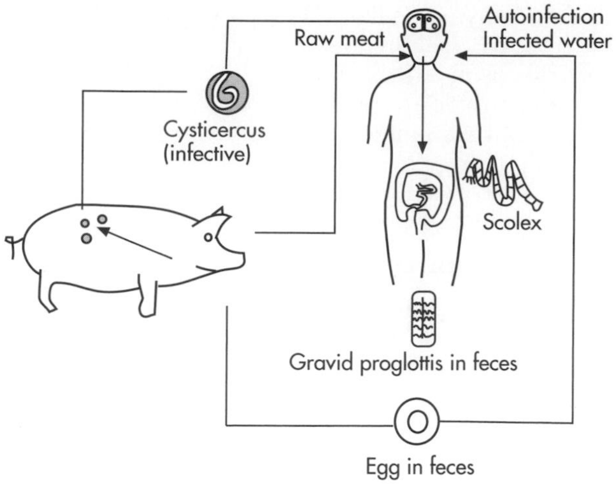

FIGURE 6-65

Caused by *Taenia solium* (pork tapeworm). Epidemiology: Central and South America, Hispanic population in United States. Source: ingestion of contaminated water or pork. Ingested eggs penetrate intestine, disseminate hematogenously, and encyst in muscle, brain, and ocular tissue. Cysts first contain a living larva, which ultimately dies, causing inflammation (contrast enhancement) and calcifications. 75% of infected patients have CNS involvement. Seizures are the most common presentation. Treatment: praziquantel, albendazole, VP shunting for obstructive hydrocephalus. Evolution of lesions:

- Nonenhancing cyst: live larvae
- Ring-enhancing lesion: dying larvae cause inflammatory reaction.
- Calcification: old lesion

Imaging Features

Four stages in brain parenchyma:

- Vesicular stage—thin-walled vesicles (<20 mm) with CSF-like fluid and a mural nodule; inflammatory response is absent
- Colloid stage—viable cyst dies, cyst fluid becomes turbid, inflammatory reaction leads to breakdown of blood-brain barrier
- Nodular granular stage—lesion undergoes involution and begins to calcify
- Calcified stage

Typical appearance of cysts:

- Multiple cystic lesions of water density
- Larvae (scolices) appear of variable signal intensity on T2W images
- Ring enhancement (inflammatory response caused by dying larvae)

Three locations:

- Parenchymal (most common)
- Intraventricular (may cause obstruction)
- Subarachnoid

Other findings:
- Hydrocephalus
- Chronic meningitis
- Calcification of skeletal muscle

LYME DISEASE

- Multisystemic inflammatory disease caused by a spirochete, *Borrelia burgdorferi*
- Single or multiple parenchymal abnormalities associated with meningeal and multiple cranial nerve enhancement
- May mimic multiple sclerosis and ADEM by imaging; lesions may or may not enhance

VIRAL INFECTIONS

HERPES SIMPLEX VIRUS (HSV) ENCEPHALITIS

Two general herpes types:
- HSV-2, genital herpes
  - Neonatal TORCH infection (see later)
  - Acquired during parturition
  - Manifests several weeks after birth
  - Diffuse encephalitis (nonfocal)
- HSV-1, oral herpes
  - Children and adults
  - Usually activation of latent virus in trigeminal ganglion
  - Altered mental status; fulminant course
  - Limbic system; frequently bilateral but asymmetrical

Imaging Features

- CT and MRI findings are usually normal early in disease.
- MRI is the imaging study of choice. The first imaging abnormalities become apparent within 2 to 3 days after onset.
- Distribution: limbic system, temporal lobe > cingulate gyrus, subfrontal region
- Acute stage: emergency because untreated acute herpes encephalitis has high mortality
- Decreased/restricted diffusion in affected areas
  - Gyral edema (T1W hypointense/T2W hyperintense)
  - No enhancement
- Subacute stage
  - Marked increase in edema
  - Bilateral asymmetrical involvement
  - Gyral enhancement
  - Hemorrhage is common in this stage.

CONGENITAL INFECTIONS

Congenital CNS infections result in brain malformations, tissue destruction, and/or dystrophic calcification; the CNS manifestations depend on both the specific infectious agent and the timing of the infection during fetal development.

Causes

TORCH
- Toxoplasmosis (second most common)
- Rubella
- CMV infection (most common)
- Herpes simplex

Other
- HIV infection
- Syphilis
- Varicella

Imaging Features (Fig. 6-66)

CMV infection
- Gestational age at time of infection predicts the nature and extent of abnormalities. In general, infection acquired during the first two trimesters causes congenital malformations, whereas infection in the third trimester manifests as destructive lesions.
- Periventricular calcification. CT is adequate for diagnosis in 40%-70% of cases with typical calcifications. However, calcifications may be in atypical locations such as basal ganglia or subcortical regions. In neonate, the calcifications may appear hyperintense on T1W and hypointense on T2W images in comparison with adjacent WM.
- Neuronal migration anomalies, especially polymicrogyria

Congenital toxoplasmosis (Fig. 6-67)
- Basal ganglia and parenchymal calcification (diffuse). Intracranial calcifications may regress or resolve over time in cases of treated toxoplasmosis.
- Hydrocephalus
- Chorioretinitis

Rubella
- Microcephaly
- Basal ganglia and parenchymal calcifications

HSV-2
- Multifocal GM and WM involvement

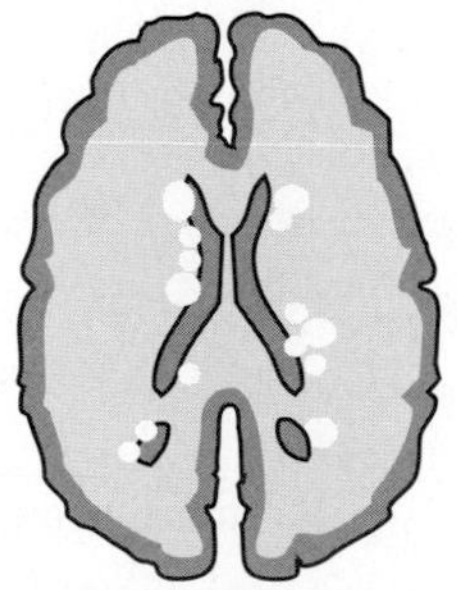

FIGURE 6-66

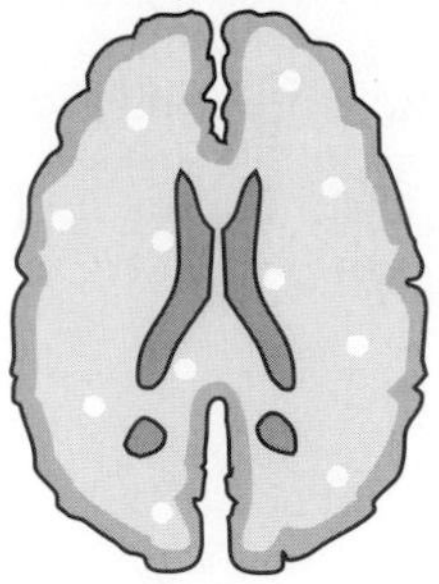

FIGURE 6-67

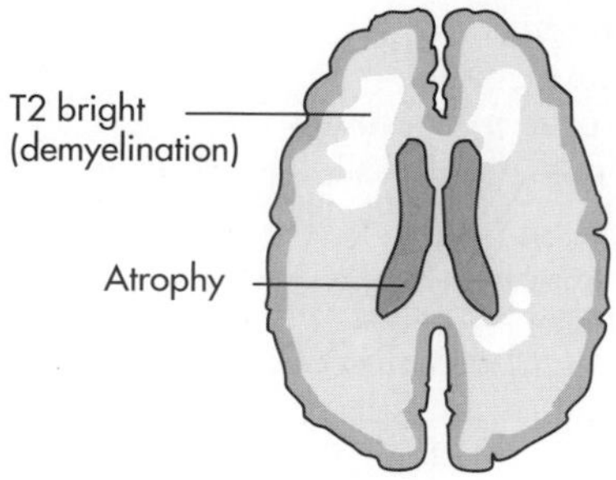

FIGURE 6-68

- Hemorrhagic infarction—consider this diagnosis in a neonate who presents in the second or third week of life with diffuse brain edema and leptomeningeal enhancement.
- Neonatal herpes encephalitis lacks the temporal and inferior frontal lobe predominance associated with adult herpes infection.

Congenital HIV (primary HIV encephalitis)
- Diffuse atrophy
- Basal ganglia calcification after 1 year

AIDS

HIV is a neurotropic virus that directly infects the CNS and is the most common CNS pathogen in AIDS. HIV-related infections include:
- HIV encephalopathy (most common)
- Toxoplasmosis: most common opportunistic CNS infection
- Cryptococcosis
- Progressive multifocal leukoencephalopathy (PML)
- TB
- Syphilis
- Varicella
- CMV

HIV ENCEPHALOPATHY

Progressive subacute subcortical dementia secondary to HIV itself. Eventually develops in 60% of AIDS patients.

Imaging Features (Fig. 6-68)
- Atrophy is the most common finding.
- T2W bright WM lesions in frontal and occipital lobes and periventricular location (gliosis, demyelination)
- No enhancement or mass effect of WM lesions

TOXOPLASMOSIS

Most common opportunistic CNS infection in AIDS. Caused by *Toxoplasma gondii* (reservoir: infected cats). Three manifestations:

Congenital
- Meningitis, encephalitis: calcification
- Encephalomalacia, atrophy
- Chorioretinitis

Immunocompetent adults
- Systemic disease with lymphadenopathy and fever
- CNS is not involved (in contradistinction to AIDS).

Immunocompromised patients
- Fulminant CNS disease
- Predilection for basal ganglia and corticomedullary junction

Imaging Features (Fig. 6-69)
- Solitary or multiple ring-enhancing lesions with marked surrounding edema
- Target appearance of lesions is common.
- Treated lesions may calcify or hemorrhage.
- Major consideration in differential diagnosis is CNS lymphoma:
  - Periventricular location and subependymal spread favors lymphoma.
  - Empirical treatment with antiprotozoal drugs followed by reassessment of lesions is often used to distinguish between the two.
- SPECT thallium or FDG PET: lymphoma appears as hot lesions, toxoplasmosis appears as cold lesions.

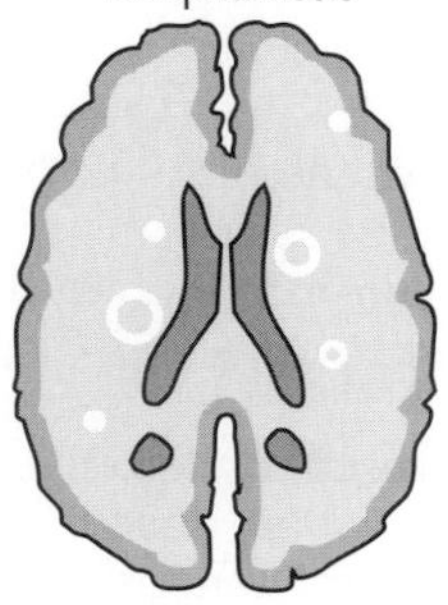

FIGURE 6-69

CRYPTOCOCCOSIS

Manifests as meningitis (more common) and intraparenchymal lesions. The most common intraparenchymal findings are multiple T2W bright foci in basal gelatinous pseudocysts in ganglia and midbrain with variable enhancement (cryptococcomas).

PROGRESSIVE MULTIFOCAL LEUKOENCEPHALOPATHY (PML)

Demyelinating disease caused by reactivation of JC virus, a polyomavirus. The reactivated virus infects and destroys oligodendrocytes.

Imaging Features (Fig. 6-70)

- Posterior centrum semiovale is the most common site.
- Bilateral but asymmetrical
- Begins in subcortical WM; spreads to deep WM
- T2W bright lesions (parietooccipital)
- No enhancement (key distinguishing feature from infections and tumors)
- May cross corpus callosum
- No mass effect

DIFFERENTIATION BETWEEN HIV ENCEPHALITIS AND PML

	HIV Encephalitis	PML
Signal intensity on T1W images	Usually isointense	Commonly isointense
Enhancement	—	May have mild enhancement
Mass effect	—	May have mild mass effect
Posterior fossa involvement	Uncommon	Common
Subcortical U fibers	Uncommon	Common
WM lesions	Symmetrical	Asymmetrical
Hemorrhage	Never	Occasional

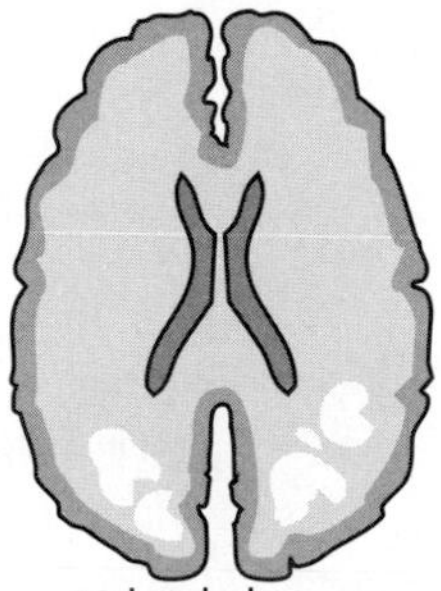

FIGURE 6-70

CMV ENCEPHALITIS

Indistinguishable imaging appearance from HIV encephalopathy. Shows periventricular hyperintensity on proton density or FLAIR images. Quantitative PCR assay of CSF may be useful in monitoring response to therapy.

Congenital Disease

GENERAL

CLASSIFICATION (Fig. 6-71)

Neural tube closure defects
- Anencephaly (most common anomaly)
- Chiari II, III
- Encephalocele

Disorders of diverticulation and cleavage
- Holoprosencephaly
- Septooptic dysplasia
- Corpus callosum anomalies

Neuronal migration and sulcation abnormalities
- Lissencephaly
- Pachygyria
- Polymicrogyria
- Schizencephaly
- Heterotopia
- Hemimegalencephaly

Posterior fossa malformations
- DW malformation
- DW variant
- Mega cisterna magna
- Chiari I

Neurocutaneous syndromes (phakomatoses)
- Tuberous sclerosis
- Neurofibromatosis
- Sturge-Weber syndrome (encephalotrigeminal angiomatosis)
- Von Hippel-Lindau (VHL) disease

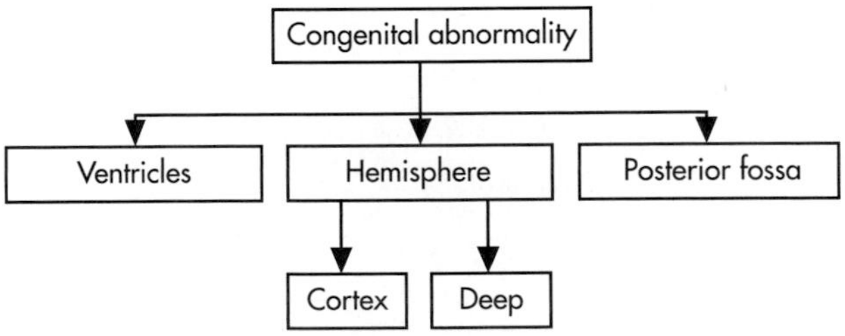

FIGURE 6-71

NEURAL TUBE CLOSURE DEFECTS

CHIARI MALFORMATIONS

Overview of Chiari Malformations

- Chiari I = downward displacement of cerebellar tonsils below foramen magnum (>5 mm); unrelated to Chiari II malformation
- Chiari II = abnormal neurulation leads to a small posterior fossa, caudal displacement of brainstem and herniation of tonsils and vermis through the foramen magnum; myelomeningocele
- Chiari III = encephalocele and Chiari II findings (rare)
- Chiari IV = severe cerebellar hypoplasia (rare)

Chiari I Malformation (Fig. 6-72)

Downward displacement of cerebellar tonsils below foramen magnum (distance C from AB line >5 mm). The 4th ventricle may be elongated but remains in a normal position. Chiari I malformation is not associated with myelomeningoceles and is unrelated to Chiari II and III malformations. Adult disease: 20 years.

Clinical Findings

- Intermittent compression of brainstem:
  - Nerve palsies
  - Atypical facial pain
  - Respiratory depression
  - Long tract signs

Associations

- Syringohydromyelia, 50%; weakness of hands, arms, loss of tendon reflexes
- Hydrocephalus, 25%
- Basilar invagination, 30%
- Klippel-Feil anomaly: fusion of 2 or more cervical vertebrae, 10%
- Atlantooccipital fusion, 5%

Imaging Features

- Tonsillar herniation (ectopia is 3 to 5 mm, herniation is >5 mm) is age dependent.
- Syringohydromyelia
- No brain anomalies

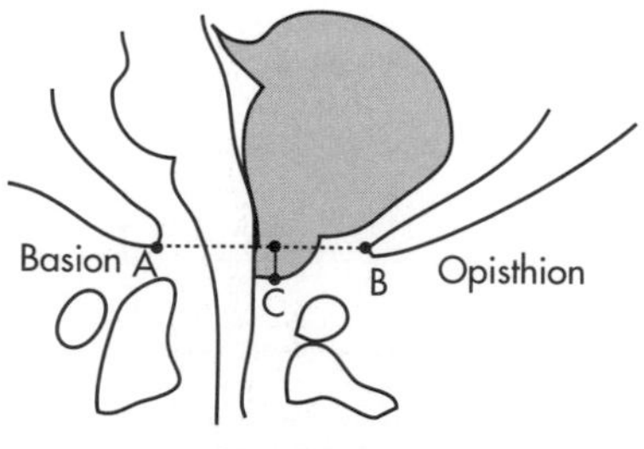

FIGURE 6-72

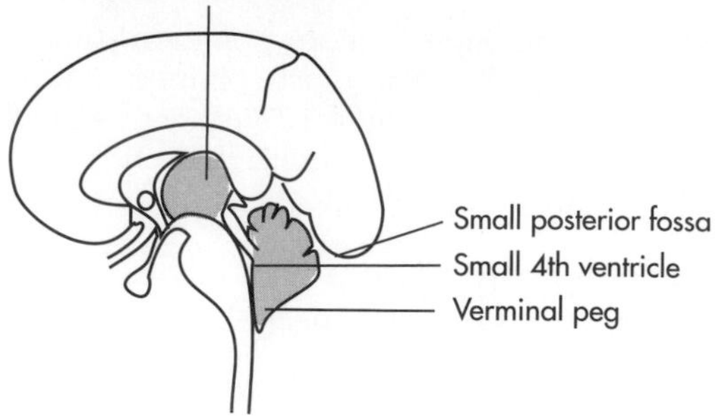

FIGURE 6-73

Chiari II Malformation

Most common in newborns

Associations

- Myelomeningocele, 90%
- Obstructive hydrocephalus, 90%
- Dysgenesis of corpus callosum
- Syringohydromyelia, 50%
- Abnormal cortical gyration
- Chiari II is not associated with Klippel-Feil anomaly or Chiari I.

Imaging Features (Fig. 6-73)

Posterior fossa

- Small posterior fossa
- Cerebellar vermis herniated through foramen (verminal peg)
- Upward herniation of cerebellum through widened incisure (towering cerebellum)
- Cerebellum wraps around pons (heart shape).
- Low, widened tentorium
  - Obliterated CPA cistern and cisterna magna
  - Nonvisualization or very small 4th ventricle

Supratentorium (Fig. 6-74)

- Hypoplastic or fenestrated falx causes interdigitation of gyri (gyral interlocking).
- Small, crowded gyri (stenogyria), 50%
- Hydrocephalus almost always present before shunting

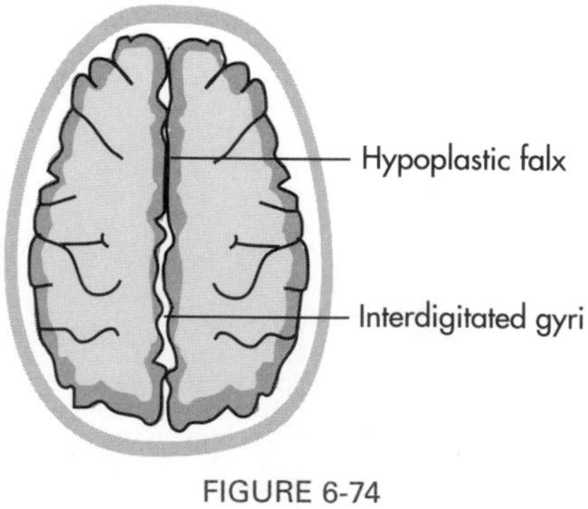

FIGURE 6-74

- Batwing configuration of frontal horns (caused by impressions by caudate nucleus)
- Small, biconcave 3rd ventricle (hourglass shape due to large massa intermedia)
- Beaked tectum

Osseous abnormalities
- Lückenschädel skull (present at birth, disappears later)
- Scalloped clivus and petrous ridge (pressure effect)
- Enlarged foramen magnum

Spinal cord
- Myelomeningocele, 90%
- Cervicomedullary kink at foramen magnum (pressure effect)
- Syringohydromyelia and diastematomyelia

CEPHALOCELE

Skull defect through which meninges, neural tissue, and/or CSF space protrude.

Usually midline and associated with other malformation (Chiari, callosal agenesis).

Location
- Occipital, 80%
- Frontal or nasoethmoidal
- Parietal, 10%
- Lateral from midline (suspect amniotic band syndrome)
- Sphenoidal (associated with sellar/endocrine anomalies)

CEREBRAL HEMISPHERE DEFECTS

AGENESIS OF CORPUS CALLOSUM (ACC)

Fibers that usually cross through corpus callosum run in longitudinal bundles (bundles of Probst) along the medial walls of the lateral ventricles (lateral displacement) and end randomly in occipital and parietal lobes. The 3rd ventricle is pathologically elevated because of this abnormality. Order of development: genu → anterior body → posterior body → splenium → rostrum. ACC may be complete or partial; when partial, the splenium and rostrum are absent. Associated CNS anomalies occur in 60%.
- DW malformation
- Lipoma (calcified in 10%)
- Chiari II
- Encephalocele
- Migration anomalies

Imaging Features (Fig. 6-75)
- Absence of corpus callosum
- Abnormal callosal bundles (bundles of Probst)
- Poor development of the WM around the atria and occipital horns: colpocephaly

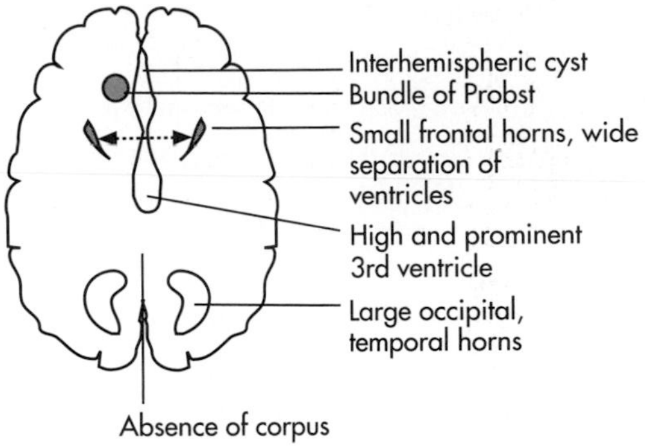

FIGURE 6-75

- Compensatory abnormalities
  - Elevated 3rd ventricle (hallmark)
  - Parallel lateral ventricles
  - Frontal horns small (bull's horn appearance), occipital horns large

HOLOPROSENCEPHALY

Failure of primitive brain to cleave into left and right cerebral hemispheres. Commonly associated with midline facial anomalies ranging from cyclopia to hypotelorism.

THREE TYPES OF HOLOPROSENCEPHALY

	Alobar	Semilobar	Lobar
Interhemispheric fissure and falx	Absent	Present posteriorly	Present*
Lateral ventricles	U-shaped monoventricle	Partially fused anteriorly	Near normal
Third ventricle	Absent	Rudimentary	Near normal
Cerebral hemisphere	One brain	Partial formation	Near normal
Thalamus	Fused	Variable fusion	Near normal
Facial anomalies	Severe	Less severe	None or mild
Septum pellucidum	Absent	Absent	Absent

* Nearly completely formed with most anteroinferior aspect absent.

Imaging Features (Fig. 6-76)

Alobar form
- No cleavage into two hemispheres: cup-shaped brain
- Single monoventricle
- Thalamic fusion
- Absent falx, corpus callosum, fornix, optic tracts, and olfactory bulbs
- Dorsal cysts common
- Midbrain, brainstem, and cerebellum are structurally normal.

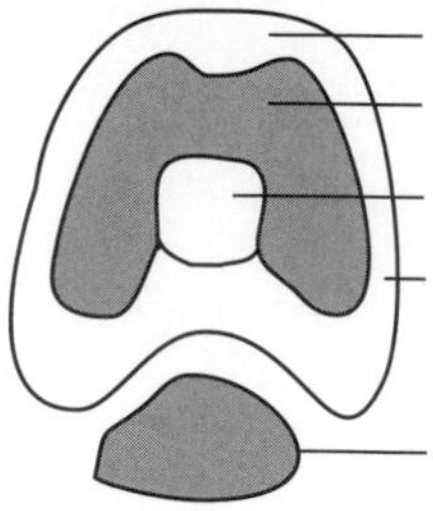

FIGURE 6-76

Semilobar form
- Partial cleavage into hemispheres
- Partial occipital and temporal horns

Lobar form (Fig. 6-77)
- Complete cleavage into two hemispheres, except for fusion in the rostral portion
- Lateral ventricles are normal or slightly dilated; frontal horns may be "squared."
- Absent septum pellucidum

Differential diagnosis
- Hydranencephaly
- Callosal agenesis with dorsal interhemispheric cyst
- Severe hydrocephalus

Facial Abnormalities
- Facial abnormalities usually correlate with severity of brain abnormalities but not vice versa.
- Hypotelorism (eyes too close together)
- Midline maxillary cleft
- Cyclopia (single eye)
- Ethmocephaly, cebocephaly

Pearls
- 50% of patients with holoprosencephaly have trisomy 13.
- Presence of a septum pellucidum excludes the diagnosis of holoprosencephaly.
- Lobar holoprosencephaly is the anteroinferior fusion of frontal lobes and absence of septum pellucidum and can thus be differentiated from severe hydrocephalus.
- Hydranencephaly has no anterior cerebral mantle or facial anomalies; falx and thalami are normal.

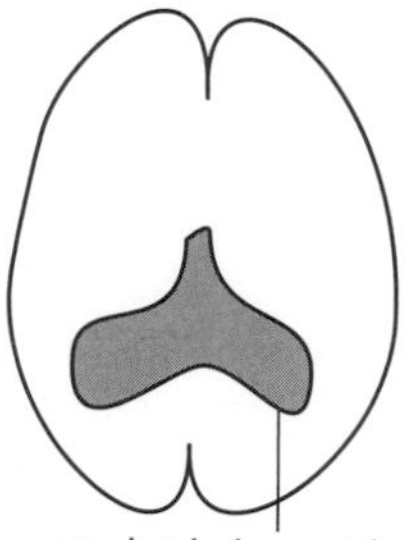

FIGURE 6-77

CEREBRAL HEMIATROPHY (DYKE-DAVIDOFF)

Intrauterine and perinatal ICA infarction leads to hemiatrophy of a cerebral hemisphere.

Imaging Features
- Atrophy of a hemisphere causes midline shift.
- Compensatory ipsilateral skull thickening (key finding)
- Ipsilateral paranasal and mastoid sinus enlargement

INTERHEMISPHERIC LIPOMA

Collection of primitive fat within or adjacent to corpus callosum.

Associations
- Absence of corpus callosum, 50%
- Midline dysraphism
- Agenesis of cerebellar vermis
- Encephalocele, myelomeningocele, spina bifida

Imaging Features
- CT: pure fat (-50 to -100 HU; no associated hair/debris) is pathognomonic.
- T1W hyperintense
- Most common location is splenium and genu.
- Curvilinear calcifications are common.

SEPTOOPTIC DYSPLASIA

Absence of septum pellucidum and optic nerve hypoplasia (mild form of lobar holoprosencephaly). 70% have hypothalamic/pituitary dysfunction.

Imaging Features
- Absence of septum pellucidum
- Squared frontal horns of lateral ventricles
- Hypoplasia of optic nerve and chiasm

MIGRATION AND SULCATION ABNORMALITIES (FIG. 6-78)

Group of disorders that result from abnormal migration of neuroblasts from subependymal germinal matrix to their cortical location.

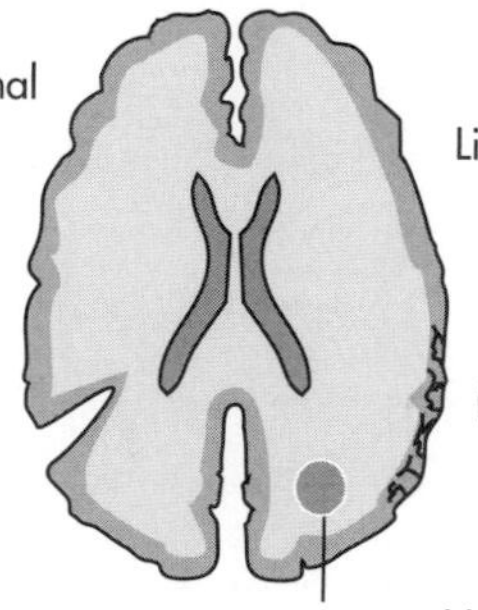

FIGURE 6-78

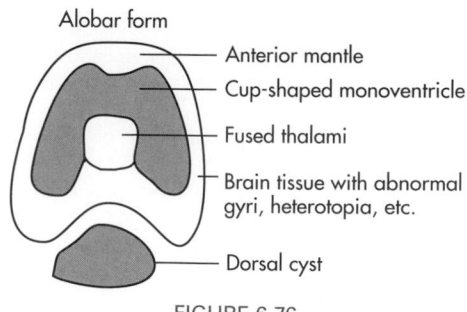

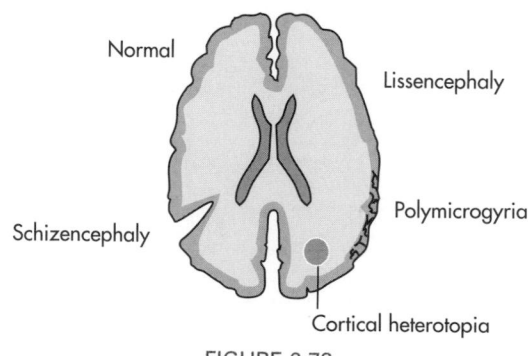

LISSENCEPHALY (SMOOTH BRAIN SURFACE)

Lack of sulcation leads to agyria (complete lissencephaly) or agyria-pachygyria (incomplete lissencephaly). May be secondary to in utero infections, especially CMV.

SCHIZENCEPHALY (SPLIT BRAIN)

GM-lined CSF cleft extends from ependyma to pia; frequent association with ACC. Open- and closed-lip variants.

POLYMICROGYRIA

Excessive cerebral convolutions with increased cortical thickness. May be distinguished from pachygyria (thick flat cortex) by MRI.

CORTICAL HETEROTOPIA

Islands of normal GM in abnormal locations due to arrest of neuronal migration. May be nodular or laminar (bandlike). Follows gray matter on all sequences. Occurs most commonly in periventricular location and centrum semiovale (anywhere along path from germinal matrix to cortex). Clinical: childhood seizures.

HEMIMEGALENCEPHALY

Diffuse migrational anomaly involving the entire cerebral hemisphere, with disorganized parenchyma
- With intractable seizures, the treatment is hemispherectomy.
- Differential diagnosis includes polymicrogyria, pachygyria, and diffuse gliomatosis.

POSTERIOR FOSSA MALFORMATIONS

DANDY-WALKER MALFORMATION

Exact etiology unknown: (1) insult to developing cerebellum and 4th ventricle, (2) congenital atresia of foramina of Magendie and Luschka. Mortality rate, 25%-50%.

Clinical Findings
- Large posterior fossa cyst
- Hydrocephalus, 75%
- Varying degrees of cerebellar hemispheric and vermian hypoplasia

Associations
- Agenesis of corpus callosum, 25%
- Lipoma of corpus callosum
- Malformation of cerebral gyri
- Holoprosencephaly, 25%
- Cerebellar heterotopia, 25%
- GM heterotopia
- Occipital cephalocele
- Tuber cinereum hamartoma
- Syringomyelia
- Cleft palate
- Polydactyly
- Cardiac abnormalities

Imaging Features (Fig. 6-79)
- Enlarged posterior fossa
- Large posterior fossa cyst communicates with the 4th ventricle.
- Absent or abnormal inferior cerebellar vermis (key finding)
- Elevation of vermian remnant
- Hypoplastic cerebellar hemispheres
- Hydrocephalus
- Elevation of torcular heterophils and tentorium

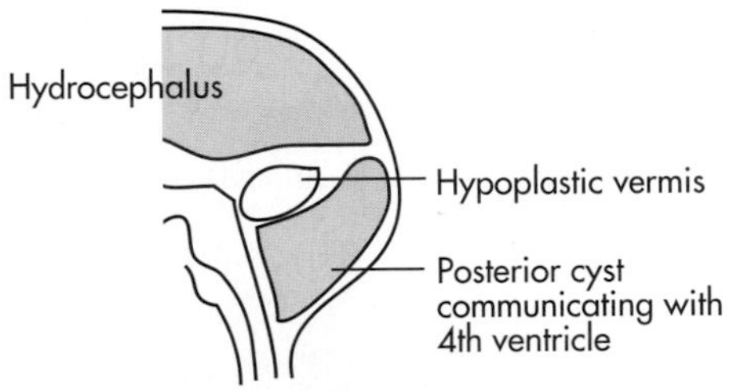

FIGURE 6-79

DANDY-WALKER VARIANT

Posterior fossa cyst with partially formed 4th ventricle and mild vermian hypoplasia. The 4th ventricle is not as dilated as in the DW malformation because it communicates freely with the basal cistern through a patent foramen of Magendie. The DW variant is more common than the DW malformation.

Imaging Features (Fig. 6-80)
- 4th ventricle communicates dorsally with enlarged cisterna magna: keyhole deformity
- Hydrocephalus not common
- Posterior fossa not enlarged

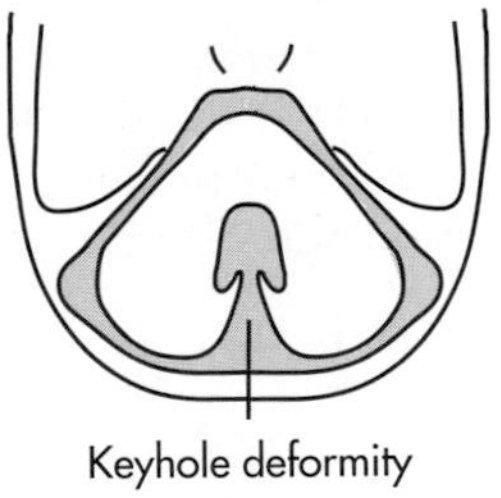

FIGURE 6-80

PHAKOMATOSES

Group of neuroectodermal disorders characterized by coexisting skin and CNS tumors:

Common phakomatoses:
- Neurofibromatosis
- Tuberous sclerosis

- VHL disease
- Sturge-Weber syndrome

Uncommon syndromes:
- Gorlin syndrome
- Osler-Weber-Rendu disease
- Ataxia-telangiectasia
- Klippel-Trénaunay syndrome
- Blue rubber bleb nevus syndrome

NEUROFIBROMATOSIS

Most common phakomatosis (1: 3000). 50% autosomal dominant, 50% spontaneous mutations. Dysplasia of mesodermal and neuroectodermal tissue.

TYPES OF NEUROFIBROMATOSIS

Feature	NF1	NF2
Name	von Recklinghausen disease	Bilateral acoustic neuroma
Defect	Chromosome 17	Chromosome 22
Frequency	90%	10%
Skin (nodules, café-au-lait)	Prominent	Minimal
Tumors	Hamartomas, gliomas, malignant nerve sheath tumor	Meningiomas, schwannoma, ependymoma
Spinal	Neurofibroma	Schwannoma

Diagnostic Criteria

NF1 (need ≥ 2 criteria)
- ≥ 6 café-au-lait spots
- ≥ 2 pigmented iris hamartomas (Lisch nodules)
- Axillary, inguinal freckling
- ≥ 2 neurofibroma (or 1 plexiform neurofibroma)
- Optic nerve glioma
- First-degree relative with NF1
- Dysplasia of greater wing of sphenoid

NF2 (need ≥ 1 criterion)
- Bilateral acoustic neuromas
- First-degree relative with NF2 and unilateral acoustic neuroma or meningioma, glioma, schwannoma, neurofibroma (any two)

Imaging Features of NF1

CNS
- Optic nerve gliomas, 15%
  - Low-grade pilocytic astrocytoma
  - Variable enhancement
- Low-grade brainstem gliomas
- Nonneoplastic hamartomas, 80%-90%
  - T2W hyperintense, T1W not visible
  - No mass effect or enhancement in 90%
  - Basal ganglia, WM, dentate nuclei
- Moyamoya cerebral occlusive disease
- Aneurysms

Spinal cord/canal
- Neurofibromas of exiting nerves
  - Enlarged neural foramen
  - Intradural extramedullary tumors (classic "dumbbell tumors")
- Dural ectasia
  - Enlarged neural foramen
  - Posterior vertebral scalloping
- Low-grade cord astrocytomas
- Lateral meningoceles

Skull
- Hypoplastic sphenoid wing
- Macrocrania
- Lambdoid suture defect

Plexiform neurofibromas, 33%
- Diagnostic of NF1
- Common along cranial nerve V peripherally
  - Head and neck
  - Intense enhancement
  - Sarcomatous degeneration, 10%

Skeletal, 50%-80%
- Erosion of bones and foramina by slow-growing neuromas
- Bowing of tibia and fibula; pseudarthroses
- Unilateral overgrowth of limbs: focal gigantism
- Twisted ribs (ribbon ribs)

Chest
- Progressive pulmonary fibrosis
- Intrathoracic meningoceles
- Lung and mediastinal neurofibromas

Vascular
- Renal artery stenosis
- Renal artery aneurysm
- Abdominal coarctation

Other
- Pheochromocytoma

Imaging Features of NF2

CNS
- Bilateral acoustic schwannoma diagnostic
- Other cranial nerve schwannomas (cranial nerve V)
- Meningiomas (often multiple)

Spinal cord/canal
- Intradural, extramedullary meningiomas
- Schwannomas
- Intramedullary ependymoma

Pearls

- Mnemonic: "MISME": **M**ultiple **I**nherited **S**chwannomas, **M**eningiomas, and **E**pendymomas
- Presence of mass effect and contrast enhancement help to differentiate gliomas from hamartomas. Some hamartomas enhance; over time they should not change in size.

- Contrast-enhanced scans should be acquired in all patients to detect gliomas, small meningiomas, and neuromas.
- NF1 typically has lesions of neurons and astrocytes.
- NF2 typically has lesions of Schwann cells and meninges.

VON HIPPEL-LINDAU (VHL) DISEASE

VHL disease (cerebelloretinal hemangioblastomatosis; autosomal dominant with 100% penetrance) is characterized by the presence of hemangioblastomas and renal (renal cell carcinoma [RCC] and cysts), adrenal, pancreatic, and scrotal abnormalities. Associated with chromosome 3.

Clinical Findings

Hemangioblastoma, 50%
- Cerebellum (most common location)
- Brainstem, spinal cord
- Retinal

Renal
- RCC, 50% (bilateral in 65%, multiple in 85%)
- Benign renal cysts, 60%

Adrenal glands
- Pheochromocytoma, 15%; bilateral in 40%

Pancreas
- Multiple cysts, 70%
- Cystadenocarcinoma
- Islet cell tumor

Scrotum
- Epididymal cysts, 10%

Other
- Hepatic cysts, 20%
- Splenic cysts, 10%

Imaging Features

- Hemangioblastomas: enhancing nodules in subpial location
- Multiple hemangioblastomas is diagnostic of VHL disease.
- MRI is the first study of choice.
- CT is often used to evaluate kidneys, adrenals, and pancreas.

Pearls

- Entire CNS must be imaged (brain and spinal cord).
- Most patients with solitary hemangioblastoma do not have VHL disease.
- Family screening is necessary.

TUBEROUS SCLEROSIS (BOURNEVILLE DISEASE) (Figs. 6-81 and 6-82)

Autosomal dominant (20%-50%) or sporadic (50%) or inherited (50%), neuroectodermal disorder. The clinical triad of adenoma sebaceum, seizures, and mental retardation is found in a minority.

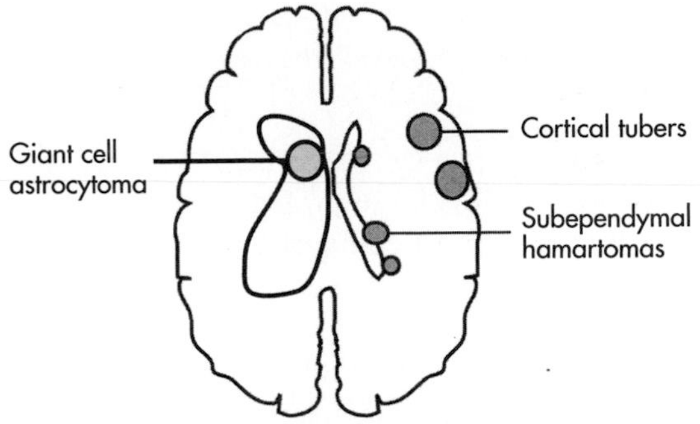

FIGURE 6-81

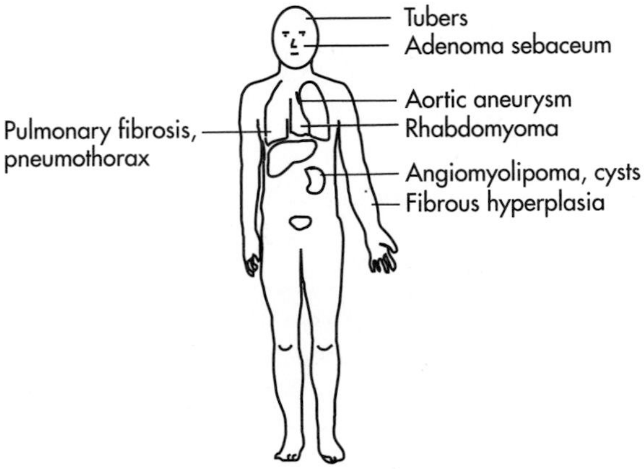

FIGURE 6-82

Imaging Features

CNS (four major CNS lesions)
- Hamartoma containing abnormal neurons and astrocytes; typical locations:
  - Cortical (GM) tubers
  - Subependymal (candle drippings), hamartomas common near foramen of Monro
- Tubers:
  - Cortical location
  - Tubers may calcify (differential diagnosis: CMV, toxoplasmosis)
  - Noncalcified tubers: T1W hypointense, T2W hyperintense; no enhancement on CT but variable enhancement on MRI
- Subependymal giant cell astrocytoma
  - Located at foramen of Monro
  - Can obstruct and cause hydrocephalus
- Disorganized/dysplastic WM lesions:
  - Wedge-shaped tumefactive and linear or curvilinear (radial bands) lesions in the cerebral hemisphere and multiple linear bands extending from a conglomerate focus near the 4th ventricle into cerebellar hemispheres. Visualization of these radial bands is specific to tuberous sclerosis, and they are usually arranged perpendicular to the ventricles.

Kidney
- Angiomyolipoma, 50%; usually multiple and bilateral
- Multiple cysts

Bone, 50%
- Bone islands in multiple bones
- Periosteal thickening of long bones
- Bone cysts

Other
- Pulmonary lymphangioleiomyomatosis
- Spontaneous pneumothorax, 50%
- Chylothorax
- Cardiac rhabdomyomas, 5%
- Aortic aneurysm

STURGE-WEBER-DIMITRI SYNDROME (ENCEPHALOTRIGEMINAL ANGIOMATOSIS)

Capillary venous angiomas of the face and ipsilateral cerebral hemisphere.

Clinical Findings
- Port-wine nevus of cutaneous distribution of cranial nerve V (V1 most frequent), unilateral
- Seizures, 90%
- Mental retardation
- Ipsilateral glaucoma
- Hemiparesis, 50%

Imaging Features
- Tramtrack cortical calcifications (characteristic) that follow cortical convolutions; most common in parietal occipital lobes
- Atrophic cortex with enlarged adjacent subarachnoid space
- Ipsilateral thickening of skull and orbit
- Leptomeningeal venous angiomas: parietal > occipital > frontal lobes; enhancement
- Enlargement and increased contrast enhancement of ipsilateral choroid plexus
- MRI: cortical calcifications may be confused with flow voids because of their hypointensity.

MESIAL TEMPORAL SCLEROSIS

Partial complex seizures in adolescents/young adults; may also be associated with infantile febrile seizures. Mesial temporal lobe contains hippocampus, amygdala, parahippocampal gyrus. Bilateral, 20%.

Imaging Features
- Volume loss of hippocampus
- Ex vacuo dilatation of temporal horn
- Hippocampal T2-hyperintensity may be present
- Atrophy of ipsilateral fornix, mammillary body

Sellar and Juxtasellar Regions

NEOPLASM

PITUITARY ADENOMA

Adenomas (10%-15% of primary brain neoplasms) originate from the anterior hypophysis. The old classification of pituitary adenomas is based on light microscopy staining (chromophobic, acidophilic, basophilic, mixed). The new classification is based on the hormones produced. Two types:
- Microadenomas (<10 mm): often (75%) endocrinologically functional
- Macroadenomas (>10 mm): often endocrinologically nonfunctional

FUNCTIONING PITUITARY MICROADENOMA

Tumor confined to the gland <10 mm.

Types
- Prolactinoma (most common; galactorrhea, amenorrhea, decreased libido)
- Growth hormone (GH) (acromegaly, gigantism)
- Adrenocorticotropic hormone (ACTH) (Cushing syndrome)
- Gonadotroph (infertility or menstrual problems in women, follicle-stimulating hormone)
- Mixed (prolactin, GH, thyroid-stimulating hormone least common)

Imaging Features (Fig. 6-83)

Sensitivity: MRI is the most sensitive imaging study to detect pituitary microadenomas.

Technique
- Obtain coronal and sagittal views before and after administration of Gd-DTPA. Small abnormalities confirmed on both planes are real, whereas those seen on one view only are likely to be artifacts.
- Use high-resolution thin slices.

T1W noncontrast appearance
- Microadenomas are hypointense/isointense relative to pituitary
- Gland asymmetry

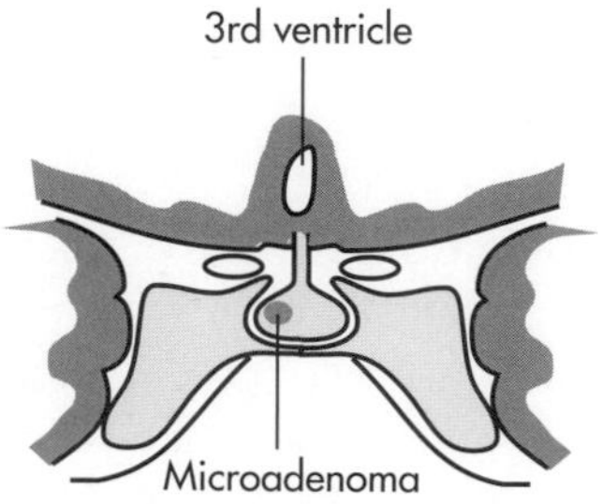

FIGURE 6-83

- Gland is convex superiorly (normal: flat or concave)
- Stalk deviation
- Depression of sella floor

Contrast enhancement (Gd-DTPA):

- Dynamic imaging is required.
- Adenoma enhances less rapidly than normal pituitary.

Differentiation of adenoma type by enhancement pattern:

- ACTH adenomas usually enhance strongly (difficult to detect).
- 70% adenomas are hypointense relative to pituitary in dynamic phase.
- Adenoma may not be seen if only delayed images are acquired.
- Petrosal sinus sampling may be helpful if MRI is nondiagnostic.

NONFUNCTIONING PITUITARY MACROADENOMA

Unlike microadenomas, macroadenomas are symptomatic because of their mass effect (e.g., hypopituitarism, visual problems). Nevertheless, they may attain very large size before cranial nerves are affected. Macroadenomas secrete hormone subunits that are clinically silent. Current nomenclature is "null-cell adenoma" or "oncocytoma."

Imaging Features (Fig. 6-84)

Large tumor extending beyond the confines of the sella

- Intrasellar expansion (ballooning of sella)
- Extension into suprasellar cistern
  - Figure-eight shape
  - Thickening of cavernous sinus
  - Encasement/narrowing of cavernous ICA flow void. Cavernous sinus involvement can be difficult to determine unless tumor surrounds the vessel/cavernous sinus.
  - Compression of optic chiasm
  - Upward displacement of third ventricle
  - Obstruction of foramen of Monro with hydrocephalus, 10%
  - Compression of frontal horn of lateral ventricles
  - Splaying of cerebral peduncles

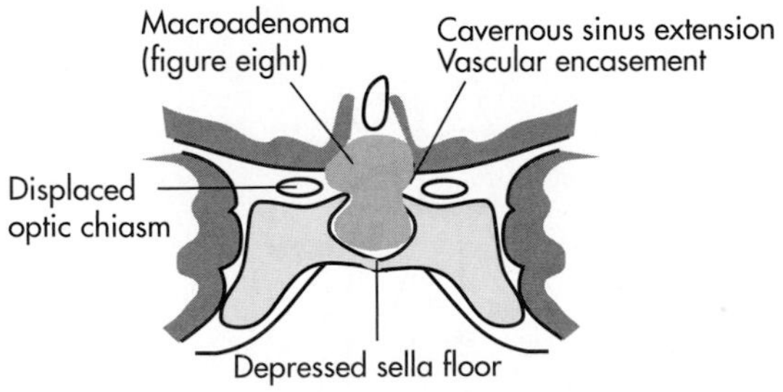

FIGURE 6-84

Morphologic features

- Calcification, uncommon (1%-8%)
- Intratumoral necrosis, hemorrhage (T1W hyperintense)
- Benign invasive adenoma cannot be distinguished from pituitary carcinoma, although malignant pituitary carcinoma is very rare (<1% of adenomas).

Enhancement

- Intense but heterogeneous

MRI features

- Heterogeneous appearance because of solid and cystic components
- Use multiplanar MRI to define relationship of tumor to surrounding anatomy.

CRANIOPHARYNGIOMA

Craniopharyngiomas are benign tumors that arise from squamous epithelial remnants along Rathke's duct/pouch. Most common tumor of the suprasellar cistern. Age: 1st to 2nd decade (>50%), with second peak in older adults. Location: 7% combined suprasellar/intrasellar; completely intrasellar craniopharyngiomas rare.

Clinical Findings

- Growth retardation (compression of hypothalamus)
- Diabetes insipidus (pituitary compression)
- Bitemporal hemianopsia
- Headaches (most common)
- Cranial nerve palsies (cavernous sinus involvement)

Types

Adamantinous (children)

- Cystic mass (90%) with mural nodule in suprasellar location
- Calcification in 90%

Papillary (adult)

- Solid lesion
- Calcification less common in adults (50%)

Imaging Features

- Enhancement of solid lesion rim, no enhancement of cystic lesion
- Variable signal intensity by MRI depending on cyst content: high protein content, blood, cholesterol. The most common MRI appearance is T1W hypointensity and T2W hyperintensity.
- Obstruction of foramen of Monro with hydrocephalus, 60%
- Usually avascular by angiography

Pearls

- A suprasellar mass in a child or adolescent is considered a craniopharyngioma until proven otherwise.

- The majority of craniopharyngiomas have cystic components; purely solid tumors are rare.
- Differential diagnosis: necrotic pituitary adenoma, cystic optochiasmic glioma, thrombosed aneurysm, Rathke's cleft cyst (no calcification, no nodular enhancement, but can have rim enhancement)
- Clinical presentations of pediatric suprasellar region lesions:
  - Diabetes insipidus most common with eosinophilic granuloma of stalk
  - Precocious puberty most common with hypothalamic hamartoma
  - Growth delay most common with craniopharyngioma

OTHER

EMPTY SELLA

Defect in sella diaphragm with extension of CSF space into the sella. An empty sella is a common anatomic variant. Incidence: 10% of adults. Clinical: incidental finding, asymptomatic, no clinical significance. Differentiate from:

- Cystic sella tumor
- Surgically removed pituitary gland
- Involuted pituitary (Sheehan syndrome)

POSTSURGICAL SELLA

Small tumors are often removed via a transsphenoidal approach (anterior wall of sphenoid sinus → sella); typically, sella and sphenoidal sinus are packed with Gelfoam, muscle, and fat; postsurgical fluid may be seen in the sphenoidal sinus.

Imaging Features

- Image sella soon after surgery to establish baseline imaging appearance for further follow-up.
- Gd-DTPA fat-suppression MRI techniques are helpful to suppress bright signal from surgical fat plug in the sella and to enhance pituitary tissue.

ECTOPIC NEUROHYPOPHYSIS

The neurohypophysis (T1W hyperintense) is located in the hypothalamic region or in the sella; frequently associated with a small or absent pituitary gland. Clinical: hypopituitarism.

PITUITARY APOPLEXY

Manifests as acute onset of terrible headache, ptosis, vision changes, diplopia, nausea/vomiting. MRI is test of choice; it may detect hemorrhage within the sella.

Causes

- Acute onset of hemorrhage into pituitary adenoma with necrosis and infarction of the pituitary gland
- Sheehan syndrome: postpartum infarction of anterior pituitary gland

Spine

CONGENITAL

SPINAL DYSRAPHISM

A group of spinal anomalies involving incomplete midline closure of bone, and neural and soft tissues.

Classification (Fig. 6-85)

Open spinal dysraphism (spina bifida aperta), 85%: posterior protrusion of spinal contents through the dorsal bone defect; neurologic defects are common.

- Myelomeningocele: protruding placode, almost 100% association with Chiari II
- Lipomyelomeningocele: protruding placode with fat
- Myelocele: neural placode flush with surface not covered by skin

Occult spinal dysraphism, 15%: no exposed neural tissue; covered by skin; neurologic defects are uncommon.

- Lipomyelomeningocele (not part of Chiari II)
- Meningocele (Fig. 6-86)
- Dorsal dermal sinus

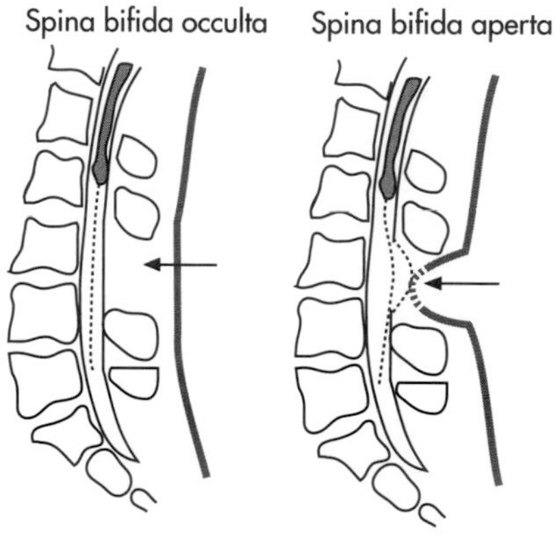

FIGURE 6-85

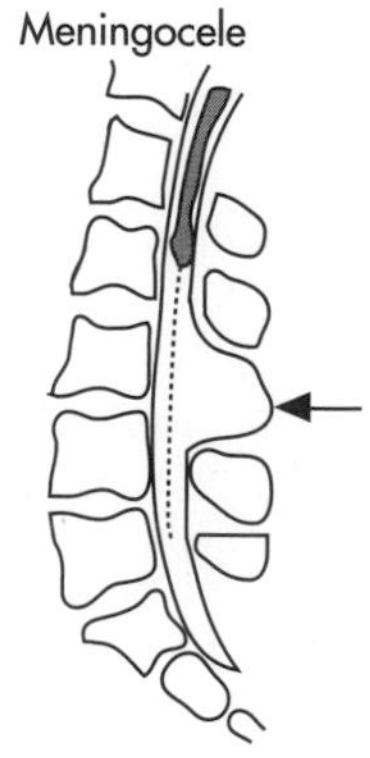

FIGURE 6-86

- Spinal lipoma
- Tethered cord
- Split notochord syndromes

Open dysraphisms are nearly always diagnosed by prenatal US. CT and MRI are most commonly used to plan surgical repair.

DORSAL DERMAL SINUS

Epithelialized sinus tract connecting the skin to the spinal canal/cord. May end in subcutaneous fat, meninges, or cord. 50% terminate in a dermoid/epidermoid. Location: lumbosacral > occipital. Clinical findings include infection, overlying hairy path, or skin abnormality.

LIPOMYELOMENINGOCELE (Fig. 6-87)

Most common occult spinal dysraphism. Female > male. Presentation: usually in infancy, some into adulthood.

Clinical Findings

- Neurogenic bladder
- Orthopedic deformities
- Sensory problems
- Not associated with Chiari II

Imaging Features

Plain film

- Incomplete posterior fusion (spina bifida)
- Widened spinal cord
- Segmentation anomalies

MRI

- Tethered cord
- Syringohydromyelia, 25%
- Extradural lipoma contiguous with subcutaneous fat
- Nerve roots from placode

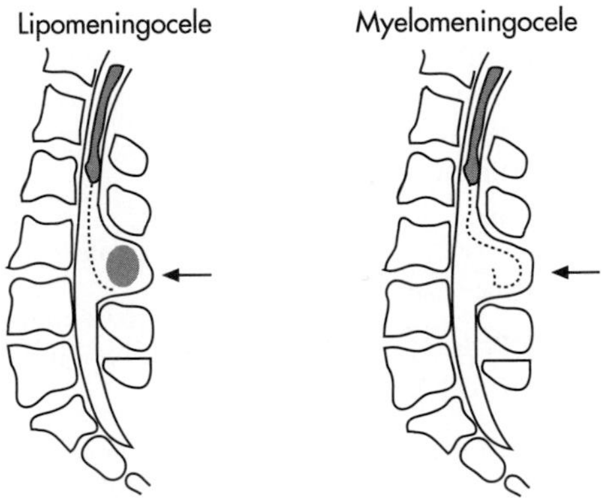

FIGURE 6-87

TETHERED SPINAL CORD (Fig. 6-88)

Neurologic and orthopedic disorders associated with a short, thick filum and an abnormally low (below L2) conus medullaris (normal location of cord at 16 weeks, L4-L5; at birth, L2-L3; later, L1-L2). Commonly a component of other spinal malformations: spinal lipoma/lipomyelomeningocele, diastematomyelia, dermal sinus. Manifests in children and young adults.

Clinical Findings

- Paresthesias
- Pain
- Neurogenic bladder
- Kyphoscoliosis
- Incontinence
- Spasticity

Imaging Features

- Plain films may or may not reveal osseous dysraphism.
- Axial MRI and CT myelography are imaging studies of choice. Sagittal views can be difficult to interpret.
- Low-lying conus (below L2)
- Enlarged thecal sac
- Lipoma, 50%
- Thick filum terminale >1.5 mm

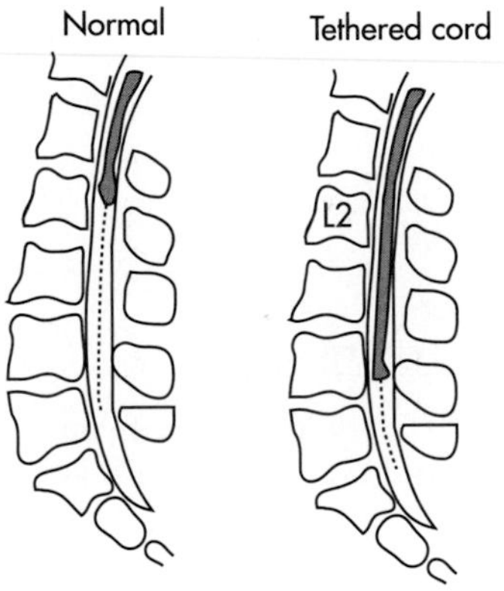

FIGURE 6-88

DIASTEMATOMYELIA (ONE OF THE "SPLIT NOTOCHORD SYNDROMES")

Sagittal division of spinal cord into two hemicords. The cords may be split by a fibrous septum or a bony spur. The two hemicords share a common thecal sac (50%) or have their own thecal sac (50%). Severe forms are associated with neurenteric cysts. Clinical presentation is similar to that of other occult spinal dysraphism. Do not confuse with diplomyelia, the true spinal cord duplication (very rare).

Associations

- Tethered cord
- Hydromyelia
- Meningocele, myelomeningocele, lipomyelomeningocele
- Abnormal vertebral bodies: hemivertebra, block vertebra, etc.
- Scoliosis, clubfoot, and cutaneous stigmata >50%
- Chiari II

Other

- Most severe but rare dorsal enteric fistula

Imaging Features

- Usually thoracolumbar (85% below T9)
- MRI is the imaging study of choice.
- Osseous abnormalities are nearly always present.
  - Segmentation anomalies (e.g., hemivertebra, block, butterfly)
  - Incomplete posterior fusion
  - Osseous spur, 50%
- Tethered cord, 75%

HYDROSYRINGOMYELIA

Term used to describe two entities that are often difficult to separate: abnormal dilatation of the central canal (hydromyelia) and short cord cavity (syrinx), which may or may not communicate with the central canal. Causes include:

Congenital (usually results in hydromyelia)

- Chiari malformation
- Myelomeningocele

Acquired (usually results in syringomyelia)

- Posttraumatic
- Tumors

INFECTION

SPONDYLITIS AND DISKITIS

Spine infections may progress from spondylitis → diskitis → epidural abscess → cord abscess. Infective spondylitis usually involves extradural components of the spine such as posterior elements, disks (diskitis), vertebral body (osteomyelitis), and paraspinous soft tissues.

Causes

- Pyogenic: *Staphylococcus aureus* > *Enterococcus* > *E. coli, Salmonella*
- TB
- Fungal
- Parasitic

Imaging Features

- Normal plain film findings for 8 to 10 days after infection onset
- T2W hyperintense disk
- Contrast enhancement
- Soft tissue mass (inflammation, abscess)

SPINAL TUBERCULOSIS (POTT DISEASE)

- Bone destruction is prominent; more indolent onset than with pyogenic bone destruction
- Loss of disk height, 80%
- Gibbus deformity: anterior involvement with normal posterior vertebral bodies
- Involvement of several adjacent vertebral bodies with disk destruction, although disk involvement may be less prominent compared to pyogenic infection
- Large paraspinous abscess
- Extension into psoas muscles (psoas abscess)

ARACHNOIDITIS

Causes

- Surgery ("failed back" syndrome)
- Subarachnoid hemorrhage
- Pantopaque myelography
- Infection

Imaging Features

- CT myelography is superior to MRI for establishing the diagnosis. Never use ionic contrast material for myelography because it may cause a fatal arachnoiditis.
- Myelographic block is seen with severe adhesive arachnoiditis.
- Intradural scarring/loculation (limited enhancement)
- Clumping of nerve roots within the thecal sac (intrathecal pseudomass); blunting of caudal nerve root sleeves; nerve roots may also clump peripherally (empty thecal sac sign)
- Intradural cysts (may be bright on T1W images)
- Irregular margins of thecal sac

GUILLAIN-BARRÉ SYNDROME

Autoimmune disease attacking the peripheral nervous system causing acute and rapidly progressive inflammatory demyelinating polyneuropathy. May have a prodromal viral illness. Can lead to complete paralysis. Respiratory support (ventilator) if the diaphragm is involved. Most patients eventually recover (70%). Diagnosis usually established from CSF and electrophysiologic criteria.

MR imaging

- Nerve root enhancement in cauda equina
- Exclude other causes

CHRONIC INFLAMMATORY DEMYELINATING POLYNEUROPATHY (CIDP)

Similar to Guillain-Barré in symptoms but chronically progressive or relapsing. However, CIDP is now considered to be a distinct disease and not a relapse or chronic form of Guillain-Barré. May have CNS involvement.

MR imaging

Nerve root enhancement

Nerve root hypertrophy, especially extra-foraminal

DEGENERATIVE ABNORMALITIES

DISK HERNIATION (Fig. 6-89)

Spectrum of Intervertebral Disk Herniation

Posterior disk herniation
- Intraspinal herniation (herniated disk)

Anterior disk herniation
- Elevation of the anterior longitudinal ligament
- May mimic anterior osteophytes

Schmorl's nodule
- Cephalocaudal extrusion of disk material
- Young adults (1 to 2 levels affected; Scheuermann disease: >3 levels affected)

Intravertebral disk herniation (limbus vertebra)
- Anterior herniation of disk material
- Triangular bone fragment

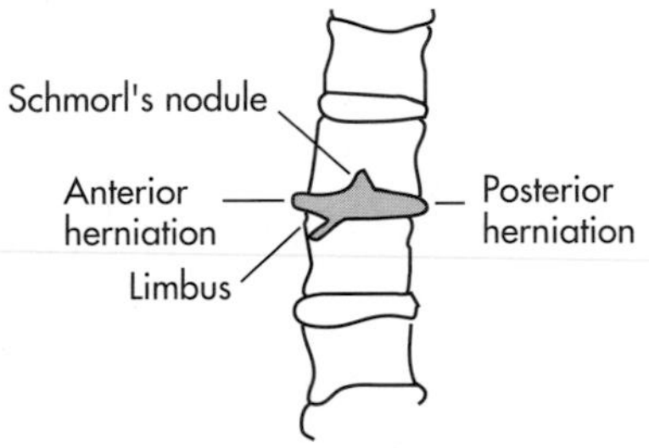

FIGURE 6-89

POSTERIOR DISK HERNIATION (Fig. 6-90)

The most important point in describing a disk herniation is the exact relationship of the disk to neural structures.

- Bulging disk: symmetrical perimeter expansion of a weakened disk; intact annulus
- Herniated disk: focal rather than diffuse bulge; annulus fibrosus is torn; disk material herniates through separation
- ASNR definitions
  - Disk bulge: >50% of circumference
  - Disk protrusion: <50% of circumference, wider than tall
  - Disk extrusion: <50% of circumference, taller than wide in any plane; some extrusions can be seen only on sagittal images

Note that there is much controversy regarding these definitions and imaging findings, especially their clinical correlation with lower back pain and need for surgery. Imaging modalities are useful mainly to guide surgery.

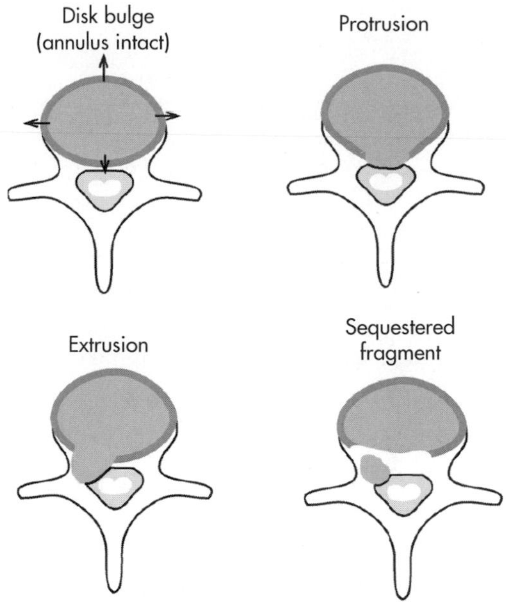

FIGURE 6-90

Imaging Features

Detection: MRI is the imaging study of choice.

CT myelography
- Permits reliable visualization of nerve roots in the thecal sac
- Disadvantage: time-consuming, invasive

Plain films
- The diagnosis of herniation is not possible by plain film.
- All findings of degenerative joint disease (e.g., narrowing of disk space, spurring, eburnation, vacuum sign) may appear in patients with or without herniation.

MRI Features (Fig. 6-91)

Techniques
- Sagittal T1W and T2W
- Axial T1W and/or FSE T2W (T1W at most institutions)
- Axial acquisitions should be angled to axis of disk space

Extruded disk material gives rise to the toothpaste sign (disk material is extruded from disk into the spinal canal like toothpaste); the material may be continuous with the disk (simple herniation) or be separated (free fragment herniation). Free fragments may have MR signal characteristics different from the native disk material.

Location of herniation

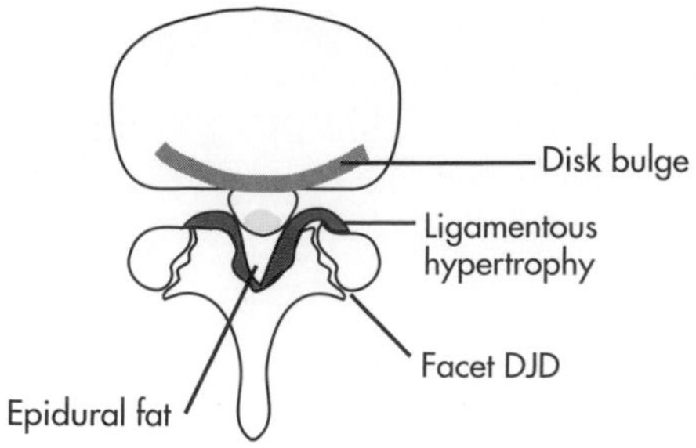

FIGURE 6-91

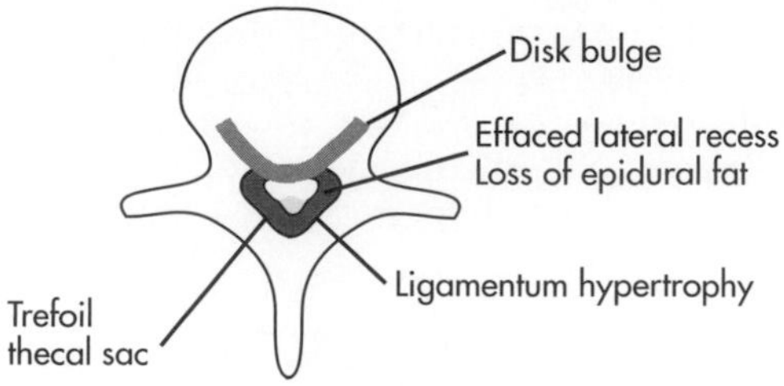

FIGURE 6-92

- Paracentral (most common)
- Posterolateral
- Central (uncommon, ligament is strongest here)
- Often missed by axial imaging:
  Lateral, extraforaminal extension
  Intraforaminal extension

Role of contrast
- Postoperation: differentiate scar from residual/recurrent disk herniation (scar enhances)
- Not as helpful in the cervical spine postoperation evaluation because the areas of abnormality are usually the levels above and below the surgery.
- Helpful for confirming extruded fragments
- Facilitates diagnosis of neuritis secondary to herniation

Secondary degenerative abnormalities
- Endplate marrow changes ("diskogenic" endplate disease)
  Modic I: T1W dark/T2W bright: vascular granulation tissue, may enhance
  Modic II: T1W bright/T2W isointense or bright: fatty marrow replacement
  Modic III: T1W dark/T2W dark: sclerosis
- Degenerated disks are T2W hypointense (loss of proteoglycans, H_2O). However, normally aging disks may also be hypointense.
- Osteophytes and facet hypertrophy contribute to neural foraminal stenosis.
- Ligamentum flavum hypertrophy

Location
- Lumbar: L4-L5 or L5-S1, 95% (the first "freely mobile" nonsacralized disk level)
- Thoracic: most common at the four lowest disk levels
- Cervical: C5-C6 and C6-C7, 90%

SPINAL STENOSIS

Narrowing of the spinal canal with or without compression of the cord and/or CSF block.

Causes (Fig. 6-92)

Acquired, most common
- Bulging or protruding disks
- Hypertrophy of ligamentum flavum
- Hypertrophy of facets
- Degenerative osteophytes
- Spondylolisthesis

Congenital
- Short pedicles, thick laminae, large facets
- Morquio syndrome
- Achondroplasia

Imaging Features

MRI is study of choice:
- T2W sequences best define the thecal sac.
- T1W sequences best define the lateral recesses (fat).
- Look for "trefoil" appearance of thecal sac and complete effacement of epidural fat.

CT myelogram useful in equivocal cases.

Associated spinal cord changes:
- T2W hyperintensity: edema or gliosis
- Atrophy: chronic

SPINAL BLOCK

Complete spinal stenosis with no communication of spinal fluid.

FORAMINAL STENOSIS

Stenosis of the intervertebral foramen that involves the exiting nerve as it passes under the pedicle. Causes include:
- Degenerative osteophytes of the facets
- Spondylolisthesis
- Lateral herniated disks
- Fracture
- Postoperative scarring
- Lateral recess masses (extradural masses)

POSTOPERATIVE SPINE

Manifests clinically as "failed back" syndrome. Common problems include:
- Recurrent disk herniation (operative site or another site)
- Scar formation
- Neural foramina stenosis
- Neuritis
- Arachnoiditis

- Lateral recess stenosis (simple laminectomy does not decompress the lateral recess)
- Dural bulge (pseudomeningocele)
- Diskitis
- Epidural hematoma or abscess
- Cord infarct: after AAA repair, conus medullaris. Restricted diffusion.

Imaging Features

Differentiation of recurrent disk herniation and epidural scar formation:
- Gd-DTPA–enhanced MRI is the study of choice.
- Scar tissue usually shows early homogeneous enhancement.
- Disk usually shows late peripheral enhancement (surrounding granulation tissue).

Detection of complications (see earlier)

ACUTE TRANSVERSE MYELOPATHY

Clinical syndrome with a variety of underlying causes:
- Acute infection
- Postinfection
  - Vaccination
  - Autoimmune
- Systemic malignancy
- Posttraumatic

Imaging Features

- MRI normal in 50% during acute phase
- T2W hyperintensity
- Focal cord enlargement
- Contrast enhancement may be present

SUBACUTE COMBINED DEGENERATION

Myelopathy involving cervical and thoracic cord, results from vitamin B_{12} deficiency. Longitudinal T2 hyperintensity is seen in the dorsal columns of the posterior cord. DDx: syphilis (tabes dorsalis).

Tumors (Fig. 6-93)

APPROACH

- MRI is the imaging study of choice.
- CT indicated for osseous lesions; CT myelography is more useful than noncontrast CT.
- Classify lesions by their location in anatomic compartments:
  - Intramedullary: within the spinal cord
  - Intradural: within the dural sac but outside cord
  - Extradural: outside the thecal sac

INTRAMEDULLARY TUMORS

Types

- Astrocytoma (most common in pediatric population)
- Ependymoma (most common in the adult population; lower spinal cord, conus medullaris and filum terminale)
- Hemangioblastoma
- Metastases (rare)

Imaging Features

- Expansion of cord
- Large cystic components, 50%
- Differentiation of different tumors is usually not possible by imaging methods, although astrocytoma tends to be less well-defined and more infiltrative.
- Describe the extent of the solid tumor and the extent of the cyst (during surgery the tumor will be removed while the cyst will be decompressed).

ASTROCYTOMA

Location: thoracic 65%, cervical 50%. Isolated conus medullaris involvement occurs in 3% of cases. Astrocytomas are rare in the filum terminale.

Imaging Features

- MRI: poorly defined margins and are isointense to hypointense relative to the spinal cord on T1W images and hyperintense on T2W images. The average length of involvement is seven vertebral segments. Cysts are a common feature, with both polar and intratumoral types being observed.
- Virtually all cord astrocytomas show at least some enhancement after the intravenous administration of contrast material.

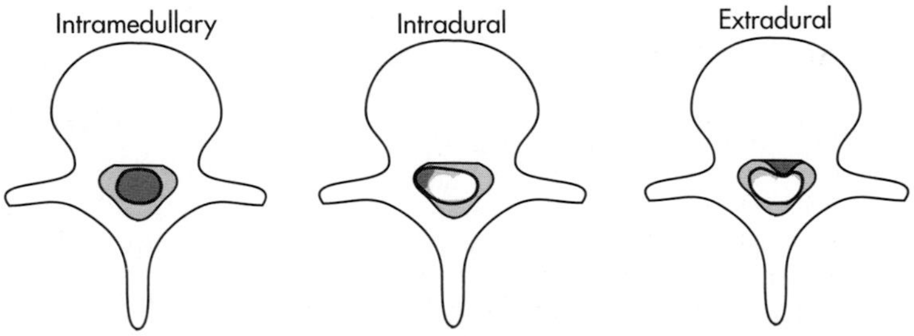

FIGURE 6-93

- Widened interpedicular distance and bone erosion may be evident on conventional radiography and CT. Patients with holocord involvement tend to present with scoliosis and canal widening.

EPENDYMOMA

Location: cervical alone, 45%; cervicothoracic, 25%; thoracic alone, 25%; conus, 5%. Myxopapillary ependymoma is, in rare cases, found in the subcutaneous tissue of the sacrococcygeal region, usually without any connection with the spinal canal. It is believed that these arise from either heterotopic ependymal cell rests or vestigial remnants of the distal neural tube during canalization and retrogressive differentiation.

Imaging Features

- T1W: isointense or hypointense relative to the spinal cord
- T2W: hyperintense. 20%-33% of ependymomas demonstrate the "cap sign," a rim of extreme hypointensity (hemosiderin) seen at the poles of the tumor on T2W images. Most cases (60%) also show evidence of cord edema around the masses.
- Cysts in 80%, most of which are the nontumoral (polar) variety
- Radiographs: scoliosis, 15%; canal widening, 10%; vertebral body scalloping, pedicle erosion, or laminar thinning
- CT: isoattenuated or slight hyperattenuated compared with the normal spinal cord. Intense enhancement with contrast. CT myelography shows nonspecific cord enlargement. Complete or partial block in the flow of contrast material.

HEMANGIOBLASTOMA

Seventy-five percent of these tumors are intramedullary but can involve the intradural space or even the extradural space. Extramedullary hemangioblastomas are commonly attached to the dorsal cord pia or nerve roots. Location: thoracic, 50%; cervical cord, 40%. Most cord hemangioblastomas (80%) are solitary and occur in patients younger than 40 years old. The presence of multiple lesions should prompt work-up for VHL disease.

Imaging Features

- Diffuse cord expansion
- T1W: isointense, 50%; hyperintense 25%
- T2W: usually hyperintense with focal flow voids
- Cyst formation or syringohydromyelia is very common.
- Only 25% of hemangioblastomas are solid.

METASTASES

Intramedullary spinal metastases are relatively rare (1% of autopsied cancer patients). Location: cervical 45%, thoracic 35%, lumbar region 8%. Most metastases are solitary, with an average length of two to three vertebral segments. Routes of spread include hematogenous (via the arterial supply) and direct extension from the leptomeninges. Primary tumors include:

- Lung carcinoma, 40%-85%
- Breast carcinoma, 11%
- Melanoma, 5%
- Renal cell carcinoma, 4%
- Colorectal carcinoma, 3%
- Lymphoma, 3%

NERVE SHEATH TUMORS

Nerve sheath tumors are the most common intradural, extramedullary mass lesions. Clinical findings may mimic those of disk herniation.

Types

- Schwannoma
- Neurofibroma
- Ganglioneuroma
- Neurofibrosarcoma (rare)

Imaging Features

Location
  - Intradural, extramedullary, 75%
  - Extradural, 15%
  - Intramedullary, <1%
  - Multiple in neurofibromatosis

Morphology
  - Dumbbell shaped, 15%
  - Enlargement of neural foramen
  - Contrast enhancement, 100%
  - T1W: isointense 75%, hyperintense 25%
  - T2W: very hyperintense, target appearance common

SYNOVIAL CYST

- Typically ovoid
- MRI: T1W hypointense; T2W hyperintense with hypointense rim
- The rim may enhance.
- Associated with the facet joint posterolaterally
- Sometimes may be difficult to distinguish from sequestered disk fragment.
- Can cause spinal stenosis and pain.

NEOPLASMS OF THE FILUM TERMINALE

Common
  - Ependymoma (especially myxopapillary)
  - Astrocytoma (especially anaplastic and pilocytic)
  - Hemangioblastoma

Less common
- Subependymoma
- Ganglioglioma
- Paraganglioma
- Metastases
- Lymphoma
- PNET
- Neurocytoma
- Oligodendroglioma
- Mixed glioma
- Glioblastoma multiforme

VERTEBROPLASTY/KYPHOPLASTY (Fig. 6-94)

Percutaneous injection of polymethylmethacrylate (PMMA) cement to prevent vertebral body collapse and pain in patients with pathologic vertebral bodies.

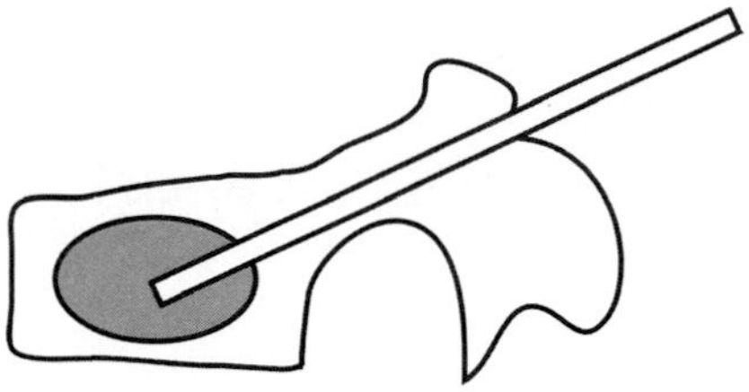

FIGURE 6-94

Indications
- Symptomatic vertebral hemangioma
- Pain due to vertebral body and acetabular tumors (multiple myeloma, metastases)
- Severely painful osteoporosis with loss of height with or without compression fractures. Sagittal STIR MRI or bone scan helpful in determining age of fractures.

Absolute Contraindications
- Hemorrhagic diathesis
- Infection

Risks
- Cement leak is the most serious complication: epidural space, disc space, vein → pulmonary embolus
- Infection
- Bleeding

Kyphoplasty
- Expansion of the vertebral body with a balloon before cement injection
- Goal is to restore height

Differential Diagnosis

TUMORS

APPROACH TO INTRACRANIAL MASS LESION (Fig. 6-95) STIR

Mnemonic: "TEACH:"
- **T**umor
  - Primary
  - Metastases
- **E**dema
- **A**bscess
- **C**yst, contusion
- **H**ematoma

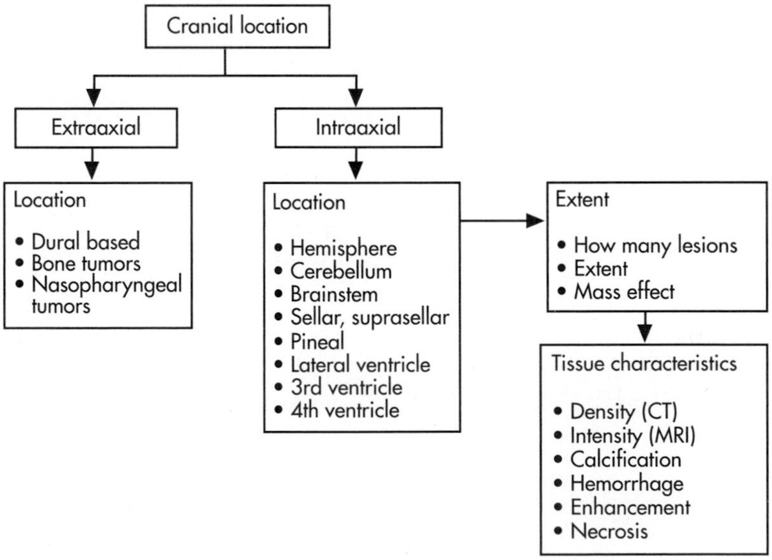

FIGURE 6-95

EXTRAAXIAL MASSES (Fig. 6-96)

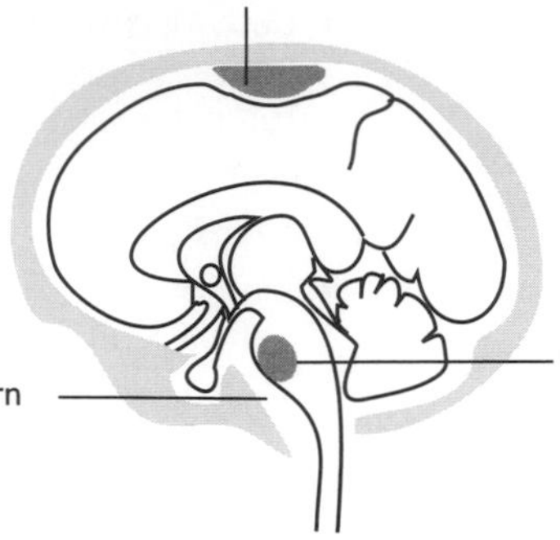
Extraaxial, hemisphere
• Meningioma
• Metastases
• Lymphoma
• Arachnoid cyst
• Dermoid/epidermoid
• Other: hemorrhagic, infectious fluid collections
Clivus, prepontine cistern
• Metastases
• Meningioma
• Chordoma
• Chondroma, chondrosarcoma
CP angle mass
• CN VIII neuroma (also CN V, CN VII)
• Meningioma
• Epidermoid
• Paraganglioma
• Petrous apex cholesterol cysts
• Aneurysm
• Metastases
• Other (arachnoid cyst, lipoma, dermoid less common)

FIGURE 6-96

INTRAAXIAL MASSES (Fig. 6-97)

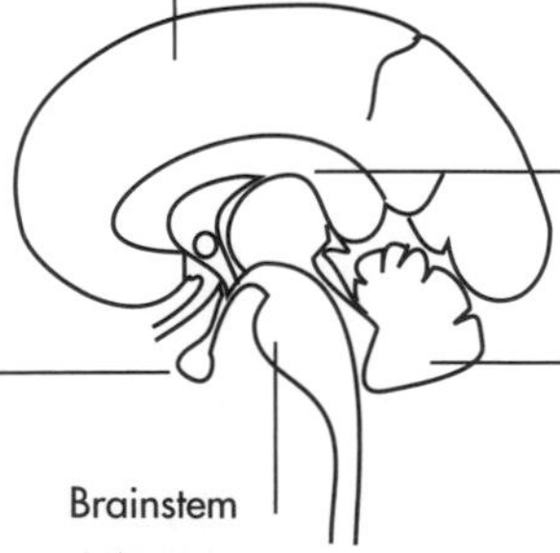
Hemisphere
• Astrocytoma
• Glioblastoma
• Oligodendroglioma
• Lymphoma
• Metastases
• PNET
• Ganglioma/cytoma
Pineal region
• Germ cell tumor
• Pineal parenchymal cell tumor
Sella
• Adenoma
• Craniopharyngioma/Rathke's cyst
• Metastases
• Abscess
• Sarcoid
• EG stalk
Brainstem
• Astrocytoma
• Glioblastoma
Cerebellum
• Astrocytoma
• Medulloblastoma
• Hemangioblastoma
• Metastases
• Ependymoma/choroid plexus papilloma or carcinoma

FIGURE 6-97

MULTIPLE LESIONS

Tumor
- Metastases
- Multicentric glioma
- Lymphoma

Infection
- Abscess
- Fungus
- Cysticercosis
- Toxoplasmosis

Vascular
- Embolic infarctions
- Multifocal hemorrhage
- Diffuse axonal injury
- Contusions
- Cavernous hemangiomas
- Vasculitis

CORPUS CALLOSUM LESIONS

Tumors
- Astrocytoma (butterfly glioma)
- Lymphoma
- Lipoma (midline)

Demyelinating disease
- Multiple sclerosis
- Marchiafava-Bignami disease (alcoholics)
- Progressive multifocal leukoencephalopathy (rarely enhances)

Infarct (always involves cingulate gyrus

INTRASELLAR MASSES (Fig. 6-98)

- Pituitary adenoma
- Pituitary apoplexy
- Craniopharyngioma
- Cysts (Rathke's cleft, pars intermedia)
- Metastasis
- Aneurysm (radiologist must exclude for the surgeon preoperatively)
- Abscess

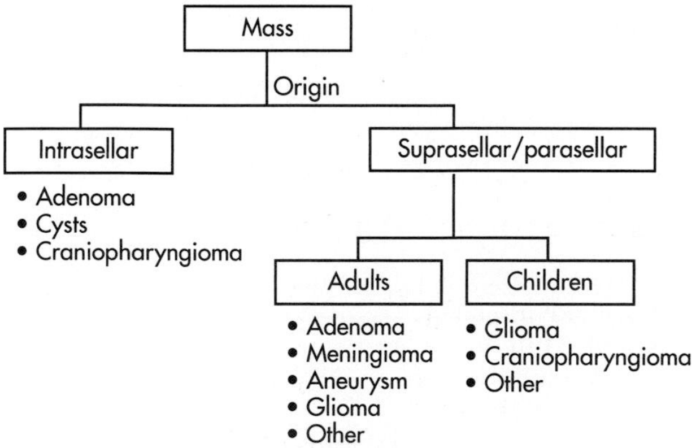

FIGURE 6-98

SUPRASELLAR MASSES

Mnemonic: "SATCHMOE":
- **S**ellar lesion with superior extension, sarcoidosis
- **A**neurysm, arachnoid cyst
- **T**eratoid lesions
  - Germ cell tumors
  - Epidermoid/dermoid
- **C**raniopharyngioma
- **H**ypothalamic glioma
- **M**etastases, meningioma
- **O**ptic nerve glioma
- **E**G

Adults
- Macroadenoma (most common)
- Meningioma
- Glioma
- Craniopharyngioma
- Aneurysm (rare, but important)

Children
- Craniopharyngioma (most common)
- Glioma (optic nerve, chiasm, hypothalamus)
- Germinoma
- Hypothalamic hamartoma
- EG

THICKENED ENHANCING PITUITARY STALK

- Adenoma
- Lymphoma
- Sarcoid
- Infection (TB)
- EG (causes diabetes insipidus, kids)
- Lymphocytic hypophysitis (if pregnant)

POSTERIOR FOSSA TUMORS

Approach

1. Intraaxial or extraaxial?
2. Location
   - Lateral (hemispheric): astrocytoma
   - Anterior: brainstem glioma
   - Posterior: medulloblastoma
   - 4th ventricle: ependymoma
3. Age
4. Spread
   - Through foramina of Luschka and Magendie: ependymoma
5. Cystic component
   - Pilocytic astrocytoma
   - Hemangioblastoma
6. Enhancement pattern
7. Dense cell packing
   - Medulloblastoma

Causes

Adults
- Metastases
- Hemangioblastoma

- Astrocytoma
- Extraaxial tumors (meningioma, schwannoma, epidermoid)

Children

- Cerebellar astrocytoma
- Medulloblastoma
- Brainstem glioma
- Ependymoma

BRAIN TUMORS IN INFANTS (≤ 2 YEARS)

- Teratoma (most common)
- PNET (primary cerebral neuroblastoma)
- Choroid plexus papilloma/carcinoma
- Anaplastic astrocytoma

INTRAVENTRICULAR TUMORS (Fig. 6-99)

Adults

- Gliomas
  - Astrocytoma (including giant cell type)
  - Subependymoma
- Meningioma
- Metastases
- Cysticercosis

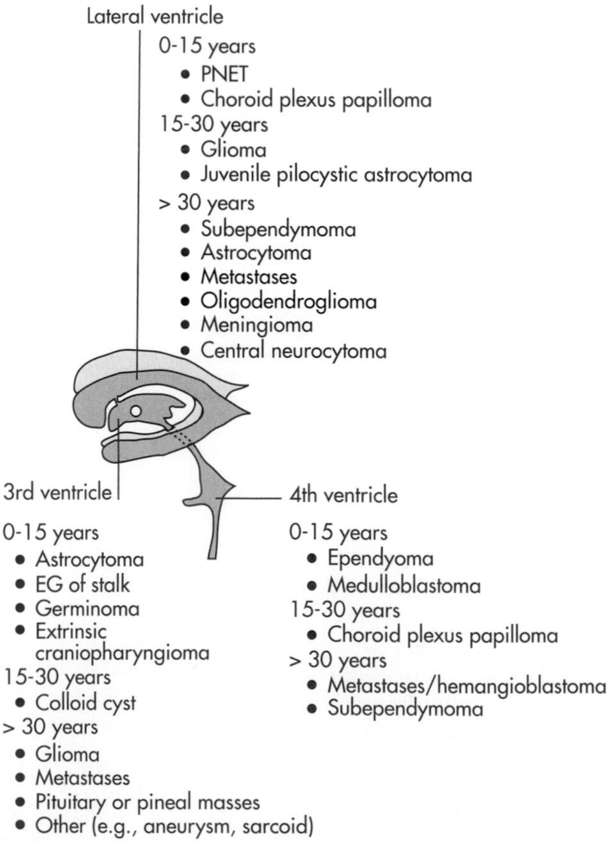

FIGURE 6-99

Children

- Choroid plexus papilloma
- Ependymoma
- PNET (medulloblastoma)
- Teratoma
- Astrocytoma

CEREBELLOPONTINE ANGLE (CPA) MASS

- Acoustic neuroma, 90%
- Meningioma, 10%
- Epidermoid, 5%
- Arachnoid cyst
- Metastases
- Vertebrobasilar dolichoectasia
- Exophytic glioma
  - Ependymoma through foramen of Luschka
  - Brainstem astrocytoma
- Lipoma

PINEAL REGION MASS

- Pineocytoma, pineoblastoma
- Germ cell tumor
- Meningioma
- Glioma
- Metastasis
- Lymphoma
- Pineal cyst
- Vein of Galen malformation

CYSTIC MASSES

Neoplastic

- Cystic astrocytoma/GBM
- Ganglioglioma
- Pleomorphic xanthoastrocytoma
- DNET
- Hemangioblastoma
- Metastases: squamous cell carcinoma

Benign (usually no peripheral enhancement)

- Dermoid/epidermoid
- Arachnoid cyst
- Colloid cyst
- Cavum variants
  - Cavum septum pellucidum
  - Cavum vergae
  - Cavum velum interpositum

TUMORS WITH CSF SEEDING

- Choroid plexus papilloma/carcinoma
- Ependymoma
- PNET tumors
  - Medulloblastoma
  - Pinealoblastoma
  - Cerebral neuroblastoma
- Germinomas
- GBM

UNDERLYING CAUSES OF HEMORRHAGE

Children
- AVM
- Cavernous malformation
- Venous thrombosis

Adults
- Metastases
- GBM
- Amyloid angiopathy

ETIOLOGY OF INTRAAXIAL (INTRAPARENCHYMAL) HEMORRHAGE

- Hypertension (most common)
- Tumor
- Trauma
- AVM
- Aneurysm
- Coagulopathy
- Amyloid angiopathy
- Emboli
- Hemorrhagic infarction (especially venous)
- Vasculitis

HYPERDENSE LESION (CT)

Tumors
- High-cell-density tumors
  - Lymphoma
  - PNETs (medulloblastoma)
  - Ependymoma
  - Germinoma
  - Other PNETs
- Hemorrhagic tumors
  - GBM
  - Metastases: kidney, lung, melanoma, choriocarcinoma (mnemonic: "CT/MR": **C**horiocarcinoma, **T**hyroid, **M**elanoma, **R**enal cell carcinoma)
- Calcified tumors (rare)
  - Mucinous metastases
  - All osteogenic tumors

Hemorrhage
- Hypertensive
- Trauma
- Vascular lesions

T2W HYPOINTENSE LESIONS (MRI)

Paramagnetic effects
- Ferritin, hemosiderin
- Deoxyhemoglobin
- Intracellular methemoglobin
- Melanin

Low spin density
- Calcification
- High nucleus/cytoplasm ratio (lymphoma, myeloma, neuroblastoma)
- Fibrous tissue (meningioma)

Other
- High protein concentration, > 35% (e.g., mucinous mets)
- Flow signal void

T1W HYPERINTENSE LESIONS (MRI)

Paramagnetic effects
- MRI contrast agent: Gd-DTPA
- Methemoglobin
- Melanin
- Ions: manganese, iron, copper, certain states of calcium

Other
- Fat: dermoid
- Very high protein concentration (i.e., colloid cyst)
- Slow flow

TEMPORAL LOBE T2W HYPERINTENSE LESIONS

- HSV encephalitis
- Limbic encephalitis (paraneoplastic)
- Mesial temporal sclerosis
- Venous infarct
- Trauma
- Lymphoma
- Tumors (low-grade glioma, ganglioglioma, DNET, pleomorphic xanthoastrocytoma)
- Status epilepticus

MULTIPLE SUSCEPTIBILITY HYPOINTENSE LESIONS (MRI)

- Amyloid angiopathy
- Multiple cavernomas
- DAI
- Hemorrhagic metastases

ABNORMAL ENHANCEMENT

LESIONS WITH NO ENHANCEMENT

- Cysts
- Tumors with intact blood-brain barrier (low-grade gliomas)

LESIONS WITH STRONG ENHANCEMENT

- Meningioma
- PNET (e.g., medulloblastoma)
- AVM
- Paraganglioma (very vascular)
- Aneurysm (nonthrombosed)
- HIV-associated lymphoma
- GBM

RING ENHANCEMENT

Tumor
- Primary brain tumors
- Metastases
- Lymphoma (AIDS)

Infection, inflammation
- Abscess
- Granuloma
- MS
- Toxoplasmosis
- Cysticercosis
- Vascular

Vascular
- Resolving hematoma
- Infarct (nonacute)
- Thrombosed vascular malformation
- Thrombosed aneurysm
- Vasculitis

DIFFUSE MENINGEAL ENHANCEMENT

- Meningitis (viral, bacterial)
- Carcinomatosis
  - Lymphoma
  - Metastases (melanoma, breast, lung)
- Postoperative/postshunt
- SAH
- Intracranial hypotension
  - CSF leak

BASILAR MENINGEAL ENHANCEMENT

Infection
- TB (most common)
- Fungal
- Pyogenic (more common on convexity)
- Cysticercosis

Tumor
- Lymphoma, leukemia
- Carcinomatosis

Inflammatory
- Sarcoid
- Rheumatoid pachymeningitis (also SLE and Wegener granulomatosis)
- Whipple disease

EPENDYMAL ENHANCEMENT (Fig. 6-100)

Tumor
- Lymphoma
- Metastases (lung, melanoma, breast)

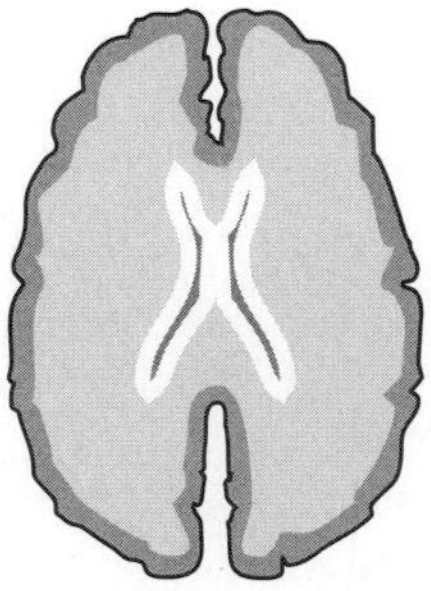

FIGURE 6-100

- CSF seeding
  - PNET
  - GBM

Infection
- Spread of meningitis
- CMV infection (rare)

Inflammatory ventriculitis
- Postshunt/instrumentation
- Posthemorrhage

NORMALLY ENHANCING STRUCTURES

- Choroid plexus
- Pineal gland
- Pituitary/stalk
- Cavernous sinus/vessels

DIFFUSE SULCAL FLAIR HYPERINTENSITY

- Hemorrhage
- Infection
- Hyperoxia

BASAL GANGLIA SIGNAL ABNORMALITIES

T2W HYPOINTENSE BASAL GANGLIA LESIONS

- Old age
- Any chronic degenerative disease
  - MS
  - Parkinsonian syndromes
- Childhood hypoxia

T2W HYPERINTENSE BASAL GANGLIA LESIONS

Mnemonic: "TINT:"
- **T**umor
  - Lymphoma
- **I**schemia
  - Hypoxic encephalopathy
  - Venous infarction (internal cerebral vein thrombosis)
- **N**eurodegenerative diseases (uncommon)
  - Huntington disease
  - Wilson disease
  - Hallervorden-Spatz disease (eye of tiger sign — gliosis (white) surrounded by iron deposit (black) on T2W images)
  - Mitochondrial encephalopathies (e.g., Leigh/Kearns-Sayre syndrome)
  - Aminoacidopathies
- **T**oxin
  - CO, CN, H_2S poisoning
  - Hypoglycemia
  - Methanol

T1W HYPERINTENSE BASAL GANGLIA LESIONS

- Dystrophic calcifications (any cause)
- Hepatic failure
- Neurofibromatosis

- Manganese (used in formulas for TPN)
- Hyperparathyroidism
- Hypoparathyroidism, pseudo(pseudo) hypoparathyroidism

BASAL GANGLIA CALCIFICATION (INCREASED CT DENSITY)

Senescent/physiologic/idiopathic calcification (most common)

Metabolic calcification
- Hypoparathyroidism (most common metabolic cause)
- Pseudohypoparathyroidism
- Pseudo-pseudohypoparathyroidism
- Hyperparathyroidism

Infection
- TORCH, AIDS
- Postinflammatory: TB, toxoplasmosis
- Cysticercosis (common)

Toxic/postanoxic
- Lead
- CO
- Radiation therapy
- Chemotherapy

Other
- Fahr disease
- Mitochondrial (common), encephalopathies (uncommon)
- Cockayne syndrome

NEURODEGENERATIVE DISEASES

VOLUME LOSS

- Diffuse
  - Aging
  - Alcoholism
  - HIV
  - Alzheimer (late)
- Focal
  - PSP (midbrain)
  - Multisystem atrophy (pons)
  - Huntington (caudate)
  - Seizure meds (cerebellum)
- Geographic
  - Pick (frontotemporal)
  - Alzheimer (temporal parietal)

FOCAL T2 ABNORMALITIES+

- Acute Wernicke
- Wilson disease
- Hallervorden-Spatz
- ALS

DWI+

- CJD
- Carbon monoxide

CONGENITAL ABNORMALITIES

SPECTRUM OF CYSTIC SUPRATENTORIAL CONGENITAL ABNORMALITIES (Fig. 6-101)

- Holoprosencephaly
- Hydranencephaly
- Aqueductal stenosis (severe obstruction hydrocephalus)
- Callosal dysgenesis (interhemispheric cyst)
- Other
  - Porencephaly
  - Arachnoid cyst
  - Cystic teratoma
  - Epidermoid/dermoid
  - Vein of Galen AVM

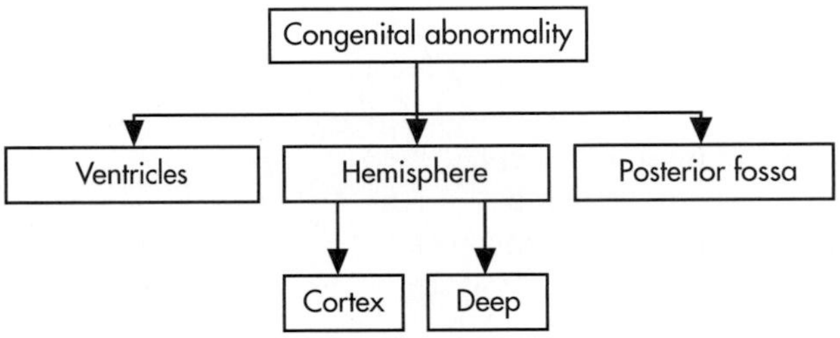

FIGURE 6-101

POSTERIOR FOSSA CYSTIC ABNORMALITIES

- DW malformation (vermian hypoplasia/aplasia and large posterior fossa)
- DW variant (normal size posterior fossa and vermian hypoplasia
- Mega cisterna magna (normal vermis)
- Retrocerebellar arachnoid cyst (must show mass effect)
- Chiari IV (near complete absence of cerebellum)
- Other
  - Epidermoid/dermoid
  - Cystic tumor

SPINE

SPINAL CORD COMPRESSION

Criteria
- No CSF seen around the cord (spinal block)
- Narrowed AP diameter of cord (<7 mm)
- Deformity of cord
- Acute compression
  - Cord edema
  - Cord swelling

Causes

- Infection (TB, pyogenic)
- Compression fracture
  - Malignancy
  - Trauma
    - Spondylosis and disk disease
  - Herniated nucleus, hypertrophy of ligaments
  - Osteophyte, facet hypertrophy
    - Primary bone disorders (Paget disease)
    - Other causes
  - Benign tumors (e.g., angioma, cysts, lipoma)
  - Epidural hematoma

INTRAMEDULLARY LESIONS

- Tumor
  - Astrocytoma (most common in pediatric population)
  - Ependymoma (most common in adult population)
  - Hemangioblastoma metastases (rare)
- Demyelinating disease/myelitis
- Syringohydromyelia
  - Tumor related
  - Chiari malformation
- AVM
- Trauma (contusion)

INTRADURAL EXTRAMEDULLARY TUMORS

- Nerve sheath tumor (most common)
  - Neurofibroma
  - Schwannoma
- Meningioma (80% thoracic)
- Drop metastases
- Lipoma
- Teratomatous lesion
- Arachnoid cyst
- Arachnoiditis/meningitis
- AVM/AVF

EXTRADURAL LESIONS

- Disk
- Metastases
- Epidural abscess
- Hematoma
- Other
  - Lipomatosis (thoracic)
  - Synovial cyst
  - Perineural cyst

CYSTIC SPINAL LESION (SYRINGOHYDROMYELIA) (Fig. 6-102)

Criteria: Syringomyelia: cavity in spinal cord; may or may not communicate with central canal; for hydromyelia: dilatation of central canal. Cannot be differentiated with imaging.

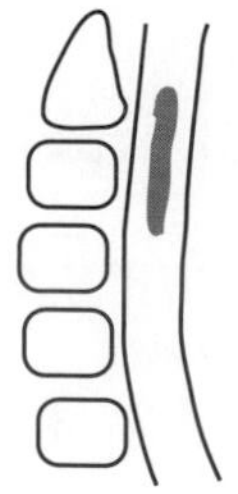

FIGURE 6-102

Causes

Primary
- Chiari malformations
- Spinal dysraphism
- DW
- Diastematomyelia

Acquired
- Tumor
  - Astrocytoma
  - Ependymoma
- Inflammatory
  - Arachnoiditis/meningitis
  - SAH
- Trauma
  - Spinal cord injury
  - Vascular insult

ENHANCING NERVE ROOTS IN THE FILUM TERMINALE

- Inflammatory
  - Arachnoiditis
  - Guillain-Barré
  - Chronic inflammatory demyelinating polyneuropathy (CIDP)
- Infection
  - Viral
  - Lyme disease
- Neoplastic
  - Lymphoma
  - Metastases

Suggested Readings

Atlas SW, ed. *Magnetic Resonance Imaging of the Brain and Spine*. Philadelphia: Lippincott Williams & Wilkins; 2008.

Barkovich AJ. *Pediatric Neuroimaging*. Philadelphia: Lippincott Williams & Wilkins; 2005.

Grossman RI, Yousem DM. *Neuroradiology: The Requisites*. 2nd ed. St. Louis: Mosby; 2004.

Morris P. *Practical Neuroangiography*. Philadelphia: Lippincott Williams & Wilkins; 2006.

Osborn AG. *Diagnostic Neuroradiology*. St Louis: Mosby; 1994.

Osborn AG. *Handbook of Neuroradiology*. St. Louis: Mosby; 1996.

Osborn AG, Blaser S, Salzman K. *Diagnostic Imaging: Brain*. Philadelphia: WB Saunders; 2004.

Taveras JM, Ferrucci JT. *Radiology: Diagnosis, Imaging, Intervention*. Philadelphia: Lippincott Williams & Wilkins; 2002.

Yock D. *MRI of CNS Disease: A Teaching File*. 2nd ed. St. Louis: Mosby; 2002.

CHAPTER 7

Head and Neck Imaging

CHAPTER OUTLINE

Temporal Bone

GENERAL

The temporal bone is divided into 5 portions:

- Mastoid (mastoid process: insertion for sternocleidomastoid muscle)
- Petrous portion (inner ear structures, skull base)
- Squamous portion (lateral inferior skull)
- Tympanic portion with tympanic cavity
- Styloid portion

EXTERNAL AUDITORY CANAL (EAC) (Fig. 7-1)

- Cartilaginous portion
- Bony portion

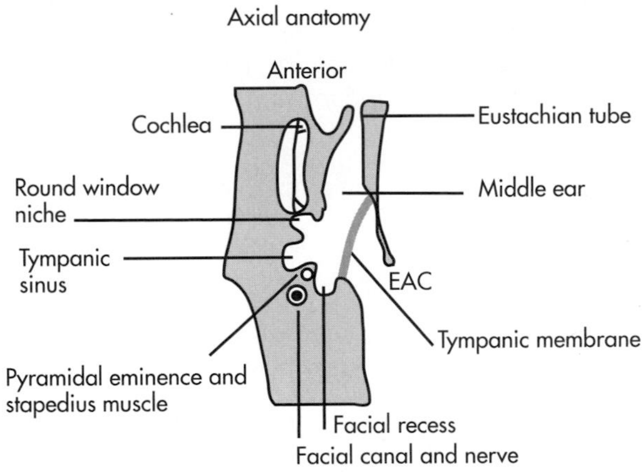

FIGURE 7-1

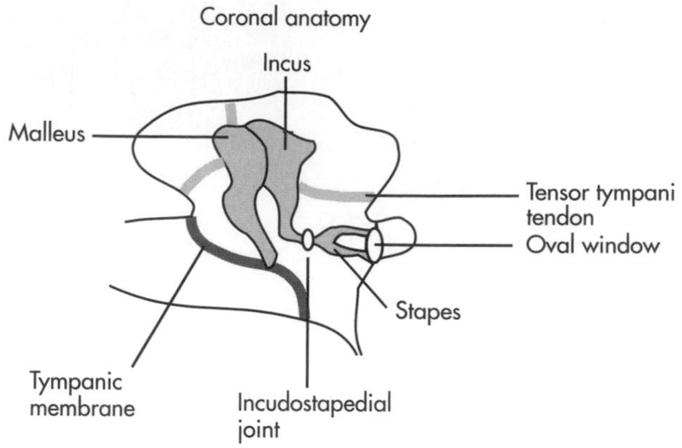

FIGURE 7-2

MIDDLE EAR (Fig. 7-2)

Composed of air-filled spaces that contain the ossicles and are divided into:
- Epitympanum
- Mesotympanum
- Hypotympanum

Boundaries of the middle ear are tympanic membrane laterally, the tegmen superiorly, and the inner ear (promontory) medially. The eustachian tube (pressure equalization) connects the middle ear with the nasopharynx. Three ossicles transmit sound waves from the tympanic membrane to the oval window in the vestibule:
- Malleus
- Incus
- Stapes (2 crura, 1 footplate)

INNER EAR (Fig. 7-3)

The inner ear (labyrinth) consists of:
- 3 semicircular canals, which connect to vestibule
- Vestibula with utricle and saccule
- Cochlea (sensorineural hearing), which connects to:

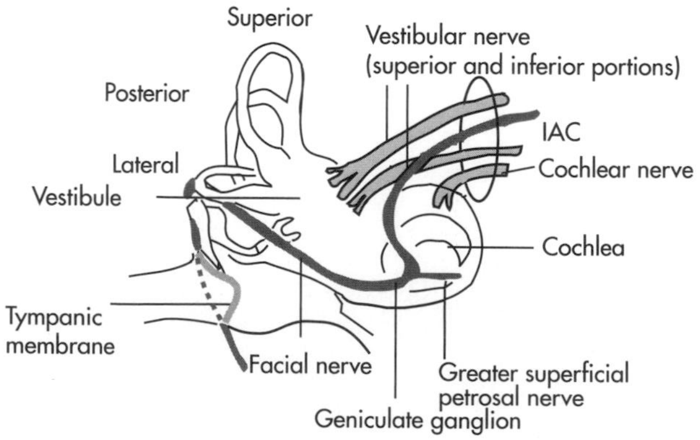

FIGURE 7-3

  Stapes → oval window
  Round window (allows for counterpulsation of fluid)

INTERNAL AUDITORY CANAL (IAC) (Fig. 7-4)

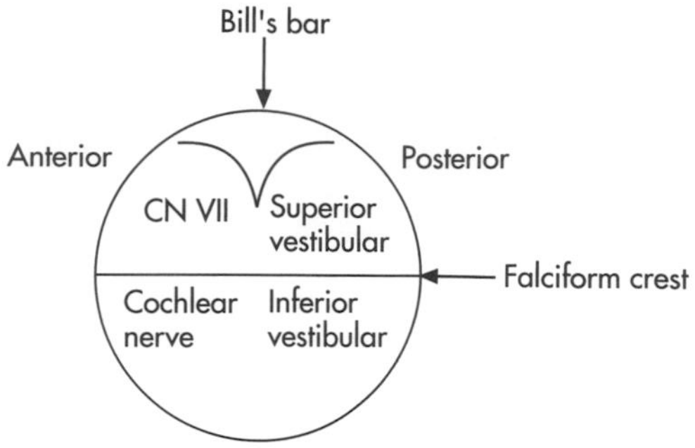

FIGURE 7-4

Left and right IAC should not differ >2 mm in diameter. Contents of IAC are divided by the falciform crest and "Bill's" bar:
- Facial nerve (anterior superior): CN VII ("7 up")
- Cochlear part (anterior inferior): CN VIII ("Coke down")
- Superior vestibular nerve (posterior) with superior and inferior divisions: CN VIII
- Inferior vestibular nerve (posterior): CN VIII

FACIAL NERVE (Fig. 7-5)

3 main portions of the facial nerve:
- Intracranial (extracanalicular) portion
  - Cerebellopontine angle (CPA) segment
  - Meatal segment

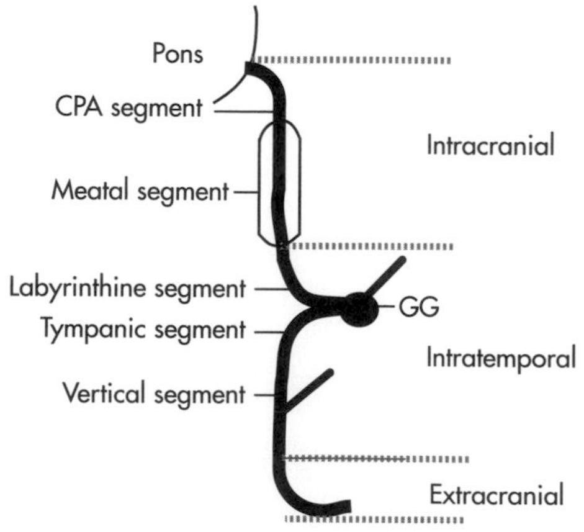

FIGURE 7-5

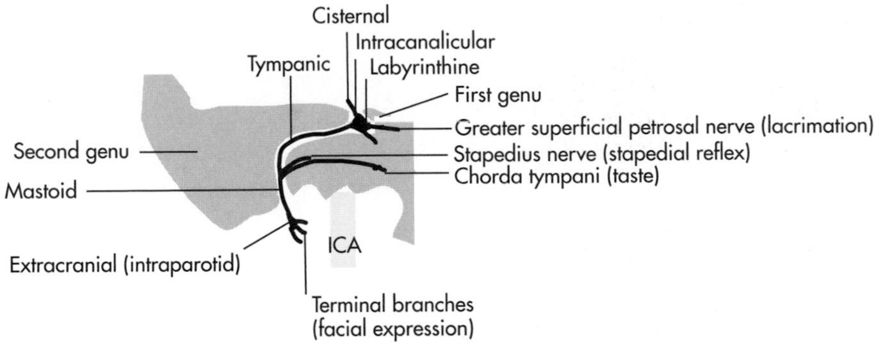

FIGURE 7-6

- Intratemporal (intracanalicular) portion (30 mm)
  - Labyrinthine segment
  - Tympanic (horizontal)
  - Mastoid (vertical)
- Extracranial portion with 5 branches

The facial nerve gives rise to 4 branches: (Fig. 7-6)
- Greater superficial petrosal nerve
- Stapedius nerve
- Chorda tympani
- Terminal branches (total of 5 extracranial branches)

SKULL BASE (Fig. 7-7)

OVERVIEW OF FORAMINA

Opening	Cranial Nerve	Artery	Vein
Jugular foramen pars nervosa	IX		Inferior petrosal sinus
Jugular foramen pars venosa	X, XI		Internal jugular vein
Foramen rotundum	V2	Artery of foramen rotundum	Emissary veins
Foramen ovale	V3	Accessory meningeal artery	Emissary veins
Foramen spinosum	Recurrent meningeal branch of mandibular nerve, lesser superficial petrosal nerve	Middle meningeal artery	Middle meningeal vein
Foramen lacerum	Nerve of the pterygoid canal	Meningeal branches of ascending pharyngeal artery	
Superior orbital fissure	III, IV, V, VI	Orbital branches of middle meningeal artery Recurrent meningeal branches of lacrimal artery	Ophthalmic veins
Stylomastoid foramen	VII		
Hypoglossal canal	XII		
Carotid canal	Sympathetics	ICA	
Vidian canal		Vidian artery	
Optic canal	II	Ophthalmic artery	

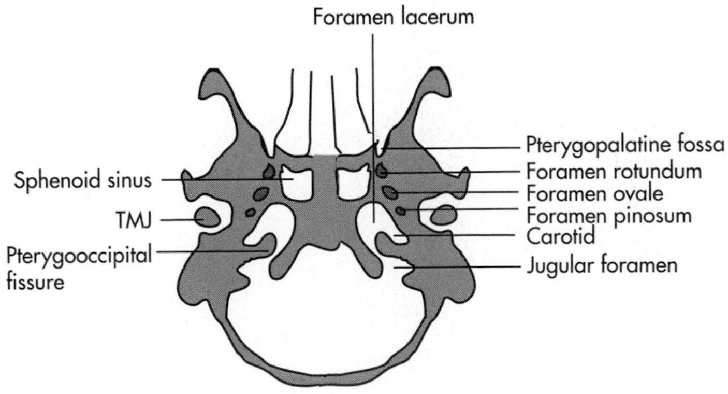

FIGURE 7-7

CRANIAL NERVES

- CN I: olfactory nerve
- CN II: optic nerve
- CN III: oculomotor nerve
- CN IV: trochlear nerve
- CN V: trigeminal nerve
- CN VI: abducens nerve
- CN VII: facial nerve
- CN VIII: auditory nerve
- CN IX: glossopharyngeal nerve
- CN X: vagus nerve
- CN XI: spinal accessory nerve
- CN XII: hypoglossal nerve

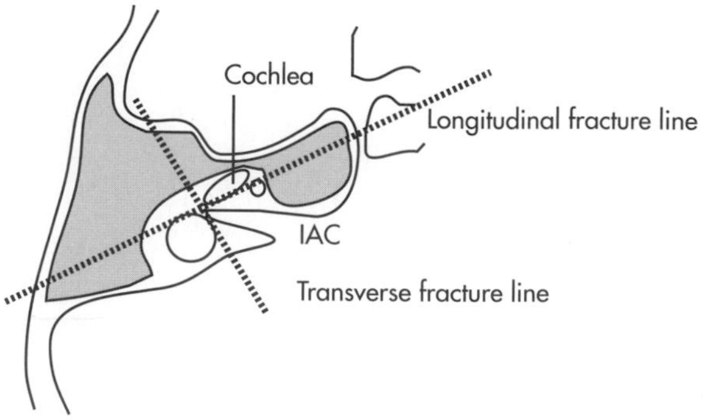

FIGURE 7-8

TRAUMA

TEMPORAL BONE FRACTURES

Clinical Findings

- Hearing loss
- Tinnitus
- Vertigo
- Bleeding into EAC
- Cerebrospinal fluid (CSF) leak
- Facial paresis

Radiographic Features

TEMPORAL BONE FRACTURES

Parameter	Longitudinal Fractures (Middle Ear Fracture)	Transverse Fractures (Inner Ear Fracture)
Frequency	80%	20%
Fracture line	Parallel to long axis	Perpendicular to long axis
Labyrinth	Spared	Involved: vertigo, sensorineural hearing loss
Ossicles	Involved: conductive hearing loss	
Tympanic membrane	Involved	Spared
Facial paralysis	20%	50%

Fracture Complications (Fig. 7-8)

- Ossicular fractures or dislocations
- Tympanic membrane perforation
- Hemotympanum
- CN VII paralysis
- CSF otorrhea
- Meningitis, abscess
- Sinus thrombosis, rare
- Labyrinthitis ossificans (late)

Indications for Surgery in Temporal Bone Fractures

- Ossicular fracture or dislocation
- Decompression of the facial nerve
- Labyrinthine fistulae
- CSF leaks

INFLAMMATION

ACUTE INFLAMMATION

- Otitis media (edema fills middle ear cavity): acute, subacute, chronic forms
  - Children: common
  - Adults: less common; exclude nasopharyngeal carcinoma, which causes serous otitis media.
- Mastoiditis (bony destruction has to be present to make diagnosis; fluid-filled mastoid cells are also often present)
- Labyrinthitis
  - Serous
  - Toxic
  - Suppurative

Complications

- Meningitis
- Sinus thrombosis
- Epidural abscess
- Petrositis (infection of petrous air cells)

BELL PALSY

Acute onset. Unilateral peripheral facial nerve palsy. Bell palsy resolves in 6 weeks to 3 months. By MRI there is enhancement along the facial nerve involving intracanalicular and labyrinthine segments that normally do not enhance in normal individuals. The facial nerve can normally enhance in its tympanic and mastoid segments due to arterial supply. Facial nerve enhancement is nonspecific and can occur in other inflammatory and neoplastic conditions. Perineural spread of a tumor should also be considered.

MASTOIDITIS

Types

Uncomplicated forms:
- Edema and/or fluid only

Complicated forms:
- Bone demineralization
- Coalescent mastoiditis (cell breakdown)
- Thrombophlebitis
- Bezold abscess
- Gradenigo syndrome (petrositis)
- Sigmoid sinus thrombosis
- Epidural
- Subdural empyema
- Meningitis
- Focal encephalitis, brain abscess, otitic hydrocephalus

ACQUIRED CHOLESTEATOMA (Fig. 7-9)

Mass of keratin debris lined by squamous epithelium. Etiology: epithelial cells move into the middle ear via a perforation of the tympanic membrane. Secondary to eustachian tube dysfunction. Types:
- Acquired: chronic middle ear infection (common). Either in attic (Prussak's space) or sinus location
- Congenital (epidermoid): cholesteatoma arises from epithelial nests in middle ear, mastoid, or petrous bone, including the labyrinth (uncommon).

Radiographic Features

- Soft tissue mass in middle ear
- Borders may be well- or ill-defined.
- Erosion of incus and otic spur (scutum) common
- Bone resorption (collagenase) is typical and occurs most commonly in:
  - Ossicles
  - Lateral semicircular canal (fistula)
  - Tegmen tympani
  - Facial canal
- Mastoid air cells are typically underpneumatized and sclerotic.

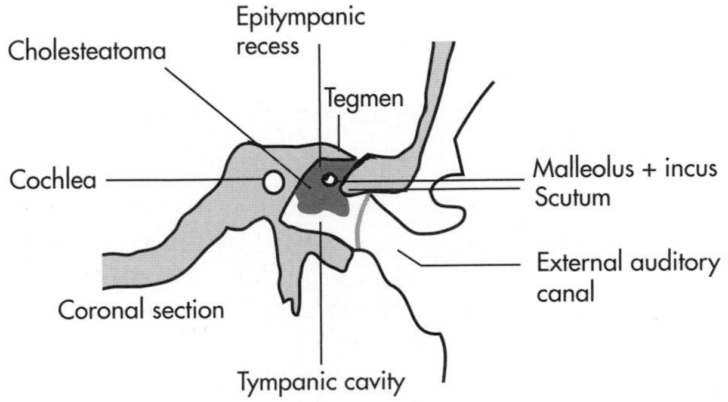

FIGURE 7-9

- Labyrinthine fistula formation in lateral semicircular canal is less common.
- It is often impossible to distinguish chronic middle ear infection from cholesteatoma in cases with little bone destruction.

LOCATION OF ACQUIRED CHOLESTEATOMA

Parameter	Attic Cholesteatoma	Sinus Cholesteatoma
TM perforation	Pars flaccida	Pars tensa
Location	Prussak's space	Sinus tympani
Ossicles displaced	Medially	Laterally
Bone erosion	Lateral tympanic wall (erosion of scutum is an early finding)	Initially subtle
Ossicle erosion	Head of malleus and long process of incus	Short process of incus and stapes

Complications of Acquired Cholesteatoma

- Labyrinthine fistula (dehiscence of semicircular canals—most frequently lateral canal)
- Facial nerve paralysis (involvement of facial nerve canal)
- Sinus thrombosis
- Meningitis
- Encephalitis
- Abscess
- Petrous apex syndrome (Gradenigo syndrome)

CONGENITAL CHOLESTEATOMA (EPIDERMOID)

Rare lesions that may occur in middle ear, mastoid, EAC, jugular fossa, labyrinth, petrous apex, CPA, and jugular fossa. The most common location is anterosuperior portion of the middle ear. Histologically, the cholesteatoma is made up of squamous cell lining, keratin debris, and cholesterol.

Radiographic Features

SIGNAL CHARACTERISTICS RELATIVE TO BRAIN

	Epidermoid (Congenital Cholesteatoma)	Cholesterol Granuloma (Cholesterol Cyst)	Mucocele
CT	≤	Isodense, no calcium, no enhancement	<
T1W	≤ (lamination)	> (cholesterol)	≤
T2W	>	> (methemoglobin)	>

CHOLESTEROL GRANULOMA (CHOLESTEROL CYSTS)

Subtype of granulation tissue that may be present anywhere in the middle ear, including the petrous apex. Clinical symptoms occur when the granuloma expands and causes bone erosion, such as in the petrous apex, leading to hearing loss, tinnitus, and cranial nerve palsies. Histologically, cholesterol granulomas contain hemorrhage and cholesterol crystals.

Radiographic Features

- Bone erosion of petrous apex
- Expansion of petrous apex
- CT: isodense relative to brain, no enhancement, no calcification
- MRI: hyperintense relative to brain on T1-weighted images because of cholesterol content

MALIGNANT EXTERNAL OTITIS

Severe, life-threatening *Pseudomonas aeruginosa* infection in elderly diabetics.

The aggressive infection spreads via cartilaginous fissures of Santorini and extends into:

- Middle ear
- Base of temporal bone
- Petrous apex (osteomyelitis)
- Parapharyngeal space
- Nasopharynx
- Meninges
- Central nervous system
- Bone (osteomyelitis)

Radiographic Features

- Mastoiditis
- Osteomyelitis of base of skull (jugular, sigmoid) and at bony/cartilaginous junction of EAC
- Sinus phlebitis, thrombosis
- Multiple cranial nerve paralyses

LABYRINTHITIS OSSIFICANS

Causes: chronic labyrinthitis, meningitis, trauma. HRCT may detect ossification within the cochlea. MRI (T2W) may be helpful if fibrous obliteration has occurred.

HEARING LOSS

Types

Conductive
- 3 main locations of abnormalities: tympanic membrane, ossicles, hyperostosis of oval window
- Common underlying causes: otitis, cholesteatoma, otosclerosis, trauma

Sensorineural
- Evaluate inner ear, IAC
- Common underlying causes: idiopathic, hereditary, acoustic neuroma, enlargement of vestibular aqueduct (most common cause in inner ear), labyrinthitis ossificans, otosclerosis

PULSATILE TINNITUS

Causes

Normal vascular variants
- Aberrant ICA
- Jugular bulb anomalies (high or dehiscent megabulb, diverticulum)
- Persistent stapedial artery

Vascular tumors
- Glomus jugulare
- Glomus tympanicum

Vascular abnormalities
- Arteriovenous malformation (AVM)
- Atherosclerosis
- ICA dissection or aneurysm at petrous apex
- Fibromuscular hyperplasia

Other causes of tinnitus
- Paget disease
- Otosclerosis
- Ménière disease

TUMORS

GLOMUS TUMORS

Glomus tumors (chemodectoma = nonchromaffin paraganglioma) arise from chemoreceptor cells in multiple sites in the head and neck. Most tumors are benign, but 10% of glomus tumors are associated with malignant tumors elsewhere in the body. Ten percent are multiple; thus, it is important to check other common locations in the head and neck during imaging (glomus jugulare, vagale, and carotid body tumor). Glomus tumors represent the most common middle ear tumor.

Types

- Glomus jugulare: origin at jugular bulb; more common
- Glomus tympanicum: origin at cochlear promontory; less common, rises from paraganglia along Jacobson's and Arnold's nerves within the tympanic cavity

Clinical Findings

- Pulsatile tinnitus (most common)
- Hearing loss
- Arrhythmias
- Sudden blood pressure (BP) fluctuations

Radiographic Features

- Glomus tympanicum typically presents as a small soft tissue mass centered over the cochlear promontory. Glomus tympanicum is usually indistinguishable from other soft tissue masses in the tympanic cavity.
- Glomus jugulare is centered in the region of the jugular foramen and rarely extends below

the level of hyoid bone. It is accompanied by permeative bone changes in the jugular foramen. Characteristic findings by MRI are multiple low-signal-intensity areas that represent flow voids in the tumor. This has a salt-and-pepper appearance.
- Intense contrast enhancement by CT, MRI, angiography
- Large tumors erode bone.

BENIGN TEMPORAL BONE TUMORS

- Meningioma
- Facial neuroma may arise anywhere along the course of CN VII. In the IAC, the tumor is indistinguishable from an acoustic neuroma.
- Osteoma
- Adenoma (ceruminoma = apocrine adenoma) in the EAC, benign but locally aggressive, rare
- Epidermoid (primary cholesteatoma)
- Petrous apex cholesterol granuloma

MALIGNANT TEMPORAL BONE TUMORS

- Carcinoma (most common tumors)
  - Squamous cell carcinoma (SCC) arising from the EAC
  - Adenocarcinoma
- Lymphoma
- Metastases: breast, lung, melanoma
- Chondrosarcoma, other primary bone tumors
- Rhabdomyosarcoma in children

CONGENITAL ANOMALIES

OVERVIEW OF SYNDROMES

CONGENITAL ABNORMALITIES OF THE INNER EAR

- Cochlear malseptation (Mondini's deafness) results in <2.5 cochlear turns and an "empty cochlea." Direct connection to CSF results in leaks and meningitis.
- Single cochlear-vestibular cavity (Michel's deafness) results in <2.5 cochlear turns. Hypoplastic petrous pyramid.
- Small IAC
- Cochlear aplasia
- Large vestibule or aqueduct

PETROUS MALFORMATIONS ASSOCIATED WITH RECURRENT MENINGITIS

- Lamina cribrosa/spiralis defect at lateral end of IAC: perilymphatic hydrops develops, with secondary displacement of stapes.
- Dehiscence of tegmen tympani
- Wide cochlear aqueduct

OTODYSTROPHIES AND DYSPLASIAS

OTOSCLEROSIS

The osseous labyrinth (otic capsule) normally has a dense capsule. In otosclerosis, the capsule is replaced by vascular, irregular bony trabeculae and later by sclerotic bone. Unknown etiology; inherited. Bilateral, 90%. Patients (female > male) present with hearing loss.

Types

- Fenestral otosclerosis: sclerosis or spongiosis around oval window, including fixation of stapes. Diagnosis is usually made from clinical and

SYNDROMES ASSOCIATED WITH VARYING DEGREES OF DEAFNESS

Syndrome/Disease	Inner Ear	Middle Ear	Outer Ear	Other Abnormalities
Otocraniofacial				
Treacher Collins syndrome	+++	+++	0	Coloboma, mandibular hypoplasia ("fishmouth")
Crouzon disease	+++	+++	0	Exophthalmos, craniosynostosis
Otocervical				
Klippel-Feil syndrome	++	++	+++	Cervical fusion, short neck
Cleidocranial dysostosis	+	+	++	Large head, underdeveloped facial bones, absent clavicles
Otoskeletal				
Osteogenesis	0	+	+++	Deformity, fractures, blue sclera
Osteopetrosis	++	++	+++	Increased bone density
Other				
Thalidomide	+++	+++	+++	Short limbs, cardiac abnormalities, GI, hemangiomas

audiometric findings (conductive hearing loss). Imaging is usually not required for diagnosis.
- Cochlear (retrofenestral) otosclerosis: involves cochlea and otic capsule. CT findings:
  - Deossification around cochlea (lucent halo)
  - Sclerosis occurs later in disease

SUPERIOR SEMICIRCULAR CANAL DEHISCENCE SYNDROME (TULLIO SYNDROME)

CT shows a small defect in the bony wall of the superior semicircular canal. Clinically presents with dizziness and vertigo with loud sound or pressure. Can also be associated with conductive hearing loss and upward and torsional nystagmus evoked by sound pressure. Most patients do not need treatment if they avoid provocative stimuli.

Causes
- Postsurgical treatment of otosclerosis
- Cholesteatoma
- Syphilis
- Trauma
- Ménière disease
- Perilymphatic fistula
- Lyme disease

OTHER OTODYSTROPHIES AND DYSPLASIAS

- Paget disease
- Fibrous dysplasia
- Osteogenesis imperfecta
- Osteopetrosis resulting in cupulolithiasis
- Craniometaphyseal dysplasia (Pyle disease)
- Craniodiaphyseal dysplasia (Engelmann disease)
- Cleidocranial dysostosis

Orbit

GENERAL

Orbital Spaces (Figs. 7-10 and 7-11)

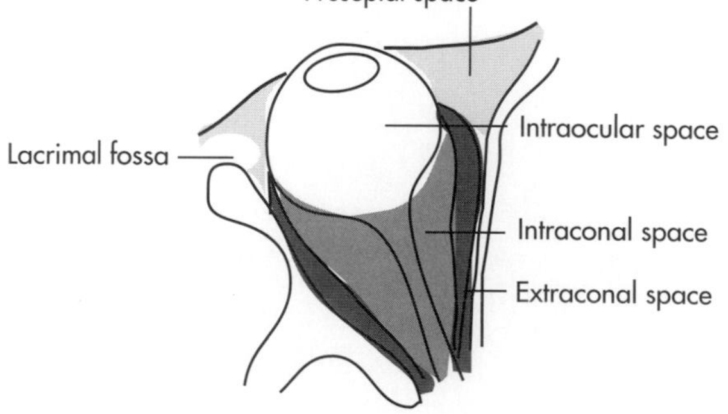

FIGURE 7-10

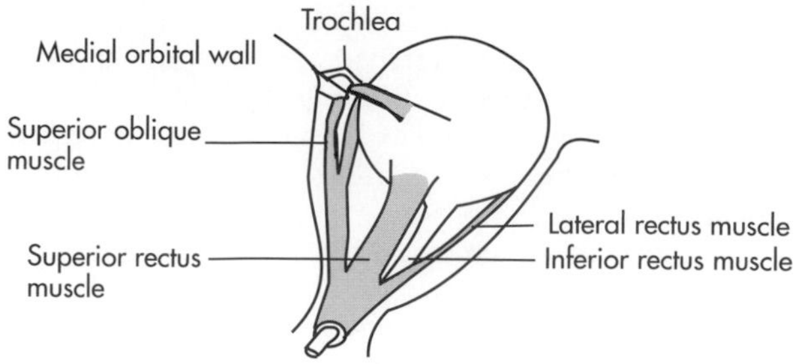

FIGURE 7-11

- Intraconal space: space inside the rectus muscle pyramid
- Extraconal space: space outside the rectus muscle pyramid
- Preseptal space
- Postseptal space
- Lacrimal fossa

Orbital Structures
- Globe (lens, anterior chamber, posterior chamber, vitreous, sclerouveal coat)
- Intraconal, extraconal fat
- Optic nerve and sheath
- Ophthalmic artery and vein
- Rectus muscles

Orbital Septum
- Represents condensed orbital rim periosteum
- Attaches to outer margins of bony orbit and deep tissues of lids
- Separates all the structures in the orbit from soft tissues in the face (preseptal versus postseptal)

GLOBE

RETINOBLASTOMA

Malignant tumor that arises from neuroectodermal cells of retina. Clinical: leukocoria (white mass behind pupil). Age: <3 years (70%)
- 30% bilateral, 30% multifocal within one eye
- 10% of patients have a familial history of retinoblastoma

Radiographic Features
- Intraocular mass
- High density (calcification, hemorrhage)
- Dense vitreous, common
- Calcifications (Fig. 7-12) are common (90%); in absence of calcifications suspect other mass lesions:
  - Persistent hyperplastic primary vitreous
  - Retrolental fibroplasia
  - Toxocariasis
  - Coats disease

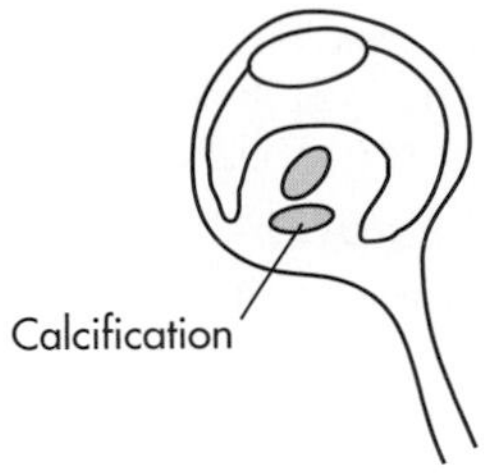

FIGURE 7-12

- Primary role of imaging is to determine tumor spread:
  - Optic nerve extension, 25%
  - Scleral breakthrough
  - Metastases: meninges, liver, lymph nodes

Pearls

- Tumors may occur bilaterally or trilaterally, counting pineoblastoma
- Associated with other malignancies (osteosarcoma most common) later in life; postradiation sarcoma at 10 years: 20%, 20 years: 50%, 30 years: 90%

MELANOMA

Most common (75%) ocular malignancy in adults. Arises from pigmented choroidal layer; retinal detachment is common.

Radiographic Features (Fig. 7-13)

- Thickening or irregularity of choroid (localized, polypoid, or flat)
- Exophytic, biconvex mass lesion
- Usually unilateral, posterior location
- Retinal detachment, common
- Contrast enhancement
- MRI: T1W hyperintense, T2W hypointense

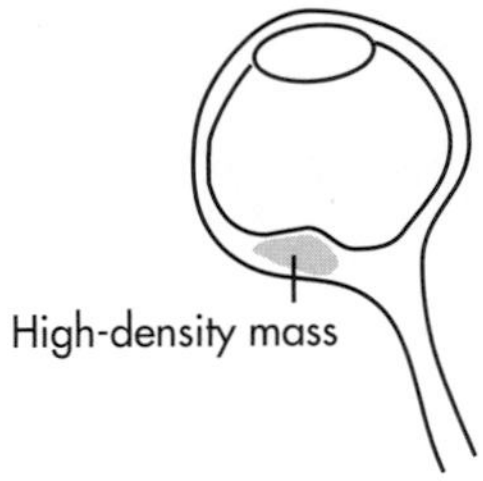

FIGURE 7-13

- Poor prognostic indicators:
  - Large tumor size
  - Heavy pigmentation
  - Infiltration of the angles, optic nerve, sclera, ciliary body

PERSISTENT HYPERPLASTIC PRIMARY VITREOUS (PHPV)

Caused by persistence of portions of the fetal hyaloid artery and primary vitreous. Associated with ocular dysplasias (e.g., Norrie disease = PHPV, seizures, deafness, low IQ). Clinical findings of blindness, leukocoria, and microphthalmia. Usually unilateral. Rare.

Radiographic Features

- Small globe (microphthalmia)
- Vitreous body hyperdensity along the remnant of the hyaloid artery
- No calcification (in contrast to retinoblastoma)
- Complications:
  - Retinal detachment
  - Chronic retinal hemorrhage

RETROLENTAL FIBROPLASIA

Toxic retinopathy caused by oxygen treatment (e.g., for hyaline membrane disease). A retinal vasoconstriction leads to neovascularization of the posterior vitreous and retina. Hemorrhage with scarring, retraction, and exudate formation follows. Bilateral.

COATS DISEASE

Primary vascular abnormality (exudative retinitis) causing lipoprotein accumulation in retina, telangiectasia, neovascularization, and retinal detachment (pseudoglioma). Age: 6 to 8 years, males. Rare.

Radiographic Features

- Dense vitreous with focal mass or calcium
- Unilateral

DRUSEN

Focal calcification in hyaline bodies in the optic nerve head. Usually bilateral and asymptomatic. Blurred disk margins may be mistaken for papilledema.

GLOBE-SHAPE ABNORMALITIES (Fig. 7-14)

- Coloboma: focal outpouching involving retina, choroid, iris; caused by deficient closure of fetal

FIGURE 7-14

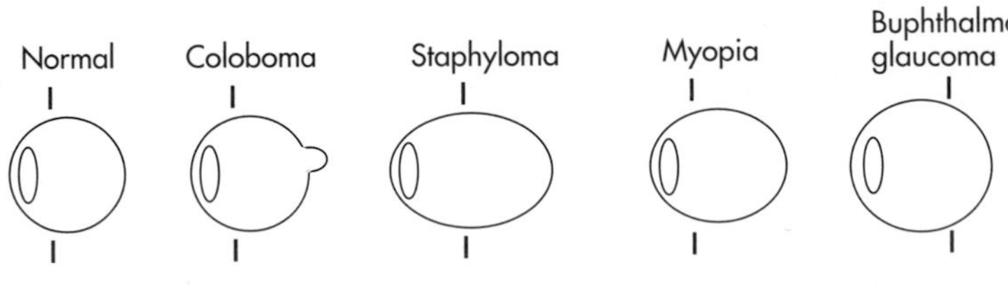

optic fissure; located in region of optic disc; associated with:
  - Morning glory anomaly
  - Microphthalmos with cyst
- Staphyloma: acquired defect of globe wall with protrusion of choroid or sclera
- Axial myopia: AP elongation but no protrusion
- Buphthalmos: congenital glaucoma; anterior ocular chamber drainage problem

LEUKOKORIA

Leukokoria refers to a white pupil. Clinical, not a radiologic, finding. Underlying causes:

- Retinoblastoma
- PHPV
- Congenital cataract
- Toxocariasis
- Other
  - Sclerosing endophthalmitis
  - Coats disease
  - Retrolental fibroplasia
  - Trauma
  - Chronic retinal detachment

RETINAL DETACHMENT (Fig. 7-15)

Separation of the sensory retina from the retinal pigment epithelium. Appears in a characteristic V shape, with the apex of the detachment at the optic disc. The presence of retinal or choroidal detachment may be caused by an ocular mass.

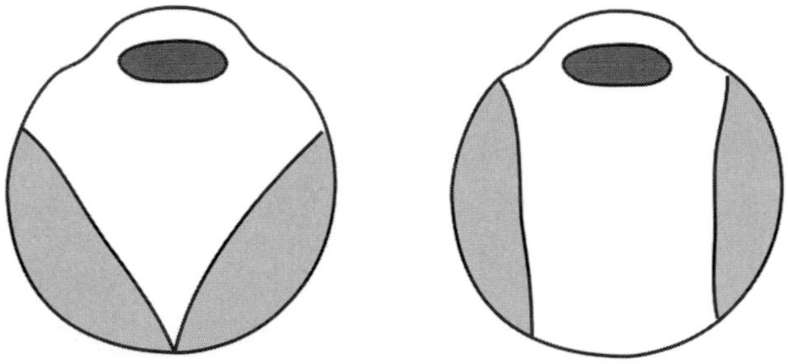

FIGURE 7-15

CHOROIDAL DETACHMENT

Usually results after ocular surgery, trauma, or uveitis, causing fluid to accumulate in the subchoroidal space. Characteristic appearance spares the posterior third of the globe (region of the optic disc) in contradistinction with retinal detachment.

OPTIC NERVE

OPTIC NERVE GLIOMA

Most common cause of diffuse optic nerve enlargement, especially in childhood. Pathology: usually well-differentiated, pilocytic astrocytoma. Clinical findings include loss of vision, proptosis (bulky tumors). 80% occur in first decade of life. In neurofibromatosis (NF-1) the disease may be bilateral.

Radiographic Features

- Types of tumor growth: tubular, excrescent, fusiform widening of optic nerve
- Enlargement of optical canal; >1 mm difference between left and right is abnormal.
- Lower CT density than meningioma
- Contrast enhancement variable
- Calcifications rare (but common in meningioma)
- Tumor extension best detected by MRI: chiasm → optic tracts → lateral geniculate body → optic radiation

OPTIC NERVE MENINGIOMA

Optic nerve sheath meningiomas arise from arachnoid rests in meninges covering the optic nerve. Age: 4th decade (80% female); younger patients typically have NF. Progressive loss of vision.

Radiographic Features

Mass
- Tubular, 60%
- Fusiform, surrounding the optic nerve, 25%
- Eccentric, 15%
- Calcification (common)

Enhancement
- Intense contrast enhancement
- Linear bands of enhancement (nerve within tumor): "tramtrack sign"

Other
- Sphenoid bone and/or optical canal hyperostosis

OPTIC NEURITIS

Clinical Findings

- Visual loss
- Pain on eye movement
- Afferent papillary defects.

Causes

- Multiple sclerosis (most common cause; occurs in 80% of MS patients)
  - Devic syndrome: optic neuritis (bilateral) with transverse myelitis (MS or ADEM may be the cause)
- Ischemia
- Vasculitis

Radiographic Features

- Fat-suppressed T2W or postgadolinium with fat suppression best for diagnosis
- T2W: obliteration of the perioptic space; increased T2 signal of the affected optic nerve
- Enhancement of the optic nerve

EXTRAOCULAR TUMORS

HEMANGIOMA

Common benign tumor of the intraconal space.

Types

Capillary hemangioma (children; strawberry nevus): no capsule
- Represents 10% of all pediatric orbital tumors, most common pediatric vascular orbital tumor
- Infiltrates conal and extraconal spaces
- Grows for <1 year and then typically involutes
- 90% are associated with cutaneous angioma.

Cavernous hemangioma (adults): true capsule, benign, most common vascular orbital mass in adults, affecting more women (60%-70%)
- Large, dilated venous channels with fibrous pseudocapsule
  - Dense enhancement with contrast
  - Signal intensity similar to fluid (e.g., CSF) on T2W
- Well-delineated, round
- Expansion of orbit
- Calcified phleboliths, rare
- Hemosiderin deposition
- No bone destruction but remodeling in large hemangiomas

DERMOID CYST

Common orbital tumor in childhood. Age: 1st decade.

Radiographic Features
- Low CT attenuation and T1 hyperintensity (fat) are diagnostic.
- Contiguous bone scalloping or sclerosis is common.
- May contain debris (inhomogeneous MRI signal)

LYMPHANGIOMA

2% of orbital childhood tumors. Age: 1st decade. Associated with other lymphangiomas in head and neck. Lymphangiomas of the orbit do not involute spontaneously.

Radiographic Features
- Variable CT appearance because of different histologic components (lymphangitic channels, vascular stroma)
- Multiloculated
- Rim enhancement
- Signal intensity similar to fluid (e.g., CSF) on T2W

LACRIMAL GLAND TUMORS

Lymphoid, 50%
- Benign reactive lymphoid hyperplasia
- Lymphoma

Epithelial tumors, 50%
- Benign mixed (pleomorphic) tumor (75% of epithelial tumors)
- Adenoid cystic carcinoma
- Mucoepidermoid carcinoma
- Malignant mixed tumor

RHABDOMYOSARCOMA

Most common malignant orbital tumor in childhood. Mean age: 7 years.

RADIOGRAPHIC FEATURES
- Large, aggressive soft tissue mass (intraconal or extraconal)
- Metastases to lung and cervical nodes

METASTASES

Children: Ewing tumor, neuroblastoma, leukemia. Adults: breast, lung, renal cell, prostate carcinoma. Direct extension of SCC from paranasal sinus.

INFLAMMATORY AND INFILTRATIVE LESIONS

ORBITAL INFECTION

The orbital septum represents a barrier to infectious spread from anterior to posterior structures. Common causes of orbital infection include spread from infected sinus and trauma.

Radiographic Features
- Periorbital cellulitis: soft tissue swelling
- Postseptal infection (true orbital cellulitis)
  - Subperiosteal infiltrate or abscess
  - Stranding of retrobulbar fat
  - Lateral displacement of enlarged medial rectus muscle
  - Proptosis

THYROID OPHTHALMOPATHY (Fig. 7-16)

Orbital pathology (deposition of glycoproteins and mucopolysaccharides in the orbit) caused by long-acting thyroid-stimulating factor (LATS) in Graves

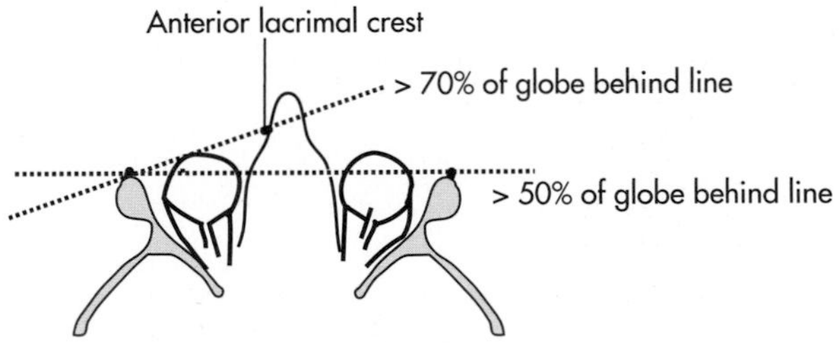

FIGURE 7-16

disease. Clinical: painless proptosis; patients may be euthyroid, hypothyroid, or hyperthyroid. Grades:

- Grade 1: lid retraction, stare, lid lag (spasm of upper lid due to thyrotoxicosis)
- Grade 2: soft tissue involvement
- Grade 3: proptosis as determined by exophthalmometer measurement
- Grade 4: extraocular muscle involvement; affects muscles at midpoint
- Grade 5: corneal involvement
- Grade 6: optic nerve involvement: vision loss

Treatment: prednisone → radiation therapy → surgical decompression; surgery or ^{131}I for thyroid.

Radiographic Features (Fig. 7-17)

Exophthalmos
Muscle involvement

- Mnemonic for involvement: "**I'M SL**ow":
  Inferior (most common)
  Medial
  Superior
  Lateral
- Enlargement is maximal in the middle of the muscle and tapers toward the end (infiltrative, not inflammatory disease).
- Spares tendon insertions
- Often bilateral, symmetrical

Other

- Optic nerve thickening
- Expansion of orbital fat

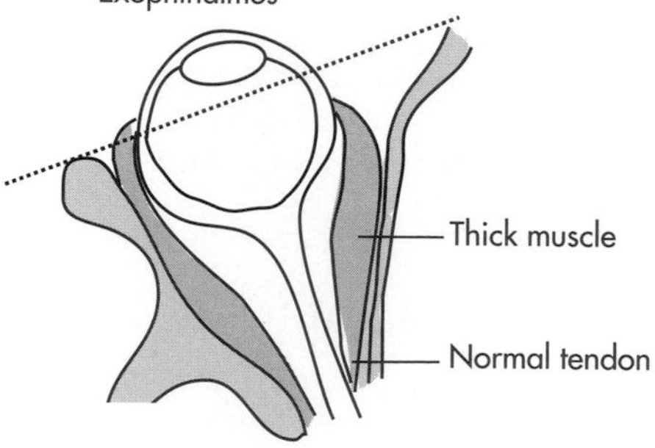

FIGURE 7-17

ORBITAL PSEUDOTUMOR

Inflammation of orbital soft tissues of unknown origin

Clinical Findings

- Painful proptosis
- Unilateral
- Steroid responsive

Causes

- Idiopathic
- Systemic disease: sarcoid, endocrine
- Unrecognized focal infections, foreign bodies

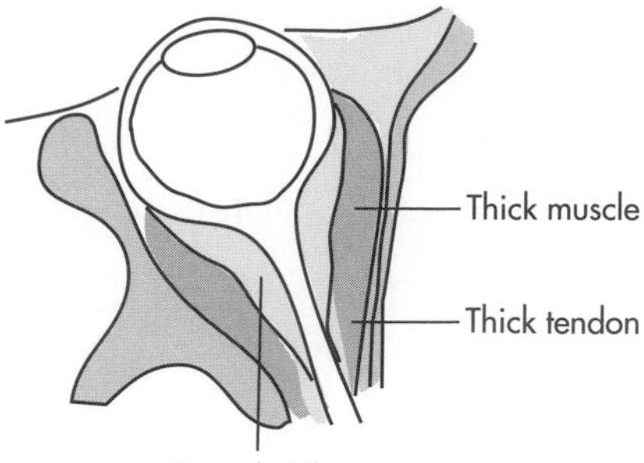

FIGURE 7-18

Radiographic Features (Fig. 7-18)

- Infiltrating intraconal or extraconal inflammation presenting as ill-defined infiltrations or less commonly as a mass
- Typical features:
  Unilateral
  Unlike thyroid ophthalmopathy, pseudotumors involve tendons of muscles (because it is an inflammatory disease).
  Muscle enlargement
- Stranding of orbital fat (inflammation)
- Enlarged lacrimal gland
- May involve orbital apex including superior orbital fissure (Tolosa-Hunt syndrome)

DIFFERENTIATION

	Pseudotumor	Thyroid Ophthalmopathy
Involvement	Unilateral, 85%	Bilateral, 85%
Tendon	Involved	Normal
Muscle	Enlargement	Enlargement: I > M > S > L
Fat	Inflammation	Increased amount of fat
Lacrimal gland	Enlarged	
Steroids	Good response	Minimal response

ACUTE INFECTIONS

Bacterial infection (extraconal > intraconal) are often due to sinusitis complicated by cavernous sinus thrombosis.

TRAUMA

Types:

- Blunt trauma with orbital blow-out fractures, 50%
- Penetrating injury, 50%

Detection of ocular foreign bodies:
- Metal: objects $>0.06\,mm^3$
- Glass: objects $>1.8\,mm^3$
- Wood: difficult to detect because wood density is similar to that of soft tissue

OTHER

ERDHEIM-CHESTER DISEASE

Lipid granulomatosis (non-Langerhans histiocytosis) with retroorbital deposition or mass, xanthelasma of eyelids, skeletal manifestations (medullary sclerosis, cortical thickening), and cardiopulmonary manifestations due to cholesterol emboli. Rare.

OCULAR MANIFESTATIONS OF PHAKOMATOSES

NF1
- Lisch nodules
- Sphenoid bone dysplasia
- Choroidal hamartoma
- Optic glioma
- Plexiform neurofibroma

NF2
- Meningioma
- Schwannoma

Sturge-Weber
- Choroidal angioma
- Buphthalmos
- Glaucoma

Tuberous sclerosis
- Retinal astrocytic hamartoma

Von Hippel-Lindau (VHL)
- Retinal angioma

Pharynx, Larynx

GENERAL

ANATOMY

The upper aerodigestive tract consists of the pharynx and the larynx. The larynx connects pharynx and trachea.

The pharynx is divided into:
- Nasopharynx: extends to inferior portion of soft palate
- Oropharynx: extends from soft palate to hyoid bone
- Hypopharynx (laryngeal part of pharynx): contains pyriform sinuses and posterior pharynx

The larynx contains:
- Laryngeal surface of epiglottis
- Aryepiglottic folds
- Arytenoid cartilage
- False cords
- True cords (glottis is the space between vocal cords)
- Subglottic larynx

AXIAL CT ANATOMY (Fig. 7-19, A-C)

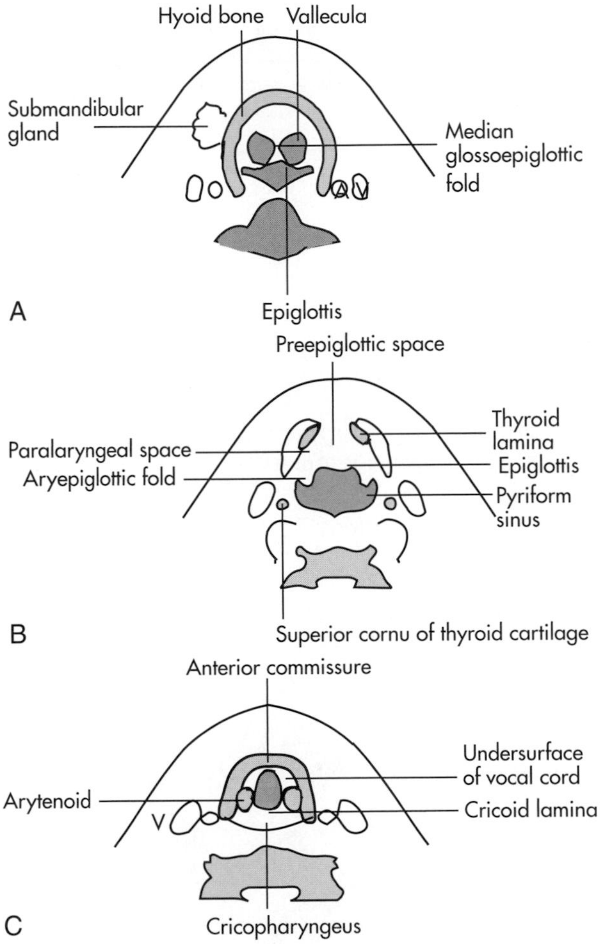

FIGURE 7-19

PARAPHARYNGEAL SPACE (Fig. 7-20)

Potential space filled with loose connective tissue. Space is pyramidal, with the apex directed toward the lesser cornua of the hyoid bone and the base toward the skull base. Extends from skull base to midoropharynx. Borders:
- Lateral: mandible, medial pterygoid muscle
- Medial: superior constrictor muscles of pharynx, tensor and levator veli palatini
- Anterior: buccinator muscle, pterygoid, mandible
- Posterior: carotid sheath

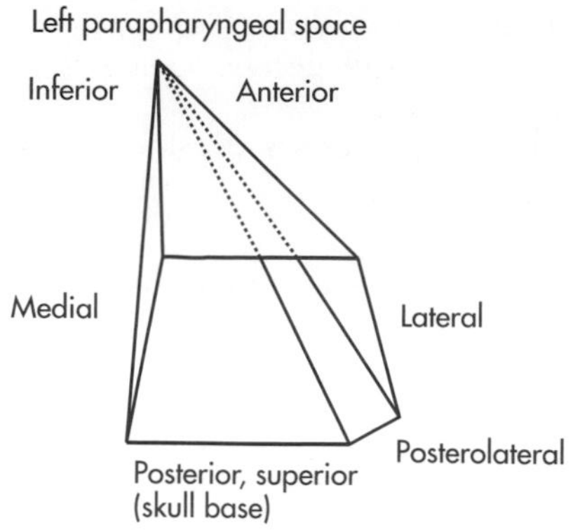

FIGURE 7-20

Contents (Fig. 7-21)

Anterior (prestyloid) compartment
- Internal maxillary artery
- Interior alveolar, lingual, auriculotemporal nerves

Posterior (retrostyloid) compartment
- ICA, internal jugular vein (IJV)
- CNs IX, X, XII
- Cervical sympathetic chain lymph nodes

Medial (retropharyngeal) compartment
- Lymph nodes (Rouvière)

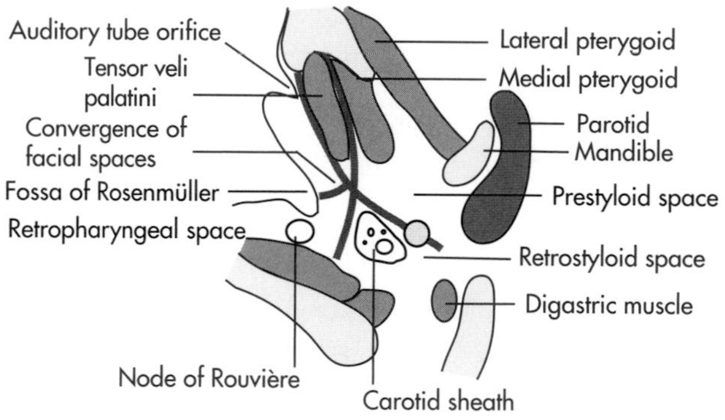

FIGURE 7-21

Lymphatics (Fig. 7-22)

The parapharyngeal space has abundant lymph node groups.
- Lateral pharyngeal node (Rouvière)
- Deep cervical nodes
- Internal jugular chain, including jugulodigastric node
- Chain of spinal accessory nerve
- Chain of transverse cervical artery

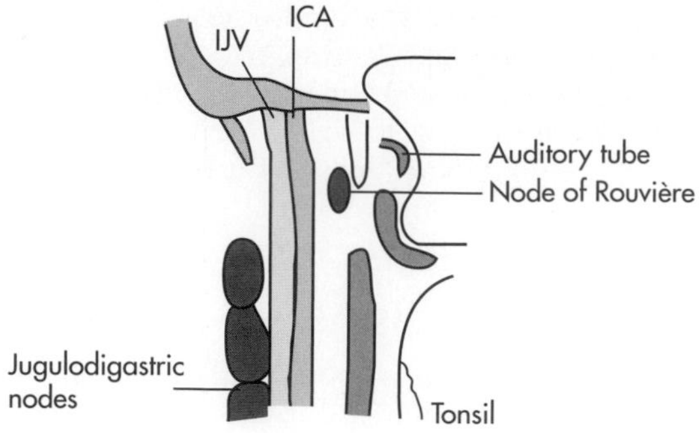

FIGURE 7-22

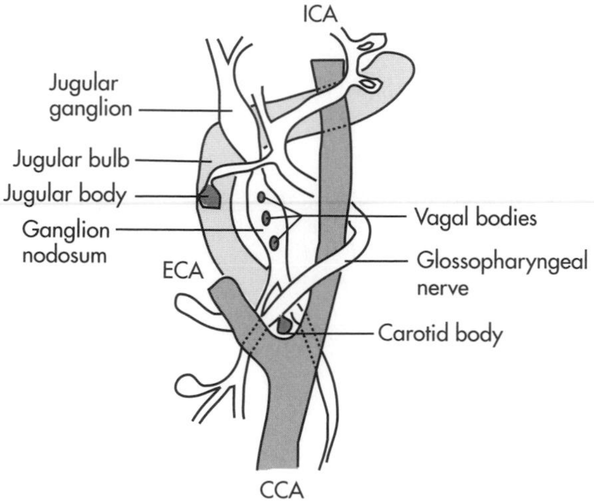

FIGURE 7-23

Paraganglia (Fig. 7-23)

Cells of neuroectodermal origin that are sensitive to changes in oxygen and CO_2. Types:
- Carotid body (at carotid bifurcation)
- Vagal bodies

Neoplastic transformation of the jugular bulb ganglion produces the glomus jugulare.

FLUOROSCOPIC VOCAL CORD EXAMINATION (Fig. 7-24)

Occasionally performed to evaluate the subglottic region (Valsalva maneuver), invisible by laryngoscopy.
- Phonation of "E" during expiration: adducts cords

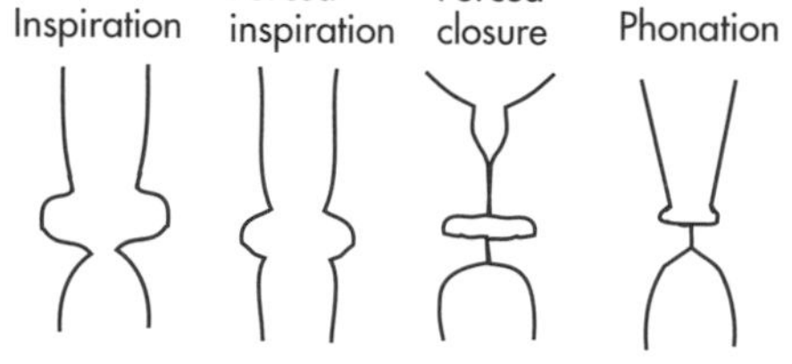

FIGURE 7-24

- Phonation of "reversed E" during inspiration; distends laryngeal ventricles
- Puffed cheeks (modified Valsalva): distends pyriform
- Valsalva: distends subglottic region
- Inspiration: abducts cords

NODAL STATIONS (Fig. 7-25)

- IA: between anterior margins of the anterior bellies of the digastric muscles, above the hyoid bone and below the mylohyoid muscle (submental)
- IB: below mylohyoid muscle, above hyoid bone, posterior to anterior belly of digastric muscle, and anterior to a line drawn tangential to the posterior surface of the submandibular gland (submandibular)
- Levels II, III, IV: internal jugular nodes
  - II: (jugulodigastric) from skull base to lower body of the hyoid bone, through posterior edge of the sternocleidomastoid muscle and posterior edge of the submandibular gland. *Note:* A node medial to the carotid artery is classified as a retropharyngeal node.
  - III: hyoid bone to cricoid cartilage
  - IV: cricoid to clavicle
- Level V: skull base to clavicle, between anterior edge of trapezius muscle and posterior edge of sternocleidomastoid muscle

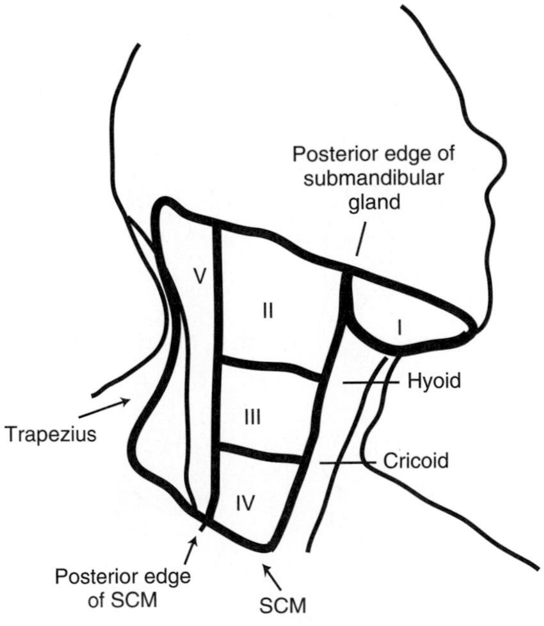

FIGURE 7-25

- Level VI: visceral nodes; from hyoid bone, top of manubrium, and between common carotid arteries on each side
- Level VII: caudal to top of the manubrium in superior mediastinum (superior mediastinal nodes)

Pathologic Adenopathy Size Criteria

Neck lymphadenopathy by size has poor specificity, and no universal standard exists for determination of adenopathy.

Nonetheless, two methods are commonly used:

- Long axis: 15 mm in levels I and II, 10 mm elsewhere
- Short axis: 11 mm in level II, 10 mm elsewhere

Retropharyngeal nodes should not exceed 8 mm (long) or 5 mm (short). Emerging technologies such as MRI lymph node imaging with iron nanoparticles (see Chapter 13) or PET may prove to be more specific and sensitive.

NASOOROPHARYNX

THORNWALDT CYST

Cystic midline nasopharyngeal notochordal remnant (3% of population). May occasionally become infected. Age: 15 to 30 years.

Radiographic Features

- Hemispherical soft tissue density seen on lateral plain films
- Typical cystic appearance by CT and MRI
- Location: midline; same level as adenoids

RETROPHARYNGEAL ABSCESS (Fig. 7-26)

Cause: dental disease, pharyngitis, penetrating trauma, vertebral osteomyelitis. Organism: *Staphylococcus, Streptococcus,* anaerobes, *Mycobacterium tuberculosis* (TB).

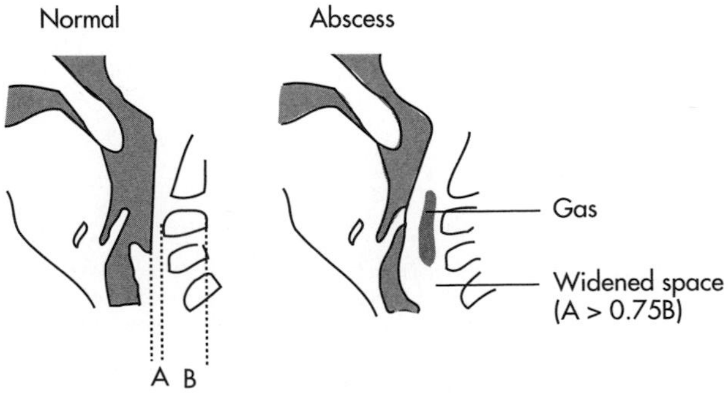

FIGURE 7-26

Radiographic Features

- Widened retropharyngeal space
- May involve retropharyngeal, parapharyngeal, prevertebral, submandibular, or masticator space or spread to mediastinum via the danger space
- CT appearance
  - Gas
  - Necrotic tissue and edema appear hypodense.
  - Stranding of fat
  - Rim enhancement with contrast

JUVENILE ANGIOFIBROMA

Vascular tumor of mesenchymal origin. Most frequent benign nasopharyngeal tumor in adolescents (age: 10 to 20, males only).

Clinical Findings

- Epistaxis (very vascular tumor)
- Mass in the pterygopalatine fossa
- Extension to infratemporal fossa, nasal cavity

Radiographic Features

Usually large soft tissue mass causing local bony remodeling

- Pterygopalatine fossa, 90%; with extension causing displacement of posterior wall of maxillary sinus
- Sphenoidal sinus, 65%
- Pterygomaxillary fissure, infratemporal fossa, intracranial cavity via superior orbital fissure

Highly vascular:

- Intense enhancement by CT and MRI
- MRI: very hyperintense on T2W, flow voids
- Angiography: tumor blush

Embolization before resection

- Main supply from ECA particularly maxillary artery
- May have supply from ICA

Pearls

- Do not biopsy (hemorrhage).
- Recurrent if incompletely resected; recurrence rate today is low because of early diagnosis.

SQUAMOUS CELL CARCINOMA (SCC)

SCC accounts for 80%-90% of malignant tumors in the nasooropharynx (lymphoma: 5%; rare tumors: adenocarcinoma, melanoma, sarcoma).

Location

Nasopharynx

- Tumors most commonly arise from lateral pharyngeal recess (fossa of Rosenmüller).
- Possibly associated with Epstein-Barr virus
- Common in Chinese persons

Oropharynx

- Palate
- Tonsil
- Tongue, pharyngeal wall
- Lips, gingiva, floor of mouth

Radiographic Features

- Asymmetry of soft tissues; primarily infiltrating carcinomas produce only slight asymmetry
- Mass, ulceration, infiltrating lesion

Staging of Nasopharyngeal SCC (Fig. 7-27)

Primary tumor

- Tis: carcinoma in situ
- T1: tumor confined to 1 site of nasopharynx or no tumor visible
- T2: tumor involving 2 sites (both posterosuperior and lateral walls)
- T3: extension of tumor into nasal cavity or oropharynx
- T4: tumor invasion of skull, cranial nerve involvement, or both

Adenopathy

- N0: clinically positive node
- N1: single clinically positive homolateral node ≤ 3 cm in diameter
- N2: single clinically positive homolateral node >3 cm but not >6 cm in diameter
- N3: node >6 cm

Distant metastasis

- M0: no evidence of metastasis
- M1: distant metastases present

Pearls

- Elderly patients with serous otitis media have nasopharyngeal carcinoma until proved otherwise.
- 20% of tumors are submucosal and cannot be seen by the clinician.
- Schmincke tumor: undifferentiated cancer
- 80%-90% of patients with nasopharyngeal SCC have positive lymph nodes at presentation.

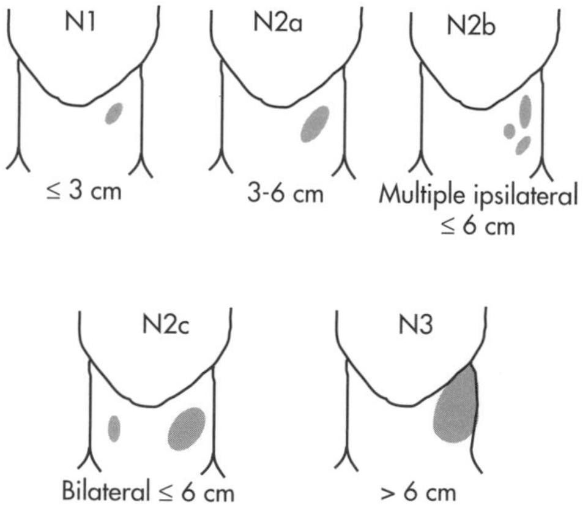

FIGURE 7-27

OTHER NEOPLASMS

OVERVIEW OF OTHER HEAD AND NECK NEOPLASMS BY SITE

Space	Congenital	Benign	Malignant
Prestyloid/parapharyngeal	2nd branchial cleft cyst	Mixed tumor Neuroma	SCC of tonsil Salivary/parotid carcinoma Sarcoma Lymphoma
Poststyloid/ parapharyngeal		Paraganglioma Neuroma Chordoma	SCC Nodal metastases Lymphoma Neuroblastoma
Infratemporal fossa, masticator space	Lymphangioma Cystic hygroma	Odontogenic cyst Neural tumor Hemangioma	SCC Sarcoma (MFH, rhabdomyosarcoma) Lymphoma Salivary/parotid carcinoma
Floor of mouth, sublingual	Epidermoid, dermoid Teratoma Lymphangioma Cystic hygroma	Ranula Pleomorphic adenoma Neural tumor Hemangioma	Salivary/parotid SCC Sarcoma Lymphoma
Retropharyngeal	Meningocele	Chordoma Neural tumor Fibroma Teratoid	Sarcoma (muscle, nerve, liposarcoma) Vertebral metastases Primary bone tumor Neuroblastoma

MFH, malignant fibrous histiocytoma.

HYPOPHARYNX, LARYNX

VOCAL CORD PARALYSIS (Fig. 7-28)

Innervation of vocal cord muscles is through the recurrent laryngeal nerve of the vagus (CN X). The left recurrent laryngeal nerve is more commonly injured. Causes of paralysis include:

- Idiopathic
- Traumatic, surgical
- Tumor: mediastinum, left hilum, or lung apex
- Arthritis (degenerative changes of cricoarytenoid cartilage)

Radiographic Features

- Abnormal movement of the involved cord
- Widening of laryngeal ventricle
- Expansion of pyriform sinus
- Flattening of false vocal cords
- Flattened subglottic angle

LARYNGOCELE (Fig. 7-29)

Dilatation of the laryngeal ventricle. Most commonly seen in glassblowers or patients with chronic obstructive pulmonary disease (COPD). May extend through the thyrohyoid membrane and into the neck. May be fluid or air filled.

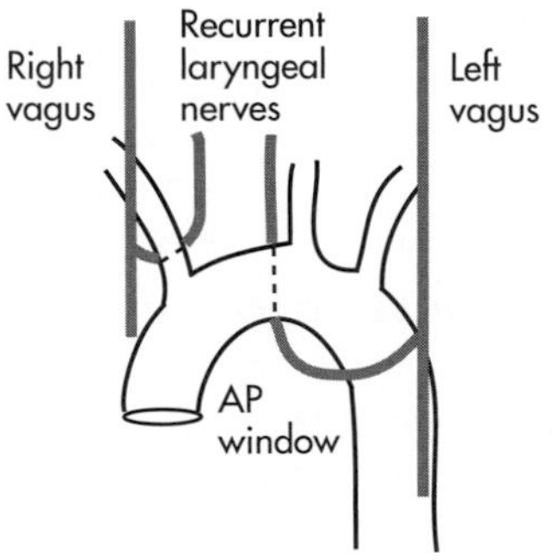

FIGURE 7-28

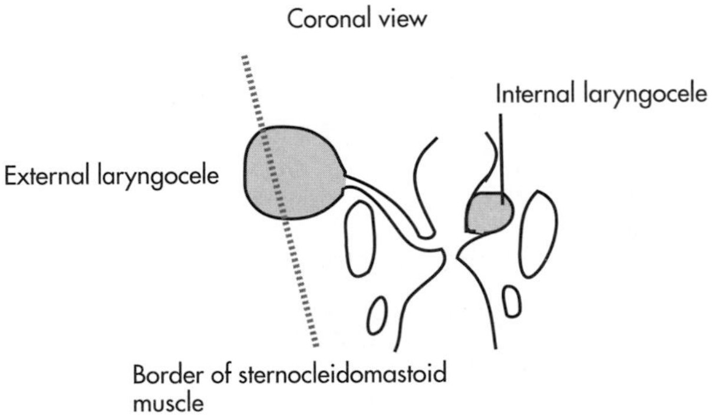

FIGURE 7-29

LARYNGEAL TRAUMA

Cause

Intubation: erosions, laryngomalacia, stenosis
Direct force: fractures. The main goal of CT is to demonstrate the presence of:
- Displaced fractures of thyroid or cricoid cartilage
- Arytenoid dislocation
- A false passage
- Displacement of epiglottis

Types
- Thyroid: longitudinal, paramedian, transverse, or comminuted fractures
- Cricoid: always breaks in 2 places; the posterior component is often not clinically recognized.
- Epiglottis: may be avulsed posteriorly and superiorly.
- Arytenoids: anterior and posterior dislocation

BENIGN LARYNGEAL TUMORS

- Papilloma and hemangioma are the most common tumors.
- Less common tumors: chondroma, neurofibroma, fibroma, paraganglioma, rhabdomyoma, pleomorphic adenoma, lipoma
- Vocal cord polyps (not true tumors) are the most common benign lesions of the larynx.

LARYNGEAL CARCINOMA

Histology

SCC, 90%
Others, 10%
- Adenocarcinoma
- Metastases
- Tumors arising from supporting tissues of larynx (chondrosarcoma, lymphoma [rare])
- Carcinosarcoma
- Adenocystic carcinoma

Types

Supraglottic, 30%
- Tumor arises from false cords, ventricles, laryngeal surface of epiglottis, arytenoids, and aryepiglottic folds.
- Usually large when discovered
- Treated by supraglottic laryngectomy or radiation therapy

Glottic, 60%
- Tumor arises from true vocal cords, including anterior commissure.
- Usually small when discovered (hoarseness is an early finding)
- Early symptoms, good prognosis
- T1 tumors treated with cordectomy, hemilaryngectomy, or radiation therapy
- T3 tumors treated with total laryngectomy

Subglottic, 10%
- Uncommon as an isolated lesion and usually seen as an extension of glottic tumors
- Poor prognosis because of early nodal metastases

Radiographic Features

Common locations of mass lesions:
- Pyriform sinus (most common)
- Postcricoid
- Posterolateral wall

Determine mobility of cords (fluoroscopy); locate the cause of cord fixation:
- Cricoarytenoid joint arthritis
- Vocalis muscle invasion from tumor
- Paralaryngeal space tumor
- Recurrent laryngeal nerve paresis
- Idiopathic (virus infection?)

Invasion
- Fat spaces become obliterated; >2 mm soft tissue indicates tumor spread to contralateral side of cord
- Thickening of anterior commissure
- Cartilage invasion: erosion, distortion (bowing, bulging, buckling), sclerosis (microinvasion)
- Adenopathy

Staging
- T1: confined to true vocal cords, normal mobility
- T2: confined to true vocal cords, limited mobility but no fixation of cords
- T3: fixation of cords

Pearls

- 25%-50% of supraglottic tumors have metastasized at time of surgery.
- Subglottic tumors metastasize most frequently.
- Glottic tumors confined to cords metastasize infrequently but spread locally to contralateral cord via anterior commissure or posterior interarytenoid area. Masses may also be due to hemorrhage, inflammation, edema, or fibrosis.

POSTSURGICAL LARYNX

Vertical Hemilaryngectomy

- True vocal cord, laryngeal ventricle, false cord, and ipsilateral thyroid lamina are removed.
- Used to treat limited true vocal cord tumors or supraglottic tumors

Horizontal Hemilaryngectomy (Supraglottic)

- Epiglottis, aryepiglottic folds, false vocal cords, preepiglottic space, superior portion of thyroid cartilage, and portion of hyoid bone are removed.
- Used for selected tumors of epiglottis, aryepiglottic folds, and false vocal cord

Total Laryngectomy

- Entire larynx and preepiglottic space, hyoid bone, strap muscles, and part of the thyroid gland are removed; permanent tracheostomy
- A neopharynx (extending from the base of the tongue to the esophagus) is created using muscular, mucosal, and connective tissue layers.
- Used for extensive laryngeal tumors

Radical Neck Dissection

- Sternocleidomastoid muscle, IJV, lymph nodes, and submandibular salivary gland are removed.
- Myocutaneous flaps are used for repair.

PARAPHARYNGEAL SPACE

BRANCHIAL CLEFT CYST (Fig. 7-30)

Embryologic cysts derived from 1st or 2nd (most common) cervical pouch. Mass in anterior triangle; may be infected.

Radiographic Features

- Cyst location
  - Type 1: EAC or parotid
  - Type 2: anterior triangle, angle of mandible
- Signal intensity
  - Water density (<20 HU) unless infected (debris)
    - Intense rim enhancement in infected cysts
- Cleft sinus passes between internal and external carotid arteries

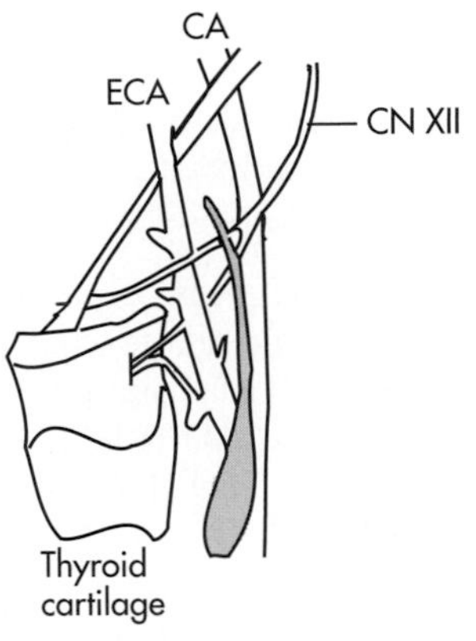

FIGURE 7-30

THYROGLOSSAL DUCT CYST

Extends from thyroid to foramen cecum. Palpable midline mass (80%). Represents 70% of congenital neck lesions.

Location

- Suprahyoid, 20%
- At hyoid bone, 15%
- Infrahyoid, 65%

Radiographic Features

- Thin-walled cystic structure
- Water density (<20 HU)
- Thickening and enhancement of wall indicate infection.

GLOMUS TUMORS (PARAGANGLIOMA, CHEMODECTOMA)

Benign tumors that arise from paraganglion cells of the sympathetic system. Tumors are very vascular and thus enhance extensively (CT, dense blush with angiography). Location:

- Skull base (glomus jugulare)
- Below skull base (glomus vagale)
- At carotid bifurcation (carotid body tumor)

GLASSCOCK-JACKSON GLOMUS TUMOR CLASSIFICATION

Type	Findings
Glomus Tympanicum	
Type I	Tumor limited to promontory
Type II	Tumor completely filling middle ear space
Type III	Tumor filling middle ear, extending into mastoid or through tympanic membrane
Type IV	Tumor filling middle ear, extending into mastoid or through tympanic membrane to fill EAC; may extend anterior to internal carotid artery
Glomus Jugulare	
Type I	Tumor involving jugular bulb, middle ear, and mastoid
Type II	Tumor extending under internal auditory canal; may have intracranial extension
Type III	Tumor extending into petrous apex; may have intracranial extension
Type IV	Tumor extending beyond petrous apex into clivus or infratemporal fossa; may have intracranial extension

Sinuses, Nasal Cavity

GENERAL

SINUSES (Fig. 7-31)

- Frontal
- Ethmoidal
- Sphenoidal
- Maxillary

Osteomeatal Complex (OMC)

- Control point for drainage from 3 sinuses: frontal, anterior ethmoidal, maxillary
- Medial wall of OMC is formed by uncinate process.

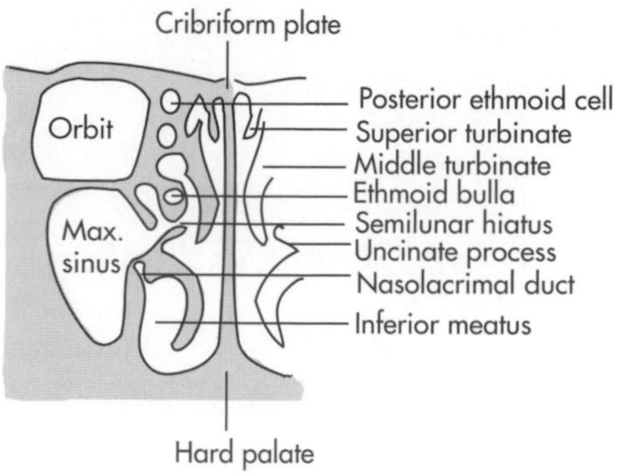

FIGURE 7-31

- Superolateral wall of OMC is formed by inferior orbital wall and may also be formed by low-lying ethmoid air cells.
- The infundibulum leads to the hiatus semilunaris.
- The middle turbinate may contain an air cell (concha bullosa).
- Ostia for sinuses vary in size (depending on PO_2, mucus stasis).

Cells

- Haller cells: posterior ethmoid cells invading the medial floor of the orbit; can obstruct ostia, can be source of infection
- Onodi cells: most posterior ethmoid cells that surround optic canal and optic nerve
- Agger nasi cells: most anterior ethmoid air cells frequently pneumatize adjacent bones such as frontal bone, maxilla, middle turbinate, sphenoid, and/or lacrimal bone

Anatomic Variation (may potentially lead to obstruction)

- Concha bullosa, 35%
- Septal deformity, 20%
- Paradox middle turbinate, 15%
- Reversed uncinate process
- Inferiorly migrated ethmoid bullae

Nasofrontal Duct

- Frontal sinus drains directly into the frontal recess of the nasal cavity, 85%.
- In 15% a nasofrontal duct drains frontal sinus into the ethmoid infundibulum.

ANATOMIC SPACES

Pterygopalatine Fossa (Fig. 7-32)

Pyramidal space between upper pterygoid process and posterior wall of maxillary antrum. Fossa continues superiorly with the inferior orbital fissure and laterally with the infratemporal fossa. Pterygopalatine fossa is the crossroad of foramina

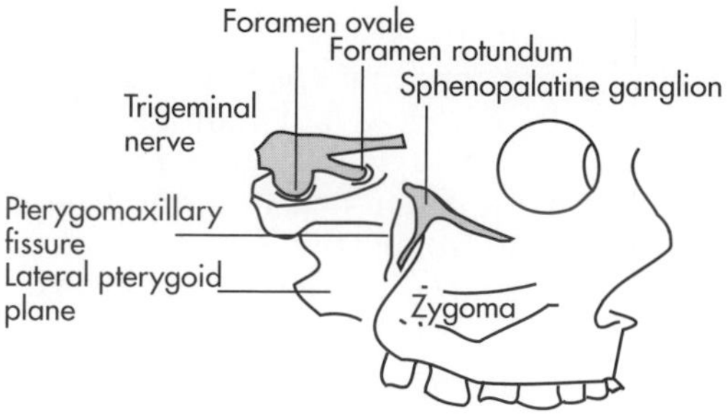

FIGURE 7-32

and from which pathology can spread. Connections to other spaces:

- Foramen rotundum leads to middle cranial fossa.
- Sphenopalatine foramen connects to posterior nasal cavity.
- Pterygoid (vidian) canal inferior and lateral to foramen rotundum (vessels and nerves)

Sphenopalatine Foramen

The foramen extends from the pterygopalatine fossa to the posterior nasal cavity. It contains pterygopalatine vessels and nerves and is the favored pathway of least resistance for tumor spread from nasal cavity to pterygopalatine fossa, inferior orbital fissure, and infratemporal fossa.

Pterygoid (Vidian) Canal

Located at the base of pterygoid plates below and lateral to foramen rotundum in the sphenoid bone. Connects pterygopalatine fossa and foramen lacerum. Contains nerve of the pterygoid canal (vidian nerve = continuation of greater superficial petrosal nerve) and the vidian artery (branch of the internal maxillary artery).

Foramen Lacerum

Plugged with fibrocartilage during life; only branches of the ascending pharyngeal artery and some sympathetic nerves go through this foramen. Located at the base of the medial pterygoid plate. Favored site of nasopharyngeal carcinoma. Pathways to skull base:

- Fossa of Rosenmüller lies subjacent to foramen lacerum.
- Prestyloid parapharyngeal space lies anterior.
- Tensor and levator veli palatini take origin from this region.
- Carotid artery rests on the foramen lacerum.

SINUSES

ACUTE SINUSITIS

Frequency of involvement: maxillary > ethmoidal, frontal > sphenoidal sinus. Sinusitis is frequently associated with upper respiratory tract infections due to occlusion of draining ostia.

Types

- Infectious sinusitis
  - Acute
  - Subacute
  - Chronic
- Noninfectious (allergic)
- Dental infection and sinusitis (20% maxillary antrum)

Radiographic Features (Figs. 7-33 and 7-34)

- Opacified sinus partial, complete
- Mucosal thickening
- Air-fluid levels
- Chronic sinusitis: mucosal hyperplasia, pseudopolyps, hyperostosis of bone
- Complications
  - Mucus retention cyst
  - Mucocele
  - Osteomyelitis
  - Cavernous sinus thrombosis
  - Intracranial extension
  - Empyema
  - Cerebritis
  - Abscess
  - Orbital complications
- Recurrent sinusitis: hyperostosis, bone erosion (rare), mucosal hypertrophy

Pearls

- Plain film diagnosis of opaque sinus is nonspecific.
- Obtain CT to assess bone detail and OMC anatomy for recurrent sinusitis.
- Contrast-enhanced CT: tumors, polyps, and mucosa enhance; secretions do not enhance.
- T2W: benign lesions are usually very bright; tumors have intermediate brightness.

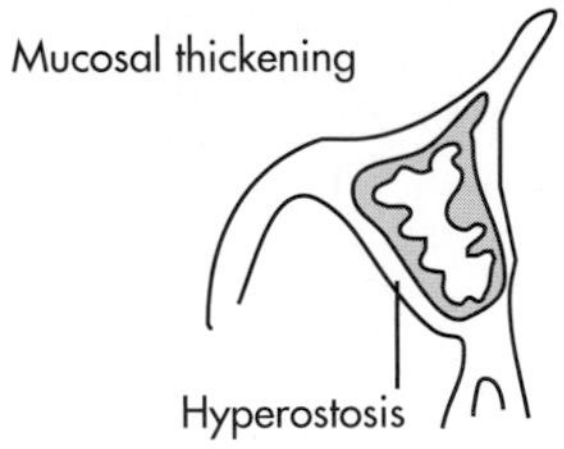

FIGURE 7-33

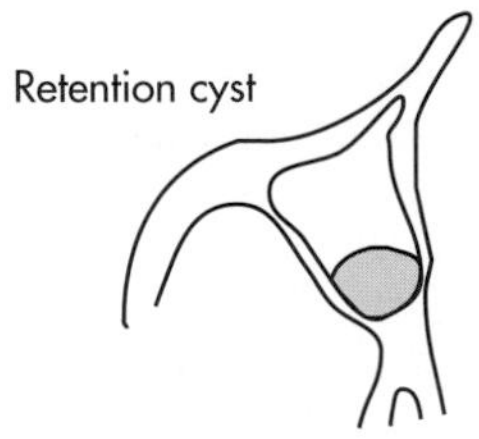

FIGURE 7-34

MUCUS RETENTION CYST (Fig. 7-35)

Incidence: 10% of population. Cysts occur from blockage of duct draining glands. Most commonly in maxillary sinus (floor).

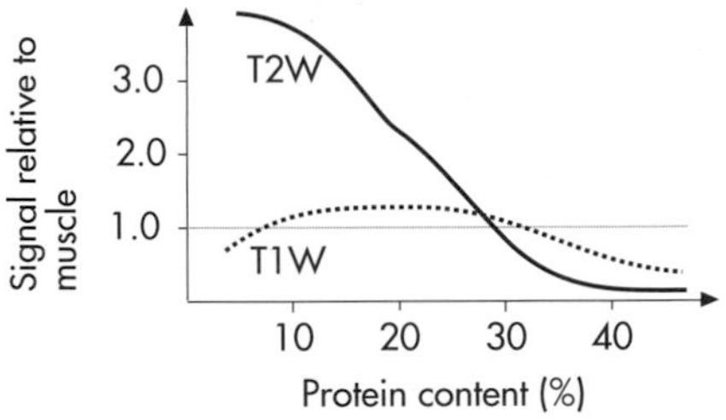

FIGURE 7-35

Radiographic Features

- Cysts adhere to sinus cavity wall without causing bony expansion (in contradistinction to mucocele).
- Rounded soft tissue mass on T1W
- MRI signal intensity depends on pulse sequence used and protein content (see graph).

POLYPS (Fig. 7-36)

Most common tumors of sinonasal cavity. Diseases associated with sinonasal polyps include:

- Polypoid rhinosinusitis (allergy)
- Infection
- Endocrine disorders
- Rhinitis medica (aspirin)
- Cystic fibrosis

Radiographic Features

- Location: ethmoidal sinus > nose
- Soft tissue polyps are typically round.
- Bony expansion and remodeling
- Very hyperintense on T2W
- Mucoceles may form as a result of blocked draining ostia.

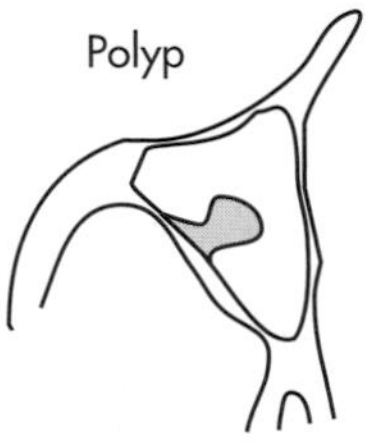

FIGURE 7-36

DESTRUCTIVE SINUSITIS

Causes

- Mucormycosis
- Aspergillosis
- Wegener granulomatosis
- Neoplasm

FUNGAL SINUSITIS

Predisposing factors: diabetes, prolonged antibiotic or steroid therapy, immunocompromised patient

Radiographic Features

- Bony destruction and rapid extension into adjacent anatomic spaces
- Indistinguishable from tumor: biopsy required
- Main role of CT/MRI is to determine extent of disease
- Aspergillosis may appear hyperdense on CT and hypointense on T1W
- If sphenoidal sinus alone is involved, consider aspergillosis.

MUCOCELE (Fig. 7-37)

True cystic lesion lined by sinus mucosa. Mucoceles occur as a result of complete obstruction of sinus ostium (inflammation, trauma, tumor). The bony walls of the sinus are remodeled as the pressure of secretions increases. In pediatric patients, consider cystic fibrosis. Location: frontal 65% > ethmoidal 25% > maxillary >10%. Sphenoidal (rare). Patients with polyposis may have multiple mucoceles.

Radiographic Features

- Rounded soft tissue density
- Typically isodense on CT
- MR signal intensity:
    - Low T1W, high T2W: serous content
    - High T1W, high T2W: high protein content
    - Dark T1W and T2W: viscous content
- Differential diagnosis signal voids within paranasal sinuses
    - Aerated sinus
    - Desiccated secretions
    - Calcifications
    - Fungal concretions (mycetoma)
    - Foreign body
    - Ectopic (undescended) tooth
    - Dentigerous cyst
    - Acute blood
- Distortion and expansion of bony sinus walls
- Nonenhancement unless infected (mucopyocele): rim enhancement

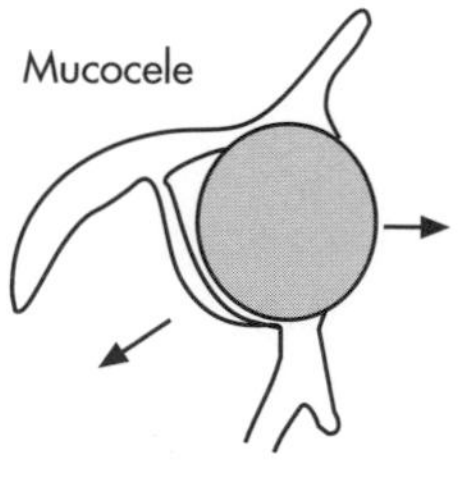

FIGURE 7-37

- Complication: breakthrough into orbit or anterior cranial fossa

INVERTED PAPILLOMA

- Unilateral polypoid lesion of the nasal cavity and paranasal sinuses
- Associated with HPV and malignancy
- Treatment: surgical resection
- Differential diagnosis
    - Antral choanal polyp (young male adults)
    - Allergic polyposis
    - Allergic fungal sinusitis
    - Juvenile angiofibroma
    - Mycetoma
    - Mucocele
    - SCC
    - Adenocarcinoma

BENIGN TUMORS

- Osteoma (most common paranasal sinus tumor)
- Papilloma
- Fibroosseous lesions
- Neurogenic tumors
- Giant cell granuloma

MALIGNANT TUMORS

Types

SCC, 90%
- Maxillary sinus, 80%
- Ethmoidal sinus, 15%

Less common tumors, 10%
- Adenoid cystic carcinoma
- Esthesioneuroblastoma
    - Arises from olfactory epithelial cells
    - Commonly extends through cribriform plate
- Lymphoepithelioma
- Mucoepidermoid carcinoma
- Mesenchymal tumors: fibrosarcoma, rhabdomyosarcoma, osteosarcoma, chondrosarcoma
- Metastases from lung, kidney, breast

Tumor Spread

Direct invasion
- Maxillary sinus:
    - Posterior extension: infratemporal fossa, pterygopalatine fossa
    - Superior extension: orbit
- Ethmoidal or frontal sinus: frontal lobe

Lymph node metastases
- Submandibular, lateral pharyngeal, jugulodigastric nodes

Perineural spread
- Pterygopalatine fossa
- Connection to middle cranial fossa via foramen rotundum

ENDOSCOPIC SINUS SURGERY

The goal of endoscopic sinus surgery is to relieve obstructions of the sinus ostia. Endoscopic surgery replaces the more invasive procedures, such as Caldwell-Luc, for maxillary sinus access. Complications include:

- Recurrent inflammatory disease due to adhesions, synechiae, incomplete removal, 10%
- Orbital complications, 5%
  - Hematoma
  - Abscess
  - Optic nerve injury
- Intraoperative hemorrhage
- CSF leak, 1%
- Intracranial injury
- ICA dissection

NOSE

COCAINE SEPTUM

Cocaine use can lead to nasal septal erosions and perforations because of its vasoconstrictive properties causing ischemia.

RHINOLITH

Calcification of foreign body or granuloma in nasal cavity can lead to nasal obstruction.

SINCIPITAL ENCEPHALOCELE (Fig. 7-38)

Brain tissue trapped in the nose during embryologic development, most common in Asia and Latin America (occipital encephalocele more common in North America). Connects to the intracranial brain.

Types

- Nasoethmoidal: through the foramen cecum into the ethmoid sinuses and nose
- Frontonasal: anteriorly between the nasal and frontal bones
- Nasoorbital: between nose and orbit

Management

- Potential site for meningitis and abscess
- Connection to intracranial cavity needs to be obliterated

NASAL GLIOMA

Hamartomatous trapped brain tissue, which unlike encephalocele, has no connection to the intracranial brain. Two types: intranasal (40%) and extranasal (60%).

Glands and Periglandular Region

GENERAL

FLOOR OF MOUTH (Figs. 7-39 and 7-40)

- Formed by mylohyoid muscle
- Mylohyoid muscle extends from mandible to hyoid.
- Above the mylohyoid muscle the floor is subdivided by different tongue muscles (genioglossus, geniohyoid).

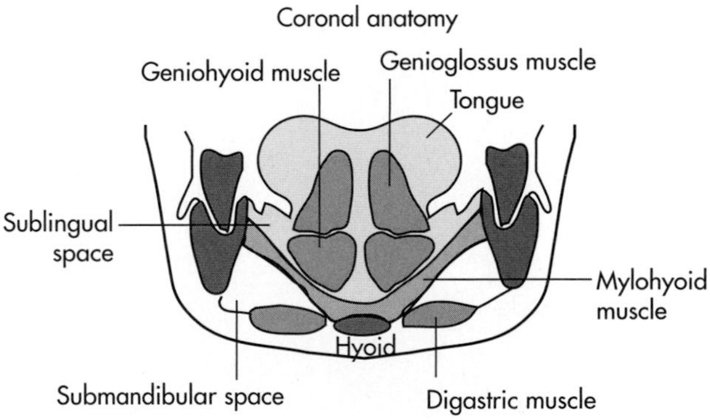

FIGURE 7-39

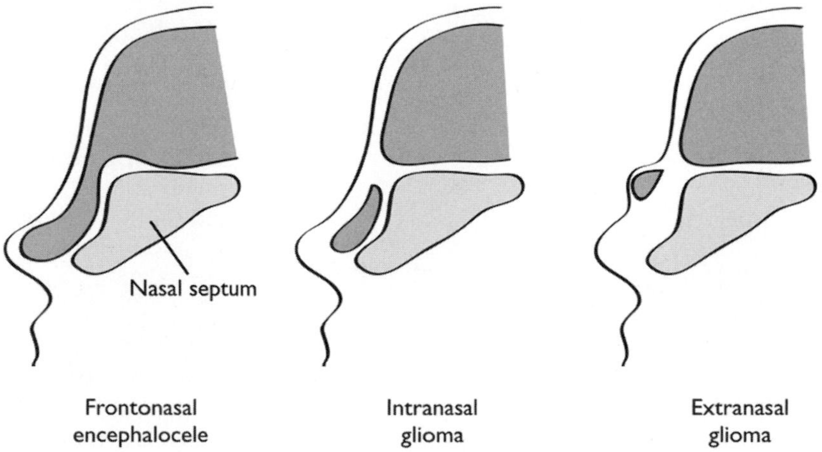

FIGURE 7-38

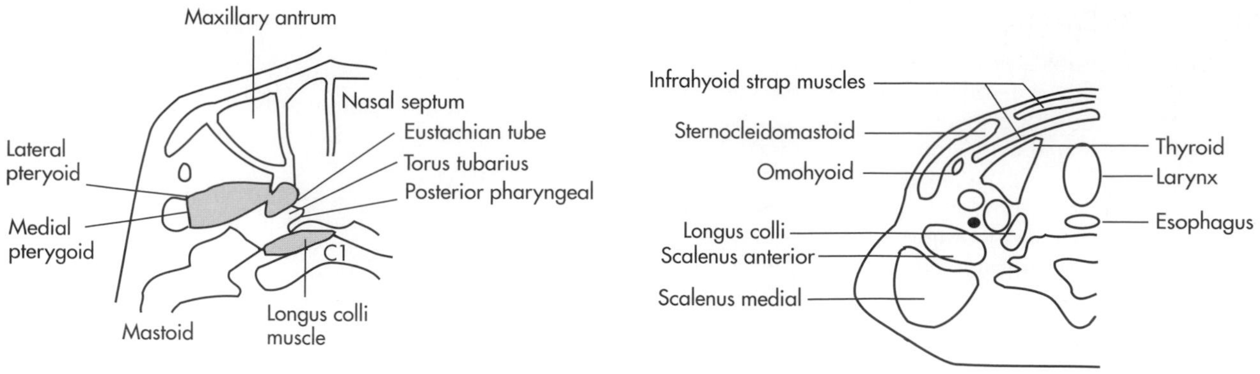

FIGURE 7-40

- Sublingual space refers to the space between the mylohyoid and genioglossus-geniohyoid complex.
- Submandibular space refers to space below mylohyoid. Not limited posteriorly; disease may spread to masticator or parapharyngeal space.

SUPERFICIAL NECK ANATOMY (Fig. 7-41)

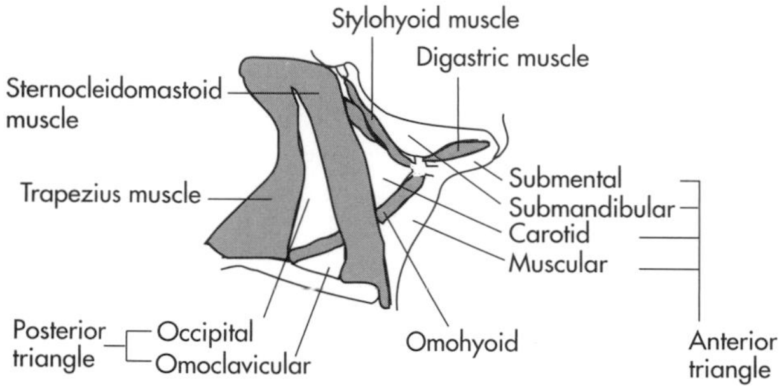

FIGURE 7-41

GLANDULAR STRUCTURES IN NECK

Salivary glands
- Parotid glands (inferior to external ear; Stenson's duct)
- Submandibular glands (medial to body of mandible; Wharton's duct)
- Sublingual glands (posterior to mandibular symphysis; Bartholin's duct)

Thyroid gland
Parathyroid gland

SALIVARY GLANDS

SIALOLITHIASIS (CALCULI)

Calculi are often composed of hydroxyapatite and are multiple in 25% of patients. Total duct obstruction is usually due to calculi >3 mm. Location:

Submandibular gland, 80%
- Most calculi are radiopaque (80%-90%). The higher incidence of submandibular calculi is due to (1) more alkaline pH of submandibular gland, which tends to precipitate salts; (2) thicker, more mucous submandibular saliva; (3) higher concentration of hydroxyapatite and phosphatase; (4) narrower Wharton's orifice compared with main lumen; and (5) slight uphill course of salivary flow in Wharton's duct when patient is in upright position.

Parotid, 20%
- 50% of calculi are radiopaque.

Radiographic Features

- Radiopaque calculi can often be seen on plain films or CT.
- Radiolucent calculi are best demonstrated by sialography. Sialography typically shows a contrast filling defect and ductal dilatation.
- On contrast CT, there may be strong and persistent enhancement. It is important not to mistake calcification in the stylohyoid ligament for a calculus.
- Complications of large stones:
  Obstruction
  Strictures

SIALOSIS

Recurrent, noninflammatory enlargement of parotid gland (acinar hypertrophy, fatty replacement). Causes:
- Cirrhosis
- Malnutrition, alcoholics
- Drugs (thiourea, reserpine, phenylbutazone, heavy metal)

SIALOADENITIS

Acute Sialoadenitis

- Bacterial, viral
- Abscess may form.

Chronic, Recurrent Sialoadenitis

- Recurrent infection due to poor oral hygiene
- Sialography: multiple sites of peripheral ductal dilatation
- Small gland

Granulomatous Inflammation

- Causes: sarcoid, TB, actinomycosis, cat-scratch disease, toxoplasmosis
- Produces intraglandular masses indistinguishable from tumors; biopsy is therefore required.

SJÖGREN DISEASE

Autoimmune disease causing inflammation of secretory glands (e.g., lacrimal, parotid, submandibular, tracheobronchial tree). Male:Female = 1:9 (most common in menopausal women).

Clinical Findings

- Sicca complex: dry eyes (keratoconjunctivitis sicca), dry mouth, xerostomia (dry mouth)
- Systemic disease: rheumatoid arthritis

Radiographic Features

Parotid gland enlargement (lymphoepithelial proliferation), 50%

Sialography patterns:

- Punctate: normal central and peripheral ductal system, punctate (1 mm) parenchymal contrast collections
- Globular: normal central system, peripheral duct system does not opacify, larger (>2 mm) extraductal collections
- Cavitary: >2 mm extraductal collections
- Destructive: ductal structures not opacified

MRI findings are similar to those seen by CT: parenchymal heterogeneity, cystic degeneration (microcysts), and fatty replacement.

CYSTIC SALIVARY LESIONS

- Mucus retention cyst: true cyst with epithelial lining
- Ranula: retention cyst from sublingual glands in floor of mouth
- Mucocele (extravasation cyst): results from ductal rupture and mucus extravasation. Not a true cyst; composed of granulation tissue
- Benign lymphoepithelial cysts (BLCs)
  - HIV-positive patients (early), precursor to AIDS
  - Associated adenopathy and lymphoid hyperplasia may be clues to HIV seropositivity.
  - They typically present as bilateral parotid cysts, superficial in location, in lymph nodes.
  - With parotid enlargement, it may be indistinguishable from Sjögren disease, where the lesions are parenchymal.
  - In absence of HIV infection, parotid cysts are rare.
  - Warthin tumor must be considered in the differential diagnosis.
- Cystic tumors (Warthin)
  - Bilateral in 10%
  - Accumulation of pertechnetate
  - Well-defined, lobulated, intermediate-signal-intensity mass with cystic areas

PAROTID TUMORS

Types

Benign, 80%

- Pleomorphic adenoma (most common), 70%
- Warthin tumor (papillary cystadenoma lymphomatosum), 5% (of these, 5%-20% are bilateral), male > female
- Rare: oncocytoma, hemangioma, adenoma

Malignant, 20%

- Mucoepidermoid carcinoma, 5%
- Carcinoma arising from pleomorphic adenoma, 5%
- Adenoid cystic carcinoma (cylindroma), 2%
- Adenocarcinoma, 4%
- SCC, 2%
- Oncocytic carcinoma, 1%

PLEOMORPHIC ADENOMA (MIXED TUMOR) (Fig. 7-42)

Most common (75%) benign salivary neoplasm. Unifocal mass, slow growing, well demarcated.

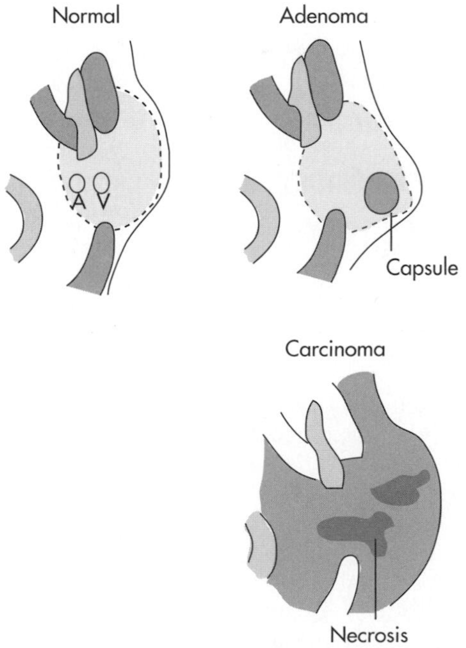

FIGURE 7-42

Radiographic Features

- Well-circumscribed, encapsulated mass
- Superficial posterior glandular location, 80%
- Lesions are hypoechoic by ultrasound (US)
- Moderate enhancement by CT
- Calcification in a parotid mass is very suggestive of pleomorphic adenoma.
- Malignant transformation, 5%
- T1W hypointense, T2W hyperintense moderate enhancement
- MRI characteristics that suggest malignancy include:
  - Irregular margins
  - Heterogeneous signal
  - Lymphadenopathy
  - Adjacent soft tissue or bone invasion
  - Facial perineural spread
- The deep lobe of the parotid gland extends between the mandibular ramus and styloid process into the parapharyngeal space. For ideal surgical planning, masses arising from deep lobe (transparotid approach) must be differentiated from other parapharyngeal space masses (transcervical approach). In deep lobe masses there will be an absence of fatty tissue plane on some or all axial slices. Normal parotid tissue partially wrapped around the mass or extension of mass laterally into stylomandibular tunnel further suggests deep parotid lobe origin of mass.

MALIGNANT TUMORS

Radiographic Features

- Areas of necrosis due to infarction (rapid growth)
- Locally invasive and aggressive
- Lymph node metastases

PARATHYROID

HYPERPARATHYROIDISM

Usually detected by increased serum calcium during routine biochemical screening. Incidence: 0.2% of the general population (female > male).

Types

Primary hyperparathyroidism:
- Adenoma, 80%
- Hyperplasia, 20%
- Parathyroid carcinoma, rare

Secondary hyperparathyroidism:
- Renal failure
- Ectopic parathormone (PTH) production by hormonally active tumors

Tertiary hyperparathyroidism: results from autonomous glandular function after long-standing renal failure

Clinical Findings

- GI complaints
- Musculoskeletal symptoms
- Renal calculi

Effect of PTH

- Increases vitamin D metabolism
- Increases renal calcium reabsorption (hypercalcemia)
- Increases bone resorption
- Decreases renal PO_4 resorption (hypophosphatemia)

Radiographic Features

Parathyroid
- Single parathyroid adenoma, 80%
- Hyperplasia of all 4 glands, 20%

Bone
- Osteopenia
- Subperiosteal resorption (virtually pathognomonic)
- Brown tumors
- Soft tissue calcification

Renal
- Calculi (due to hypercalciuria)

PARATHYROID ADENOMA

Adenomas may consist of pure or mixed cell types, with the most common variant composed principally of chief cells. Some cases are associated with the multiple endocrine neoplasia (MEN) I syndrome. 80% single, 20% multiple.

Radiographic Features

Detection
- US and scintigraphy are the best screening modalities.
- Adenomas are hypoechoic on US.
- If US is negative, further evaluation with CT or MRI may be helpful.
- Angiography is reserved for patients with negative neck explorations and persistent symptoms.
- Location:
  - Adjacent to thyroid lobes
  - Thoracic inlet
  - Prevascular space in mediastinum (not in posterior mediastinum); the inferior glands follow the descent of the thymus (also a 3rd pouch derivative).

Angiography
- Adenomas are hypervascular.
- Arteriography is most often performed after unsuccessful surgery and has a 60% success rate in that setting.
- Venous sampling and venography: 80% success rate after unsuccessful neck explorations

TYPES OF HYPOPARATHYROIDISM

Type	Calcium	PO_4	PTH	Comments
Hypoparathyroidism	↓	↑	↓	Surgical removal (most common cause)
Pseudohypoparathyroidism	↓	↑	Ø↑	End-organ resistance to PTH (hereditary)
Pseudo-pseudohypoparathyroidism	Ø	Ø	Ø	Only skeletal abnormalities (Albright hereditary osteodystrophy)

HYPOPARATHYROIDISM

Cause

Idiopathic
- Rare; associated with cataracts, mental retardation, dental hypoplasia, obesity, dwarfism

Secondary
- Surgical removal (most common)
- Radiation
- Carcinoma
- Infection

Radiographic Features

- Generalized increase in bone density, 10%
- Calcifications in basal ganglia
- Other calcifications: soft tissues, ligaments, tendon insertion sites

THYROID (Fig. 7-43)

THYROID NODULE

Palpable thyroid nodules are found in 4%-7% of the population, and nonpalpable nodules are found in 50% of persons >60 years. 2%-5% of the thyroid nodules are malignant.

Thyroid US is usually performed with a 5- to 10-MHz transducer. Images are obtained in transverse and longitudinal sections. Look for enlargement of lobes, cysts, and hypoechoic or hyperechoic focal lesions and describe them as such.

Detection
- Allows precise localization of neck nodules (intrathyroid vs. extrathyroid)
- Differentiation of solid and cystic nodules
- Detection of nonpalpable nodules in high-risk groups (e.g., prior neck radiation, MEN II)

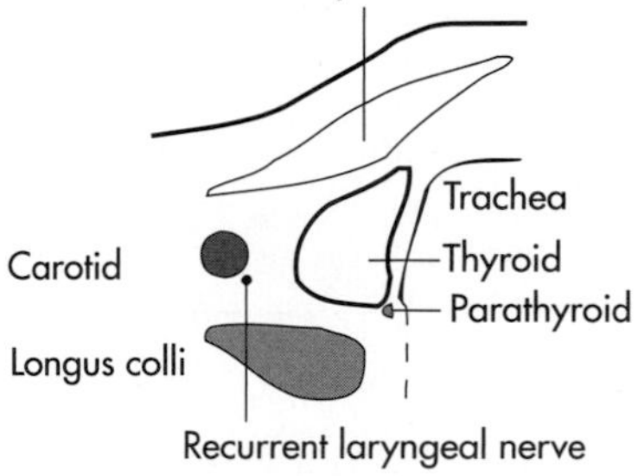

FIGURE 7-43

- Extent of disease (nodes, vessel invasion)
- Postsurgical follow-up

Differentiation
- US cannot reliably differentiate benign from malignant nodules (sensitivity 87%-94%)
- US features suggestive of malignancy include:
  - Solid mass
  - Ill-defined margins
  - Microcalcification rather than large or peripheral calcification
  - Intranodular blood flow

US guidelines for thyroid nodules:
- 80% of nodular disease is due to hyperplasia (pathologically they are referred to as hyperplastic, adenomatous, or colloid nodules).
- Malignant and benign nodules present simultaneously in 10%-20% of cases; thus multiplicity is not a sign of a benign condition.
- Nodules with large cystic components are usually benign; however, 20% of papillary cancers are cystic.
- Comet-tail artifacts are seen in colloid cysts.
- In a solid hyperechoic nodule, the incidence of malignancy is 5%.
- In a solid isoechoic nodule, the incidence of malignancy is 25%.
- In a solid hypoechoic nodule, the incidence of malignancy is 65%.
- A complete halo usually indicates a benign lesion; malignant lesions may be associated with an incomplete halo.
- Halos usually form around follicular lesions.

Types of Doppler color flow in thyroid nodules:
- Type 1: no flow
- Type 2: perinodular flow
- Type 3: intranodular flow (usually malignant)

Fine-needle aspiration (FNA) biopsy of focal nodules:
- Usually recommended for nodules larger than 1 to 1.5cm
- 25-gauge needle, US guidance
- FNA with little suction from 10-mL syringe
- Cytology interpretation
  - Nondiagnostic
  - Benign (usually macrofollicular)
  - Malignant (papillary, occasionally medullary)
  - Suspicious (FNA cannot diagnose follicular or Hürthle cell cancers → surgical biopsy)

Surgical Removal

- High-risk group
- Cytologic findings are positive or equivocal
- Nodule grows despite suppressive T_4 therapy

THYROID FOLLICULAR ADENOMA

- Represents 5% of thyroid nodules
- Appears as solid masses with surrounding halo
- Difficult to differentiate from follicular cancer by cytology; thus, these lesions need to be surgically resected.

THYROIDITIS

OVERVIEW

Type	Etiology	Clinical Findings
Subacute granulomatous thyroiditis (de Quervain)	Postviral HLA-B35	Pain Hypothyroidism Systemic: fever, chills ESR>50
Subacute lymphocytic thyroiditis	Autoimmune	No pain
	Postpartum	Hypothyroidism
Hashimoto thyroiditis*	Autoimmune	Early disease: hyperthyroidism, 5%
	HLA-DR3	Late disease: hypothyroidism
	HLA-B8	Antimicrosomal antibodies

*Hashimoto thyroiditis is associated with pernicious anemia, SLE, Sjögren, Addison. Hashimoto + Addison = Schmidt syndrome. Most thyroiditis shows gallium uptake.

Radiographic Features

- Enlargement of thyroid
- Hypoechogenicity

GRAVES DISEASE (DIFFUSE GOITER)

The etiology of Graves disease is unknown but is associated with HLA-B8, DR3 (white patients), and HLA-Bw35, Bw46 (Asian patients). Pathogenetically it is an autoimmune disease in which T lymphocytes become sensitized to antigens within the thyroid gland and stimulate B lymphocytes to synthesize antibodies: thyroid-stimulating Ig (TSI). Graves disease consists of one or more of the following:

- Thyrotoxicosis
- Goiter
- Ophthalmopathy
- Dermopathy: pretibial myxedema: accumulation of glycosaminoglycan in pretibial skin
- Rare findings:
  - Subperiosteal bone formation (osteopathy of phalanges)
  - Clubbing (thyroid acropathy)
  - Onycholysis = separation of the nail from its bed
  - Gynecomastia in males
  - Splenomegaly, 10%
  - Lymphadenopathy

Radiographic Features

Scintigraphy

- Uniform distribution of increased activity by scintigraphy (Hashimoto thyroiditis can mimic this appearance, but patients are usually euthyroid)
- Elevated ^{131}I uptake: 50%-80%

US

- Enlarged thyroid
- Prominent pyramidal lobe

THYROID CANCER

Thyroid cancer is common (in 5% of all autopsies), but death due to thyroid cancer is uncommon (only 1200 deaths/year in the United States; the total of cancer deaths/year in the United States is >500,000). Most common presentation of thyroid cancer is a solitary thyroid nodule. Incidence of thyroid cancer:

- In hot nodule, very uncommon (benign >99%)
- In cold nodule, 5%-15% are malignant.

Risk Factors

- Male patient
- Young adult or child
- Palpable nodule
- Family history of goiter, thyroid cancer
- Prior head, neck irradiation

Poor Prognostic Factors

- Poor differentiation
- Male
- Advanced age
- Pain
- Lesion >4 cm
- More than 4 adjacent structures involved

TYPES OF THYROID CANCER

Type	Frequency	Comment
Papillary	60%	Metastases to cervical nodes, good prognosis
Follicular	25%	Aggressive, higher mortality (5-year survival is 50%)
Medullary	5%	Arises from C-cells (calcitonin); MEN association
Anaplastic	10%	Very aggressive, occurs in older patients
Epidermoid	<1%	—
Other (lymphoma, metastases)	<1%	—

Staging

T1: Nodule <4 cm (=T1a) or >4 cm (=T1b)
T2: Nodule with partial fixation
T3: Nodule with complete fixation

N1: Regional nodes (ipsilateral 1a; contralateral 2b; bilateral 2c)
N2: Fixed regional lymph nodes
M1: Metastases

Radiographic Features

- Cancers are most commonly detected during routine workup of nodules and multinodular goiter.
- ^{131}I is used for detection of metastases.
- Because normal hormone production can blunt TSH stimulation and prevent tumor detection, residual postsurgical thyroid tissue is usually ablated with ^{131}I.
- Anaplastic and medullary cancers do not concentrate ^{131}I and are therefore not detectable by iodine scanning.

Medullary Thyroid Cancer

- Thyroid mass
- Calcification, 10%
- Early spread to adjacent organs and chest
- Adenopathy
- Bullae formation; pulmonary fibrosis may occur as part of a desmoplastic reaction.

Mandible and Maxilla

CYSTIC MASSES

OVERVIEW

Odontogenic Cysts (Fig. 7-44)

- Periapical (radicular) cysts: caused by caries and infection; <1 cm; round/pear-shaped unilocular periapical lucency with sclerotic margins; can become periapical abscess. Usually asymptomatic. No malignant potential.
- Dentigerous cyst
- Odontogenic keratocyst (basal cell nevus syndrome)
- Developmental lateral periodontal cyst (botryoid cyst)

Nonodontogenic cysts

- Fissural cysts
    - Nasopalatine duct cyst
    - Globulomaxillary cyst
    - Nasolabial cyst
- Solitary simple hemorrhagic bone cyst
- Static bone cavity (Stafne cyst)

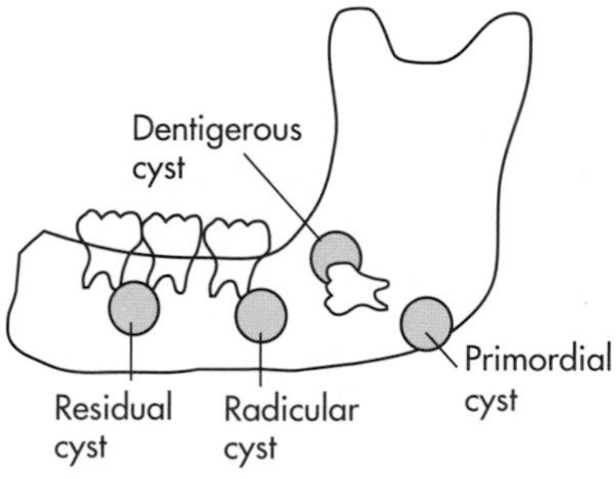

FIGURE 7-44

DENTIGEROUS CYST (FOLLICULAR CYST)

Most common pericoronal radiolucency; formed by excessive accumulation of fluid between enamel and dental capsule. Most frequently seen in mandible (80%) with unerupted 3rd molars or maxilla (20%).

Radiographic Features

- Well-corticated pericoronal radiolucency
- May become very large and occupy entire ramus
- Expansion of mandibular cortex
- May displace teeth with roots of the tooth often outside the lesion.
- Complications:
    Common: infection, pathologic fractures
    Rare: ameloblastoma, SCC, mucoepidermoid carcinoma

ODONTOGENIC KERATOCYST

Aggressive cystic jaw lesion in mandible (70%) or maxilla (30%).

Associated with basal cell nevus (Gorlin) syndrome. High rate of recurrence.

Radiographic Features

- Scalloped, corticated border (typical)
- Large size, rapid growth
- Perforation of bone cortex
- Displacement of teeth

OSTEORADIONECROSIS

Develops months to years following radiation therapy. May see both sclerotic and lytic components with ill-defined borders and enlarged trabecular spaces. A sequestered bone may also be present.

BENIGN TUMORS

OVERVIEW

- Ameloblastoma
- Odontoma
- Odontogenic myxoma
- Cementoma

AMELOBLASTOMA (ADAMANTINOMA)

Multilocular, expansile, radiolucent lesion most commonly located in ramus area. Locally aggressive and may perforate the lingual cortex. May also appear unilocular and associated with an impacted tooth, thus indistinguishable from an odontogenic keratocyst and dentigerous cyst.

ODONTOMA

Hamartomatous malformation. Most common odontogenic tumor. Two types: compound (more common), contains multiple teeth or toothlike structures; complex: well-defined lesions with amorphous calcifications. May be associated with a follicle/cyst. 1-3 cm in size.

ODONTOGENIC MYXOMA

Uncommon benign neoplasma that is locally aggressive and can destroy adjacent bone and infiltrate soft tissue. Painless. May appear multilocular with internal osseous trabeculae and honeycomb-like internal structure, as well as with irregular calcifications.

CEMENTOMA

Self-limited lesion around the apices of teeth. More common in women. Can be solitary or multiple. Usually <1 cm. Initially lucent but becomes mineralized over time. May have a thin lucent halo around the radiopaque lesion. No treatment is needed.

BASAL CELL NEVUS (GORLIN) SYNDROME

This syndrome, a phakomatosis, consists of multiple basal cell nevi of the skin, odontogenic jaw cysts (derived from odontogenic epithelium), and a variety of other abnormalities. Evolution of basal cell carcinoma at the age of 30 years.

Skin
- Multiple nevoid basal cell carcinoma, palmar plantar dyskeratosis, sebaceous cysts, cutaneous fibroma

Oral
- Multiple jaw cysts (odontogenic keratocysts), mandibular prognathism, cleft lip or palate, ameloblastoma, SCC

Other
- CNS: agenesis of corpus callosum, congenital hydrocephalus, medulloblastoma, meningioma, cerebellar astrocytoma, craniopharyngioma, dural calcification
- Skeletal: rib anomalies, short 4th metacarpal (50%), vertebral anomalies, polydactyly, clavicular and scapular deformities
- Eyes: congenital blindness, cataracts, glaucoma, coloboma
- Genital: uterine and ovarian fibromas (often with calcification), hypogonadism, cryptorchism

MALIGNANT TUMORS

OVERVIEW

Primary odontogenic tumors, rare
- Odontogenic carcinoma
- Odontogenic sarcoma

Primary nonodontogenic tumors
- Osteosarcoma
- Chondrosarcoma
- Ewing sarcoma
- Multiple myeloma
- Others

Metastases
- Carcinomas, 85% (breast, lung, renal)
- Sarcomas, 5%
- Other

PRIMARY ODONTOGENIC MALIGNANCIES

Extremely rare tumors. Always rule out primary nonodontogenic bone tumors, which are more common.

Classification

Odontogenic carcinoma
- Malignant ameloblastoma
- Primary intraosseous carcinoma
- Other carcinomas arising from odontogenic epithelium

Odontogenic sarcoma
- Ameloblastic fibrosarcoma
- Ameloblastic odontosarcoma

TEMPOROMANDIBULAR JOINT

ANATOMY (Fig. 7-45)

Joint is composed of two synovial compartments separated by a fibrocartilage disk. Posterior capsular attachment is very elastic (bilaminar zone). In the open mouth position, the condyle and disk translate anteriorly.

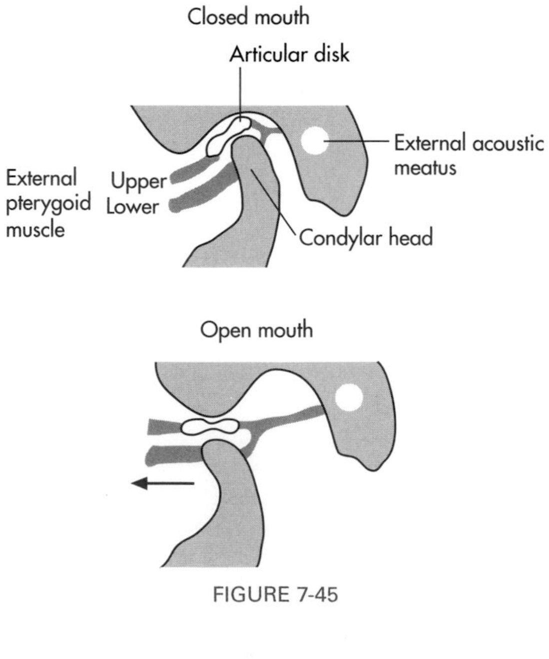

FIGURE 7-45

DISK DISPLACEMENT

Pain, clicking, and locked jaw occur.

Types

- Anteromedial displacement with reduction (most common type); disk is displaced anteriorly in the open-mouth view and recaptured in the closed-mouth view.
- Persistent anterior displacement; disk does not reduce closed lock
- Rotational displacement
- Medial displacement (uncommon)

DEGENERATIVE CHANGES OF TMJ

Radiographic findings are similar to those of osteoarthritis in other joints:

- Joint space narrowing
- Subchondral sclerosis, spurring, pseudocyst formation
- Deformity
- Avascular necrosis

Differential Diagnosis

TEMPORAL BONE (Fig. 7-46)

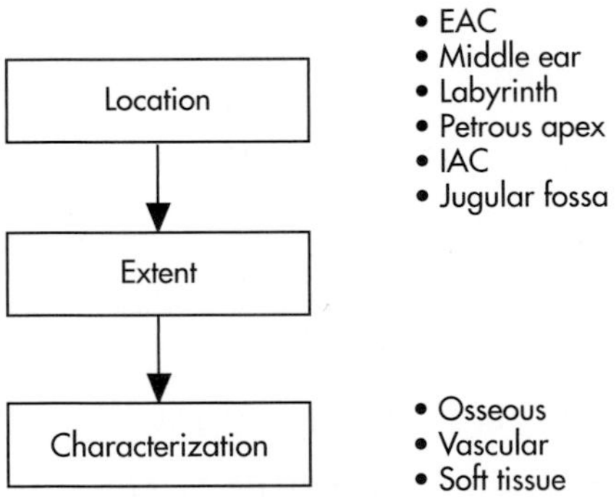

FIGURE 7-46

APPROACH

SOFT TISSUE MASS IN MIDDLE EAR

- Cholesteatoma
- Chronic otitis media
- Granulation tissue
- Cholesterol granuloma
- Glomus tympanicum tumor
- Aberrant internal carotid artery
- High or dehiscent jugular bulb

VASCULAR MASS IN MIDDLE EAR

- Glomus tympanicum
- Aberrant carotid artery
- Carotid artery aneurysm
- Persistent stapedial artery
- Exposed jugular bulb
- Exposed carotid artery
- Hemangioma
- Extensive glomus jugulare

INTRACANALICULAR INTERNAL AUDITORY CANAL MASSES

Exclusively intracanalicular lesions

- Acoustic neuroma (CN VIII), common
- Facial neuroma (CN VII), rare
- Hemangioma
- Lipoma

Not primarily intracanalicular

- Meningioma
- Epidermoid

JUGULAR FOSSA MASS

- Glomus jugular tumor, most common
- Neurofibroma, second most common
- Schwannoma
- Chondrosarcoma
- Metastases

MASTOID BONE DEFECT

- Neoplastic bone destruction
- Cholesteatoma
- Postoperative simple mastoidectomy
- Postoperative radical mastoidectomy
- Posttraumatic deformity

PETROUS APEX LESIONS

- Cholesterol granuloma (T1W hyperintense)
- Mucocele (T1W hypointense but may be T1W hyperintense if proteinaceous, then indistinguishable from cholesterol granuloma)
- Epidermoid (restricted diffusion)
- Chondrosarcoma
- Chordoma (if central extending to petrous)
- Endolymphatic sac tumor (rare, more posterior; L > R; if bilateral, think VHL)

ORBIT

APPROACH TO ORBITAL MASSES (Fig. 7-47)

ORBITAL MASSES BY ETIOLOGY

Tumors

- Hemangioma (adults: cavernous; children: capillary)
- Lymphoma
- Metastases
- Lymphangioma
- Less common
  - Rhabdomyosarcoma

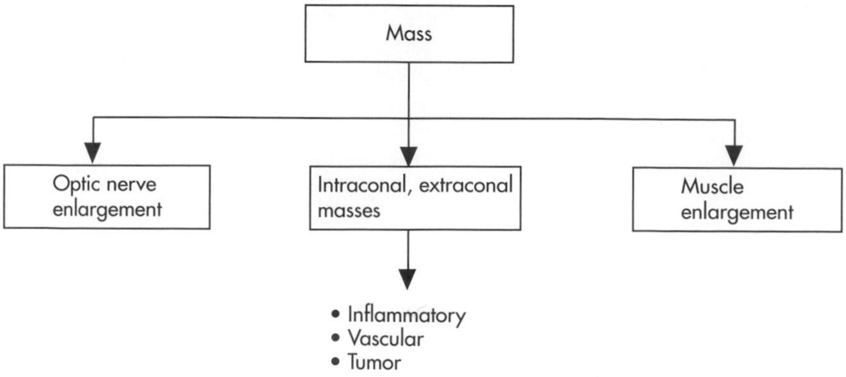

FIGURE 7-47

Hemangiopericytoma
Neurofibroma

Inflammatory
- Pseudotumor, common
- Thyroid ophthalmopathy common
- Cellulitis, abscess
- Granulomatous: Wegener disease

Vascular
- Carotid-cavernous fistula
- Venous varix
- Thrombosis of superior ophthalmic vein

Trauma
- Hematoma
- Foreign body

EXTRACONAL DISEASE

Nasal disease
- Infection
- Neoplasm

Orbital bone disease
- Subperiosteal abscess
- Osteomyelitis
- Fibrous dysplasia
- Tumors
- Trauma

Sinus disease
- Mucocele
- Invasive infections
- Neoplasm

Lacrimal gland disease
- Adenitis
- Lymphoma
- Pseudotumor
- Tumor

INTRACONAL DISEASE

Well-defined margins
- Hemangioma
- Schwannoma
- Orbital varix
- Meningioma

Ill-defined margins
- Pseudotumor
- Infection
- Lymphoma
- Metastases

Muscle enlargement
- Pseudotumor
- Graves disease (thyroid ophthalmopathy)
- Myositis
- Carotid cavernous fistula

VASCULAR ORBITAL LESIONS

Tumor
- Hemangioma, hemangioendothelioma, hemangiopericytoma
- Lymphangioma
- Meningioma

Vascular (with enlarged superior ophthalmic vein)
- Carotid cavernous fistula
- Cavernous thrombosis
- Orbital varix
- Ophthalmic artery aneurysm

OPTIC NERVE SHEATH ENLARGEMENT

Tumor
- Optic nerve glioma
- Meningioma
- Meningeal carcinomatosis
- Metastases, lymphoma, leukemia

Inflammatory
- Optic neuritis
- Pseudotumor
- Sarcoid

Increased intracranial pressure
Trauma: hematoma

TRAMTRACK ENHANCEMENT OF ORBITAL NERVE

- Optic nerve meningioma
- Optic neuritis

- Idiopathic
- Pseudotumor
- Sarcoidosis
- Leukemia, lymphoma
- Perioptic hemorrhage
- Metastases
- Normal variant

THIRD NERVE PALSY

- Compression
  - Intracranial aneurysm (do not miss)
  - Uncal herniation
  - Tumors (neurofibroma, metastases, primary)
  - Granuloma (Tolosa-Hunt, sarcoid)
- Infection
  - Encephalitis
  - Meningitis
  - Herpes zoster
- Vasculitis, dural cavernous sinus fistula
- Demyelination
- Trauma
- Infiltration (leptomeningeal carcinomatosis)

OCULAR MUSCLE ENLARGEMENT

- Thyroid ophthalmopathy (most common cause); painless
- Pseudotumor; painful
- Infection from adjacent sinus
- Granulomatous: TB, sarcoid, cysticercosis
- Rare causes: high flow (dural AVM, carotid cavernous sinus fistula [CCF], lymphangioma), hemorrhage, tumor (lymphoma, rhabdomyosarcoma, leukemia, metastases), trauma, acromegaly, apical mass

OVERVIEW OF ORBITAL MASSES

Mass	Children	Adults
Tumor	Retinoblastoma	Hemangioma
	Rhabdomyosarcoma	Schwannoma
	Optic nerve glioma	Melanoma
	Lymphoma	Meningioma
	Hemangioma	Lymphoma
Other	Dermoid cyst	Pseudotumor
		Trauma

Mnemonic for childhood orbital masses: "LO VISON:"

- **L**eukemia
- **O**ptic nerve glioma
- **V**ascular malformation (hemangioma, lymphangioma)
- **I**nflammation
- **S**arcoma, rhabdomyosarcoma
- **O**phthalmopathy, orbital pseudotumor
- **N**euroblastoma

CYSTIC LESIONS OF THE ORBIT

- Dermoid
- Epidermoid
- Teratoma
- Aneurysmal bone cyst
- Cholesterol granuloma
- Colobomatous cyst

T1W HYPERINTENSE ORBITAL MASSES

Tumor
- Melanotic melanoma
- Retinoblastoma
- Choroidal metastases
- Hemangioma

Detachment
- Coats disease
- Persistent hyperplastic primary vitreous
- Trauma

Other
- Hemorrhage
- Phthisis bulbi
- Intravitreal oil treatment for detachment

GLOBE CALCIFICATIONS

Tumor
- Retinoblastoma (95% are calcified, 35% are bilateral)
- Astrocytic hamartoma (associated with tuberous sclerosis, NF)
- Choroidal osteoma

Infection (chorioretinitis)
- Toxoplasmosis
- Herpes
- CMV
- Rubella

Other
- Phthisis bulbi
  - Calcification in end-stage disease
  - Shrunken bulb
- Optic nerve drusen
  - Most common cause of calcifications in adults
  - Bilateral

SUDDEN ONSET OF PROPTOSIS

- Orbital varix (worsened by Valsalva maneuver)
- Hemorrhage into cavernous hemangioma
- CCF
- Hemorrhage into lymphangioma
- Thrombosis of superior orbital vein

LACRIMAL GLAND ENLARGEMENT

Lymphoid lesions, 50%
- Benign lymphoid hyperplasia
- Pseudotumor
- Sjögren syndrome

- Mikulicz disease
- Lymphoma

Epithelial neoplasm
- Pleomorphic adenoma, 75%
- Adenoid cystic carcinoma

DIFFUSE BONE ABNORMALITY

Signs: bony enlargement (fibrous dysplasia), expansion, sclerosis
- Fibrous dysplasia
- Paget disease
- Thalassemia
- Congenital (rare): osteopetrosis, craniometaphyseal and diaphyseal dysplasia

SINUSES

RADIOPAQUE SINUS

Normal variant
- Hypoplasia
- Unilateral thick bone

Sinusitis (acute: AFL; chronic: mucosal thickening, retention cysts)
- Allergic
- Fungal: aspergillosis, mucormycosis
- Granulomatous: sarcoid, Wegener disease

Solid masses
- SCC
- Polyp, inverted papilloma
- Lymphoma
- Juvenile angiofibroma; most common tumor in children
- Mucocele: expansile, associated with cystic fibrosis in children

Postsurgical
- Caldwell-Luc operation

NASOOROPHARYNX

MUCOSAL SPACE MASS

Tumors
- SCC
- Lymphoma
- Rhabdomyosarcoma
- Melanoma

Benign masses
- Adenoids
- Juvenile angiofibroma
- Thornwaldt cyst

PARAPHARYNGEAL AND CAROTID SPACE MASSES

Tumors
- Salivary gland tumors; 80% are benign, 20% are malignant
- Neurogenic tumor (schwannomas, glomus vagale)
- Nasopharyngeal carcinoma
- Lymphadenopathy: benign, malignant

Abscess, cellulitis

PREVERTEBRAL MASS

- Metastases
- Chordoma
- Osteomyelitis, abscess
- Hematoma

NECK

CYSTIC EXTRATHYROID LESIONS

Neck
- Branchial cleft cyst (lateral to carotid artery)
- Thyroglossal duct cyst (midline mass)
- Ranula (retention cyst) of sublingual glands
- Retention cysts of mucous glands (parotid)
- Cystic hygroma (lymphangioma): most common <2 years of age
- Rare lesions: cervical thymic cysts, dermoid, teratoma, hemangioma

Nasoorophyarynx
- Thornwaldt cyst
- Mucus retention cyst (obstructed glands)
- Necrotic SCC (thick wall)

Larynx, paralaryngeal space
- Laryngocele
- Mucus retention cyst

CYSTIC THYROID LESIONS

- Colloid cysts
- Cystic degeneration
- Cystic tumor
  - Papillary cancer
  - Cystic metastases (papillary cancer)

SOLID NECK MASS

Tumors
- SCC of larynx or nasooropharynx (common)
- Lymphadenopathy
  - Reactive hyperplasia
  - Malignant
- Parotid tumors
- Neural tumors
  - Neurilemoma
  - Neurofibroma
  - Glomus tumors
- Other rare tumors
  - Mesenchymal, dermoid, teratoma

Inflammatory
- Infection (abscess, fungal, TB)
- Granulomatous inflammation (sarcoid, TB lymphadenitis = scrofula)

Congenital
- Ectopic thyroid

VASCULAR HEAD AND NECK MASSES

- Glomus tumor
  - Carotid body tumor
  - Glomus vagale
  - Glomus jugulare
  - Glomus tympanicum
- Hemangioma
- AVM
- Aneurysm (often ICA)
  - Pseudoaneurysm
  - Posttraumatic

AIDS

ENT complications occur in 50% of patients.

Parotid
- Multiple intraparotid cystic masses (benign lymphoepithelial lesion)
- Lymphadenopathy

Sinonasal
- Sinusitis *(Staphylococcus, Streptococcus, Pseudomonas > Legionella, Cryptococcus, Pneumocystis carinii,* CMV)
- Kaposi sarcoma (uncommon)

Oral cavity
- *Candida*
- Periodontal and gingival infections

Pharynx/larynx
- Opportunistic infections
- Epiglottitis
- Lymphoma (tonsils)

Temporal bone (rare)
- Otitis media: *P. carinii*
- Otitis externa: *Pseudomonas*

Suggested Readings

Ahuja AT, Evans RM, King AD, van Hasselt CA. *Imaging of Head and Neck Cancer.* Cambridge: Cambridge University Press; 2003.

Baert AI, Sortor K. *Imaging in Treatment Planning of Sinonasal Disease.* New York: Springer; 2004.

Bailey B, ed. *Head and Neck Surgery—Otolaryngology.* Philadelphia: Lippincott Williams & Wilkins; 2001.

Brockstein B, Masters G. *Head and Neck Cancer.* New York: Springer; 2003.

Delbalso AM. *Maxillofacial Imaging.* Philadelphia: WB Saunders; 1990.

Harnsberger R. *Handbooks in Radiology: Head and Neck Imaging.* St. Louis: Mosby; 1994.

Harnsberger R, Hudgins P, Wiggins R, et al. *Diagnostic Imaging: Head and Neck.* Philadelphia: WB Saunders; 2004.

Harnsberger R, Koch B, Phillips C, et al. *EXPERTddx: Head and Neck.* Philadelphia: Lippincott Williams & Wilkins; 2009.

Lufkin R, Borges A, Villablanca P. *Teaching Atlas of Head and Neck Imaging.* New York: Thieme Medical Publishers; 2000.

Mukherji S. *Head and Neck Radiology: Text and Atlas.* New York: Thieme Medical Publishers; 2004.

Nadich DP, Webb WR, Grenier PA. *Imaging of the Airways: Functional and Radiologic Considerations.* Philadelphia: Lippincott Williams & Wilkins; 2005.

Som PM, Curtin HD. *Head and Neck Imaging.* 4th ed. St. Louis: Mosby; 2004.

Swartz H, Harnsberger R. *Imaging of the Temporal Bone.* New York: Thieme Medical Publishers; 1998.

Vogl TJ, Balzer J, Mack M, et al. *Differential Diagnosis in Head and Neck Imaging.* New York: Thieme Medical Publishers; 1999.

CHAPTER 8

Vascular Imaging

CHAPTER OUTLINE

Techniques

GENERAL

PREPROCEDURE EVALUATION

1. What is the indication for the procedure?
    - Diagnosis
    - Preoperative staging
    - Therapy
2. Define the problem.
    - What is the diagnostic question that is to be answered?
    - What study can best answer the question (ultrasound [US], computed tomography [CT], magnetic resonance imaging [MRI], angiography)?
3. Patient history, interview, examination
    - Review chart
    - Key data: signs and symptoms
      Prior vascular surgery/interventions
      Prior studies
      Laboratory values
      Other medical illnesses
      Pulse examination
    - Explanation of the procedure to the patient
    - Obtain informed consent
4. Assess risk versus benefit (there are no absolute contraindications to angiography).
    - Approach and access
    - Coagulopathy?
    - Renal insufficiency?
    - What are alternative options?
5. Preprocedural orders
    - Appropriate laboratory samples drawn (i.e., PT/PTT)?
    - Appropriate medication withheld (i.e., Coumadin)?
    - IV access present?
    - Hydration
    - Clear liquids only
    - Premedication if necessary

ACCESS

Types of Arterial Approaches

- Right femoral artery
- Left femoral artery
- Left axillary artery
- Right axillary artery
- Translumbar aorta
- Brachial arteries
- Antegrade femoral artery
- Through a surgical graft

Right Femoral Approach (Preferred)

- Easily accessible for manipulations and hemostasis
- Large-caliber vessel
- Well-defined landmarks exist.
- Most angiographers are right-handed.
- Low complication rate compared with other approaches

Standard Femoral Approach: Seldinger Technique

- Double-wall technique is preferred.
- Advantages of "single-wall" puncture are only theoretical.
- Use fluoroscopy to determine puncture level.
  - Artery entry: midfemoral head
  - Skin entry: inferior margin of femoral head
- Local anesthesia at skin entry site: 1%-2% lidocaine
- Palpate artery above site
- Advance 18-gauge Seldinger needle (45° to 60° angle) to bone.
- Remove central stylet and withdraw slowly.
- Advance guidewire through needle while good pulsatile flow jets out of the hub.
- Always use fluoroscope when advancing a guidewire.
- Never advance guidewire against resistance.
- Exchange needle over wire for dilator or catheter.

Advantage of Puncturing Symptomatic Extremity

- Inflow can be assessed by obtaining pull-down pressures.
- Should complications arise (i.e., emboli, thrombosis), they will affect the already compromised extremity.
- Conversion to antegrade approach is possible if necessary.

Disadvantage of Puncturing Symptomatic Extremity

- May interfere with surgical procedure if complication develops (e.g., hematoma)
- If a severe stenosis is present, a catheter may obturate the vessel completely.

Axillary Artery Approach

- Main indication for this approach is nonpalpable femoral pulses (i.e., aortic occlusion)
- Left-sided approach is preferred.
  - Easier to access descending aorta
  - Left-sided approach crosses fewer central nervous system (CNS) arteries.
- 3J wire is preferred.
- Disadvantages:
  - Difficult to compress
  - Relatively high incidence of complications (e.g., stroke, bleeding, thrombosis)
  - Brachial plexus injury
- Always check for blood pressure differential to detect occult arterial disease.

Translumbar Approach (TLA)

- Main indication for this approach is nonpalpable peripheral pulses.
- High TLA is preferred: above abdominal aortic aneurysm, grafts, diseased distal aorta
- Disadvantages:
  - Patient must lie prone for entire study.
  - Higher incidence of bleeding (debatable)
  - More difficult to manipulate catheters
- Use an 18-gauge needle/sheath system.

Antegrade Femoral Approach

- The main indication for this approach is a distal extremity intervention (e.g., percutaneous transluminal angioplasty [PTA] of the superficial femoral artery [SFA]).
- Retrograde catheterization may be converted to antegrade access with a Simmons 1 catheter and a 3J or angled guidewire.
- Difficult to manage in obese patients

ANGIOGRAPHY COMPLICATIONS

There are four types of complications:

- Puncture site complications (e.g., groin hematoma)
- Contrast agent complications (e.g., anaphylactoid reaction)
- Catheter-related complications (e.g., vessel dissection)
- Therapy-related complications (e.g., CNS bleeding during thrombolysis)

Problems with the puncture site and contrast media are the most frequent complications during angiography. Puncture site problems depend on coagulation status, size of catheter, patient body habitus, and compliance issues. The overall incidence of death related to angiography is very low (<0.05%).

Puncture Site Complications

- Minor hematoma, >5%
- Major hematoma that requires surgical therapy, <0.5%
- Arteriovenous fistula (AVF), 0.05%

- Pseudoaneurysm, 0.01%
- Vessel thrombosis, 0.1%
- Neuritis
- Infection

Contrast Complications (see also Chapter 13)

- Renal failure
- Cardiac failure
- Phlebitis (venography)
- Anaphylactoid reactions (rare with arteriography)

Catheter-Related Complications

- Cholesterol emboli
- Thromboembolism
- Cerebrovascular accident
- Arterial dissection

Pearls

- Complications can be limited by:
  - Careful preangiography assessment (e.g., correct coagulopathies)
  - Appropriate approach (e.g., history and pulse examination)
  - Good technique (e.g., trained angiographer)
- Risk factors for development of AVF or pseudoaneurysm:
  - Low puncture
  - Heparinization
  - Large catheters
- Most puncture site complications can be prevented by good manual compression and correction of coagulopathies before angiography.
- Always reassess patient after the procedure.

HARDWARE

CATHETERS

Generic Types

Diagnostic catheters
- High-flow catheters with side holes are used for central vessels (>10 mL/sec).
- Low-flow catheters with end holes are used for selective arterial work.

Therapeutic catheters
- Balloon catheters (PTA and balloon occlusion)
- Atherectomy catheters
- Coaxial infusion catheters
- Embolization catheters

Measurements

- Outer diameter (OD): catheter size is determined by the OD and given in "French" size. French (Fr) = the circumference in millimeters. Divide French size by 3 to obtain OD in millimeters.
- Inner diameter (ID): measured in 1/1000 of an inch
- Length: measured in centimeters. 65 cm is commonly used for abdominal studies. 100 cm is usually used for arch and carotid studies.

SPECIFIC CATHETERS

Catheter Type	Use
Pigtail	Aorta, pulmonary
Cobra (c)	Mesenteric, renal, contralateral iliac
Simmons (s)	Mesenteric, arch vessels
Headhunter (H)	Carotid, arch vessels
Berenstein	Carotid
Davis	Arch, carotids, upper extremity
Tracker	Coaxial subselection

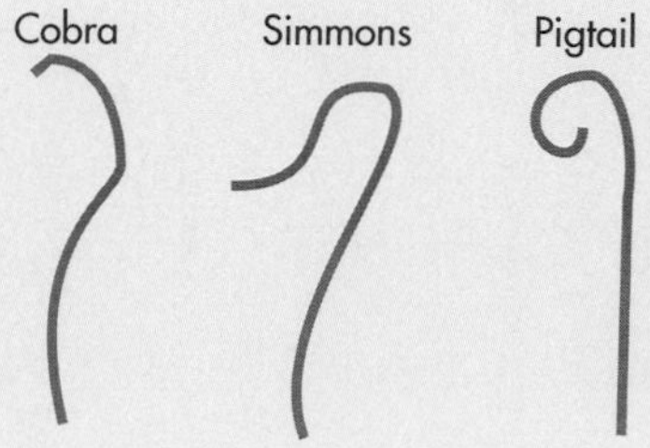

FLOW RATES OF INJECTIONS (MGH)

Location	Catheter	Injection*	Comments
Thoracic aorta	Pigtail	25/50	
Abdominal aorta	Pigtail/tip occluded straight	20/40	Tip occluded straight catheter for iliac pressures
Celiac	C2, S2	5/50	Variations in anatomy common
Renals	C2, S2	4/8	Multiple vessels in 25%
SMA	C2, S2	5/50	IA tolazoline (Priscoline) for venous phase
CT portography	In SMA	3/120	Helical CT

Continued

FLOW RATES OF INJECTIONS (MGH)—cont'd

Location	Catheter	Injection*	Comments
IMA	S2, C2	3/30	
Splenic	Variable	5/50	Good splenic vein opacification
Hepatic	Variable	5/50	Dual (artery, portal) blood supply; variable anatomy
Aortic bifurcation/pelvic	Pigtail	10/20	Position above bifurcation
Internal iliac	C2, S2	5/25	
One leg runoff	Straight tip	4/48	Positioned in external iliac
Two leg runoff	Pigtail	6/72	Position above bifurcation
Arm	H1	Variable	LOCA (reduces pain)
IVC	Pigtail	20/30	
Pulmonary	Pigtail	20/40	
Aortic arch	Pigtail	30/60	Higher injections in young patients
CCA	Davis A1	8/10	60% HOCA or LOCA
ICA	Davis A1	6/8	60% HOCA or LOCA
ECA	Davis A1	2/4	60% HOCA or LOCA
Vertebral	Davis A1	6/8	60% HOCA or LOCA
Coronary	Judkins	4/8	LOCA

* Flow rate (mL/sec)/total volume of injection (mL).

Material

- Thermoplastic materials (polyurethane and polyethylene) are very commonly used for catheter manufacturing.
- Nylon: combined with polyurethane to manufacture high-flow, small French catheters
- Teflon: very stiff, low-friction material
- Braided catheters: internal wire mesh improves torquability.

Pearls

- Rate and volume of contrast are reduced for digital subtraction angiography (DSA).
- Rate and volume always depend on rate of blood flow and size of vessel observed under fluoroscopy.
- Shorter catheters allow for higher flow rates and easier exchangeability.
- The larger the ID, the better the flow dynamics.
- It is good practice to size catheters, sheaths, and wires before their use; considerable discrepancy of dimensions may occur (variable among manufacturers).
- Maximum flow rate and pressure tolerance of catheters are specified by manufacturer on package or insert.

GUIDEWIRES

All nonspecialty guidewires have a similar construction:

- Central stiff steel core with a distal taper
- Wire coil spring wound around core
- Thin filamentous safety wire holding the other two components together
- Most wires are coated with Teflon to decrease friction.

Measurements

- Length: 145 cm is the standard length and allows exchanges of 65-cm catheters. “Exchange length” wires are 220 to 250 cm in length and are used for long catheters.
- OD: guidewires are designated by OD in 1/1000 of an inch: 0.018 to 0.038 is the most common size range.
- J tip: refers to the radius of wire curvature in millimeters (i.e., a 3J wire has a 3-mm distal curvature)

SPECIFIC GUIDEWIRES

Wire	Major Use/Comments
3J	Tortuous and diseased vessels, avoids selecting branch vessels
15J	Large vessels: femoral, aorta, IVC
Straight wire	Dissection is more common
Rosen	Exchanges/PTA
Amplatz stiff	Exchanges, tortuous iliac arteries
Bentson	Long, flexible taper (floppy end)
Terumo	Slippery hydrophilic coating; glides well, torque guide

PHARMACOLOGIC MANIPULATION

DRUGS COMMONLY USED

	Dosage*	Use	Comments
Vasodilator			
Papaverine	1 mg/min infusion	Mesenteric ischemia	Smooth muscle relaxant
Tolazoline (Priscoline)	25 mg IA	Peripheral spasm	Direct muscle relaxant
Nitroglycerin	100 μg IA or IV	Peripheral spasm	Direct muscle relaxant
Nifedipine	10 mg SL	Peripheral spasm	Calcium channel blocker
Vasoconstrictor			
Vasopressin (Pitressin)	0.2-0.4 U/min	GI bleeding	Contraindication: CAD, HTN, arrhythmias
Epinephrine	5 μg	Renal vasoconstriction	Differentiate tumor from normal renal vessels

*See manufacturer's package insert for specific rates of administration.
CAD, coronary artery disease; GI, gastrointestinal; HTN, hypertension; IA, intraarterial; IV, intravenous; SL, sublingual.

ANGIOGRAPHIC INTERVENTIONS

EMBOLIZATION

Indication

Hemorrhage
- GI bleeding
- Varices
- Traumatic organ injury
- Bronchial artery hemorrhage
- Tumors
- Postoperative bleeding

Vascular lesions
- Arteriovenous malformation (AVM) or fistula (AVF)
- Pseudoaneurysms

Preoperative devascularization
- Renal cell carcinoma
- AVM
- Vascular bone metastases

Other
- Hypersplenism
- Gonadal varices
- Hepatic chemoembolization

General Principles

- Proximal occlusion is equivalent to surgical ligation. It does not compromise collateral flow. For this reason, it may be ineffective to control bleeding if collaterals continue to supply the bleeding site.
- Distal embolization usually infarcts tissue and is followed by necrosis.
- Temporary versus permanent embolization: tumors, vascular lesions, varices, and preoperative embolizations are usually permanent occlusions. GI bleeding is best treated with Gelfoam at first (if vasopressin has failed).
- Be as selective as possible (i.e., use tracker catheter).
- Prevent reflux of embolic material into other vessels.
- Document preangiographic and postangiographic appearance.

Embolic Agents

Temporary
- Surgical gelatin (Gelfoam): not FDA approved for embolization. Pledgets are cut to size or occlude large vessels; Gelfoam powder occludes distal vessels and causes infarction.

Permanent
- Steel coils of variable sizes are commercially available; coils obstruct proximal vessels.
- Microcoils (platinum) are used to occlude more distal vessels.
- Detachable balloons are used for large vessel occlusion. FDA restricted. Useful for pulmonary AVF, carotid cavernous fistula.
- Polyvinyl alcohol (Ivalon): small particles for distal occlusion. 200 to 1000 μm. Suspend in albumin–contrast agent mixture.
- Absolute ethanol: causes tissue necrosis. Used with proximal balloon occlusion to minimize shunting and reflux. Useful for solid organ necrosis (i.e., malignant tumors).
- Plastic polymers: glue, tissue adhesives

EMBOLIZATION MATERIALS

Material	Occlusion	Primary Use
Temporary Agents		
Autologous blood clot	6-12 hr	Rarely used currently
Gelfoam	Weeks	Upper GI, hemorrhage, pelvic, trauma
Permanent Agents		
Ethyl alcohol (1 mL/kg)	Permanent	Tumors (causes coagulative necrosis)
Steel coils	Permanent	Large vessel, aneurysm, tumor
Polyvinyl alcohol (200-1000 m)	Permanent	Tumors
Balloons	Permanent	High-output AVF
Cyanoacrylate (glue)	Permanent	AVM

Complications

- Postembolization syndrome (fever, elevated WBC), 40%
- Infection of embolized area (administer prophylactic antibiotics)
- Reflux of embolic material (nontarget embolization)
- Alcohol causes skin, nerve, and muscle infarction if used in the periphery; its use should be restricted to parenchymal organs.

HEPATIC CHEMOEMBOLIZATION

- Palliative only; prolonged survival or relief of endocrine symptoms
- Dual hepatic/portal supply allows for arterial embolotherapy
- Agents: Gelfoam or Ethiodol mixed with chemotherapeutic agents; drug-eluting microspheres
- Tumors: hepatocellular carcinoma, ocular melanoma, metastatic endocrine tumors

HEPATIC RADIOEMBOLIZATION

- Ytrium-90 radioembolization of hepatic artery is an effective treatment for unresectable HCC. It is a form of brachytherapy.
- Y-90 is a pure beta emitter with a short half-life (64 hr). The size of the microspheres ranges between 20 and 40 μm (sufficient for local trapping).
- Basic requirements
  - Absent surgical or ablative options
  - Absent other conventional treatment options
  - Preserved liver function
  - Adequate general condition
  - Liver dominant tumor burden
  - Life expectancy >3 months

THROMBOLYSIS

Indication

- Arterial graft thrombosis
- Native vessel acute thrombosis
- Before percutaneous intervention
- Hemodialysis AVF or graft
- Venous thrombosis
  - Axillosubclavian
  - Portal vein, SMV
  - IVC

General Principles (Fig. 8-1)

- Always obtain a diagnostic angiogram before thrombolysis.
- Streptokinase is no longer used (antigenic side effects).
- r-tPA is no more effective than UK but is much more expensive.
- Favorable prognostic factors for thrombolysis:
  - Recent clot (<3 months)
  - Good inflow/outflow
  - Positioned in thrombus
- End points of thrombolytic therapy:
  - No lysis present after 12 hours of infusion
  - Major complication develops
  - Severe reperfusion syndrome
  - Progression to irreversible ischemia
- Successful thrombolysis is defined as:
  - >95% lysis of thrombus
  - Clinical reperfusion
- Always treat underlying lesions.
- Overall success:
  - Grafts, 90%
  - Native arteries, 75%
- Heparinize concomitant with UK infusion
- Monitor in ICU
- No good correlation among success, complications, and blood tests

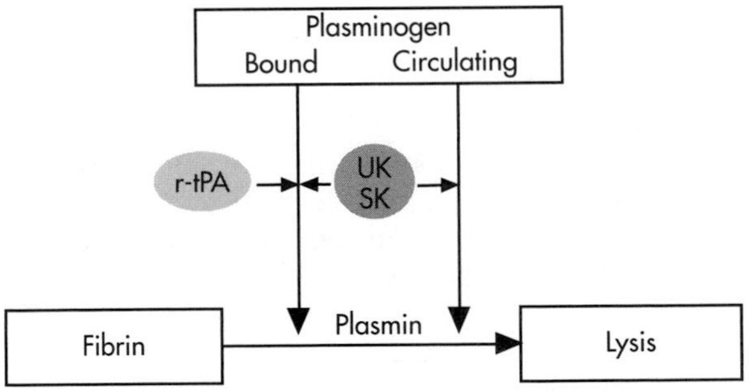

FIGURE 8-1

THROMBOLYTIC AGENTS

	SK	UK	r-tPA
Source	*Streptococcus* culture	Renal cell culture	DNA technology
Dosage	5000 U/hr	100,000 U/hr	0.001-0.02 mg/kg/hr*
Half-life	20 min	10 min	5 min
Treatment time	24-48 hr	24 hr	6 hr
Bleeding cost	20%	10%	10%
Cost	Inexpensive	Expensive	Very expensive

*Dosage not to exceed 10 mg for a single bolus; total dose should be <40 mg.

Techniques

Low-dose technique (constant)
- 100,000 U/hr of UK
- Repeat angiogram after 12 hours

High-dose technique (graded)
- 250,000 U/hr x 4 hours of UK
- Repeat angiogram and then 125,000 U/hr

Pulse spray ultra-high dose
- 600,000 U/hr in 5000 U of UK bolus doses
- Aliquots every 30 seconds

Catheter placement
- Coaxial dual infusion is best.
- 5-Fr catheter lodged in proximal thrombus
- T3 or infusion wire (Katzen) coaxially into distal thrombus
- Split infusion of UK into proximal and distal catheters
- Secure skin entry site

tPA infusion
- tPA (arterial): Infuse at 1 mg/hr total dose divided among infusion sites. Total maximum dose per patient is 100 mg. tPA has half-life of 6 minutes.
- tPA (venous): Same infusion rate as arterial, lower bleeding complication rate
- tPA (line clearance): 0.5 mg/hr x 3 to 4 hours

Contraindications

Absolute
- Active bleeding
- Intracranial lesion (stroke, tumor, recent surgery)
- Pregnancy
- Nonviable limb
- Revascularization of nonviable limb will cause acute renal failure and cardiovascular collapse due to lactic acid and myoglobin
- Infected thrombus

Relative
- Bleeding diathesis
- Cardiac thrombus
- Malignant hypertension
- Recent major surgery
- Postpartum

Complications
- Major hemorrhage requiring termination of UK, surgery, or transfusion (e.g., intracranial hemorrhage, massive puncture site bleed), 7%
- Minor hemorrhage, 7%
- Distal embolization
- Pericatheter thrombosis
- Overall, termination of therapy is required in 10%.

ANGIOPLASTY

PTA is a method to fracture the vascular intima and stretch the media of a vessel by a balloon (Fig. 8-2). Atherosclerotic plaques are very firm and are fractured by PTA. Healing occurs by intimal hyperplasia.

Indication

- Claudication or rest pain
- Tissue loss
- Nonhealing wound
- Establish inflow for a distal bypass graft
- Hemodialysis AVF or grafts

General Principles

- Premedication with aspirin and 10 mg of nifedipine
- Ipsilateral approach is preferred.
- Heparinize (5000 to 10,000 U) after the lesion is crossed.
- Diagnostic angiogram is obtained before PTA.
- Measure pressure gradients with borderline lesions.

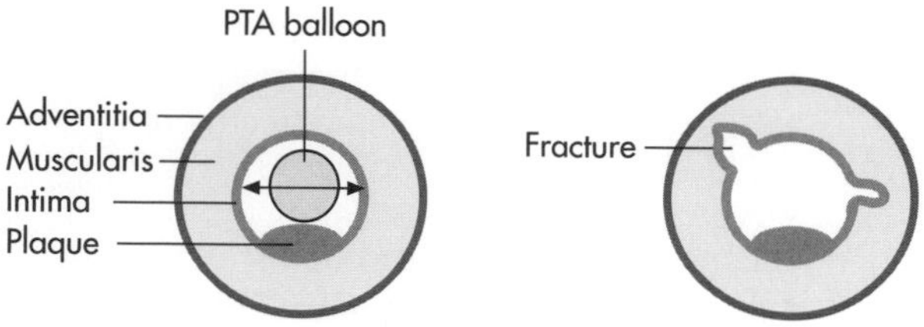

FIGURE 8-2

- Significant gradient >10 mm Hg at rest; >20 mm Hg after vasodilator; >10% systolic blood pressure
- Pharmacologic adjuncts
  - IA nitroglycerin or tolazoline for vasospasm and provoked pressure measurements
- Balloon size: sized to adjacent normal artery
  - Common iliac artery: 8 to 10 mm
  - External iliac artery: 6 to 8 mm
  - Superficial femoral artery: 4 to 6 mm
  - Renal artery: 4 to 6 mm
  - Popliteal artery: 3 to 4 mm
- Wire should always remain across lesion
- Repeat angiogram and pressure measurements after angioplasty.
- Postprocedure heparin with "limited flow" results (dissection, thrombus)

Prognostic Indicators

- Large vessels/proximal lesions respond better than small vessel/distal lesions.
- Stenoses respond better to PTA than occlusions.
- Short stenoses respond better to PTA than long stenoses.
- Isolated disease responds better to PTA than multifocal disease.
- Poor inflow or poor outflow decreases success.
- Limb salvage interventions have a poor prognosis.
- Diabetics have a poorer prognosis than nondiabetic patients.

PTA Results

Iliac system
- 95% initial success
- 70%-80% 5-year patency

Femoral popliteal
- 90% initial success
- 70% 5-year patency

Renal artery
- 95% initial success
- Fibromuscular dysplasia: 95% 5-year patency
- Atherosclerosis: 70%-90% 5-year patency
- Ostial lesions have a poorer prognosis.

Acute failures are due to thrombosis, dissection, or inability to cross a lesion.

Recurrent stenosis
- Intimal hyperplasia (3 months to 1 year)
- Progression of disease elsewhere (>1 year)

Complications

- Groin complications (same as diagnostic angiography)
- Distal embolism
- Arterial rupture (rare)
- Renal infarction or failure (with renal PTA)

INTRAVASCULAR STENTS

Metallic stents have an evolving role in interventional angiography. Two major types of stents:

Balloon-expandable stent (Palmaz, Genesis, Omniflex, Herculink, Crown)
- Balloon mounted; usually made of nitinol
- Placement is precise; shortens slightly
- Less flexible (minimal elastic deformation due to hoop strength), limited by balloon size
- Should not be placed at sites where extrinsic forces could crush the stent
- Thoracic outlet veins
- Dialysis graft

Self-expandable (Wallstent, Protégé, Luminex, Symphony, SMART, Dynalink)
- Bare; usually made of stainless steel
- Placement is less precise; can have large diameters
- Considerable elastic deformity (flexible)
- Useful in tortuous vessels and tight curves

Gianturco zigzag stent (Cook)

Stent grafts (metallic stents combined with synthetic graft material) are used in aortic aneurysms and dissections (AneuRx, Ancure, Gore [descending thoracic] are FDA approved).

Indications for Metallic Stents

- Unsuccessful PTA
- Recurrent stenosis
- Venous obstruction, thrombosis
- Transjugular intrahepatic portosystemic shunt

Indications for Stents in Revascularization Procedures

- Long-segment stenosis
- Total occlusion
- Ineffective or unsuccessful PTA:
  - Residual stenosis >30%
  - Residual pressure gradient >5 mm Hg rest, >10 mm Hg post hyperemia
  - Hard, calcified plaque
  - Large post-PTA dissection flap
- Recurrent stenosis after PTA
- Ulcerated plaque
- Renal ostial lesions

Stent Results

- Iliac artery: over 90% 5-year patency (better than PTA)
- Renal artery and other vessels: limited long-term data

TRANSJUGULAR INTRAHEPATIC PORTOSYSTEMIC SHUNT (TIPS)

Established Indications

- Portal hypertension with variceal bleeding that has failed endoscopic treatment
- Refractory ascites

Possible Future Indications

- Budd-Chiari syndrome
- Pretransplant

General Principles

- Confirm portal vein patency before procedure (US, CT, or angiography).
- Preprocedure paracentesis may be helpful.
- Right internal jugular vein (IJV) is the preferred access vessel.
- Goal: portosystemic gradient <10 mm Hg, decompression of varices

Contraindications

- Absolute
  - Severe right-sided heart failure with elevated central venous pressure
  - Polycystic liver disease
- Relative
  - Active infection
  - Severe encephalopathy
  - Portal vein thrombosis
  - Large liver hypervascular tumor
  - Hepatic failure

Technique (Fig. 8-3)

- Right IJV approach
- Obtain wedged hepatic pressure and venogram
- Create tract from right hepatic vein to portal vein with 16-gauge needle
- Advance catheter over wire into portal venous system
- Obtain portal venogram
- Measure portal pressures
- Dilate tract with PTA balloon (8 mm)
- Deploy metallic stent (Palmaz or Wallstent) or stent graft
- Dilate stent until gradient <10 mm Hg
- Coil embolization of varices optional

Results

- Patency: 50% at 1 year
- Recurrent bleeding in 10%

Complications

- Hepatic encephalopathy 10%; more likely when residual gradient is less than 10 mm Hg
- Bleeding
- Shunt thrombosis or stenosis
- Right-sided heart failure
- Renal failure

Signs of Malfunction

- No flow
- Low-velocity flow (<50 to 60 cm/sec) at portal venous end of shunt
- Reversal of flow in hepatic vein away from IVC
- Hepatopedal flow in intrahepatic portal vein
- Reaccumulation of ascites; varices; recanalized umbilical vein

TRANSJUGULAR LIVER BIOPSY

May be preferred over percutaneous liver biopsy in patients with bleeding disorders and when a hepatic venous pressure gradient (= wedged – free hepatic venous pressure) is desired.

Technique

- Right IJV approach preferred
- Right hepatic vein is selected with wire/catheter, and sheath advanced.
- Core biopsy device (18 to 19 G) is advanced into the liver parenchyma.

TYPES OF VENOUS ACCESS

Device	Purpose/Situation
External tunneled catheter (silicone or polyurethane)	Continuous use, multiple simultaneous uses
Implantable port	Intermittent use; immunocompromised patient
High-flow catheter	Temporary hemodialysis; pheresis
Peripherally inserted central catheter	Short-term use, usually <2-3 months; infrequent blood drawing

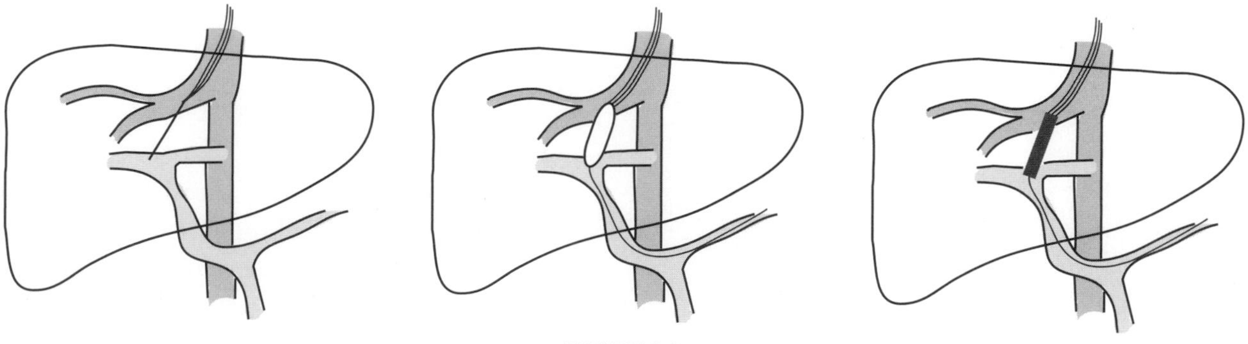

FIGURE 8-3

VENOUS ACCESS

CENTRAL VENOUS ACCESS CATHETERS

The catheters are typically inserted through axillary (subclavian), internal jugular, or arm vein. Pneumothorax, symptomatic vein stenosis, and thrombotic complications are less common with jugular than subclavian vein approaches. IJ approach preserves subclavian for future fistula/graft. For the axillary vein puncture, the entry site should be lateral to the ribs in the subcoracoid region (Fig. 8-4). This approach eliminates the possibility of pneumothorax and also ensures that the catheter is well within the subclavian vein as it passes through the costoclavicular space. If the catheter is extravascular at this site, chronic compression may occur and lead to catheter erosion and fracture—"pinch-off syndrome." For IJV puncture, a site on the midneck above the clavicle is selected. The vein is punctured under transverse US guidance, ensuring that the carotid artery is avoided.

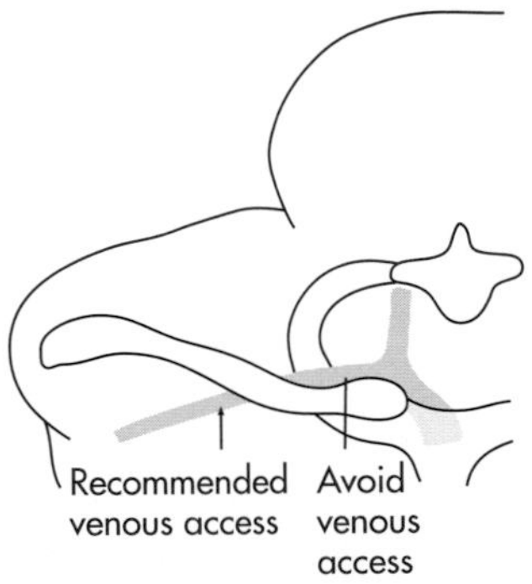

FIGURE 8-4

COMPLICATIONS OF CENTRAL VENOUS CATHETER PLACEMENT

- Pneumothorax
- Arterial puncture
- Hemorrhage or hematoma
- Occlusion
- Mechanical problems
- Air embolism

This usually occurs when venous dilator is removed from peel-away sheath to be replaced with the catheter.

The embolism can be avoided by covering the opening with a gloved finger and removing the dilator with patient in suspended deep inspiration.

If air does get sucked in, perform fluoroscopy of the chest. If there is air in the pulmonary artery do the following:

- Place patient in left lateral decubitus position to keep air in the right chamber.
- Suck out air with Swan-Ganz balloon catheter.
- Administer supplemental O_2 and monitor patient.

VASCULAR ULTRASOUND

GENERAL

Frequency shift = 2 x transducer frequency × velocity of blood × cosine of angle × 1/speed of sound (1540 m/s). Cos of 90° = 0 and cos of 0° = 1. The optimal angle between the probe and the vessel is <60° (Fig. 8-5).

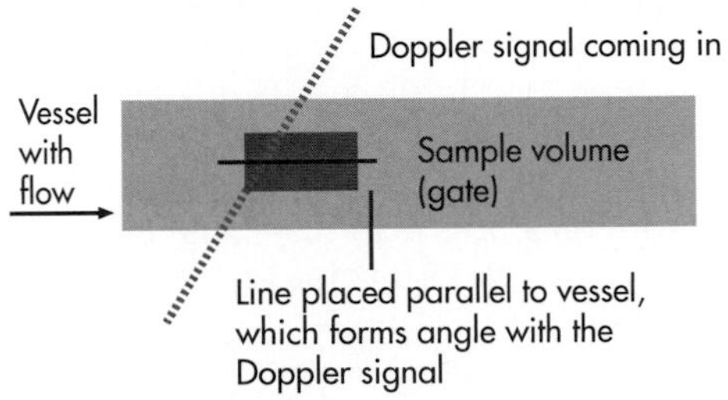

FIGURE 8-5

CONTINUOUS WAVE DOPPLER

- Performed with a pencil probe. No static image is produced, as the machine does not stop to listen. If one vessel is located behind the other, one cannot use continuous wave Doppler because it will reveal both waveforms.

PULSED WAVE DOPPLER

- Frequently used for interrogating arteries and veins; duplex Doppler refers to the fact that one gets gray scale and Doppler images.
- The operator can set the machine to listen only to those Doppler shifts coming from a particular depth. This is called *Doppler gate* or *sample volume.*
- Color flow is used to determine the direction of flow (by convention, red is toward the transducer and blue is away), as well as magnitude of shift.
- Color machines do not display velocity, because angle of insonation is not used to assign color; the color indicates magnitude of frequency shift. The greater the shift, the lower the saturation of color. In simple terms, in a tortuous vessel the frequency shifts and angle of insonation changes; thus, change in color is due to frequency shift even though velocity is the same.
- The color image is a display of average frequency shift and not peak frequency shift. Calculations of stenosis from Doppler data are based on peak frequency shift or peak velocity.

POWER DOPPLER US

- The signal is related to the number of moving targets (usually red blood cells).
- This technique ignores velocity and direction of flow. Used to detect flow and has high sensitivity.

ALIASING

Aliasing is the result of flow velocity exceeding the measuring ability of pulsed wave Doppler. By Doppler imaging, this is seen as a wraparound with high velocity below the bottom of the scale rather than on the top. By color imaging, aliasing becomes evident by inversion of color (blue within an area of red and vice versa). Ways for reducing aliasing:

- Pulse repetition frequency (PRF) can be increased by raising the scale.
- The Doppler shift can be reduced by manipulating variables of equation—thus, either a greater angle (reduced cosθ value) or a lower frequency can be used.
- Color aliasing refers to wrapping of signal displayed as areas of color reversal.
- Changes due to vessel tortuosity can also change colors, but in that case color changes are marked by a band of black, thus red to blue with black (no signal) in between. Artifacts due to $0 = 90°$.
- Because the ultrasound machine typically only displays either gray scale or color information, there is competition as to which signal is displayed. If gray scale gain setting is high, the color image is suppressed when flow is low, giving the impression of absent flow or smaller lumen.

MRI

NONCONTRAST IMAGING TECHNIQUES

Two main noncontrast MR angiography (MRA) techniques: time of flight (TOF) MRA and phase contrast (PC) MRA. Both techniques can be acquired in either two dimensions (2D) or three dimensions (3D).

TOF-MRA

- Maximizes contrast between flowing blood and stationary tissue; flow-related enhancement
- TR < T1
- 3D has higher signal-to-noise ratio (SNR) and shorter imaging times than 2D.
- Works well for high-flow arterial systems
- Limitations for imaging: slow flow vessels (especially venous system), tortuous vessels, poor background resolution

PC-MRA

- Flowing spins encoded with a bipolar gradient
- Velocity Encoding Gradient setting critical
- Speed or flow images
- 2D good for slow flow
- 3D has better spatial resolution
- Less saturation effects
- Flow velocity information
- Longer imaging times

GADOLINIUM-ENHANCED MRA

A perfectly timed gadolinium contrast agent injection with 3D spoiled gradient-echo (SPGR) produces high SNR MRA covering extensive regions of vascular anatomy within a breathhold. Compared with noncontrast techniques, signal does not depend on inflow of blood, is not subject to problems of flow saturation, and reduces intravoxel dephasing. The IV-administered Gd shortens the T1 of blood to <270 msec (T1 of fat), so all bright signal essentially originates from vessels. Images are reconstructed as maximum-intensity projections (MIPs). Technique:

- Dose: Two or three bottles (20 mL each) of the gadolinium (about 0.3 mmol/kg Gd)
- Timing: Perfect contrast agent bolus timing is crucial to ensure that the maximum arterial Gd occurs during the middle of the acquisition, when central k-space data are acquired. Begin injecting Gd immediately after starting the scan. Finish the injection just after the midpoint of the MR acquisition. To ensure full use of the entire dose of contrast, flush the IV tubing with 20 mL of normal saline.

SPINAL GD-MRA

Spinal AVF/AVM is a potentially devastating disease that is often overlooked. MRA can be an excellent screening examination in suspected patients and for preangiographic planning. Patients usually present with pain and weakness of the extremities. On MRI, there is often an abnormal T2W signal change in the cord, most commonly near the conus (congestive phenomenon), which can be reversible if the AVF/AVM is treated. Small flow voids can also be seen on T2W sagittal images. MRA protocol:

- Acquire MRA in the coronal plane unless there is extensive scoliosis; then, the sagittal plane is preferred.
- Timing run: axial image, one slice centered on the aorta at L2; 2 mL of gadolinium bolus (usually about 17 seconds)
- Acquisition: 30 mL of contrast followed by 30 mL of saline push with NEX = 1 (no repetition) to ensure arterial phase
- Look for early enhancing tortuous venous structures usually posterior to the spinal cord.

MRA RECONSTRUCTION TECHNIQUES

Technique	Application
Multiplanar reformation	Routine
MIP	Overall survey; identify areas of further interest
Targeted MIP	Isolate vessel of interest; reduce background signal
Curved reformations	Obtain vessel measurements
Shaded surface display	Convey depth perception
Volume rendering	Convey anatomic relationship
Subtraction	Eliminate background; produce pure venous images

OTHER TECHNIQUES

DIGITAL SUBTRACTION ANGIOGRAPHY (DSA)

Venous DSA

- Catheter in central venous structure; a combined large volume and high concentration of contrast agent is given as a bolus.
- Adequate results in only 70% of patients
- Invasive study

Arterial DSA

- Advantages: lower iodine concentration required than that for cut film, less pain, speedy
- Disadvantages: less resolution, motion, and bowel gas artifacts

PETROSAL VEIN SAMPLING

Venous blood is obtained from bilateral inferior petrosal veins (which drain the cavernous sinus) to detect lateralization of hormones produced by pituitary tumors (very sensitive test). Simultaneous tracker catheters are advanced into the inferior petrosal veins. Simultaneous samples are obtained to distinguish paraneoplastic/endocrine production of hormones from pituitary sources and localize the abnormality to left or right.

LYMPHOGRAPHY

- Isosulfan blue, 1 mL, injected between 1st-2nd and 4th-5th toes; wait 10 minutes for lymphatic uptake.
- Cutaneous cutdown to the fascia (dorsum of foot)
- Isolate a lymphatic; pass a silk suture above and below.
- Milk the blue dye into the vessel.
- Puncture lymphatic with a 30-gauge needle lymphography set.
- Hook up needle to pump and inject oily contrast medium (Ethiodol)
- Obtain initial images of lymphatic vascular phase and later of the nodal phase.

CONSCIOUS SEDATION

Form of sedation in which the patient is given sedation and pain medication but should remain easily arousable. The following parameters are continuously monitored:

- BP
- Oxygenation using a pulse oximeter
- ECG and heart rate

Conscious sedation is usually achieved by small aliquot dosing of midazolam and fentanyl.

COMMON MEDICATIONS AND DOSAGES*

	IV Dosage	Total Dose	Duration (hr)	Comments
Benzodiazepines				
Diazepam	1-5 mg	10-25 mg	6-24	Long-acting
Lorazepam	0.5-2.0 mg	2-4 mg	6-16	
Midazolam	0.5-2.0 mg	<0.15 mg/kg	1-2	Good amnesic effect; short-acting
Flumazenil	0.2 mg	May repeat q 1 min up to 1 mg	0.5 - 1	For benzodiazepine reversal
Narcotic Analgesics				
Morphine	1-5 mg	<0.2 mg/kg	3–4	Histamine release
Meperidine	12.5-25 mg	0.5-1 mg/kg	2-4	MAOI interaction
Fentanyl	15-75 μg	1-3 μg/kg	0.5-1	Immediate onset
Naloxone	0.4-0.8 mg	Repeated as needed	0.3-0.5	For narcotic overdose
Antiemetics				
Metoclopramide	10 mg	0.5-1 mg/kg	1-2	Stimulates GI motility
Ondansetron	4 mg	8 mg	4-8	
Prochlorperazine	2.5-10 mg	10 mg	4-6	Adjust dosage for age
Promethazine	12.5-25 mg	25 mg	4-6	CNS depressant effects
Droperidol	0.625-1.25 mg	Higher dose: sedation	4-6	Potent antiemetic at low doses

*See manufacturer's packet insert for specific rates of administration.
MAOI, monoamine oxidase inhibitor.

COAGULATION

GENERAL (Fig. 8-6)

- Coumadin interferes with vitamin K-dependent synthesis of clotting factors.
- Heparin inactivates thrombin by combining with antithrombin III.
- Partial thromboplastin time (PTT) is the time required for 1 mL of recalcified whole blood to clot. It therefore reflects the intrinsic clotting axis.
- Prothrombin time (PT) is the time required for 1 mL of recalcified whole blood to clot in the presence of thromboplastin (phospholipid extract); it therefore reflects the extrinsic clotting axis.

OVERVIEW

Clotting Parameter	Normal Value	Causes of Abnormal Values
Prothrombin time (extrinsic coagulation system)	<3 sec of control	Warfarin, heparin Liver disease
		Coagulopathy (DIC, thrombolytic therapy) Vitamin K deficiency (parenteral nutrition, biliary obstruction, malabsorption, antibiotics)
PTT (intrinsic coagulation system)	<6 sec of control	Lupus anticoagulant
		Hemophilia
Bleeding time	<8 min	platelet count <50,000/mm^3 Qualitative: uremia, NSAIDs von Willebrand disease

DIC, disseminated intravascular coagulation.

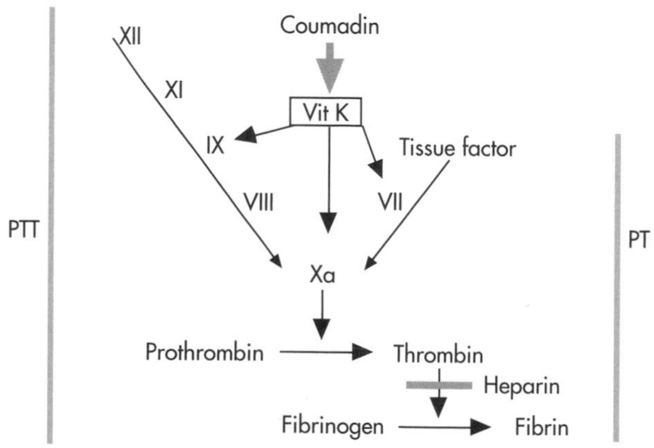

FIGURE 8-6

NORMALIZATION OF PROLONGED COAGULATION TIMES

Interventions (biopsy, aspiration, drainage) should not be performed if coagulation times are markedly prolonged (i.e., beyond above values); correction of coagulopathies (see table) can often be achieved in several hours.

CORRECTING PROLONGED COAGULATION TIMES

Anticoagulant	PT/PTT	Antidote	Normalization
Heparin	Both prolonged	Stop heparin	3-6 hr
		IV protamine titration	Minutes
Coumadin	Both prolonged	IV vitamin K for 3 doses	Days
		Fresh frozen plasma	Minutes
Aspirin	Normal (platelet aggregation reduced)	Platelet concentrates	Minutes
		Stop aspirin	Week

Monitoring Heparin Therapy

- Activated clotting time (ACT) is the method of choice for monitoring heparin therapy.
  - Preheparin administration: <120 sec
  - Heparin drip: <300 sec
  - Catheter and PTCA: >200 sec
  - Postprocedure/sheath removal: <200 sec

ANTICOAGULATION DRUGS AND PROCEDURES

Heparin

Mechanism of Action: Potentiates the action of antithrombin III and thereby inactivates thrombin (as well as activated coagulation factors IX, X, XI, XII, and plasmin) and prevents the conversion of fibrinogen to fibrin; heparin also stimulates release of lipoprotein lipase (lipoprotein lipase hydrolyzes triglycerides to glycerol and free fatty acids). Half-life: 1 to 2 hr, depending on route. Stop 2 hr before procedure.

Coumadin (Warfarin)

Mechanism of Action: Interferes with hepatic synthesis of vitamin K–dependent coagulation factors (II, VII, IX, X). Duration of action is 2 to 5 days. Stop 4 days before procedure.

Fragmin (Dalteparin)

Low-molecular-weight heparin. SC dose, OD after the loading dose. Duration: >12 hr; half-life: 2 to 5 hr. Stop the dose 24 hr before procedure.

Argatroban

Direct thrombin inhibitor, IV infusion; half-life: 39 to 51 minutes. Stop 4 hr before procedure.

Arixtra (Fondaparinux)

Factor X inhibitor; half-life: 17 to 21 hr, SC dose OD. Stop 24 hr before procedure.

Plavix (Clopidogrel)

Platelet aggregation inhibitor. Pharmacodynamic/kinetic peak effect: 75 mg/day; bleeding time: 5 to 6 days. Platelet function: 3 to 7 days; half-life: ~8 hr. Discontinue 7 days before procedure.

ReoPro (Abciximab)

Glycoprotein IIb/IIIa inhibitor. IV dosage. Pharmacodynamic/kinetic half-life: ~30 min. Takes 24 to 48 hr for platelet function to return to normal after discontinuation of infusion. Antiplatelet effects can be reversed with platelet transfusions.

Other Antiplatelet Agents

Aspirin, cilostazol, dipyridamole, eptifibatide, ticlopidine, tirofiban. Stop most of the antiplatelet agents 5 days before procedure.

ANTIBIOTICS

Recommended

- All biliary, renal and other nonvascular interventions
- Stent placements, TIPS, ports
- (Chemo)embolizations
- Patients with increased risks: endocarditis, transplant
- G-tube in patients with head and neck cancer
- Solid organ biopsies

Not recommended

- Diagnostic angiography
- Vena cava filter
- Regular G-tube (non-head and neck cancer patients)
- Simple biopsies: thyroid, subcutaneous
- Paracentesis and thoracentesis

Thoracic Aorta and Great Vessels

GENERAL

ANATOMY (Fig. 8-7)

- The normal ascending aorta is always larger in diameter than the descending aorta.
- Branches:
  - Great vessels
  - Intercostal arteries
  - Bronchial arteries
- Normal great vessel configuration, 70% (see diagram). Variants occur in 30%:
  - Bovine arch, 20%: common origin of brachiocephalic and left CCA
  - Left vertebral artery (LVA) comes off aortic arch between left CCA and subclavian artery (SA), 5%
  - Common carotid trunk, 1%
  - Arteria thyroidea IMA to thyroid isthmus
- Intercostal arteries are usually paired from 3rd to 11th intercostal spaces; these arteries may give rise to spinal arteries.

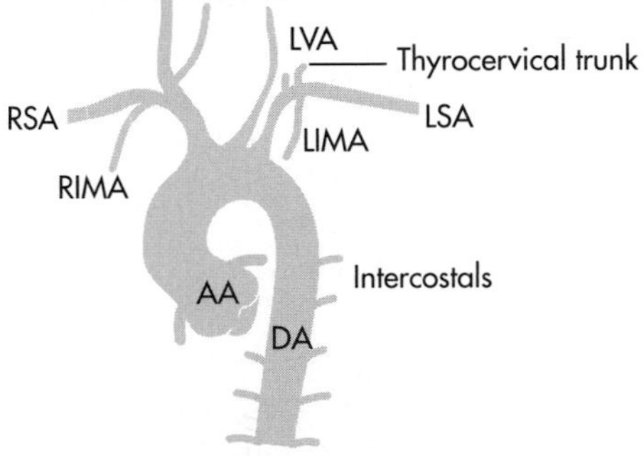

FIGURE 8-7

Procedure	Antibiotic
All routine procedure	Ampicillin (1 g IV) and gentamicin (80 mg IV or 40 mg IV if creatinine elevated)
Ampicillin allergy (low cost)	Clindamycin (Clindacin, 600 mg IV) and gentamicin (80 mg IV or 40 mg IV if creatinine elevated)
Ampicillin allergy (higher cost)	Levofloxacin (Levaquin, 500 mg IV or 250 mg if creatinine elevated)
Septic patients	Consider adding metronidazole (Flagyl, 500 mg IV) to above combination of ampicillin and gentamicin
Tube injection	Levofloxacin (Levaquin, 500 mg PO)
G-tube (HN cancer)	Cefazolin (Ancef, 1 g, IV) followed by 5 days cephalexin (Keflex 500 mg BID PO)
Prostate biopsy	Gentamicin (80 mg IM on day of procedure) and ciprofloxacin (Cipro, 500 mg PO for 7 days including day before procedure)
Transplant patients	Piperacillin and tazobactam (Zosyn, 3,375 mg IV)
Indwelling catheter and continued resistant growth	Consider giving vancomycin (500 mg IV) instead of gentamicin. Consult resistance tests.

- Bronchial artery configuration is quite variable. Most common configurations are:
  - Single right bronchial artery
  - Multiple left bronchial artery

IMAGING PRINCIPLES

CT

- Indications:
  - Diagnosis and surveillance of aneurysms
  - Aneurysm rupture
  - Aortic dissection
- Spiral CT is currently expanding CT indications.
- CT is not yet validated as the sole evaluation of traumatic arch injuries.

MRI

- Indications:
  - Diagnosis and surveillance of aneurysms
  - Aortic dissection
- Allows evaluation of the aortic root better than CT
- MRA of great vessels is gaining in diagnostic importance.

Aortography

- Indications:
  - Preoperative aneurysm assessment
  - Traumatic arch injury
  - Equivocal CT or MRI
- Remains the gold-standard diagnostic tool but is rarely the initial diagnostic examination for the thoracic aorta

Transesophageal Echocardiography

- Indications:
  - Aortic dissection
  - Associated cardiac disease (AI, LV dysfunction)
- Not validated to evaluate traumatic aortic injury

Thoracic Aortography Technique

- Catheter: 7- to 8-Fr pigtail
- Contrast: Hypaque 76 or nonionic equivalent
- Rate: 30 to 40 mL/sec × 2 sec (total: 60 to 80 mL)
- Fast filming: 3/sec × 3. Higher rate for DSA.
- Always perform imaging in at least two orthogonal views.

THORACIC AORTIC ANEURYSM

GENERAL

True aneurysms contain all three major layers of an intact arterial wall. False aneurysms lack one or more layers of the vessel wall; false aneurysms are also called *pseudoaneurysms*. Most thoracic aortic aneurysms are asymptomatic and are detected incidentally. Clinical symptoms usually indicate large size, expansion, or contained rupture.

Causes

- Atherosclerosis (most common)
- Connective tissue diseases (Marfan, Ehlers-Danlos)
- Syphilis
- Posttraumatic pseudoaneurysm
- Mycotic aneurysm
- Aortitis
  - Takayasu arteritis
  - Giant cell aortitis
  - Collagen vascular diseases (rheumatoid arthritis, ankylosing spondylitis)

Pearls

- True aneurysms tend to be fusiform.
- False aneurysms tend to be saccular.
- Posttraumatic, mycotic, and postsurgical aneurysms are false aneurysms.

ATHEROSCLEROTIC ANEURYSM

90% of these aneurysms are fusiform because thoracic atherosclerosis is usually circumferential; 10% are saccular. A saccular shape should therefore raise the suspicion of a false aneurysm (pseudoaneurysm). Atherosclerotic thoracic aneurysm is more common in the descending aorta and has a high incidence of concomitant abdominal aortic aneurysm.

Complications

Expansion
- Pain
- Hoarseness, dysphagia
- Aortic insufficiency

Rupture (uncommon if <5 cm)
- Rupture into pericardial or pleural space, trachea, mediastinum, esophagus
- Rupture into superior vena cava (SVC) (aortocaval fistula), pulmonary artery (aortopulmonary fistula)

Radiographic Features

Angiography (Fig. 8-8)
- Most useful in preoperative assessment of asymptomatic patients
- Appearance
  - Fusiform > saccular

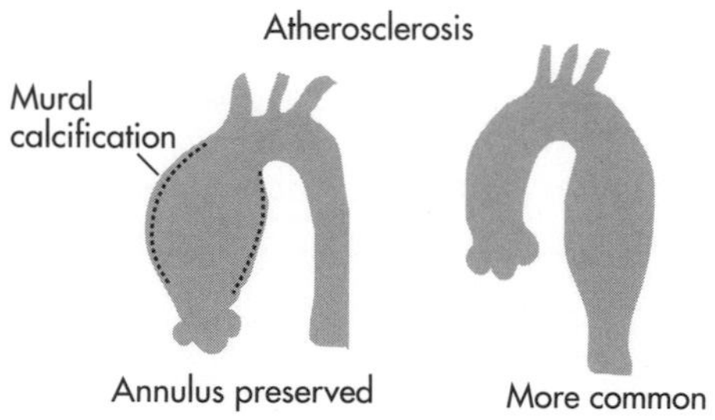

FIGURE 8-8

Determine proximal and distal extent (often thoracoabdominal)
Determine branch involvement
Coexistent aneurysmal or occlusive disease
- Not accurate in determining aneurysm size because of
  Magnification
  Layering of contrast
  Thrombus in the lumen
- An indicator of an impending rupture is focal ectasia (so-called pointing aneurysm, or nipple of aneurysm)

CT
- Mural thrombus well seen
- Extraluminal extent and contained rupture better seen than by angiography

CYSTIC MEDIAL NECROSIS

Degenerative process of the aortic muscular layer (media) causing aneurysms of the ascending aorta. Commonly involves aortic sinuses and sinotubular junction, resulting also in aortic insufficiency. Causes:
- Hypertension
- Marfan, Ehlers-Danlos, homocystinuria (structural collagen diseases)

Radiographic Features (Fig. 8-9)
- Symmetrical sinus involvement ("tulip bulb")
- Ascending aorta is most commonly involved.
- Dissection is a frequent complication.
- Calcifications are rare.

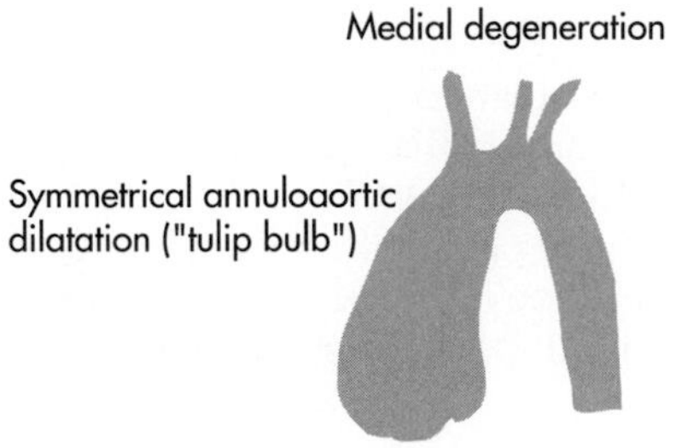

FIGURE 8-9

SYPHILITIC ANEURYSMS

Syphilitic aneurysms are a delayed manifestation of tertiary syphilis 10 to 30 years after primary infection. Infectious aortitis occurs via vasa vasorum. 80% of cases involve the ascending aorta or the aortic arch.

Radiographic Features (Fig. 8-10)
- Asymmetrical saccular sinus involvement
- Tree bark calcification is common.
- Dissections are rare.

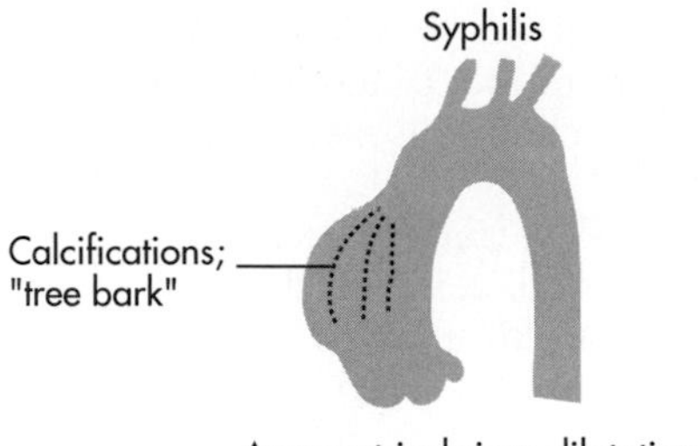

FIGURE 8-10

MYCOTIC ANEURYSMS

Mycotic aneurysms are saccular pseudoaneurysms located in ascending aorta or isthmus. Organisms: *Staphylococcus, Streptococcus, Salmonella*. CT often reveals perianeurysmal inflammation. Associations include:
- Immunocompromised patients
- Intravenous drug abuse
- Endocarditis
- Postsurgical
- Idiopathic

Treatment with resection and extraanatomic bypass.

AORTIC DISSECTION

GENERAL

Aortic dissection represents a spectrum of processes in which blood enters the muscular layer (media) of the aortic wall and splits it in a longitudinal fashion. Most dissections are spontaneous and occur in the setting of acquired or inherited degeneration of the aortic media (medial necrosis). Medial necrosis occurs most commonly as an acquired lesion in middle-aged to elderly hypertensive patients. Dissections (spontaneous) almost exclusively originate in the thoracic aorta and secondarily involve the abdominal aorta by extension from above. Aortic dissection results in the separation of two lumens by an intimal flap. The false lumen represents the space created by the splitting of the aortic wall; the true lumen represents the native aortic lumen. "Dissecting aortic aneurysm" is somewhat of a misnomer because many dissections occur in normal-caliber aortas. In chronic dissections the false channel may become aneurysmal.

Clinical Findings
- Chest pain or back pain, 80% to 90%
- Aortic insufficiency
- Blood pressure discrepancies between extremities
- Neurologic deficits
- Ischemic extremity
- Pulse deficits
- Silent dissections are very rare.

Causes

Medial degeneration is a pathologic finding associated with many diseases that predispose to dissection.

- Hypertension (most common)
- Structural collagen disorders
  - Marfan syndrome
  - Ehlers-Danlos syndrome
- Congenital
  - Aortic coarctation
  - Bicuspid or unicuspid valve
- Pregnancy
- Collagen vascular disease (very common)

Types (Fig. 8-11)

Classification is based on location because treatment and prognosis depend on the portion of aorta involved.

Stanford classification
- Type A, 60%: involves at least ascending aorta; surgical treatment
- Type B, 40%: limited to descending aorta; medical treatment

DeBakey classification
- Type I, 50%: involves ascending and descending aorta
- Type II, 10%: confined to ascending aorta
- Type III, 40%: same as a Stanford B

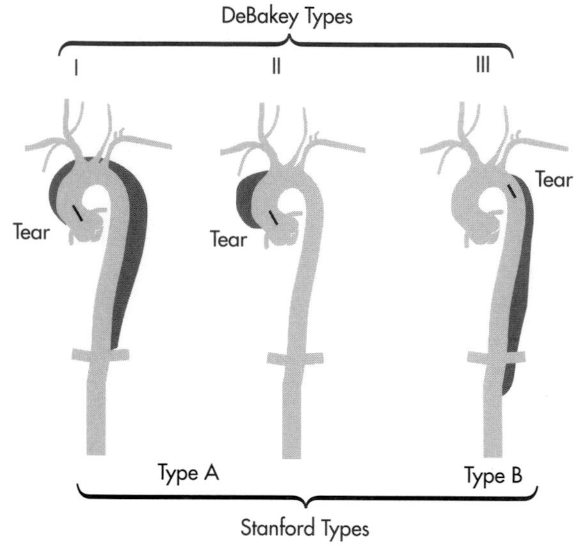

FIGURE 8-11

Treatment

Stanford B: medical control of hypertension is the Standard therapy. Surgery is indicated in complicated type B dissections.
- Ischemic extremity
- Mesenteric ischemia or renal artery compromise
- Rupture
- Aneurysmal enlargement of false lumen

Stanford A: requires surgery because of involvement of aortic root
- Pericardial tamponade
- Coronary artery occlusion
- Aortic insufficiency

Indications for Imaging (Fig. 8-12)

- Diagnosis
- Preoperative evaluation (aortography ± coronary angiography)
- Follow-up of postoperative and chronic dissections (CT or MRI)

Goals of Imaging Studies

- To determine if ascending aorta is involved
- To determine origin and extent of dissection
- To define branch vessel involvement: coronary arteries, great vessels, mesenteric and renal vessels, iliac arteries
- To determine if there is aortic regurgitation
- To find the intimal flap and entry/reentry points
- To evaluate patency of false lumen
- To determine if there is an extraaortic hematoma (pericardial, paraaortic, wall thickening)

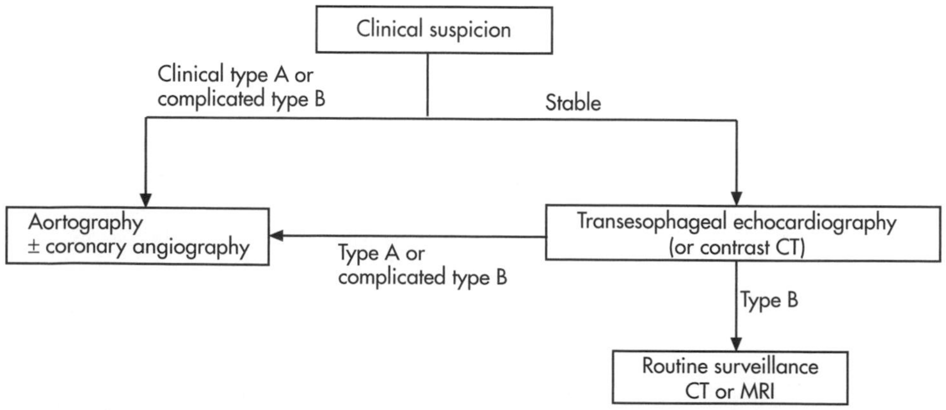

FIGURE 8-12

Angiographic Features

- Key diagnostic finding: intimal flap
- Intimal flap or false and true lumens are detectable in 85%-90%.
- Delayed opacification of false lumen
- Compression of true lumen by false lumen
- Occlusion of branch vessels
- Soft tissue companion shadow adjacent aorta (hematoma, thrombosed false lumen)
- Abnormal catheter position
  - Displaced from aortic wall by false lumen
  - Inability to opacify true lumen (catheter in false lumen)
- Differentiation of true and false lumens
  - Location: false lumen is anterolateral in ascending aorta and posterolateral in descending aorta
  - Size: false lumen is larger and compresses true lumen
  - Opacification: slower flow leads to delayed opacification of false lumen

CT Features (Fig. 8-13)

- Same hallmark findings as angiography
  - Intimal flap
  - Two lumens (true and false)
- CT is more accurate in detection of:
  - Thrombosed false channels
  - Periaortic hematoma and pericardial/pleural blood
  - Isolated aortic wall hematoma (hyperdense wall)
- CT is not accurate in evaluation of:
  - Coronary arteries or great vessels
  - Aortic valve
  - Entry or exit sites
- Dynamic contrast-enhanced helical CT is the technique of choice.
  - Precontrast scan (to detect wall hematoma)
  - Dynamic contrast-enhanced helical CT (to detect intimal flap)
  - Delayed contrast-enhanced helical CT (occasionally needed)
- Role of CT
  - Triage patients with equivocal clinical findings
  - Surveillance of chronic dissections

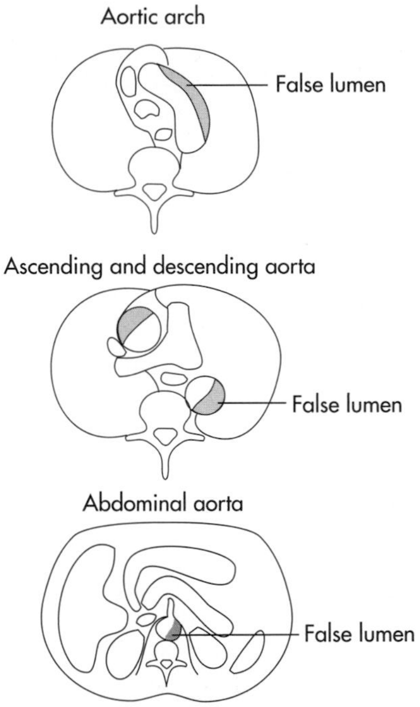

FIGURE 8-13

MRI Features

- Conventional spin echo: excellent for detecting intimal flaps and wall hematoma
- Phase-contrast gradient echo detects differential flow velocities in true and false lumens.
- Cine MR sequences allow detection of aortic insufficiency.

DIFFERENTIATION OF THROMBOSED ANEURYSM AND DISSECTION

	Thrombosed Aneurysm	Dissection
Longitudinal extent	Usually focal	Extensive, >6 cm
Calcification	Outside aortic shadow	Inside aortic shadow
Size of aorta	Large	Normal in acute phase, may become very large in chronic dissection
Aortic lumen	Large	Normal
Involved branches	Lumbar, IMA	Renal, SMA
	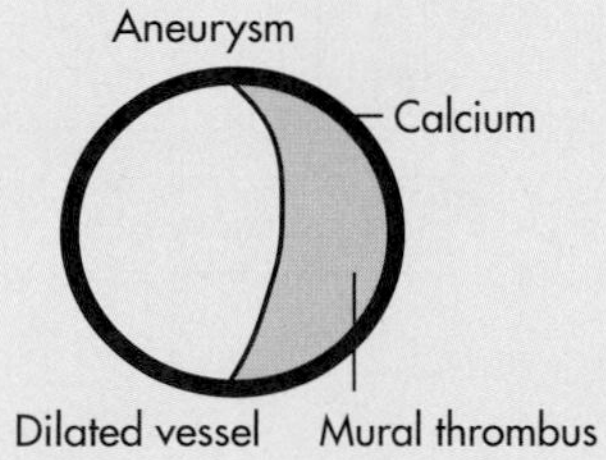	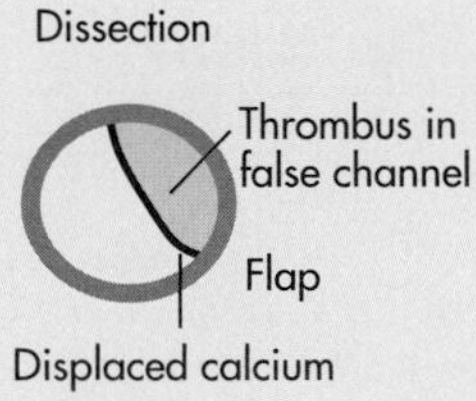

IMA, inferior mesenteric artery; SMA, superior mesenteric artery.

Pearls

- CXR is normal in 25% of aortic dissections.
- Abnormal CXRs in aortic dissection are nonspecific; clinical findings are usually much more helpful.
- CTA may be used as a triage exam in suspected acute aortic syndrome
- Do not confuse dissection with transection (traumatic aortic injury).
- Most aortic dissections are spontaneous; minor trauma may precipitate dissection in predisposed patients (Marfan syndrome), but this is the exception.

VARIANTS

Aortic Wall Hematoma (Fig. 8-14)

Hemorrhage within the aortic wall with no identifiable intimal flap or false lumen. This entry is caused by bleeding from the vasa vasorum into the media. Not detected by angiography; noncontrast CT is the study of choice (hyperdense aortic wall).

Penetrating Aortic Ulcer

Found usually in association with an atherosclerotic aneurysm. An ulcer ruptures into the media and results in a contained rupture or focal dissection. Not a true dissection but has a similar presentation. High mortality because of rupture.

Chronic Dissection

Type B or repaired dissections may persist with true and false lumens (double-barrel aorta). These dissections are compatible with long survival. Surveillance imaging with CT or MRI is used to detect an enlarging false lumen (dissecting aortic aneurysm) or extension.

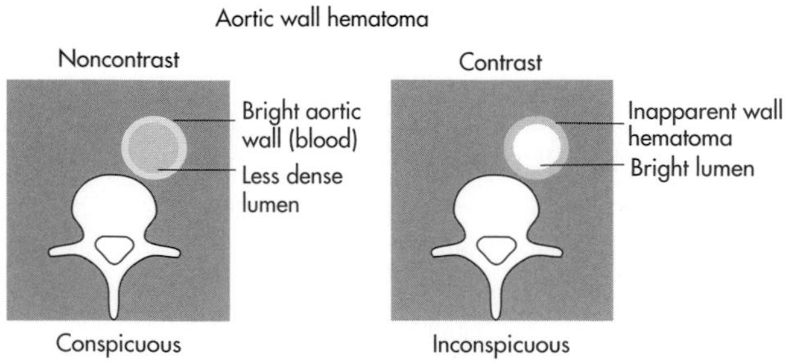

FIGURE 8-14

TRAUMATIC AORTIC INJURY

GENERAL

Exact mechanisms are unknown, but shear forces of deceleration injury are postulated to be the main cause of traumatic aortic injury. Only 15%-20% of patients who sustain traumatic aortic injury survive and present for imaging evaluation. Aortic injury typically results in a false aneurysm involving disruption of either intima or intima and media or of all wall layers. Only 5% of untreated patients are surviving at 4 months.

Location

- Aortic isthmus, 95%: between left subclavian artery and ligamentum arteriosum
- Proximal ascending aorta
- Descending aorta (at hiatus)
- Associated great vessel injury, 5%-10%

Approach

A history of appropriate mechanism of injury is a sufficient reason to evaluate a patient for aortic tear. The goal is to diagnose the injury as expeditiously as possible so that surgical repair can be undertaken (Fig. 8-15). Angiography remains the most accurate imaging examination for the detection and preoperative staging, although CTA now plays a more dominant role. CT may be used to accurately determine the absence or presence of mediastinal hematoma in low-risk patients with equivocal CXR and high-risk patients with normal chest radiograph.

Chest Radiograph

- Routinely obtained in all patients
- Look for signs of mediastinal hematoma:
  - Widened mediastinum or right paratracheal widening
  - Loss of aortic contour
  - Left apical cap
- Secondary signs are not specific:
  - Rightward displacement of nasogastric tube
  - Downward displacement of left bronchus
  - Fracture of first and second ribs
  - Hemothorax
- Only 15% of patients with mediastinal hematoma will have an aortic tear.
- Aortic injury rarely occurs in a normal mediastinum CXR.

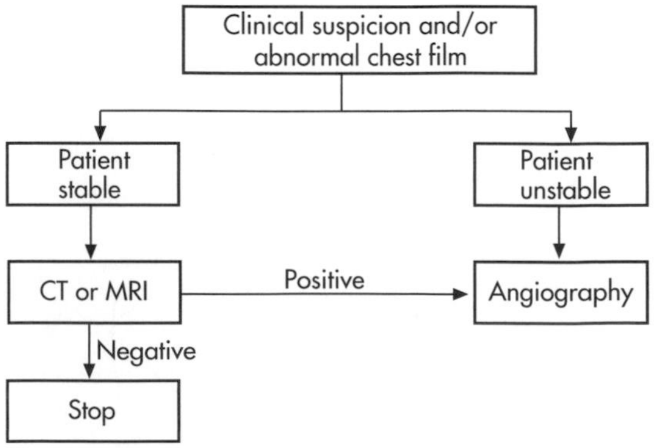

FIGURE 8-15

CT

- Noncontrast CT to determine absence or presence of mediastinal hematoma, rupture
- Patients with any appearance other than normal mediastinal fat should go straight to angiography.
- Pitfalls:
  - Young patients with residual thymus
  - Ventilated patients (motion artifact)
  - Patients with little mediastinal fat

Angiography

- Intimal tear: linear filling defect or irregularity or aortic contour
- Pseudoaneurysm at isthmus, 80%
- Associated great vessel injuries, 5%
- False-positive studies are very rare: ductus bump or diverticulum (remnant of the embryonic double arch)
- Always obtain at least 2 views
- Sensitivity, 100%

Pearls

DIFFERENTIATION OF DUCTUS KNOB FROM AORTIC TEAR

Ductus Knob	Aortic Tear
Smooth	Sharp
Round	Irregular
Broad neck	Narrow neck
No companion shadow	Companion shadow
Ductus diverticulum	Traumatic pseudoaneurysm

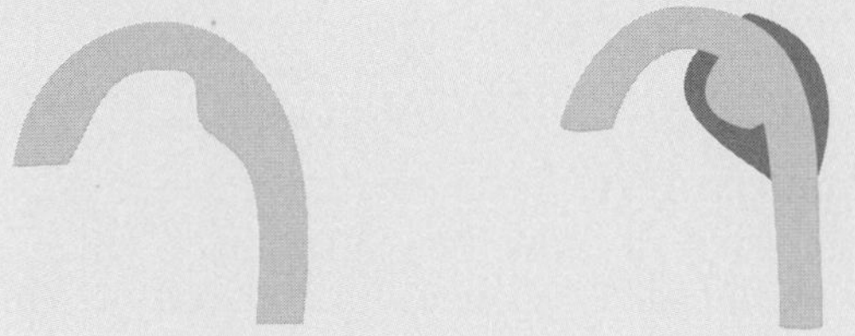

- Some clinicians still consider the mechanism of injury alone (regardless of CXR findings) as an indication for aortography.
- CTA is increasingly replacing aortography in the initial evaluation of traumatic aortic injury.

AORTITIS

TAKAYASU ARTERITIS (PULSELESS DISEASE)

Marked intimal proliferation and fibrosis lead to occlusion and narrowing of aorta and involved arteries; aneurysms may also be found. Age: 90% <30 years (in contradistinction to all other arteritis types). More common in females.

Types (Fig. 8-16)

Type 1: aortic arch
Type 2: abdominal aorta
Type 3: entire aorta
Type 4: pulmonary arteries

Radiographic Features

- Smooth long-segment stenoses of arch vessels (most common)
- Stenosis and occlusion of aorta (may mimic coarctation)
- Thickening of aortic wall
- Pulmonary artery involvement, 50%
- Abdominal coarctation and renal artery stenoses

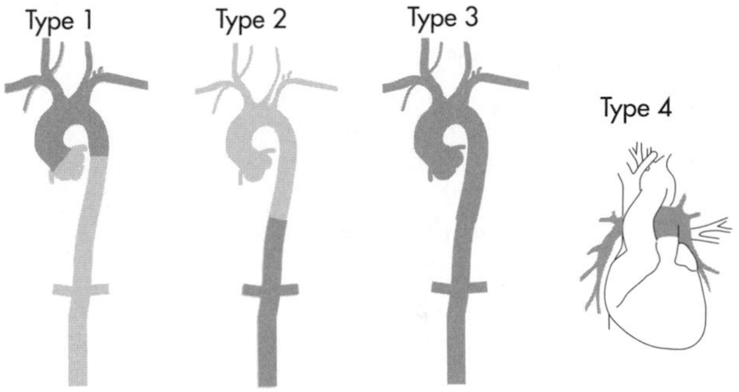

FIGURE 8-16

GIANT CELL ARTERITIS

- Older patients >50 years
- Diagnosis: biopsy of temporal artery
- Most commonly involves medium-size arteries; skip lesions
- Aorta is involved in 10%, most commonly ascending aorta
- Complications: aneurysm, dissection

SYPHILITIC AORTITIS

Syphilitic aortitis occurs 10 to 30 years after infection as the aorta becomes progressively weakened by inflammation and fibrosis (wrinkling of the intima), ultimately leading to aneurysm formation. Organism: *Treponema pallidum*. Diagnosis: positive FTA-ABS, VDRL. Treatment is with high-dose penicillin and resection of enlarging aneurysm.

Complications

- Aneurysm, 10%
- Aortic valve disease
- Coronary artery narrowing at ostium, 30%
- Gummatous myocarditis (rare)

Radiographic Features

- Involvement: ascending aorta (60%) > aortic arch (30%) > descending thoracic aorta (10%)
- Tree-bark appearance
- Saccular aneurysm of ascending aorta
- Heavy calcification of the ascending aorta is typical (but not common).

Abdomen and Pelvis

ABDOMINAL AORTA

ANATOMY (Fig. 8-17)

ABDOMINAL AORTIC ANEURYSM (AAA)

Atherosclerotic aneurysms are most commonly located in the abdominal aorta. 90% of AAAs are infrarenal. The major risk of an abdominal aneurysm is rupture, but other complications occur.

- Expansion and/or leakage: pain
- Aortocaval fistula: congestive heart failure (CHF), leg swelling
- Distal embolization: blue-toe syndrome
- Aortoenteric fistula
- Infection

The risk of rupture is small in aneurysms <5 cm but increases for aneurysms >5 cm. Associated with other aneurysms, especially popliteal artery aneurysm.

Radiographic Features (Fig. 8-18)

Plain film

- Determine size by atherosclerotic calcification.
- Lateral projection is most helpful.

CT

- AAA is defined as vessel diameter ≥ 3 cm.
- Contrast-enhanced helical CT may provide preoperative assessment in simple cases.
- Most accurate imaging study to determine the size of aneurysm

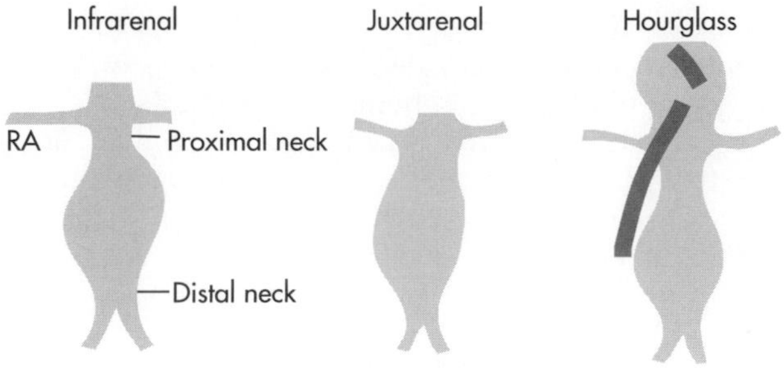

FIGURE 8-18

- Suspected rupture:
  - Retroperitoneal hematoma is the most common finding
  - Draped aorta sign: posterior wall of the aorta either is not identifiable or closely follows vertebral bodies
  - Hyperattenuation crescent sign: well-defined peripheral crescent of increased attenuation within the thrombus of a large aneurysm indicates acute or impending rupture

Angiography

- Routinely used for preoperative staging
- Yields more accurate data regarding status of mesenteric and renal vessels than CT does
- Not reliable for size determination
- Allows mapping of pelvic and leg arterial anatomy
- Always define:
  - Proximal and distal neck of aneurysm
  - Patency of mesenteric vessels
  - Presence of aberrant vessels

OTHER ABDOMINAL AORTIC ANEURYSMS

Inflammatory AAA

Represents 5% of all AAAs. The inflammatory mantle surrounding the AAA enhances on contrast CT. This entity must be differentiated from leaking or ruptured AAAs.

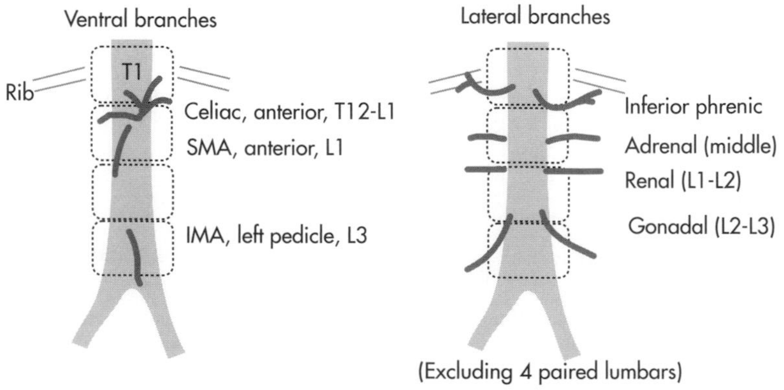

FIGURE 8-17

Mycotic AAA

The aorta is a common site for infected aneurysms. Mycotic aneurysms are typically eccentric saccular aneurysms in a location atypical for atherosclerotic AAAs. Organisms: *Salmonella, Staphylococcus*. Fever of unknown origin (FUO) occurs.

Risk Factors

- Arterial trauma
- Sepsis
- Immunosuppression
- Bacterial endocarditis
- IV drug abuse (IVDA)

AORTOILIAC OCCLUSIVE DISEASE

Multiple patterns exist (Fig. 8-19):

- Infrarenal aortic occlusion: occlusion up to the level of renal arteries
- Distal aortoiliac disease: involves bifurcation and iliac arteries
- Small aorta syndrome: focal atherosclerotic stenosis of distal aorta; occurs most commonly in younger female smokers
- Multisegment disease: often associated with infrainguinal occlusive disease

Common clinical symptoms include thigh, hip, and buttock claudication; impotence; and diminished femoral pulses (Leriche syndrome in men). In general, aortoiliac occlusive disease responds well to percutaneous interventions such as PTA and endovascular metallic stents.

Radiographic Features

- Arteriography is the imaging study of choice once the decision is made to intervene.
- Collateral arterial pathways:
  - Internal mammary arteries → external iliac arteries via superior and inferior epigastric arteries
  - IMA → internal iliac arteries via hemorrhoidal arteries
  - Intercostal/lumbar arteries → external iliac arteries via deep circumflex iliac arteries
  - Intercostals/lumbar arteries → internal iliac arteries via iliolumbar and gluteals
- Always measure pressure gradients across stenoses to determine their hemodynamic significance and to assess response to intervention.
- Role of MRA:
  - 2-D TOF and Gd-DTPA 3-D SPGR are commonly used techniques.
  - Diagnostic study of choice in patients with high risk for contrast reactions or renal failure
  - Good for visualizing distal "runoff" when aorta is occluded

ABDOMINAL AORTIC COARCTATION

Abdominal aortic coarctation may be congenital or acquired. Most commonly affects young adults and children. Clinical: renovascular hypertension (common), claudication, abdominal angina. Associations include:

Congenital
- Thoracic aortic coarctation
- Idiopathic hypercalcemia syndrome (Williams syndrome)
- Congenital rubella
- Neurofibromatosis (NF)

Acquired
- Takayasu arteritis
- Fibromuscular dysplasia
- Radiation therapy

Radiographic Features

- Segmental coarctation is most common.
- Coarctation usually involves the renal arteries.
- IMA serves as major collateral vessel to lower extremities.
- Diffuse hypoplasia is a less common form of presentation.

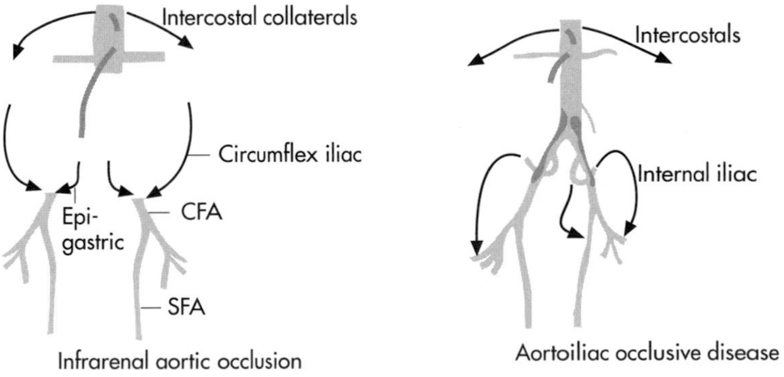

FIGURE 8-19

AORTIC INTERVENTIONS AND SURGERY

ENDOVASCULAR STENT GRAFTS

Endovascular stent graft implantation is an alternative to open surgery for the treatment of aortic aneurysm. Advantages of endovascular procedures are lower blood loss, shorter stay in intensive care and hospitalization, and quicker recovery. Common complications that can be discerned by imaging include:

- Graft thrombosis
- Graft kinking
- Pseudoaneurysm caused by graft infection
- Graft occlusion
- Shower embolism
- Colonic necrosis
- Aortic dissection
- Hematoma at arteriotomy site
- Endoleak (see below for classification)

Endoleak Classification (White)

- Type I endoleak is present when a persistent perigraft channel with blood flow develops. This can be due to an inadequate or ineffective seal at the graft ends (either the proximal or distal graft) or attachment zones (synonyms: "perigraft endoleak" or "graft-related endoleak").
- Type II endoleak occurs when there is persistent collateral retrograde blood flow into the aneurysm sac (e.g., from lumbar arteries, the IMA, or other collateral vessels). There is a complete seal around the graft attachment zones, so the complication is not directly related to the graft itself (synonyms: "retrograde endoleak" or "non–graft-related endoleak").
- Type III endoleak arises at the midgraft region and is due to leakage through a defect in the graft fabric or between the segments of a modular, multisegmental graft. This subgroup of endoleak is primarily due to mechanical failure of the graft (early component defect or late material fatigue). In some cases, hemodynamic forces or aneurysm shrinkage may be contributory (synonyms: "fabric tear" or "modular disconnection").
- Type IV endoleak is detected by angiography or other contrast studies as any minor blush of contrast that is presumed to emanate from contrast diffusion across the pores of the highly porous graft fabric or perhaps through the small holes in the graft fabric caused by sutures or stent struts, etc. This is usually an intentional design feature rather than a form of device failure. In practice, differentiation of type IV endoleak from type III can often be difficult, perhaps requiring postoperative, directed angiography (synonym: "graft porosity").
- Endoleak of undefined origin. In many cases, the precise source of endoleak will not be clear from routine follow-up imaging studies, and further investigation may be required. In this situation, it may be appropriate to classify the condition as "endoleak of undefined origin" until the type of endoleak is elucidated by further studies.
- Nonendoleak aneurysm sac pressurization (endopressure). In this situation, no endoleak is demonstrated on imaging studies, but pressure within the aneurysm sac is elevated and may be very close to systemic pressure (unpublished data). The seal is formed by semiliquid thrombus, and the pressure in the sac is similar to the pressures measured in the endoleak. The aneurysm is pulsatile; wall pulsatility also may be detected and monitored by specialized US techniques.

TYPES OF GRAFTS

- Bifurcation grafts are used mainly for AAA repair and aortoiliac occlusive disease.
  - End-to-side (used only for aortoiliac occlusive disease)
  - End-to-end
- Tube grafts are used mainly for AAA repair.
- Endarterectomy is usually used for aortoiliac occlusive disease.
- Aortofemoral bypass is used mainly in aortoiliac occlusive disease.
- Extraanatomical grafts
  - Axillofemoral
  - Axillobifemoral
  - Femorofemoral

These grafts are preferred in patients with unilateral iliac disease, high surgical risk, severe scarring from prior vascular procedures, abdominal or groin infections, or chronic occlusion of one limb and those with AFB.

AORTIC BIFURCATION GRAFTS (ONLAY GRAFTS, INVERTED Y GRAFTS)

Aortic Onlay Graft (Figs. 8-20 and 8-21)

The end of the graft is anastomosed to the ventral wall of the aorta. The distal lines are anastomosed to both CFAs. Only used for occlusive disease.

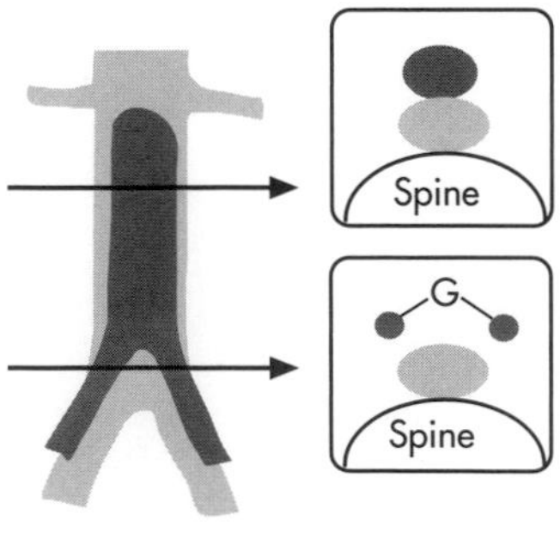

FIGURE 8-20

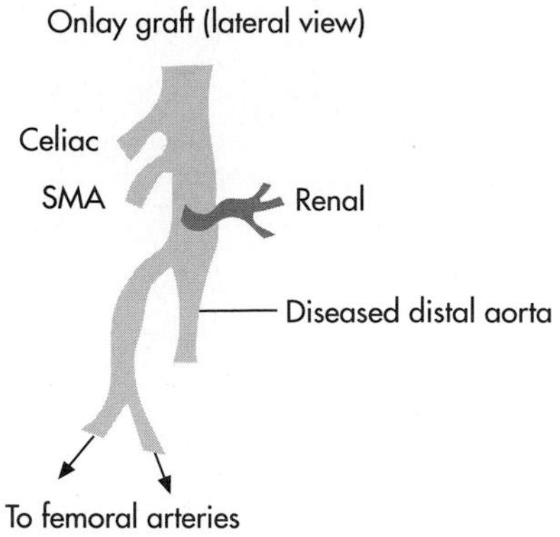

FIGURE 8-21

- Preserves flow to native pelvic arteries, especially internal iliac arteries
- Impotence is less common.
- Higher incidence of graft occlusion

End-to-End Y Graft

Hemodynamically better than end-to-side anastomosis. Used for AAA and occlusive disease. May be bifurcated to iliac arteries or extended distally to CFAs. Advantages include:

- More physiologic flow at anastomosis
- Lower risk of aortoduodenal fistula
- Higher patency

WRAPPED GRAFT (TUBE GRAFT) (Fig. 8-22)

The graft is positioned within the aneurysm. The native aortic wall is sutured around the graft.

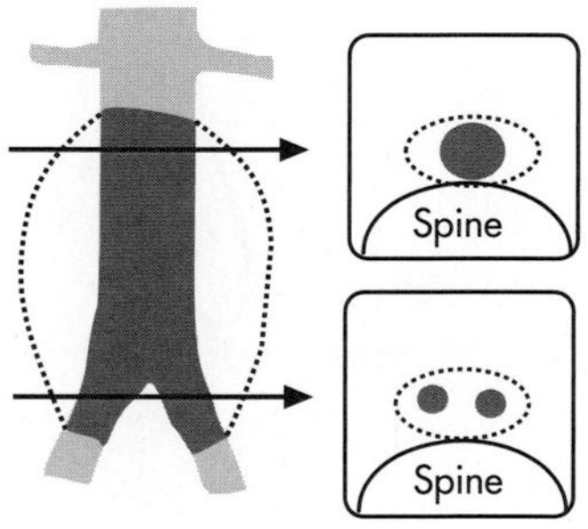

FIGURE 8-22

SURGICAL GRAFT COMPLICATIONS

CT is the study of choice for detecting:

- Perigraft infection
- Anastomotic pseudoaneurysm
- Hematoma, lymphocele
- Aortoenteric fistula

^{111}In-WBC may be helpful in detecting graft infection.

OVERVIEW

Complication	Incidence (%)
Perigraft abscess	40
Groin infection	25
Pseudoaneurysm	20
Hematoma, lymphocele	10
Aortoenteric fistula	10
Other	10
Bowel infarction	
Abscess	

INFRAINGUINAL GRAFT FAILURE

Causes of early or subacute infrainguinal bypass graft failure

- Scarred vein segments
- Anastomotic stricture
- Retained valve cusps (in situ grafts)
- Clamp injury
- Nonligated vein graft tributaries that divert flow away from the graft

Late infrainguinal graft failure

- Graft stenosis from intimal hyperplasia
- Progression of atherosclerosis
- Poor runoff

MESENTERIC VESSELS (FIG. 8-23)

CELIAC AXIS

Arises at T12-L1. Branches:

- 1st branch: left gastric artery (LGA)
- 2nd branch: splenic artery
- 3rd branch: common hepatic artery (CHA)

FIGURE 8-23

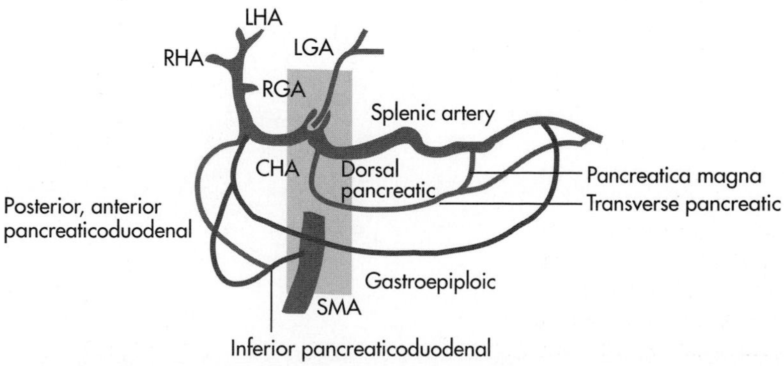

HEPATIC VASCULATURE

Hepatic Arteries

The CHA represents the segment from the origin to take-off of GDA. The proper hepatic artery divides into LHA and RHA. Aberrations, 40%:

- RHA from SMA, 15%
- LHA from LGA, 10%
- Accessory LHA from LGA, 8%
- Accessory RHA from SMA, 5%
- RHA and LHA from SMA with no supply from celiac axis, 2%

Hepatic Veins

- Hepatic venous drainage occurs via 3 hepatic veins that drain into the IVC.
- Hepatic veins define hepatic anatomic segments (8 segments; see Chapter 3).

SPLENIC ARTERY

Branches

- Dorsal pancreatic artery arises from splenic artery in 40%.
- Pancreatica magna arises in midportion.
- Short gastric arteries
- Left gastroepiploic artery
- Splenic polar branches

SUPERIOR MESENTERIC ARTERY (SMA) (Fig. 8-24)

The SMA arises at L1 at 1 to 20 mm below the celiac axis. The first part lies immediately posterior to the body of the pancreas; it then passes ventral to the uncinate process (CT landmark).

Branches

- Inferior pancreaticoduodenal artery (1st branch)
- Middle colic artery (2nd branch)
- Jejunal and ileal arteries
- Right colic artery
- Ileocolic artery

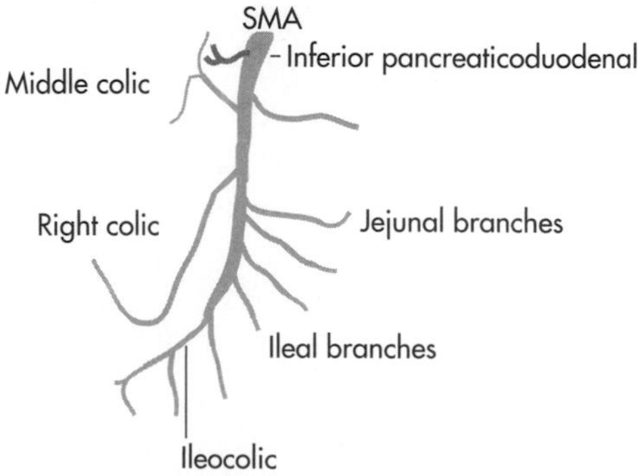

FIGURE 8-24

INFERIOR MESENTERIC ARTERY (IMA) (Fig. 8-25)

Originates below renal arteries at left pedicle of L3.

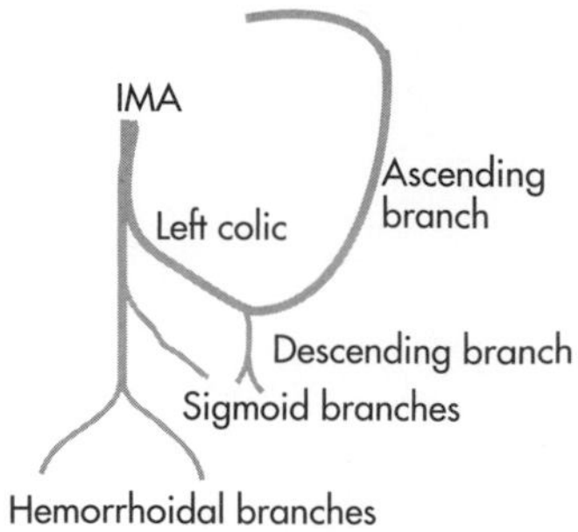

FIGURE 8-25

Branches

- Left colic artery: separate vessel in 40%; arises as a trunk with some sigmoid branches in 60%
- Sigmoid arteries: supply the sigmoid; marginal arteries (complex of arcades)
- Superior hemorrhoidal artery: continuation of IMA or sigmoid artery; becomes hemorrhoidal artery after passing over common iliac vessel

MESENTERIC COLLATERALS (Figs. 8-26 and 8-27)

Celiac artery to SMA

- Arc of Buehler: embryonic ventral communication of celiac artery to SMA
- Pancreaticoduodenal arcade

SMA to IMA

- Arc of Riolan: middle colic artery → left colic artery

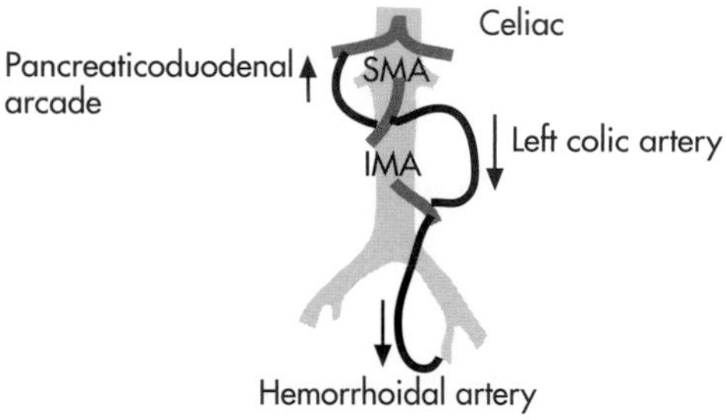

FIGURE 8-26

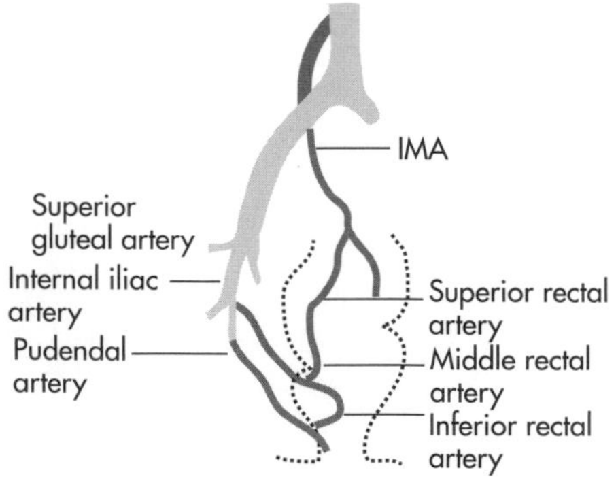

FIGURE 8-27

- Marginal arteries of Drummond: arcades along the mesenteric border of the colon

IMA to internal iliac artery

- Via superior hemorrhoidal artery

Rectal arcades

- Superior rectal artery from IMA
- Middle rectal artery from internal iliac artery
- Inferior rectal artery from pudendal artery

PELVIC ARTERIES (Fig. 8-28)

Internal iliac artery

- Superior gluteal artery
- Inferior gluteal artery
- Obturator artery
- Internal pudendal artery
- Iliolumbar artery
- Cystic artery
- Uterine artery
- Hemorrhoidal artery

External iliac artery

- Deep circumflex and inferior epigastric arteries are the first branches of the common femoral artery, thus marking the end of external iliac vessels and the inguinal ligament.

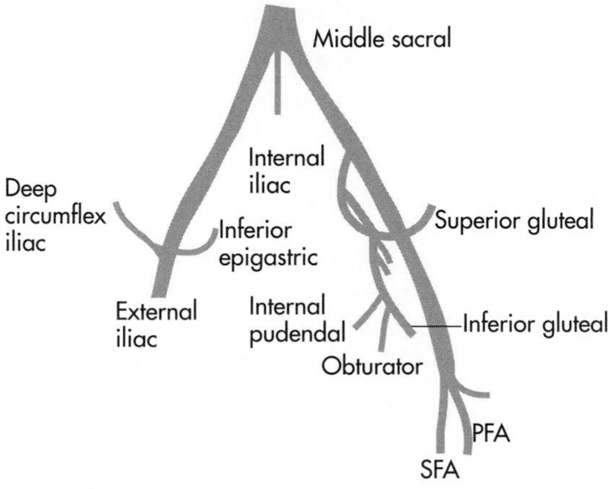

FIGURE 8-28

UPPER GI HEMORRHAGE

Endoscopy and conservative therapy are the primary forms of treatment.

Angiography is used after failure of primary therapies. Rarely, massive upper GI bleeding can present as hematochezia.

Causes

- Gastritis (most common)
- Peptic ulcer disease
- Gastroesophageal varices
- Mallory-Weiss tear
- Aortoduodenal fistula
- GI malignancy

Radiographic Features

- Confirm active bleeding by a selective arteriogram.
- The most common bleeding vessel in upper GI hemorrhage is the left gastric artery (LGA), 85%-90%.
- Extravascular contrast extravasation is the hallmark of active bleeding.
    - Accumulation in bowel lumen
    - Gastric "pseudovein" sign (contrast between rugal folds)
    - Filling of pseudoaneurysm or pooling
- Normal variants of LGA origins:
    - Celiac trunk (most common)
    - Directly from aorta
    - Common trunk with splenic artery from aorta
- Alternative sources of gastric bleeding:
    - Right gastric artery (RGA)
    - Left and right gastroepiploic arteries
    - Short gastric arteries
- Common sources of duodenal bleeding:
    - GDA and/or its branches
    - Pancreaticoduodenal arcade
    - Bleeding scans are not usually helpful for evaluating upper GI bleeding.

Angiographic Intervention

- Vasopressin
    - Usually successful in gastritis, esophagogastric tears
    - Proceed to embolization if no response after 30 minutes
    - Contraindications: CAD, severe HTN, renal failure
- Embolization is more successful with tumors, peptic ulcer disease, and duodenal hemorrhages.
- Gelfoam embolization is used for self-limited lesions (e.g., benign ulcers), because recanalization will occur after initial cessation of bleeding.

SUCCESS RATES OF TREATMENTS FOR UGI BLEEDING

Type of Hemorrhage	Treatment	Success (%)
Esophagogastric Hemorrhage		
Mallory-Weiss tear	Vasopressin	90
Diffuse gastric bleeding*	Vasopressin	80
Esophageal varices	IV (not IA) vasopressin	
	Endoscopic sclerosis	
	TIPS	
Pyloroduodenal Hemorrhage		
Ulcer	Vasopressin	35
	Vasopressin and embolization	60

*Related to stress, trauma, surgery, burns, NSAIDs, etc.

- Permanent embolization (polyvinyl alcohol, coils) is reserved for major arterial injury (e.g., tumor, duodenal ulcers, pseudoaneurysm).
- Embolization of upper GI does not result in ischemia because of rich collateral supply.

LOWER GI HEMORRHAGE (Fig. 8-29)

Defined as bleeding distal to ligament of Treitz. 98% of hemorrhages are located in large bowel, and 2% are located in small bowel. Endoscopy is performed to exclude rectal bleeding. Unlike the outcome with UGI hemorrhage, endoscopy is often technically not successful because bleeding obscures visualization.

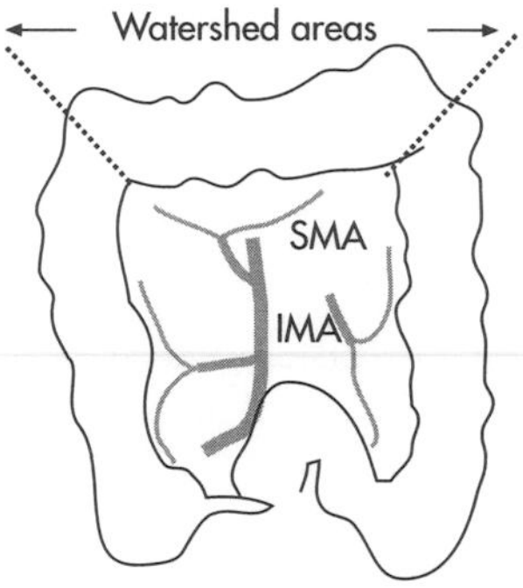

FIGURE 8-29

Causes

Large bowel, 98%
- Diverticulosis (most common)
- Angiodysplasia
- Colon carcinoma
- Polyps
- Inflammatory bowel disease, other colitis
- Rectal disease
  - Ulcer or tear
  - Hemorrhoids
  - Tumor

Small bowel, 2%
- Leiomyoma
- Arteriovenous malformation
- Ulcer (steroid therapy or transplant patients)
- Small bowel varices
- Other
  - Inflammatory bowel disease (IBD)
  - Diverticulosis, Meckel's diverticulum
  - Small bowel tumors (e.g., metastases, Kaposi sarcoma)

Radiographic Features

Scintigraphic scans are sensitive and often helpful.
- Threshold of detection is 0.1 mL/min.
- If scintigraphy is negative, the angiographic likelihood of a positive study is very low.
- Prolonged imaging can detect intermittent bleeding.

Selective SMA and IMA arteriograms
- Multiple runs should be obtained to cover entire vascular bed (colonic flexures, rectum).
- Anomalous arteries (e.g., middle colic) may require celiac arteriogram.

Angiographic Intervention (Fig. 8-30)

- Intraarterial vasopressin is successful in 90%. Abdominal pain may indicate ischemia.
- Rebleed rate, 30%
- Compared with embolization of the upper GI tract, embolization of the lower GI tract has a higher rate of complications because of less collateralization. Bowel ischemia and/or infarction occurs in 25%.

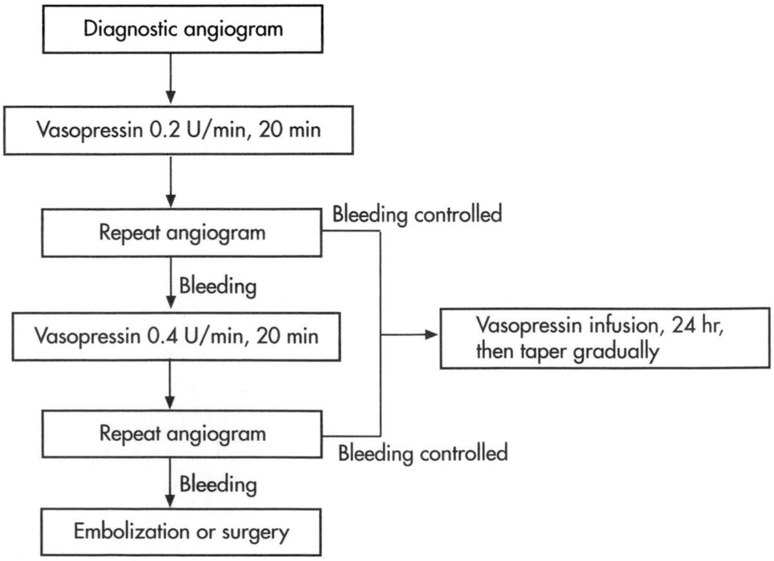

FIGURE 8-30

INTESTINAL ISCHEMIA

May be acute or chronic. Chronic ischemia occurs when progressive occlusive disease involves all three mesenteric arteries. Patients are usually not very ill and present with abdominal angina and weight loss. Patients with acute ischemia, in contradistinction, usually present with an acute abdomen and often have a deranged metabolic status and other concomitant medical conditions (e.g., shock, cardiac disease, sepsis).

Causes

Arterial occlusion

- Embolization
- In situ thrombosis
- Aortic dissection
- Primary mesenteric artery dissection (fibromuscular dysplasia, iatrogenic)
- Vasculitis

Nonocclusive arterial ischemia (most common)

- Atherosclerosis and low cardiac output/hypotension

Mesenteric venous thrombosis

Other

- Incarcerated hernia
- Volvulus
- Intussusception

Radiographic Features

Angiography

- Helical CT often used for triage; angiography remains the study of choice.
- Filling defects or occlusions: thrombus, embolus
- In situ thrombosis occurs proximally (origin of SMA)
- Emboli tend to be peripheral and/or located at vascular branch points.
- Late phase: lack of veins, collaterals, filling defects (venous thrombosis)
- Diffuse vasospasm may accompany nonocclusive or occlusive etiology.

Angiographic interventions

- Intraarterial or venous thrombolysis
- Nonocclusive ischemia: IA papaverine, 30 to 50 mg/hr

ANGIODYSPLASIA

Thought to represent an acquired vascular anomaly, most commonly located in cecum or right colon. Associated with aortic valvular stenosis. Angiodysplasia is a common cause of chronic lower GI bleeding in patients > age 50; rarely presents as acute GI hemorrhage. Treat with surgery/embolization, not vasopressin.

Radiographic Features

- Only detectable by mesenteric arteriography
- Vascular tuft on antimesenteric border
- Early or persistent draining vein
- Active bleeding usually cannot be seen.

MEDIAN ARCUATE LIGAMENT SYNDROME

Median arcuate ligament is a fibrous band formed at the base of the diaphragm, along the anterior aspect of the aortic hiatus, and normally above the celiac artery. When the band passes in front of the celiac artery, it may lead to celiac artery compression. Treatment: surgery.

Radiographic Features

- Indentation along superior aspect of the celiac artery; expiration may exaggerate appearance.
- Hooked appearance of celiac artery on conventional or CT angiography.

VARICOCELE

Incompetent or absent valves in the spermatic vein may lead to dilated pampiniform plexus, which may cause infertility, pain, and scrotal enlargement. Treatments: surgery or coil embolization along length of spermatic vein, including collaterals.

LIVER

ARTERIAL IMAGING

HEPATIC TUMORS

Lesion	Arterial Vascularity	Other Findings
Hemangioma pools	Normal	Dense peripheral stain; small, multiple (cotton wool)
FNH	++	Spokewheel appearance, 35%
Adenoma	+	Paradoxically not very vascular
Regenerating nodules	–	Often hypovascular, seen with cirrhosis
HCC	++, AV shunting	Portal vein invasion, 75%

VENOUS IMAGING (Figs. 8-31 and 8-32)

Indications

- Portal vein thrombosis
- Hepatic vein thrombosis (Budd-Chiari syndrome)
- Portal hypertension
- Evaluation of hepatic transplants
- TIPS evaluation
- Evaluation of portosystemic shunts

Imaging Modalities

US

- Cannot reliably diagnose intrahepatic venoocclusive disease

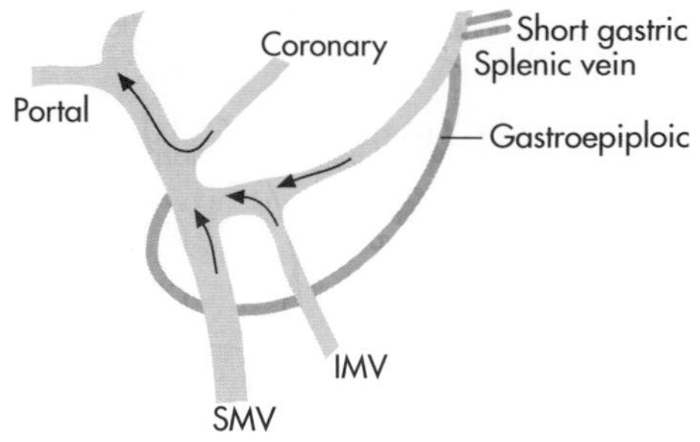

FIGURE 8-31

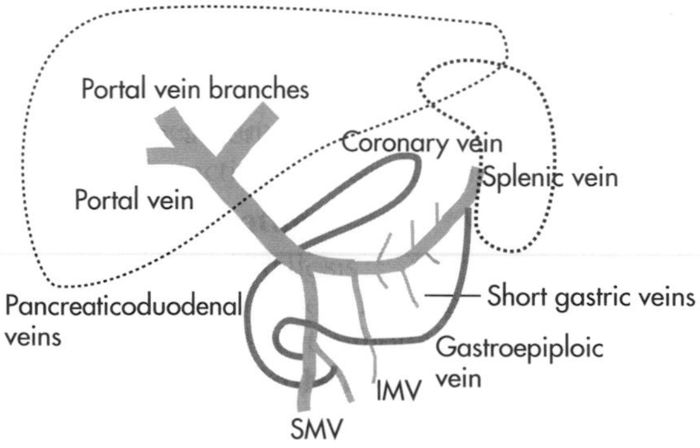

FIGURE 8-32

- Useful for most other indications

Angiography
- Hepatic and wedged hepatic venography
- Portal venography
    - Arterial portography (late-phase celiac/SMA arteriography)
    - Transhepatic direct portal venography
    - Transjugular direct portal venography
    - Percutaneous splenoportography
    - Umbilical vein catheterization

CT angiography and MRA
- Evolving roles

PORTAL HYPERTENSION

Defined as a portal pressure >10 mm Hg. Most commonly caused by hepatic cirrhosis. Clinical manifestations occur because of altered flow dynamics; GI variceal bleeding is the most common presentation.

Causes

Presinusoidal
- Portal vein obstruction
    - Thrombosis
    - Tumor (pancreatic cancer, metastases)
- Schistosomiasis (most common cause worldwide)

Sinusoidal
- Cirrhosis

Postsinusoidal
- Budd-Chiari syndrome
- Hepatic vein or IVC occlusion

High flow states
- Traumatic AVF
- AVM (Osler-Weber-Rendu, HCC)

Physiology (Fig. 8-33)
- Elevated portal pressures
- Increased hepatic arterial flow to liver
- Biphasic or hepatofugal portal flow
- Decompression of portal venous system occurs via systemic collaterals.
    - Coronary vein to azygos or hemiazygos veins: esophageal varices
    - SMV/IMV to iliac veins: mesenteric varices, stomal varices
    - IMV to inferior hemorrhoidal veins: hemorrhoids
    - Umbilical vein to epigastric veins: caput medusae
    - Splenic vein to azygos veins: gastric fundal varices
    - Splenic vein to retroperitoneal veins: duodenal/retroperitoneal varices

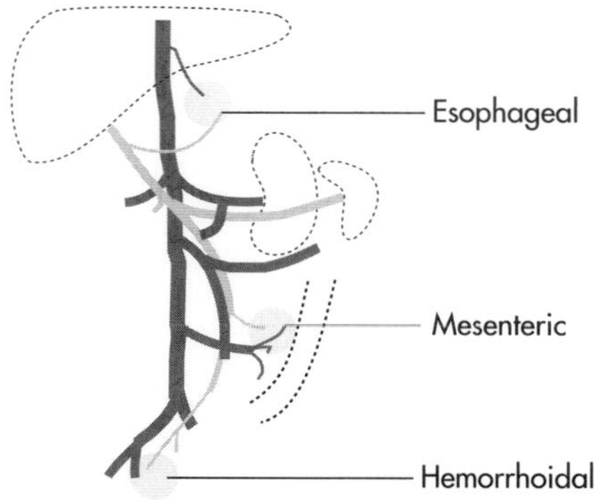

FIGURE 8-33

Radiographic Features

US
- Recanalized umbilical vein or hepatofugal flow is diagnostic.
- Always demonstrate portal and splenic vein patency to determine treatment options.
- Portal collaterals
- Splenomegaly
- Ascites

Angiography
- Elevated portal pressure
    - Corrected sinusoidal pressure (CSP) = hepatic wedge pressure – IVC pressure
    - CSP < 5 mm Hg is normal.
    - Direct portal vein pressure <5 mm Hg is normal.

SURGICAL SHUNT TYPES

Shunt Type	Use
Portacaval	
Portal vein → IVC	Performed for immediate decompression
Splenorenal	
Splenic vein → renal vein	—
Warren (distal)	Common elsewhere
Linton (proximal)	Common at MGH
Mesocaval	
SMV → IVC	—

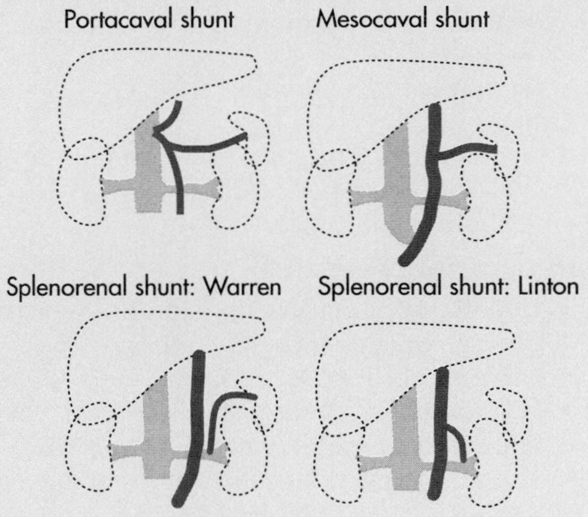

- Portal flow away from liver
- Portosystemic collaterals or varices
- Corkscrew hepatic arteries
- Always exclude presinusoidal and postsinusoidal causes.

Treatment

- TIPS is the treatment of choice after conventional endoscopic techniques fail to control bleeding.
- Variceal embolization is adjunctive.
- Surgical portosystemic shunts

PORTAL VEIN THROMBOSIS

Causes

- Idiopathic (most common)
- Tumor (HCC, pancreatic cancer, metastases)
- Postoperative (splenectomy transplant)
- Blood dyscrasias
- Coagulopathies
- Sepsis, pylephlebitis
- Pancreatitis
- Cirrhosis, portal hypertension

Complications

- Hepatic infarction
- Bleeding varices
- Mesenteric thrombosis
- Presinusoidal portal hypertension

Radiographic Features

US

- Best screening imaging modality
- Thrombus appears echogenic
- Collaterals and varices

CT

- Hyperdense thrombus on noncontrast CT
- Low-density filling defect on contrast CT
- Cavernous transformation: occurs in setting of subacute/chronic portal vein thrombosis: multiple portal tubular collaterals are present in porta hepatis

MRI

- T1 hyperintense portal vein thrombus
- Numerous portal flow voids (collaterals)

Angiography

- May be treated with intraarterial (SMA) or portal venous thrombolysis

Splenic Vein Occlusion (Isolated)

- Segmental portal hypertension with gastric fundal varices
- Esophageal varices are absent.
- Normal portal venous pressure
- Cannot be treated by TIPS

BUDD-CHIARI SYNDROME (BCS)

Obstruction of hepatic venous outflow resulting in hepatic enlargement, portal hypertension with varices, and ascites. Venous obstruction may be at the level of intrahepatic venules, the hepatic veins, or the IVC.

Causes

Hepatic vein thrombosis

- Hematologic disorders
- Coagulopathies
- Pregnancy

- Oral contraceptives
- Phlebitis
- Idiopathic

Tumor growth in hepatic veins and/or IVC
- Renal cell carcinoma
- HCC
- Adrenal carcinoma

Other
- IVC membrane or web (common in Asians)
- Constrictive pericarditis
- Right atrial tumor

Radiographic Features
- Hepatic venography and inferior venacavography are diagnostic studies of choice
- Spider web hepatic veins
- IVC narrowing ("steeple" or "pencil point" configuration of intrahepatic IVC) or webs
- Stretched, straight hepatic arteries on arteriography

Treatment
- Temporize with TIPS
- Ultimately may require transplantation

KIDNEYS

ANATOMY

Arteries (Fig. 8-34)

Single vessel, 65%; multiple vessels, 35% (aberrant vascular supply is common in malrotated or horseshoe kidneys). Branches of renal artery:
- Anterior and posterior divisions
- Segmental arteries (5 segments)
- Interlobar arteries (each supplies one renal column)
- Arcuate arteries → interlobular arteries → afferent glomerular arterioles

Variants
- Gonadal arteries arise from renal arteries in 20%.
- Inferior phrenic artery may occasionally arise from renal artery.

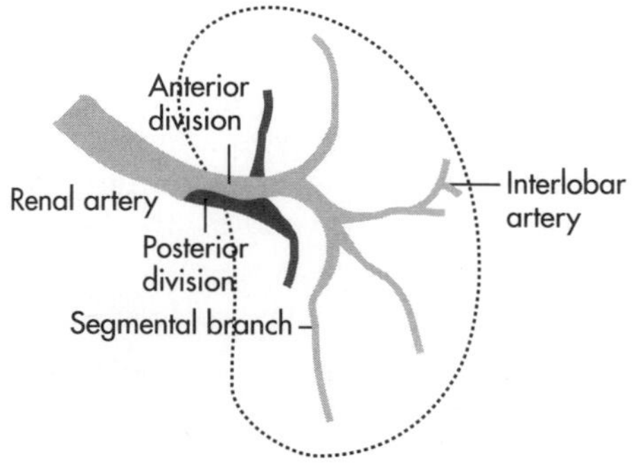

FIGURE 8-34

- Inferior adrenal arteries often arise from renal artery.

Veins
- Left renal vein is 3 times longer than the right; therefore, the left kidney is used for transplants.
- Left renal vein passes anterior to the aorta (3% retroaortic) and inferior to the SMA.
- Left renal vein receives left adrenal and gonadal veins.
- Multiple renal veins in 35%

INDICATIONS FOR RENAL ANGIOGRAPHY

Diagnostic Renal Arteriography
- Renovascular hypertension (detection of renal artery stenosis)
- Trauma
  - AVF or pseudoaneurysm
  - Traumatic bleeding, hematuria
  - Devascularization injury
- Tumors (determine vascular supply)
- Transplant donors
  - Number and location of renal arteries
  - Complicating normal variants
  - Detect unsuspected pathology

Renal Venography
- Renin sampling in renovascular hypertension
- Diagnosis of renal vein thrombosis
- Evaluation for tumor extension into IVC or renal veins
- Unexplained hematuria (renal varices)

Angiographic Interventions
- Renovascular hypertension: PTA or stents
- Embolization
  - Preoperative tumor embolization to reduce blood loss
  - Aneurysm
  - Posttraumatic AVF
  - Active bleeding (trauma, iatrogenic causes)

RENAL ARTERY STENOSIS (RAS) (Fig. 8-35)

Significant clinical entity because it is a potentially treatable cause of hypertension and, when advanced, of renal insufficiency. Renal artery stenosis may cause hyperreninemic HTN. Not all patients with RAS have HTN (thus, RAS is not synonymous with renovascular HTN).

Causes
- Atherosclerosis, 70%
- FMD, 25%
- NF
- Arteritis
  - Takayasu arteritis
  - Polyarteritis nodosa

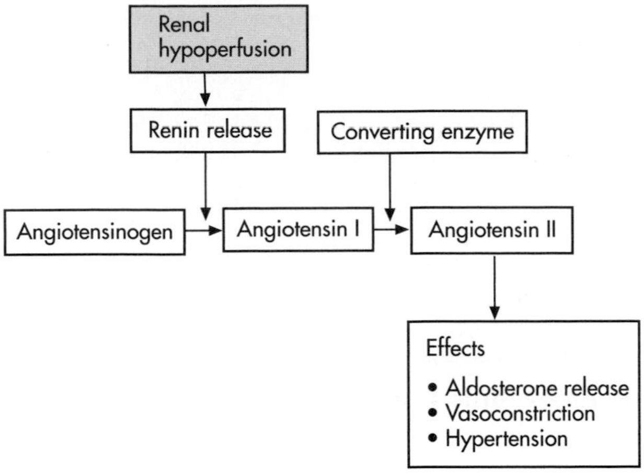

FIGURE 8-35

Abdominal aortic coarctation
- Other
  - Radiation therapy
  - Aortic dissection
  - Pheochromocytoma

Radiographic Features

- Radionuclide scan is often the first imaging study (see Chapter 12).
- RAS is hemodynamically significant if there is/are:
  - Lumen stenosis of ≥ 50%
  - Peak systolic pressure gradient >15%
  - Poststenotic dilatation
  - Collaterals
- Renin vein sampling is helpful in some cases. Lateralizing renins (ratio >1.5:1) indicate that revascularization will be beneficial.
- Pitfalls in angiographic diagnosis of RAS
  - Renal artery spasm (pseudostenosis)
  - Standing waves may simulate FMD but unlike FMD do not persist.
  - Multiple views are usually required to unmask the entire renal artery.
- Renal MRA
  - In comparison with angiography, MRA has sensitivity and specificity of greater than 90% for detecting renal artery stenosis (>50%).
  - Technique:
    - Phased-array coils are typically used
    - Breathhold technique to avoid respiratory artifacts
    - Right arm vein preferred for IV access because this provides direct path to central circulation
    - Injector used: dose of gadolinium is 0.2 mmol/kg (~30 mL) with 40 mL of saline flush
    - Protocol: sagittal black-blood sequence; axial and coronal T2W, single-shot fast spin-echo sequence; coronal 3-D dynamic Gd acquisition repeated during arterial and venous phases (recommended matrix is 512 × 192, with 2- to 3-mm-thick slices zero filled down to 1 to 1.5 mm)
    - 3-D images reconstructed using MIP and volume rendering

RENAL ARTERY ATHEROSCLEROSIS

Most common cause of renovascular HTN. Occurs in older patients (over 50) and usually involves the proximal artery. Does not respond as well to percutaneous PTA as FMD does.

Radiographic Features (Fig. 8-36)

- Ostial stenosis is usually associated with aortic stenosis plaque.
  - Poor PTA response, 30% patency
  - Metallic stents might improve patency rates.
- Main renal artery stenoses: 80% respond to PTA.
- Distal and peripheral RAS may also occur
- Frequently bilateral
- Two indications for revascularization:
  - Control HTN
  - Preserve renal function

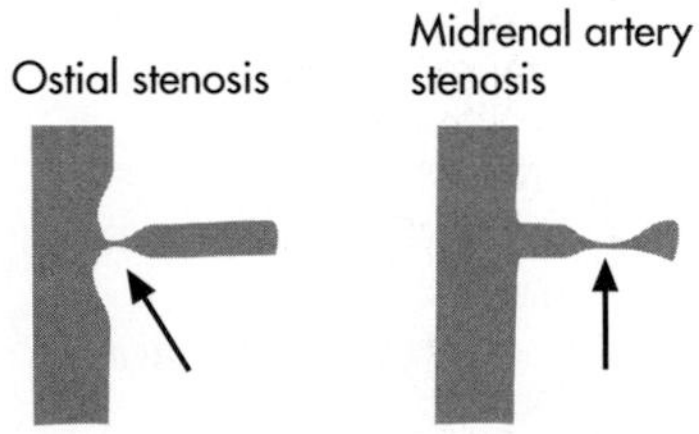

FIGURE 8-36

FIBROMUSCULAR DYSPLASIA (FMD)

Proliferation of muscular and fibrous elements in middle-and large-sized arteries. Unknown etiology. Five types exist and are classified by the layers of the arterial wall involved.

- Intimal fibroplasia (rare)
- Medial fibroplasia: most common type, 85%; causes classic stenoses alternating with aneurysms
- Perimedial fibroplasia; no aneurysms
- Medial hyperplasia (rare)
- Periadventitial fibroplasia (rare)

Distribution

- Renal arteries, 60%: most common site
- ICA or vertebral arteries, 35%
- Iliac arteries, 3%
- Visceral arteries, 2%

Radiographic Features

- Most commonly located in middle and distal renal artery
- "String of beads" appearance most common (85%)
- Smooth stenoses less common (10%)
- Bilateral in 50%
- Excellent response to PTA (treatment of choice)

Pearls

- Most common cause of RAS in children
- Spontaneous renal artery dissection is due to FMD until proved otherwise.
- Always look for visceral vessel involvement and/or other aneurysms.
- Complications:
  - Spontaneous dissection
  - Aneurysm rupture, emboli
  - HTN
  - Renal insufficiency (rare)

RENAL ARTERIAL ANEURYSM

- FMD (common)
- Atherosclerosis (common)
- NF
- Angiomyolipoma
- Lymphangioleiomyomatosis
- Rare
  - Congenital
  - Inflammatory
  - Infectious
  - Posttraumatic

Intraparenchymal arterial aneurysm occurs in:

- Polyarteritis nodosa
- Speed kidney (amphetamine abuse)

POLYARTERITIS NODOSA (PAN)

Vasculitis of small- and medium-sized arteries. Autoimmune origin and associated with hepatitis B virus. Presents as systemic illness but renal manifestations are common: hematuria, hypertension, and perinephric hematoma.

Radiographic Features

- Multiple small aneurysms of interlobar and arcuate arteries
- Aneurysms tend to be smaller and more peripheral than in FMD
- Renal infarctions
- Always evaluate visceral arteries.

RENAL VEIN THROMBOSIS

Most cases occur in children <2 years of age. Variable clinical presentation; many patients are asymptomatic.

Causes

Children
- Dehydration
- Sepsis
- Maternal diabetes

Adults
- Glomerulopathies (membranous type most common)
- Collagen vascular disease
- Diabetes
- Trauma
- Thrombophlebitis

Radiographic Features

IVP
- Poor or absent nephrogram
- Enlarged kidney
- Ureteral notching

US
- Cannot accurately diagnose partial thrombosis
- More accurate in pediatric than in adult patients

CT/MRI
- Helpful to depict thrombus in main renal vein segment

Venography
- Protruding thrombus or lack of inflow on cavogram
- Selective renal venography is the most definitive study.
- Left renal vein has more collaterals (gonadal, adrenal, ureteral).

Complications
- Pulmonary embolism
- Loss of renal function

SPLEEN

SPLENIC ARTERY ANEURYSM

Treat if >2.5 cm, pregnancy, symptomatic, rapidly expanding. May treat with coils placed proximal and distal to the aneurysm or exclude with stent graft.

Chest

GENERAL ANATOMY

PULMONARY ARTERIES (Fig. 8-37)

THORACIC VEINS (Figs. 8-38 and 8-39)

LIJV = left internal jugular vein
LEJV = left external jugular vein
LSCV = left subclavian vein
LTV = lateral thoracic vein
LSICV = left superior intercostal vein

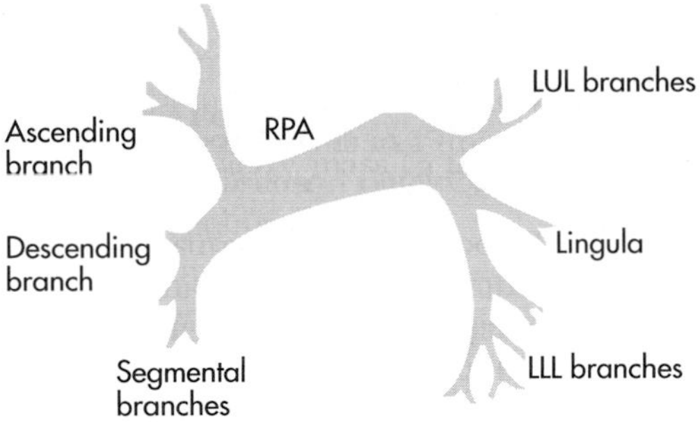

FIGURE 8-37

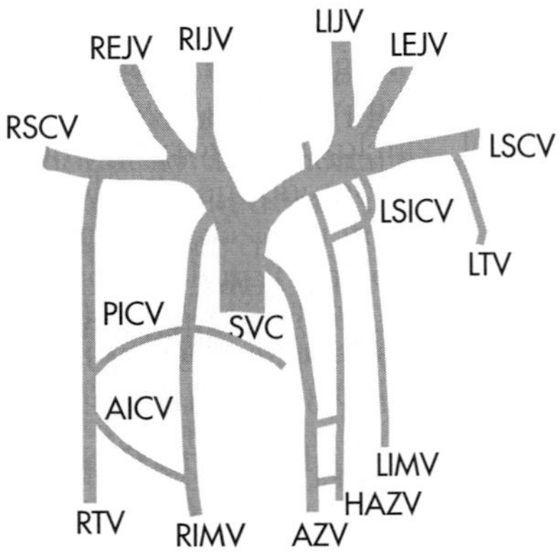

FIGURE 8-38

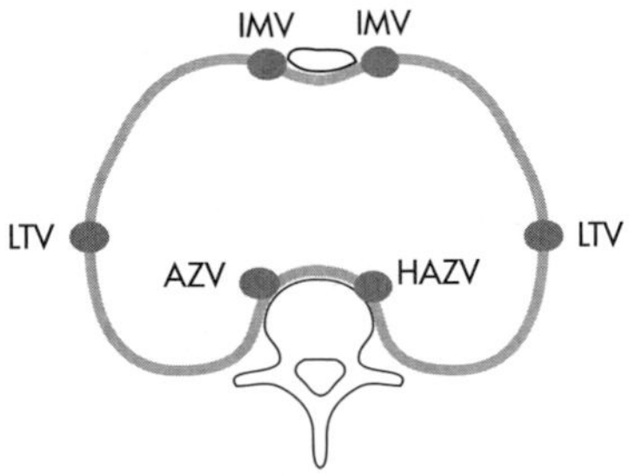

FIGURE 8-39

LIMV = left internal mammary vein
HAZV = hemiazygos vein
AZV = azygos vein
RIJV = right internal jugular vein
REJV = right external jugular vein
RSCV = right subclavian vein
PICV = posterior intercostal vein
AICV = anterior intercostal vein
RTV = right thoracic vein
RIMV = right internal mammary vein
SVC = superior vena cava
Left-sided SVC: More often duplicated SVC than isolated; drains into coronary sinus > left atrium. Associated with CHD.

ANGIOGRAPHIC TECHNIQUES

PULMONARY ANGIOGRAPHY

CATHETERS

Type	Comment
Pigtail	Requires tip-deflecting device; maintains a stable position during high-volume injections
Grollman	Secondary multipurpose curvature obviates need for tip-deflecting device
NIH catheter	Perforations possible
Balloon float catheter	Whips back with contrast injection because of floppiness

Indications

- Suspected pulmonary thromboembolism
- Diagnosis and treatment of pulmonary pseudoaneurysms and AVM
- Workup of pulmonary arterial hypertension

Technique

- Common femoral vein lies medial to artery
- Hand injection of IVC (cavogram) is performed to exclude IVC thrombus.
- Tip deflector directs catheter into right ventricle. Inability to advance the wire from the RA into the RV can be due to primary placement in the coronary sinus.
- Ventricular ectopy is common when catheter is in RV.
- Tip deflector is needed to catheterize right PA but usually not left PA.
- Measure pulmonary arterial pressures.
- Hand-inject contrast agent to evaluate flow rate.
- Views
  Right: PA and RPO magnified base
  Left: PA and LPO magnified base
  Additional views as needed
- Always pull catheter back through heart under fluoroscopy.

PULMONARY PRESSURES

Location	$P_{systolic}$	$P_{diastolic}$	P_{mean}
RA	—	—	0-5 mm Hg
RV	20-25 mm Hg	0-7 mm Hg	
PA	20-25 mm Hg	8-12 mm Hg	15 mm Hg
LA	—	—	5-10 mm Hg
LV	110-130 mm Hg	5-12 mm Hg	
Aorta	110-130 mm Hg	75-85 mm Hg	100 mm Hg

Pearls

- Pulmonary hypertension: mean PA pressure >15 mm Hg, systolic >30 mm Hg

- All injections should be selective or subselective.
- Arterial flow with fluoroscopic hand injection determines rate of injection.
  - Normal flow: 22 mL/sec for 44 mL total
  - Slow flow: reduce injection rate.
  - Fast flow: increase injection rate up to 30 mL/sec for 60 mL total.
- No absolute contraindications
- Relative contraindications:
  - Severe pulmonary hypertension
  - LBBB (catheter irritation may induce RBBB → complete heart block)—place transvenous pacemaker
  - CHF

Complications

- Acute right-sided heart failure (in pulmonary arterial hypertension)
- Cardiac arrhythmias
- Death, <0.3%

BRONCHIAL ARTERIOGRAPHY (Fig. 8-40)

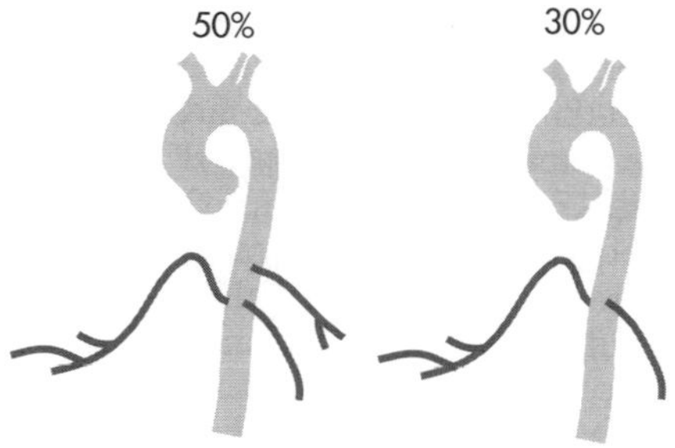

FIGURE 8-40

Indication

Hemoptysis, usually in patients with TB, cystic fibrosis, carcinoma.

Technique

- Descending thoracic aortogram is initially obtained as a road map.
- 90% of bronchial arteries originate from T4-T7 posterolaterally.
- Selective catheterization with Cobra or Simmons catheters
- DSA is preferred over cut film.
- Embolization may be performed if active hemorrhage is present.

Complications

- Spinal cord injury
- Pain

BRONCHIAL ARTERY EMBOLIZATION

Indication

Hemoptysis. Massive hemoptysis defined as >300 mL/day.

Technique

- Right femoral artery approach
- Descending aortogram to document takeoff of bronchial arteries
- Simmons, Cobra, or Berenstein for selective catheterization
- Use tracker to superselect bleeding vessel
- Use polyvinyl alcohol or Gelfoam. Proximal coil embolization not desired as may impair future treatments.
- Beware collaterals from internal mammary, intercostal, lateral thoracic, thyrocervical trunk, inferior phrenic arteries.
- Systemic antibiotics are usually given.

Complications

- Reflux of embolization material
- Spinal artery injury, paralysis (characteristic hairpin loop appearance of spinal artery branch)

PULMONARY THROMBOEMBOLISM

Pulmonary embolism (PE) is a common complication of DVT. Despite the extrapolative and speculative nature of the medical literature concerning PE, a few generalizations apply.

- PE has high morbidity and mortality if not treated.
- Treatment significantly reduces morbidity and mortality.
- Subclinical PE is common and goes unrecognized.
- The clinical presentation of PE is most commonly nonspecific.
- Risk factors play an important role in the development of PE.
- Pulmonary arteriography is the gold standard for the detection of PE.

One or more preliminary diagnostic examinations are usually performed (Fig. 8-41):

- Chest radiograph
  - Exclude other causes of signs/symptoms (e.g., pneumonia)
  - Triage to $\dot{V}/\dot{Q}$ scan/ CT
  - Required to optimally interpret $\dot{V}/\dot{Q}$ scan
- CTA: becoming the first line of examination in the diagnosis of PE
- $\dot{V}/\dot{Q}$ scan (see Chapter 12)
  - Useful with "clear" CXR
- Venous US

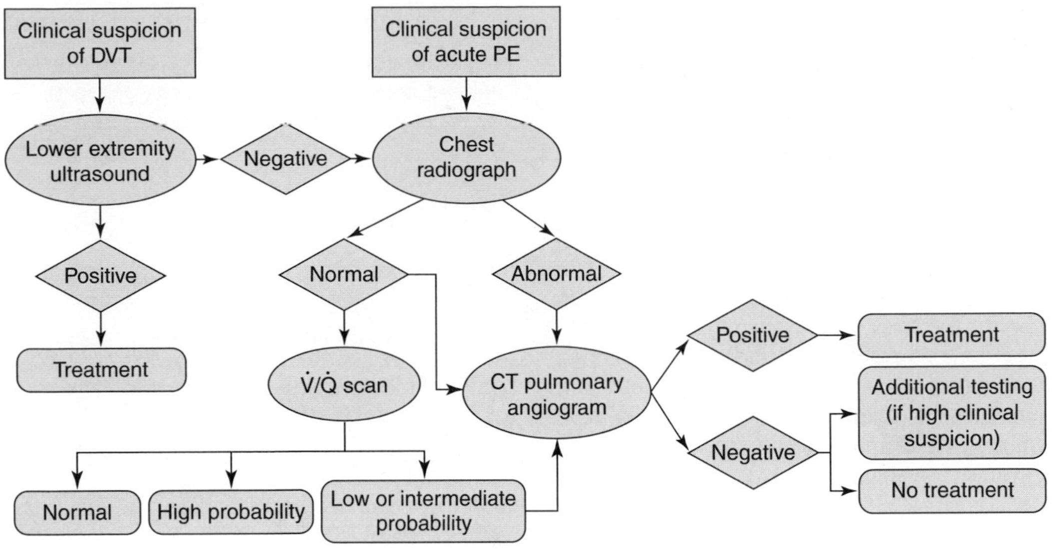

FIGURE 8-41

- Used to diagnose underlying DVT

Suggested diagnostic algorithm for suspected pulmonary embolism

Risk Factors (same as for DVT)

- Postoperative patients, especially neurosurgical, orthopedic, and gynecologic
- Trauma and burn patients
- Malignancy
- History of PE or DVT
- Immobility
- Obesity
- Congestive heart failure
- Neurologic event
- Hormonal:
  - Hormone therapy
  - Oral contraceptives
  - Pregnancy
- Coagulopathies, blood dyscrasias:
  - Lupus anticoagulant
  - Protein C, protein S, or antithrombin III deficiency
  - Polycythemia vera

CT Pulmonary Angiography (CTPA)

Direct findings of PE

- Direct visualization of filling defect
- Vessel cutoff sign: distal artery is not opacified due to occlusive embolus
- Occluded artery is larger than the normal artery on the opposite side
- Partial occlusion can cause rim sign on axial and tramtrack sign on long axis view

Indirect findings of PE

- Pulmonary hemorrhage; usually resolves in a week
- Pulmonary infarction in lower lobes; wedge-shaped peripheral areas of consolidation with central low attenuation areas that do not enhance and represent uninfarcted secondary pulmonary lobules
- Air bronchograms typically not seen in areas of infarction
- Vascular sign; acute embolus in a dilated vessel leading to apex of consolidation
- Linear parenchymal bands
- Focal oligemia
- Atelectasis
- Small pleural effusion
- Dilatation of right ventricle from strain

Artifacts that mimic acute PE

- Respiratory motion artifact can mimic filling defect in vessels
- Poor contrast opacification of pulmonary arteries due to poor cardiac function
- A soft tissue reconstruction algorithm should be used to avoid high attenuation around vessels that may mimic PE
- Lymph nodes in the intersegmental region can be confused for emboli
- Low-density mucus-filled bronchi and pulmonary veins might also mimic filling defects

INDICATIONS FOR PERFORMING PULMONARY ANGIOGRAPHY

Performed when noninvasive diagnostic tests (CTA, ultrasound, $\dot{V}/\dot{Q}$ scan) are inconclusive.

Prior $\dot{V}/\dot{Q}$ scan

- Intermediate or indeterminate $\dot{V}/\dot{Q}$ scan

- Discrepancy between $\dot{V}/\dot{Q}$ scan and clinical assessment (e.g., low-probability scan and high clinical suspicion)

Without $\dot{V}/\dot{Q}$ scan

- Complex therapeutic issues
- Hemodynamically unstable patient (may need embolectomy, lysis, etc.)
- Contraindication to anticoagulation
- A high likelihood of having a nondiagnostic $\dot{V}/\dot{Q}$ scan

RADIOGRAPHIC FEATURES

Acute PE

- Embolus seen as intraluminal filling defect
- Tramtracking of contrast
- Abrupt cutoff of artery
- "Missing" vessels
- Angiographic findings do not always correlate with signs, symptoms, or $\dot{V}/\dot{Q}$ scan findings.

Chronic PE

- Eccentric filling defects: "muralized" embolus
- Synechia or webs
- Smooth cut-offs
- "Missing" vessels
- Elevated pulmonary arterial pressures

OTHER PULMONARY VASCULAR DISEASES

PULMONARY ARTERIOVENOUS MALFORMATION (AVM) OR FISTULA (AVF)

Most patients with pulmonary AVM/AVF are asymptomatic. Symptoms depend on size and number of lesions and when present include epistaxis, dyspnea, cyanosis, and clubbing. Paradoxical embolization: CVA, brain abscess.

Causes

Congenital

- Isolated, 50%
- Osler-Weber-Rendu syndrome, 50%

Acquired

- Trauma
- Infection
- Hepatogenic angiodysplasia

Radiographic Features

CT, CXR

- Lung mass or nodule with feeding artery and draining vein angiography
- Most lesions are direct AVFs
- Lesions may be embolized with coils.

Multiple in 35%

Most lesions occur in lower lobes.

May be treated with transcatheter embolization with coils or Amplatzer occluder.

PULMONARY ARTERY PSEUDOANEURYSM

Posttraumatic or iatrogenic pseudoaneurysms are most common cause. Hemoptysis occurs. Treatment is with transcatheter embolization (coils).

Extremities

ANATOMY

LOWER EXTREMITY ARTERIES

Branches (Fig. 8-42)

Common femoral artery (CFA)

- Superficial femoral artery (SFA)
- Profunda femoral artery (PFA)
  - Medial circumflex artery
  - Lateral circumflex artery
  - Descending branch

Popliteal artery

- Superior and inferior medial and lateral genicular arteries
- Anterior tibial artery: first trifurcation
- Posterior tibial artery
- Peroneal artery

Foot (Fig. 8-43)

- Dorsal arteries (from anterior tibial artery): dorsalis pedis
  - Medial and lateral malleolar artery
  - Arcuate artery → metatarsal arteries → digital arteries
- Plantar arteries (from posterior tibial)
  - Medial and lateral malleolar arteries
  - Medial and lateral plantar → plantar arch → metatarsal arteries → digital arteries

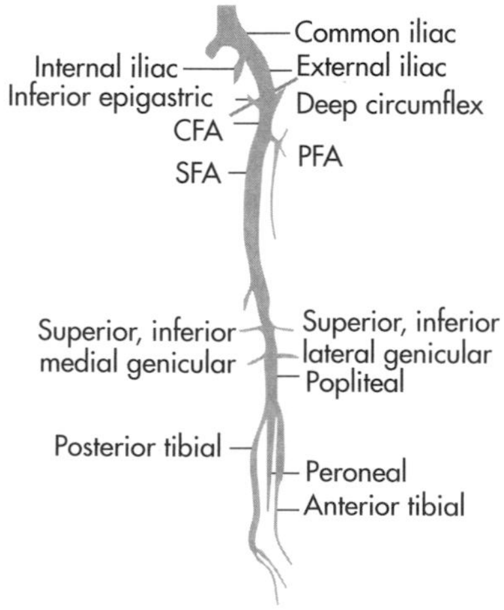

FIGURE 8-42

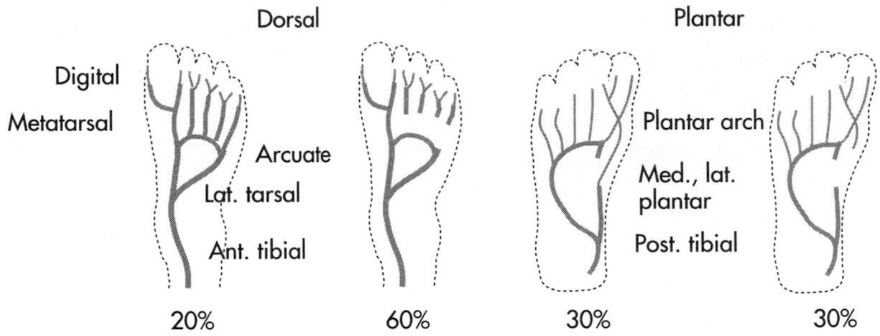

FIGURE 8-43

Collaterals

Collaterals develop in the setting of occlusive iliac and lower extremity disease.

- Internal mammary artery → inferior epigastric artery → CFA
- Lumbar/iliolumbar artery → circumflex iliac artery → PFA
- Lumbar/iliolumbar artery → lateral circumflex artery→ PFA
- Gluteal/obturator artery → lateral and medial circumflex artery → PFA
- PFA branches
- Geniculate branches

Persistent Sciatic Artery

- An embryonic sciatic artery remains the dominant flow inflow vessel to the leg; rare
- The aberrant vessel comes off the internal iliac artery, passes through the greater sciatic foramen, and runs deep to the gluteus maximus muscle.
- The aberrant artery joins the popliteal artery above the knee.
- The anomaly is usually bilateral.
- The artery is prone to intimal injury and aneurysm formation in the ischial region, owing to its superficial location.

LOWER EXTREMITY VEINS (Fig. 8-44)

Calf veins are duplicated and follow the course of the arteries.

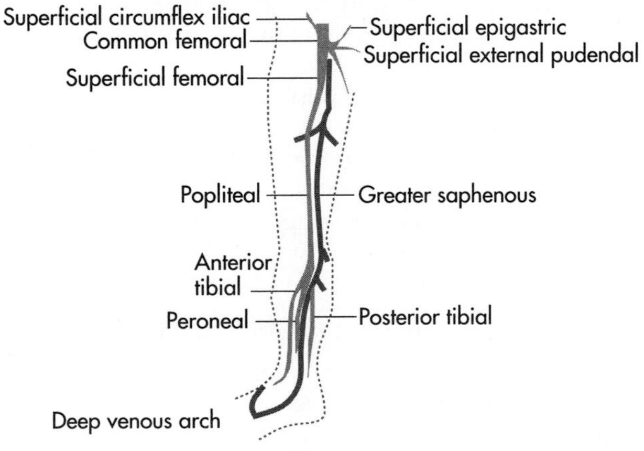

FIGURE 8-44

Common femoral vein
- Profunda vein
- Superficial femoral vein (receives blood from deep system via popliteal veins)

Deep calf system
- Anterior tibial veins (small)
- Peroneal veins
- Posterior tibial veins

Superficial calf system
- Greater saphenous vein (medial)
- Lesser saphenous veins (posterior calf)
- Many superficial collaterals connect the 2 saphenous veins.

UPPER EXTREMITY ARTERIES (Fig. 8-45)

Branches

Subclavian artery
- Vertebral artery
- Internal mammary artery
- Thyrocervical trunk
- Costocervical artery

Axillary artery
- Supreme thoracic artery
- Thoracoacromial artery
- Lateral thoracic artery

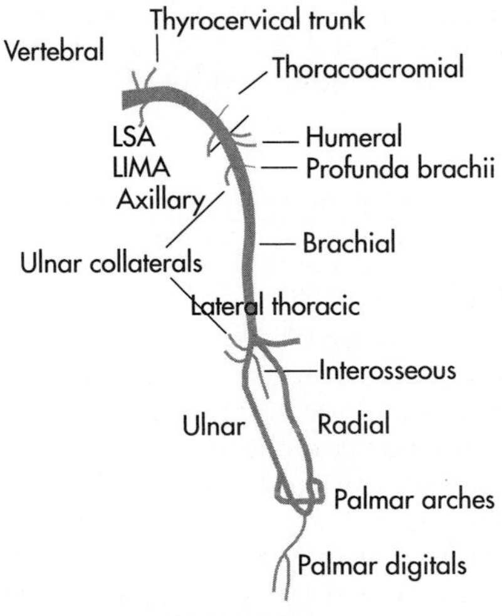

FIGURE 8-45

- Subscapular artery
- Humeral circumflex arteries

Brachial artery
- Profunda brachial artery
- Radial artery
- Ulnar artery
- Ulnar collaterals

Forearm
- Radial artery
  - Deep palmar arch
- Ulnar artery
  - Recurrent ulnar arteries
  - Common interosseous artery
  - Superficial palmar arch
  - Wrist, hand
- Deep palmar arch
- Superficial palmar arch

LOWER EXTREMITY

LOWER EXTREMITY OCCLUSIVE DISEASE

CAUSE OF LOWER EXTREMITY OCCLUSIVE DISEASE BY AGE

Younger Patients
Inflammatory diseases
Takayasu arteritis
Collagen vascular disease, autoimmune diseases, Buerger disease
Older Patients
Atherosclerosis
Embolism
Drugs
Ergotism (long, smooth narrowing)
Amphetamine: speed kidney
Other
Spasm due to trauma (standing waves)
Popliteal artery entrapment
Radiation

ATHEROSCLEROTIC OCCLUSIVE DISEASE

Intimal plaque formation leads to symptoms that depend on:
- Specific artery involved
- Severity of disease (degree of stenosis, multifocality)
- Superimposed complications:
  - Plaque ulceration or subintimal hemorrhage
  - Acute thrombosis
  - Distal embolization

Sudden changes in symptomatology usually indicate an acute complication.

Clinical presentation is variable:
- Diminished pulses
- Claudication
- Hair loss, skin changes
- Tissue loss
- Rest pain
- "Cadaveric extremity:" pale, paralyzed, pulseless, painful
- Gangrene

Risk factors for atherosclerosis of extremities are the same as those for atherosclerosis elsewhere:
- Diabetes
- Hypertension
- Smoking
- Genetic predisposition, family history
- Hypercholesterolemia

Radiographic Features

- Atherosclerotic disease is usually symmetrical and commonly affects arterial bifurcations.
- Location of involvement: SFA > iliac artery > tibial artery > popliteal artery > CFA
- Suspect diabetes if tibioperoneal disease > femoral arteries; profunda femoris > SFA
- Role of arteriography:
  - Preoperative staging
  - Percutaneous intervention: PTA, stent, atherectomy, lysis
- Assess hemodynamic significance of stenosis:
  - >50% narrowing of luminal diameter
  - Presence of collaterals
  - Peak systolic pressure gradient across lesion >10 mm Hg
- Role of MRA is still in evolution.
- May perform limited DSA runoff using gadolinium chelate as contrast agent

Treatment

Angiographic (often used in conjunction with surgery)
- PTA
- Metallic stents (kissing stents if extends to aortoiliac junction)
- Atherectomy (less commonly used)

Surgical
- In situ autologous saphenous vein graft
- Reversed vein graft
- Synthetic (polytetrafluoroethylene) grafts: usually not used below the knee
- Xenografts are no longer used.
- Endarterectomy
- Amputation

ATHEROSCLEROTIC ANEURYSMAL DISEASE

Atherosclerosis in extremities may result in aneurysmal as well as occlusive disease. Location: popliteal artery (most common) > iliac artery > femoral artery. Frequently associated with AAA.

Clinical Findings

- Popliteal aneurysm: Most common peripheral arterial aneurysm. 50% of aneurysms are bilateral, and 80% are associated with aneurysm elsewhere. Commonly due to atherosclerotic disease or trauma. Angiography may show luminal dilatation or mural calcification. 25% of popliteal artery aneurysms may not be associated with visible arterial dilatation by angiography. In these cases, secondary signs such as the "dog-leg sign" (acute bend in lumen of the popliteal artery) may be helpful. Complications of aneurysm include distal embolization and thrombosis, resulting in ischemia. Rupture is uncommon.
- Iliac aneurysms have a high incidence of rupture. Nearly all cases are associated with AAA.
- Common femoral aneurysm: distal embolization and/or thrombosis

ARTERIOMEGALY

- Diffusely enlarged vessels without focal aneurysms
- Usually in aortoiliac and femoral-popliteal systems
- Sluggish flow

ARTERIAL THROMBOEMBOLISM

Results in acute arterial occlusion and threatened limb. Clinical "5 Ps:" pain, pallor, pulselessness, paresthesias, paralysis. Minimizing time from diagnosis to intervention is crucial to prevent limb loss.

Causes

- Cardiac: mural thrombus (most common)
    - Ventricular aneurysm
    - Myocardial infarction
    - Atrial fibrillation
- Aneurysms
- Iatrogenic
- Paradoxical embolus (DVT and right-to-left shunt)

Radiographic Features

- Multiple lesions
- Emboli frequently lodge at bifurcations.
- Lack of collateral vessels
- Severe vasospasm
- Filling defects with menisci
- Bilateral lesions

Treatment

- Surgical embolectomy
- Always differentiate arterial thromboembolism from in situ thrombosis secondary to atherosclerosis because therapy is different.

BUERGER DISEASE

Nonnecrotizing panarteritis of unknown etiology (thromboangiitis obliterans); venous involvement occurs in 25%. Nearly all patients are smokers, and 98% are male. Age: 20 to 40 years. Claudication is common. Associated with migratory thrombophlebitis. Treatment: smoking cessation (arrests but does not reverse process).

Location

- Calf and foot vessels (most common)
- Ulnar and radial arteries
- Palmar and digital arteries

Radiographic Features

- Abrupt segmental arterial occlusions
- Intervening normal-appearing arteries
- Multiple corkscrew collaterals
- Sparing of larger inflow arteries (e.g., iliac, femoral arteries)
- More than 1 limb affected. Lower extremity > upper extremity.

SMALL VESSEL ATHEROSCLEROSIS

Pattern of atherosclerosis in diabetics, with preponderance of calf and foot involvement. High frequency of gangrene requiring amputation.

CHOLESTEROL OR ATHEROMA EMBOLI

Microemboli to distal small arteries result in painful ischemic digits, livedo reticularis, "blue-toe syndrome," and/or irreversible renal insufficiency. Source of emboli is most commonly atherosclerotic plaque from more proximal arteries. Emboli may occur spontaneously or after catheterization.

ERGOTISM

Bilateral, symmetrical, diffuse, and severe vasospasm. Primarily seen in young females on ergot medications for migraines. Reversible after discontinuation of medication.

POSTCATHETERIZATION GROIN COMPLICATIONS

Iatrogenic complications of femoral artery catheterization include most commonly:

- Hematoma
- Pseudoaneurysm
- AVF

Risk Factors

- Anticoagulation
- Large catheters or sheaths
- Inadequate compression
- Poor access technique

Radiographic Features

- US is the imaging study of choice to evaluate the patient for complications.
- Hematoma: mass of variable echogenicity. No color flow within hematoma.
- Pseudoaneurysm:
  - Communicates with femoral artery
  - Swirling flow in pseudoaneurysm ("yin-yang") by color Doppler
  - To-and-fro flow at site of communication by pulse wave Doppler
  - Compression thrombosis with US transducer
  - May be treated with percutaneous injection of thrombin by US guidance (prefer narrow neck, inject body not neck of PSA)
- AVF:
  - More common with low entries (artery on top of vein)
  - Arterialized flow in the vein
  - Loss of high-resistance triphasic arterial waveform
  - Low-resistance diastolic flow in artery

MAY-THURNER SYNDROME

Compression of left common iliac vein by crossing of the right common iliac artery. Angiography may demonstrate lumbar collaterals. Treatment: stent.

UTERINE ARTERY EMBOLIZATION

Alternative to surgery for symptomatic uterine fibroids of any size; also indicated for postpartum hemorrhage. Results in more rapid recovery and a shorter period for pain control than those achieved with surgery.

- Embolize uterine arteries with particles (e.g., PVA). All fibroids are treated at once. Normal myometrium is unharmed because it is supplied by multiple collateral arteries. Results in gradual shrinkage of fibroids (64%-93% relief after 3 months, 91%-92% after 1 year).
- Effect on fertility uncertain and may precipitate menopause, so perform only in women over childbearing age.
- Preoperative MRI with follow-up MRI in 6 months to assess size of fibroid. May be useful in adenomyosis.
- Failed treatment may be due to incomplete embolization of uterine arteries (spasm may be mistaken for stasis during microsphere delivery) or collateral supply from ovarian arteries.

ENDOVENOUS LASER TREATMENT (EVLT) OF VARICOSE VEINS

Minimally invasive treatment of greater saphenous vein and saphenofemoral junction varicose veins. Thermal destruction of the venous tissues is by means of an 810-nm diode laser along the course of the vein.

- Performed under local anesthesia and US guidance
- Entry point just above or below the knee
- Seldinger technique with long introducer sheath (25 to 45 cm)
- Diluted local anesthetic injected into the tissues surrounding the greater saphenous vein within the fascial sheath
- Postprocedure compression reduces bruising and tenderness, risk of DVT
- Follow-up with US at 1 week should show closure of vessels.

DEEP VEIN THROMBOSIS (DVT)

Lower extremity DVT is a medically important disease because it is the source of PE in 90% and because a high morbidity is associated with postphlebitic syndrome. Risk factors are related to Virchow's triad: stasis, hypercoagulability, and venous injury. Most DVT begin in the calf.

Locations

- Femoral-popliteal veins
- Pelvic veins
- Calf veins
- Intramuscular branches

Radiographic Features (Figs. 8-46, *A* and *B*, and 8-47, *A* and *B*)

- US is the initial imaging study of choice for studying femoral-popliteal veins and has a high sensitivity (93%) and specificity (98%) for DVT.
- US is not nearly as accurate in calf or iliac veins.
- Dynamic compression US criteria:

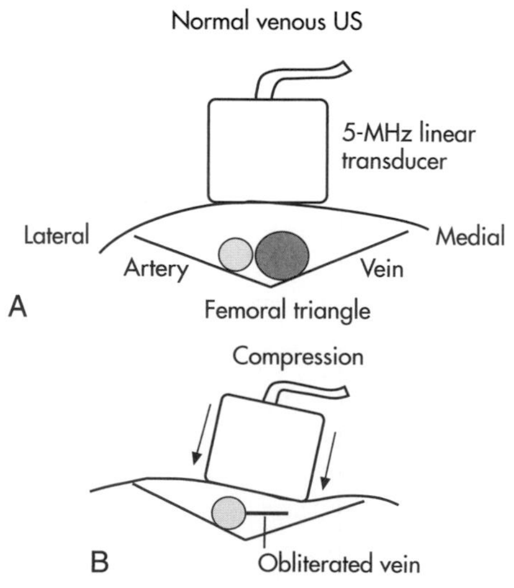

FIGURE 8-46

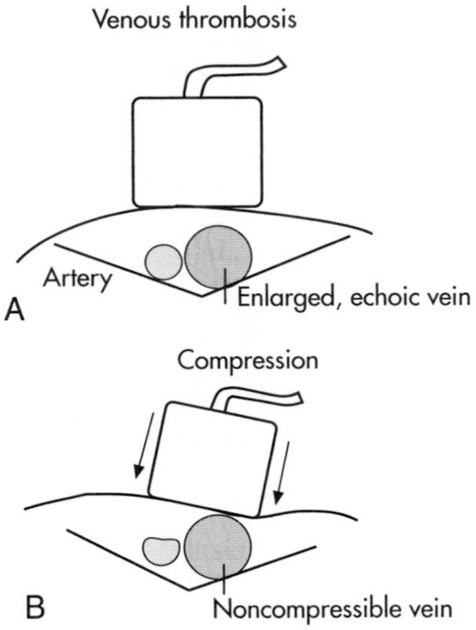

FIGURE 8-47

Noncompressibility of vein (loss of "wink" sign)
Echogenic lumen
Enlarged vein

- Color Doppler allows differentiation of occlusive and nonocclusive thrombi.
- Indirect iliac evaluation is possible by evaluating the pulse wave Doppler form. The waveform changes with respiration, augmentation, and Valsalva.
- US "misses":
  - DVT in small veins (e.g., calf)
  - DVT of intramuscular veins
  - Profunda femoral vein
  - Iliac thrombus
  - Acute DVT superimposed on chronic venous disease
- Venography is used when US is not definitive (Fig. 8-48).
  - Superior evaluation of calf veins
  - Allows differentiation of acute from chronic thrombosis
- CTV from the caval bifurcation to the popliteal vein may be performed concurrently with pulmonary CTA and can increase the detection of thromboembolic disease.?

Pearls

- Traditionally, infrapopliteal calf DVT is usually not treated medically. However, it is often followed serially with US to determine if there is proximal extension that would require treatment.
- More recently, there has been a trend toward treating calf DVT to prevent postphlebitic syndrome; this concept, however, is evolving.

IVC FILTERS

Indications: DVT and/or PE and one of the following:

- Contraindication to anticoagulation
- Failure of anticoagulation
- Complications of anticoagulation
- Prophylaxis
  - Marginal cardiopulmonary reserve
  - Preoperative protection
  - Prophylactic filter placements are performed at some institutions; this indication is controversial, however.
- Documented DVT

Types

All filters have the same efficacy.

- Bird's nest (Cook) is the only filter to accommodate a "megacava" (>28-mm diameter); for > 40 mm diameter, may place filter into each common iliac vein
- Titanium or Stainless Steel Greenfield (Medi-Tech)
- LGM filter (Vena-Tech)
- Simon nitinol filter (Bard) has the smallest delivery system. May be placed via brachial vein.

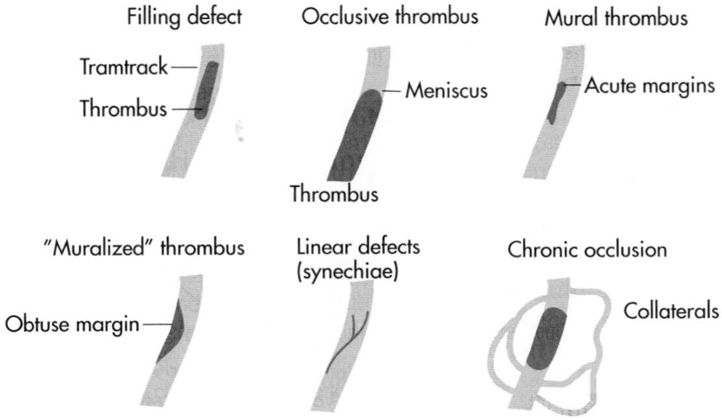

FIGURE 8-48

Technique

- Single-wall aspiration technique for right femoral vein
- IVC venogram is performed to document patency at level of renal veins (usually at L1-2), to determine cava diameter and establish that there is no preexisting IVC thrombus, and to assess variants: duplicated IVC (filters in both IVCs or suprarenal), circumaortic renal vein (place inferior to circumaortic renal vein or suprarenal vein), and retroaortic left renal vein (no change in placement).
- Consider placing suprarenal IVC filter in pregnancy or if duplicated IVC
- Because caval thrombosis is a complication of filter placement, filters are usually below the renal veins and only suprarenally in select cases.
- Large-bore left femoral vein introducer sheath

Complications

- Filter migration, <1%
- Filter failure (recurrent PE), 3%
- IVC thrombosis, 10%
- Groin complications
- PE after IVC filter may be due to filter thrombosis, collaterals, upper extremity DVT, or unrecognized left circumaortic renal vein

UPPER EXTREMITY

GENERAL

Diseases

- Atherosclerosis
- Vasculitis (Takayasu, giant cell arteritis)
- Emboli
- Trauma (stabbing, gunshot), iatrogenic (cardiac catheterization)
- Thoracic outlet syndrome

Technique

- Transfemoral angiographic approach is preferred.
  - More flexibility
  - Minimizes arterial spasm (also use spasmolytic drugs)
- Use LOCA to reduce pain and complications, especially to the carotid-vertebral system.
- Arch aortogram is obtained before selective work.
- Magnification, filtration, and subtraction are useful for hand arteriography.

THORACIC OUTLET SYNDROME

Compression of brachial plexus or subclavian vessels at the thoracic outlet. Three common sites of compression include:

- Scalene triangle
- Costoclavicular space
- Pectoralis tunnel

Causes

- Brachial plexus compression (most common), causing neurologic symptoms
- Subclavian artery: ischemia from distal emboli, claudication
- Subclavian vein thrombosis (any etiology)

SUBCLAVIAN STEAL SYNDROME

Stenoocclusive disease of the subclavian artery proximal to the vertebral artery, with reversal of flow in the vertebral artery. The syndrome should be reserved only for symptomatic steal, because steal phenomenon may be asymptomatic and incidentally identified on US.

- Transient neurologic deficits (dizziness, vertigo, visual changes, motor or sensory deficits, dysphasia) secondary to cerebral ischemia, characteristically caused by ipsilateral arm exercise (rare)
- Neck movement may provoke symptoms.
- In most patients, there is a clear provoking or reproducible event.
- Diagnosis: angiography, US, phase-contrast MRA
- Treatment: angioplasty, stent; surgery (carotid-subclavian bypass)

GIANT CELL ARTERITIS

- Classically bilateral axillary artery stenosis, DDx: radiation, crutch injury
- Treat with steroids

PRIMARY SUBCLAVIAN VEIN THROMBOSIS

Primary thrombosis is also known as spontaneous (or effort) thrombosis or Paget-Schroetter disease (treatment: anticoagulation or surgery; stent not effective). Thrombosis is caused by mechanical compression as the vein is impinged between the anterior scalene muscle, the first rib, and the subclavius tendon or the costoclavicular ligament.

Radiographic Features

- CXR may demonstrate cervical ribs, old fractures, etc.
- MRI is indicated if neurologic symptoms are present.
- Arteriography:
  - Subtle subclavian artery aneurysm (most common)
  - Mural thrombus
  - Distal emboli (forearm and hand)
  - Arterial stenosis
  - Arterial compression with hyperabduction

- Venography:
  - Dilatation or stenosis
  - Obstruction with hyperabduction

Treatment

For patients with thoracic outlet syndrome, an integrated approach that combines catheter-directed therapy with delayed surgery is now the accepted treatment and includes the following:

- Thrombolysis as initial treatment
- A short course of anticoagulation with warfarin (Coumadin)
- Conservative therapy when no extrinsic compression is detected after thrombolysis
- Surgical decompression for axillary or subclavian vein compression detected after thrombolysis
- Angioplasty or surgery for residual postoperative stenosis

HYPOTHENAR HAMMER SYNDROME

- Results from chronic repetitive trauma to the hand
- Trauma to distal ulnar artery as it crosses the hook of the hamate
- Aneurysm formation, occlusion, and distal embolization

AV FISTULAS FOR HEMODIALYSIS ACCESS

The ideal hemodialysis access is an endogenous arteriovenous fistula. Types

Native fistula
- Brescia-Cimino fistula is side-to-side anastomosis of radial artery and cephalic vein at the wrist
- Brachial artery and cephalic vein
- Brachial artery and basilic vein
- Femoral artery and saphenous vein

Synthetic bridge graft
- Manufactured out of PTFE
- Placed in forearm in straight configuration from radial artery to brachial vein or in looped configuration from brachial artery to brachial vein
- Can also be placed in upper-arm brachial or axillary artery to high brachial vein
- Can be used earlier than native fistulas
- Generally does not have the longevity of the native graft

Major Disorders for AV Fistulas

Failing dialysis graft
- Low flow rates or high recirculation at dialysis raises suspicion.
- Venous anastomotic stenosis; most likely to occur within first few centimeters of the anastomosis. Treated by dilatation with balloon angioplasty. Indications for stenting include restenosis, elastic recoil, and vein rupture.
- Arterial stenosis: responsible for graft failure in <15% of cases
- Intragraft stenosis is relatively uncommon.

Thrombosed dialysis graft
- In most cases, graft thrombosis occurs from progressive narrowing in the graft circuit (usually at the venous end). Treatment options: percutaneous therapy pulse spray pharmacomechanical thrombolysis (PSPMT), mechanical thrombectomy.

Ischemia and steal syndrome

TRAUMA

INDICATIONS FOR ANGIOGRAPHY IN EXTREMITY TRAUMA

- Blunt trauma with pulsatile bleeding, expanding hematoma, pulse deficits, digital ischemia, or a bruit or thrill at trauma site
- High-velocity missile
- Low-velocity missile and clinical findings (expanding hematoma, loss of pulses)
- Crush injury
- Iatrogenic trauma
- Reconstructive surgery planned (e.g., free flaps, bone grafts)

TRAUMATIC INJURIES

Many possible injuries can occur:
- Intimal tear: linear defect in lumen; may progress to pseudoaneurysm
- Pseudoaneurysm: may be amenable to transcatheter embolization
- Mural hematoma
- Laceration
- Transection
- Dissection
- AVF of early-draining vein
- Distal embolization: may occur from proximal injuries
- Vasospasm

Pearls

- All patients with posterior knee dislocations should undergo arteriography because of:
  - High incidence of popliteal artery injury and thrombosis
  - High rate of limb loss
- Hemorrhage secondary to pelvic fractures rarely requires arteriography.
- Vasospasm and compartment syndrome cannot be distinguished by arteriography in many instances.

Differential Diagnosis

GENERAL

ANEURYSM

Atherosclerosis
- Aorta
    - Abdominal aorta (most common)
    - Descending thoracic aorta
- Peripheral vasculature (popliteal > iliac > femoral)

Infection (mycotic)
- Bacterial *(Staphylococcus, Salmonella)*
- Syphilis

Inflammation
- Takayasu arteritis
- Giant cell arteritis
- Collagen vascular diseases
    - Polyarteritis nodosa

Congenital
- Structural collagen diseases
    - Marfan syndrome
    - Homocystinuria
    - Ehlers-Danlos syndrome
- Fibromuscular dysplasia
- Neurofibromatosis
- Pseudoxanthoma elasticum
    - Trauma

ISCHEMIA

Arterial
- Dissection
- Embolus
- Thrombosis, thrombosed aneurysm
- Vasculitis
- Drugs

Venous
- Thrombosis
    - Phlegmasia alba dolens: acute occlusion of deep system with venous stasis and edematous "white leg;" drainage through superficial system
    - Phlegmasia cerulean dolens: acute occlusion of deep and superficial systems, cyanosis. Arterial insufficiency may result in gangrene. Treat with thrombolysis.

Low flow
- Hypovolemia, shock
- Hypoperfusion

PERIPHERAL VASCULAR DISEASE

- Occlusive atherosclerosis
- Aneurysmal atherosclerosis
- Small vessel atherosclerosis (diabetics)
- Embolic disease
    - Thromboemboli
    - Cholesterol emboli
    - Plaque emboli
- Vasculitis
- Other
    - Buerger disease
    - Medication (e.g., ergot)

POPLITEAL "DOG-LEG" SIGN (ACUTE BEND IN THE LUMEN OF THE POPLITEAL ARTERY)

- Popliteal aneurysms (if bilateral, 80% also have AAA)
- Tortuous artery
- Popliteal artery entrapment syndrome (accentuated arterial narrowing with passive dorsiflexion or active plantar flexion at arteriography)
- Adventitial cystic disease (no flow on US)
- Baker's cyst (no flow on US)

EMBOLI

Cardiac emboli
- Atrial fibrillation
- Recent acute myocardial infarction
- Ventricular aneurysm
- Bacterial endocarditis
- Cardiac tumor (myxoma)

Atherosclerotic emboli
- Aortoiliac plaque
- Aneurysm (AAA, popliteal)

Paradoxical emboli (R-L shunt)
- DVT

ANGIOGRAPHIC TUMOR FEATURES

Mnemonic: "BEDPAN:"
- **B**lush
- **E**ncasement of arteries
- **D**isplacement of arteries
- **P**uddling of contrast
- **A**rteriovenous shunting
- **N**eovascularity

"MANY VESSELS"

DIFFERENTIATION OF HYPERVASCULAR LESIONS

	Early-Draining Vein	Mass Effect
Arteriovenous malformation	Yes	No (only in brain)
Extensive collaterals	No	No
Tumor neovascularity	Yes in AV shunting	Yes from tumor

THORAX

AORTIC ENLARGEMENT

- Aneurysm
- Dissection
- Poststenotic dilatation due to turbulence:

Coarctation
Aortic valvular disease
Sinus of Valsalva aneurysm

AORTIC STENOSIS

Congenital
- Coarctation
- Pseudocoarctation
- Williams syndrome (supravalvular aortic stenosis)
- Rubella syndrome

Aortitis
- Takayasu arteritis (most common arteritis to cause stenosis)

Other
- Neurofibromatosis
- Radiation

PULMONARY ARTERY STENOSIS

- Williams syndrome (infantile hypercalcemia)
- Rubella syndrome
- Takayasu arteritis
- Associated with congenital heart disease (especially tetralogy of Fallot)
- Fibrosing mediastinitis
- Radiation
- PE
- Extrinsic mass (tumor or nodes)

ASYMMETRICAL PULMONARY ARTERY ENLARGEMENT

- Pulmonary valve stenosis
- Pulmonary artery aneurysm

PULMONARY VENOUS HYPERTENSION

- Congenital narrowing of the pulmonary veins
- RF ablation
- Mediastinal fibrosis
- Left atrial obstruction

DIMINISHED PULMONARY ARTERY

- Hypoplasia
- Interruption of the pulmonary artery
- Bronchiolitis obliterans/Swyer-James
- PE

PULMONARY (PSEUDO)ANEURYSMS

- Swan-Ganz catheterization (most common)
- Infection
  TB (Rasmussen aneurysm), syphilis, fungus, bacteria
- Congenital heart disease
- Atherosclerosis
- Cystic medionecrosis
- Marfan syndrome

SUBCLAVIAN STEAL

- Atherosclerosis
- Takayasu arteritis
- Congenital
- Postsurgical
- Trauma
- NF1
- Radiation

SVC OBSTRUCTION

- Malignancy
- Radiation
- Central venous catheter
- Pacemaker

ABDOMEN

HYPERRENINEMIC HYPERTENSION

Decreased renal perfusion
- Atherosclerosis
- Fibromuscular dysplasia

Renin-secreting tumors
Renal compression
- Large intrarenal masses (cysts, tumors)
- Subcapsular hemorrhage (Page kidney)

RENAL TUMORS

Renal cell carcinoma
- 80% hypervascular
- Neovascularity
- AV shunting
- Parasitization

Angiomyolipoma
- Aneurysms
- Fat content

Oncocytoma
- Spokewheel, 30%
- Most hypovascular

RENAL ARTERIAL ANEURYSM

Main artery aneurysm
- FMD (common)
- Atherosclerosis (common)
- Neurofibromatosis
- Mycotic
- Trauma
- Congenital

Distal intrarenal aneurysms
- Polyarteritis nodosa
- IVDA (septic)
- Other vasculitides (Wegener granulomatosis, collagen vascular disease)
- Traumatic pseudoaneurysm
- Radiation therapy
- Amphetamine abuse (speed kidney)

SOFT TISSUE DENSITY AROUND AORTA

- Hematoma
- Rupture/penetrating ulcer
- Aortitis
- Mycotic blowout
- Angiosarcoma/tumor

IVC TUMOR THROMBUS

- Hepatocellular carcinoma
- Renal cell carcinoma
- Adrenocortical carcinoma
- Adrenal pheochromocytoma
- IVC leiomyosarcoma

Suggested Readings

Abrams HL, ed. *Abrams Angiography: Vascular and Interventional Radiology*. Boston: Little, Brown; 2005.

Bakal CW, Sillerzweig JE, Cynamon J, Sprayregen S. *Vascular and Interventional Radiology: Principles and Practice*. New York: Thieme Medical Publishers; 2002.

Castaneda-Zuniga WR. *Interventional Radiology*. Philadelphia: Lippincott Williams & Wilkins; 1997.

Cope C, Burke DR, Meranze SG. *Atlas of Interventional Radiology*. New York: Gower Medical Publishers; 1990.

Dyer R, ed. *Handbook of Basic Vascular and Interventional Radiology*. London: Churchill Livingstone; 1993.

Gedgaudas E, Moller JH, Castaneda-Zuniga WR, et al. *Cardiovascular Radiology*. Philadelphia: WB Saunders; 1985.

Johnsrude IS, Jackson DC, Dunnick NR. *A Practical Approach to Angiography*. Baltimore: Williams & Wilkins; 1987.

Kadir S. *Atlas of Normal and Variant Angiographic Anatomy*. Philadelphia: WB Saunders; 1990.

Kadir S. *Current Practice of Interventional Radiology*. New York: BC Decker; 1991.

Kadir S. *Diagnostic Angiography*. Philadelphia: WB Saunders; 1986.

Kadir S. *Teaching Atlas of Interventional Radiology: Diagnostic and Therapeutic Angiography*. New York: Thieme Medical Publishers; 1999.

Kaufman JA, Lee MJ. *Vascular and Interventional Radiology: The Requisites*. St. Louis: Mosby; 2003.

LaBerge JM. *Interventional Radiology Essentials*. Philadelphia: Lippincott Williams & Wilkins; 2000.

Valji K. *Vascular and Interventional Radiology*. Philadelphia: Elsevier; 2006.

Wojtowycz MM. *Handbook of Interventional Radiology and Angiography*. St. Louis: Mosby; 1995.

CHAPTER 9

Breast Imaging

CHAPTER OUTLINE

Breast Imaging Techniques

MAMMOGRAPHY TECHNIQUES

Mammography is primarily a screening and not a diagnostic tool. The mediolateral oblique and craniocaudal views are standard screening views, whereas additional views described below are used mainly for further evaluation of lesions.

MAMMOGRAPHIC VIEWS (Fig. 9-1)

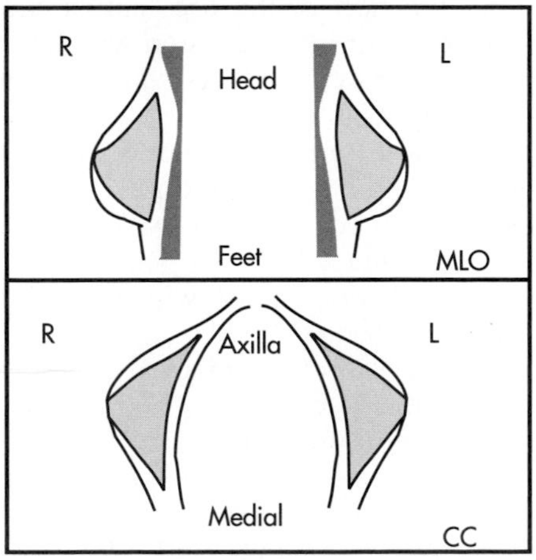

FIGURE 9-1

Mediolateral Oblique (MLO) View

This standard view is a projection parallel to the pectoralis major muscle (C-arm of mammographic unit is 40° to 60°). The pectoralis should be seen to the level of or below the axis of the nipple and appear convex (never concave toward the nipple).

Craniocaudal (CC) View

Projection with slight rotation toward the sternum to detect posteromedial tumors that may be missed on the MLO view. In general, better breast compression is achieved with the CC view than with the MLO view.

Exaggerated Craniocaudal (XCCL) View

This view is done to evaluate the lateral tissue (axillary tail of Spence). The patient is asked to rotate so the film holder can be placed at the midaxillary line.

Lateral Views: Mediolateral (ML) and Lateromedial (LM)

These views are a true lateral projection (x-ray beam parallel to floor). Used commonly to evaluate lesions for triangulation and needle localization. The direction of the x-ray beam is defined by the name of the view.

Axillary Tail View (Cleopatra View)

This view allows imaging of the axillary tail of the breast. It resembles the mediolateral view but allows evaluation of breast tissue more laterally oriented.

Cleavage Valley View

Modified CC view that improves visualization of area between breasts. Both breasts are positioned on the detector.

Spot Compression Views

With or without microfocus magnification. For evaluation of margins and morphology of lesions. Spreads structures; useful to determine if densities are real or not.

Magnification Views

Provides additional information on margins, satellite lesions, and microcalcifications. Can also be useful for asymmetrical tissue or architectural distortion.

Tangential View

Performed to demonstrate dermal location of lesions.

Rolled Views (Fig. 9-2)

- Roll breast laterally: superior lesion moves laterally.
- Roll breast medially: superior lesion moves medially.

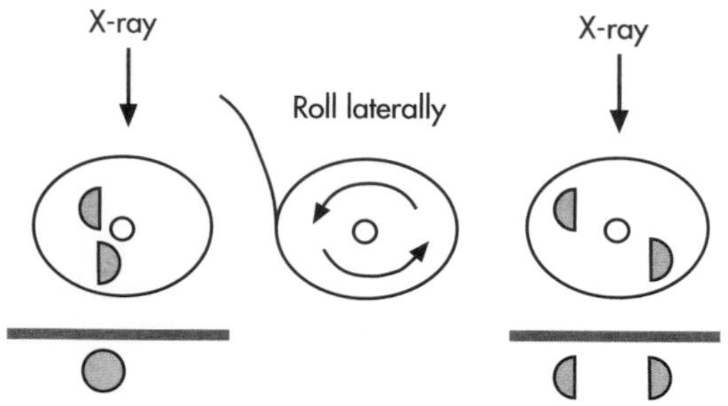

FIGURE 9-2

PROPER POSITIONING

Proper positioning is crucial for lesion detection. A cancer not imaged will not be detected. For both the CC and MLO views, the mobile border of the breast (CC: inferior border, MLO: lateral border) should be moved as far as possible toward the fixed border before placing the breast on the bucky. Check for correct positioning on CC and MLO views:

- Pectoralis muscle: On the MLO view, the pectoralis major should be convex anteriorly (never concave) and be seen to or below the level of the axis of the nipple. On the CC view, the muscle is seen approximately 35% of the time. The perpendicular distance from the nipple to the pectoralis on the MLO is used as a reference for adequacy of the CC view. The measurement on the CC view (taken as the distance from the nipple to the pectoralis or the back of the image) should be within 1 cm of the MLO measurement.
- The nipple should be in profile on at least one view. This may require an extra view in addition to the screening CC and MLO views.
- Retroglandular fat should usually be seen behind all fibroglandular tissue.
- Improper positioning on the MLO results in sagging, which is manifested by low nipple position and skin folds near the inframammary fold. The breast should be pulled up and out.
- Skin folds are usually not problematic in the axilla but can obscure lesions elsewhere. Repeat such views.
- Although the CC view is taken to include all of the medial breast tissue, exaggerated positioning is not desired. To check for this, make sure the nipple is near midline and not off to one side.
- On the MLO view, check for "cutoff" of inferior breast or axillary tissue resulting from placing the breast too low or too high on the bucky.
- Problems with compression or cutoff may be related to the image receptor size. Both 18 × 24-cm and 24 × 30-cm sizes are available. Too small a size results in cutoff. Too large a size can impair compression by impinging on other body parts.
- Motion is best detected by checking the septations located inferiorly and/or posteriorly or calcifications, which will be blurred by motion.

Pearls

Lesion localization: Start with the view in which the lesion is best seen, and modify it. If a finding is seen only on

- CC view: ask for rolled CC views (top-rolled medially and laterally)
  - Lesion in superior breast will now project in the direction to which the top half of the breast was rolled: e.g., a superior lesion will move laterally if top half of breast is rolled laterally.
  - Lesion in inferior breast will move opposite the direction of the top half of the breast roll: e.g., an inferior lesion will move medially compared with its starting point in a top-rolled lateral CC.
- MLO view: ask for straight lateral. This is a quick version of nipple triangulation.
  - Lesion in medial breast will move up on straight lateral (ML)
  - Lesion in lateral breast will move down on straight lateral (ML)
  - Mnemonic: "Muffins (medial) rise, Lead (lateral) sinks"

To better evaluate difficult areas:

- Outer breast → exaggerated CC lateral and Cleopatra (axillary tail) view
- Inner breast → exaggerated CC medial and cleavage ("valley") view
- Retroareolar area → nipple in profile view

- Skin lesions: tangential views and skin localization procedure
  - Place calcifications in center of alphanumeric paddle
  - Place marker
  - Release compression and go tangential; calcifications should be right below marker

COMPRESSION

Compression should always be symmetrical. Breast compression is used to reduce patient dose and improve image quality:

- Reduction of motion artifacts by immobilization of breast
- Reduction of geometric blur
- Reduction in change of radiographic density (achieve uniform breast thickness)
- Reduction of scattered radiation by decreasing breast thickness

PATIENT INTERACTION

The comparable radiation risk of mammography (~200 mR/breast per view with grid) is very low; in a population of 1 million, one would expect 800 occult, naturally occurring cancers and only 1 to 3 cancers (absolute risk model) induced by mammography. This risk of concern or injury is similar to that for:

- Breathing Boston air for 2 days
- Riding a bicycle for 10 miles
- Driving a car for 300 miles
- Eating 40 tablespoons of peanut butter

OBTAIN HISTORY

- Family history
- Risk factors for breast cancer
- Complaints
  - Mass, thickening
  - Pain
  - Nipple discharge

MAMMOGRAPHY INTERPRETATION

VIEWING CONDITIONS

Ideally, dedicated mammography viewing equipment is used. Minimal requirements include:

- Adequate view box luminescence
- Low ambient light
- Masking of mammograms to exclude peripheral view box light
- Magnifying glass: each film should be reviewed with a magnifying glass after initial inspection

IMAGE LABELING

American College of Radiology (ACR) requirements:

- Markers identifying the view and side are required and are to be placed near the axilla to guide orientation.
- An identification label must include the patient's name (first and last), ID number, facility name and location, and technologist's initials if not included elsewhere on the film.
- Cassette number (Arabic numeral)

Optional

- Technical factors
- Mammography unit number (Roman numeral)

DOUBLE READING

Although it is not the standard of practice, institutions performing double readings of screening mammograms report increases in cancers detected, ranging from 6.4%-15%. At Massachusetts General Hospital (MGH) it is 7.7%.

EVALUATION OF THE MAMMOGRAM (Fig. 9-3)

Each mammogram should be systematically evaluated for:

- Adequate quality of study; additional views required?
- Adequate penetration of fibroglandular breast tissue
- Skin, nipple, trabecular changes
- Presence of masses
- Calcifications
- Axillary nodes
- Asymmetry (usually a variant of normal)
- Architectural distortion

Comparison with prior films is mandatory. Breast cancers can grow slowly, and minimal progressive changes need to be documented. All masses and calcifications need to be further characterized. If the initial views are not adequate, additional views have to be obtained.

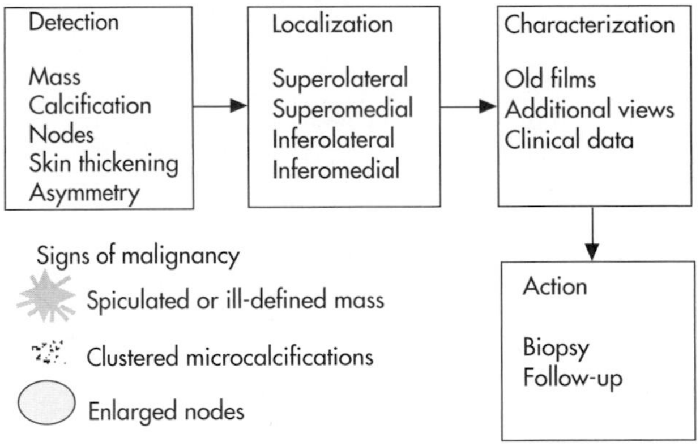

FIGURE 9-3

QUALITY CONTROL

ACR requirements:

- Daily: processor, darkroom cleanliness
- Weekly: screen cleanliness, view box

- Monthly: replenishment rates, phantom, visual checklist. Some mammographers advocate more frequent evaluation of phantom images because such images evaluate the entire imaging system.
- Quarterly: fixer retention, repeat/reject, light x-ray field alignment analysis
- Semiannually: darkroom fog, screen-film contact, compression, view box luminance

MAMMOGRAPHY REPORTING (Fig. 9-4)

MASS

A mass is a 3-D structure demonstrating convex outward borders on two orthogonal views. Due to confusion with the term *density*, a potential mass seen on a single view only is now called an "asymmetry," which lacks a convex outward border and conspicuity of a mass.

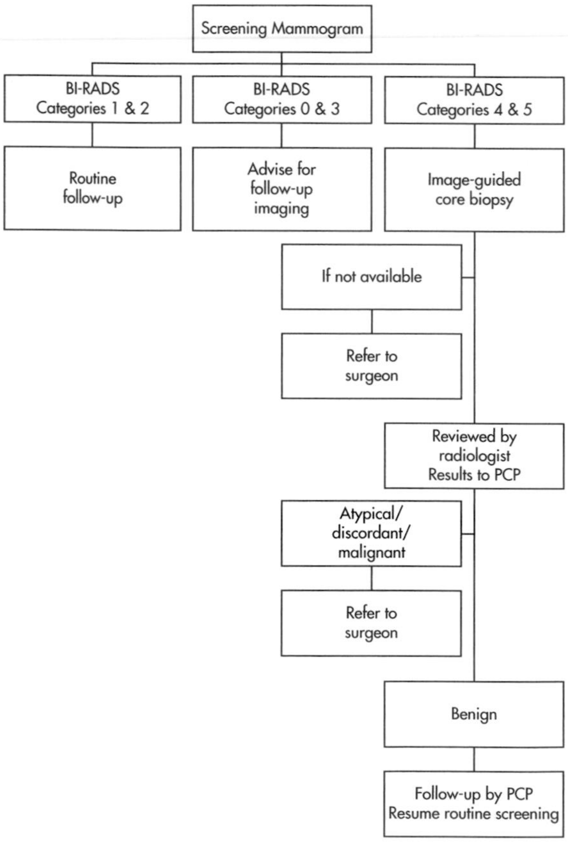

FIGURE 9-4

Margins

- Spiculated: a spiculated tumor margin is the only specific sign of malignancy; however, not all spiculated masses are cancers. Spiculated masses are the easiest masses to diagnose, although they may be obscured by fibroglandular tissue.

Spiculations are also seen in:
  - Scar tissue (usually resolves in 1 year if a surgical scar and in 3 years if a postradiation scar)
  - Desmoid tumors
  - Fat necrosis
- Indistinct (ill-defined): rapidly growing tumors that do not elicit significant fibrous tissue reaction. Some benign lesions may also have indistinct or fuzzy margins:
  - Fat necrosis
  - Elastosis refers to radial scar, indurative mastopathy, or sclerosing duct hyperplasia; elastosis is probably a form of sclerosing adenosis.
  - Infection/abscess
  - Spontaneous hematomas
- Microlobulated: small lobulations are more worrisome for malignancy than larger lobulations.
- Obscured: margin cannot be seen or evaluated because of overlying normal tissue.
- Circumscribed masses with well-defined borders (>75% circumference): uncommon sign of malignancy; only 2% of solitary masses with smooth margins are malignant.

Other Features

Other features of mass lesions are less useful:

- Size: the larger the tumor the worse the prognosis. Malignant tumors >1 cm are twice as likely to have spread to axillary nodes. A biopsy should be considered in any solitary noncystic lesion >8 mm. If spiculated, any size lesion should be sampled. The size of a mass does not correlate with likelihood of malignancy.
- Shape: the more irregular the mass, the greater the likelihood of malignancy. Shapes are classified as round, oval, lobular, or irregular.
- Density: malignant lesions are usually very dense for their size; lucent, fat-containing lesions, on the contrary, are benign (posttraumatic oil cyst, lipoma, galactocele). Lesions are described as high-density equal (isodense), or low-density or as fat-containing.
- Location: distinguish parenchymal mass from skin lesion. Small lesions in the periphery of the upper outer quadrant are most likely lymph nodes.
- Multiplicity: multiple, well-circumscribed masses are commonly benign fibroadenomas (younger patients) or cysts after 35 years of age, neurofibromatosis. In older patients, metastases from other primaries should be excluded.

CALCIFICATIONS

50% of all malignant tumors are discovered by mammography because of the presence of suspicious calcifications. Once detected, calcifications should be categorized as definitively benign, malignant, or suspicious (i.e., biopsy is necessary). In asymptomatic women, 75% of sampled clustered calcifications are benign and 25% are associated with cancer.

EVALUATION OF CALCIFICATIONS

Parameter	Malignant	Benign
Size	<1 mm	>1 mm
Number per cm³	>5	<5
Distribution	Clustered	Scattered (not clustered)
Morphology	Wild, unordered, fine linear branching	Round, lucent center; solid rods

Malignant Calcifications (Fig. 9-5)

- A "cluster of microcalcifications" is usually defined as >5 calcifications per cm^3 of tissue.
- Each particle size is invariably <2 mm (except comedocarcinoma); most malignant calcifications are less than 0.5 mm in diameter; lower limit of detectability is 0.2 to 0.3 mm.
- Calcifications within a cluster typically vary in size and shape (fine pleomorphic).
- Malignant calcifications are almost always located in ducts (intraductal component), even when the tumor is not.
- Dot-dash branching pattern (fine linear branching) and irregular shapes are typical of malignant calcification.
- The use of microfocal spot magnification improves the diagnostic accuracy in the evaluation of calcification.
- Always biopsy suspicious calcifications.
- Distribution patterns
  - Diffuse: usually benign
  - Regional: in >2 mL of volume not conforming to ductal distribution; malignancy less likely
  - Clustered/group: >5 calcifications in <1 mL of volume; high suspicion
  - Linear: increased suspicion (in ducts)
  - Segmental: increased suspicion, may require bracketed localization

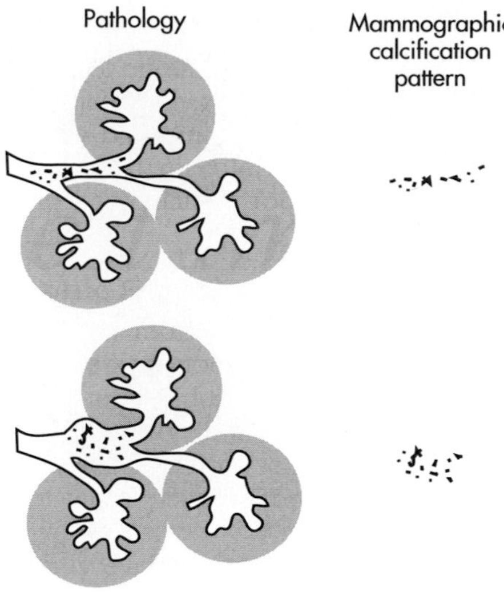

FIGURE 9-5

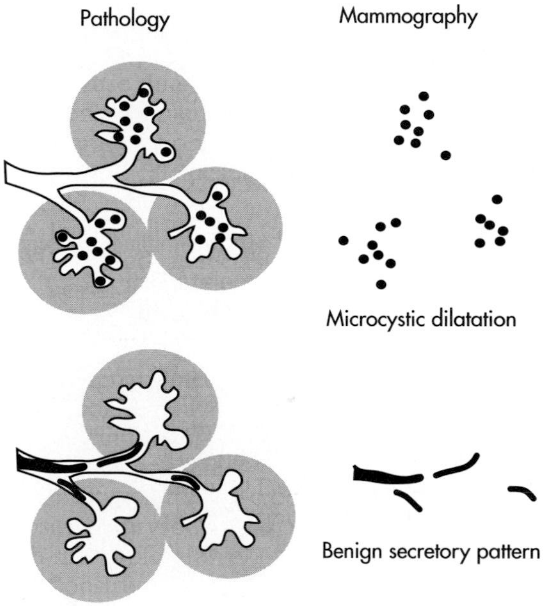

FIGURE 9-6

Benign Calcifications (Fig. 9-6)

Round/punctate
- May vary in size; classified as punctate if <0.5 mm
- Probably clustered benign; 6-month follow-up for 2-year interval

Coarse heterogeneous
- Calcifications of intermediate concern >0.5 mm and variable in size and shape but smaller than those that usually occur in response to injury

Dystrophic
- Irregular, >0.5 mm, often lucent centers

Indistinct/amorphous
- If diffuse/scattered: likely benign
- If clustered/regional/linear/segmental: biopsy

Large rodlike calcification
- >1 mm continuous rods, may branch
- Benign secretory disease (plasma cell mastitis) or duct ectasia

Skin calcifications
- Polyhedral shape with lucent centers

- Appearance is usually typical, so no further workup is required; occasionally a "skin localization" with tangential views will be useful.

Vascular calcifications—if seen in those <50 years old, high correlation with CAD
- Parallel tracks

Coarse/"popcorn"-like
- Involuting fibroadenoma

Rim/eggshell calcification
- Cyst
- Fat necrosis

Milk of calcium (Fig. 9-7)
- Layering calcification in microcysts
- Fuzzy, amorphous on CC view
- Semilunar on linear or MLO view

Suture calcification
- Linear or tubular with shape of knot

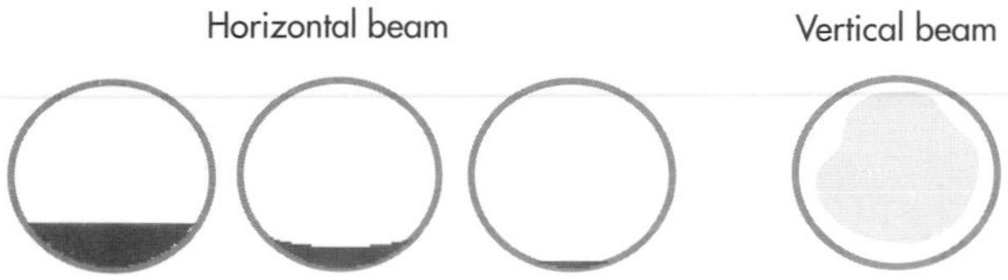

FIGURE 9-7

ARCHITECTURAL DISTORTION

Architectural distortion refers to a tumor-associated desmoplastic response that results in a focal change of breast parenchyma. Architectural distortion should always be seen on at least 2 views. Mammographic signs of a desmoplastic response include:
- Abnormal arrangement of Cooper's ligaments
- Ducts and periductal fibrosis
- "Pulling in" of superficial structures

SKIN, NIPPLE, AND TRABECULAR CHANGES

- Skin retraction due to fibrosis and shortening of Cooper's ligaments (skin becomes flat or concave); the tumor itself is almost always palpable if skin retraction is present on the mammogram.
- Skin thickening (>3 mm) may be a sign of malignancy or benign conditions.

Types:

Focal: local tumor

Diffuse: sign of edema; may be due to inflammatory cancer

- Nipple retraction is worrisome when acute and unilateral.
- Fine linear nipple calcification obliges one to rule out Paget disease (other causes of nipple calcification are benign).

ABNORMAL DUCTAL PATTERNS

Cancer may cause shortening, dilatation, or distortion of ducts. Mammography:
- Ducts >2 mm in diameter extending >2 cm into the breast are usually due to benign ductal ectasia.
- Asymmetrical-appearing ducts are usually a normal variation, although this can be a very rare indication of malignancy.
- Symmetrical ductal ectasia is a benign condition.

BREAST LESIONS THAT ARISE IN MAIN SEGMENTAL DUCTS

- Papillomas
- Papillary cancer

BREAST LESIONS ARISING IN TERMINAL DUCTS

- Peripheral papillomas
- Epithelial hyperplasia
- Ductal carcinoma in situ (DCIS)
- Invasive ductal carcinoma

LYMPH NODE ABNORMALITIES

Normal intramammary lymph nodes are usually visible only in the upper outer quadrant. Nodes may occasionally be seen below the medial plane. There have been rare reports of lymph nodes in the medial breast. An increase in size, number, or density of axillary lymph nodes is abnormal: axillary nodes >2 cm or intramammary nodes >1 cm without lucency or hilar notch are suspicious (if lucent fat center is present, even larger nodes may be benign). Nodes that contain tumor lose the radiolucent hilum and appear dense, although benign hyperplasia may appear similar. Nodal calcification implies:
- Metastasis (most common)
- Lymphoma
- Rheumatoid arthritis and previous gold injections

ASYMMETRY OF BREAST TISSUE

Asymmetrical, dense tissue is seen in 3% of breasts, usually in the upper outer quadrant, and is considered a normal variant (caused by fibrosis). The mammographic finding of asymmetrical breast tissue is suspicious only if it is *palpable* or if there are associated abnormalities (mass, calcifications, architectural distortion, or asymmetry that has developed over time). The following are the criteria that an opacity has to fulfill to be called asymmetrical tissue:
- Not a mass (i.e., changes morphology on different views)
- Contains fat

- No calcifications
- No architectural distortion
- If asymmetrical tissue is palpable, ultrasound may be useful for further workup.

SKIN CALCIFICATIONS

- Suspect skin calcification if superficial in location.
- Periareolar, axillary, or medial location
- Tiny hollow spherical calcifications
- Plaquelike on one view and linear on another view
- Tangential view for confirmation

DICTATION

Reports are organized by a short description of breast composition, description, and location of significant findings, as well as any interval changes, and an overall impression. The ACR categorizes reports into 7 categories according to the Breast Imaging Reporting and Data System (BI-RADS):

0 = Needs additional mammographic evaluation and/or prior mammogram for comparison. This is almost always used in a screening situation. Category 0 should be used only for old film comparison when such comparison is *required* to make a final assessment.

1 = Negative: breasts are symmetrical and normal; return to annual screening

2 = Benign finding: includes typical nodes, calcified fibroadenomas, lucent lesions (implants), and scattered benign calcifications; return to annual screening

3 = Probably benign: initial short-interval follow-up suggested: <2% risk of malignancy. Noncalcified circumscribed solid mass, focal asymmetry, and cluster of round/punctate calcifications are considered in this category. Lesions should not be palpable. → 6 month follow-up

4 = Suspicious: abnormality; biopsy should be considered:

- 4a = findings needing intervention but with low suspicion for malignancy
- 4b = lesions with intermediate suspicion for malignancy
- 4c = lesions with moderate concern but not classic for malignancy

5 = Cancer with >95% certainty: spiculated lesions → biopsy/excision

6 = Known biopsy-proven malignancy: findings that have been confirmed by biopsy but the patient has not undergone definitive therapy

The use of categories 4a, 4b, and 4c is optional.

Pearls

- Short-term follow-up <6 months is almost never useful because most processes will not change over such a short interval. The rare exception is a suspected hematoma, which would be expected to show signs of regression at 3 months.
- Heterogeneously and extremely dense parenchymal patterns lower the sensitivity of mammography, and a short statement to this effect may be included in the report.
- BIRADS categorization is not employed in male patients

REASONS FOR MISSING BREAST CANCER

- Failure to detect lesions
- Faulty technique
  - Underexposure on mammogram
  - Patient motion
  - Poor film screen contact
  - Dense or nodular parenchymal pattern
  - Subthreshhold size
- Misdiagnosis of lesions

COMMONLY MISSED LESIONS

- Invasive lobular carcinoma. Mammographically this lesion appears as architectural distortion and asymmetrical density. Lack of a discrete mass or clustered microcalcifications can make this lesion difficult to detect. 10%-15% bilateral.
- Invasive ductal carcinoma—most common well-circumscribed lesion
- DCIS coexistent with atypical ductal hyperplasia (ADH) on core needle biopsy; if core biopsy returns ADH, excisional biopsy is performed as may be upgraded to DCIS ⅓ of time
- Palpable mass: palpable masses not seen on mammography must be investigated further. Spot films or tangential films over the palpable mass may disclose a mass that is otherwise occult.

ULTRASOUND

Indications

- Women < age 28 (MGH threshold) with a palpable lump should be evaluated with US because the palpable lesion most likely represents a fibroadenoma. The decision to biopsy a solid mass in a young woman must be made by the patient and her physician because the risk of malignancy is very low.
- Differentiation of cyst from solid structure (use 7.5- or 10-MHz transducer): no internal echoes;

through-transmission; thin, imperceptible wall. Abscess and hematoma may mimic a solid mass. If there are low-level echoes, a mass lesion has to be excluded by biopsy/aspiration.
- Not a screening modality

Interpretation

- BI-RADS
  Shape: oval, round, irregular
  Margin: circumscribed, indistinct, angular, microlobulated, spiculated
  Orientation of long-axis of lesion to chest wall: Parallel, antiparallel
  Border: echogenic halo, abrupt transition
  Echogenicity relative to fat: anechoic, hypoechoic, hyperechoic, isoechoic, complex
  Posterior acoustic enhancement, shadowing, or combined
  Calcifications
- Ultrasound cannot detect most small calcifications.
- Fibroadenomas are usually hypoechoic and well circumscribed.
- Lymphomas are usually hypoechoic.
- Lipomas are difficult to differentiate from surrounding tissue.
- Oil cysts are hypoechoic and have poor through-transmission.
- Benign lymph nodes may have a characteristic central echogenic center due to fat in the lymph node hilum.
- Cysts and solid lesions often cannot be differentiated from one another on mammograms, particularly well-circumscribed mammographic densities.
- Complex cyst contains solid component, from which a biopsy needs to be taken. Complicated cysts contain internal echoes.
- Malignant lesions tend to be taller than they are wide and have posterior acoustic shadowing.
- Vascularity of a lesion is not helpful.

GALACTOGRAPHY

Indications

- Workup of solitary and spontaneous duct discharge
- Identifies deep lesions that might be missed by surgery
- May be used to identify proximal lesions because papilloma and cancer have a similar appearance; take a biopsy to distinguish
- Multiple filling defects may be due to papillomatosis

Technique

1. Patient sitting or lying down
2. Express secretions to identify duct origins.
3. Prep breast
4. Blunt pediatric sialogram needle
5. Inject 0.1 to 2 mL of water-soluble contrast agent.
6. Avoid air bubbles.
7. Obtain mammogram. Look for filling defects, distorted ducts, and/or extravasation.

MRI

Indications

- Staging
- High-risk patients
- Suspected multiple or bilateral cancers
- Occult breast cancer
- Preoperative surgical planning
- Positive surgical margins
- Response to therapy
- Postoperative scar versus recurrence
- Breast implants

Advantages

- Images breast implants and ruptures
- Highly sensitive to small abnormalities
- Used effectively in dense breasts
- Evaluation of inverted nipples for cancer
- Determines the extent of breast cancer
- Determines what type of surgery is indicated (lumpectomy or mastectomy)
- Evaluation of breast cancer recurrence and residual tumors after lumpectomy
- Evaluation of axillary lymph nodes
- Can be useful in cutaneous disorders such as neurofibromatosis
- Characterization of small abnormalities
- May be useful in screening women at high risk for breast cancer according to recent studies

Limitations

- MRI takes 30 to 60 minutes compared with 10 to 20 minutes for screening mammography.
- The cost of MRI is several times that of mammography.
- MRI requires the use of a contrast agent.
- MRI can be nonspecific; often it cannot distinguish between cancerous and noncancerous tumors.
- Minimally invasive breast biopsy techniques need to be further developed to evaluate abnormalities detected with MRI.
- Advanced MRI techniques may not be available at many outpatient centers.

Technique

- Prone position
- Dedicated bilateral surface coils are usually receive-only coils but can be transmit/receive coils.
- MGH protocol
  - Axial T1 3-D GRE precontrast and postcontrast (dynamic)
  - Axial T2 spin-echo
  - Sagittal SPGR with fat saturation
  - Sagittal T2 with fat saturation
- Postprocessing:
  - Subtraction images
  - Maximum-intensity projection 3-D reconstruction
- 1.5 T for optimal MRI

BI-RADS

- Foci: <5 mm, usually benign
- Mass
  - Shape: round, oval, lobulated, irregular
  - Margins: smooth, irregular, spiculated
  - Enhancement: homogeneous, heterogeneous, rimlike, nonenhancing septae, enhancing septae, central
  - Nonmasslike enhancement
    - Distribution: focal, linear, ductal, segmental, regional, multiple regions, diffuse
    - Pattern: homogeneous, heterogeneous, clumped, stippled, punctuate, reticular
- Associated findings: nipple retraction, skin thickening, pectoralis/chest wall invasion (must see enhancement within muscle; obliteration of fat plane insufficient evidence of invasion)
- Enhancement kinetics: initial upslope first 2 minutes classified as slow, medium rapid; delayed phase: persistent, plateau, washout
- Rapid upslope with plateau or washout on delayed phase more likely malignant

Contrast Enhancement by MRI

- Cancer
- Benign masses
- Regional enhancement: usually implies benign etiology
- Patchy enhancement (i.e., enhancement in one part of the breast that seems to be confined to one ductal system): reasonable likelihood of underlying obstructive malignancy
- Diffuse enhancement is believed to be a benign pattern (fibrocystic or proliferative changes)

Evaluation of Implants (see later section on implants in this chapter)

- Silicone has long T1W and long T2W.
- Proton signal is from methyl groups in the dimethyl polysiloxane polymer.
- The silicone shell is of lower signal intensity than the silicone within the implant because of greater cross-linking of methyl groups.
- Fast spin-echo T2W, as well as orthogonal silicone-sensitive (fat-suppressed) inversion recovery sequences, are obtained. Chemical H_2O suppression will yield a silicone-only image.
- MRI of implant rupture: 94% sensitivity, 97% specificity (compared with US: 70% sensitivity, 92% specificity)

Evaluation of Malignancy

- MRI is useful in patients with dense breasts not well evaluated with mammography or with known multicentric lesions (i.e., in different quadrants).
- Most protocols use a dynamic contrast enhancement pattern of breast lesion on fat-suppressed images, usually a volume acquisition.
- Most protocols use fat suppression on dynamic enhanced sequences.
- Subtraction may increase sensitivity.
- Cancer enhances more rapidly than benign lesions, and the critical period is in the first 3 minutes.
- For lesions ≥ 1 cm: 88%-100% sensitivity, 30%-97% specificity
- DCIS generally enhances more slowly than invasive cancers, and findings overlap significantly with hyperplasia. May not enhance. MRI should not be used to evaluate malignant character of microcalcification.
- The use of MRI for monitoring postsurgical or postradiation patients for recurrence or for screening of patients with implants is questionable because a trend toward a more advanced stage at diagnosis is known (although the risk of malignancy is the same as in patients without implants).

BIOPSY

MGH statistics: between 1978 and 1988, 3000 biopsies were performed. Of those, 25% proved to be malignant (25% positive predictive value). Breast biopsies do not seed tumors in the needle tract.

NEEDLE LOCALIZATION FOR SURGICAL BIOPSY/EXCISION (Fig. 9-8)

1. Identify lesion (use 90° films to direct needle parallel to chest wall); choose shortest distance to lesion.
2. Obtain view with breast in compression device; clean skin with iodine 3 times and then once with alcohol; pass needle tip in direction of x-ray beam past lesion.

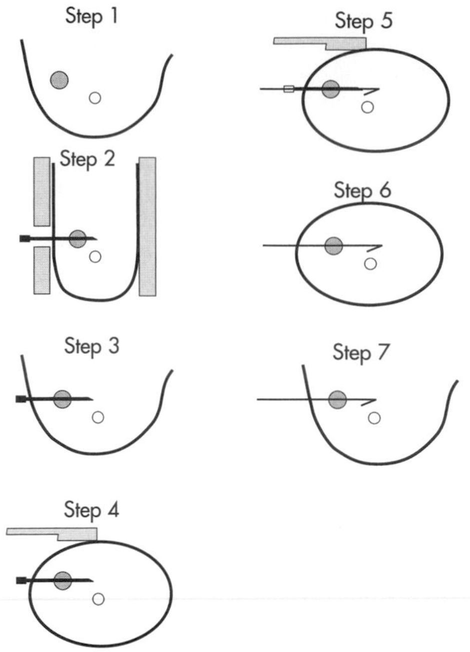

FIGURE 9-8

3. Obtain a second film; if the needle is in good position, take a 90° opposed film.
4. If needle is in appropriate location (tip 1 cm beyond lesion), pass hook wire through needle. Pull needle back to engage hook; the wire may back out somewhat when patient stands up.
5. Take a third mammogram perpendicular to wire with wire in place.
6. A mammogram of the postbiopsy specimen should be obtained to ensure that the lesion is included in the specimen.

TECHNIQUE FOR LOCALIZING LESION SEEN ONLY ON A SINGLE VIEW (TRIANGULATION) (Fig. 9-9)

Same as above technique with the following modifications:

1. Place the breast in compression in the position in which the lesion is seen.
2. Pass the needle tip deep to the lesion (TLN: true length of needle; PLN: projected length of needle; TLPN: true length to pull back needle; PLPN: projected length to pull back needle; TDL: true depth of lesion).
3. With slight repositioning to slant the needle, its projection allows use of similar triangles to calculate the distance of pull back.

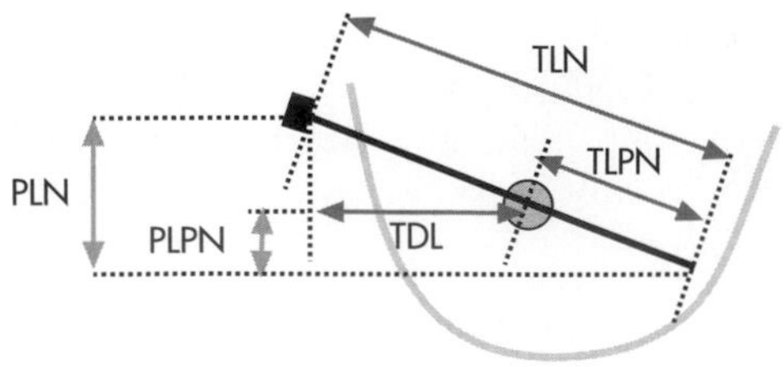

TLPN = (TLN × PLPN) / PLN

FIGURE 9-9

4. The needle is adjusted accordingly and the wire deployed after confirming needle position.
5. Take a mammogram with the wire in place in the orthogonal position.

Alternative Technique (Fig. 9-10)

This technique allows localization of an unseen lesion on the CC view if it is visible only on the straight lateral and MLO views.

1. Align straight lateral, oblique, and CC views from left to right.
2. Nipple should be on a horizontal line.
3. Connect the lesion on any two views by a straight line.
4. Lesion should be located along path of the line on the 3rd view.
5. When describing the location of a lesion, the breast is seen as the face of a clock, and the location in this plane is given as clock position (Fig. 9-11). Depth is then indicated as anterior, middle, or posterior.
6. Additional descriptions are subareolar, central, and axillary tail areas.

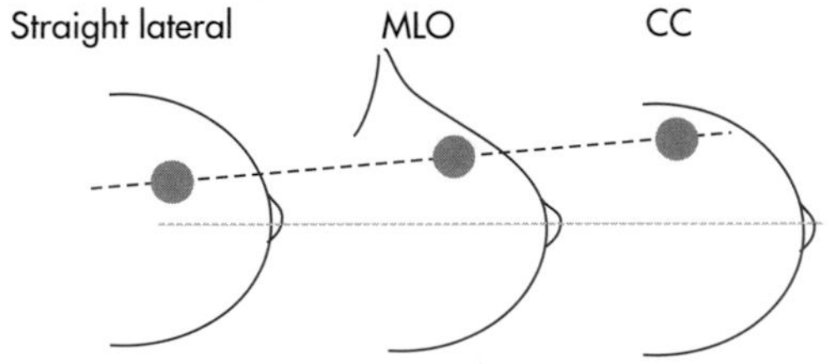

FIGURE 9-10

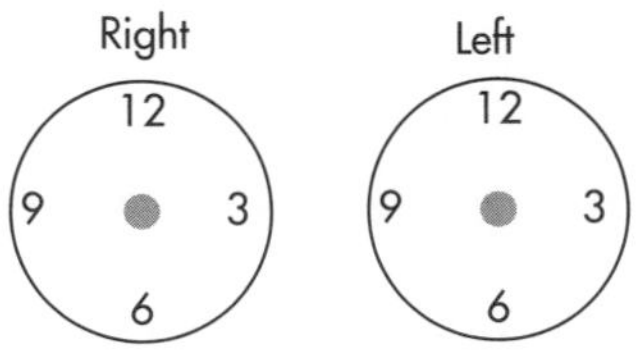

FIGURE 9-11

LESION SEEN ON CT BUT NOT EASILY SEEN MAMMOGRAPHICALLY

These are usually lesions near the chest wall.

1. Place a linear marker or localization grid over the lesion and scan.
2. Once the lesion is scanned, determine the percutaneous puncture site with the linear marker or grid.
3. Because of breast mobility, the patient is left in the gantry and the needle is advanced. Caution is necessary not to advance the needle through the chest wall.
4. Confirm needle position with CT and deploy wire.

CORE BIOPSY

Indications

- Solid mass lesion in young patient that is most likely benign (i.e., core biopsy thus avoids an excisional biopsy)
- Solid mass lesion that is most likely malignant (i.e., patients would go directly to radical mastectomy, avoiding an excisional biopsy)
- Some mammographers also biopsy suspicious calcifications; however, this is not universally accepted.

Technique

- 11- to 14-G needle as well as vacuum-assisted devices may be used
- US guidance. Trajectory parallel to chest wall, avoiding muscle and pleura
- Stereotactic guidance
    - Contraindications: Body weight, compressible thickness <2 to 3 cm, unable to lie prone for 45 minutes
    - Select trajectory with shortest distance, compress breast with fenestrated pad
    - Stereo pair of 15° images to right and left of midline
    - Target on pair of images selected on monitor; computer calculates horizontal and vertical distances as well as depth
    - Sterilize skin, apply local anesthetic, make small skin incision with blade
    - Needle advanced to predetermined depth and prefire stereo films obtained to verify on target
    - Needle is fired. Sampling may be performed; a vacuum-assisted device may be used
    - Obtain radiographs of the specimen and breast after clip placement
- MRI guidance
    - Commercial systems are available
    - Example: pad with square-shaped fenestrations. After preliminary images, computer selects square and a smaller insert containing multiple holes inserted into that square. Computer selects hole.
    - Advance introducer and trocar through hole to predetermined depth, biopsy, and place clip.

SPECIMEN RADIOGRAPHY

Specimen radiography confirms that a mammographically visible mass, area of architectural distortion, microcalcifications, etc., have been sampled. Occasionally, microcalcifications are not detectable by pathology. Polarized light may better demonstrate calcium oxalate crystals. In addition, radiography of the sectioned paraffin block may be helpful.

Breast Cancer

GENERAL

INCIDENCE

11% of women age 20 in the United States will develop breast cancer if they live to age 85 (4% if the high-risk groups are excluded). Breast cancer is the second leading cause of cancer death (lung is first) in women. There are approximately 45,000 deaths/year from breast cancer in the United States and over 185,000 new cases each year. The presumed etiology of breast cancer is DNA damage, with estrogen playing a key role. 25% have *TP53* mutations (tumor-suppressor gene located on chromosome 17). 40% of inherited breast cancers (5%-10% of all breast cancers) have *BRCA1* mutations (tumor-suppressor gene located on chromosome 17); 40% have *BRCA2* mutations (chromosome 13). 75% of breast cancers occur in women with no risk factors.

Risk Factors

Older women

Family history (1st degree: mother or sister)

Other

- Early menarche, late menopause, late first pregnancy, nulliparity
- Atypical proliferative changes
- Lobular neoplasia (previously known as lobular carcinoma in situ, LCIS) is not in itself considered malignant but carries a 30% risk of breast cancer (15% in each breast).
- Prior history of breast cancer (in situ or invasive) increases the risk for a second cancer by 1% per year.

SCREENING

General

- Early screening campaigns have led to the detection of 75% of malignancies in stage 0 (in situ) or stage 1.
- All palpable lesions should be referred for a mammogram in appropriately aged women; the mammogram aids in detection of multifocal disease and bilateral disease (4% of cancers are bilateral).
- Screening has led to a nearly 30% reduction in mortality compared with the unscreened group.
- More than 40% of cancers are detected by mammography only.
- Approximately 10% of cancers are palpable but not seen on mammography.
- There is decreased lead time in finding cancers in females <50 (lead time 2 years), such that yearly screening is more important at this age than in patients >50 (lead time 3 to 4 years).
- Radiation risk of screening is higher in young females (teens to early 20s) but is negligible after 35 to 40 years of age.

Health Insurance Plan (HIP) Study, New York

A total of 62,000 patients were offered screening: 31,000 by mammography and physical examination and 31,000 by physical examination only; patients were then followed for the development of breast cancer. After 18 years of follow-up, there was a 23% lower mortality rate from breast cancer in patients who had a mammogram.

Breast Cancer Detection Demonstration Program (BCDDP)

- 88% of cancers are detected by mammogram.
- 42% of cancers are detected by mammogram only.
- 20% of cancers were not detected by mammogram or physical examination within 1 year.
- 9% of cancers are detected by physical examination only.

It was concluded from this study that physical examination and mammography are two complementary studies that do not replace each other, although mammography is the more sensitive study for detection of small lesions.

SCREENING RECOMMENDATIONS (ACR JANUARY 2010)

Asymptomatic women
- MGH follows ACR recommendations of yearly screening after age 40.
- Monthly breast self-examination to begin at age 20
- Medical examination every 3 years between 20 and 40 years (yearly after 40)
- Stop screening when life expectancy is <5 to 7 years or when abnormal results would not be acted on because of age or comorbid conditions

High-risk women
- *BRCA1* or *BRCA2* mutation carriers, untested first-degree relatives of BRCA mutation carrier – annual mammogram and annual MRI by age 30 but not before age 25
- Women with ≥ 20% lifetime risk for breast cancer on the basis of family history – annual mammogram and MRI by age 30 but not before age 25, or 10 years before the age of the youngest affected relative, whichever is later
- History of chest irradiation between ages 10 to 30 – annual mammogram and MRI starting 8 years after treatment; mammogram not recommended before age 25
- Personal history of breast cancer, ovarian cancer, or biopsy diagnosis of lobular neoplasia or ADH; annual mammogram from time of diagnosis, annual MRI or ultrasound may be considered
- Dense breast only; may add ultrasound to screening mammogram

Mammography at any age over 28 to 30 for the following:
- Palpable mass (if not a simple cyst by US)
- Bloody discharge
- Planned breast surgery (unless <25 years of age)

PROGNOSIS

Annual incidence of breast cancer has increased 1% per year since 1940. A recent larger increase may be due to earlier detection. Mortality may be decreasing. Survival rates decrease with positive nodal involvement. The involvement of nodes correlates with primary tumor size (cancers >1 cm have nodal involvement in 30%; cancers <1 cm have nodal involvement in only 15%). Doubling time of breast cancer is 100 to 180 days.

BREAST CANCER SURVIVAL RATE

BREAST CANCER 5-YEAR SURVIVAL RATE

Stage	5-Year Relative Survival Rate
0	100%
I	100%
IIA	92%
IIB	81%
IIIA	67%
IIIB	54%
IV	20%

STAGING

Lymph Nodes (Fig. 9-12)

Axillary lymph nodes are divided into 3 levels:

- Level I: low axilla
- Level II: more medial under pectoralis minor
- Level III: most medial under clavicle

Positive supraclavicular and internal mammary nodes are considered distant metastases.

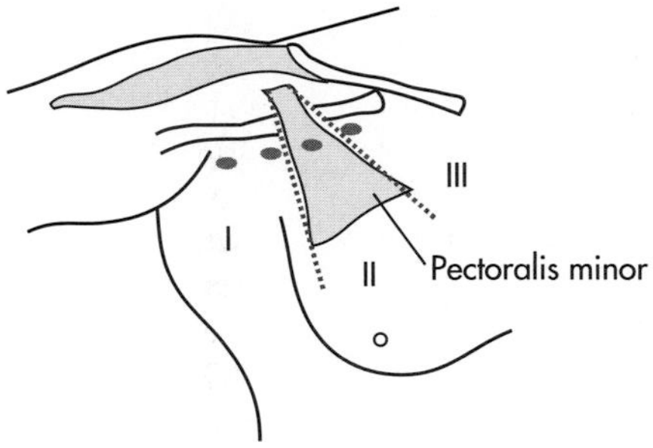

FIGURE 9-12

Staging System

- Stage 0: ductal carcinoma in situ (DCIS)
- Stage I: small cancers
  - Cancers <2 cm in diameter
  - No axillary or distant disease
- Stage II: large cancers
  - Cancers 2 to 5 cm in diameter, or
  - Axillary node involvement
  - No distant metastases
- Stage III: extensive local/regional spread
  - Cancers >5 cm, or
  - Cancers fixed to pectoralis, or
  - Cancers with lymph nodes fixed together in a matted axillary mass
- Stage IV: distant metastases

STAGING SYSTEM

Stage	Tumor (T)	Node (N)	Metastasis (M)
Stage 0	Tis	N0	M0
Stage 1	T1	N0	M0
Stage IIA	T0	N1	M0
	T1	N1	M0
	T2	N0	M0
Stage IIB	T2	N1	M0
	T3	N0	M0
Stage IIIA	T0	N2	M0
	T1	N2	M0
	T2	N2	M0
	T3	N1, N2	M0
Stage IIIB	T4	any N	M0
	any T	N3	M0
Stage IV	any T	any N	M1

Metastatic Spread

- Axillary lymph nodes
- Bones
- Lungs
- Liver
- Opposite breast
- Skin

SENSITIVITY OF DETECTION

- 20% of cancers that appear within 1 year of a negative screen are missed by the combination of mammography and physical examination.
- 10% of cancers missed on initial mammography may be seen with additional views.
  - 50% of mammography misses are unavoidable due to truly normal findings.
  - 30% of mammography misses are due to observer oversight or poor positioning.

SPECIFIC NEOPLASM

PATHOLOGY

99% of all malignant breast tumors are epithelial tumors (adenocarcinomas) that have their origin in the terminal duct lobular unit (TDLU). Of these, 90% are ductal and 10% are lobular in origin.

Classification (Fig. 9-13)

1. Tumors of ductal epithelial origin
   - Carcinoma in situ (DCIS)
   - Invasive carcinoma:
     - Not otherwise specified (NOS)
     - Medullary carcinoma (extensive lymphocytic infiltrate; good prognosis)
     - Mucinous or colloid carcinoma (extensive mucin production; well differentiated)
     - Papillary carcinoma (related to small duct papillomas; low lethality, can be intracystic)
     - Tubular carcinoma (attempts to form ducts, well differentiated; most benign and slow growing of all breast carcinomas)
     - Inflammatory carcinoma (aggressive with early dermal lymphatic invasion)
     - Paget disease (tumor cells involve the nipple)
2. Tumors of lobular origin
   - Lobular carcinoma
     - Lobular neoplasia (not malignant)
     - Invasive lobular carcinoma
3. Tumors of stromal origin
   - Sarcoma: fibrosarcoma, liposarcoma
   - Lymphoma
4. Rare tumors
   - Phyllodes tumor
   - Carcinosarcoma

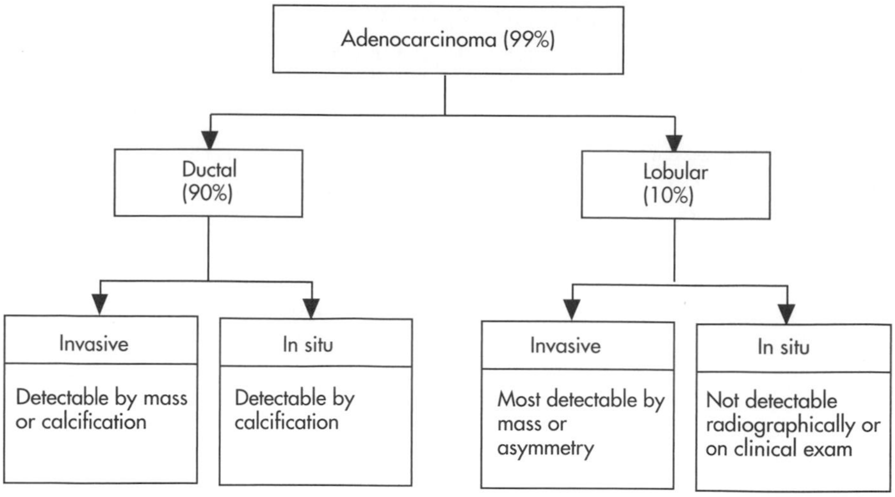

FIGURE 9-13

5. Metastases to breast
   - Melanoma (most common)
   - Lymphoma
   - Lung, renal, primary tumor

Pearls

- Tubular, mucinous, and medullary carcinomas are the three tumors with the best prognosis.
- Phyllodes tumors and cysts are the two fastest-growing breast lesions.
- Lobular neoplasia does not produce calcifications
- Most of the tumors cannot be differentiated by mammography; the tissue-specific diagnosis is usually made by histology.

OVERVIEW OF INFILTRATING-TYPE BREAST CANCERS

Type	Frequency (%)	Positive Node (%)	5-Year Survival (%)
Ductal (NOS) carcinoma	80	60	55
Lobular carcinoma	8	60	50
Medullary carcinoma	4	40	65
Colloid carcinoma	3	30	75
Comedocarcinoma	5	30	75
Papillary carcinoma	1	20	85

DCIS (COMEDOCARCINOMA, CRIBRIFORM)

Noninfiltrating, intraductal carcinoma is confined to ducts, which it fills and plugs. The centers of the tumor may undergo necrosis, and cheesy material can usually be expressed (hence the term *comedocarcinoma*). Typically, exuberant calcification (heterogeneous and irregular) is produced in the necrotic debris. Low grade forms: micropapillary, cribriform, solid; high grade: comedocarcinoma.

INVASIVE DUCTAL CARCINOMA (NOS)

Most common form of breast cancer (80%). Probably arises from DCIS and typically measures about 2 cm at diagnosis (in the absence of screening). Microscopically, the tumor has extensive collagen. Calcifications are common. Infiltration of tumor occurs into:

- Dermal lymphatics, which leads to inflammation and skin thickening
- Perivascular and perineural spaces

Desmoplastic response of breast tissue causes radiographically visible spiculations.

MEDULLARY CARCINOMA

Uncommon (4%), well-differentiated tumor that may get very large (5 to 10 cm) before discovery. Histologically the tumor is highly cellular with little stroma. Typically there is a striking lymphocytic infiltration. Tumor has high thymidine labeling. It is soft to palpation due to lack of desmoplastic reaction.

Mammographically the tumor presents as a mass as opposed to calcifications (typically absent). By US the tumor may show posterior enhancement rather than shadowing.

PAPILLARY CARCINOMA

Uncommon (1%) tumor that usually occurs near menopause. Tumors are usually not palpable but rather present as bloody discharge. At the time of diagnosis, tumors are usually large (>5 cm). They have a slower growth rate and better prognosis than infiltrative ductal carcinoma (NOS).

TUBULAR CARCINOMA

Rare, well-differentiated, most benign of all breast carcinomas. Histologically characterized by tubule formation. Mammographically the tumor is indistinguishable from other malignant tumors (e.g., spiculated margins), although tumors tend to be small (1 to 2 cm) due to slow growth.

INFLAMMATORY CARCINOMA

Uncommon (<1%), aggressive tumor with early dermal lymphatic invasion. The diagnosis is based on clinical findings of inflammation (usually there is no mass seen by mammography):

- Increased warmth (inflammation)
- Diffuse, brawny induration of breast skin
- Erysipeloid edge (peau d'orange)
- Nipple usually retracted and crusted
- Axillary lymphadenopathy common
- Mammographically there is typical skin thickening (due to carcinomatosis of dermal lymphatics).

PAGET DISEASE

Represents 5% of mammary carcinomas and typically occurs in older patients. Paget disease is a lesion of the nipple that is caused by epidermal infiltration of a ductal carcinoma. Clinically, there are eczematoid nipple changes and occasionally serous or bloody nipple discharge. Because of the early clinical signs, this cancer leads to early detection and thus has a good prognosis.

LOBULAR NEOPLASIA (LOBULAR CARCINOMA IN SITU, LCIS)

Does not produce gross morphologic changes on clinical or mammographic examination (LCIS is a histologic diagnosis). LCIS tends to occur in younger women. Not considered a cancer, but patients have 30% risk of eventually developing breast cancer (15% each breast), which may be ductal or lobular.

INFILTRATING LOBULAR CARCINOMA

Eighty percent of patients have additional foci of LCIS.

PHYLLODES TUMOR

Rare fibroepithelial tumor that is usually benign; however, 25% will recur and 10% metastasize. Tumor is partially or completely encapsulated. Pleural metastases, pleural effusion. Histologically the tumor resembles a giant fibroadenoma. Age at onset: 40 to 50 years.

METASTASES

- Melanoma is the most common metastasis to the breast, followed by sarcoma, lymphoma, lung cancer, and gastric cancer.
- Usually round, multiple, well-defined lesions
- Calcifications are not a typical feature of metastases (in contradistinction to primary breast tumors).

LYMPHOMA

- Secondary lymphoma (non-Hodgkin > Hodgkin) of the breast is more common than primary lymphoma, although both are rare (0.3% of all breast malignancies).
- Presents as palpable mass or diffuse thickening with large axillary nodes

MAMMOGRAPHIC SIGNS OF MALIGNANCY

Primary signs (due to the tumor itself; most reliable signs). 20%-30% with these findings will have breast cancer:

- Mass with spiculated or ill-fined margin
- Malignant calcifications

Secondary signs (occur as a result of the tumor; less specific signs):

- Architectural distortion
- Skin, nipple, trabecular changes (thickening, retraction)
- Abnormal ductal patterns
- Lymphadenopathy
- Asymmetry of breast tissue

Noncancerous Lesions

NORMAL BREAST

ANATOMY

The mammary gland overlies the fascia of the pectoralis major and is attached to the overlying skin by bands of connective tissue (Cooper's ligament) (Fig. 9-14). Lymphatic drainage:

- Axillary nodes, 75%
- Internal mammary nodes, 25%
- Posterior intercostal nodes (rare)
- Contralateral nodes (uncommon unless ipsilateral obstruction present)

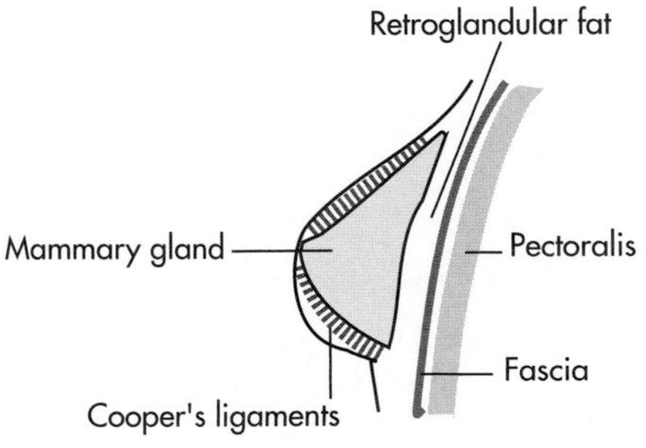

FIGURE 9-14

The gland is divided into 15 to 20 lobes that are arranged in a radial pattern. Each lobe drains separately into the nipple via a lactiferous duct. However, some ducts may join before ending in the nipple; usually there are 5 to 10 openings.

The collecting ducts terminate proximally in TDLUs, which are composed of an extralobular terminal duct, intralobular terminal duct, and ductules (Figs. 9-15 and 9-16). The ductules are the most peripheral structures. The lobule (500 μm) is the smallest structural unit of the breast.

Ducts are surrounded by cellular connective tissue, including lymphatics. The epithelium of the TDLU comprises two layers:

- Luminal true epithelial layer
- Deep myoepithelial layer

Most malignant tumors and fibrocystic changes arise from the TDLU (i.e., are epithelial in origin), but some arise from supporting stroma.

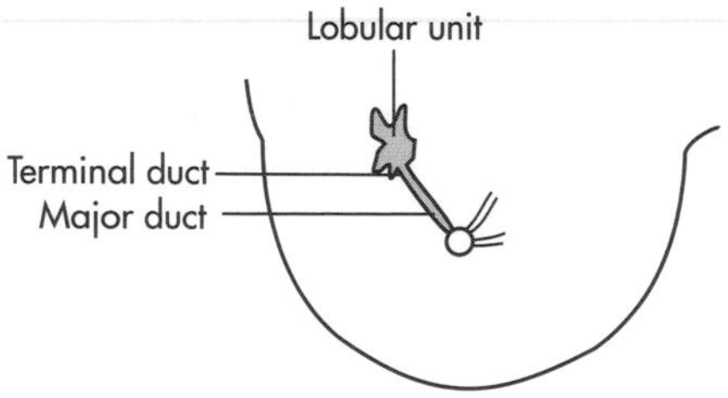

FIGURE 9-15

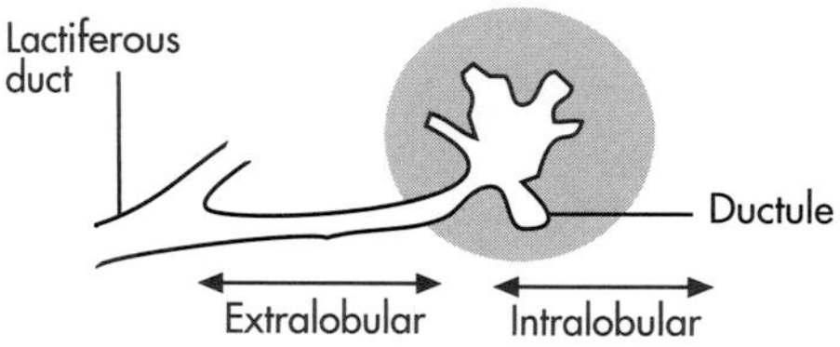

FIGURE 9-16

DENSENESS OF BREAST TISSUE

After the age of 30, the parenchymal pattern of the breast does not vary much except for changes in body habitus and/or estrogen levels (which cause parenchyma to become denser). Menopause does not change the breast pattern. Most commonly the density of breast tissue is categorized as:

- Mostly fat
- Fat with some fibroglandular tissue
- Extensively and heterogeneously dense, with fibroglandular tissue
- Extremely dense breast tissue

BENIGN PROCESSES

FIBROCYSTIC CHANGES (Fig. 9-17)

Fibrocystic changes refer to cellular proliferation in terminal ducts, lobules, and connective tissue, with development of fibrosis. Within this spectrum are changes that are symptomatic or asymptomatic, are or are not associated with increased risk for developing cancer (see list), and can be seen by mammography (fibrosis) or cannot be (epithelial proliferation).

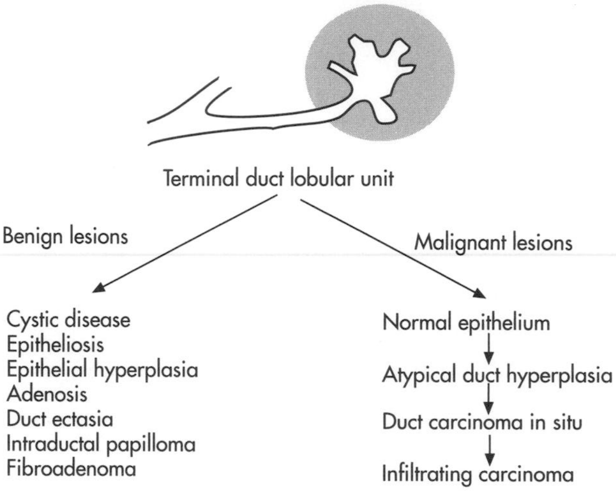

FIGURE 9-17

Risk

Increased risk for developing cancer (5 times)
- Atypical hyperplasia (lobular or ductal)

Increase risk for developing cancer (2 times)
- Hyperplasia, moderate or florid, solid or papillary
- Sclerosing adenoma

No increased risk
- Cysts
- Fibroadenoma
- Fibrosis
- Adenosis
- Duct ectasia
- Mild hyperplasia (<4 cell layers in depth)
- Mastitis
- Metaplasia (squamous, apocrine)

CYSTIC DISEASE (Fig. 9-18)

Cysts arise from terminal acini and enlarge because of obstruction or secretion imbalance. Cysts are classified according to their size:

- Microcyst (<3 mm), believed to be a normal finding
- Macrocyst (>3 mm), present in up to 50% of adult population

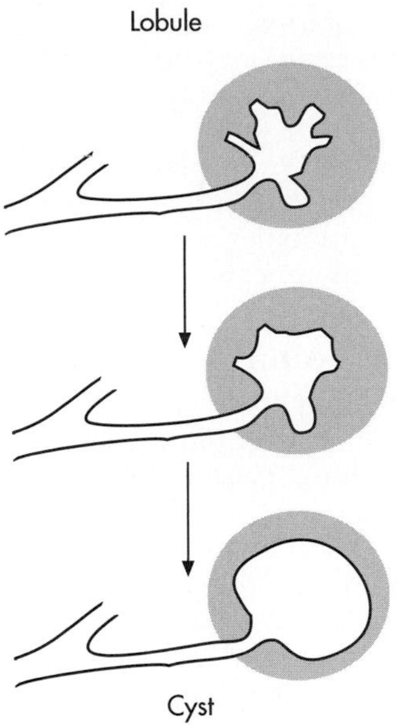

FIGURE 9-18

Histologically, cysts have an epithelial lining. Spectrum of clinical presentations includes:

- Asymptomatic presentation
- Palpable mass
- Pain from enlargement or rupture

Radiographic Features

Mammography

- Multiple rounded densities may be lobulated.
- Cysts may leak and cause inflammation and pericystic fibrosis.
- Cyst wall may calcify or the cysts may contain precipitated milk of calcium. In the mediolateral views, the x-ray beam is horizontal, allowing visualization of calcium fluid level within the cyst.
- Some cysts recur and should be reaspirated; if recurrent after second aspiration, many surgeons prefer to take a biopsy of the cyst (although the data supporting this approach are obscure).
- Tumor within a cyst is very rare but if seen usually represents a papilloma (papillary carcinoma would be the most common intracystic malignancy).
- The presence of cysts does not exclude cancer elsewhere in the breast.

US

- Cyst appearance:
  Anechoic with enhanced through-transmission
  Sharply defined anterior and posterior margins
  Round or oval
- A cyst with classic US appearance does not require aspiration.
- Thinly septated cysts are not worrisome.

FIBROADENOMA

Fibroadenomas are the most common benign solid breast lesion. They are characterized by the presence of glandular and fibrous components (focal glandular hypersensitivity to estrogen?) and proliferation of connective tissue of the lobule. They are commonly found from adolescence to age 40.

Clinical Spectrum

- Malignancy is reported to occur within fibroadenomas because they contain epithelium, but this is very rare.

Radiographic Features (Fig. 9-19)

- Well-defined, often lobulated masses
- Halo often surrounds the mass (Mach effect)
- Often contain typical popcorn calcification, a result of myxoid degeneration
- Multiple, 20%
- Rarely, fibroadenomas contain microcalcifications and are then indistinguishable from malignancy.
- Well-circumscribed and relatively hypoechoic by US
- MRI: T1-hypointense, T2-hyperintense, enhancing mass with non-enhancing dark septae

Giant Fibroadenoma

Giant fibroadenoma, or juvenile fibroadenoma, is a more cellular variant that occurs at 10 to 20 years. Most commonly solitary.

Giant fibroadenoma is indistinguishable from a phyllodes tumor by imaging. In adolescent patient, surgery may be performed for cosmesis; biopsy if no surgery to rule out phyllodes tumor.

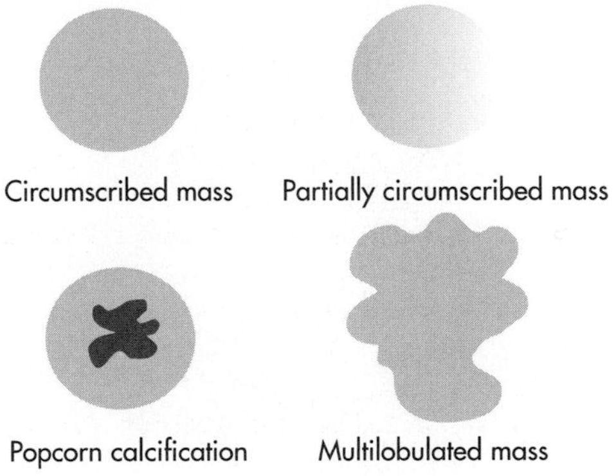

FIGURE 9-19

Complex Fibroadenoma

May contain proliferative changes such as:
- Cysts greater than 3 mm
- Sclerosing adenosis
- Epithelial calcification
- Papillary apocrine changes

PHYLLODES TUMOR

- Similar to fibroadenoma
- Large, rapidly growing breast mass
- Majority of lesions are benign. 10%-15% are malignant, with lung metastases.
- Patients are typically older than those with fibroadenomas.
- Large round or oval masses with smooth borders
- US: solid mass with low-level internal echoes
- Small fluid-filled spaces or cysts may be present.
- Biopsy required for definite diagnosis

FIBROSIS

Dense fibrosis (focal, diffuse) arises from unknown etiology. Focal forms can mimic cancer and are diagnosed by biopsy.

ADENOSIS (Fig. 9-20)

Benign entity characterized by a proliferation of glandular structures:
- Formation of new ductules and lobules
- Terminal intralobular ducts accompanied by proliferation of epithelium
- Overgrowth of myoepithelial cells

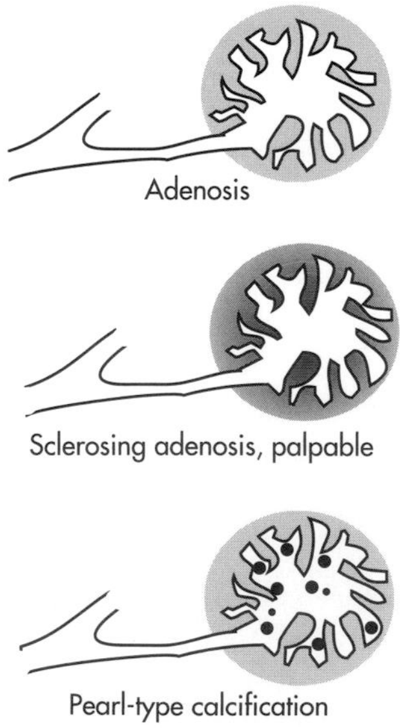

FIGURE 9-20

- May be combined with sclerosis (sclerosing adenosis); this entity may be palpable and may contain diffuse calcifications. Associated with 1.5 to 2 times higher risk for breast cancer.
- Cystic lobular hyperplasia refers to a process that is similar to adenosis but typically has cystic dilatation of lobules. Calcium within these cystic spaces often appears as milk of calcium (teacup configuration).

Radiographic Features

- Adenosis rarely forms a visible mass.
- May contain round, diffuse, segmental, or malignant-appearing, clustered microcalcifications

DUCTAL ECTASIA

Benign entity that represents accumulation of cellular debris in enlarged subareolar ducts. Patients typically present with nonsanguineous discharge and/or pain (inflammatory response). Plasma cell mastitis refers to an inflammatory component associated with extensive secretory calcifications

Radiographic Features

- Enlarged ducts can occasionally be seen by mammography.
- Often associated with extensive benign secretory calcifications

PAPILLOMA WITH FIBROVASCULAR CORE

Solitary Intraductal Papillomas

Benign lesions (hyperplastic epithelium on a stalk) usually found in an ectatic subareolar major duct. A papilloma is the most common cause of bloody or serous nipple discharge (duct ectasia is the second most common cause). Mammographic appearance:
- Occasionally seen as small mass lesion (subareolar)
- May be detected because of dilated duct
- Rarely contains benign calcifications (raspberry type)
- Galactography confirms diagnosis.
- Unlike papillomatosis, there is no increased risk of cancer.

Papillomatosis

Refers to multiple peripheral papillomas that are located in the duct lumen just proximal to the lobule. Increased risk for malignancy.

RADIAL SCAR

Idiopathic scarring process, not related to a surgical scar. Pathologically, there is sclerosing ductal hyperplasia. Has the same mammographic findings as a spiculated tumor or postsurgical scar. Usually does not have a central mass. Usually not palpable. Excise as it may be associated with ADH, DCIS, and tubular carcinoma.

PSEUDOANGIOMATOUS STROMAL HYPERPLASIA (PASH)

Benign proliferative lesion of mammary stroma, particularly of myofibroblasts. Ranges from incidentally detected microscopic foci to mammographically visible circumscribed, noncalcified mass. Hypoechoic on US. May grow and recur after excision.

BENIGN MASSES

TUBULAR ADENOMA

Uncommon, benign tumor consisting of tubular structures. The lactating adenoma is a variant.

LIPOFIBROADENOMA (HAMARTOMA)

Uncommon, large (3- to 5-cm) breast tumor that is palpable in 75% of cases. Typically the tumor is surrounded by a pseudocapsule (displaced surrounding trabeculae). Tumors contain varying amounts of fat that may occasionally be difficult to differentiate from fat in the remainder of the gland.

LIPOMA

Common tumor of the breast. Usually slow growing and seen in older patients. Easily detected mammographically because of the thin capsule (may be calcified) and lucency of the mass. Lipomas are most common in women >40 years of age.

TENSION CYSTS

Develop as a result of an obstructed apocrine cyst. The obstruction may be caused by epithelial hyperplasia, fibrosis, kinking of duct, cancer, and so on.

GALACTOCELE

Most common benign breast lesion in lactating women. Milk-containing cysts caused by inspissated milk obstructing a duct. Galactoceles typically occur in 20- to 30-year-old patients postlactation. Because milk contains fat, these lesions may be entirely lucent. A horizontal beam may show a fat-fluid level.

DESMOID

Extraabdominal desmoids are very rare breast lesions. Desmoids are usually in close proximity to the pectoralis muscle. May have spiculated borders, thus mimicking cancer. Never contain microcalcifications.

SEBACEOUS CYST

Keratin-filled sac below skin, which may become inflamed. US may demonstrate superficial hypoechoic mass with thin hypoechoic linear connection to skin.

INFLAMMATION

MASTITIS

Types

- Acute mastitis (puerperal mastitis): staphylococcal infection related to lactation (pain, erythema, clinical diagnosis)
- Mastitis in older patients (nonpuerperal mastitis): secondary to infection of sebaceous glands; may proceed to abscess
- Plasma cell mastitis: rare aseptic inflammation of subareolar region; in elderly women it is often bilateral and symmetrical; thought to result from extravasation of intraductal secretions with subsequent reactive inflammation
- Granulomatous mastitis (rare): TB, sarcoid

Radiographic Features

Density
- Areas of diffusely increased density
- May mimic inflammatory cancer (especially in older patients)
- Abscess appears as focal mass.

Nodes
- Axillary adenopathy is common.

Skin
- Skin thickening
- Nipple retraction

FAT NECROSIS

Results from blunt trauma, surgery, or radiation therapy. Lipocytes necrose, fat liquefies (oil cysts), and fibrosis develops before healing.

Radiographic Features

- Poorly defined mass with ill-defined, hazy borders; may be spiculated (may mimic cancer)
- Unlike cancer, fat necrosis decreases in size over time.
- May form a lucent oil cyst
- Rim calcifications are common.
- Coarse calcifications
- Microcalcifications indistinguishable from breast cancer (rare)

IMPLANTS

Implants used for breast augmentation include most commonly Silastic bags filled with silicone or saline. Implant leakage occurs in 1%-2%. Old silicone injections (no longer used) present as multiple curvilinear calcifications near the skin surface (0.5 to 2 cm; differential diagnosis: scleroderma). There are 2 locations for surgical implants (without clear-cut evidence of which one is superior):

- Subpectoral implants
- Retroglandular implants

There are many types of implants:
- Single lumen: silicone or saline
- Double lumen: inner silicone/outer saline
- Reverse double-lumen: inner saline/outer silicone
- Other: expander, foam
- Multiple stacked implants

To diagnose breast cancer in patients with implants, the entire remaining glandular tissue has to be imaged. The screening mammographic examination for patients with implants consists of four views:
- Routine CC and MLO
- Implant displaced CC and MLO (Ecklund)

If the implant is not freely movable so that adequate displacement is not possible, a straight lateral view is added to image the posterior tissue above and below the implant.

Radiographic Features (Fig. 9-21)

Contour abnormalities
- Breast forms a fibrous capsule around the implant.
- Rupture can be intracapsular (implant shell only) or extracapsular (implant shell and fibrous capsule).
- Gel bleed: microscopic silicone leaks through intact shell. A gel bleed usually cannot be detected by imaging.
- Flaps ("linguini sign" by MRI) may represent intracapsular rupture.
- Radiating folds: normal findings are not to be confused with rupture.
- Crenulated margins indicate capsular contracture.
- Focal bulges: may represent a rupture or a herniation through the fibrous capsule
- Inverted teardrop: nonspecific sign seen with extensive gel bleed or focal intracapsular rupture; occurs when silicone enters radial fold and then leaks between internal and external capsules

Calcifications
- Silicone-induced tissue calcifications may have a variety of sizes and shapes.
- Capsular calcification is due to an inflammatory response.

US
- Implants are normally hypoechoic.
- Echogenic implants are abnormal ("snowstorm" or "stepladder" appearance of ruptured implants).

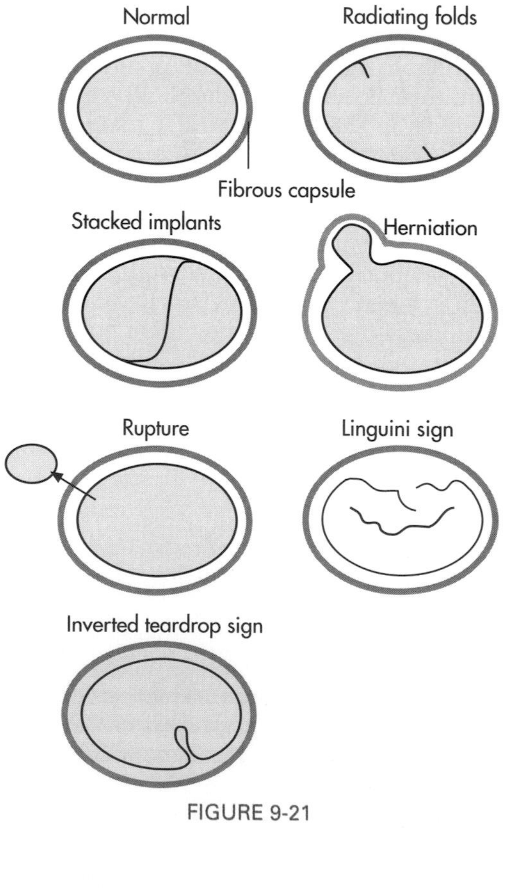

FIGURE 9-21

POSTSURGICAL BREAST

IMAGING FINDINGS IN THE POSTSURGICAL BREAST

Finding	0-6 mo (%)	7-24 mo (%)	>2 yr (%)
Skin changes	95	55	25
Architectural distortion	85	35	15
Loss of tissue	10	10	5
Parenchymal scar	30	5	3
Calcification	5	5	5
Fat necrosis	5	1	1
Foreign body	1	1	1

Postsurgical scars and spiculated tumors have the same mammographic appearance and usually cannot be separated reliably without knowledge of the clinical findings. Findings suggestive of scars include:
- Involution with time (should be gone by 1 year)
- Long curvilinear spicules extending to skin

Postreduction Mammography

Mammograms may show any of the findings listed above, as well as a swirling appearance of the parenchyma in the inferior breast. The retroareolar ducts may be interrupted.

Transverse Rectus Abdominis Musculocutaneous (TRAM) Reconstruction

Palpable abnormality after TRAM reconstruction may be due to fat necrosis or cancer and may be evaluated with mammography.

POSTRADIATION BREAST

Typical radiation dose is 50 Gy to the breast and boosting 60 to 75 Gy at lumpectomy site. The postradiation mammograms should be performed 6 months after initiation of therapy and followed annually. Women with diffuse intraductal disease may be at increased risk of recurrence after radiation therapy. Mastectomy, not breast conservation therapy, is performed in cases of local recurrence.

Radiographic Features

- Diffuse density of entire breast, unilateral (edema); most pronounced at 6 months, nearly gone at 24 months
- Thickening of skin and trabecula usually resolves within months but may progress to permanent fibrosis. Persistent distortion or scarring after 1 year is difficult to differentiate from tumor.
- Calcifications after radiation therapy may represent:
  - Residual tumor calcifications (although all should have been removed by surgery)
  - Benign dystrophic calcifications, which arise 2 to 4 years after radiation (usually large with central lucency)

MALE BREAST

The normal male breast is predominantly composed of fat that has no lobules and only rudimentary ducts. Therefore, male breasts do not develop fibroadenomas.

GYNECOMASTIA

Gynecomastia refers to an enlargement of the male breast (most common male breast abnormality). It occurs most commonly in adolescent boys and men >50 years.

Gynecomastia is usually asymmetrical. There are two types.

- Florid type (usually pubertal type): predominantly epithelial proliferation, edema, and cellular stroma
- Fibrous type (usually older men): predominantly fibrosis

Causes

Drugs
- Reserpine
- Spironolactone
- Cimetidine
- Marijuana
- Estrogens

Secreting testicular tumors (increased estrogen production)
- Seminoma
- Embryonal cell carcinoma
- Choriocarcinoma

Hepatic cirrhosis
- Inadequate estrogen degradation

Klinefelter syndrome

Cryptorchidism

Radiographic Features

- Subareolar increased density, which is typically flame shaped (the normal male breast is predominantly fatty)
- Unilateral or bilateral, symmetrical or asymmetrical
- Secretions may be present especially in gynecomastia secondary to estrogens.
- US appearance may be "volcano-like"

MALE BREAST CANCER

Very rare tumor (0.2% of male malignancies). Mean age: 70 years. Risk factors include exposure to ionizing radiation, occupational exposure to electromagnetic field radiation, cryptorchidism, testicular injury, Klinefelter syndrome, liver dysfunction, family history of breast cancer, previous chest trauma, and advanced age. Mammographic findings in male breast cancer are similar to those in female cancer. For mammography of the male breast, bilateral studies are performed routinely, even if the symptoms are only unilateral. Spot film, US, and biopsy may be performed for suspected cancer. Histology: infiltrating ductal carcinoma or DCIS (even in men with gynecomastia, lobule formation is rare). Gynecomastia does not increase a man's risk for developing breast carcinoma.

Male breast cancer usually occurs in a subareolar location or is positioned eccentric to the nipple. The lesions can have any shape but are frequently lobulated. Calcifications are fewer, coarser, and less frequently rod shaped than those seen in female breast cancer. Secondary features include skin thickening, nipple retraction, and axillary lymphadenopathy.

Differential Diagnosis

MASS LESIONS

SPICULATED MASSES

All spiculated masses are suggestive of neoplasm and should be sampled. Causes include:
- Malignancy
- Radial scar (benign sclerosing adenosis)

- Fat necrosis
- Postsurgical scar
- Superimposed tissue mimicking a lesion
- Desmoid

MASS WITH MICROLOBULATION

- Cancer

MASS WITH MACROLOBULATION

- Phyllodes tumor
- Fibroadenoma
- Simple cyst
- Intramammary lymph node

WELL-CIRCUMSCRIBED MASSES (ROUNDED DENSITIES)

- Cysts (common lesion <40 years; less common in postmenopausal women)
- Fibroadenoma (most common lesion in the 10- to 40-year age group)
- Hematoma (seat belt injury, biopsy)
- Lymph nodes are common in upper outer quadrant. However, they are suspicious if:
  - >1 cm without fat
  - No lucent center or hilar notch
- Skin
  - Seborrheic keratosis is most common skin lesion seen by mammography. Nipple imaged out of profile
- Malignant tumors
  - Primary tumors rarely present as well-circumscribed mass lesions; however, the following types can occur:
    - Invasive (NOS)
    - Papillary cancer
    - Medullary cancer
    - Mucinous cancer
    - Metastasis (rare)
- Other
  - Fibrosis (may be isolated, dense, and sharply marginated; never distorts architecture)
  - Trauma (hematoma): usually resolves weeks after trauma; scars can persist.
  - Phyllodes tumor: rare lesion, usually benign (15% malignant), variant of fibroadenoma (benign giant fibroadenoma, very dense)

Approach

- Lesions <8 mm: follow-up in 6 months (US is less accurate in these small lesions)
- Lesions >8 mm: US to determine whether the lesion is a cyst

DEVELOPING DENSITY ON MAMMOGRAM

- Carcinoma
- Hematoma
- Cysts
- Hormonal changes in fibroglandular tissue

LUCENT LESIONS (FATTY LESIONS)

- Hamartoma (lipofibroadenomas; usually large)
- Lipoma
- Traumatic oil cysts
- Steatocystoma multiplex: multiple calcified and noncalcified oil cysts, autosomal dominant
- Galactocele (rare; may have fat-fluid level, lactating breasts)

GIANT MASSES (>5 CM)

Tumors
- Hamartoma (in older patients)
- Cystosarcoma phyllodes
- Giant fibroadenoma (young patients: 10 to 20 years old)

Abscess

BREAST MASS DURING PREGNANCY/LACTATION

- Lactating adenoma
- Galactocele
- Fibroadenoma
- Focal mastitis
- Cancer

OTHER

ARCHITECTURAL DISTORTION

- Cancer
- Radial scar
- Postbiopsy, surgery
- Sclerosing adenosis

NIPPLE RETRACTION

- Acquired with age (usually bilateral and symmetrical)
- Hamartoma or seroma
- Congenital
- Tumor
- Inflammatory

NIPPLE DISCHARGE

- Papilloma (most common cause)
- Duct ectasia (2nd most common cause)
- Only 5% of cancers (especially intraductal carcinoma) present with nipple discharge as a solitary finding.
- Others
  - Papillomatosis
  - Fibrocystic changes

PROMINENT DUCTS

- Duct ectasia (bilateral)
- Intraductal papilloma (unilateral)
- Intraductal carcinoma (unilateral)
- Vascular structures mimicking ducts

TRABECULAR THICKENING

- Mastitis (always obtain a follow-up view to exclude an underlying mass)
- Inflammatory carcinoma
- Postradiation
- Postreduction mammoplasty
- Lymphatic or SVC obstruction, including metastases to local lymph nodes
- Metastases

MALE BREAST ENLARGEMENT

- Gynecomastia (most common cause)
- Abscess
- Lipoma
- Sebaceous cysts
- Breast cancer (uncommon)

SHRINKING BREAST

- Surgery
- Diabetic mastopathy
- Diffuse invasive lobular carcinoma

SKIN

DIFFUSE SKIN THICKENING (>2.5 MM)

Tumor
- Inflammatory breast cancer
- Lymphoma
- Leukemia

Inflammation
- Acute mastitis
- Abscess
- Radiation
- Postsurgery

Lymphatic obstruction
- Lymphatic spread of tumor to axilla (breast, lung)

Generalized edema
- Right-sided heart failure
- Central venous obstruction
- Nephrotic syndrome

RINGLIKE PERIPHERAL CALCIFICATION IN MASS

- Fibroadenoma
- Calcified cyst
- Oil cyst
- Fat necrosis

FOCAL SKIN THICKENING

Tumor
- Carcinoma
- Intradermal metastases
- Skin lesions (usually have radiolucent rim around them): seborrheic keratitis, moles, warts

Inflammation
- Plasma cell mastitis
- Dermatitis
- Prior trauma, biopsy
- Fat necrosis
- Mondor disease (thrombosis of superficial veins)

BASIC WORKUP FOR COMMON FINDINGS

Palpable lump
- Old films
- Inquire about history of surgery or trauma
- Spot compression magnification views (to better define borders)
- Targeted ultrasound (unless the area of interest shows *complete* fat density on mammogram)

Nonpalpable mass on mammogram/ultrasound
- Core biopsy (ultrasound or stereotactic) or needle localization for surgical excision

Calcifications
- Old films
- Localize on two views
- Spot magnification CC and ML (straight lateral rather than MLO to identify benign layering/teacup calcifications, if present)
- Tangential if skin calcifications are suspected

Asymmetrical density (also known as global asymmetry)
- Must be nonpalpable *and* in typical location (upper outer breast)
- If stable from prior exams (i.e., not a new or enlarging density), no mass-forming borders or architectural distortion, and no calcifications → BI-RADS 2
- In the absence of the criteria above, work up as for any palpable or mass lesion.

Architectural distortion without prior surgery
- Conservative approach: needle localization for surgical excision
- More practical approach: attempt stereotactic biopsy and *leave clip*. If pathology shows cancer, surgeon can proceed to single comprehensive surgery. Any other pathology diagnosis (e.g., radial scar) requires needle localization of clip for surgical excision and definitive diagnosis.

Complex mass (old term: complex cyst) on US: needle localization of solid component of complex mass for surgical excision.

Simple cyst on ultrasound → BI-RADS 2

Nipple discharge

- Worrisome discharge: bloody, clear, unilateral, spontaneous
- Benign discharge color: green or brown
- Workup: mammogram with nipple in profile and targeted retroareolar ultrasound. Galactography may be helpful, depending on local surgeon's preferences.

Unilateral axillary lymphadenopathy with negative diagnostic mammograms

- Biopsy lymph node: if pathology shows adenocarcinoma, obtain breast MRI to search for occult primary breast lesion; if pathology shows lymphoma, stage patient with CT.

Suggested Readings

Breast Imaging Reporting and Data System (BI-Rads). 4th ed. Reston, VA: American College of Radiology; 2003.

Egan RL. *Breast Imaging: Diagnosis and Morphology of Breast Diseases*. Philadelphia: WB Saunders; 1988.

Homer MJ. *Mammographic Interpretations: A Practical Approach*. Philadelphia: WB Saunders; 2000.

Kopans D. *Breast Imaging*. Philadelphia: Lippincott Williams & Wilkins; 2006.

Peters ME, Voegeli CM. *Breast Imaging*. London: Churchill Livingstone; 1989.

Sickles EA, Destouet JM, Eklund GW, et al. *Breast Disease (test and syllabus)*. 2nd ed. Reston, VA: American College of Radiology; 1993.

CHAPTER 10

Obstetric Imaging

CHAPTER OUTLINE

First Trimester

GENERAL

REFERENCE

All ages in this section refer to the menstrual age or gestational age based on the last menstrual period (LMP) and not the embryonic age based on day of conception. A 4-week pregnancy by the LMP method thus corresponds to a 2-week pregnancy by the conception method. All measurements given in this section are for transvaginal sonography (TVS) unless otherwise stated.

ROLE OF IMAGING

1st Trimester

1. Confirm an intrauterine pregnancy (IUP)
2. Date an IUP (confirm gestational age)
3. Determine fetal number and placentation
4. Evaluation for an ectopic pregnancy
5. Evaluation of 1st trimester bleeding: assess viability
   - Normal IUP
   - Abortion: impending, in progress, incomplete, missed
   - Ectopic pregnancy
   - Subchorionic hemorrhage

2nd Trimester

1. Determine fetal number and viability
2. Placental evaluation and location
3. Estimate amount of amniotic fluid
4. Assess gestational age and growth
5. Fetal survey
6. Evaluate adnexa and cervix

3rd Trimester

1. Fetal presentation (vertex, breech) (Fig. 10-1)
2. Type of placenta
3. Membranes
4. Cervical os
5. Biophysical profile, growth

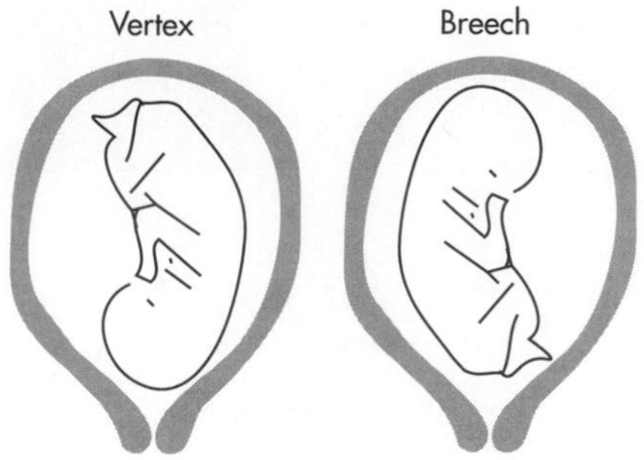

FIGURE 10-1

PRENATAL SCREENING

Screening Tests

- Ultrasound (US)
- α-Fetoprotein (AFP)
- β-Human chorionic gonadotropin (β-HCG)
- Amniocentesis
- Chorionic villous sampling (CVS)
- Fetal blood sampling

Reasons for Prenatal Screening

- Advanced maternal age (most common) (age ≥ 35 years)
- Prior children with chromosomal abnormalities or structural defects
- Family history of genetic or metabolic disorder
- Exposure to teratogens (drugs, infections)

α-Fetoprotein (AFP) (Fig. 10-2)

- AFP is formed by the fetal liver, yolk sac, and gut and is found at different concentrations in fetal serum, amniotic fluid, and maternal serum (MSAFP).
- In the normal fetus, AFP originates from fetal serum and enters amniotic fluid through fetal urination, fetal GI secretions, and transudation from membranes (amnion and placenta).

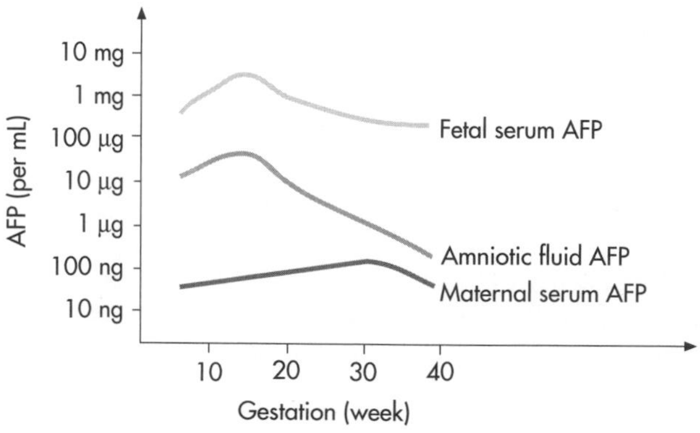

FIGURE 10-2

- Elevated MSAFP levels occur if there is transudation of AFP into the maternal serum, such as in open neural tube defects (AFP screening has an 80%-90% sensitivity for detection) or in fetal swallowing problems (abdominal wall defect).
- MSAFP is best measured at 16 weeks.
- False-positive causes of elevated AFP include:
  - Gestational age 2 weeks≥ that estimated clinically
  - Multiple gestations
  - Fetal death
- In case of elevated AFP, test for acetylcholinesterase in amniotic fluid, which is present in neural tube defects.

β-HCG

Normal β-HCG levels correlate with size of gestational sac until 8th to 10th week. Thereafter, β-HCG levels decline. Initially, the doubling time for the β-HCG is 2 to 3 days. Third International Reference Preparation = 1.84 × Second International Reference Preparation.

FOUR PATTERNS OF β-HCG IN PREGNANCY

β-HCG (mIU/ML)*	US	Outcome
<1000	Gestational sac present	Abortion likely
<1000	Gestational sac absent	Not diagnostic, repeat
>1000-2000	Gestational sac present	Normal pregnancy
>2000	Gestational sac absent	Ectopic pregnancy likely

*Second International Standard. As a general rule, values measured according to the Second International Standard are equivalent to half that of the Third International Standard (e.g., 500 mIU/mL [2IS] = 1000 mIU/mL [3IS]).

QUAD SCREEN MARKERS

Risk Category	AFP	β-HCG	Estriol	Inhibin A
NTD/abdominal wall defect	Increased	Normal	Normal	Normal
Trisomy 21	Decreased	Increased	Decreased	Increased
Trisomy 18	Decreased	Decreased	Decreased	Normal

NTD, neural tube defect.

AMNIOCENTESIS

Performed at 15 to 16 weeks using a US-guided transabdominal approach. Desquamated cells of amniotic fluid are cultured and then karyotyped 2 to 3 weeks later. In twin pregnancies, indigo carmine is injected into the amniotic cavity punctured first to ensure sampling of both cavities. The main complication is fetal loss (0.5%).

Indications

- Advanced maternal age ≥ 35 years
- Abnormal MSAFP
- History of genetic or chromosomal disorders

- Fetal anomalies: central nervous system (CNS) lesions, large choroid plexus cyst (controversial), cystic hygroma, nuchal thickening, heart defects, congenital dislocation of the hip (CDH), duodenal atresia, omphalocele, cystic kidneys, hydrops, pleural effusions, ascites, clubfoot, two-vessel umbilical cord, facial anomalies, short femur

CHORIONIC VILLUS SAMPLING (CVS)

- Performed earlier than amniocentesis: 10 to 12 weeks
- Transcervical or transabdominal approach under US guidance

FETAL BLOOD SAMPLING

- Allows rapid chromosomal analysis within 2 to 3 days
- Percutaneous US-guided sampling of umbilical vessels

NUCHAL LUCENCY THICKENING

- 1st trimester: measure inner to inner margin (midsagittal neck)
- >3 mm is abnormal
- Associated with
  - Chromosomal abnormalities (21, 18, 13), 20%
  - Cardiac anomalies
  - Skeletal dysplasia
- Second trimester: measure outer to outer margin (suboccipital-bregmatic plane at the level of the cavum septum pellucidum, cerebellum, and cisterna magna);
  - >6 mm is abnormal
  - Aneuploidy risk increased by 2× the normal maternal age risk

FIRST-TRIMESTER IMAGING

APPROACH TO 1ST-TRIMESTER SONOGRAM (Fig. 10-3)

NORMAL PREGNANCY

EARLY DEVELOPMENT (Fig. 10-4)

- Fertilization occurs in fallopian tubes.
- Oocyte + sperm cell = zygote.
- Cleavage occurs in the fallopian tube.
- Morula enters the uterine cavity.
- Blastocyst implants into the endometrial wall.
- Corpus luteum develops from ruptured graafian follicle (usually <2 cm), secretes progesterone, and induces decidual reaction.
- Corpus luteum regresses at 10 weeks, when its function is taken over by the placenta.

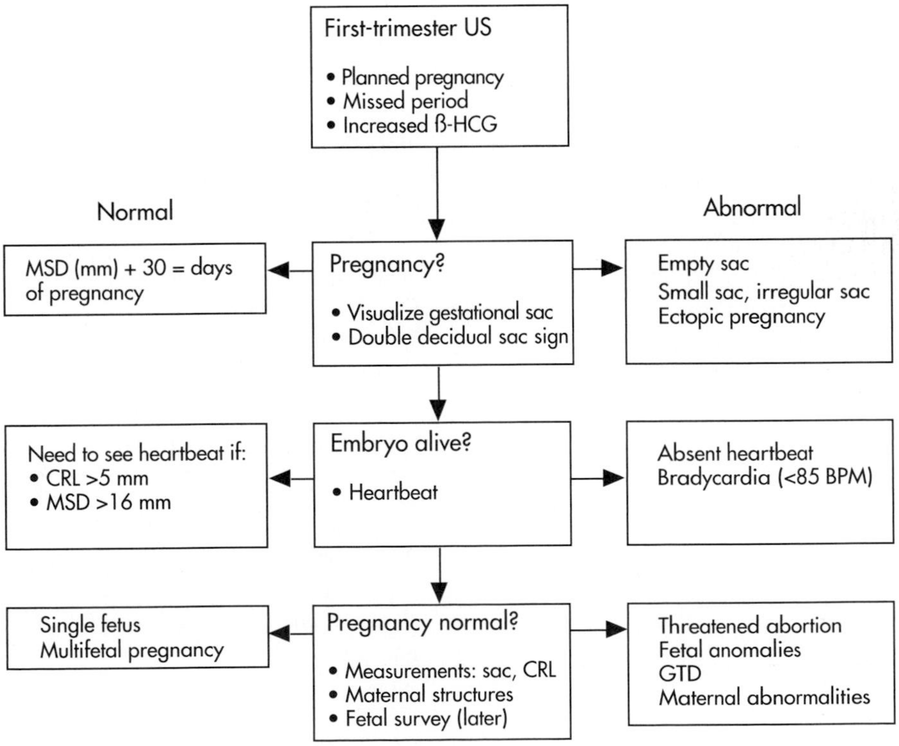

FIGURE 10-3

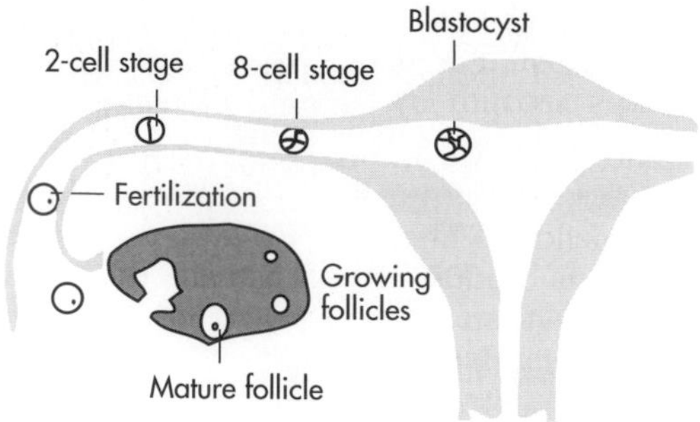

FIGURE 10-4

AMNIOTIC AND CHORIONIC MEMBRANES (Fig. 10-5)

- Amniotic cavity is initially small.
- Embryo lies within the amniotic cavity.
- Amniotic cavity enlarges and ultimately fuses with the chorion (14 to 16 weeks).
- Yolk sac is located outside the amniotic cavity but within the chorionic cavity; it is connected to primitive gut by the omphalomesenteric duct.

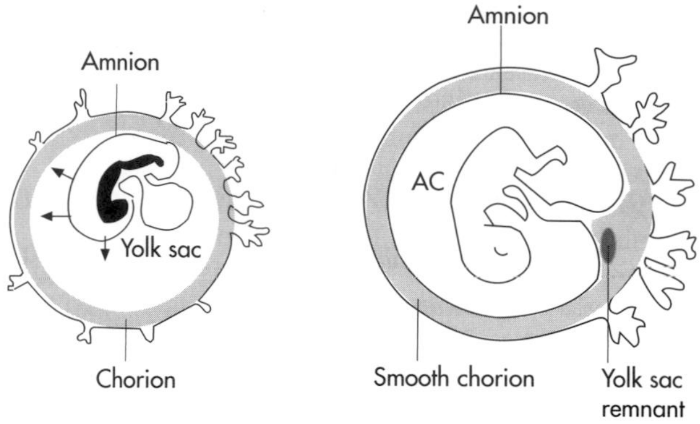

FIGURE 10-5

Double Decidual Sac Sign (Fig. 10-6)

The double decidual sac sign is a useful early sign of IUP. It is based on the demonstration of three layers of different echogenicity:

- Decidua parietalis (hyperechoic)
- Fluid in the uterine cavity (hypoechoic)
- Decidua capsularis (hyperechoic)

The double-bleb sign refers to the presence of an amnion and yolk sac at 5 to 6 weeks. The embryo lies between these two structures.

YOLK SAC

- Provides nutrients to the embryo until placental circulation is established
- Angiogenesis and hematopoiesis occur in the wall of the yolk sac.

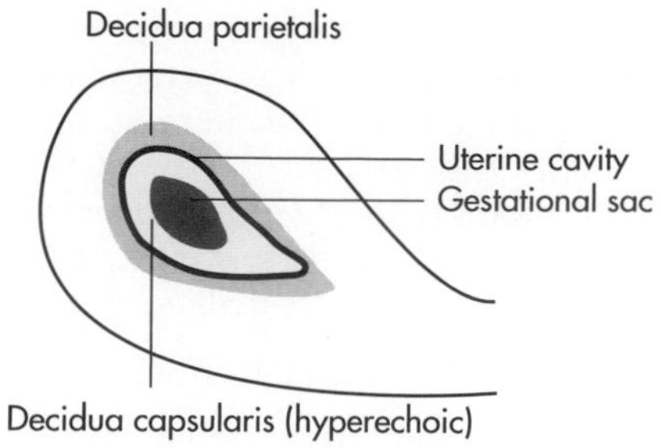

FIGURE 10-6

- Dorsal part is later incorporated into the primitive gut and remains connected by the omphalomesenteric (vitelline) duct

FETAL HEART

A fetal heartbeat should always be detectable if the crown-rump length (CRL) is ≥ 5 mm by TVS. Absence of cardiac activity in embryos >5 mm is indicative of fetal demise.

Pearls

- Occasionally, embryonic cardiac activity may be seen before a distinct embryo is visualized.
- In patients with threatened abortion, demonstration of cardiac activity is the single most important role of US.

GESTATIONAL SAC

NORMAL GESTATIONAL SAC

The gestational sac is the implantation product that occurs in the uterus on approximately day 21. At that time the blastocyst is approximately 0.1 mm in size and cannot be seen by US. Normal sacs become visible when they reach 2 to 3 mm. Measurements:

$$\text{Mean sac diameter (MSD)} = \frac{(\text{length} + \text{width} + \text{height})}{3}$$

Normal MSD (mm) + 30 = days of pregnancy

After the gestational sac has developed, a yolk sac, the fetal heartbeat, and the embryo will become visible.

TVS LANDMARKS (ACCURACY ± 0.5 WEEK)

Age	β-HCG	Gestational Sac	Yolk Sac	Heart-beat	Embryo (Fetal Pole)
5 wk	500-1000	+	–	–	–
5.5 wk	>3600	+	+	–	–
6 wk	>5400	+	+	+	–
>6 wk		+	+	+	+

Order of appearance of structures: gestational sac → yolk sac → embryo (fetal pole) → amnion (Fig. 10-7)

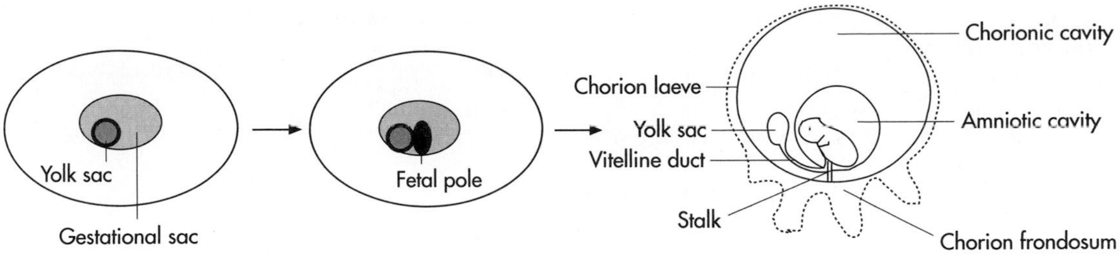

FIGURE 10-7

CORRELATION OF MSD AND β-HCG LEVELS (Fig. 10-8)

- β-HCG and MSD increase proportionally until the 8th week (25-mm MSD).
- β-HCG doubles every 2 to 3 days.
- β-HCG levels decline after 8 weeks.
- Normal MSD growth: 1.1 mm/day
- Discordance between MSD and β-HCG indicates an increased probability of demise.

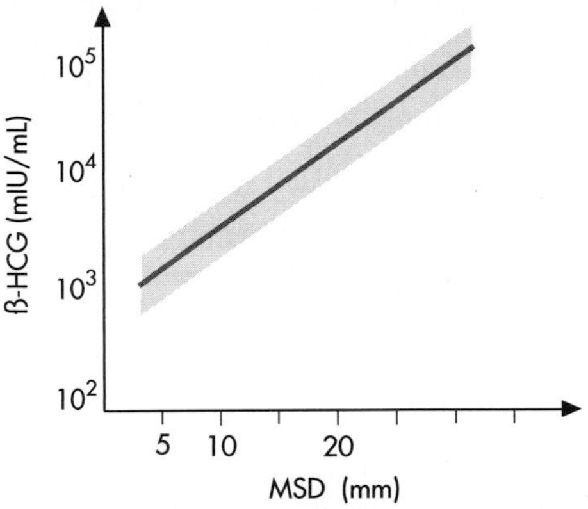

FIGURE 10-8

CRITERIA FOR THE DIAGNOSIS OF ABNORMAL GESTATIONAL SACS

MAJOR CRITERIA (POSITIVE PREDICTIVE VALUE 100%)

Finding*	MSD
Abnormal Finding by TVS	
No yolk sac	≥ 8 mm
No heartbeat	≥ 16 mm
Abnormal Finding by TAS	
No yolk sac	≥ 20 mm
No heartbeat	>25 mm
Low β-HCG for a given MSD†	

*For example, a yolk sac should always be demonstrated by TAS if the MSD is >20 mm or by TVS if the MSD is >8 mm.
†Consult a normogram.

Minor Criteria

- Irregular contour of sac
- Decidual reaction <2 mm
- Choriodecidual reaction not echogenic
- Absent double decidual sac
- Low position

SMALL GESTATIONAL SAC

Patients with small sac size have a high likelihood (>90%) of pregnancy loss. Rule of thumb:
MSD (in mm) – CRL (in mm) <5 mm indicates loss of pregnancy.

EMPTY GESTATIONAL SAC

Refers to a gestational sac that does not contain a yolk sac or embryo. An empty gestational sac may represent:

- An early normal IUP (if MSD <8 mm)
- An anembryonic pregnancy: blighted ovum (if MSD >8 mm)
- Pseudogestational sac of ectopic pregnancy

Blighted ovum refers to an abnormal IUP with developmental arrest occurring before formation of the embryo.

PSEUDOGESTATIONAL SAC

Twenty percent of patients with ectopic pregnancies have an intrauterine pseudogestational sac (i.e., intrauterine fluid collection rimmed by endometrium). Differentiation from gestational sac:

- Pseudogestational sacs are located centrally in uterine cavity, not eccentrically like a true sac.
- Pseudogestational sacs do not have a yolk sac.
- Pseudogestational sacs have an absent double decidual sign.

THREATENED ABORTION

Threatened abortion is a clinical term encompassing a broad spectrum of disease that occurs in 25% of pregnancies and results in true abortion in 50%. It includes:

- Blighted ovum
- Ectopic pregnancy
- Inevitable abortion

- Incomplete abortion
- Missed abortion

Signs and symptoms of threatened abortion include bleeding, pain, contractions, and open cervix. If a live embryo is identified, predictors of poor outcome are:

- Bradycardia (<85 beats/min)
- Small gestational sac size (if MSD − CRL <5 mm)
- Subchorionic hemorrhage (large > two thirds of the circumference)
- Large yolk sac (>6 mm)
- Irregular, crenated, or calcified yolk sac
- Abnormal gestational sac location
- Irregular sac shape
- Absence or thinning of the decidual reaction surrounding the sac

TERMINOLOGY OF ABORTION

Threatened abortion
- Vaginal bleeding with closed cervical os during the first 20 weeks of pregnancy
- Occurs in 25% of 1st-trimester pregnancies
- 50% survival

Inevitable abortion
- Vaginal bleeding with open cervical os; an abortion in progress
- Incomplete abortion
- Retained products of conception causing continued bleeding
- Spontaneous abortion
- Vaginal bleeding, passage of tissue
- Most common in 1st trimester
- No US evidence of viable IUP; ectopic pregnancy must be excluded.
- High percentage have chromosomal abnormalities.
- Missed abortion
- Retention of a dead pregnancy for at least 2 months

EMBRYONIC DEMISE (DEAD EMBRYO)

The most common cause of embryonic death is a chromosomal abnormality that leads to arrested development. Any of the following indicate embryonic demise:

- CRL >5 mm and no cardiac activity
- MSD ≥ 8 mm and no yolk sac
- MSD ≥ 16 mm and no embryo
- Absent yolk sac in presence of an embryo
- Absent cardiac activity in embryo seen by TAS. If early, need to confirm with TVS.

BRADYCARDIA

If the heart rate is ≤ 85 beats/min at 5 to 8 weeks, spontaneous abortion will nearly always occur. Follow-up US is recommended to assess for viability.

NORMAL FETAL HEART RATES

Time	Mean (beats/min)
5-6 weeks	101
8-9 weeks	143
>10 weeks	140

The presence of cardiac activity indicates a good but not a 100% chance that a pregnancy will progress to term. There is still a 20% chance of pregnancy loss during the first 8 weeks even if a positive heartbeat is present. During the 9th to 12th weeks, the chance of fetal loss decreases to 1%-2% in the presence of a positive heart beat.

SUBCHORIONIC HEMORRHAGE

Venous bleeding causing marginal abruption with separation of the chorion from the endometrial lining extending to the margin of the placenta. Usually (80%) occurs in the late 1st trimester and presents as vaginal bleeding. Prognosis: generally good if there is a fetal heart beat and bleeding is minimal. Hemorrhage greater than two thirds of the chorionic sac circumference is associated with more than a 2-fold increase in risk of pregnancy loss.

PERCENTAGE OF PREGNANCY LOSS IN 1ST TRIMESTER WITH AND WITHOUT VAGINAL BLEEDING

Week	Bleeding (%)	No Bleeding (%)
<6	35	20
7-8	20	5
9-11	5	1-2

US Features (Fig. 10-9)
- Associated with marginal separation of placenta

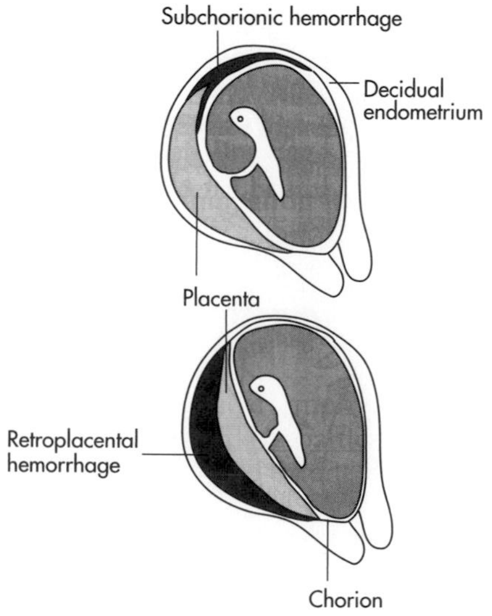

FIGURE 10-9

- Hypoechoic or hyperechoic blood separates chorion from endometrium
- Distinguish from retroplacental bleed and abruption by location and extent of placental involvement

Ectopic Pregnancy

GENERAL

LOCATION (Fig. 10-10)

- Tubal, 97%
    - Ampullary (most common)
    - Isthmus
- Interstitial (cornual), 3%
- Ovarian, 1%
- Cervical (very rare)
- Fimbria (very rare)

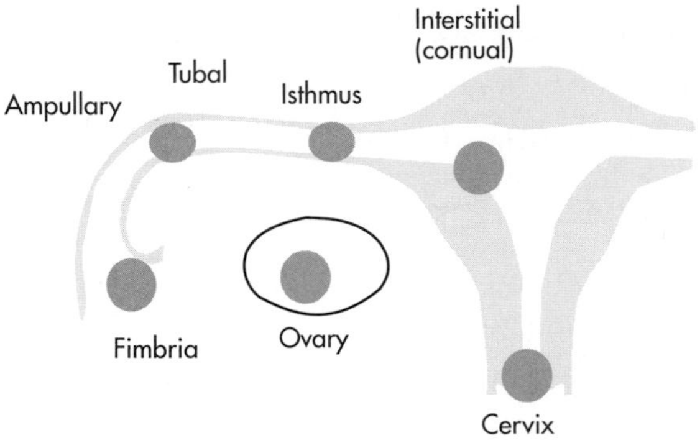

FIGURE 10-10

CLINICAL FINDINGS

Incidence: 0.5%-1% of all pregnancies. Triad:

- Pain, 95%
- Hemorrhage, 85%
- Palpable adnexal mass, 40%

RISK FACTORS

- Prior ectopic pregnancy
- History of pelvic inflammatory disease
- Tubal surgery or other tubal abnormalities
- Endometriosis
- Previous pelvic surgery
- Infertility and infertility treatments
- Uterotubal anomalies
- History of in utero exposure to diethylstilbestrol
- Cigarette smoking
- IUD is not a risk factor but has been associated with ectopic pregnancy because IUD prevents intrauterine pregnancy but not ectopic pregnancy.

DIAGNOSIS

DIAGNOSTIC TESTS

Serum markers

- Normal β-HCG doubling time depends on the age of the pregnancy but on average is 2 days.
- Ectopic pregnancies usually have a slower increase in β-HCG than normal pregnancies.
- Low levels of β-HCG suggest ectopic pregnancy.
- Reduced levels of progesterone P4 suggest ectopic pregnancy.

Culdocentesis

- Considered to be positive if >5 mL of non-clotted blood is aspirated; clotted blood indicates that a vessel has been entered; dry tap is nondiagnostic.
- Culdocentesis is preferred to detect ectopic pregnancy of <6 weeks; at later time points, US is preferred.

US

- Always use TVS. If negative, also perform TAS.
- Doppler US can be used to detect peritrophoblastic flow.

US FEATURES

Uterus

- May be normal
- Thick decidual cast with no gestational sac (Fig. 10-11)
- Pseudogestational sac (Fig. 10-12)
- Fills endometrial cavity symmetrically
- May be large
- No double decidual sign but rather a single rim of echoes around pseudogestational sac

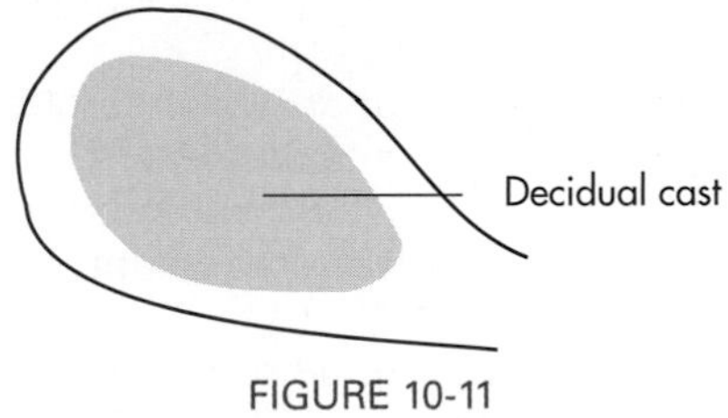

FIGURE 10-11

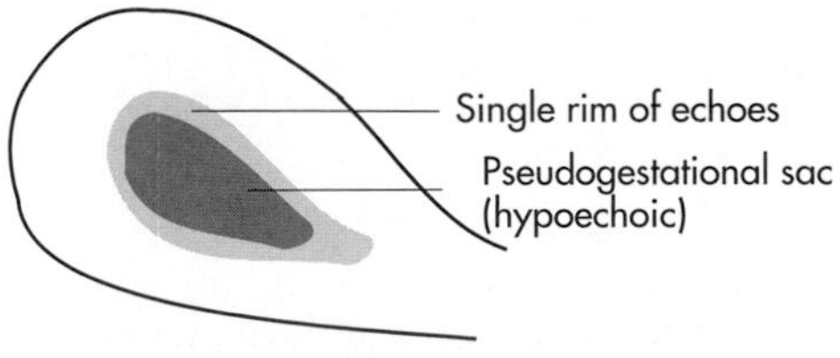

FIGURE 10-12

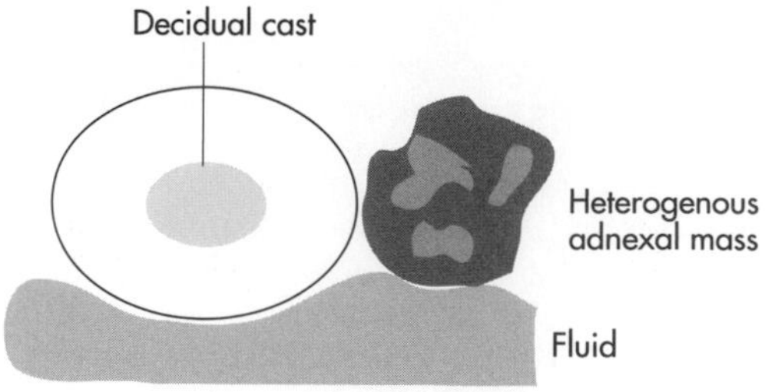

FIGURE 10-13

Extrauterine structures (Fig. 10-13)
- Free fluid in cul-de-sac (bleeding); may be anechoic or echogenic
- Simple adnexal cyst (10% chance of pregnancy)
- Complex adnexal mass (95% chance of ectopic)
- Tubal ring sign (95% chance of ectopic): echogenic rim surrounding an unruptured ectopic pregnancy
- Live embryo outside uterus; 100% specific but only seen in 25%

Pearls
- A normal TVS does not exclude an ectopic pregnancy.
- A normal IUP virtually excludes the presence of an ectopic pregnancy. The likelihood of a coexistent ectopic pregnancy is 1:7,000 in pregnancies with risk factors or 1:30,000 in pregnancies with no risk factor.
- Heterotopic pregnancy: Presence of an intrauterine and ectopic pregnancy. Associated with assisted reproduction, pelvic inflammatory disease.
- Cornual ectopic pregnancy
  - Symptoms occur later than with ectopic pregnancies in other locations.
  - Hemorrhage is more severe (uterus more hypervascular, erosion of uterine artery).
  - Higher morbidity and mortality. Look for complete rim of myometrium around gestational sac.
  - <5 mm myometrium between sac and external uterine margin
  - Interstitial line sign: hyperechoic endometrial line abuts but does not surround sac
- Cervical ectopic pregnancy
  - Requires evacuation

Treatment
- Surgery if ruptured or >2.5 cm
- Methotrexate
- Direct instillation of potassium chloride
- If dilatation and curettage planned, uterine artery embolization may be helpful to reduce the risk of bleeding

SONOGRAPHIC CATEGORIES

Class	Finding	Likelihood of Ectopic Pregnancy (%)
1	Normal IUP	Virtually none*
2	Normal or single ovarian cysts	5
3	Complex adnexal mass, free pelvic fluid, tubal ring	95
4	Live extrauterine embryo	100

*Likelihood of a coexistent ectopic pregnancy is 1 in 7000 pregnancies; more common with ovulatory induction and in vitro fertilization

Multifetal Pregnancy

GENERAL

Incidence: 1% of live births.

TYPES

Dizygotic twins (fraternal), 70%
- Independent fertilization of 2 ova
- Always dichorionic, diamniotic; each ovum has its own placenta and amnion. Overall, 80% of twins are dichorionic, diamniotic.
- Risk factors:
  - Advanced maternal age
  - Family history of twins
  - Ethnicity (e.g., Nigerian)

Monozygotic twins (identical), 30%
- Duplication of single fertilized ovum
- May be monochorionic or dichorionic
- Independent of maternal age, heredity, and race

PLACENTAL UNIT (Fig. 10-14)
- Amnionicity: number of amniotic sacs
- Chorionicity: number of placentas
- Dizygotic twins are always diamniotic, dichorionic (i.e., have 2 sacs and 2 placentas). The 2 placentas may fuse but do not have vascular connections.
- Monozygotic twins have different amnionicity and chorionicity depending on the stage of cleavage of the single fertilized ovum.
- The amnionicity/chorionicity determines the risk of complications:
  - Monoamniotic: > monochorionic, diamniotic > dichorionic
  - Monoamniotic: cord entanglement
  - Monochorionic: intraplacental vascular communication

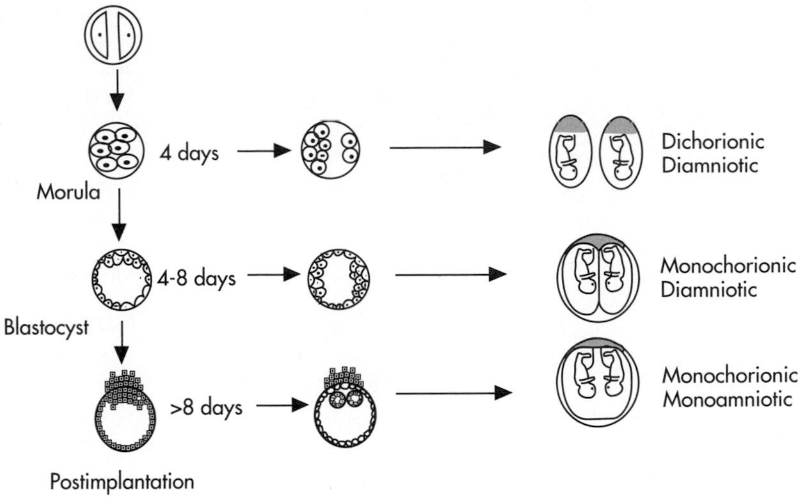

FIGURE 10-14

US IMAGING

Approach

1. Define the presence and number of twins.
2. Determine amnionicity and chorionicity.
3. Growth estimation: determine the fetal weight for each twin.
4. Are there complications or anomalies?

US FEATURES

Findings definitely indicating dichorionicity:

- Separate placentas
- Different fetal sex
- Thick (≥ 2 mm) membrane separating twins in 1st trimester
- Lambda sign: chorion extending into inter-twin membrane

Findings indicative of diamnionicity:

- Thin membrane in 1st trimester
- 2 yolk sacs

In the 2nd trimester, the sensitivity for finding an amnion is only 30%. In 70% of cases, an amnion is present but not visible.

Pearls

- Dichorionicity is easiest to establish in 1st trimester
- Different genders of fetuses always indicates dichorionicity
- Failure to identify a separating amnion is not a reliable sign to diagnose monoamnionicity.
- Twin peak sign

COMPLICATIONS

OVERVIEW OF COMPLICATIONS IN TWIN PREGNANCIES (Fig. 10-15)

All twins

- Increased incidence of premature labor
- Fetal mortality 3 times higher than for single pregnancy
- Neonatal mortality 7 times higher than that for single pregnancy

Dichorionic, diamniotic twins

- Perinatal mortality, 10%

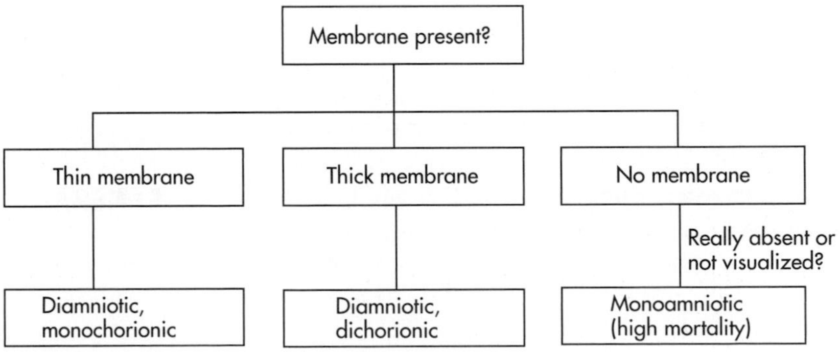

FIGURE 10-15

Monochorionic, diamniotic twins (MD twins)
- Perinatal mortality, 20%
- Twin-twin transfusion
- Acardia
- Demise of co-twin
- Twin embolization syndrome
- Structural abnormalities

Monochorionic, monoamniotic (MM) twins
- Perinatal mortality, 50%
- Entangled cords
- Conjoined twins
- All the MD complications as well

TWIN-TWIN TRANSFUSION SYNDROME (Fig. 10-16)

Only occurs in monochorionic twins (25%). Results from AV communications in placenta. Very poor prognosis.

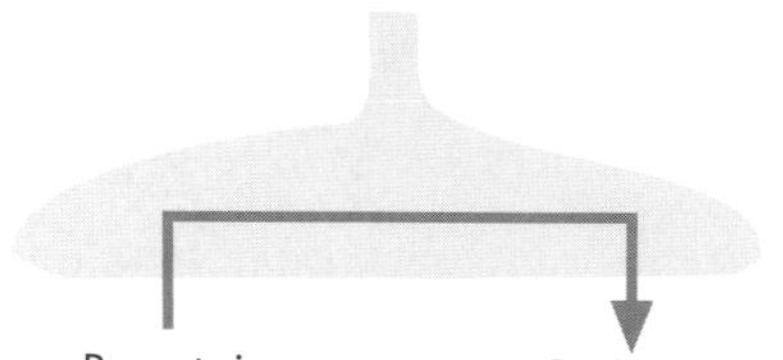

FIGURE 10-16

US Features

Recipient twin
- Large twin (increased estimated fetal weight [EFW])
- Polyhydramnios
- Polycythemia
- Fetal hydrops

Donor twin (pump twin)
- Small twin pinned to side of gestational sac (decreased EFW) "stuck twin"
- Oligohydramnios

CONDITIONS ASSOCIATED WITH DEMISE OF A TWIN

Vanishing Twin ("Blighted Twin")

Demise of a twin in the early 1st trimester (<15 weeks) and subsequent resorption of the dead fetus. Risk to the surviving twin is minimal, especially if dichorionic.

Fetus Papyraceus

Demise of a twin in the 2nd or 3rd trimester and persistence of the dead fetus as an amorphous mass or flattened structure along the uterine margin. Complications: premature labor, obstruction at labor, embolization.

Twin-Twin Embolization Syndrome

Occurs only in monochorionic twins because they share a common placenta. Demise of one twin leads to passage of thromboplastic material into the circulation of the live twin. Results in thrombosis and multiorgan failure in the live twin and maternal disseminated intravascular coagulation (DIC).

Acardiac Parabiotic Twin

- Twin reversal arterial perfusion sequence (TRAPS)
- Most extreme manifestation of twin transfusion syndrome
- Occurs in monochorionic pregnancy
- Reversal of flow in umbilical artery of the acardiac twin with blood entering via the vein and leaving via the artery
- Poor development of acardiac twin above thorax

Fetal Structural Abnormalities

All fetal structural abnormalities occur with higher frequency in twins (monozygotic > dizygotic). Most defects are not concordant and occur in only one twin. Some abnormalities are secondary to in utero crowding.

Conjoined Twins

Only occurs in MM twins. 75% are females. Prognosis is related to degree of joining and associated anomalies:
- Thoracopagus (most common, 70%): thorax is fused
- Omphalopagus, xiphopagus: anterior abdomen is fused
- Pygopagus: sacrococcygeal fusion
- Craniopagus: cranium is fused

Ectopic Twin Pregnancy

There may be an increase in this condition because of more widespread use of ovulation induction and in vitro fertilization techniques. Incidence: 1 in 7000; consider if the patient has previously mentioned risk factors.

Second and Third Trimesters

GENERAL

Some pathologic entities in this section are described in more detail in Chapter 11.

FETAL SURVEY

Organ/Views	Normal Appearance	Common Anomalies
Supratentorium Ventricular view Thalamic view	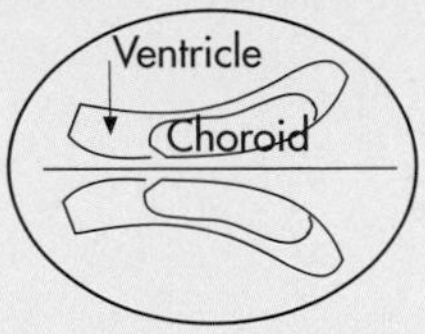	Hydrocephalus Holoprosencephaly Hydranencephaly Agenesis corpus callosum Anencephaly (lethal) Encephalocele Spina bifida Abnormal contour Scalp edema Cystic hygroma Cystic masses Hemorrhage
Posterior fossa Cerebellar view	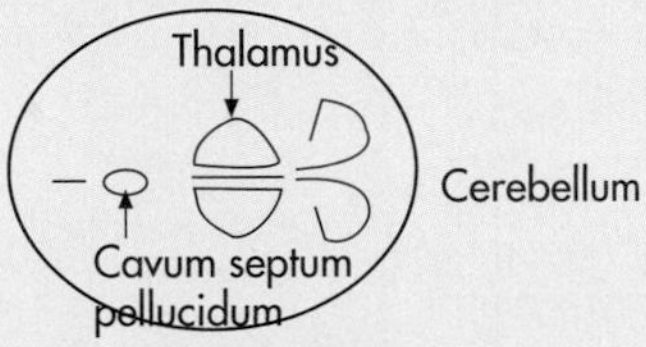	Large cisterna magna Dandy-Walker malformation Banana sign (spina bifida)
Orbits Axial view	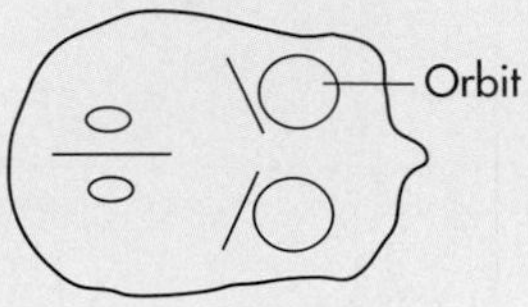	Anophthalmia Proptosis Hypertelorism, hypotelorism (orbital spacing)
Nose and lip Sagittal profile Coronal view Axial view	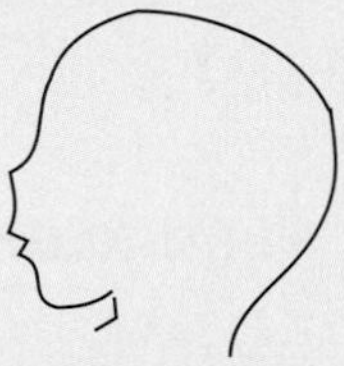	Facial cleft Proboscis Micrognathia Facial mass
Spine Longitudinal view (coronal and sagittal) Axial view (posterior and lateral)	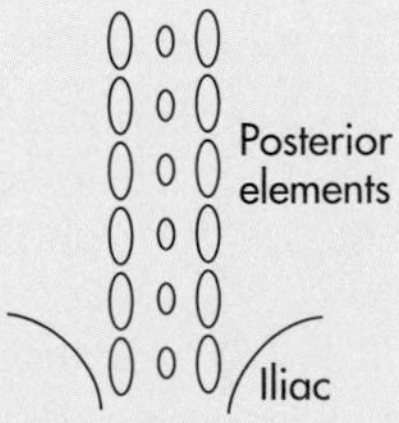	Spina bifida Scoliosis Sacral agenesis Sacrococcygeal teratoma
Heart, lungs 4-chamber view Short-axis view Outflow tract view	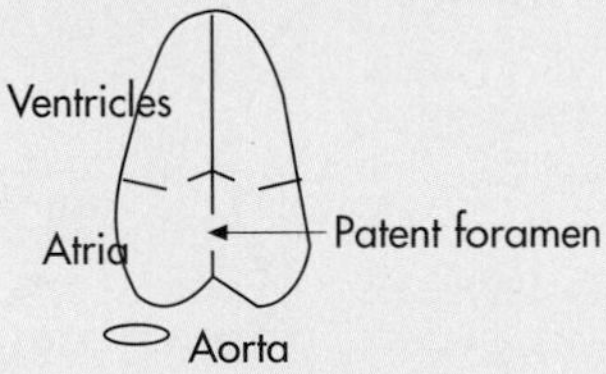	CHD: VSD, TA, TGA, DORV, tetralogy of Fallot Dextroposition Cardiac masses Lung masses Effusion
Gastrointestinal	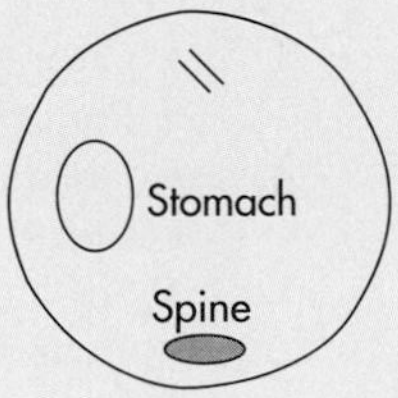	Esophageal atresia Duodenal atresia Small bowel atresia Ascites Meconium peritonitis Situs

Continued

FETAL SURVEY—cont'd

Organ/Views	Normal Appearance	Common Anomalies
Kidneys (K)	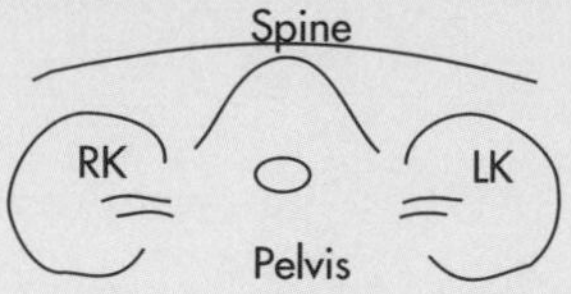	Renal agenesis Hydronephrosis MCDK APCKD Hydroureter Ectopic kidney
Bladder		Outlet obstruction Exstrophy
Cord, abdominal wall	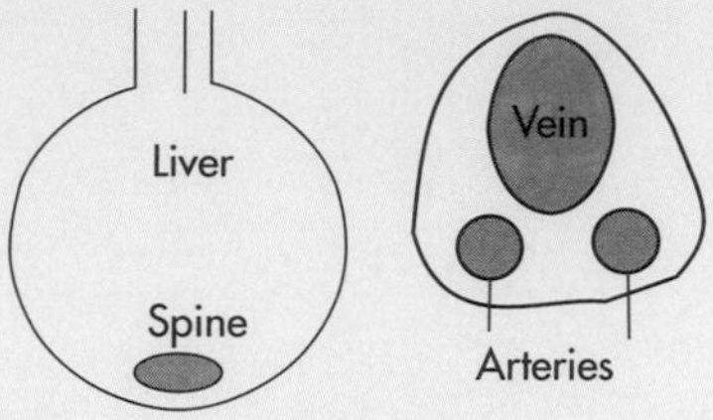	Gastroschisis Omphalocele Limb-body wall complex 2-vessel cord
Extremities		Dwarfism Clubfoot Hands, fingers Polydactyly

ARPCKD, autosomal recessive polycystic kidney disease; CHD, congenital heart disease; DORV, double-outlet right ventricle; MCDK, multicystic dysplastic kidney; TA, truncus arteriosus; TGA, transposition of great arteries; VSD, ventricular septal defect.

Pearls

- A normal cavum septum pellucidum, ventricular atrium (<10 mm), and cisterna magna (2 to 10 mm) virtually exclude all neural axis abnormalities.
- The 2 most common forms of neural tube defects are:
  - Anencephaly (missing cranial vault)
  - Myelomeningocele (most are associated with Chiari malformation). A normal cisterna magna excludes nearly all cases of myelomeningocele.
  - Risk reduction of neural tube defects with supplemental maternal folic acid intake.
- Always obtain a 4-chamber view and 2 views of cardiac outflow tracts (LV → aorta, RV → PA).
- In the 4-chamber view, chamber closest to anterior wall is right ventricle.
- Bladder and stomach should be visualized by 14 weeks. If they are not seen, rescan the patient in 2 hours: bladder should fill within this time frame. Doppler shows iliac arteries "splayed" by bladder.
- Any structure or mass that touches the fetal spine most likely originates from the genitourinary (GU) tract.

FETAL NEURAL AXIS

ANATOMY

Normal CNS Structures (Fig. 10-17)

- Ventricles: <10 mm at atrium
  - Choroid plexus in atria of lateral ventricles should occupy 60%-90% of atrium. It is easier to see the far field atrium as reverberation artifacts that may obscure near field atrium.
  - Choroid absent in anterior or occipital horns
- Cisterna magna: 4 to 10 mm
- Thalami are in midline
- Cavum septum pellucidum

Signal Intensities (Fig. 10-18)

Hyperechoic structures

- Choroid plexus
- Pia-arachnoid
- Dura
- Cerebellar vermis
- Specular reflections from ventricles

Hypoechoic structures

- Brain white matter
- Cerebrospinal fluid (CSF)

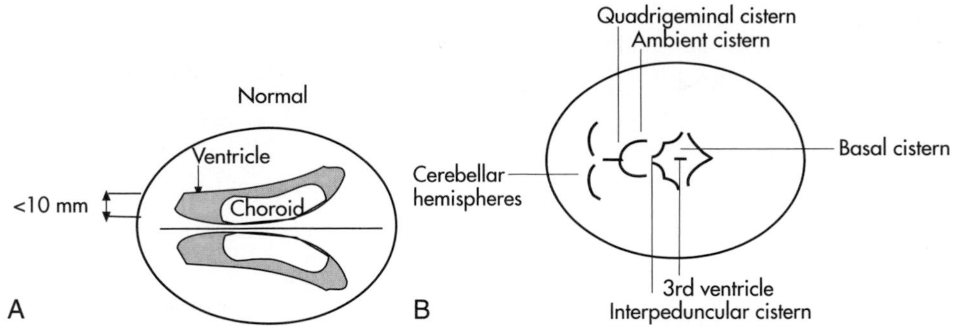

FIGURE 10-17

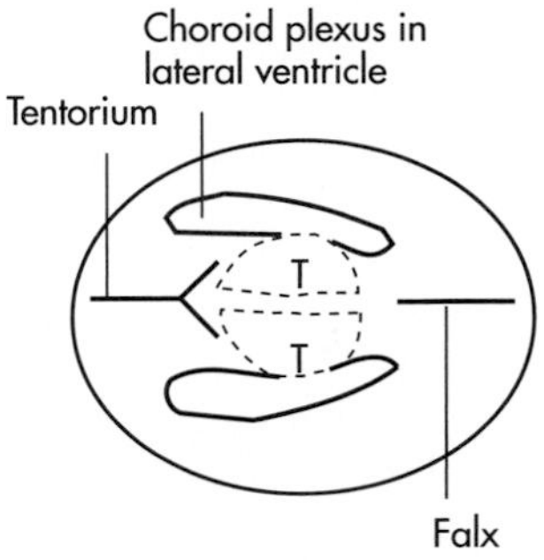

FIGURE 10-18

Spine (Fig. 10-19)

- 3 hyperechoic ossification centers
  Posterior ossification centers: 2 neural arches
  Anterior ossification center: vertebral body
- Spinal cord is hypoechoic

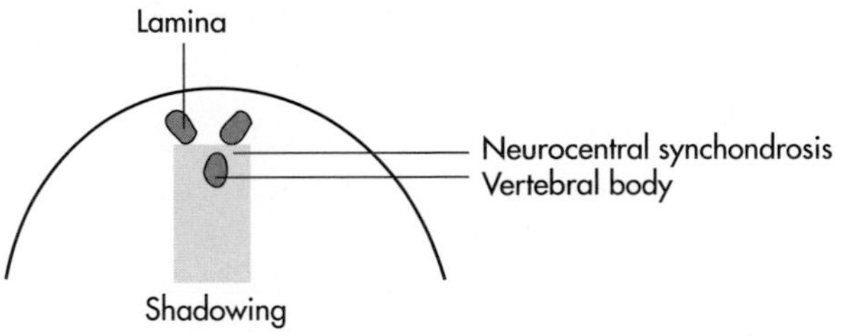

FIGURE 10-19

HOLOPROSENCEPHALY

Failure of midline cleavage of the forebrain:

- Alobar form: no cleavage
- Semilobar form: partial cleavage
- Lobar form: almost complete cleavage

US Features (Fig. 10-20)

Alobar holoprosencephaly

- Monoventricle communicates with dorsal cyst
- Thin anterior mantle of brain tissue: "horseshoe" or "boomerang"
- Fused thalami
- No falx, corpus callosum, or septum pellucidum
- No brain tissue around dorsal cyst

Semilobar holoprosencephaly

- Monoventricle with rudimentary occipital horns
- Posterior brain tissue is present (no dorsal cyst).
- Fused thalami
- Partial falx posteriorly
- No corpus callosum or septum pellucidum

Lobar holoprosencephaly

- Very difficult to make specific diagnosis

All types have:

- Absent septum pellucidum and corpus callosum

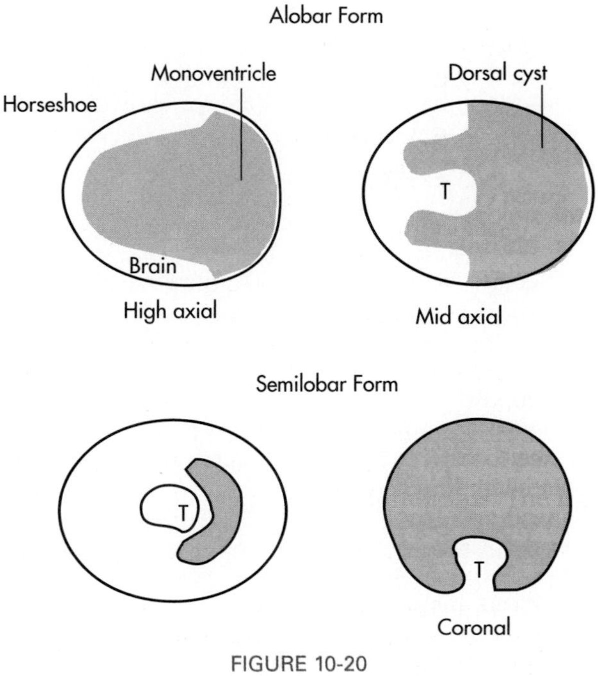

FIGURE 10-20

- Thalamic fusion
- Associated midline facial anomalies: clefts, cyclopia, hypotelorism

Pearls

- Identification of septum pellucidum excludes all types of holoprosencephaly.
- Fused thalami exclude severe hydrocephalus.
- Anterior cerebral mantle (horseshoe) excludes hydranencephaly.
- Look for midline facial abnormalities (clefts, hypotelorism, cyclopia, proboscis).
- Associated with trisomy 13

AGENESIS OF CORPUS CALLOSUM (ACC)

The normal development of the corpus callosum begins anterior (genu) and progresses to posterior (splenium). Agenesis may be partial (affects dysgenesis posterior aspects) or complete.

US Features

- The corpus callosum is not visible in complete agenesis.
- Colpocephaly
- Lateral ventricles are displaced laterally (parallel lateral ventricles).
- Enlarged 3rd ventricle expands superiorly (high riding third ventricle).
- Angulated frontal horns (coronal view)
- Abnormal (sunburst) gyral pattern in interhemispheric fissure is a late feature.
- The presence of a cavum septum pellucidum excludes complete ACC.
- Common associations include:
  Dandy-Walker (DW) syndrome
  Holoprosencephaly
  Heterotopias
- TVS scanning is often helpful for early diagnosis.
- Associated with pericallosal lipoma (hyperechoic)

HYDRANENCEPHALY

- Near-total absence of cerebrum with intact cranial vault, thalamus, and brainstem
- Secondary to occlusion of supraclinoid arteries

PORENCEPHALY

- Less severe vascular insult than in hydranencephaly
- Cystic lesions are often in free communication with the ventricle or subarachnoid cisterns

VENTRICULOMEGALY (Fig. 10-21)

Refers to dilated (>10 mm) ventricles (measured at level of atrium). Associated with other anomalies in 75% of cases. Types:

- Hydrocephalus (noncommunicating, obstructive > communicating)

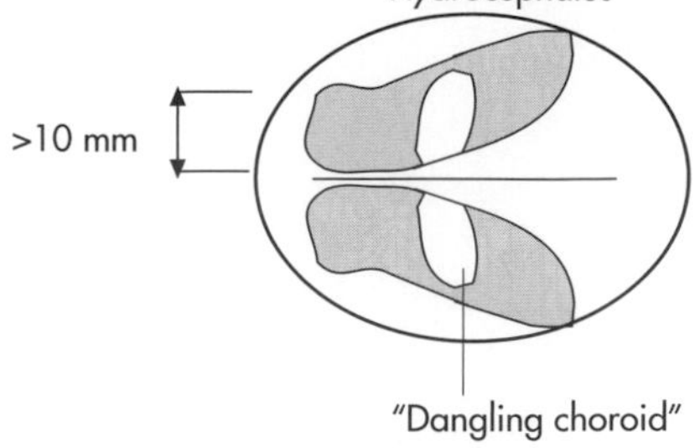

FIGURE 10-21

- Brain atrophy (enough brain tissue developed but it regresses later)
- Colpocephaly (not enough brain tissue developed)

Hydrocephalus is the most common CNS abnormality. Causes include:

Obstructive (common)
- Spina bifida is the most common cause of hydrocephalus.
- Aqueductal stenosis
- Dandy-Walker syndrome
- Encephalocele
- Arnold-Chiari malformation

Nonobstructive (uncommon)
- Hemorrhage
- Infection: cytomegalovirus (CMV), *Toxoplasma* (calcification)

US Features

- Enlarged ventricles (>10 mm)
- Dangling choroid plexus in the lateral ventricle
- The presence of colpocephaly should prompt search for possible callosal agenesis.

CYSTIC STRUCTURES

Cystic Teratoma

- Most common congenital intracranial tumor
- Solid and cystic components

Choroid Plexus Cysts

- Very common between 12 and 24 weeks (2nd trimester); most resolve by 3rd trimester
- Usually multilocular, 5 to 20 mm; may be bilateral
- Most cysts <10 mm are of no consequence.
- Cysts >10 mm may indicate trisomy 18, and amniocentesis is often performed, although controversial. Look for other findings of trisomy 18.

Arachnoid Cysts

- Cystic space within the pia-arachnoid has a ball valve communication with the subarachnoid space.
- Congenital or acquired (after hemorrhage, infection)

- No communication with ventricle
- Must differentiate from cystic teratoma, porencephaly, and arteriovenous malformation (AVM)

HEMORRHAGE

Similar imaging features and classification (Papile grades 1 to 4) to germinal matrix hemorrhage in fetuses born prematurely but different etiology. In utero hemorrhage is very common. Causes:
- Maternal hypertension, eclampsia
- Isoimmune thrombocytopenia
- Maternal hemorrhage
- Nonimmune hydrops

DANDY-WALKER (DW) SYNDROME (Fig. 10-22)

Abnormal development of posterior fossa structures characterized by:
- Posterior fossa cyst that communicates with the 4th ventricle
- Hypoplasia of the cerebellar vermis
- Variable hydrocephalus
- Variant form does not have enlargement of posterior fossa

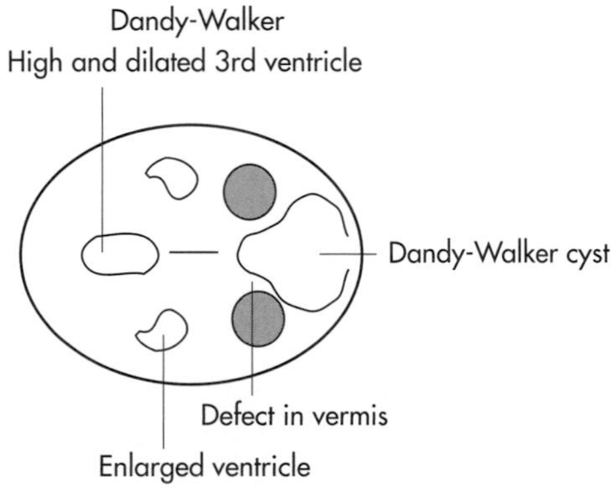

FIGURE 10-22

US Features
- Posterior fossa cyst separates the cerebellar hemispheres and connects to the 4th ventricle
- Absence or hypoplasia of vermis
- Other associations
  - Hydrocephalus
  - ACC
  - CHD

LARGE CISTERNA MAGNA (Fig. 10-23)

Diagnosis of exclusion; must exclude DW complex.

US Features
- AP diameter >10 mm
- No communication with 4th ventricle

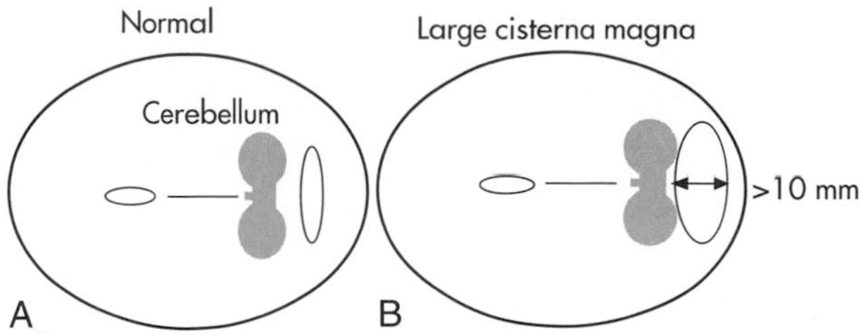

FIGURE 10-23

NEURAL TUBE DEFECT (NTD)

Incidence: 1:600 births in the United States.

Increased risk (3%) in parents with prior NTD child. Screening: amniotic fluid and MSAFP are increased because of transudation of fetal serum AFP across the NTD. Spectrum of disease:
- Anencephaly (most common)
- Spina bifida and meningomyelocele
- Face and orbits usually intact
- Encephalocele (least common)

ANENCEPHALY (Fig. 10-24)

- Complete absence of cranial vault (acrania) and cerebral hemispheres; should be symmetrical. Asymmetrical absence should raise the suspicion of amniotic band syndrome (ABS).
- Angiomatous tissue covers base of the skull
- Some functioning neural tissue is nearly always present.
- Polyhydramnios, 50%
- Should not be diagnosed before 14 weeks of age (skull is not ossified)

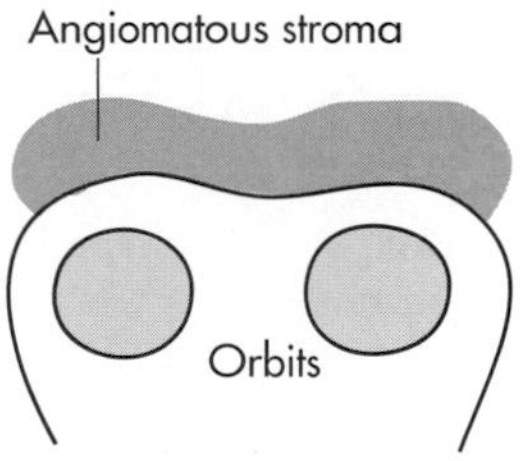

FIGURE 10-24

ENCEPHALOCELE (Fig. 10-25)

Herniation of intracranial structures through a cranial defect. Cephalocele = meninges; encephalocele = brain and meninges. Most defects are covered by skin, and MSAFP levels thus are normal. Location: occipital, 70%; frontal, 10%. Lesions are typically midline. Asymmetrical lesions should raise the suspicion of ABS. Prognosis depends on the amount of herniated brain. Mortality, 50%; intellectual impairment, 50%-90%.

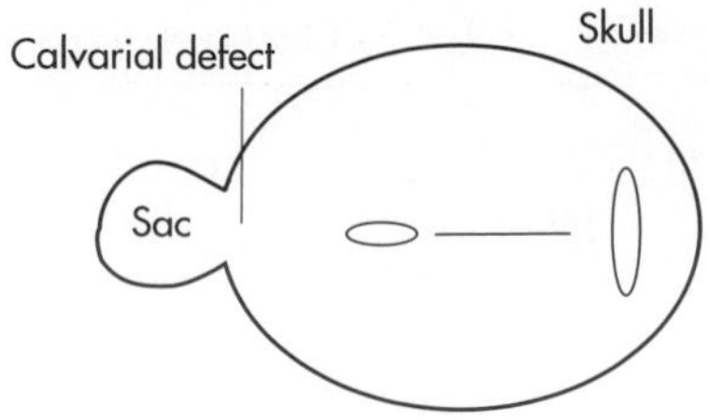

FIGURE 10-25

Associations

- Other intracranial anomalies
- ABS
- Meckel-Gruber syndrome

US Features

- Extracranial mass lesion (sac)
- The sac may contain solid (brain tissue), cystic (CSF space), or both components; absence of brain tissue in the sac is a favorable prognostic indicator.
- Bony defect
- Lemon sign (skull deformity)

SPINA BIFIDA AND MYELOMENINGOCELE (Fig. 10-26)

Location: lumbosacral > thoracic, cervical spine. MSAFP is elevated unless the myelomeningocele is covered with skin. Incidence: 0.1% of pregnancies.

Associations (due to imbalanced muscular activity):
- Clubfoot
- Hip dislocations

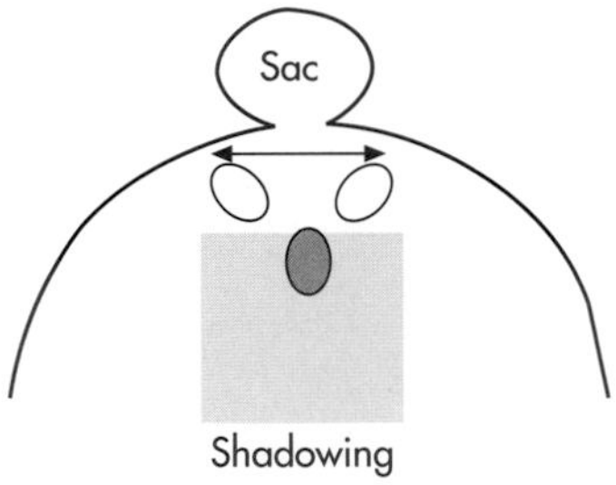

FIGURE 10-26

US Features

Spine
- Complex mass outside spinal canal
- Sac is best seen when surrounded by amniotic fluid.
- Sac may be obscured if oligohydramnios is present.
- Separation of posterior lamina

Indirect signs
- Lemon sign (Fig. 10-27): bifrontal indentation. In 90% of fetuses with spina bifida <24 weeks.

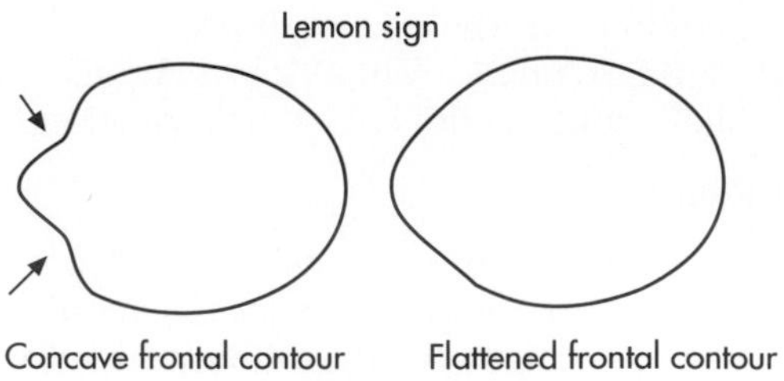

FIGURE 10-27

In older fetuses (24 to 37 weeks), lemon sign disappears. Lemon sign is rarely seen in a normal fetus.
- Banana sign (Fig. 10-28): represents the cerebellum wrapped around the posterior brainstem secondary to downward traction of the spinal cord as part of Arnold-Chiari malformation
- Hydrocephalus, 90%

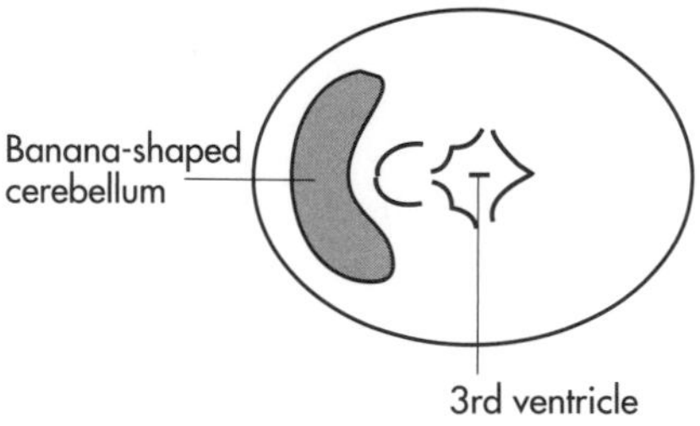

FIGURE 10-28

Pearls

- Most cases of spina bifida are suspected because of head abnormalities (e.g., banana sign).
- Spina bifida is almost always associated with a Chiari malformation.
- A normal cisterna magna excludes spina bifida.
- Spina bifida is the most common cause of ventriculomegaly.

ALGORITHM FOR INTRACRANIAL MALFORMATIONS (Fig. 10-29)

FACE, NECK

CYSTIC HYGROMA

Fluid-filled structures with spokewheel appearance caused by lymphatic malformation. Location: neck, upper thorax. Prognosis depends on size: high incidence of hydrops and in utero death in large lesions. Cystic hygromas in noncervical location do not carry a significant risk of chromosomal anomalies and have

FIGURE 10-29

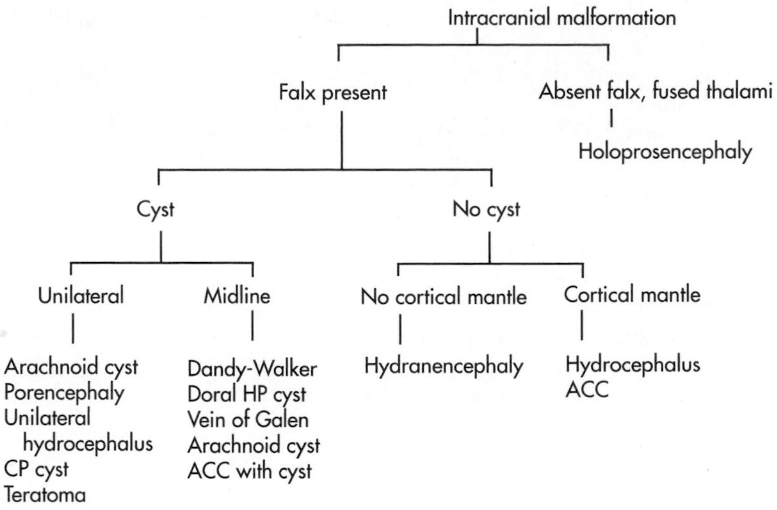

a favorable outcome. Amniocentesis is performed in cervical cystic hygromas because of frequently associated syndromes:

- Turner, 45XO (most common, 50%)
- Trisomies (21, 18, 13)
- Noonan syndrome
- Fetal alcohol syndrome

US Features

- Bilateral, posterolateral cystic head and neck masses
- Cysts are usually multiple.
- Cysts may become very large and extend to thorax.
- Generalized lymphedema (nonimmune hydrops)
- Cyst multiplicity and intact skull exclude encephalocele.

OTHER ANOMALIES OF THE FACE AND NECK

Types

- Anophthalmia: no orbits
- Arrhinia: absent nose
- Cebocephaly: hypotelorism and rudimentary nose
- Cyclopia: usually one eye, with supraorbital proboscis
- Ethmocephalus: hypotelorism and proboscis
- Facial clefts (lip, palate, or face)
- Flattened nose
- Hypotelorism: distance between eyes is decreased.
- Hypertelorism: distance between eyes is increased.
- Macroglossia: large tongue
- Micrognathia: small mandible
- Nuchal thickening (>5 mm)
- Proptosis: eye protrudes from skull
- Proboscis: cylindrical appendage near the orbits
- Single nostril

Associations

- Holoprosencephaly: cyclopia, ethmocephalus, cebocephaly, clefts, hypotelorism
- Cloverleaf skull: proptosis
- Craniosynostoses: hypertelorism
- Frontal encephalocele: hypertelorism
- Median cleft face syndrome: hypertelorism and clefts
- Beckwith-Wiedemann: large tongue
- Trisomy 21: nuchal thickening

HEART

DETECTION

Cardiac abnormalities are often difficult to detect because of small heart size, complex anatomy, and rapid heart rate. Because cardiac abnormalities may be associated with chromosomal abnormalities (15%-40%), amniocentesis is indicated in all patients with cardiac defects.

Cardiac abnormalities best detected on 4-chamber view:

- Septal defect–ventricular septal defect (VSD), AV canal
- Endocardial cushion defect
- Hypoplastic left heart: absent or small LV
- Ebstein anomaly (associated with maternal lithium use): large RA and small RV; tricuspid valve within RV
- Critical aortic stenosis: RV < LV. Coarctation: LV < RV

Cardiac abnormalities best detected on outflow tract views:
- Tetralogy of Fallot: large aorta overriding a small PA
- Transposition of great arteries: large vessels run in a parallel plane
- Truncus arteriosus: single truncal vessel overriding the septum
- Pentalogy of Cantrell
  - Omphalocele
  - Sternal cleft
  - Cardiac exstrophy
  - CVS malformations
  - Anterior diaphragmatic hernia

Cardiac abnormalities often missed:
- Isolated atrial septal defect (ASD)
- Isolated VSD
- Aortic or pulmonic stenosis
- Coarctation of the aorta
- Total anomalous pulmonary venous connection (TAPVC)

Other detectable abnormalities:
- Rhabdomyoma: most common prenatal and neonatal cardiac tumor (commonly associated with tuberous sclerosis)
- Endocardial fibroelastosis: markedly echogenic myocardium
- Ectopia cordis: heart is outside thoracic cavity
- Cardiomyopathy: dilated heart, poor contractility

MATERNAL RISK FACTORS FOR CHD

- Diabetes
- Infection: rubella, CMV
- Collagen vascular disease: systemic lupus erythematosus (SLE)
- Drugs: alcohol, trimethadione, phenytoin, lithium
- Family history of heart disease

FETAL ARRHYTHMIAS (USE M-MODE OR DOPPLER US FOR EVALUATION)

- Premature atrial contractions (PACs) are the most common fetal arrhythmia.
- PACs and premature ventricular contractions (PVCs) are benign (most disappear in utero).
- Supraventricular tachycardia (HR ≥ 180) is the most common tachyarrhythmia:
  - 10% incidence in CHD: structural abnormalities uncommon
  - May lead to hydrops. Treatment is with digoxin or verapamil.
- Fetal bradycardia (HR <100 for >10 seconds) usually indicates fetal hypoxia distress.
- Fetal heart block: 40%-50% have structural abnormality.
  - 40% incidence in CHD
  - Associated with maternal SLE

THORAX

PULMONARY HYPOPLASIA

Types

- Primary pulmonary hypoplasia (idiopathic)
- Secondary hypoplasia:
  - Bilateral
    - Oligohydramnios (Potter's sequence)
    - Restricted chest cage (skeletal dysplasias)
  - Unilateral
    - Congenital cystic adenoid malformation (CCAM)
    - Congenital diaphragmatic hernia (CDH)
    - Hydrothorax

US Features

- Small thorax
- Low thoracic circumference (below 2 SD of normal) is suggestive but not diagnostic of pulmonary hypoplasia.
- Fetal lung maturity is most accurately determined by the lecithin:sphingomyelin ratio in amniotic fluid samples (normal ratio >2). The echogenicity pattern of lung is an unreliable indicator of lung maturity.

CONGENITAL CYSTIC ADENOID MALFORMATION

Hamartomatous malformation of the lung. Usually unilateral, involving one lobe.

Types

Macroscopic types: includes types I and II; cysts >5 mm
- Hydrops uncommon
- Overall good prognosis

Microscopic type: small cysts with solid US appearance
- Hydrops common
- Very poor prognosis

US Features

Solid or cystic pulmonary mass
- Macroscopic type appears cystic (hypoechoic)
- Microscopic type appears solid (echogenic)

Mass effect on normal lung determines prognosis:
- Pulmonary hypoplasia
- Mediastinal shift: impaired swallowing → polyhydramnios
- Cardiac compromise

BRONCHOPULMONARY SEQUESTRATION

Only the extralobar type is usually detected prenatally.

Types

- Intralobar: pulmonary venous drainage
- Extralobar: systemic venous drainage

Associations (Extralobar, 65%; Intralobar, 10%)

- Congenital diaphragmatic hernia (most common)
- Foregut abnormalities
- Sternal abnormalities

US Features

- Well-defined, homogeneous, echogenic mass
- Most common location (90%) is left lung base.
- May mimic microcystic CCAM
- Complications (mass effect on esophagus → impaired swallowing)
    - Polyhydramnios
    - Fetal hydrops

CONGENITAL DIAPHRAGMATIC HERNIA (BOCHDALEK HERNIA)

90% are on the left side; 95% are unilateral. Mortality: 50%-70% (because of pulmonary hypoplasia). Because of commonly associated anomalies, all patients with CDH should have an amniocentesis.

US Features (Fig. 10-30)

Chest
- Stomach and/or bowel adjacent to heart (key finding) on 4-chamber view
- Herniation into chest may occur intermittently
- Peristaltic movements in chest
- Shift of heart and mediastinum

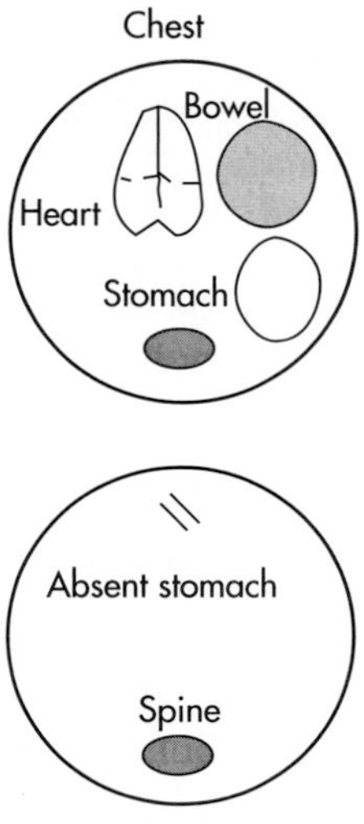

FIGURE 10-30

Abdomen
- Absent stomach in abdomen
- Small abdominal circumference (because of herniation of organs into chest)

Other
- Polyhydramnios (impaired swallowing)
- Always look for associated anomalies (anencephaly is most common).

MEDIASTINAL MASSES

Anterior and middle mediastinum
- Teratoma
- Cystic hygroma
- Normal thymus

Posterior mediastinum
- Neurogenic tumors
- Enteric cysts

PLEURAL EFFUSION

Causes

- Fetal hydrops
- Underlying chest mass (CCAM, CDH, sequestration)
- Chromosomal anomalies (21, Turner): consider karyotyping
- Infection
- Idiopathic
- Pulmonary lymphangiectasia
- Chylothorax
- 10% resolve spontaneously
- May require thoracentesis or thoracoamniotic shunt if large and recurrent

US Features

- Crescentic fluid around lung ("bat-wing appearance")

ABDOMEN

NORMAL ANATOMY

Umbilical Vessels (Fig. 10-31)

- 1 umbilical vein (UV) connects to either portal system:
    - UV → left portal vein → ductus venosus → IVC
    - UV → left portal vein → right portal vein → liver
- 2 umbilical arteries (UAs) connect to internal iliac arteries

Stomach

- Always visible by 14 weeks
- Anechoic because it contains swallowed amniotic fluid

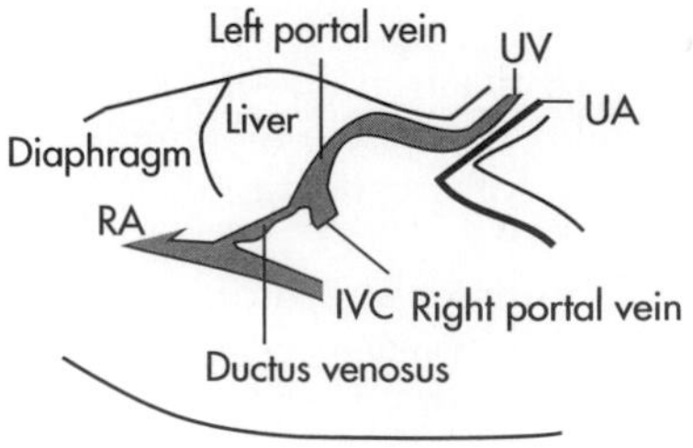

FIGURE 10-31

Bowel

- Small bowel is meconium filled and appears echogenic (pseudomass).
- Meconium is passed only during fetal distress.
- 95% of infants born with meconium-stained amniotic fluid are older than 37 weeks.
- Large bowel is fluid filled and appears hypoechoic.

Adrenal Glands

- Usually well seen because they initially are 20 times their adult size relative to the kidney
- Adrenal glands can be mistaken for kidneys (hypoechoic rim, echogenic center: Oreo cookie sign).

Other

The gallbladder is seen in nearly all fetuses by 20 weeks. The spleen is seen from 18 weeks on; it appears isoechoic to kidneys and hypoechoic relative to liver. The pancreas is not routinely seen.

GASTRIC ABNORMALITIES

Echogenic material in the stomach (gastric pseudomass):

- Debris
- Blood clot
- Vernix

Failure to visualize stomach:

- Oligohydramnios (not enough fluid to swallow; most common cause)
- Esophageal atresia (always look for other VACTERL associations)
- Diaphragmatic hernia
- Swallowing abnormality (cranial defect)
- Situs abnormality: look on both sides

DUODENAL ATRESIA

Associated anomalies occur in 50% of patients with duodenal atresia. Therefore, a chromosomal analysis and detailed fetal survey are indicated:

- Down syndrome, 30%
- Malrotation, 20%
- Heart disease, 20%
- Other: renal anomalies, tracheoesophageal fistula, VACTERL

Radiographic Features

- Double-bubble sign (can be seen as early as 24th week of gestation)
- Polyhydramnios

MECONIUM

Echogenic material within the bowel may represent:

- A normal finding if present in 2nd trimester
- Cystic fibrosis (carrier testing of parents performed)

There are 3 meconium-associated problems during pregnancy:

Meconium peritonitis (10% have cystic fibrosis)

- Sterile chemical peritonitis develops after bowel perforation.
- Calcification, 85%
- Ascites, 55%
- Polyhydramnios
- Causes (can be determined in only 50% of cases)
- Volvulus
  - Atresia
  - Intussusception
  - Meconium ileus

Pseudocyst

- Inflammatory response around walled-off peritoneal meconium

Ileus (100% have cystic fibrosis)

- Inspissation of thick meconium in distal ileum
- Bowel dilatation, 25%
- Polyhydramnios, 65%

ASCITES

Ascites is always an abnormal finding.

Causes

Isolated ascites

- Urinary ascites
- Meconium peritonitis, bowel rupture
- Ruptured ovarian cyst

Hydrops

Pseudoascites: the hypoechoic anterior abdominal wall musculature may be mistaken for ascites

ADRENAL GLAND

NEUROBLASTOMA

- Most common antenatal tumor (arises from adrenal gland)
- Usually unilateral
- Hyperechoic
- Often metastasizes to placenta, liver, subcutaneous tissues
- Often associated with hydrops

ABDOMINAL WALL

ANATOMY

- Midgut elongation and umbilical herniation: 8 weeks
- Rotation and peritoneal fixation: 12 weeks

Pearls

- 20% of normal pregnancies may show herniated bowel at 12 weeks.
- Bowel outside of fetal abdomen beyond 14 weeks is always abnormal.

ANTERIOR WALL DEFECTS

OVERVIEW

	Gastroschisis	Omphalocele	LBWC
Location	Right-sided defect	Midline defect	Lateral
Size of defect	Small (2-4 cm)	Large (2-10 cm)	Large
Umbilical cord insertion	Anterior abdominal wall	On omphalocele	Variable
Membrane	No	Yes (3 layers)	Contiguous with placenta
Liver involved	No	Yes	Yes
Bowel involved	Common	Uncommon	Uncommon
Ascites	No	Yes	Yes
Other anomalies	Rarel	Common (50%-70%)	Always

ALGORITHM FOR ANTERIOR ABDOMINAL WALL DEFECTS (Fig. 10-32)

GASTROSCHISIS

Gastroschisis is a defect involving all 3 layers of the abdominal wall. MSAFP is elevated. Incidence 1:3000. Mortality 10%. Gastroschisis has a better prognosis than omphalocele because of the lower incidence of associated anomalies. Associated anomalies are usually limited to the GI tract and result from bowel ischemia:

- Intestinal atresia or stenosis
- Bowel perforation
- Meconium peritonitis

US Features (Fig. 10-33)

- Wall defect is usually small, <2 cm
- Defect located to the right side of the umbilical cord, 90%
- Bowel outside abdominal cavity. By definition, the bowel is nonrotated.
- Externalized structures appear disproportionately large relative to abdominal wall defect.
- Bowel wall thickening and dilatation may indicate ischemia and potential for perforation.

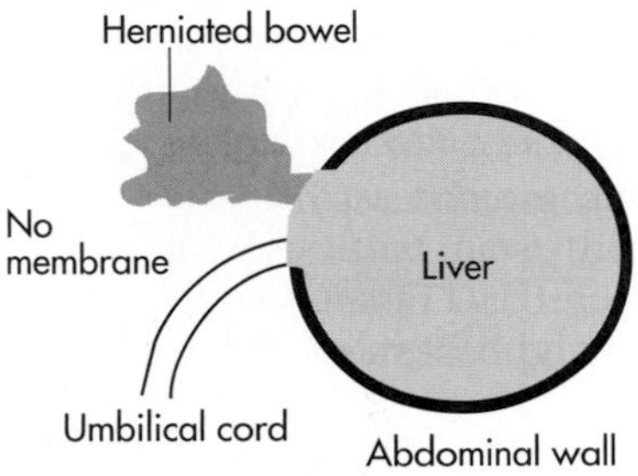

FIGURE 10-33

OMPHALOCELE

A large midline abdominal wall defect is covered by a membrane consisting of peritoneum (inside layer), amnion (outside layer), and Wharton's jelly (between the 2 layers). Rupture of the membrane occurs in 10%-20%. Mortality is 80%-100% depending on severity of concurrent abnormalities. In contrast to gastroschisis, MSAFP levels are normal if the membrane is intact. Diagnosis after

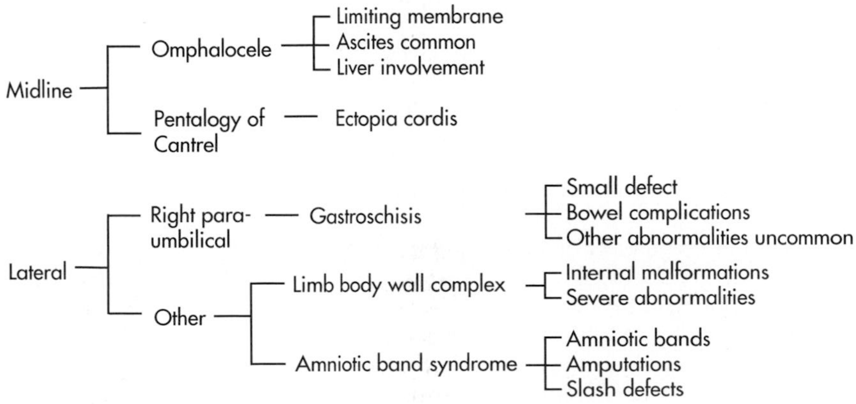

FIGURE 10-32

12 weeks when physiologic gut herniation complete. Unlike gastroschisis, omphaloceles are frequently (50%-70%) associated with other severe malformations:

- GU, GI, CNS, cardiac anomalies
- Pentalogy of Cantrell: omphalocele, CDH, sternal cleft, ectopia cordis, CHD
- Beckwith-Wiedemann: omphalocele, macroglossia, gigantism, pancreatic hyperplasia with hypoglycemia
- Trisomies (13 > 18 > 21)
- Turner syndrome

US Features (Fig. 10-34)

- Umbilical cord enters centrally into herniated sac
- Layers of the covering membrane (peritoneum, amnion, Wharton's jelly) may occasionally be distinguished.
- Defect may contain any intraabdominal organ but most commonly liver with or without bowel
- If bowel loops lie within the omphalocele, it indicates a higher incidence of karyotypic anomalies.
- Allantois cyst is often present.
- Ascites
- Associated cardiac anomalies, 40%

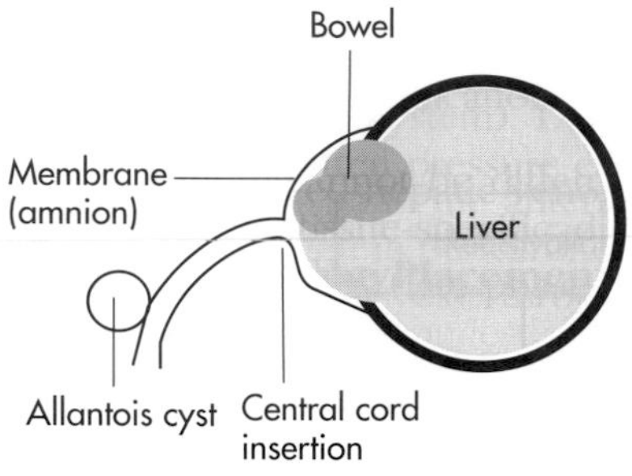

FIGURE 10-34

AMNIOTIC BAND SYNDROME (ABS)

The amnion is ruptured and multiple bands form within the amniotic fluid. Amniotic bands result in amputation defects of abdominal wall, trunk, and extremities.

US Features (Fig. 10-35)

- Limb entrapment in bands
- Multiple asymmetrical limb amputations or facial defects
- Asymmetrical encephalocele (adherence of fetus to "sticky" chorion)
- Gastropleural schisis
- Abdominal wall defects similar in appearance to gastroschisis
- Bands are occasionally visualized.

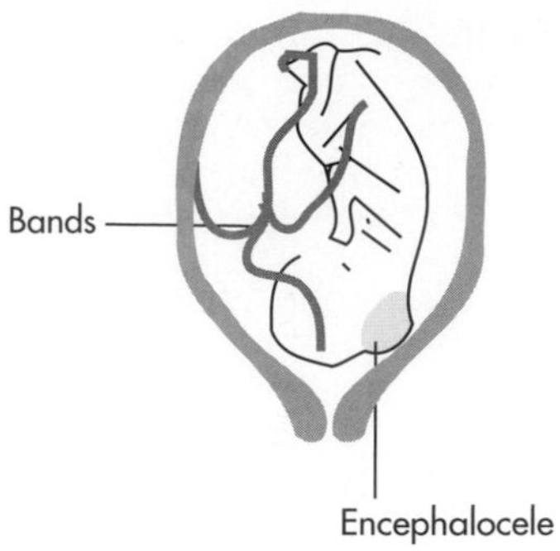

FIGURE 10-35

- Associated anomalies: syndactyly, clubfoot
- Amniotic band syndrome must be differentiated from chorioamniotic separation, normal unfused amnion in 1st trimester, uterine synechiae (also called amniotic sheets), and fibrin strands that occur after amniocentesis.

LIMB/BODY WALL COMPLEX (LBWC)

Complex malformation characterized by eccentric body wall defect involving thorax and abdomen, extremities, cranium, and face. Thought to represent a severe form of ABS; incompatible with life.

US Features

Thoracoabdominal defect
- Defects are usually large.
- Fetal membranes are contiguous with defect.

Neurologic abnormalities
- NTD common: encephaloceles, meningomyeloceles
- Scoliosis (common)
- Anencephaly

Other abnormalities
- Cardiovascular anomalies
- Single umbilical artery
- The constellation of omphalocele and scoliosis suggests the presence of LBWC.

URINARY TRACT

NORMAL DEVELOPMENT

Renal morphology
- Kidneys are routinely seen at 16 weeks of age.
- Pyramids and medulla can be differentiated at 23 to 26 weeks of age.
- Normal renal pelvis is normally <10 mm in diameter. Measurement is a function of gestational age.
- Ratio of renal to abdominal area on cross section is constant (0.3 ± 0.03).
- Ratio of renal pelvis to kidney on cross section is normally <0.5.

- Length of kidney: +1 mm for every week of gestation

Renal function can be estimated by evaluation of:

- Urine in bladder: routinely seen at 16 weeks; the normal urinary bladder fills and empties every 30 to 45 minutes. Fetal urine becomes major source of amniotic fluid by 16 weeks.
- Amniotic fluid volume: a normal amniotic fluid volume is an indicator of good prognosis.
- Amount of amniotic fluid: oligohydramnios is an indicator of bad prognosis.

Amniotic fluid

- Fetal urine accounts for almost all amniotic fluid in 2nd half of pregnancy.

POTTER SYNDROME (Figs. 10-36 and 10-37)

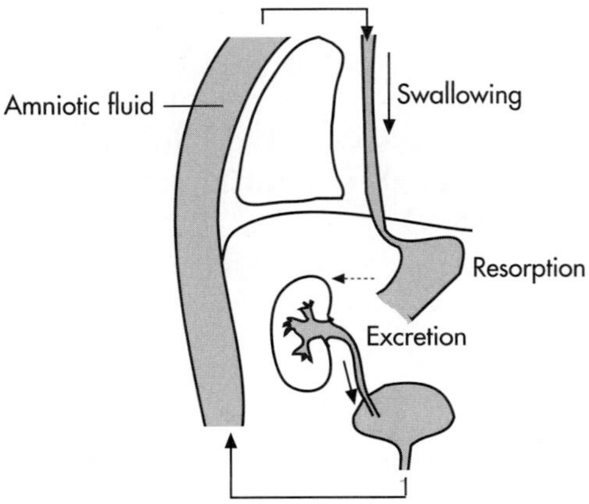

FIGURE 10-36

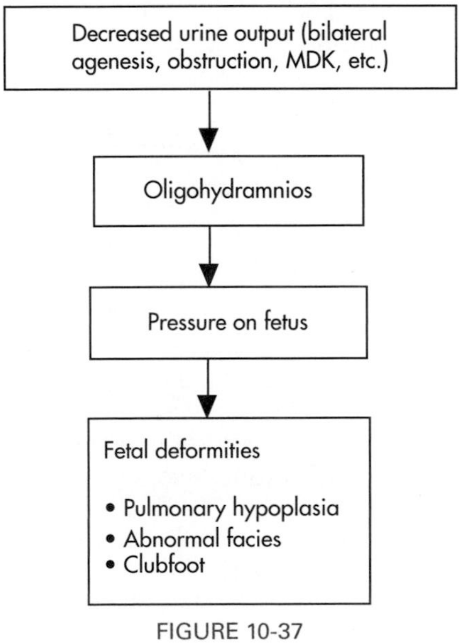

FIGURE 10-37

Also referred to as Potter's sequence. Renal failure causes decreased urine output, which results in oligohydramnios. Pulmonary hypoplasia, contractures, and Potter's facies result. Underlying renal causes include:

- Bilateral renal agenesis
- Posterior urethral valves
- Infantile polycystic dysplastic kidney (PCDK)
- Multicystic dysplastic kidney (MCDK)

RENAL AGENESIS

Unilateral renal agenesis is 4 times more common than bilateral agenesis. Bilateral agenesis is always fatal at birth because of associated pulmonary hypoplasia.

US Features

- Kidneys are not visualized; do not mistake adrenal glands or bowel loops for kidneys.
- Fetal bladder does not fill during a 2-hour US examination.
- Severe oligohydramnios
- Small fetal thorax (pulmonary hypoplasia)
- Potter's facies and limb deformity

URINARY TRACT OBSTRUCTION

Approach

1. Upper or lower obstruction?
2. Renal function impaired (oligohydramnios?)
3. Associated anomalies?
4. Surgical decompression required to improve prognosis?
   - Normal amniotic fluid indicates excellent prognosis.
   - Oligohydramnios indicates poor outcome.
   - Renal dysplasia indicates poor outcome.

Ureteropelvic Junction (UPJ) Obstruction

(Figs. 10-38 and 10-39)

- Most common antenatal cause of hydronephrosis
- Bilateral UPJ, 20%
- Severe hydronephrosis can greatly distend the abdomen and compress the thorax.
- Associated renal anomalies, 25%: contralateral renal agenesis, UVJ obstruction
- Paranephric urinoma
- Amniotic fluid is usually normal.

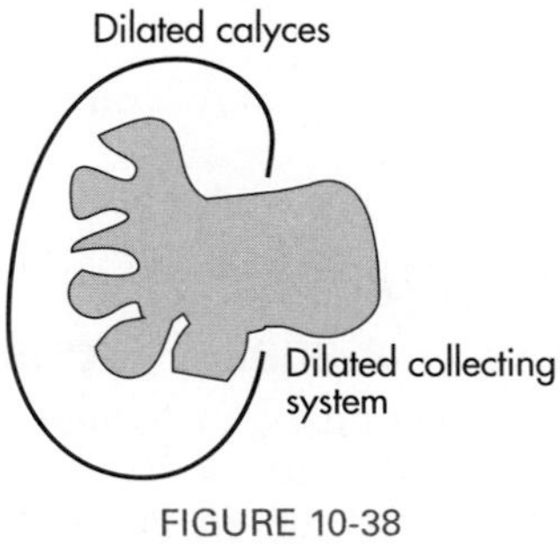

FIGURE 10-38

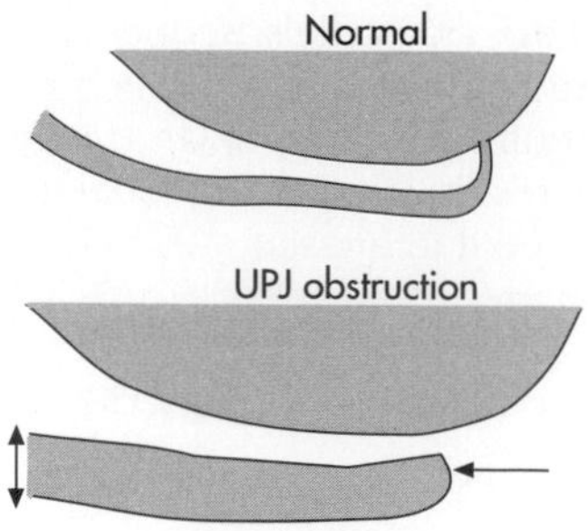

FIGURE 10-39

Ureterovesical Junction (UVJ) Obstruction

- Less common than UPJ obstruction
- Common causes:
  - Duplex system (ectopic upper pole ureter obstructed)
  - Primary megaureter
  - Distal ureteral atresia
- A dilated ureter may mimic large bowel.
- Most obstructions are unilateral.
- As with UPJ, amniotic fluid quantity is usually normal, and definitive diagnosis can be made in neonatal period.
- Associated renal anomalies: UPJ obstruction, MCDK

Bladder Outlet Obstruction

- Most common cause: posterior urethral valves in males (much less common: caudal regression syndrome, megacystis microcolon–intestinal hypoperistalsis, which is very rare)
- Dilated bladder and posterior urethra ("key hole" appearance)
- Thickened bladder wall (>2 mm)
- Dystrophic bladder wall calcification
- Pyelocaliectasis, 40%
- Urine ascites
- Oligohydramnios, 50%

ANTENATAL PREDICTORS OF POOR POSTNATAL RENAL FUNCTION

US
- Severe oligohydramnios
- Increased renal echogenicity
- Renal cortical cysts
- Slow bladder refilling after emptying

Fetal urine
- Increased Na^+, Ca^{2+}, and osmolality

Fetal blood
- Increased β_2-microglobulin

RENAL CYSTIC DISEASE

Multicystic Dysplastic Kidney (MCDK) Disease

Cystic dysplasia secondary to in utero obstruction. Severity related to degree of obstruction and time of occurrence. Most common neonatal renal mass. Usually unilateral; incompatible with life if bilateral.

US Features (Fig. 10-40)

- Paraspinal mass with numerous macroscopic cysts of varying sizes
- Cysts are usually noncommunicating (differentiation from hydronephrosis is thus possible).
- Ureter and renal pelvis are atretic and not visualized.
- Contralateral renal anomalies, 40%:
  - UPJ obstruction common
  - Agenesis (lethal)
  - MCDK (lethal if bilateral)

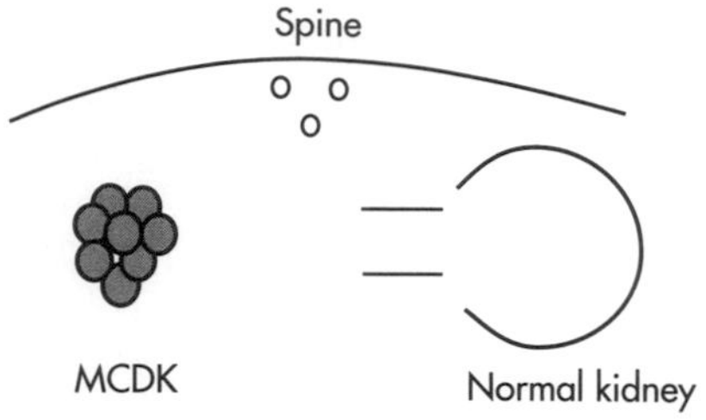

FIGURE 10-40

Autosomal Recessive Polycystic Kidney Disease (ARPCKD) (Infantile Polycystic Kidney Disease)

A heterogeneous spectrum of renal and liver disease. Renal disease predominates in the severe perinatal form; inverse relationship occurs between hepatic and renal disease.

US Features (Fig. 10-41)

- Bilaterally enlarged, hyperechoic kidneys
- Enhanced renal through-transmission
- Individual cysts cannot be visualized by US
- Associated with liver fibrosis
- Potter syndrome: absent bladder, oligohydramnios, small thorax

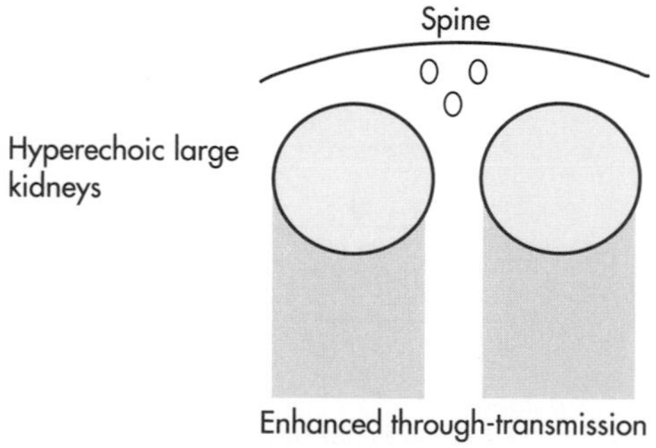

FIGURE 10-41

Cystic Renal Dysplasia

Nonspecific dysplasia secondary to collecting system obstruction
- Small bilateral renal cortical cysts

- Prognosis depends on residual renal function
- Search for oligohydramnios and cause of obstruction (e.g., UPJ, UVJ obstruction)

Meckel-Gruber Syndrome

- Characteristic features (need 2 of the 3 features for diagnosis):
  - Bilateral MCDK, 95%
  - Occipital encephalocele, 80%
  - Polydactyly 75%
- Fatal at birth because of pulmonary hypoplasia
- Autosomal recessive; 25% recurrence risk in subsequent pregnancies

Megacystis Microcolon—Intestinal Hypoperistalsis Syndrome

Rare nonobstructive cause of megacystis. Female preponderance.

- Normal or increased amniotic fluid
- Dilated small bowel may be present but is rare.

EXSTROPHY

Difficult to detect prenatally. Most cases are suspected because of failure to visualize a normal bladder. Some are suspected because of associated infraumbilical omphaloceles.

Bladder Exstrophy

Defect of lower abdominal and anterior bladder wall. Associated findings include:

- Epispadia, always
- Cryptorchidism
- Bilateral inguinal hernias
- Infraumbilical omphalocele
- Anorectal atresia
- OEIS complex (omphalocele, exstrophy, imperforate anus, spinal anomalies)

Cloacal Exstrophy

Two hemibladders are separated by intestinal mucosa. Each hemibladder has its own ureters. Associated with multiple GI and GU anomalies.

HYDROPS FETALIS

GENERAL

Hydrops refers to excessive accumulation of serous fluid within body cavities and fetal soft tissues. Need to involve three different spaces for diagnosis (pericardial, pleural, peritoneal, skin, placenta, cord). Incidence: 1:700 to 1000.

US Features

- Effusions
  - Ascites (fluid around urinary bladder) is the first and most reliable sign.
  - Pleural effusions (in advanced disease)
  - Pericardial effusions
- Subcutaneous edema (skin thickening >5 mm)
  - Localized: lymphatic obstruction, vascular abnormalities
  - Neck, upper thorax: suspect Down syndrome, Turner syndrome
  - Generalized: often associated with cardiovascular anomalies
- Placental edema (placenta is >4 cm thick)
- Polyhydramnios (75%) is more common than oligohydramnios.

Types

- Immune hydrops fetalis, 10%
- Nonimmune hydrops fetalis, 90%

Approach

Hydrops is a fetal emergency. Immediate steps to be taken:

1. Determine maternal immune status.
2. Prepare for fetal transfusion.
3. Search for structural abnormalities and determine the cause of hydrops.
4. Obtain a biophysical profile.

IMMUNE HYDROPS FETALIS (IHF)

Pathophysiology

- Rh-negative mother develops immunoglobulin G (IgG) antibodies to fetal Rh-antigen after first exposure (e.g., delivery, abruption). Production of maternal antibodies can be tested with the indirect Coombs' test.
- In second fetus, antigen-antibody interaction causes anemia → extramedullary hematopoiesis → hepatomegaly → portal-venous hypertension → hydrops.
- Prophylaxis: administer anti-Rh antigen immunoglobulin (RhoGAM) to all Rh-negative mothers at 28 weeks. This effectively blocks maternal sensitization.
- Good prognosis

Role of Prenatal US

Establish and monitor severity of IHF

- Effusions, anasarca, placental edema, polyhydramnios

US-guided therapeutic interventions

- Blood transfusions via the umbilical cord
- Fetal blood sampling through umbilical vessel puncture

NONIMMUNE HYDROPS FETALIS (NIHF)

NIHF represents 90% of fetal hydrops. The overall prognosis is poor because of the frequent inability to treat underlying causes or even the failure to identify an underlying cause. Mortality: 50%-90%.

Concomitant oligohydramnios indicates very poor prognosis. In many instances, the pathophysiology of NIHF is poorly understood.

Causes

- Cardiac, 25%
  - Tachyarrhythmias (most common; most treatable)
  - Structural defects
- Idiopathic, 20%
- Chromosomal anomalies, 10%
  - Turner syndrome
  - Trisomies 21, 18
- Twin-twin transfusion, 10%
- Anemias
- Infections (CMV, toxoplasmosis, parvovirus)
- Other, 25%
  - Chest masses: CCAM, CDH, sequestration
  - Skeletal dysplasia: dwarfism, osteogenesis imperfecta, arthrogryposis
  - GU anomalies
  - Lymphatic anomalies: cystic hygroma, lymphangiectasia, lymphedema
  - Placental chorioangioma
  - GI anomalies: meconium peritonitis
  - Vein of Galen malformation

Complications of Fetal Hydrops

- Neonatal death from pulmonary hypoplasia or structural anomalies
- Maternal hypertension, 30%
- Maternal anemia, 20%
- Maternal hydrops (mirror syndrome)

EXTREMITIES

SKELETAL DYSPLASIAS (DWARFISM)

Approach (see also Chapter 11)

1. Measure long bones and place the abnormality in one of the following categories:
   - Rhizomelic: disproportionate shortening of proximal limb (humerus, femur)
   - Mesomelic: disproportionate shortening of distal long bones (tibia, radius, ulna)
   - Micromelia: entire limb shortened. Subclassify:
     - Mild
     - Severe
     - Bowed
2. Look for associated findings: bowing, fractures, ossification, skull shape.
3. Obtain family history.
4. Consult nomograms and reference texts.

Thanatophoric Dwarf

Most common lethal dysplasia. Sporadic:

- Cloverleaf skull (trilobed) is the key finding, 15%
- Severe micromelia
- Polyhydramnios, 75%
- Nonimmune hydrops
- Small thorax

Homozygous Achondroplasia

Autosomal dominant lethal dysplasia that resembles thanatophoric dwarf. Both parents are achondroplasts (key observation). Similar US features as in thanatophoric dwarfs.

Achondrogenesis (Type I)

Autosomal recessive lethal dysplasia.

- Severe micromelia
- Absent vertebral body ossification
- Ossified calvarium (feature distinguishing from hypophosphatasia)

Osteogenesis Imperfecta (Type II)

Autosomal recessive lethal condition with severe hypomineralization.

- Unossified skull, skull compressible with transducer
- Multiple fractures and long bone angulation/thickening

Congenital Lethal Hypophosphatasia

Autosomal recessive lethal condition with imaging features similar to osteogenesis imperfecta type II.

- Fractures are less common.
- Long bones are thin and delicate.

Short Rib/Polydactyly Syndromes

Spectrum of inherited disorders:

- Severe micromelia differentiates this condition from Jeune and Ellis-van Creveld syndromes.
- Short ribs and narrow thorax
- Polydactyly

Camptomelic Dysplasia

Lethal dysplasia with mild micromelia and anterior bowing of long bones.

Chondrodysplasia Punctata

Lethal autosomal recessive dysplasia that is not frequently diagnosed in utero.

- Stippled epiphyses (only specific feature)

Heterozygous Achondroplasia

- Decreased femur after 27 weeks is sensitive indicator of this dysplasia.
- Narrow lumbosacral interpedicular distance

Asphyxiating Thoracic Dysplasia (Jeune Syndrome)

Autosomal recessive dysplasia that is usually lethal.

- Small thorax
- Polydactyly
- May be indistinguishable from Ellis-van Creveld syndrome

Chondroectodermal Dysplasia (Ellis-van Creveld Syndrome)

Appears similar to Jeune syndrome except that 50% of fetuses have ASD and it is usually nonlethal.

Diastrophic Dysplasia

Nonlethal autosomal recessive dwarfism.
- Hitchhiker thumb: abducted thumb
- Flexion contractures
- Clubfoot

CLUBFOOT (TALIPES)

Types

Idiopathic (good prognosis, more common)
Secondary (worse prognosis)
- Trisomy 18
- Amniotic band syndrome
- Meningocele

US Features

- Foot is at right angle to tibia
- Abnormal position of a foot has to persist (i.e., a permanent flexion has to be differentiated from temporary flexion)
- Metatarsal bones are seen in the same plane as the tibia-fibula plane.

EXTREMITY ABNORMALITIES

Short Radial Ray (Radial Hypoplasia)

Radius and ulna normally end at the same level. In radial hypoplasia, the radius is shorter. Associated conditions include:
- Fanconi anemia
- Thrombocytopenia-absent radius (TAR) syndrome
- Holt-Oram syndrome
- VACTERL
- Klippel-Feil syndrome
- Mental retardation (Cornelia de Lange syndrome)

Limb Anomalies

- Acromelia: shortening of distal extremity
- Adactyly: absence of digits
- Amelia: absence of extremity
- Camptomelia: bent limb
- Hemimelia: absence of distal limb
- Mesomelia: shortening of middle segments (forearm)
- Polydactyly: supernumerary digits

Sirenomelia

Severe manifestation of caudal regression syndrome (mermaid syndrome). Etiology unclear but some cases are caused by alteration in early vascular development diverting blood flow from the caudal region. Associated with infants of diabetic mothers.
- Fusion of lower extremities
- Oligohydramnios
- Bilateral renal agenesis or MCDK
- Sacral agenesis
- Imperforate anus
- Absent external genitalia
- Single umbilical artery

ARTHROGRYPOSIS MULTIPLEX

Neural motor unit defect that results in deformities and disability. Rare. Diseases with similar imaging appearance include:
- Oligohydramnios
- Fetal akinesia syndrome
- Pena-Shokeir syndrome

US Features

- Fetus presents as "Buddha" (no movement)
- Hydrops
- Clubfoot, 75%
- Flexion deformities, 50%
- CDH, 40%

SYNDROMES

Trisomy 21 (Down syndrome)

13%-50% may not have any sonographically detectable abnormalities. Most common anomaly is CHD (40%-50%); AV canal defect is usually mentioned, but ASD and VSD are most common. Other anomalies:
- Duodenal atresia (rarely identified before 25 weeks), 50%
- Hydrothorax
- Hydrops
- Omphalocele
- Increased nuchal thickness, 40%
  - Nuchal translucency: ≥ 3 mm at 11 to 14 weeks; can resolve after 14 weeks. Measure AP diameter on axial image at level of cerebellum
  - Nuchal fold: ≥ 6 mm at 15 to 21 weeks; measure on sagittal image of neck
- Echogenic bowel: other causes of echogenic bowel (similar or increased echogenicity compared with adjacent bone):
  - Trisomy 21
  - Cystic fibrosis
  - CMV
  - Intrauterine growth restriction (IUGR)
  - Intraamniotic bleeding normal
- Short femur length
- Shorter humeral length
- Widening of iliac angle (normal angle of iliac crests on axial view, 60°)
- Pyelectasis
  - >4 mm before 33 weeks
  - >7 mm after 33 weeks
- Echogenic (= bone) intracardiac focus (papillary muscle):
  - Most commonly in LV
  - Can also be seen in RV

5% of normal
More common in Asians
Minimally increased risk of Down, no amniocentesis if isolated
- Small frontal lobes
- Separation of great toe from second toe ("sandal gap")
- Hypoplasia of fifth digit and clinodactyly (incurving of fifth digit to fourth)
- Absence of nasal bone
- Simian crease

Trisomy 18 (Edwards Syndrome)

- CHD, 90%
- IUGR, 60%
- Single umbilical artery, 80%
- Choroid plexus cysts, 30% (1%-2% of normal population)
  - All CP cysts resolve, but resolution does not alter association
  - Normal if no other abnormality
- Polyhydramnios
- Characteristic face:
  - Dolichocephaly strawberry skull
  - Micrognathia
  - Low-set ears
- Skeletal abnormalities
  - Clenched hand with overlap of 2nd and 3rd digits, 80%
  - Rockerbottom feet
- GI anomalies (hernia, omphalocele, atresias)
  - If omphalocele contains liver, it is less likely to be associated with trisomy 18.

Trisomy 13 (Patau Syndrome)

- CHD, 80%
- CNS abnormalities, 70%
  - Holoprosencephaly
  - Microcephaly
  - Agenesis of the corpus callosum
  - Dandy-Walker malformation
  - Hydrocephalus
- IUGR
- Abnormal face
  - Cleft defects
  - Microphthalmia/hypotelorism
- Skeletal abnormalities
  - Polydactyly, 70%
  - Rockerbottom feet
- GU anomalies
  - Hyperechoic kidney
  - Bladder exstrophy

Meckel-Gruber Syndrome

- Bilateral MCDK, 95%
- Occipital encephalocele, 80%
- Postaxial polydactyly 75%

Measurements and Growth

MEASUREMENTS

RECOMMENDATIONS

Fetal measurements become less accurate as a pregnancy progresses. Therefore, the gestational age assigned at the initial scan should be considered a baseline and later age determinations should be based on the initial scan. Best measurements:

1st trimester
- MSD
- CRL

2nd and 3rd trimesters
- Biparietal diameter (BPD) and occipitofrontal diameter (OFD)
- Head circumference (HC)
- Femur length (FL)
- Abdominal diameter (AD)
- Abdominal circumference (AC)
- Composite (BPD, HC, AC, FL)

CONFIDENCE LIMITS OF MEASUREMENTS

Time	US Finding/Measurement	Confidence Limits
TVS		
5 wk	MSD	
5.5 wk	MSD + yolk sac	± 1.0
6 wk	MSD + yolk sac, fetal heart, CRL	± 0.5
TAS		
6-13 wk	CRL	± 0.5
2nd trimester	Corrected BPD	± 1.5
3rd trimester	Corrected BPD or composite	± 3.2

ESTIMATED GESTATIONAL AGE (EGA)

- EGA in days (±1 week) = MSD + 30
- EGA in weeks = CRL + 6.5

GESTATIONAL SAC (Fig. 10-42)

- Accurate size measurements are possible up to 5 to 6 weeks.
- Sac measurements are made from inside to inside border of hypoechoic sac.
- In ovoid sacs, determine 3 diameters:

$$MSD = \frac{(L + W + H)}{3}$$

- Only need to measure 1 diameter in perfectly round sacs

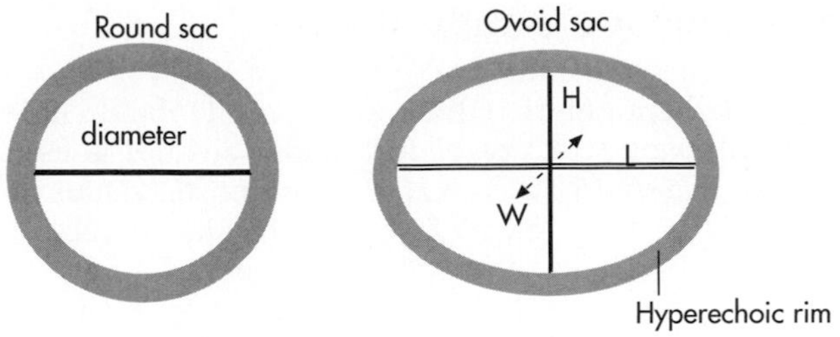

FIGURE 10-42

CROWN-RUMP LENGTH (CRL)

- Accurate size measurements are possible from 6 to 12 weeks (1st trimester).
- The CRL is the most accurate estimation of fetal age (± 0.5 week).
- Measure longest longitudinal diameter of fetal axis, excluding yolk sac.
- After 13 weeks, CRL measurements are not reliable because of fetal flexion.

HEAD MEASUREMENTS

Biparietal Diameter (BPD)

- BPD = inner-to-outer wall measurement (Fig. 10-43)
- OFD = mid-to-mid wall measurement (Fig. 10-44)
- BFD and OFD are measured at the widest portion of the skull at the level of the thalami.

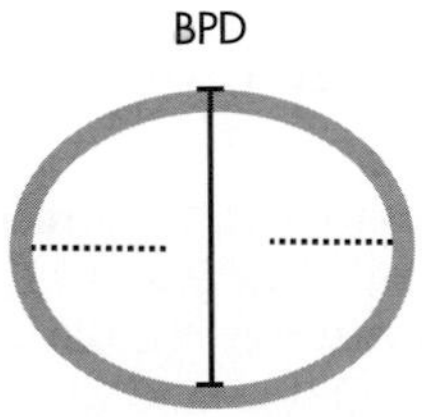

FIGURE 10-43

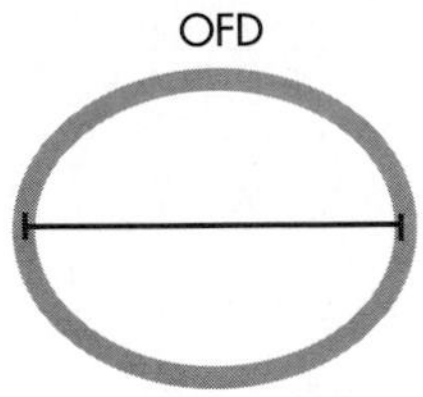

FIGURE 10-44

Cephalic Index (Fig. 10-45)

- Used to determine whether head shape is normal or whether it needs correction
- Cephalic index: (A/B) × 100
- Normal index: 70 to 86
- Note that A and B are outer-to-outer wall measurements.

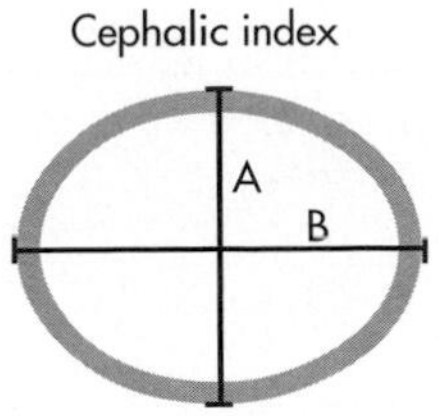

FIGURE 10-45

Corrected Biparietal Diameter

- Most accurate predictor of age in 2nd trimester
- Corrects for shape abnormalities of the head
- Corrected BPD = (BPD × OFD) ÷ $\sqrt{1.265}$
- Rough estimation of age: BPD (cm) × 4 + 2 weeks = age in weeks

Head Circumference (Fig. 10-46)

- Same accuracy as BPD measurements
- HC = 1.57 × (outer BPD + outer OFD)

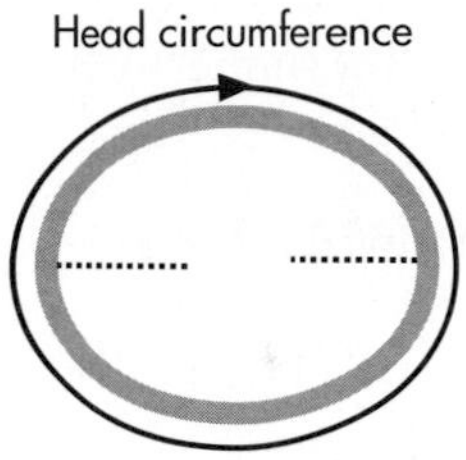

FIGURE 10-46

ABDOMINAL MEASUREMENTS (Fig. 10-47)

- Measurements are performed at the level of the liver.
- Intrahepatic umbilical vein serves as a landmark and should be equidistant from lateral abdominal walls.
- All measurements are outer edge measurements.
- Types of measurements:
  Abdominal diameter (AD)
  Abdominal circumference
  (AC) = 1.57 × (AD_1 + AD_2)

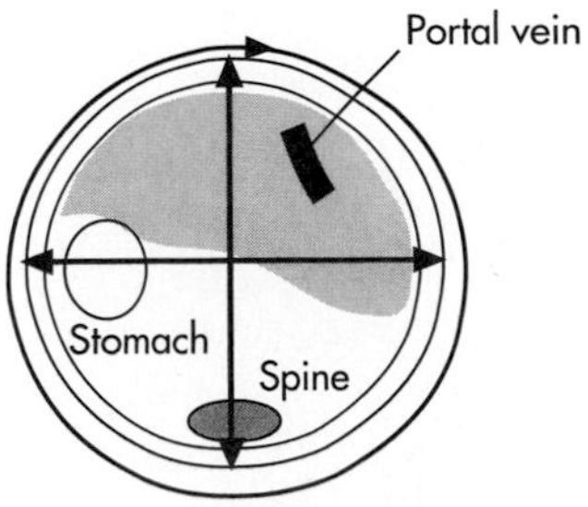

FIGURE 10-47

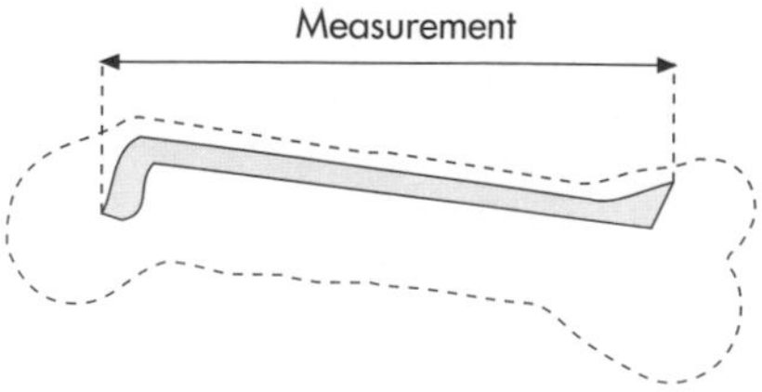

FIGURE 10-48

FEMUR LENGTH MEASUREMENT (Fig. 10-48)

- Only the hyperechoic diaphysis is included in the measurement.
- The epiphyseal cartilage is not calcified and therefore appears hypoechoic.

ESTIMATED FETAL WEIGHT (EFW)

- Use 3 body measurements (head, abdomen, femur length) to compute EFW.
- Correlate EFW to gestational age; 95% confidence interval is ± 15% (2 standard deviations) of the determined value (approximately ± 15%-20%).

GROWTH ABNORMALITIES

ABNORMALLY SMALL FETUS (IUGR)

Intrauterine growth restriction = IUGR. Definition: EFW is present if weight is <10th percentile of normal. Best time for screening is 34 ± 1 week. Two forms: asymmetric and symmetric.

Asymmetric IUGR (90%)

- Abdominal circumference more affected than head or extremities/femur, until severe
- Oligohydramnios
- Often detected in 3rd trimester
- Due to maternal/placental causes:
    - Primary placental insufficiency
    - Secondary placental insufficiency
        - Hypertension
        - Collagen vascular disease, vasculitis
- Nutrition or toxin related
    - Alcohol or drug abuse
    - Smoking
    - Starvation
    - Teratogenic medications

Symmetric IUGR (10%)

- Head and body equally affected
- Normal amniotic fluid volume
- May be detected in first trimester
- Due to fetal causes:
    - Chromosomal anomaly
    - Infection (TORCH)
    - Normal small infant

Sonographic Determination

- No single parameter best defines IUGR.
- Different criteria (BPD, EFW, AD, FL) and clinical signs (e.g., placental grade, alcohol abuse, hypertension) have varying prognostic value.
- HC/AC ratio detects 70% of all IUGRs but misses 30% of IUGRs that appear symmetrical.
- The most reliable criterion to determine the presence of IUGR is the combination of EFW + amniotic fluid volume (AFV) + presence of maternal hypertension. Doppler of umbilical cord systolic/diastolic ratio is elevated.

ABNORMALLY LARGE FETUS

Large for gestational age (LGA): EFW is present if weight is >90th percentile. Macrosomia is a subset of LGA defined as fetal weight >4000 g at birth. It is important to recognize this because a large fetus has increased morbidity and mortality.

Risk Factors

- Maternal diabetes (most common)
- Maternal obesity
- Prior LGA infant
- Prolonged pregnancy

Complications

- Asphyxia
- Meconium aspiration
- Neonatal hypoglycemia
- Trauma (shoulder dystocia, brachial plexus palsy)

BIOPHYSICAL PROFILE (BPP)

Method for assessing antepartum risk of fetal asphyxia. Goal of the BPP is to identify a fetus at risk for perinatal death or complications, thus directing obstetric management and altering perinatal outcome. More sensitive and specific than a non–stress test alone.

MANNING CRITERIA FOR FETAL VIABILITY

Parameters	Criterion of Normal	Indicator of
1. Fetal heart acceleration	≥ 2 episodes of ≥ 15 beats/min in 20 min	Acute hypoxia
2. Breathing movements	≥ 1 episode ≥ 30 sec in 30 min	Acute hypoxia
3. Gross body movements	≥ 3 movements in 30 min	Acute hypoxia
4. Muscular tone	≥ 1 flexion and extension of extremity	Acute hypoxia
5. Amniotic fluid volume	≥ 2 cm in perpendicular plane	Chronicity

Binary assignment: 2 points for normal, 0 points for abnormal. The score is the sum of all points.

Clinical Relevance

- Score 8-10: retest after periodic interval
- Score 4-6:
  - Mature lung: deliver now
  - Immature lung: close monitoring
- Score 0-2: delivery indicated

Mortality

- Score 8-10: 0.1%
- Score 6: 1%
- Score 4: 3%
- Score 2: 10%
- Score 0: 30%

Fetomaternal Structures

GENERAL

APPROACH (Fig. 10-49)

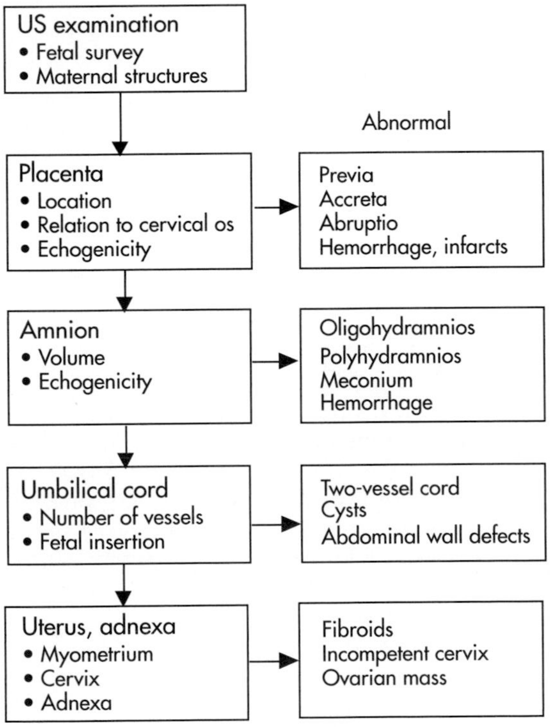

FIGURE 10-49

PLACENTA

NORMAL DEVELOPMENT (Fig. 10-50)

Placenta is derived from 2 units:

- Maternal decidua basalis
- Fetal chorion frondosum

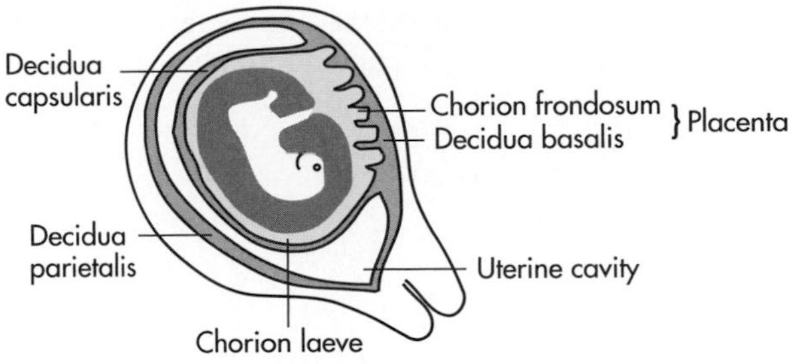

FIGURE 10-50

Decidua (maternal endometrium)

- Decidua capsularis: layer that covers implanted embryo
- Decidua parietalis: layer lining the uterine cavity
- Decidua basalis: layer between embryo and myometrium

Chorion (Fetal Component)

- Chorion results from fusion of trophoblast and extraembryonic mesenchyme.
- Layers
  - Chorion laeve: smooth portion of chorion surrounds embryo
  - Chorion frondosum: forms primordial placenta, adjacent to decidua basalis
- *Chorion* and *placenta* are terms used interchangeably later in pregnancy.

Placental Unit (Fig. 10-51)

- First, the trophoblast differentiates into 2 layers: an inner layer of cytotrophoblasts and an outer layer of syncytiotrophoblasts.
- Syncytiotrophoblasts erode endometrium, and a lacunar network of maternal blood develops around the syncytiotrophoblast.
- Villi form from columns of syncytiotrophoblasts and proliferate.

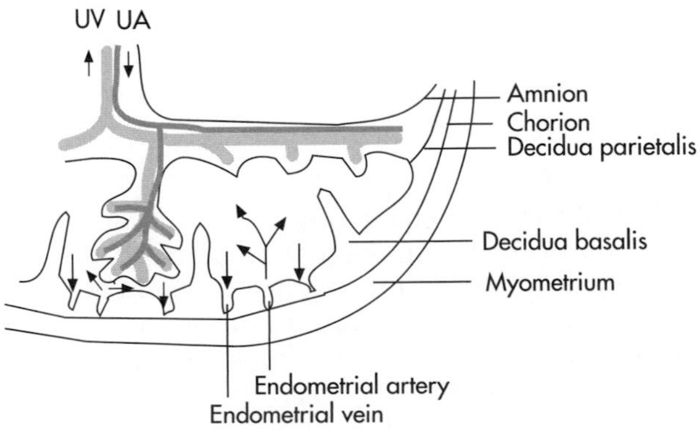

FIGURE 10-51

- The functional unit of the placenta is the cotyledon; the entire placenta consists of 10 to 30 cotyledons.
- Measurements of final placenta:
  Diameter: 15 to 20 cm
  Weight: 600 g
  Thickness <4 cm

US features (Fig. 10-52)

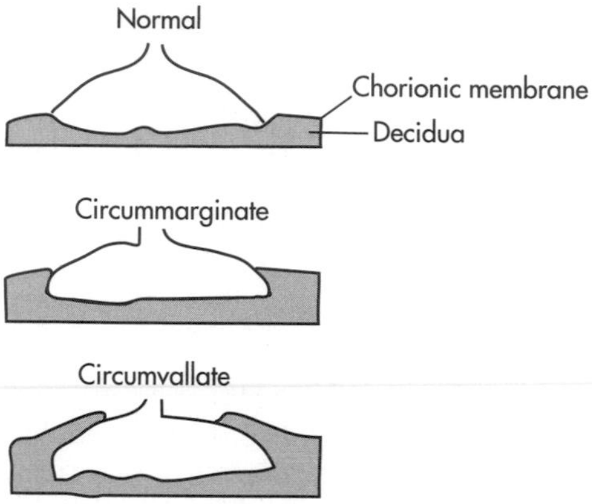

FIGURE 10-52

Normal Placenta

- Appears hyperechoic relative to adjacent myometrium
- Draining veins can be seen in the basal plate.
- Spiral arterioles are too small to be seen by US.
- Placental calcifications are physiologic and have no clinical significance; calcifications occur primarily along basal plate and septa.
- Normal hypoechoic or anechoic foci in placenta may represent fibrin, thrombus, maternal lakes, and cysts.

Placental Variants

- Succenturiate lobe: an accessory placental lobe
  Complication: hemorrhage from connecting vessels
- Extrachorial placenta: fetal membranes do not extend to the edge of the placenta. Types:
  Circummarginate: no clinical significance
  Circumvallate: predisposes to hemorrhage

Placental Grading

Grading system originally described by Grannum to reflect the normal maturation of the placenta. Grade 3 placentas are most mature and usually indicate term. Classification is generally of no clinical use.

- Grade 0: smooth surface, homogeneous
- Grade 1: scattered calcification
- Grade 2: calcification in chorionic plate and basal plate
- Grade 3: calcification extends continuously from chorionic plate to basal surface, dividing placenta into cotyledons; posterior shadowing

PLACENTA PREVIA

A placenta previa covers the internal cervical os. Incidence: 1:200. Incidence increases with age, multiparity prior cesarean sections, and smoking. A pregnancy with placenta previa should be delivered by cesarean section. Diagnose after 20 weeks. Complications include:

- 3rd-trimester bleeding, 90%
- Premature delivery
- Perinatal death
- Maternal death

Types (Fig. 10-53)

- Marginal: placenta extends to os
- Complete: complete coverage of os
- Low-lying placenta: placental edge within 2 cm of os

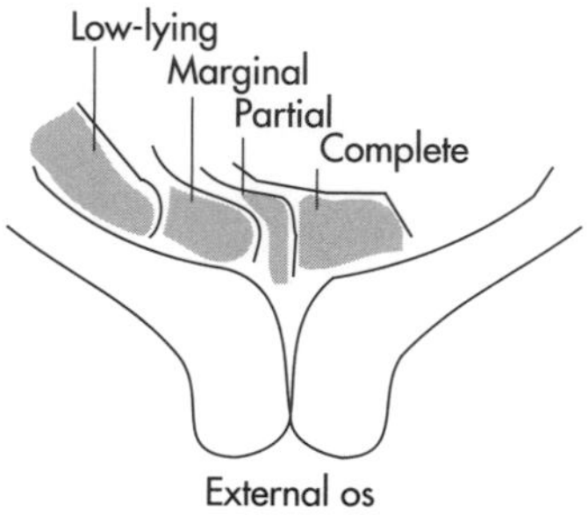

FIGURE 10-53

US Features

- Transperineal or endovaginal US often useful to establish diagnosis
- Determine the subtype of placenta previa
- Placental position can change during pregnancy (regressing placenta previa) because of differential growth of lower uterine segment; 60%-90% of patients with 2nd-trimester placenta previa will have a normal placenta at term.
- Placenta previa can be mimicked by (false positive):
  Overdistended bladder (rescan with empty bladder after 20 to 30 minutes)
  Focal myometrial contractions

PLACENTAL SEPARTION

Premature separation of a normal placenta from the myometrium results in hemorrhage and hematomas. Incidence: 1% (may be as high as 4% because a separation often goes undiagnosed). Recurrence rate: 5%-10%. Increased risk of abruption with:

- Higher parity
- Older age

- Preeclampsia, eclampsia
- Trauma
- Uterine anomalies
- Cocaine abuse

Complications

- 3rd-trimester bleeding (abruptio placentae)
- IUGR
- DIC
- Fetal death

Types (Fig. 10-54)

Placental separation constitutes a spectrum of abnormalities with different clinical presentations and outcomes. Subchorionic hematoma (marginal hemorrhage) usually occurs early in pregnancy and has a good outcome. Large retroplacental hematomas (abruptio placentae) commonly present as catastrophic 3rd-trimester events with pain, bleeding, and fetal death.

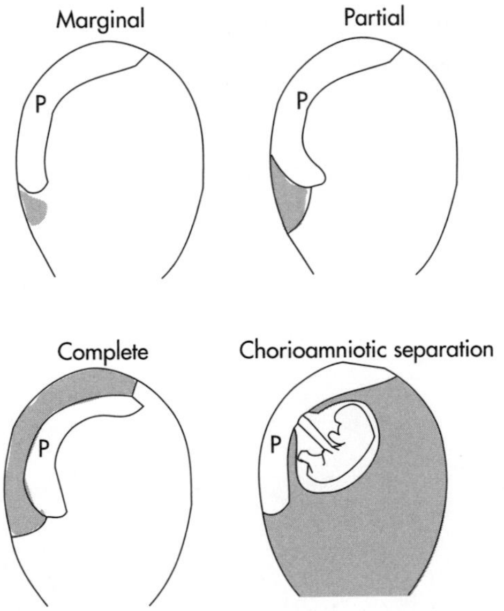

FIGURE 10-54

US Features

Specific
- Retroplacental hematoma
- Elevation of fetal membranes (subchorionic hematoma)

Suggestive
- Focal placental thickening
- Edge abnormalities

Nonspecific
- Subchorionic hypoechoic areas
- Placental hypoechoic areas

Appearance of hemorrhage
- Hyperechoic acute hemorrhage may mimic an echogenic placenta (false negative).

CLINICAL SIGNS OF PLACENTAL SEPARATION

	Retroplacental Hematoma	Marginal Separation
Time	Late, >20 Weeks	Early, <20 weeks
Type of hemorrhage	Arterial (spiral arteries)	Venous
Vaginal bleeding	Occasionally	Yes
Symptoms	Major	Minor
Prognosis	Worse	Better
Common terminology	Abruption placentae	Subchorionic hemorrhage

PLACENTA ACCRETA

The normal decidua forms a barrier to deep invasion of chorionic villi into the uterus. In placenta accreta, there is loss of the normal placenta/myometrium border. The risk of placenta accreta is higher in patients with a prior cesarean section.

Types (Fig. 10-55)

- Placenta accreta, 80%: chorionic villi adhere to myometrium
- Placenta increta, 15%: villi invade myometrium
- Placenta percreta, 5%: villi completely penetrate myometrium (usually into bladder)

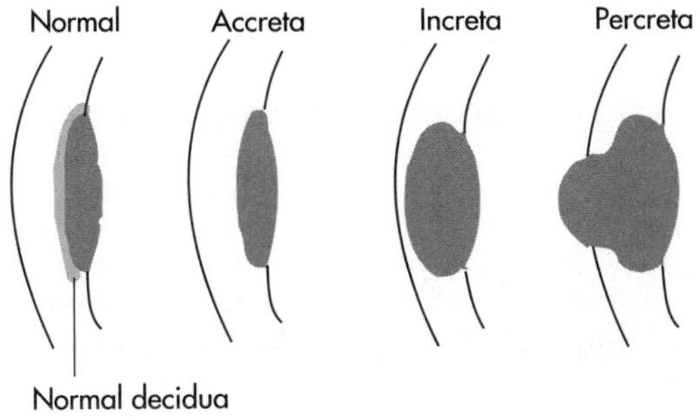

FIGURE 10-55

Complications

- Maternal hemorrhage after delivery
- Postpartum infection (retained placenta)

Imaging Features

- Very difficult to diagnose by US
- MRI findings include:
  - Placenta previa
  - Uterine bulging
  - Heterogeneous signal intensity within the placenta
  - Dark intraplacental bands on T2-weighted images
  - Focal interruptions in the myometrial wall
  - Tenting of the bladder
  - Placental tissue invades pelvic structures

NORMAL INTRAPLACENTAL LESIONS

All of the following lesions except infarcts appear as anechoic or hypoechoic foci within the placenta and have no pathologic significance:

- Fibrin depositions in 25% of pregnancies
- Intervillous thrombosis
- Maternal lakes
- Septal cysts
- Small infarcts are of no clinical significance (if the infarct area is >10% of placental area, IUGR commonly results from hypoxia). Infarcts are usually not detected unless they hemorrhage.

CHORIOANGIOMA

Benign vascular malformation of the placenta. Most chorioangiomas are small and are of no significance. Complications of large lesions are related to shunting:

- Polyhydramnios
- Hydrops
- IUGR
- Premature labor
- Fetal death

US Features

- Chorioangioma may appear as a mixed hyperechoic/hypoechoic solid mass.
- Flow in lesions can be demonstrated by Doppler US (in contrast to hemorrhage).
- Polyhydramnios

GESTATIONAL TROPHOBLASTIC DISEASE

CLASSIFICATION

Gestational trophoblastic disease (GTD) is a proliferative disease of the trophoblast that may present as:

- Hydatidiform mole (partial or complete)
- Invasive mole
- Choriocarcinoma

Modified NIH Classification

Nonmetastatic trophoblastic disease
- Hydatidiform mole
- Persistent mole (>8 weeks)
- Invasive mole or choriocarcinoma confined to uterus

Metastatic trophoblastic disease
- Low risk
  - <4 months
  - β-HCG <100,000 mIU/mL
  - Lung or vaginal metastases
- Intermediate risk
  - 4 months
  - β-HCG >100,000 mIU/mL
  - Lung or vaginal metastases
- High risk
  - CNS or liver metastases

KARYOTYPES

Type	Malignant Potential	Karyotype*	Fetal Tissue
Complete mole	Yes (20%)†	46 XX > 46 XY	No
Partial mole	No	69 (triploidy)	Yes

*DNA in all hydatidiform moles is paternal in origin.
†15% invasive mole, 5% choriocarcinoma.

HYDATIDIFORM MOLE

Most benign and most common form of GTD. Incidence 1:1500 (geographic variation). Risk factors: increased age, prior GTD, Asian.

Clinical Findings

- Uterus too large for dates
- Elevated β-HCG (levels can be used to monitor treatment and regression of disease)
- Molar vesicles passed per vagina
- Hemorrhage (common)
- Hyperemesis gravidarum

US Features (Fig. 10-56)

- Hyperechoic soft tissue mass fills uterine cavity (snowstorm appearance).
- Cystic degeneration of mole (vesicular appearance)
- Large, usually multiseptated theca lutein adnexal cysts, 50%
- Absence of fetal parts

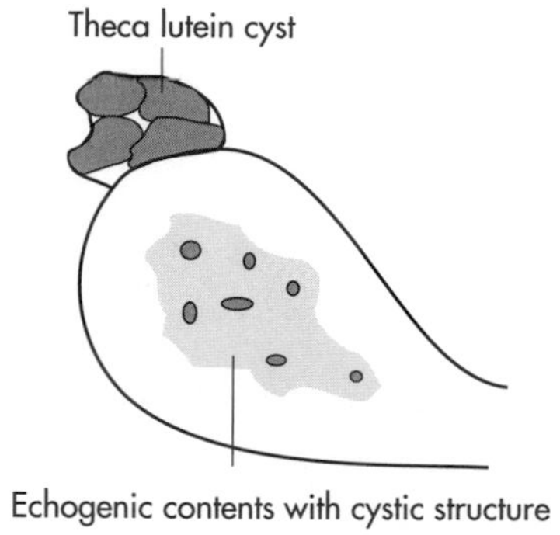

FIGURE 10-56

Prognosis

- Resolution after evacuation, 80%
- Locally invasive mole, 15%
- Metastatic choriocarcinoma, 5%

VARIANTS

Incomplete or Partial Mole

A pregnancy with a formed but abnormal placenta (cystic spaces) and an abnormal dysmorphic fetus. Genetic triploidy (69 chromosomes). May develop persistent GTD but has no malignant potential.

Coexistent Trophoblastic Disease and a Living Fetus

Very rare. May be seen in a twin pregnancy with GTD of one placenta.

Hydropic Degeneration of the Placenta

Hydropic degeneration of the placenta does not represent GTD. There is enlargement of chorionic villi, but β-HCG is low. Most frequently seen with a missed abortion.

CHORIOCARCINOMA

Malignant form of GTD. Incidence 1:40,000 pregnancies; only 5% of moles progress to choriocarcinoma. Choriocarcinoma is preceded by:
- Mole, 50%
- Abortion, 25%
- Normal pregnancy, 20%
- Ectopic pregnancy, 5%

Metastases

- Lung
- Brain
- Liver
- Bone
- GI tract

AMNION

NORMAL AMNIOTIC FLUID

Volume

Several methods are used for assessment of fluid; there is no evidence that any method is better than the other:
- Subjective assessment (recommended by most sonographers)
  - Anterior uterine wall displaced away from fetal body (good sign)
  - Fetal extremities readily visible because of excessive fluid
  - Umbilical cord readily visible
  - Oligohydramnios: bad image, crowded (increased fetal-uterine contact), small pockets
  - Polyhydramnios: fetus not touching uterine wall, placental compression, large pockets
- Single deepest pocket measurement; <2 cm oligohydramnios; >8 cm polyhydramnios; >16 cm tense polyhydramnios
- 4-quadrant amniotic fluid index (AFI): need to adjust for age
  - Sum of largest vertical measures in centimeters in four quadrants
  - <5 cm: oligohydramnios (any age)
  - 5-8: borderline
  - 8-18: normal
  - >18: polyhydramnios (>28 at 35 weeks)

Echogenicity

Normal amnion is anechoic. Low-level echoes may be due to:
- Vernix
- Hemorrhage
- Meconium

Pearls

- Amniotic fluid volume is dynamic because of constant production (fetal urination) and consumption (fetal swallowing and lung absorption).
- The greater the degree of polyhydramnios, the greater the likelihood that a major malformation and a chromosomal abnormality are present.

POLYHYDRAMNIOS

Amniotic fluid volume more than expected for gestational age and defined as (1) amniotic fluid index >18 to 28; (2) largest fluid pocket greater than 8 cm, or (3) fluid volume larger than 1500 to 2000 cm^3.

Causes

Idiopathic, 40%

Maternal, 40%
- Diabetes
- Hypertension

Fetal, 20%
- CNS lesions (neural tube defect)
- Proximal GI obstruction
- Chest masses
- Twin-twin transfusion
- Nonimmune hydrops

OLIGOHYDRAMNIOS

Amniotic fluid volume less than expected for gestational age. 1st-trimester oligohydramnios results in failure of pregnancy in 95% of cases (pulmonary hypoplasia, limb contractures). Criteria:
- 4-quadrant amniotic fluid index <5
- Largest pocket method: <2 cm

Causes

Mnemonic: "DRIPPC":
- **D**emise
- **R**enal abnormalities (decreased urine output)
- **I**UGR, 80%
- **P**remature rupture of membranes
- **P**ost dates
- **C**hromosomal anomalies

UMBILICAL CORD

CORD ANATOMY (Fig. 10-57)

The normal umbilical cord measures 1 to 2 cm in diameter. The cord contains 2 arteries and 1 vein. Placental insertion:

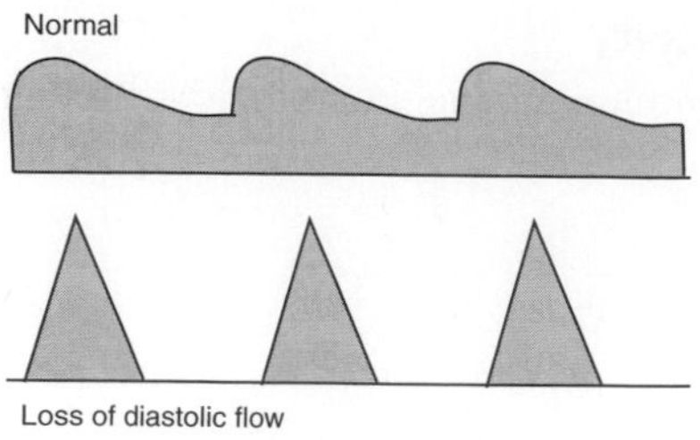

FIGURE 10-57

- Central insertion, 90%
- Marginal insertion, 5% (no clinical significance)
- Insertion on membranes at distance from placenta (velamentous insertion); may cause loss of diastolic flow, bleeding in antenatal period, 5%
- Normal cord Doppler waveform is low resistance with relatively large diastolic flow; loss of or reversal of diastolic flow indicates fetal stress.
    - The peak systolic to end diastolic (A/B or S/D) ratio decreases from 4.25 at 16 weeks to 2.5 at term due to increased diastolic flow; abnormal (increased resistance) if >90th percentile.
    - Pulsatility index (PI) of middle cerebral artery: (peak systolic − end diastolic)/area under Doppler waveform; remains stable in IUGR until severe → decreasing PI indicates loss of autoregulation.

VASA PREVIA

Velamentous insertion of the umbilical cord with vessels traversing the internal cervical os. Use Doppler US to confirm vessels at the os. Complication: hemorrhage at delivery.

TWO-VESSEL CORD

Umbilical cord containing only 1 artery and 1 vein. Incidence: 1%. Associated with structural (holoprosencephaly, skeletal dysplasia, hydrocephalus, omphalocele, hydrothorax, diaphragmatic hernia) and chromosomal abnormalities in 50% of cases.

- Should prompt fetal survey and possibly karyotyping
- Associated with IUGR, premature delivery, and perinatal mortality
- Normal variant in multiple gestations

STRAIGHT CORD

A normal cord appears twisted by US (coiled cord), a result of fetal movement. Straight cords are commonly associated with other anomalies. Mortality: 10%.

MASSES

- Localized deposition of Wharton's jelly
- Hematomas, variable echogenicity depending on age of hematomas
- Hemangioma: echogenic or complex mass; increased AFP; associated with umbilical cord edema, fetal hydrops, and hemorrhage
- Cystic masses
    - Allantoic cyst: may be associated with omphalocele
    - Amniotic inclusion cyst
    - Omphalomesenteric duct cyst

UTERUS AND ADNEXA

INCOMPETENT CERVIX

Premature dilatation of cervical canal before start of labor. Treatment: cerclage.

Clinical Findings

- Painless cervical dilatation
- Prolapse of membranes into vagina
- Recurrent 2nd-trimester abortions

Causes

Prior injury (most common)

- Abortion, ectopic
- Prior pregnancy
- Curettage, conization, dilatation
- Fetal anatomic variants

Congenital

- Prior diethylstilbestrol (DES) exposure in utero
- Inadequacy of lower uterine segment?

US Features (Fig. 10-58)

Technique

- TAS: bladder should not be fully distended
- TVS: insert probe 3 to 4 cm into vagina to visualize cervix
- Translabial US

Criteria

- Shortening of cervix <2.5 cm
- Cervical canal width >8 mm
- Prolapse of:
    - Membrane
    - Cord
    - Fetal parts

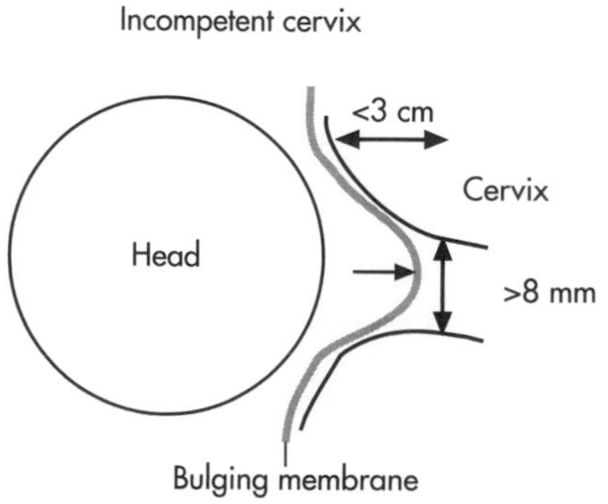

FIGURE 10-58

- Funneling of lumen beginning at internal os
- Change in length of configuration of cervix with application of fundal pressure

Management Issues

- Serial imaging should be performed if incompetent cervix is suspected but not shown by the first US; an incompetent cervix is a dynamic process.
- Serial assessment of the efficacy of surgical cerclage should be monitored by US; sutures usually appear as hyperechoic structures with posterior shadowing.
- Main complication of incompetent cervix: 2nd-trimester abortion

UTERINE FIBROIDS

Most common uterine mass identified during pregnancy. Most fibroids do not change size during pregnancy; however, some may enlarge due to elevated estrogen levels. Focal myometrial contractions (FMCs) may be mistaken for fibroids. FMCs are transient and usually disappear within 10 minutes.

DIFFERENTIATION OF FIBROID VERSUS FMC

	Fibroid	FMC
Echogenicity	Hypoechoic	Isoechoic
Attenuation of beam	Yes	No
Heterogeneous	Yes	No
Persistence	Yes	Resolves

ADNEXAL MASSES

Corpus Luteum Cyst (CLC)

Most common adnexal mass during 1st trimester. CLC secretes progesterone to support the pregnancy until placental progesterone secretion is established.

US Features

- Most masses are <5 cm and unilocular.
- May contain septations and/or debris
- Typically resolve by 16 weeks
- CLCs are physiologic structures. Do not mention them in report unless:
  - Very big
  - Symptomatic
  - Hemorrhagic

Other Adnexal Masses

- Benign cystic teratoma
- Cystadenoma
- Endometriosis
- Appendicitis

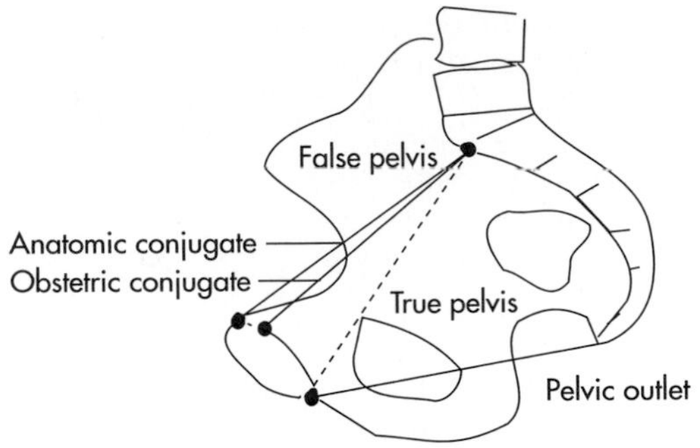

FIGURE 10-59

PELVIMETRY

MEASUREMENTS (Fig. 10-59)

Can be obtained from plain films, CT, or MRI. MRI is now the modality of choice for pelvimetric measurements. Pelvimetry is used to determine pelvic dimensions in breech presentations.

- Obstetric conjugate (>10 cm), sacral promontory to superior symphysis pubis
- Anatomic conjugate, sacral promontory to superior symphysis pubis
- Diagonal conjugate (>11.5 cm), sacral promontory to subpubic angle
- Bispinous diameter (>10.5 cm), distance between ischial spines

FETAL MRI

Emerging as an adjunct to ultrasound for problem solving to evaluate specific fetal anomalies.

Advantages

- Not limited by maternal obesity, fetal position, or oligohydramnios
- Better visualization of fetal brain (not limited by skull)
- Superior soft tissue contrast; distinguish individual organs (e.g., gray and white matter, lung, liver, kidney, bowel)
- Multiplanar imaging is easier.
- Large field of view

Disadvantages

- Expensive
- Claustrophobia
- Less spatial resolution
- Sensitive to fetal motion
- Safety not yet established, although no adverse events have been reported

Technique

- Gadolinium contrast not used: crosses placenta and may be teratogenic at high doses
- Imaging >18 weeks to avoid exposure during peak organogenesis

- US should be performed before MRI, especially to establish the presence of fetal cardiac activity.
- No sedation needed in routine imaging
- Body coil or larger phase-array coils usually used
- Sequences
    - Single-shot fast spin echo (SSFSE) for T2W images; each sequence acquired in 20 to 25 seconds
        - Assess major thoracic and abdominal structures
    - Inversion recovery single-shot fast spin echo for T1W images 4- to 7-mm thickness
        - Detect bowel loops

Applications

- Most studies are performed to evaluate CNS abnormalities.
- Most common indication is ventriculomegaly: to evaluate associated abnormalities.
- Thorax: evaluate chest masses, lung maturation (lungs normally T2 hyperintense from alveolar fluid).
- Abdomen: location of liver, especially when CDH is present for prognosis

Differential Diagnosis

FIRST TRIMESTER

FIRST-TRIMESTER BLEEDING (Fig. 10-60)

Pregnancy Related (Common)

- Normal intrauterine pregnancy (implantation hemorrhage)
- Abortion (impending, in progress, incomplete)
- Ectopic pregnancy
- GTD
- Subchorionic hemorrhage

Unrelated to Pregnancy (Rare)

- Polyp
- Cancer
- Vaginal ulcers

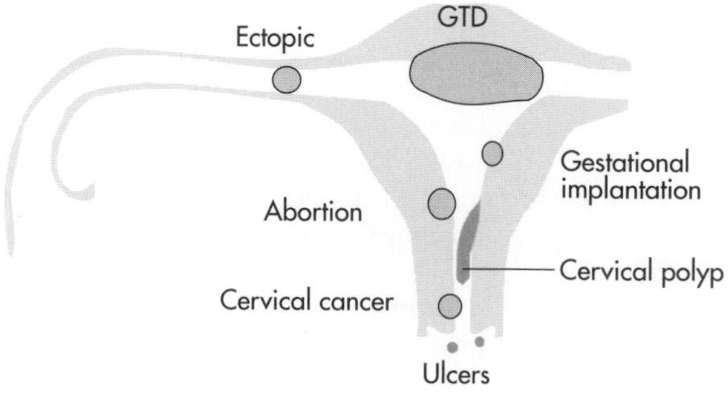

FIGURE 10-60

EMPTY SAC

- Normal early IUP
- Blighted ovum (anembryonic gestation)
- Ectopic pregnancy (pseudogestational sac)

ECHOGENIC CENTRAL CAVITY

Normal pregnancy
- Decidua in early, not yet visible IUP
- Hemorrhage

Ectopic pregnancy
- Decidual reaction

Abortion
- Retained products after an incomplete abortion

COMPLEX INTRAUTERINE MASS

- Missed abortion with placental hydropic degeneration
- Fetal demise with retained tissue
- Molar pregnancy
- Degenerated uterine fibroid
- Endometrial carcinoma

AFP ABNORMALITIES (Fig. 10-61)

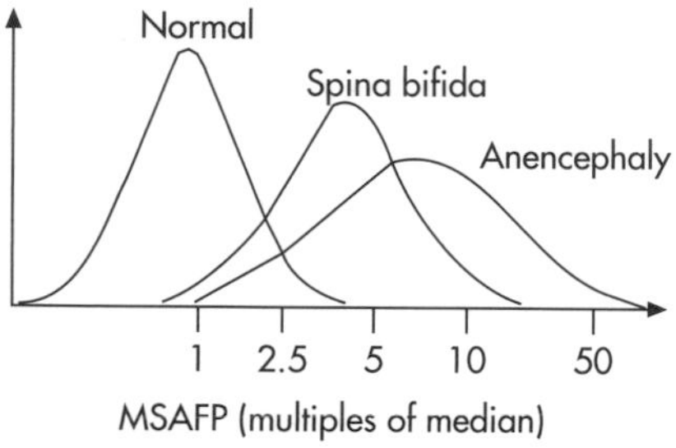

FIGURE 10-61

Elevated MSAFP (2 multiples of median)

- Fetal abnormalities, 60%
    - NTD
    - Abdominal wall defects
    - Cystic hygroma
    - Gastrointestinal obstruction, atresia
    - Liver disease: hepatitis
    - Renal disease: congenital nephrosis
- Incorrect dates, 20%
- Multiple gestation, 15%
- Fetal demise, 5%
- Low birth weight
- Placental abnormalities (abruption, mole)

Low MSAFP (<0.5 multiples of median)

- Down syndrome
- Trisomy 18
- Incorrect dates

PREDICTORS OF POOR OUTCOME

- Fetal heartbeat not seen with CRL >5 mm.
- MSD ≥ 8 mm and no yolk sac (TVS)

- MSD ≥ 16 mm and no fetal pole (TVS)
- β-HCG > 1000 mIU/mL and no gestational sac (Fig. 10-62)
- β-HCG >3600 mIU/mL and no yolk sac
- Heart rate <90 beats/min
- MSD – CRL <5 mm
- Irregular gestational sac
- Abnormal yolk sac (>6 mm, calcified, irregular)
- Absent double decidual sign with MSD >10 mm
- Empty sac, large sac
- Large subchorionic hematoma
- <2 mm choriodecidual reaction

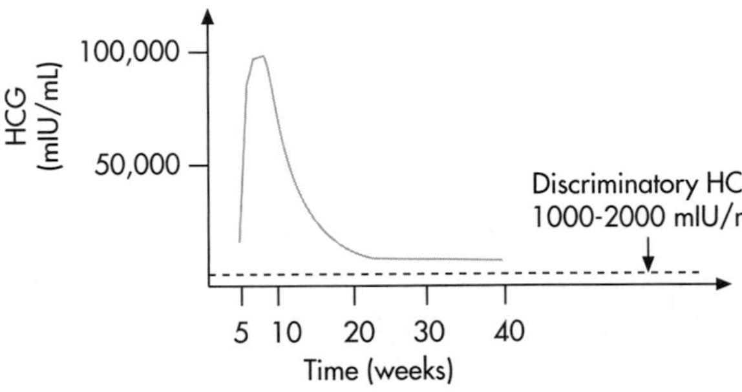

FIGURE 10-62

SECOND AND THIRD TRIMESTERS

PLACENTA SIZE

Diffusely Enlarged Placenta (>4 cm thick)

- Hydrops fetalis
- Maternal diabetes
- Maternal anemia
- Congenital infection (TORCH)
- Intraplacental hematoma
- Molar change, partial mole

Small Placenta (Hypoperfusion)

- Maternal hypertension
- Toxemia
- Severe diabetes
- IUGR

ABNORMAL PLACENTAL ECHOTEXTURE

- Partial mole
- Hydropic placenta
- Hemorrhage or abruption
- Chorioangiomas
- Common but insignificant findings (venous lakes, fibrin, intervillous thrombosis, septal cysts, infarcts)

UMBILICAL CORD ABNORMALITIES

Solitary Umbilical Artery

- Trisomies 13, 18
- Structural anomalies (holoprosencephaly, skeletal dysplasia, hydrocephalus, omphalocele, hydrothorax, diaphragmatic hernia)

Enlargement of Umbilical Cord

- Edema
- Hematoma
- Cysts (allantoic, omphalomesenteric)
- Mucoid degeneration of Wharton's jelly

Other

- Knots
- Varices

RISK FACTORS FOR PRETERM DELIVERY

- Prior preterm delivery
- Multiple gestation (triplets > twins)
- Uterine anomaly, 25%
- DES exposure of mother in utero, 25%
- Incompetent cervix, 25%
- Large fibroid, 20%
- Polyhydramnios, 20%

ABNORMAL LOWER UTERINE SEGMENT

- Prolapse of cord (emergency; put patient in Trendelenburg position and call obstetrician)
- Incompetent cervix
- Placenta previa
- Cerclage
- Low fibroid

THIRD-TRIMESTER BLEEDING

- Placenta previa, 10%
- Abruptio placentae
- Cervical lesions
- Idiopathic (occult abruptio)

MASSES DURING PREGNANCY

Uterus
- Fibroid
- Focal myometrial contractions
- GTD
- Hemorrhage

Adnexal
- Corpus luteum cyst
- Dermoid (fat)
- Theca lutein cysts
- Other ovarian neoplasms

Other
- Pelvic inflammatory disease
- Other organs: appendiceal abscess, diverticulitis

FREQUENTLY MISSED LESIONS

- NTD
- Facial anomalies
- Head anomalies in near field
- Heart defects
- Limb anomalies
- Difficulties with imaging in oligohydramnios

FETAL DEATH

- No fetal heart beat
- Absent fetal movement
- Occasional findings:
  - Overlapping skull bones (Spalding's sign)
  - Gross distortion of fetal anatomy (maceration)
  - Soft tissue edema: skin >5 mm
- Uncommon findings:
  - Thrombus in fetal heart
  - Gas in fetal heart

FETAL HEAD AND SPINE

CYSTIC CNS STRUCTURES

Supratentorial
- Choroid plexus cysts
- Ventriculomegaly, hydrocephalus
- Hydranencephaly
- Porencephaly
- Holoprosencephaly
- Arachnoid cyst
- Teratoma

Posterior fossa
- DW complex
- Arachnoid cyst
- Mega cisterna magna

Midline cysts
- Cavum septum pellucidum
- Dorsal cyst in ACC
- Vein of Galen AVM (check Doppler)

HYDROCEPHALUS

Noncommunicating
- NTD: Chiari II malformation, meningocele, meningomyelocele, encephalocele, spina bifida
- Dandy-Walker complex
- Aqueduct stenosis
- ACC (colpocephaly)

Communicating (rare prenatally)
- Hemorrhage
- Infection

CYSTIC HEAD AND/OR NECK MASSES

- Cystic hygroma
- Encephalocele (bony calvarial defect)
- Hemangioma
- Teratoma (solid elements)
- Branchial cleft cyst (anterolateral) or thyroglossal (midline) duct cyst
- Umbilical cord tangled around neck

CYSTIC BACK MASSES

- NTD
- Cystic teratoma

HYPERECHOIC BRAIN MASS

- Hemorrhage
- Teratoma
- Lipoma of corpus callosum

INCOMPLETE MINERALIZATION OF THE SKULL

- Osteogenesis imperfecta
- Achondrogenesis, type 1 (skull usually partially ossified)
- Hypophosphatasia

SKULL DEFORMITIES

Lemon Sign
- Chiari II, myelomeningocele
- Encephalocele

Cloverleaf Skull
- Craniosynostosis
- Thanatophoric dwarfism
- Other rare skeletal dysplasias

Strawberry Skull
- Trisomy 18

KYPHOSCOLIOSIS

Isolated finding: hemivertebra, butterfly vertebra

Complex anomalies
- VACTERL complex
- Limb/body wall complex
- Any skeletal dysplasia

FETAL CHEST

CYSTIC THORACIC MASSES

- Diaphragmatic hernia (stomach adjacent to heart)
- CCAM, types 1, 2
- Cysts: bronchogenic, enteric duplication, pericardial
- Cystic hygroma

SOLID (ECHOGENIC) MASSES

- Diaphragmatic hernia
- CCAM, type 3
- Pulmonary sequestration
- Tumors
  - Teratoma
  - Rhabdomyoma of the heart

DIFFUSELY ECHOGENIC LUNGS

- Laryngotracheal obstruction
- Bilateral CCAM

PLEURAL EFFUSION

Unilateral usually due to lung masses
- CHD
- Sequestration
- CCAM

Bilateral
- Fetal hydrops (any cause)
- Pulmonary lymphangiectasia (rare)

Unilateral or bilateral
- Idiopathic
- Infection
- Chromosomal anomalies

FETAL ABDOMEN

ABNORMAL STOMACH

Absent Stomach Bubble (Fig. 10-63)

- Oligohydramnios
- Swallowing abnormality (CNS defect)
- Esophageal atresia
- Congenital diaphragmatic hernia
- Situs abnormality
- Risk of chromosomal abnormalities (trisomy 18)

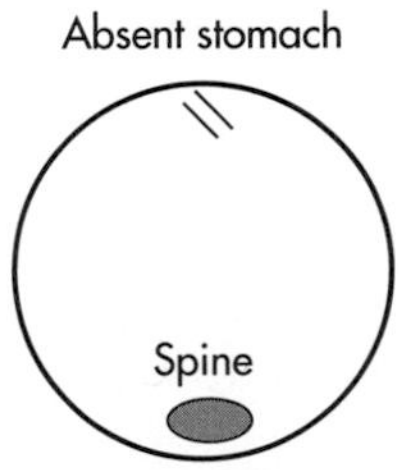

FIGURE 10-63

Double Bubble (Associated with Polyhydramnios) (Fig. 10-64)

Mnemonic: "LADS:"
- **L**add's bands
- **A**nnular pancreas
- **D**uodenal atresia (Down syndrome)
- **S**tenosis of the duodenum

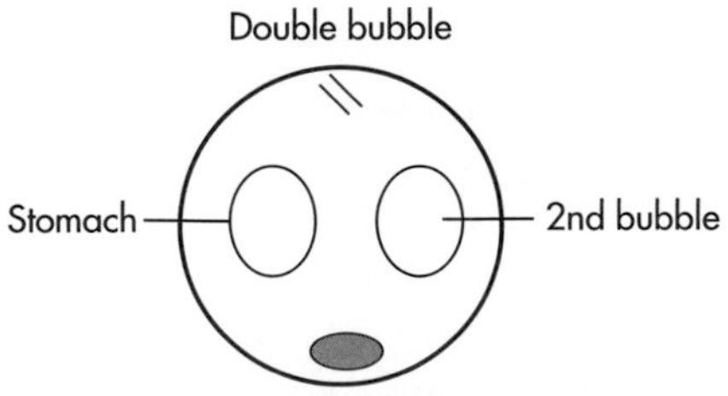

FIGURE 10-64

DILATED BOWEL (Fig. 10-65)

- Atresia
- Stenosis
- Volvulus
- Meconium ileus
- Enteric duplication
- Hirschsprung disease

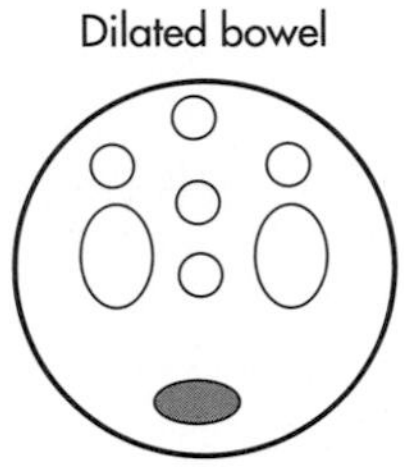

FIGURE 10-65

Pearls

- Proximal obstructions are usually associated with polyhydramnios.
- Distal obstructions are usually associated with normal amniotic fluid volume (colon absorbs fluid).

ECHOGENIC BOWEL CONTENT

Criteria: bowel content as bright as iliac bone.
- Normal variant during 2nd trimester (transient inspissation)
- Cystic fibrosis (most common cause)
- Down syndrome (rare but has been reported)
- IUGR
- CMV infection

ABDOMINAL CALCIFICATION

Bowel related (usually occurs with obstruction)
- Meconium peritonitis (most common cause)
- Meconium ileus
- Atresias
- Volvulus

Related to other organs
- Renal
- Liver: infections (TORCH)
- Neuroblastoma
- Teratoma
- Fetal gallstones (usually resolve without consequences)

HYDRONEPHROSIS

The most common causes are:
- UPJ obstruction
- UVJ obstruction (primary megaureter)
- Duplicated collecting system with obstruction of upper pole
- Bladder outlet obstruction: males
- PUV (thick bladder wall)
- Prune-belly syndrome (normal bladder wall): females and males

- Caudal regression syndrome
- Megacystis microcolon–intestinal hypoperistalsis
- Ureteral agenesis
- Maternal drugs
- Ectopic ureterocele

COMMON RENAL ANOMALIES

- Agenesis
- Ectopic kidney
- Hydronephrosis
- Cystic disease
    - ARPCKD (infantile form): enlarged hyperechoic kidneys
    - Multicystic dysplastic kidney: large, noncommunicating hypoechoic cysts

ECHOGENIC KIDNEYS

- Reflux
- Medical renal disease
- MCDK

CYSTIC ABDOMINAL STRUCTURES

- Hydronephrosis, bladder outlet obstruction
- Fluid-filled dilated bowel
- Ascites
- Meconium pseudocyst
- Fetus in fetus
- Hydrometrocolpos
- Urinoma
- Teratoma
- Cysts
    - Mesenteric cysts
    - Urachal cysts
    - Duplication cysts
    - Ovarian cysts
    - Choledochal cysts

LIVER

Hepatic Calcifications

- Infection: TORCH

Hepatic Cysts

- Simple cyst
- Polycystic disease
- Choledochal cyst, Caroli disease
- Hamartoma

Hepatic Masses

- Teratoma
- Hepatoblastoma
- Hemangioma, hemangioendothelioma
- Hamartoma

SPLENOMEGALY

- Rh immune hydrops
- Premature rupture of membranes
- TORCH infection

ASCITES

- Hydrops (any cause)
- Urine ascites
- Meconium peritonitis
- Infection
- Pseudoascites

ANTERIOR WALL DEFECTS

Midline
- Omphalocele
- Pentalogy of Cantrell

Lateral
- Gastroschisis
- Limb/body wall complex
- Amniotic band syndrome

Infraumbilical
- Bladder or cloacal exstrophy

ANOMALIES IN SACRAL REGION

- Teratoma
- Meningocele (anterior or posterior)
- Caudal regression syndrome (e.g., sacral agenesis, sirenomelia)

FETAL EXTREMITIES

FRACTURES

- Osteogenesis imperfecta
- Hypophosphatasia

POLYDACTYLY

- Familial
- Trisomies 18, 13
- Meckel-Gruber syndrome
- Jeune syndrome
- Short-rib polydactyly syndromes

Suggested Readings

Bianchi DW, Crombleholme TM, D'Alton ME, et al. *Fetology: Diagnosis and Management of the Fetal Patient*. New York: McGraw-Hill Professional; 2010.

Callen PW. *Ultrasonography in Obstetrics and Gynecology*. Philadelphia: WB Saunders; 2007.

Fleischer AC, Manning FA, Jeanty P, et al. *Sonography in Obstetrics and Gynecology: Principles and Practice*. New York: McGraw-Hill Professional; 2001.

Nyberg DA, McGahan JP, Pretorius D, et al. *Diagnostic Ultrasound of Fetal Anomalies: Text and Atlas*. Philadelphia: Lippincott Williams & Wilkins; 2002.

Rumack CM. *Diagnostic Ultrasound*. St. Louis: Mosby; 1998.

Sanders RC. *Structural Abnormalities: The Total Picture*. Philadelphia: Mosby; 2002.

Sauerbrei EE, Nguyen KT, Nolan RL. *A Practical Guide to Ultrasound in Obstetrics and Gynecology*. Philadelphia: Lippincott Williams & Wilkins; 1998.

Woodward PJ, Kennedy A, Sohaey R, et al. *Diagnostic Imaging—Obstetrics*. Salt Lake City: Amirsys; 2005.

CHAPTER 11

Pediatric Imaging

CHAPTER OUTLINE

Respiratory Tract

UPPER AIRWAY

APPROACH

Inspiratory stridor is the most common indication for radiographic upper airway evaluation. The main role of imaging is to identify conditions that need to be treated emergently and/or surgically (e.g., epiglottitis, foreign bodies). Technique:

1. Physician capable of emergency airway intervention should accompany child
2. Obtain 3 films:
   - Lateral neck: full inspiration, neck extended (Fig. 11-1)
   - Anteroposterior (AP) and lateral chest: full inspiration, include upper airway (Fig. 11-2)
3. Fluoroscope the neck if radiographs are suboptimal or equivocal
4. Primary diagnostic considerations:
   - Infection (epiglottitis, croup, abscess)
   - Foreign body (airway or pharyngoesophageal)
   - Masses (lymphadenopathy neoplasms)
   - Congenital abnormalities (webs, malacia)
5. If upper airway is normal, consider:
   - Pulmonary causes (foreign body, bronchiolitis)
   - Mediastinal causes (vascular rings, slings)
   - Congenital heart disease (CHD)

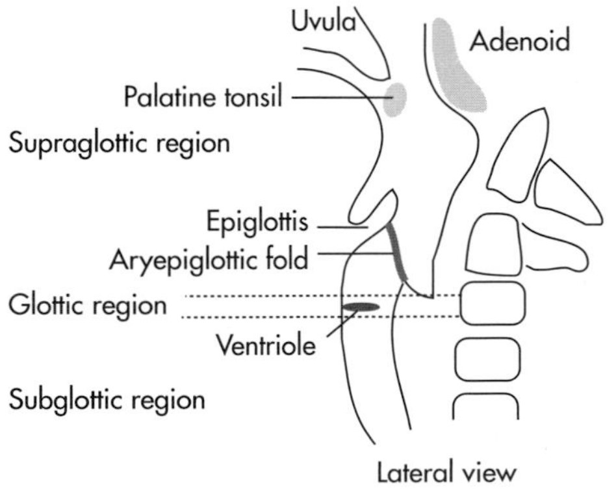

FIGURE 11-1

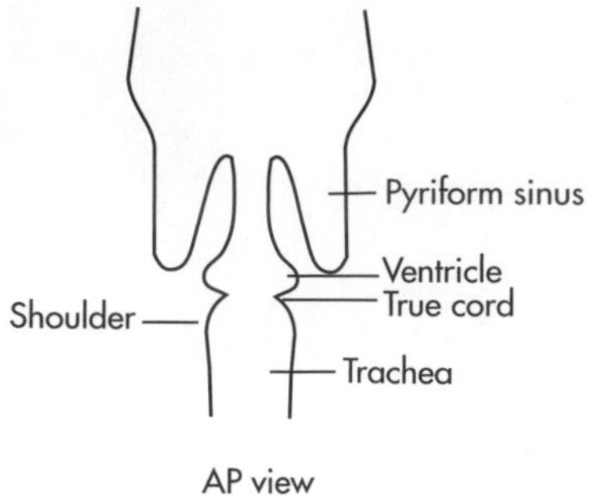

FIGURE 11-2

NORMAL APPEARANCE

- 3 anatomic regions:
  - Supraglottic region
  - Glottic region: ventricle and true cords
  - Subglottic region
- Epiglottis and aryepiglottic folds are thin structures.
- Glottic shoulders are seen on AP view.
- Adenoids are visible at 3 to 6 months after birth.
- Normal retropharyngeal soft tissue thickness (C1-C4) = three-fourths vertebral body width

LARYNGOMALACIA

Common cause of stridor in the 1st year of life. Immature laryngeal cartilage leads to supraglottic collapse during inspiration. Stridor improves with activity and is relieved by prone positioning or neck extension. Self-limited course. Diagnosis is established by fluoroscopy (laryngeal collapse with inspiration).

TRACHEOMALACIA (Fig. 11-3)

Collapse of trachea with expiration. May be focal or diffuse; focal type is usually secondary to congenital anomalies that impress on the trachea, such as a vascular ring.

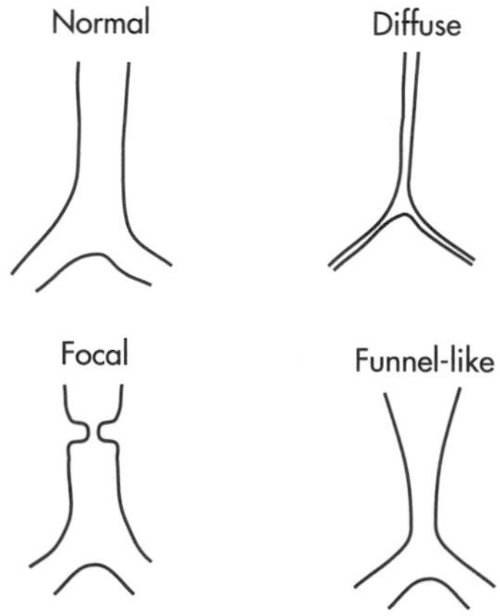

FIGURE 11-3

WEBS

Most common in larynx.

TRACHEAL STENOSIS

- Diffuse hypoplasia, 30%
- Focal ringlike stenosis, 50%
- Funnel-like stenosis, 20%

SUBGLOTTIC STENOSIS

Fixed narrowing at level of cricoid. Failure of laryngeal recanalization in utero.

EPIGLOTTITIS

Life-threatening bacterial infection of the upper airway. Most commonly caused by *Haemophilus influenzae*. Age: 3 to 6 years (older age group than with croup). Treatment is with prophylactic intubation for 24 to 48 hours and antibiotics.

Clinical Findings

- Fever
- Dysphagia
- Drooling
- Sore throat

Radiographic Features (Figs. 11-4 and 11-5)

- Thickened aryepiglottic folds (hallmark)
- Key radiographic view: lateral neck
- Thickened epiglottis
- Subglottic narrowing due to edema, 25%: indistinguishable from croup on AP view
- Distention of hypopharynx

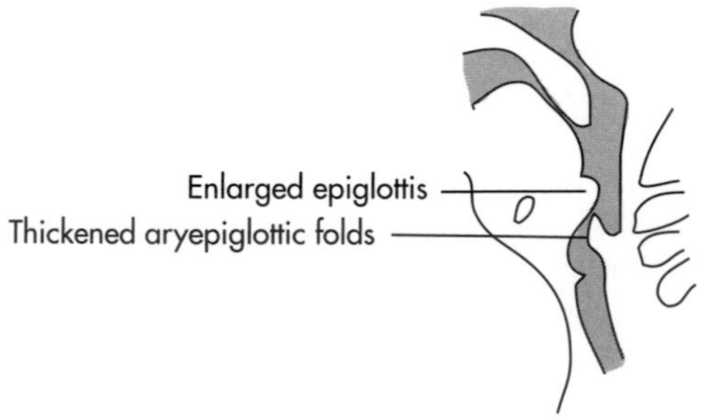

FIGURE 11-4

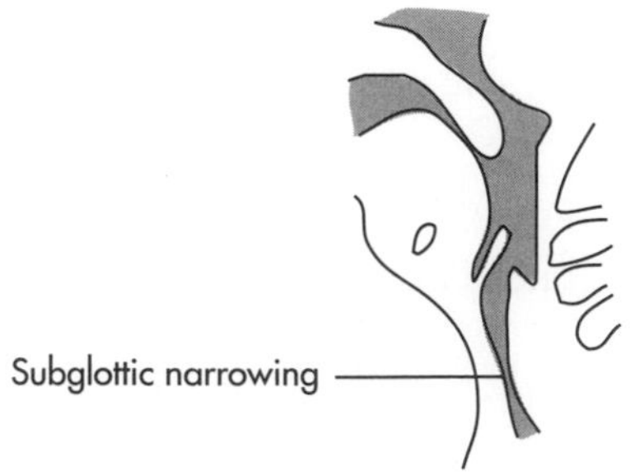

FIGURE 11-5

Pearls

Other causes of enlarged epiglottis or aryepiglottic folds:

- Caustic ingestion
- Hereditary angioneurotic edema
- Omega-shaped epiglottis (normal variant with normal aryepiglottic folds)
- Stevens-Johnson syndrome

CROUP

Subglottic laryngotracheobronchitis. Most commonly caused by parainfluenza virus. Age: 6 months to 3 years (younger age group than epiglottitis).

Clinical Findings

- Barking cough
- Upper respiratory tract infection
- Self-limited

Radiographic Features (Fig. 11-6)

- Subglottic narrowing (inverted "V" or "steeple sign")
- Key view: AP view
- Lateral view should be obtained to exclude epiglottitis.
- Steeple sign: loss of subglottic shoulders

Pearls

- Membranous croup: uncommon infection of bacterial origin *(Staphylococcus aureus)*. Purulent membranes in subglottic trachea.
- Epiglottitis may mimic croup on AP view.

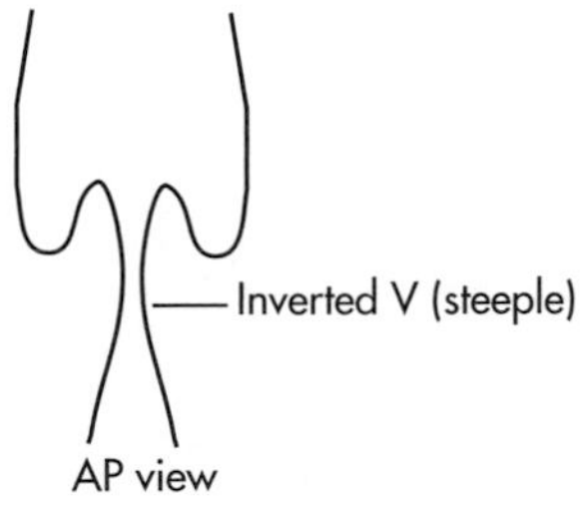

FIGURE 11-6

RETROPHARYNGEAL ABSCESS

Typically due to extension of a suppurative bacterial lymphadenitis, most commonly *S. aureus*, group B streptococci, oral flora. Age: <1 year. Other causes include foreign body perforation and trauma.

Clinical Findings

- Fever
- Stiff neck
- Dysphagia
- Stridor (uncommon)
- Most cases present as cellulitis rather than true abscess.

Radiographic Features

- Widened retropharyngeal space (most common finding)
- Air in soft tissues is specific for abscess.
- Straightened cervical lordosis
- Computed tomography (CT) is helpful to define superior and inferior mediastinal extent.
- Plain film findings are usually nonspecific.
- Main differential diagnosis:
  - Retropharyngeal hematoma
  - Neoplasm (i.e., rhabdomyosarcoma)
  - Lymphadenopathy

TONSILLAR HYPERTROPHY

The tonsils consist of lymphoid tissue that encircles the pharynx. Three groups: pharyngeal tonsil (adenoids), palatine tonsil, and lingual tonsil. Tonsils enlarge secondary to infection and may obstruct nasopharynx and/or eustachian tubes. Rarely, bacterial pharyngitis can lead to a tonsillar abscess (quinsy abscess), which requires drainage. Specific causes include:

- Mononucleosis (Epstein-Barr virus)
- Coxsackievirus (herpangina, hand-foot-mouth disease)
- Adenovirus (pharyngoconjunctival fever)
- Measles prodrome (rubeola)
- β-Hemolytic *Streptococcus* (quinsy abscess)

Radiographic Features (Fig. 11-7)

- Mass in posterior nasopharynx (enlarged adenoids)
- Mass near end of uvula (palatine tonsils)
- CT is useful to determine the presence of a tonsillar abscess.

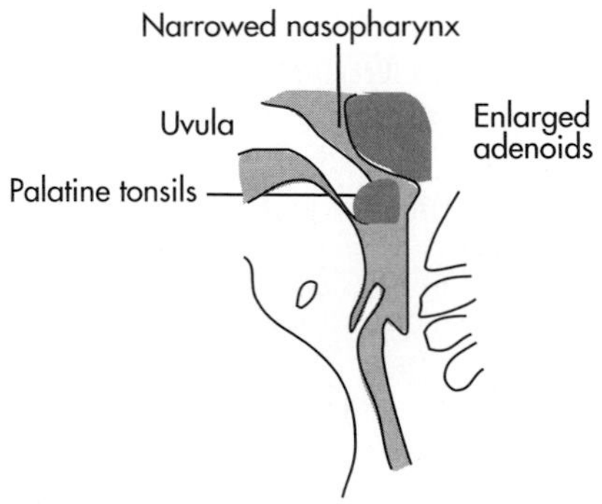

FIGURE 11-7

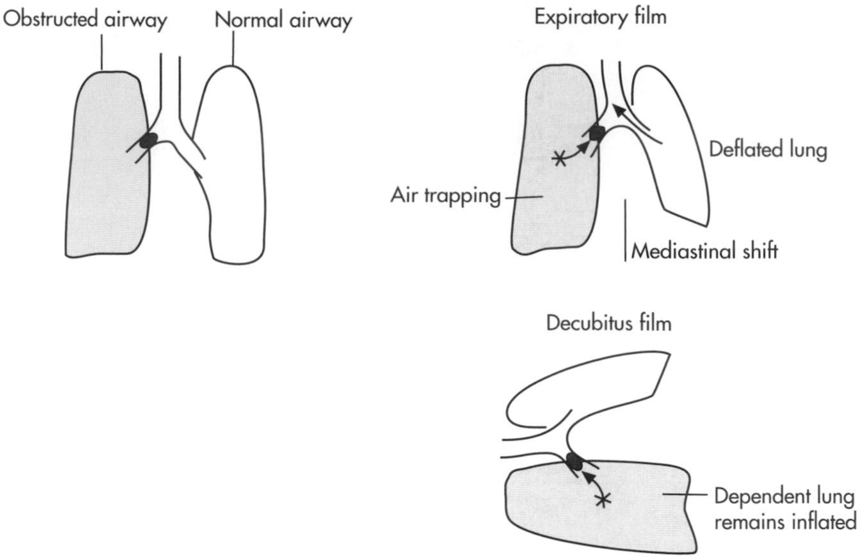

FIGURE 11-8

AIRWAY FOREIGN BODY

Common cause of respiratory distress. Age: 6 months to 4 years. Acute aspiration results in cough, stridor, wheezing; chronic foreign body causes hemoptysis or recurrent pneumonia. Location: right bronchi > left bronchi > larynx, trachea.

Radiographic Features (Fig. 11-8)

Bronchial foreign body

- Unilateral air tapping causing hyperlucent lung, 90%
- Expiratory film or lateral decubitus makes air trapping more apparent.
- Atelectasis is uncommon, 10%
- Only 10% of foreign bodies are radiopaque.
- Chest fluoroscopy or CT should be performed if plain film findings are equivocal.

Tracheal foreign body

- Foreign body usually lodges in sagittal plane
- CXR is usually normal.

CONGENITAL PULMONARY ABNORMALITIES

BRONCHOPULMONARY FOREGUT MALFORMATION

Arise from a supernumerary lung bud that develops below the normal lung bud. Location and communication with GI tract depend on when in embryonic life the bud develops. Most malformations present clinically when they become infected (communication with GI tract).

OVERVIEW OF BRONCHOPULMONARY MALFORMATIONS

Malformation	Location
Sequestration	
Intralobar	60% basilar, left
Sequestration	80% left or below diaphragm
Bronchogenic cyst	Mediastinum, 85%; lung, 15%
CCAM	All lobes
Congenital lobar emphysema	LUL, 40%; RML, 35%; RUL, 20%

CCAM, congenital cystic adenoid malformation of the lung; LUL, left upper lobe; RML, right middle lobe; RUL, right upper lobe.

PULMONARY SEQUESTRATION

Clinical Findings

- Recurrent infection
- Lung abscess
- Bronchiectasis
- Hemoptysis during childhood

Pathology

- Nonfunctioning pulmonary tissue (nearly always posteromedial segments of lower lobes)
- Systemic arterial supply: anomalous arteries from the aorta (less common branch of the celiac artery)
- No connection to bronchial tree

TYPES OF PULMONARY SEQUESTRATION*

Feature	Intralobar Sequestration	Extralobar Sequestration
Age	Older children, adults	Neonates
Pleura	Inside lung (intralobar)	Outside lung (extralobar, own pleura)
Forms	Airless (consolidation) and air-containing, cystic type	Always airless (pleural envelope) unless communication with GI tract
Venous return	Pulmonary vein	Systemic: IVC, azygos, portal
Arterial supply	Thoracic aorta > abdominal aorta	Thoracic aorta > abdominal aorta
Associations	In 10% of patients: Skeletal anomalies, 5% Foregut anomalies, 5% Diaphragmatic anomalies Other rare associations	In 65% of patients: Diaphragmatic defect, 20% Pulmonary hypoplasia, 25% Bronchogenic cysts Cardiac anomalies

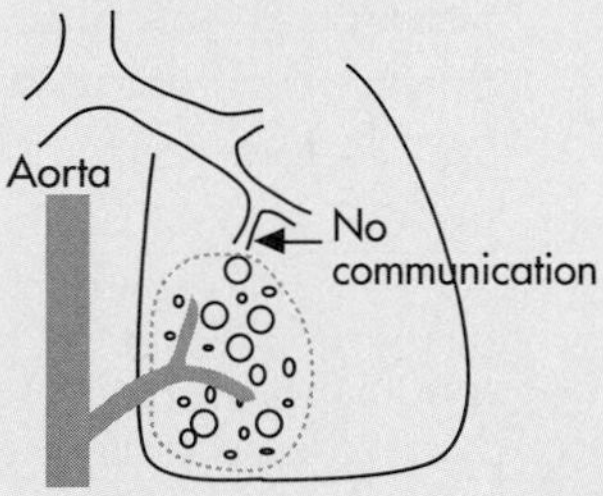

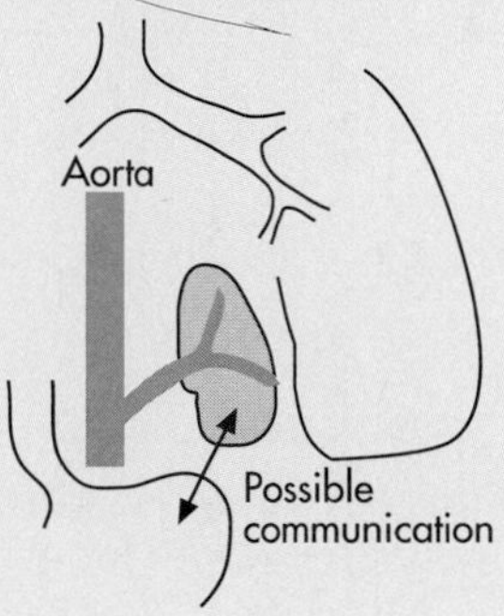

*Location of all sequestrations: posterobasal, L > R.
IVC, inferior vena cava.

Radiographic Features

- Large (>5 cm) mass near diaphragm
- Air-fluid levels if infected
- Surrounding pulmonary consolidation
- Sequestration may communicate with GI tract.

BRONCHOGENIC CYST

Result from abnormal budding of the tracheobronchial tree. Cysts contain respiratory epithelium. Location:

- Mediastinum, 85% (posterior > middle > anterior mediastinum)
- Lung, 15%

Radiographic Features (Fig. 11-9)

- Well-defined round mass in subcarinal/parahilar region
- Pulmonary cysts commonly located in medial third of lung
- Initially no communication with tracheobronchial tree
- Cysts are thin walled.
- Cysts can be fluid or air filled.

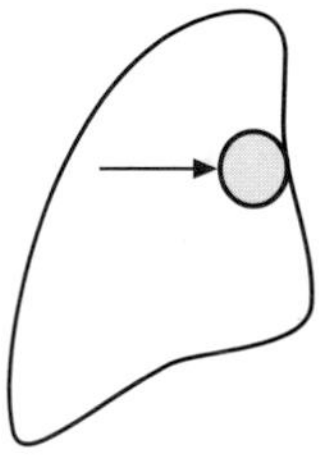

FIGURE 11-9

CONGENITAL CYSTIC ADENOID MALFORMATION (CCAM)

CCAM refers to a proliferation of polypoid glandular lung tissue without normal alveolar differentiation. Respiratory distress occurs during first days of life. Treatment is with surgical resection (sarcomatous degeneration has been described).

Types

- Macrocystic (Stocker types 1 and 2): single cyst or multiple cysts >5 mm confined to one hemithorax; better prognosis; common

- Microcystic (Stocker type 3): homogeneous echogenic mass without discernible individual cysts; closely resembles pulmonary sequestration or intrathoracic bowel from a diaphragmatic hernia; less common

Radiographic Features (Fig. 11-10)

- Multiple cystic pulmonary lesions of variable size
- Air-fluid levels in cysts
- Variable thickness of cyst wall

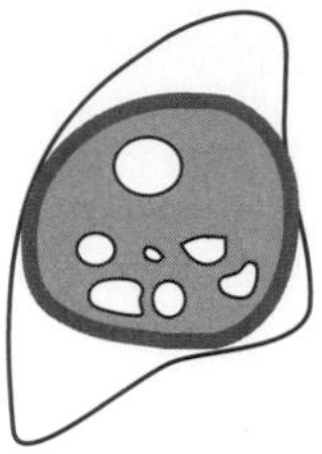

FIGURE 11-10

CONGENITAL LOBAR EMPHYSEMA

Progressive overdistention of one or more pulmonary lobes but usually not the entire lung. 10% of patients have congenital heart disease (patent ductus arteriosus [PDA] and ventricular septal defect [VSD]).

Causes

Idiopathic, 50%
Obstruction of airway with valve mechanism, 50%

- Bronchial cartilage deficiency or immaturity
- Mucus
- Web, stenosis
- Extrinsic compression

Radiographic Features (Fig. 11-11)

- Hyperlucent lobe (hallmark)
- First few days of life: alveolar opacification because there is no clearance of lung fluid through bronchi
- May be asymptomatic in neonate but becomes symptomatic later in life
- Use CT to differentiate from bronchial obstruction

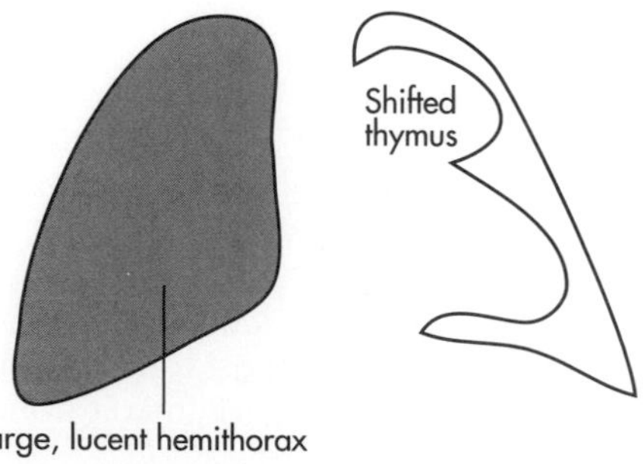

FIGURE 11-11

- Distribution
  LUL, 40%
  RML, 35%
  RUL, 20%
  2 lobes affected, 5%

PULMONARY HYPOPLASIA

Types of Pulmonary Underdevelopment

- Agenesis: complete absence of one or both lungs (airways, alveoli, and vessels)
- Aplasia: absence of lung except for a rudimentary bronchus that ends in a blind pouch
- Hypoplasia: decrease in number and size of airways and alveoli; hypoplastic PA

Scimitar Syndrome (Hypogenetic Lung Syndrome, Pulmonary Venolobar Syndrome)

Special form of hypoplastic lung in which the hypoplastic lung is perfused from the aorta and drained by the IVC or portal vein. The anomalous vein has a resemblance to a Turkish scimitar (sword). Associations include:

- Accessory diaphragm, diaphragmatic hernia
- Bony abnormalities: hemivertebrae, rib notching, rib hypoplasia
- CHD: atrial septal defect (ASD), VSD, PDA, tetralogy of Fallot

Radiographic Features (Fig. 11-12)

- Small lung (most commonly the right lung)
- Retrosternal soft tissue density (hypoplastic collapsed lung)
- Anomalous vein resembles a scimitar
- Systemic arterial supply from aorta
- Dextroposition of the heart (shift because of hypoplastic lung)

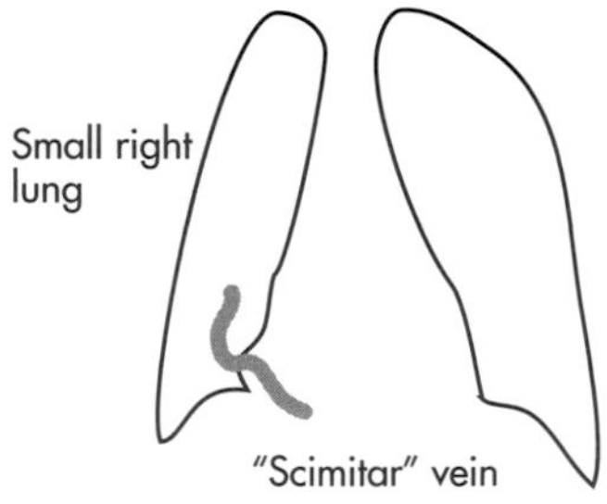

FIGURE 11-12

CONGENITAL DIAPHRAGMATIC HERNIA (CDH)

Incidence

1 in 2000 to 3000 births. Mortality rate of isolated hernias is 60% (with postnatal surgery) and higher when other abnormalities are present. Respiratory distress occurs in neonatal period. Associated abnormalities include:

- Pulmonary hypoplasia (common)

- CNS abnormalities
  - Neural tube defects: spina bifida, encephalocele
  - Anencephaly

Types

Bochdalek's hernias (90% of CDH): posterior
- 75% are on the left, 25% on right
- Right-sided hernias are more difficult to detect because of similar echogenicity of liver and lung.
- Contents of hernia: stomach, 60%; colon, 55%; small intestine, 90%; spleen, 45%; liver, 50%; pancreas, 25%; kidney, 20%
- Malrotation of herniated bowel is very common.

Morgagni hernias (10% of CDH): anterior
- Most occur on right (heart prevents development on the left).
- Most common hernia contents: omentum, colon
- Accompanying anomalies common

Eventration
- Due to relative absence of muscle in dome of diaphragm
- Associated with:
  - Trisomies 13, 18, congenital CMV, rubella arthrogryposis multiplex, pulmonary hypoplasia

Radiographic Features (Fig. 11-13)
- Hemidiaphragm not visualized
- Multicystic mass in chest
- Mass effect

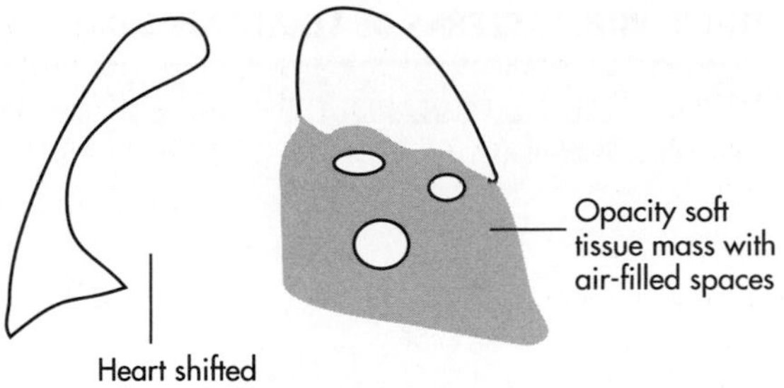

FIGURE 11-13

KARTAGENER SYNDROME

Kartagener syndrome (immotile cilia syndrome) is due to the deficiency of the dynein arms of cilia causing immotility of respiratory, auditory, and sperm cilia.

Radiographic Features
- Complete thoracic and abdominal situs inversus
- Bronchiectasis
- Sinus hypoplasia and mucosal thickening

PNEUMONIA

Childhood pneumonias are commonly caused by:
- *Mycoplasma,* 30% (lower in age group <3 years)
- Viral, 65% (higher in age group <3 years)
- Bacterial, 5%

VIRAL PNEUMONIA

Causes: respiratory syncytial virus (RSV), parainfluenza

RADIOGRAPHIC PATTERNS OF VIRAL PNEUMONIA

Pattern		Frequency	Description
Bronchiolitis	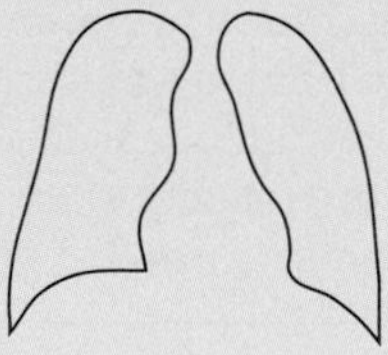	Common	Normal CXR Overaeration is only diagnostic clue Commonly due to RSV
Bronchiolitis+parahilar, peribronchial opacities	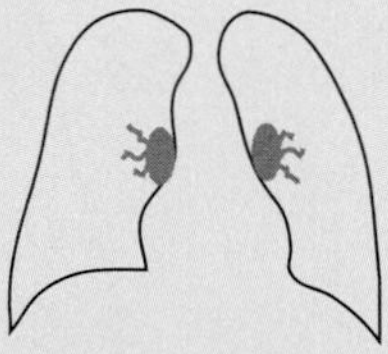	Most common	Dirty parahilar regions caused by: Peribronchial cuffing (inflammation) Hilar adenopathy
Bronchiolitis+atelectasis	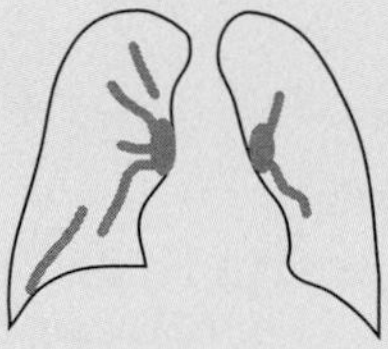	Common	Disordered pattern with: Atelectasis Areas of hyperaeration Parahilar+peribronchial opacities

Continued

RADIOGRAPHIC PATTERNS OF VIRAL PNEUMONIA—cont'd

Pattern		Frequency	Description
Reticulonodular interstitial	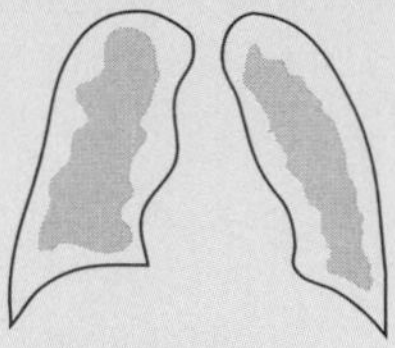	Rare	Interstitial pattern
Hazy lungs	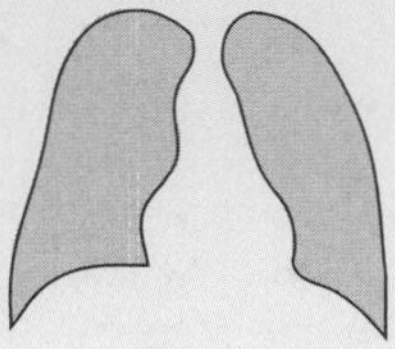	Rare	Diffuse increase in density

Pearls

- All types of bronchiolitis and bronchitis cause air trapping (overaeration) with flattening of hemidiaphragms.
- RSV, *Mycoplasma,* and parainfluenza virus are the most common agents that cause radiographic abnormalities (in 10%-30% of infected children).
- Any virus may result in any of the 5 different radiographic patterns.

BACTERIAL PNEUMONIA

The following 3 pathogens are the most common:

- Pneumococcus (ages 1 to 3)
- *Staphylococcus aureus* (infancy)
- *Haemophilus influenzae* (late infancy)

Radiographic Features

Consolidation
- Alveolar exudate
- Segmental consolidation
- Lobar consolidation

Other findings
- Effusions
- Pneumatocele

Complications
- Pneumothorax
- Bronchiectasis (reversible)
- Swyer-James syndrome (acquired pulmonary hypoplasia), radiographically characterized by small, hyperlucent lungs with diminished vessels (focal emphysema)
- Bronchiolitis obliterans

Round Pneumonia

- Usually age <8 years
- Pneumococcal pneumonia in early consolidative phase
- Pneumonia appears round because of poorly developed collateral pathways (pores of Kohn and channels of Lambert).
- With time the initially round pneumonia develops into a more typical consolidation.

Recurrent Infections

- Cystic fibrosis
- Recurrent aspirations
- Rare causes of recurrent infection:
  - Hypogammaglobulinemia (Bruton disease; differential diagnosis clue: no adenoids or hilar lymph nodes)
  - Hyperimmunoglobulinemia E (Buckley syndrome)
  - Immotile cilia syndrome (Kartagener syndrome)
  - Other immunodeficiencies
  - Bronchopulmonary foregut malformation

ASPIRATION PNEUMONIA (Fig. 11-14)

Aspiration pneumonia results from inhalation of swallowed materials or gastric content. Gastric acid damages capillaries causing acute pulmonary edema. Secondary infection or acute respiratory distress syndrome (ARDS) may ensue.

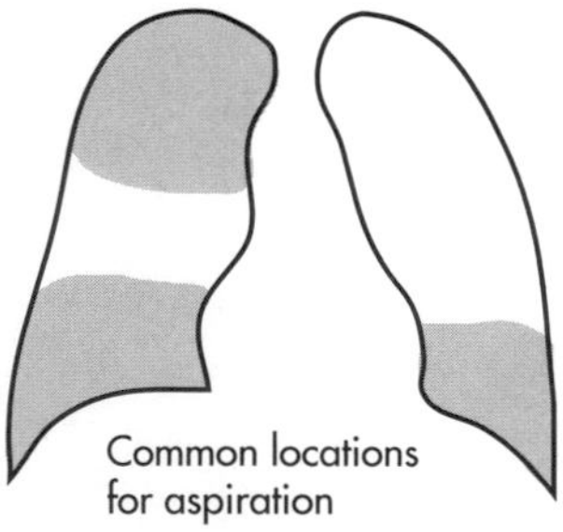

FIGURE 11-14

Causes

Aspiration due to swallowing dysfunction (most common cause)
- Anoxic birth injury (common)
- Coma, anesthesia

Aspiration due to obstruction
- Esophageal atresia or stenosis
- Esophageal obstruction
- Gastroesophageal reflux, hiatal hernia
- Gastric or duodenal obstruction

Fistula
- Tracheoesophageal fistula

Radiographic Features
- Recurrent pneumonias; distribution: aspiration in supine position: upper lobes, superior segments of lower lobes; aspiration in upright position: both lower lobes
- Segmental and subsegmental atelectasis
- Interstitial fibrosis
- Inflammatory thickening of bronchial walls

SICKLE CELL ANEMIA

Pulmonary manifestations (pneumonia, acute chest syndrome, and pulmonary fibrosis) are the leading cause of death. Children with acute chest syndrome may present with one or multiple foci of consolidation, fever, chest pain, or cough. Causes: infection (higher incidence), fat emboli originating from infracting bone, pulmonary thrombosis.

Radiographic Findings
- Consolidation
- Pleural effusion
- Fine reticular opacities (pulmonary fibrosis)
- Large heart in severe anemia
- H-shaped vertebral bodies
- Osteonecrosis, bone infarct in visualized humeri

NEONATAL RESPIRATORY DISTRESS

Respiratory distress in the newborn is usually due to one of 4 disease entities:
- Respiratory distress syndrome (RDS; hyaline membrane disease)
- Transient tachypnea of the newborn (TTN)
- Meconium aspiration
- Neonatal pneumonia

The most common complications of RDS are:
- Pulmonary interstitial emphysema (PIE)
- Persistent PDA
- Bronchopulmonary dysplasia (BPD)

RESPIRATORY DISTRESS SYNDROME (RDS)/ HYALINE MEMBRANE DISEASE (Fig. 11-15)

Evolving Terminology
- The term *hyaline membrane disease* is now less commonly used in clinical practice to describe pulmonary surfactant insufficiency in infants. Hyaline membranes are considered a byproduct, not the cause, of respiratory failure in neonates with immature lungs.
- The term *respiratory distress syndrome* is currently used to denote surfactant deficiency and should not be used for other causes of respiratory distress.
- In recognition of the underlying pathogenesis of the disease process, the alternative term *surfactant deficiency disorder* has been proposed.

RDS is caused by surfactant deficiency. Surfactant diminishes surface tension of expanding alveoli. As a result, acinar atelectasis and interstitial edema occur. Hyaline membranes are formed by proteinaceous exudate. Symptoms occur within 2 hours of life. The incidence of RDS depends on the gestational age at birth.

INCIDENCE OF RESPIRATORY DISTRESS SYNDROME

Birth at Gestational Age (wk)	Incidence (%)
27	50
31	16
34	5
36	1

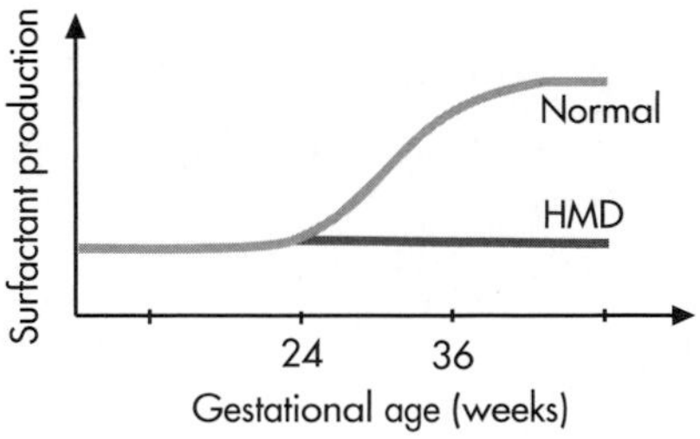

FIGURE 11-15

NEONATAL RESPIRATORY DISTRESS

Disease	Lung Volume	Opacities	Time Course	Complication
RDS	Low	Granular	4-6 days	PIE, BPD, PDA
Transient tachypnea	High or normal	Linear, streaky*	<48 hours	None
Meconium aspiration	Hyperinflation	Coarse, patchy	At birth	PFC, ECMO
Neonatal pneumonia	Anything	Granular	Variable	

*Ground-glass opacity at birth.

BPD, bronchopulmonary dysplasia; ECMO, extracorporeal membrane oxygenation; PDA, patent ductus arteriosus; PFC, persistent fetal circulation; PIE, pulmonary interstitial emphysema; RDS, respiratory distress syndrome.

Radiographic Features (Fig. 11-16)

- Any opacity in a premature infant should be regarded as RDS until proven otherwise.
- Lungs are opaque (ground-glass) or reticulogranular (hallmark).
- Hypoaeration (atelectasis) leads to low lung volumes: bell-shaped thorax (if not intubated).
- Bronchograms are often present.
- Absence of consolidation or pleural effusions
- In contrast to other causes of RDS in neonates, pleural effusions are uncommon.
- Treatment with surfactant may result in asymmetric improvement
- CXR signs of premature infants:
  - No subcutaneous fat
  - No humeral ossification center
  - Endotracheal tube present

In most cases of RDS, the diagnosis is made clinically but may initially be made radiographically. The role of the radiologist is to assess serial chest films. Treatment complication of RDS:

- Persistent PDA (signs of congestive heart failure [CHF]); the ductus usually closes within 1 to 2 days after birth in response to the high PO_2 content.
- Air-trapping: PIE and acquired lobar emphysema
- Diffuse opacities (whiteout) may be due to a variety of causes:
  - Atelectasis
  - Progression of RDS
  - Aspiration
  - Pulmonary hemorrhage
  - CHF
  - Superimposed pneumonia

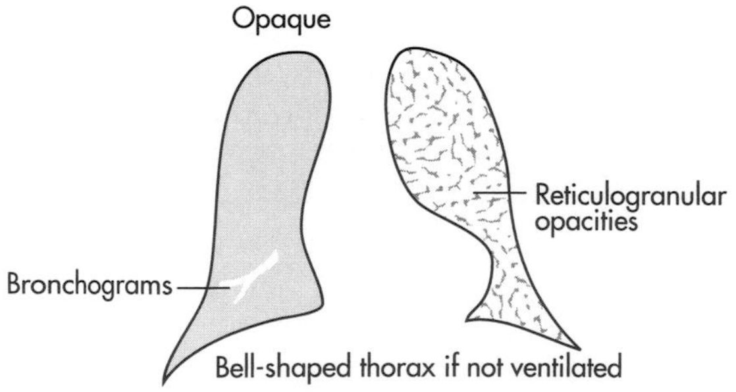

FIGURE 11-16

PULMONARY INTERSTITIAL EMPHYSEMA (PIE)

PIE refers to accumulation of interstitial air in peribronchial and perivascular spaces. Most common cause: positive-pressure ventilation. Complications:

- Pneumothorax
- Pneumomediastinum
- Pneumopericardium

Radiographic Features

- Tortuous linear lucencies radiate outward from the hilar regions.
- The lucencies extend all the way to the periphery of the lung.
- Lucencies do not change with respiration.

BRONCHOPULMONARY DYSPLASIA (BPD)

Caused by oxygen toxicity and barotrauma of respiratory therapy. BPD is now uncommon in larger and more mature infants (gestational age >30 weeks or weighing >1200 g at birth).

DEFINITION OF BPD AND DIAGNOSTIC CRITERIA

Diagnostic Criterion	Gestational Age Less than 32 wk	Gestational Age Greater than 32 wk
Time point of assessment	36 wk PMA* or discharge to home, whichever comes first; treatment with >21% oxygen for at least 28 days plus	>28 days but <56 days postnatal age or discharge to home, whichever comes first; treatment with >21% oxygen for at least 28 days plus
Mild BPD	Breathing room air at 36 wk PMA or discharge, whichever comes first	Breathing room air by 56 days postnatal age or discharge, whichever comes first
Moderate BPD	Need* for <30% oxygen at 36 wk PMA or discharge, whichever comes first	Need* for <30% oxygen at 56 days postnatal age or discharge, whichever comes first
Severe BPD	Need* for ≥30% oxygen and/or positive pressure (PPV* or nasal CPAP) at 36 wk PMA or discharge, whichever comes first	Need* for ≥30% oxygen and/or positive pressure (PPV or nasal CPAP) at 56 days postnatal age or discharge, whichever comes first

*Using a physiologic test (pulse oximetry saturation range) to confirm the oxygen requirement.
BPD, bronchopulmonary dysplasia; CPAP, continuous positive airway pressure; PMA, postmenstrual age (gestational age at birth plus chronologic age); PPV, positive-pressure ventilation.

There are 4 stages in the development; the progression of BPD through all 4 stages is now rarely seen because of the awareness of this disease entity.

STAGES OF BRONCHOPULMONARY DYSPLASIA

Stage	Time	Pathology	Imaging
1	<4 days	Mucosal necrosis	Similar to RDS
2	1 week	Necrosis, edema, exudate	Diffuse opacities
3	2 weeks	Bronchial metaplasia	Bubbly lungs*
4	1 month	Fibrosis	Bubbly lungs*

*Bubbly lungs (honeycombing): rounded lucencies surrounded by linear densities; hyperaeration.

Prognosis of Stage 4

- Mortality, 40%
- Minor handicaps, 30%
- Abnormal pulmonary function tests in almost all in later life
- Clinically normal by 3 years, 30%

MECONIUM ASPIRATION SYNDROME

Meconium (mucus, epithelial cells, bile, debris) is the first stool that is evacuated within 12 hours after delivery. In fetal distress, evacuation may occur into the amniotic fluid (up to 10% of deliveries). However, in only 1% does this aspiration cause respiratory symptoms. Only meconium aspirated to below the vocal cords is clinically significant. Meconium aspiration sometimes clears in 3 to 5 days. CXR nearly always returns to normal by 1 year of age.

Radiographic Features

- Patchy, bilateral opacities, may be "rope-like"
- Atelectasis
- Hyperinflated lungs
- Pneumothorax, pneumomediastinum, 25%

Complication

- Mortality (25%) from persistent fetal circulation

NEONATAL PNEUMONIA (NP)

Pathogenesis

Transplacental infection
- TORCH
- Pulmonary manifestation of TORCH is usually less severe than other manifestations.

Perineal flora (group B streptococci, enterococci, *Escherichia coli*)
- Ascending infection
- Premature rupture of membranes
- Infection while passing through birth canal

Radiographic Features

- Patchy asymmetrical opacities in a term infant represent neonatal pneumonia until proven otherwise.
- Hyperinflation

TRANSIENT TACHYPNEA OF THE NEWBORN (TTN)

TTN (wet lung syndrome) is a clinical diagnosis. It is caused by a delayed resorption of intrauterine pulmonary liquids. Normally, pulmonary fluids are cleared by:
- Bronchial squeezing during delivery, 30%
- Absorption, 30%: lymphatics, capillaries
- Suction, 30%

Causes

- Cesarean section, premature delivery, maternal sedation (no thoracic squeezing)
- Hypoproteinemia, hypervolemia, erythrocythemia

Radiographic Features

- Fluid overload (similar appearance as noncardiogenic pulmonary edema)
  - Prominent vascular markings
  - Pleural effusion
  - Fluid in fissure
  - Alveolar edema
- Lungs clear in 24 to 48 hours.

EXTRACORPOREAL MEMBRANE OXYGENATION (ECMO)

Technique of providing prolonged extracorporeal gas exchange. Indications: any severe respiratory failure with predicted mortality rates of >80%. Exclusion criteria for ECMO include:
- <34 weeks of age
- >10 days of age
- Serious intracranial hemorrhage
- Patients who require epinephrine

Complications

- Late neurologic sequelae; developmental delay, 50%
- Intracranial hemorrhage, 10%
- Pneumothorax, pneumomediastinum
- Pulmonary hemorrhage (common)
- Pleural effusions (common)
- Catheter complications

MEDIASTINUM

THYMUS

The ratio of thymus to body weight decreases with age. Thymus is routinely identified on CXR from birth to 2 years of age. Size and shape of the thymus are highly variable from person to person.

COMMON MEDIASTINAL TUMORS

Anterior
- Thymic hyperplasia and thymic variations in shape and size (most common)
- Teratoma
- T-cell lymphoma
- Cystic hygroma
- Thymomas are extremely rare.

Middle
- Adenopathy (leukemia, lymphoma, TB)
- Bronchopulmonary foregut malformation

Posterior
- Neuroblastoma
- Ganglioneuroma
- Neurofibromatosis
- Neurenteric cysts
- Meningoceles

Pearls
- Any pediatric anterior mediastinal mass is considered thymus until proven otherwise.
- Posterior mediastinal masses are the most common abnormal chest masses in infants.

Gastrointestinal Tract

GENERAL

EMBRYOLOGY

The GI tract develops from three embryologic precursors, each of which has a separate vascular supply: foregut, midgut, hindgut.

EMBRYONIC PRECURSORS OF GI TRACT

Origin	Vascular Supply	Derivatives
Foregut	Celiac artery	Pharynx, lower respiratory tract, esophagus, stomach, liver, pancreas, biliary tree, duodenum
Midgut	SMA	Distal duodenum, small bowel, ascending colon
Hindgut	IMA	Transverse colon, rectum, bladder, urethra

IMA, inferior mesenteric artery; SMA, superior mesenteric artery.

Bowel is formed in 3 steps (Fig. 11-17):
- Rotation
- Fixation
- Canalization

Rotation
- Duodenojejunal loop (first 270° loop) brings stomach into horizontal axis and puts liver into right and spleen into left abdomen. The common bile duct (CBD) is associated with the ventral pancreas and becomes located dorsally because of the rotation. Before the rotation, the 1st loop rotation results in the duodenojejunal junction being located to the left.
- Cecocolic loop (second 270° loop). The small bowel develops from the dorsal mesentery and then rotates 270° so that the cecum lies near the right upper quadrant (RUQ). It later descends to the right lower quadrant (RLQ).

Fixation

Fixation is incomplete at birth. Abnormal fixation of the colonic mesentery to the posterior abdominal wall results in potential spaces into which the bowel may herniate (paraduodenal hernias). Abnormalities of fixation include:
- Increased mobility (cecal bascule)
- Internal hernia (paraduodenal, paracecal)

Canalization

After forming a primitive tube, the bowel lumen solidifies and then recanalizes to form the viable lumen. Anomalies in this step may result in atresia or duplication.
- Atresia
  - Duodenal atresia results from failure of recanalization of the foregut (10 weeks) and is frequently associated with other abnormalities (malrotation, 50%; Down syndrome, 30%; esophageal atresia).
  - Jejunoileal atresia results from an ischemic insult, not a failure of recanalization; occurs later and is usually an isolated phenomenon.
- Duplication
  - Abnormal recanalization: small intramural duplication cysts may develop.
  - Notochordal adhcsion: a portion of bowel remains adherent to the notochord and a diverticulum may develop.

UMBILICAL ARTERY (UA) LINE (Fig. 11-18)

Traverses the UA, the internal iliac artery, and the infrarenal aorta. The tip of the line should be located above the renal arteries between levels T8 and T12. An alternative location of the catheter tip is below the renal arteries between levels L3 and L4.

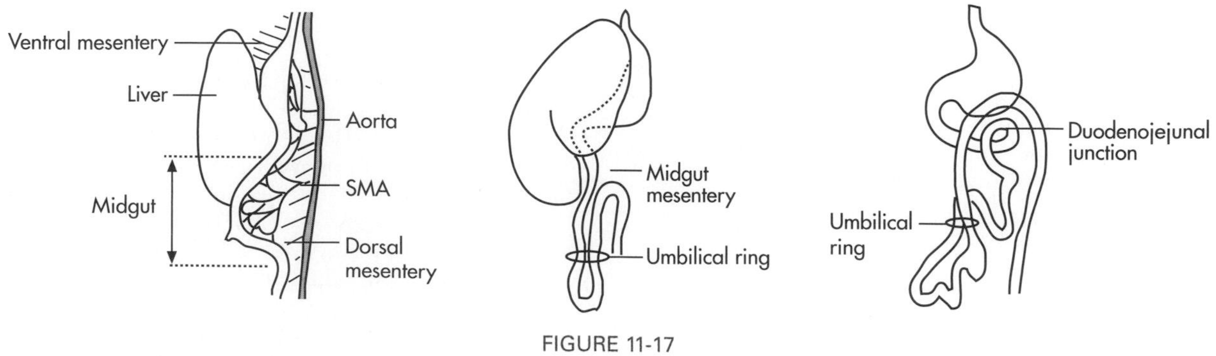

FIGURE 11-17

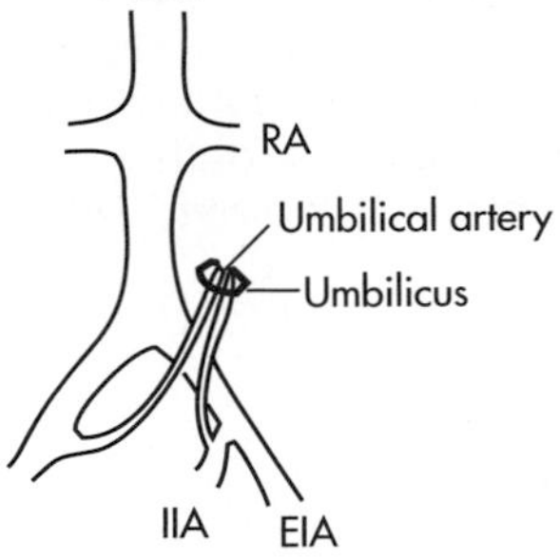

FIGURE 11-18

UMBILICAL VEIN (UV) LINE (Fig. 11-19)

The UV line should traverse the UV, portal sinus (junction of left and right portal vein), ductus venosus (which closes at 96 hours of life), and IVC and end in the right atrium. The line can easily be misplaced in a portal or hepatic branch (the tip then projects over the liver).

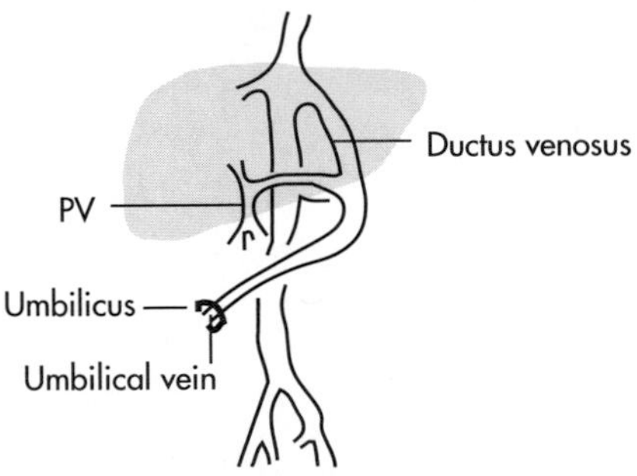

FIGURE 11-19

ESOPHAGUS

ESOPHAGEAL ATRESIA (EA) AND TRACHEOESOPHAGEAL FISTULA (TEF)

Spectrum of anomalies involving esophagus and trachea. There are two clinical presentations:

- Early presentation in EA with a pouch (N-type, 85%): vomiting, choking, difficulty with secretions
- Late presentation of recurrent pneumonias if there is a fistula between esophagus and trachea (H-type, 5%)

Types (Fig. 11-20)

- TEF, N-type fistula, 85%
- Pure EA without fistula, 10%
- TEF, H-type fistula (no atresia), 1%
- Other forms

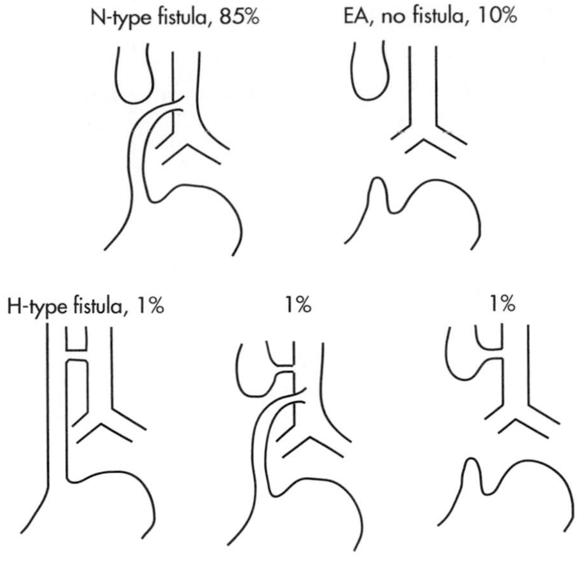

FIGURE 11-20

Associations

Mnemonic:
"VACTERL:"

- **V**ertebral anomalies
- **A**norectal anomalies
- **C**ardiovascular anomalies
- **T**racheal anomalies
- **E**sophageal fistula
- **R**enal anomalies: renal agenesis
- **L**imb anomalies: radial ray cardiac anomalies
- VSD
- Ductus arteriosus
- Right aortic arch
- EA is associated with other atresias and/or stenosis
- Duodenal atresia
- Imperforate anus

Radiographic Features

Plain film findings

- Gas-filled dilated proximal esophageal segment (pouch)
- Gasless abdomen (EA-type)
- Excessive air in stomach (H-type)
- Aspiration pneumonia

Procedures

- Pass 8-Fr feeding tube through nose to the level of atresia; distal end of tube marks level of atresia; inject air if necessary
- Definite diagnosis is established by injection of 1 to 2 mL of liquid barium; this, however, should be done only at a large referral institution.
- Videotape the injection.

Main differential diagnosis

- Traumatic perforation of posterior pharynx
- Pharyngeal pseudodiverticulum

GASTROESOPHAGEAL REFLUX

Causes

- Immaturity of lower esophageal sphincter during first 3 months of life (usually resolves spontaneously)
- Congenital short esophagus
- Hiatal hernia
- Chalasia (lower esophageal sphincter fails to contract in resting phase; differentiate from achalasia in adults)
- Gastric outlet obstruction

Radiographic Features

Barium swallow
- Determine presence of reflux
- Exclude organic abnormalities

Gastroesophageal scintigraphy
- Most sensitive technique to determine reflux and gastroesophageal emptying
- Semiquantitative method
- Anatomy only poorly visualized

ESOPHAGEAL FOREIGN BODY (Fig. 11-21)

Foreign bodies in the esophagus may cause airway symptoms by:
- Direct mechanical compression of airway
- Periesophageal inflammation
- Perforation and abscess
- Fistulization to trachea

Radiographic Features

- Foreign body lodges in coronal plane
- Esophagogram may show inflammatory mass.
- Fluoroscopic removal with Foley catheter in select instances (e.g., nonembedded)

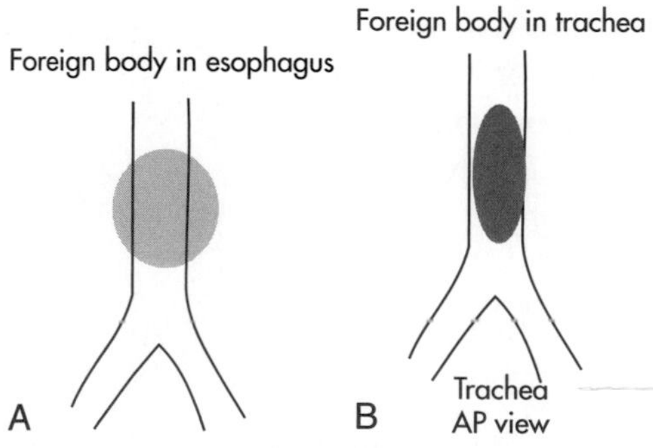

FIGURE 11-21

STOMACH

HYPERTROPHIC PYLORIC STENOSIS (HPS)

Caused by hypertrophy of the circular musculature of the pylorus. Incidence: 1:1000 births. Male:female = 4:1. Unknown etiology. Treatment is with pyloromyotomy.

Clinical Findings

- Projectile nonbilious vomiting after each feeding
- Peaks at 3 to 6 weeks after birth
- Never occurs after 3 months
- Palpable antral mass (olive sized)
- Weight loss
- Dehydration
- Jaundice
- Alkalosis

Associations

- EA, TEF, hiatal hernia
- Renal abnormalities
- Turner syndrome
- Trisomy 18
- Rubella

Radiographic Features

Plain film (Fig. 11-22)
- Gastric distention (>7 cm)
- Peristaltic waves result in a "caterpillar" appearance to the distended stomach.
- Decreased air in distal bowel
- Thick antral folds

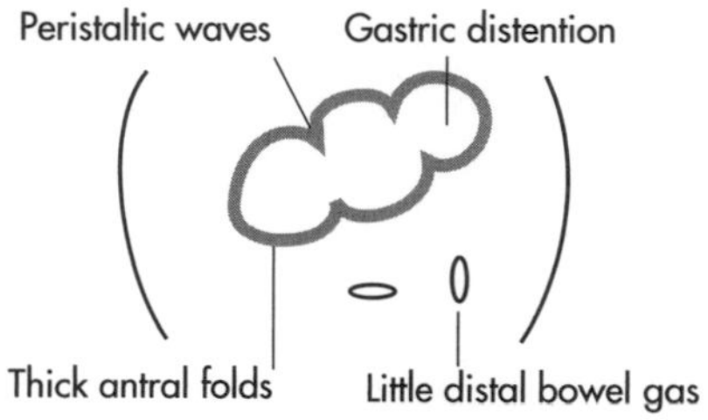

FIGURE 11-22

US
- HPS appears as target lesion (anechoic mass in RUQ with central echoes due to gas).
- Scan in RPO projection (move fluid into antrum)
- Size criteria are used to establish the diagnosis of HPS:
  - Pyloric muscle thickness >3.5 to 4 mm
  - Pyloric length >15 to 18 mm
- Useful as first imaging modality

Upper GI technique (Fig. 11-23):
1. Insert an 8-Fr feeding tube to decompress the stomach and drain gastric contents before administration of contrast agent.
2. Use RAO view (to visualize the pylorus)
3. Instill 10 to 20 mL of barium.
4. Wait for pylorus to open; obtain spot views
5. Get air contrast view by turning patient supine
6. If there is no pyloric stenosis, get lateral and AP views to exclude malrotation.

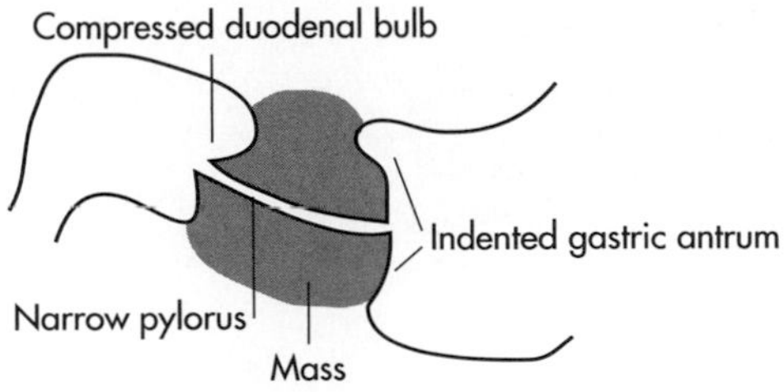

FIGURE 11-23

7. Upper gastrointestinal (UGI) findings of HPS:
   - Indented gastric antrum (shoulder sign)
   - Compression of duodenal bulb
   - Narrow and elongated pylorus: string sign

PYLOROSPASM

Intermittent findings of pyloric stenosis. Treatment is with antispasmodic drugs.

Associations include:

- Adrenogenital syndrome
- Dehydration
- Sepsis

Radiographic Features

- Pyloric musculature is of normal thickness.
- Prominent mucosa (echogenic)
- Exclude secondary causes of pylorospasm (e.g., ulcer).

VOLVULUS

Mesenteroaxial volvulus: pylorus lies above gastroesophageal (GE) junction.

- Occurs with eventration of left diaphragm or diaphragmatic hernia
- Acute syndrome: obstruction, ischemia

Organoaxial volvulus: rotation around long axis of stomach

- Rare in children
- Associated with large hiatal hernia
- Lesser curvature is inferior and greater curvature lies superior.
- Associated gastric outlet obstruction

CHRONIC GRANULOMATOUS DISEASE

Inherited genetic disorder (X-linked and autosomal recessive) leading to dysfunctional NADPH oxidase in phagocytic cells (leukocytes and monocytes), preventing normal respiratory burst. Usually presents at <5 years of age.

Clinical Findings

- Recurrent bacterial and fungal infections: Recurrent pneumonia (80%), osteomyelitis (30%, esp. small bones of the feet and hand)
- Lymphadenitis, abscess, and granuloma formation
- Hepatosplenomegaly
- GI manifestations from granuloma infiltration: esophageal strictures and antral narrowing (characteristic), which may lead to gastric outlet obstruction

DUODENUM, PANCREAS, SMALL BOWEL

CONGENITAL DUODENAL ATRESIA, STENOSIS

Results from failure of recanalization (around 10 weeks). Incidence: 1:3500 live births. Atresia : stenosis = 2:1. Common cause of bowel obstruction. Bilious vomiting occurs within 24 hours after birth. Treatment is with duodenojejunostomy or duodenoduodenostomy.

Associations

- 30% have Down syndrome.
- 40% have polyhydramnios and are premature.
- Malrotation, EA, biliary atresia, renal anomalies, imperforate anus with or without sacral anomalies, CHD

Radiographic Features

- Enlarged duodenal bulb and stomach (double-bubble sign)
- Small amount of air in distal small bowel does not exclude diagnosis of duodenal atresia (hepatopancreatic duct may bifurcate in "Y" shape and insert above and below atresia).

DUODENAL DIAPHRAGM (Fig. 11-24)

Variant of duodenal stenosis caused by an obstructive duodenal membrane. The pressure gradient through the diaphragm causes the formation of a diverticulum ("wind sock" appearance).

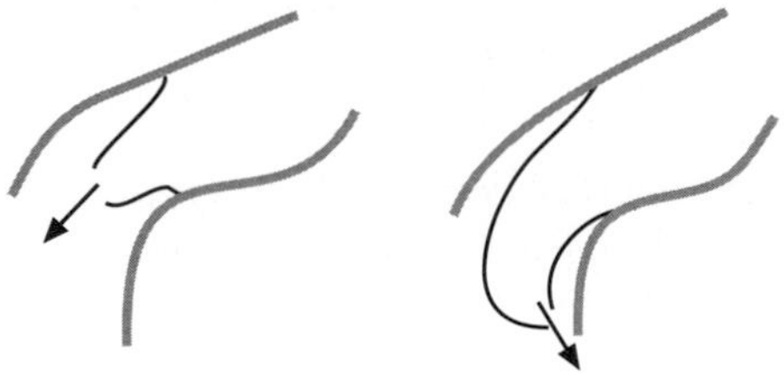

FIGURE 11-24

ANNULAR PANCREAS

Uncommon congenital ringlike position of pancreas surrounding the second portion of duodenum. Results from abnormal rotation of embryonic pancreatic tissue. The annular pancreas usually causes duodenal narrowing. Diagnosis is made by ERCP and MRCP.

PANCREATIC TUMORS

Rare. Well-defined, expansile, less infiltrative compared with adult pancreatic tumors.

Types

- Pancreatoblastoma (most common, young children <10 years old): heterogeneous large multilocular septated masses which enhance
- Solid pseudopapillary tumor (adolescent girls): low malignant potential, cystic and solid, hemorrhagic, may have calcification.
- Islet cell tumors (older children): insulinomas tend to be smaller compared with gastrinomas

MALROTATION AND MIDGUT VOLVULUS

Normally, the rotations place the ligament of Treitz to the left of the spine at level of duodenal bulb. Distal end of mesentery is in RLQ. In malrotation the mesenteric attachment is short, allowing bowel to twist around the superior mesenteric vessels (Fig. 11-25). SMV compression (edematous bowel) is followed by SMA compression (gangrene).

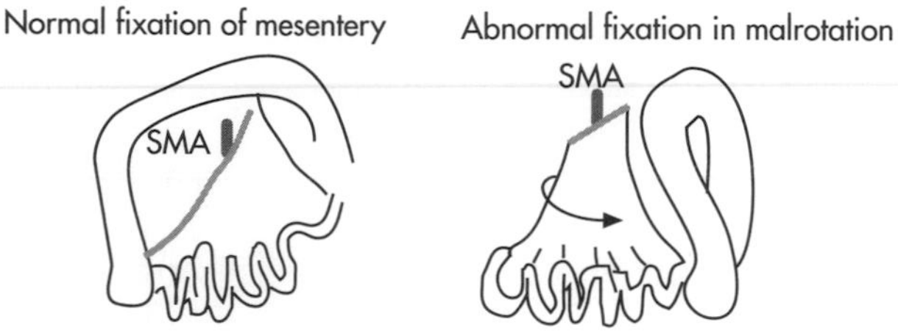

FIGURE 11-25

Associations

- Gastroschisis
- Omphalocele
- Diaphragmatic hernia
- Duodenal or jejunal atresia

Radiographic Features

Plain film

- Suspect diagnosis in the setting of bowel obstruction and abnormally positioned bowel loops.
- A normal position of the cecum does not exclude malrotation but makes it much less likely.

US

- Reversal of SMA (right) and SMV (left) location may occasionally be diagnosed by color Doppler imaging.
- Distended proximal duodenum
- Usually not useful

UGI

- Abnormal position of duodenojejunal junction because of absence of ligament of Treitz
- Beaking at site of obstruction
- Spiraling of small bowel as it twists around SMA (corkscrew) (Fig. 11-26)
- Edema of bowel wall
- Early diagnosis is essential to prevent bowel necrosis.

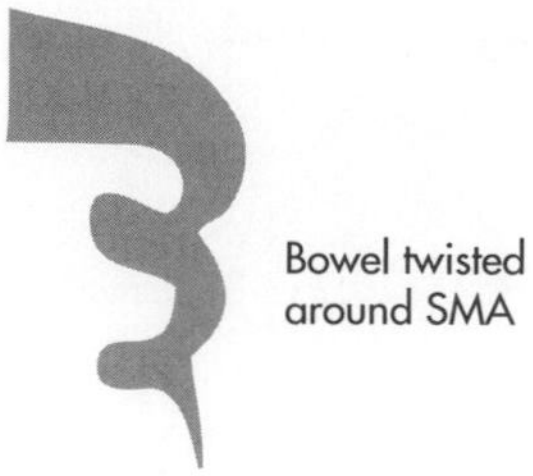

FIGURE 11-26

Barium enema

- A normal barium enema will rule out 97% of malrotation.
- Can determine if there is a concomitant cecal volvulus

CT

- SMA to right of SMV
- Gastric outlet obstruction
- Spiraling of duodenum and jejunum around SMA axis

LADD'S BANDS (Fig. 11-27)

Peritoneal bands in patients with malrotation. The bands extend from malplaced cecum to porta hepatis and may cause duodenal obstruction.

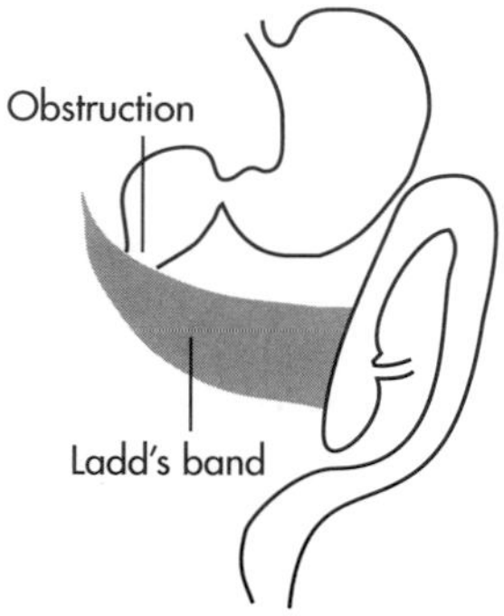

FIGURE 11-27

SMALL BOWEL ATRESIA

Due to in utero ischemia rather than recanalization failure. Ileum is most commonly affected, followed by jejunum and duodenum; may involve multiple sites. Associated with polyhydramnios in 20%-40%.

Radiographic Features

- Dilated small bowel
- Microcolon

MECONIUM ILEUS

In 10% of patients with cystic fibrosis, meconium ileus is the presenting symptom. Thick, tenacious meconium adheres to the small bowel and causes obstruction, usually at the level of the ileocecal valve.

Meconium ileus can be uncomplicated (i.e., no other abnormalities) or complicated (50%) by other abnormalities, such as:

- Ileal atresia
- Perforation, peritonitis
- Stenosis
- Volvulus

Radiographic Features (Fig. 11-28)

Plain film

- Neuhauser's sign: "Soap bubble" appearance (air mixed with meconium)
- Small bowel obstruction
- Calcification due to meconium peritonitis, 15%

Enema with water-soluble contrast medium

- Microcolon is typical: small unused colon
- Distal 10 to 30cm of ileum is larger than colon.
- Inspissated meconium in terminal ileum
- Hyperosmolar contrast may stimulate passage of meconium.

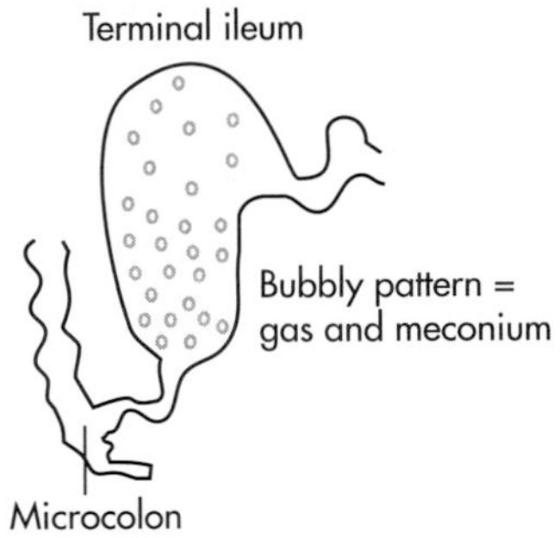

FIGURE 11-28

OTHER MECONIUM PROBLEMS

Meconium Plug Syndrome

Neonatal intestinal obstruction due to colonic inertia (in contradistinction to meconium ileus where there is accumulation of meconium in small bowel). Because of the inertia, the colon usually requires an enema to stimulate peristalsis. Usually occurs in full-term babies and infants of diabetic mothers. In the spectrum with small left colon syndrome. No association with cystic fibrosis.

Meconium Peritonitis

Due to antenatal perforation of bowel. The inflammatory response may cause peritoneal calcification as early as 12 hours after perforation. Can also observe calcifications in testes.

Meconium Ileus Equivalent

Occurs in older patients with cystic fibrosis, usually patients who do not excrete bile salts. The inspissated fecal material causes intestinal obstruction.

INTUSSUSCEPTION

Invagination of a segment of bowel into more distal bowel.

Types

- Ileocolic
- Ileoileocolic
- Ileoileal
- Colocolic

Ileocolic and ileoileocolic intussusception make up 90% of all intussusceptions. 90% of all pediatric intussusceptions have no pathologic lead point; in the remaining 10%, the lead point is due to:

- Meckel diverticulum
- Polyp or other tumors
- Cysts
- Mesenteric adenitis

Clinical Findings

- Usually in the first 2 years of life (40% from 3 to 6 months), rarely in neonates
- Pain, 90%
- Vomiting, 90%
- Mass, 60%
- Blood per rectum, 60%

Radiographic Features

Plain film

- Frequently normal (50%)
- Intraluminal convex filling defect in partially air-filled bowel loop (commonly at hepatic flexure)

Ultrasound (US)

- Target or doughnut sign

Intussusception Reduction (80% Success Rate)

1. Alert pediatric surgeon.
2. Preliminary KUB to rule out free air.
3. Dilute contrast (e.g., Cysto-Conray 17%) in bag placed 3 feet above table top. Alternatively, air reduction is commonly used; should not exceed 110mm Hg. Rectal tube may be taped to reduce air leak.
3. Avoid abdominal palpation.
4. Maintain constant hydrostatic pressure but no longer than 3 minutes against the nonmoving intussusception mass. If patient evacuates around tube, repeat filling may be performed up to 3 tries before surgery is contemplated. (Rule of 3s: bag 3 feet high, 3 minutes per try, and 3 tries)
5. Successful reduction is marked by free flow of contrast into the terminal ileum. Fluoroscopy is used to evaluate for a pathologic lead point. A postevacuation and a 24-hour film are obtained.

6. Contraindications to reduction:
   - Perforation
   - Peritonitis
   - Henoch-Schönlein purpura (predisposes to perforation)
7. Complications
   - Recurrence in 6%-10% (half within 48 hours after initial reduction)
   - Perforation during radiographic reduction is rare (incidence: 1:300 cases)

HENOCH-SCHÖNLEIN PURPURA

Small vessel vasculitis presenting with rash, subcutaneous edema, abdominal pain, bloody stools, and arthritis.

Radiographic Features

- Intramural hemorrhage of small bowel
- Intussusception, typically ileoileal
- Gallbladder hydrops
- Echogenic kidneys

DUPLICATION CYSTS

Location: small bowel (terminal ileum) > esophagus > duodenum > jejunum > stomach (incidence decreases from distal to proximal, skips the stomach). Duplication cysts typically present as an abdominal mass. Small bowel duplications are most commonly located on the mesenteric side; esophageal duplications are commonly located within the lumen.

Radiographic Features

- Round fluid-filled mass displacing adjacent bowel
- May contain ectopic gastric mucosa (hemorrhage)
- Calcifications are rare.
- Communicating vertebral anomalies (neurenteric cysts; most common in esophagus)

OMPHALOMESENTERIC DUCT ANOMALIES (Fig. 11-29)

Omphalomesenteric duct anomalies are due to persistence of the vitelline duct, which connects the yolk sac with the bowel lumen through the umbilicus. Spectrum:

- Meckel's diverticulum
- Patent omphalomesenteric duct (umbilicoileal fistula)
- Omphalomesenteric cyst (vitelline cyst)
- Omphalomesenteric sinus (umbilical sinus)

Meckel's Diverticulum

Persistence of the omphalomesenteric duct at its junction with the ileum. Rule of 2s:

- Occurs in 2% of population (most common congenital GI abnormality)
- Complications usually occur before 2 years of age

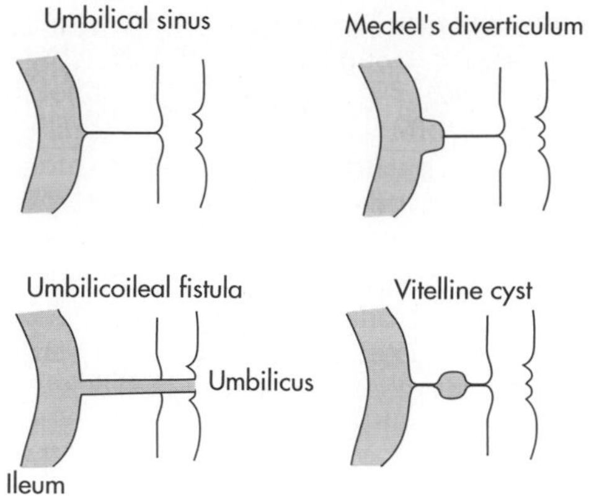

FIGURE 11-29

- The diverticulum is located within 2 feet of the ileocecal valve.
- 20% of patients have complications.
  - Hemorrhage from peptic ulceration when gastric mucosa is present within lesion
  - Inflammation and ulcer
  - Obstruction

Radiographic Features

- Difficult to detect because diverticula usually do not fill with barium
- Pertechnetate scan is the diagnostic imaging modality of choice to detect ectopic gastric mucosa (sensitivity 95%).
- False-positive pertechnetate studies may occur in:
  - Crohn disease
  - Appendicitis
  - Intussusception
  - Abscess

COLON

APPENDICITIS

Age: >4 years (most common cause of small bowel obstruction) (see also Chapter 3).

Radiographic Features

Plain film
- Mass in RLQ
- Obliterated properitoneal fat line
- Sentinel loop
- Fecalith

US
- May be useful in children
- Thickened appendiceal wall shadowing appendicolith, RLQ abscess

Barium enema (rarely done)
- A completely filled appendix excludes the diagnosis of appendicitis.

- 15% of normal appendices do not fill with contrast.
- Signs suggestive of appendicitis:
  - Beak of barium at base of appendix (mucosal edema)
  - Irregularity of barium near tip of cecum
  - Deformity of cecum (abscess, mass effect)

CT
- Helical CT with opacification of the gastrointestinal tract achieved through the oral or rectal administration of 3% diatrizoate meglumine solution is useful to diagnose or exclude appendicitis and to establish an alternative diagnosis.

NECROTIZING ENTEROCOLITIS (NEC)

Most common GI emergency in premature infants. Precise etiology unknown (ischemia? antigens? bacteria?). Develops most often within 2 to 6 days after birth.

Indication for surgery:
- Pneumoperitoneum

Increased incidence in:
- Premature infants
- Neonates with bowel obstruction (e.g., atresia)
- Neonates with CHD

Radiographic Features (Fig. 11-30)
- Small bowel dilatation: adynamic ileus (first finding), unchanging configuration over serial radiographs
- Pneumatosis intestinalis, 80% (second most common sign)
- Gas in portal vein may be seen transiently (US more sensitive than plain film); this finding does not imply as bad an outcome as it does in adults.
- Pneumoperitoneum (20%) indicates bowel perforation: football sign (floating air and ascites give the appearance of a large elliptical lucency in supine position).
- Barium is contraindicated; use water-soluble contrast if a bowel obstruction or Hirschsprung disease needs to be ruled out.

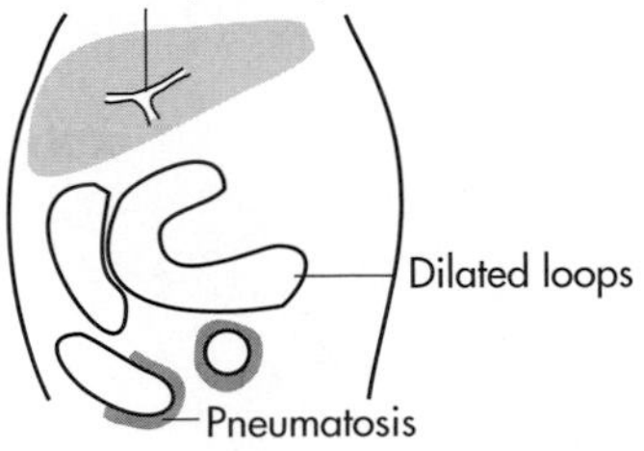

FIGURE 11-30

Complications

Acute
- Perforation

Later in life
- Bowel stricture (commonly near splenic flexure)
- Complications of surgery: short small bowel syndrome, dumping, malabsorption
- Complications of associated diseases common in premature infants:
  - Hyaline membrane disease
  - Germinal matrix hemorrhage
  - Periventricular leukomalacia

HIRSCHSPRUNG DISEASE

Absence of the myenteric plexus cells (aganglionosis, incomplete craniocaudal migration of embryonic neuroblasts) in distal segment of the colon causes hypertonicity and obstruction. Clinical: 80% (male:female = 6:1) present in the first 6 weeks of life with obstruction, intermittent diarrhea, or constipation. Diagnosis is by rectal biopsy. Treatment is with colostomy (Swenson, Duhamel, Soave operations), myomectomy. Associated with Down syndrome.

Complications
- Intestinal obstruction (in neonates)
- Perforation
- Enterocolitis 15%, etiology uncertain

Radiographic Features (Fig. 11-31)
- Bowel gas pattern of distal colonic obstruction on plain film
- Barium enema is normal in 30%
- Transition zone between normal and stenotic colonic segment
- Rectum: sigmoid diameter ratio (normal 1:0) is abnormal (<1.0) because of the narrowed segment
- Sawtooth appearance of colon on contrast enema
- Significant barium retention on the 24-hour barium enema film may be helpful.
- Transition zone in rectosigmoid, 80%

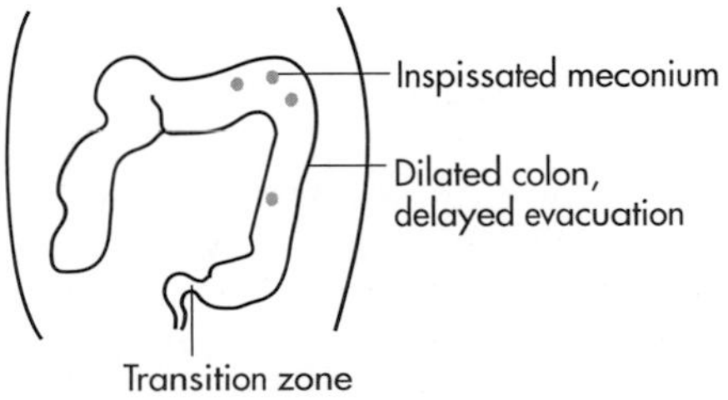

FIGURE 11-31

CONGENITAL ANORECTAL ANOMALIES (Fig. 11-32)

Failure of descent and separation of hindgut and genitourinary (GU) system in second trimester.

High (supralevator) malformations
- Rectum ends above levator sling
- High association with GU (50%) and cardiac anomalies

Low (infralevator) malformations
- Rectum ends below levator sling
- Low association with GU anomalies (25%)

OVERVIEW

	Male	Female
High malformation	Fistula to the urethra or less commonly to the bladder	Rectovaginal fistula, hydrometrocolpos
Low malformation (bowel passes through levator sling)	Anoperineal fistula	Fistula to lower portion of urethra, vagina perineum

Associated anomalies are very common:
- Sacral anomalies, 30% (tethered cord)
- Currarino's triad: anorectal anomaly, sacral bone abnormality, and presacral mass
- Genitourinary anomalies, 30%
- VACTERL
- GI anomalies: duodenal atresia, EA

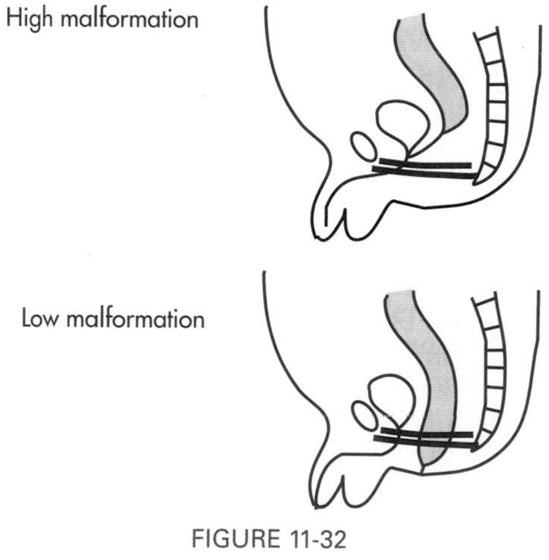

FIGURE 11-32

Radiographic Features

Plain film
- Low colonic obstruction
- Gas bubbles in bladder or vagina
- Determine location of the gas-filled rectal pouch to the M-line (line drawn through junction of upper two thirds and lower one third of ischia; line indicates level of levator sling).
- Upside-down views can be obtained to distend distal rectal pouch.

Magnetic resonance imaging (MRI)
- Determine location of rectal pouch with respect to levator and to determine if the malformation is supralevator or infralevator type.
- Facilitates the detection of associated spinal anomalies

LIVER, BILIARY TRACT

BILIARY ATRESIA

Unknown etiology (severe hepatitis, sclerosing cholangitis with vascular component?). Associated with trisomy 18 and polysplenia.

Types (Fig. 11-33)
- Correctable: portoenterostomy (Kasai procedure)
- Noncorrectable

Radiographic Features

US
- Normal gallbladder (GB) in 20%

HIDA scan
- No visualization of bowel at 24 hours
- Good hepatic visualization within 5 minutes
- Increased renal excretion
- Main differential diagnosis is neonatal hepatitis. Findings of neonatal hepatitis include:
  - Bowel activity present at 24 hours
  - Decreased and slow hepatic accumulation of tracer
  - GB may not be seen

NEONATAL HEPATITIS VERSUS BILIARY ATRESIA

Neonatal Hepatitis	Biliary Atresia
Male premature newborns	Females
TORCH syndrome	Polysplenia
Skeletal abnormality	Choledochal cyst

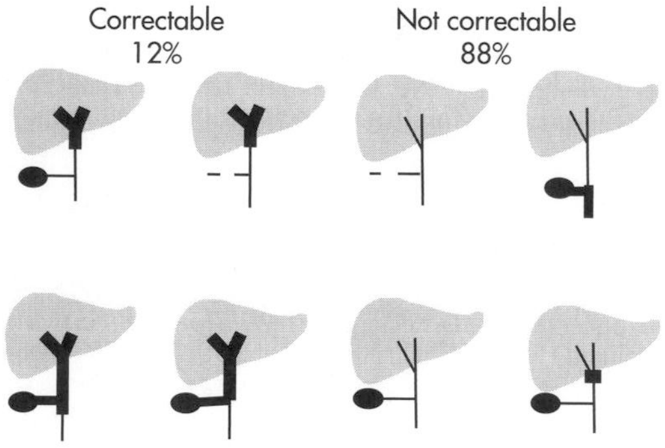

FIGURE 11-33

- Both diseases present with conjugated hyperbilirubinemia during first week of life.
- Kasai procedure for treatment of biliary atresia is often successful if the correct diagnosis is made by 40 days of age.
- One must exclude the presence of cystic fibrosis in patients thought to have biliary atresia. Inspissated bile in cystic fibrosis can be indistinguishable from biliary atresia by US or nuclear scan.
- Preprocedural phenobarbital (5 mg/kg/day × 5 days) improves sensitivity of hepatobiliary scans. The finding of normal (1.5 cm or more) or enlarged (3 cm or more) GB is more supportive of diagnosis of hepatitis.

	Hemangioma	Hemangioendothelioma
Age	Older children	<6 months
Size	<2 cm	2-15 cm
Location	Right lobe	Both lobes
Symptoms	No	Hepatomegaly, CHF
Ultrasound	Well-defined hyperechoic lesion	Variable
Malignant potential	No	Rare

HEMANGIOENDOTHELIOMA

Most common benign pediatric liver tumor. 85% present at <6 months. Associated cutaneous hemangiomas in 50%.

Complications

- CHF because of AV shunt, 15%
- Intraperitoneal hemorrhage
- Disseminated intravascular coagulopathy
- Thrombocytopenia (platelet trapping)

Radiographic Features

- Complex, hypoechoic mass by US
- Similar signal intensity/contrast characteristics as adult hemangioma

MESENCHYMAL HAMARTOMA

- Occurs during first 10 years of life
- Large multiloculated cystic lesion
- Large cysts >10 cm may be seen.
- 10% are exophytic.

HEPATOBLASTOMA

Most common primary malignant liver tumor in children. Age: <2 years.

Associations

- Beckwith-Wiedemann syndrome
- Hemihypertrophy

Radiographic Features

- Large hepatic mass
- Mixed echogenicity (US)
- Calcification, 50%
- Metastases: lungs > lymph nodes, brain

HEPATOCELLULAR CARCINOMA (HCC)

Second most common malignant primary liver tumor in children. Age: >3 years.

Associations

- Cystic fibrosis
- Autoimmune hepatitis
- Hepatitis C
- Glycogen storage disease (von Gierke)
- Galactosemia
- Tyrosinemia
- Biliary atresia

Radiographic Features

- Difficult to distinguish from hepatoblastoma other than by clinical picture
- Lower incidence of calcification than hepatoblastoma

HYPOVOLEMIC SHOCK

- Small hyperdense spleen
- Marked enhancement of bowel wall, kidneys, and pancreas
- Dilated fluid-filled bowel
- Small caliber aorta and IVC

Genitourinary Tract

GENERAL

RENAL DEVELOPMENT (Fig. 11-34)

The kidney develops in 3 stages:

- Pronephros (3rd week): tubules drain into an excretory duct that terminates in the cloaca.
- Mesonephros (4th week): serves as precursor for:
  - Male: vas deferens, seminal vesicles, ejaculatory duct
  - Female: vestigial

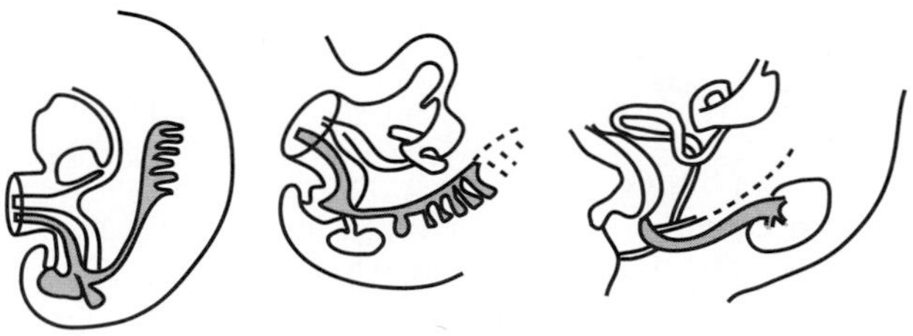

FIGURE 11-34

- Metanephros (5th week): ureteral bud develops from mesonephric duct; the ureteral bud elongates, undergoes divisions, and forms renal tubules while ascending along the posterior coelomic wall; at 12 weeks there are 7 anterior and 7 posterior renal lobes separated by a fibrous groove; at 28 weeks the boundaries between renal lobes become indistinct; persistence of fibrous groove is evident after birth.

GENITALIA (Fig. 11-35)

Wolffian Duct

- Anlage for vas deferens, seminal vesicles, epididymis
- Guides ureteral migration to bladder
- Induces kidney development and ascent
- Induces müllerian duct development in females

Müllerian Duct

- Forms entire female genitalia except distal third of vagina

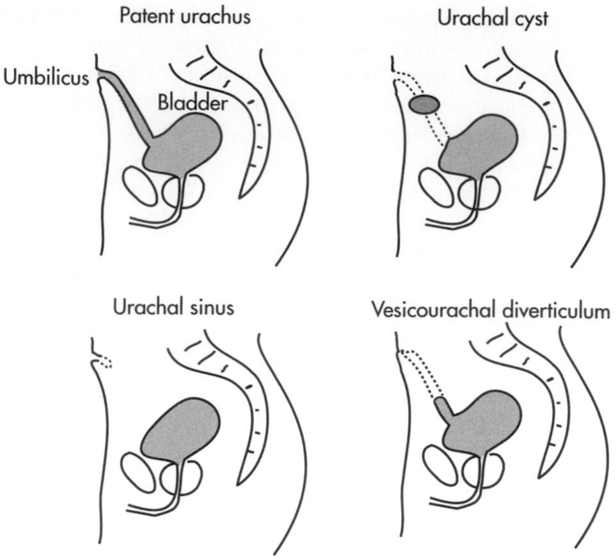

FIGURE 11-36

CLOACA

Divided by the cloacal (urorectal) septum into:

- Dorsal portion → rectum
- Ventral portion → allantois (atrophies as umbilical ligament), bladder, urogenital sinus (pelvic, phallic portions)

Wolffian and müllerian ducts drain into the ventral portion of cloaca.

URACHUS (FIG. 11-36)

The umbilical attachment of the bladder (initially allantois then urachus) usually atrophies (umbilical ligament) as the bladder descends into the pelvis. Persistent canalization of the urachus may lead to urine flow from the bladder to the umbilicus.

- Tumors: Adenocarcinoma, yolk sac tumor, adenoma, fibroma
- Urachal cyst: may splay umbilical arteries on prenatal Doppler US

UTERUS

- The prepubertal uterus has a tubular configuration (anteroposterior cervix equal to anteroposterior fundus) or sometimes a spade shape (anteroposterior cervix larger than anteroposterior fundus).

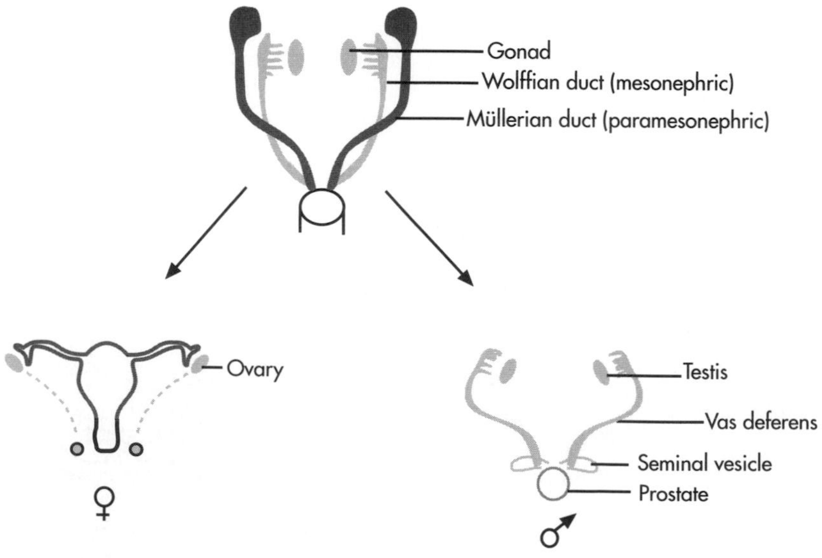

FIGURE 11-35

- The endometrium is normally not apparent; however, high-frequency transducers can demonstrate the central lining.
- The length is 2.5 to 4 cm; the thickness does not exceed 10 mm.

OVARIES

- Ovarian volume: V = half length × width × depth
- The mean ovarian volume in girls <6 years of age is ≤ 1 cm^3.
- The ovarian volume increases after 6 years of age.
- In prepubertal girls (6 to 10 years old), ovarian volumes range from 1.2 to 2.3 cm^3. In premenarchal girls (11 to 12 years old), ovarian volumes range from 2 to 4 cm^3. In postmenarchal girls, the ovarian volume averages 8 cm^3 (range, 2.5 to 20 cm^3).

CONGENITAL ANOMALIES

RENAL ANOMALIES

Anomalies of Position

- Malrotation around vertical axis (most common)
- All malpositioned kidneys are malrotated.
- Ectopic kidney
  - Usually located in pelvis
  - Most ectopic kidneys are asymptomatic, but pelvic kidneys are more susceptible to trauma and infection. Pelvic kidneys may complicate natural childbirth later in life.
  - When a single orthotopic kidney is seen on IVP, a careful search for the contralateral collecting system in the pelvis is mandated because the kidney itself may be obscured by pelvic bones.
  - An ectopic thoracic kidney is usually an acquired duplication through the foramen of Bochdalek.

Anomalies of Form

- Horseshoe kidney
- Pancake kidney results from fusion of both kidneys in the pelvis, usually near the aortic bifurcation.
- Cross-fused ectopia (Fig. 11-37)
- Congenital megacalyces: Increased number of calyces with round instead of cupped shape. May be unilateral. Increased risk of infection and stones. No obstruction. Urine empties on Lasix renogram unless associated with megaureter.
- Renal hypoplasia
  - Incomplete development results in a smaller (<50%) kidney with fewer calyces and papillae (<5) but normal function.

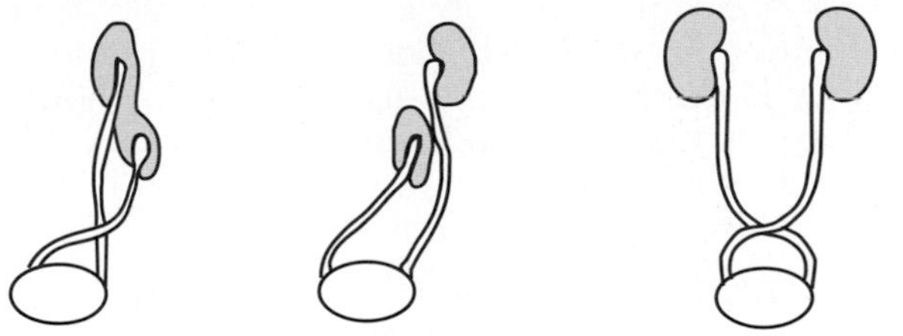

FIGURE 11-37

  - Not to be confused with dysplasia, which results from collecting system obstruction and creates a bizarre appearance of the kidney. Hypoplastic kidneys are smooth with short infundibula and sometimes have clubbed calyces.
  - Segmental hypoplasia (Ask-Upmark kidney): usually upper pole with deep transverse groove. Associated with severe hypertension.
  - Etiology is controversial (congenital versus sequelae of pyelonephritis).

Anomalies of Number

- Unilateral renal agenesis (1:1000 births); associated with hypoplasia or aplasia of testis or vas deferens, ipsilateral seminal vesicle cyst, hypospadias in males; cornuate uterus, hypoplasia or aplasia of vagina (Rokitansky-Küster-Hauser syndrome) in females; hypertrophy of contralateral kidney
- Bilateral renal agenesis
- Supernumerary kidney (very rare)

Complications of Renal Congenital Anomalies

- Infection
- Obstruction
- Calculus
- Trauma

HORSESHOE KIDNEY

Most common anomaly of renal form. In horseshoe kidneys the lower poles are fused across the midline. Incidence: 1:400 births. Associated anomalies, 50%:

- Ureteropelvic junction (UPJ) obstruction, 30%
- Ureteral duplication, 10%
- Genital anomalies
- Turner syndrome
- Other anomalies (GI, cardiac, skeletal), 30%

Radiographic Features

- Inferior fusion (isthmus)
- Abnormal axis of each kidney (bilateral malrotation)
- Variable blood supply

RENAL ECTOPIA

Crossed ectopia refers to a kidney on the opposite side from ureteral bladder insertion. The lower kidney is the one that is usually ectopic. Abnormal rotation is common, and renal pelvises may face opposite directions. In 90% there is fusion of both kidneys. Incidence: 1:1000 births. Incidence of associated anomalies is low. Slightly increased incidence of calculi.

URETERAL DUPLICATION (Fig. 11-38)

Two ureters drain one kidney (incidence 1:150). Duplications may be incomplete ("Y" ureter) or complete:

- Orthotopic ureter: drains lower pole and enters bladder near trigone
- Ectopic ureter: drains upper pole and enters bladder inferiorly and medially (Weigert-Meyer rule); the ectopic ureter may be stenotic and obstructed.

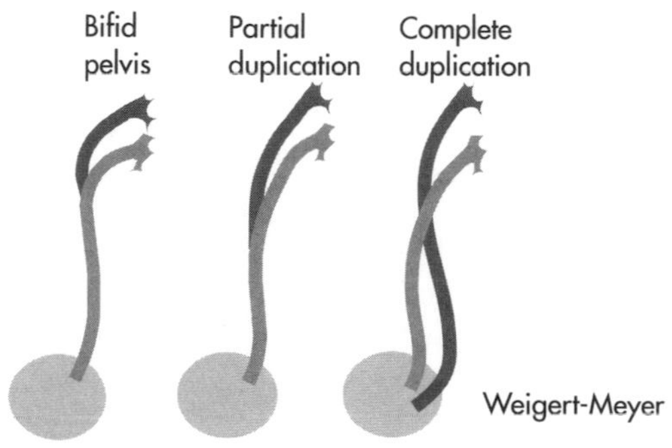

FIGURE 11-38

Complications

- Reflux in orthotopic ureter, causing urinary tract infection (UTI)
- Obstruction of ectopic ureter
- Ureterocele

Radiographic Features (Lebowitz)

(Fig. 11-39)

- Increased distance from top of nephrogram to collecting system: hydronephrotic upper pole moiety causes mass effect (1)
- Abnormal axis of collecting system (2)
- Concave upper border of renal pelvis (3)
- Diminished number of calyces compared with normal side; drooping lily sign (4)
- Lateral displacement of kidney and ureter (5)
- Spiral course of ureter (6)
- Filling defect in the bladder (ureterocele)

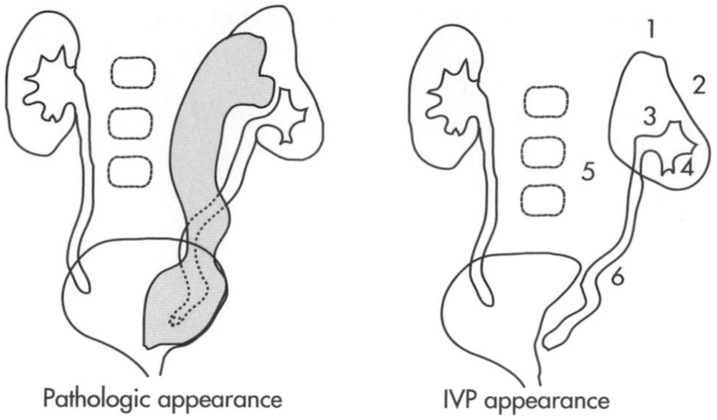

FIGURE 11-39

URETEROCELE (Fig. 11-40)

A ureterocele refers to a herniation of the distal ureter into the bladder. Two types:

Simple (normal location of ureter), 25%
- Almost always occurs in adults
- Usually also symptomatic in children

Ectopic (abnormal location of ureter), 75%
- Almost always associated with duplication
- Unilateral, 80%
- May obstruct entire urinary tract

Female incontinence (wetting) is seen with an ectopic ureter without ureterocele but not with an ectopic ureter alone

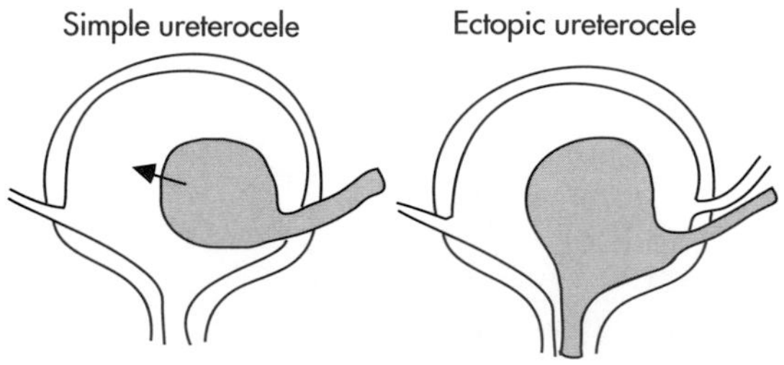

FIGURE 11-40

Radiographic Features

- Ureterocele causes filling defect in bladder on IVP.
- Typical appearance of a cystic structure by US
- Ureterocele may be distended, collapsed, or everted to represent a diverticulum.
- Complications:
  Ureteroceles may contain calculi.
  May be very large (bladder outlet obstruction)

CONGENITAL URETEROPELVIC JUNCTION (UPJ) OBSTRUCTION

Most common congenital anomaly of the GU tract in neonates. 20% of obstructions are bilateral. Treatment is with pyeloplasty.

- Intrinsic, 80%: defect in circular muscle bundle of renal pelvis
- Extrinsic, 20%: renal vessels (lower pole artery or vein)

Radiographic Features

- Caliectasis, pelviectasis
- Delayed contrast excretion of kidneys; poor opacification of renal parenchyma
- Differentiation from prominent extrarenal pelvis may require Whitaker test to determine presence and degree of obstruction.

PRIMARY MEGAURETER

Congenital dilatation of distal ureter due to functional (not mechanical) obstruction (abnormal development of muscle layers, achalasia of ureter). 20% are bilateral. Most commonly diagnosed prenatally. Clinical findings: asymptomatic (most common), pain, UTI, mass. Most commonly (95%), a megaureter is an isolated finding. Associated disorders are uncommon (5%), but if present include:

Ipsilateral
- Calyceal diverticulum
- Papillary necrosis

Contralateral
- Reflux
- Ureterocele
- Ureteral duplication
- Renal ectopia or agenesis
- UPJ obstruction

Radiographic Features

- Ureter dilated above dysfunctional distal ureteral segment
- Nonpropulsive motion in dilated ureteral segment

CIRCUMCAVAL URETER

Congenital abnormality of the IVC (not the ureter). Normally the IVC is derived from supracardinal vein, which is posterior to ureter. If the IVC is derived from the right subcardinal (most common) or postcardinal veins (both of which lie anterior to ureter), a portion of lumbar ureter becomes trapped behind the cava. Occurs mostly in males.

Radiographic Features

- Ureter passes behind IVC and emerges medial to the IVC on its course to pelvis.
- The anomaly is on the right unless patient has situs inversus.
- The anomaly can be bilateral if the IVC is duplicated.
- Types:
  - Low loop (more common)
    - Fishhook or reverse "J" course
    - Ureter is obstructed.
    - Ureter emerges between cava and aorta and descends into the pelvis.
  - High loop (less common)
    - Obstruction is mild.
    - Retrocaval segment runs obliquely at level of UPJ.
    - May simulate UPJ obstruction

BLADDER EXSTROPHY-EPISPADIAS COMPLEX (Fig. 11-41)

Defect in lower abdominal wall, pubic area, anterior wall of bladder, and dorsal aspect of urethra; the defect causes the bladder to be open and the mucosa to be continuous with skin. Most common congenital bladder abnormality; overall rare (1:50,000). Always associated with epispadias (male: urethra ends on dorsal aspect of penis; female: cleft of entire dorsal urethra). Simple epispadias without exstrophy is uncommon.

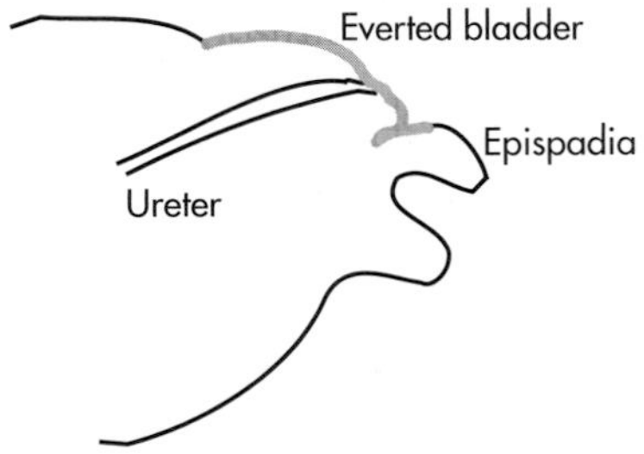

FIGURE 11-41

Radiographic Features

- Diastasis of symphysis (width correlates with severity of exstrophy)
- Omphalocele confluent with exstrophic bladder
- Cryptorchidism
- Inguinal hernia
- Acquired ureterovesical junction (UVJ) obstruction in untreated cases
- Findings after surgical repair:
  - Small bladder
  - Reflux
- Other associated anomalies
  - Rectal prolapse
  - Bifid, unicornuate uterus
  - Spinal anomalies

CLOACAL EXSTROPHY

More severe defect than isolated bladder exstrophy. Occurs earlier in embryogenesis.

Clinical Findings

Bone
- Spina bifida aperta
- Lipomyelomeningocele
- Diastasis of symphysis

Bladder
- Exstrophy

Colon
- Exstrophy

PRUNE-BELLY SYNDROME (TRIAD SYNDROME, EAGLE-BARRETT SYNDROME)

Nonhereditary disorders (1:50,000) characterized by triad:
- Widely separated abdominal rectus muscles (wrinkled appearance of skin looks like a prune)
- Hydroureteronephrosis (giant nonobstructed ureters)
- Cryptorchidism (bladder distention interferes with descent of testes)

Prognosis: lethal in most severe cases, renal failure is common in milder cases.

Severe cases are associated with other anomalies:
- Dysplastic kidneys
- Oligohydramnios
- Pulmonary hypoplasia
- Urethral atresia
- Patent urachus
- Prostatic hypoplasia

Radiographic Features

- Large distended urinary bladder is the hallmark.
- Vesicoureteral reflux (VUR) is common.
- Patent urachus (common)
- Cryptorchidism

POSTERIOR URETHRAL VALVES (PUVS) (Fig. 11-42)

PUVs represent congenital folds (thick folds > thin folds) located in the posterior urethra near the distal end of the verumontanum. These days commonly discovered on prenatal US. Treatment is with electrode fulguration.

Clinical Findings

- PUVs are the most common cause (35%) of obstructive symptoms (hesitancy dribbling, enuresis).
- UTI, 35%
- Palpable bladder or kidney in neonates, 20%
- Hematuria, 5%

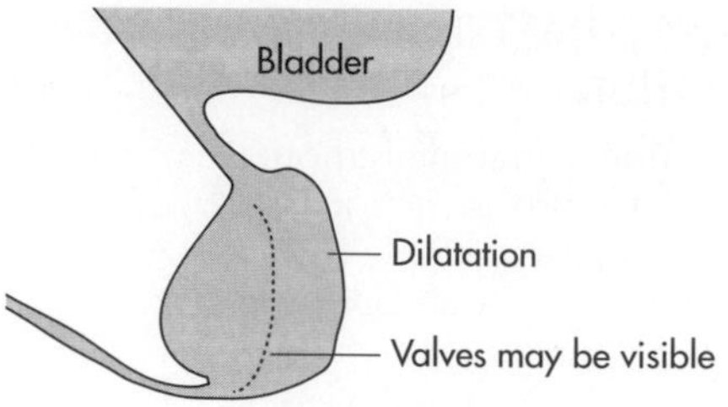

FIGURE 11-42

Types

- Type I (most common): derive from plica colliculi (normal tissue folds that extend inferiorly from verumontanum). Distal leaflets are thickened and fused at the level of membranous urethra.
- Type II: Mucosal folds extend proximally from verumontanum to the bladder neck; some no longer consider type II an obstructing valve but rather a sequela of voiding dysfunction.
- Type III: represents a diaphragm with central aperture at the distal prostatic urethra

Radiographic Features

- Verumontanum is enlarged in type I but not type III.
- Type I causes crescentic filling defect that bulges into contrast column (spinnaker sail appearance).
- Windsock appearance may be seen with type III.
- Posterior urethra above valves is dilated and elongated.
- Bladder trabeculation, saccules, and small diverticula
- VUR
- Hydroureter and hydronephrosis
- In utero complications:
  - Oligohydramnios
  - Urine leak, 15%: urinoma, urine ascites
  - Hydronephrosis
  - Prune-belly syndrome

MALE HYPOSPADIAS

Ectopic ending of the urethra on the ventral aspect of the penis, scrotum, or perineum. Hypospadias is the result of a defective midline fusion of the genital folds. Incidence: 1:300 births.

Associations

- Cryptorchidism, 30%
- Inguinal hernias, 10%
- Urinary tract abnormalities (slightly higher incidence than in general population)

Radiographic Features

- VCUG is performed in more severe cases, in patients with symptoms or other anomalies
- Enlarged utricle, 20%

CAUDAL REGRESSION

Insult to the caudal mesoderm results in spectrum of abnormalities:

- Agenesis of sacrum (20% occur in infants of diabetic mothers)
- Partial absence or underdevelopment of lower extremities
- GU and GI anomalies

Types of Sacral Agenesis

- Type 1: unilateral agenesis
- Type 2: bilateral agenesis with normal sacroiliac joint articulation
- Types 3-4: total absence of sacrum, variable fusions of vertebral bodies with ilia

RENAL CYSTIC DISEASE

AUTOSOMAL RECESSIVE KIDNEY DISEASE (ARKD)

ARKD = infantile polycystic kidney disease (IPKD) = Potter type 1 = polycystic disease of childhood. Incidence: 1:10,000 to 50,000 births.

Types (Fig. 11-43)

Antenatal form: 90% of tubules show ectasia.

- Oligohydramnios in utero
- Death from renal failure or respiratory insufficiency after birth (75% within 24 hours).

Neonatal form: 60% of tubules show ectasia, minimal hepatic fibrosis.

- Renal failure within 1st month of life
- Infants usually die within 1 year.

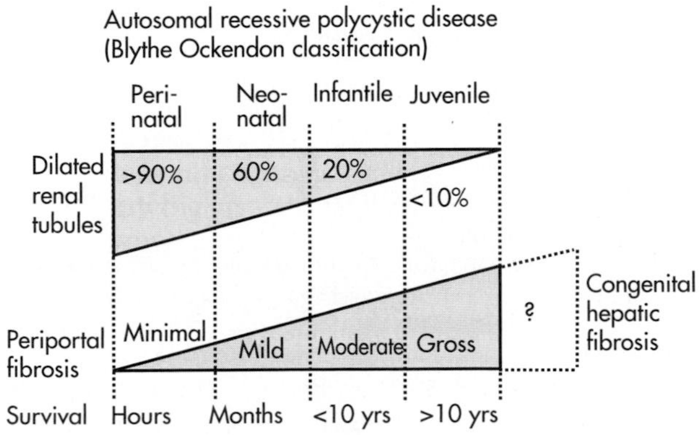

FIGURE 11-43

Infantile form: 20% of tubules show ectasia and moderate hepatic fibrosis.

- Symptoms appear at 3 to 6 months.
- Death from renal failure, portal hypertension, arterial hypertension

Juvenile form: 10% of tubules show ectasia and severe hepatic fibrosis.

- Disease appears at 1 to 5 years of age.
- Death from portal hypertension

The less severe the renal findings, the more severe hepatic periportal cirrhosis. Hepatic fibrosis is also associated with:

- Adult polycystic kidney disease
- Multicystic dysplastic kidneys
- Caroli disease
- Choledochocele

Radiographic Features

Kidneys

- Enlarged hyperechoic kidneys (hallmark)
- Cysts of 1 to 2 mm are seen only with high-resolution US equipment.
- Faint, striated nephrogram due to tubular ectasia (similar appearance as in medullary sponge kidney; IVP seldom performed today)

US findings (in utero)

- Nonvisualization of urine in bladder
- Enlarged, hyperechoic kidneys
- Oligohydramnios (nonfunctioning kidneys)

Lung

- Pulmonary hypoplasia (because of external compression)
- Pneumothorax

Liver

- Hepatic fibrosis
- Portal venous hypertension

MULTICYSTIC DYSPLASTIC KIDNEYS (MCDK)

Collection of large, noncommunicating cysts separated by fibrous tissue; there is no functioning renal parenchyma. Results from occlusion (severe UPJ obstruction) of fetal ureters before 10 weeks of gestation. Absent or atretic renal vessels and collecting system. Because MCDK is involuted, serial US follow-up is usually performed until disappearance. Associated with:

- UPJ obstruction in contralateral kidney
- Horseshoe kidney

Radiographic Features

- Cystic renal mass with no excretory function
- Hypertrophy of contralateral kidney
- Thick fibrous septa between cysts
- Calcification of cyst wall in adults
- Atretic ureter
- Absence of renal artery

MULTILOCULAR CYSTIC NEPHROMA (MLCN)

Congenital renal lesion characterized by large (>10 cm) cystic spaces. Cysts are lined by cuboidal epithelium. The lesion has biphasic age and sex distribution. It occurs in children ages 2 months to 4 years with 75% *male* predilection and in adults >40 years of age with 95% *female* predilection. May present with hematuria due to prolapse of mass into the renal pelvis. Two distinct histologic entities: cystic nephroma without blastema elements within septa and cystic, partially differentiated nephroblastoma, which has blastema elements in the septa. The two entities are indistinguishable by imaging.

Radiographic Features

- Contrast-enhanced CT scans demonstrate a well-defined intrarenal, multilocular mass that compresses or displaces the adjacent renal parenchyma. The septations enhance but the cysts do not.
- Calcifications are uncommon.
- MLCNs are surgically removed because distinction from cystic Wilms tumor is not possible by imaging modalities.

INFLAMMATION

URINARY TRACT INFECTION (UTI)

UTI is defined as >100,000 organisms/mL in a properly collected urine specimen; any bacterial growth in urine obtained by suprapubic puncture or catheterization is also abnormal. Any of the urinary structures may be involved (e.g., bladder: cystitis; prostate: prostatitis; renal tubules: pyelonephritis; urethra: urethritis). Pathogenetically UTI are most commonly ascending infections (especially in females: short urethra). Most common organism: *E. coli* (70%).

Modalities for Imaging of the UTI/VUR Complex

1. Is there a structural abnormality of the urinary tract causing stasis that predisposes to infection?
   - US is the imaging modality of first choice.
   - Structural abnormalities are frequently detected prenatally.
   - In case of abnormality, further imaging studies are usually required.
   - US should be obtained in all children after the first UTI.
2. Is there primary VUR?
   - VCUG and radionuclide cystography are the imaging modalities of first choice.
   - VCUG should be obtained in:
     All children with UTI <4 years old
     All older children with abnormal US, bladder dysfunction, or repeated UTI
3. Is there acute pyelonephritis?
   - Renal cortical scintigraphy has the highest sensitivity and specificity of imaging modalities and should be obtained if results would affect management.
   - US and IVP have a low sensitivity and specificity.
4. Is there parenchymal scarring (Fig. 11-44)?
   - Small scars are best detected with renal cortical scintigraphy.
   - Larger scars can be detected by US or IVP.
   - Wait at least 4 months after UTI to assess for scarring; earlier on, many patients have abnormalities that are not permanent.

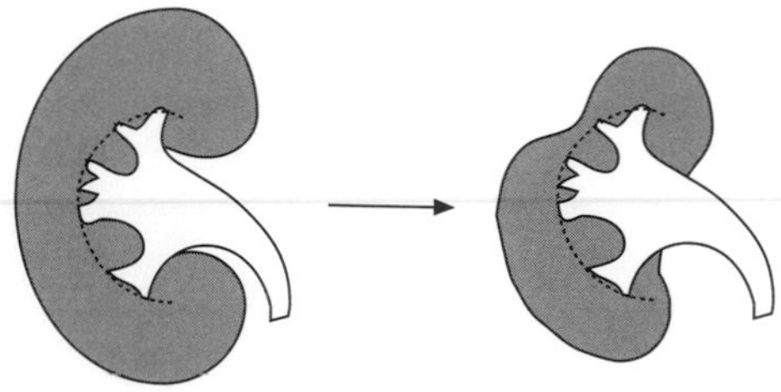

FIGURE 11-44

VESICOURETERAL REFLUX (VUR)

Primary VUR is due to immaturity or maldevelopment of the UVJ with incompetence of the antireflux flap valve action. Immaturity is due to underdeveloped longitudinal muscle of the submucosal ureter; with growth, the submucosal ureter elongates and the valve mechanism becomes competent (children with VUR often outgrow the reflux by 10 years of age, depending on grade and type of reflux).

Other causes of reflux (secondary reflux):

- Periureteral diverticulum
- Ureterocele
- Ureteral duplication
- Bladder outlet obstruction

Complications

- Cystitis
- Pyelonephritis
- Renal scarring occurs with intrarenal reflux of infected urine
- Hypertension and end-stage renal disease (in 10%-20% of renal scarring)

Incidence

Reflux seen in 30%-50% of children with UTI, in 20% of siblings (higher in younger children, lower in older children)

Radiographic Features

Grading of reflux (international grading system) (Fig. 11-45)

- Grade I: reflux to ureter but not to kidney
- Grade II: reflux into ureter, pelvis, and calyces without dilatations
- Grade III: reflux to calyces with mild dilatation, blunted fornices
- Grade IV: reflux to calyces with moderate dilatation, obliteration of fornices
- Grade V: gross dilatation, tortuous ureters

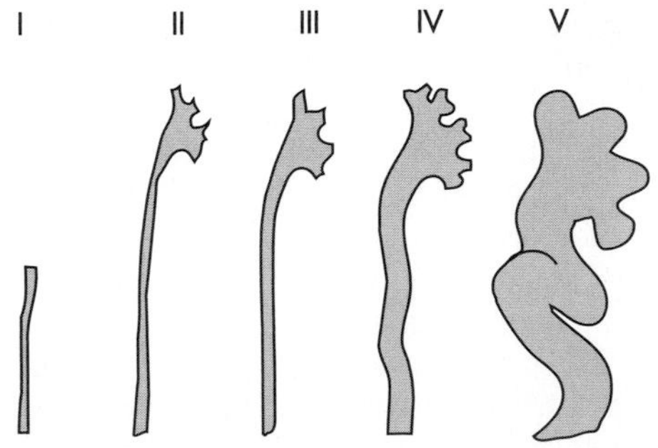

FIGURE 11-45

VOIDING CYSTURETHROGRAM (VCUG)

1. Pediatric VCUGs are performed by the radiologist, with attempts to minimize fluoroscopy time (optimally less than 15 seconds total).
2. Catheterize with an 8-Fr feeding tube (5-Fr tube in neonate).
3. Take AP spot films of the renal fossae and bladder.
4. Instill contrast by gravity drip (bottle positioned 40 cm above table).
5. When patient indicates urge to urinate or signs of imminent voiding are seen, obtain bilateral oblique spots of bladder to include urethral catheter.
6. When voiding begins, catheter is removed. In female, 2 camera spots of distended urethra are obtained with slightly oblique positioning. In the male, 2 camera high-oblique spots are obtained during voiding.
7. Quickly fluoroscope the renal fossae during voiding; if reflux is observed, obtain spot film.
8. After completion of urination, obtain AP spots of bladder and renal fossae.

TUMORS

Most renal masses are benign in infants <2 months of age; the frequency of malignancy increases with age. Approximately 87% of solid renal neoplasms in children are Wilms tumors; other tumors include clear cell sarcoma (6%); mesoblastic nephroma (2%); rhabdoid tumor (2%); lymphoma (<0.5%); renal cell carcinoma (<0.5%).

MOST COMMON AGE AT PRESENTATION FOR SOLID RENAL MALIGNANCIES

Renal Neoplasm	Age Range	Peak Age
Wilms tumor		
Unilateral form	1-11 yr	3 1/2 yr
Bilateral form	2 mo-2 yr	15 mo
Nephroblastomatosis	Any age	6-18 mo
Renal cell carcinoma	6 mo-60 yr	10-20 yr*
Mesoblastic nephroma	0-1 yr	1-3 mo
Multilocular cystic renal tumor		
Cystic nephroma	Adult female	Adult female
Cystic partially differentiated nephroblastoma	3 mo-4 yr	1-2 yr
Clear cell sarcoma	1-4 yr	2 yr
Rhabdoid tumor	6 mo-9 yr	6-12 mo
Angiomyolipoma	6-41 yr	10 yr†
Renal medullary carcinoma	10-39 yr	20 yr
Ossifying renal tumor of infancy	6 days-14 mo	1-3 mo
Metanephric adenoma	15 mo-83 yr	None
Lymphoma		
Hodgkin	>10 yr	Late teens
Non-Hodgkin	Any age child	<10 yr

*von Hippel-Lindau disease.
†Tuberous sclerosis, neurofibromatosis, von Hippel-Lindau disease.

WILMS TUMOR

Arises from metanephric blastema. Most common solid renal tumor of childhood. Third most common malignancy in children after leukemia and brain tumors and third most common cause of all renal masses after hydronephrosis and multicystic dysplastic kidney. 50% <2 years, 75% <5 years, extremely rare in the newborn. Wilms tumors are bilateral in 5%-10% and multifocal in 10%. Nephroblastomatosis is a precursor of Wilms tumor. Two loci on chromosome 11 have been implicated in the genesis of a minority of Wilms tumors. Locus 11p13 is known as the *WT1* gene, and locus 11p15 is known as the *WT2* gene. An abnormal *WT1* gene is present in patients with WAGR syndrome (Wilms tumor, aniridia, genitourinary abnormalities, mental retardation) or Drash syndrome (male pseudohermaphroditism, progressive glomerulonephritis); an abnormal *WT2* gene is present in patients with Beckwith-Wiedemann syndrome or hemihypertrophy.

Clinical Findings

- Palpable abdominal mass, 90% (12 cm mean diameter at diagnosis)
- Hypertension, 50%
- Pain, 35%

- Uncommon presentations: hematuria (5%), fever (15%), anorexia (15%)
- Wilms tumor manifests as a solid intrarenal mass with a pseudocapsule and distortion of the renal parenchyma and collecting system. The tumor typically spreads by direct extension and displaces adjacent structures but does not typically encase or elevate the aorta; such encasement or elevation is a distinguishing characteristic of neuroblastoma.

Associations

- Sporadic aniridia (35% will develop Wilms tumor)
- Hemihypertrophy
- Drash syndrome: pseudohermaphroditism, glomerulonephritis, and Wilms tumor
- Beckwith-Wiedemann syndrome: macroglossia, omphalocele, visceromegaly

Radiographic Features

Tumor

- Large (mean, 12 cm) mass arising from cortex of kidney
- Usually exophytic growth; pseudocapsule
- Cystic areas in tumor: hemorrhage, necrosis
- <15% have calcifications
- Intrarenal mass effect causes distortion of the pyelocalyceal system
- Less contrast enhancement than residual renal parenchyma
- Vascular invasion in 5%-10% (renal vein, IVC, right atrium)

Staging (similar to that of adenocarcinoma in adults)

- Stage I confined to kidney, 95% 2-year survival
- Stage II extension into perinephric space, 90%
- Stage III lymph node involvement
- Stage IV metastases to lung, liver, 50%
- Stage V bilateral renal involvement
- By MRI, Wilms tumors demonstrate low-signal intensity on T1W images and high-signal intensity on T2W images. MRI also permits assessment of caval patency and multifocal disease.
- MRI has been reported to be the most sensitive modality for determination of caval patency, but it requires sedation.

Current screening recommendations for patients at risk with Wilms include:

- US every 4 months for 1 year
- Repeat imaging every 8 months for 2 years, then every 12 months until the child is age 10
- CT every 6 months for 1 year, followed by every 12 months for 4 years, and again at age 10

NEPHROBLASTOMATOSIS

Nephrogenic rests are foci of metanephric blastemasthat persist beyond 36 weeks' gestation and have the potential for malignant transformation into Wilms tumor.

- Present in 30% of unilateral Wilms tumors
- Present in 100% of bilateral Wilms tumors

Nephrogenic rests can be classified into perilobar and intralobar on the basis of location and the syndromes with which they are associated.

- Perilobar rests lie in the peripheral cortex or columns of Bertin. They are associated with Beckwith-Wiedemann syndrome, hemihypertrophy, Perlman syndrome (visceromegaly, gigantism, cryptorchidism, polyhydramnios, characteristic facies), and trisomy 18. Malignant degeneration into Wilms tumor is most common in patients with Beckwith-Wiedemann syndrome and hemihypertrophy, occurring in 3% of cases.
- Intralobar nephrogenic rests are considerably less common but have a higher association with Wilms tumors. These rests are found in 78% of patients with Drash syndrome and nearly 100% of patients with sporadic aniridia and are also seen in patients with WAGR syndrome.

Radiographic Features

- Multiple solid, subcapsular mass lesions are virtually diagnostic.
- Lesions are hypovascular (little enhancement by CT) and hypoechoic (US). By CT, macroscopic nephrogenic rests appear as low-attenuation peripheral nodules with poor enhancement relative to that of adjacent normal renal parenchyma. By MRI, the nodules demonstrate low-signal intensity foci on both T1W and T2W images.
- Requires close follow-up to screen for Wilms tumor until 7 years of age

RENAL CELL CARCINOMA (RCC)

- RCC has been reported in patients <6 months of age. However, the tumor is rare in children, accounting for less than 7% of all primary renal tumors manifesting in the first 2 decades of life.
- RCC is associated with von Hippel-Lindau disease. The tumors tend to be multiple and manifest at a young age. This disease must be ruled out in pediatric patients diagnosed with RCC, especially when the tumor is bilateral.

CLEAR CELL SARCOMA

Represents 6% of all pediatric renal tumors. Highly malignant with worse prognosis than Wilms tumor. High propensity for skeletal metastases. Cannot be distinguished from Wilms tumor by imaging studies alone.

RHABDOID TUMOR

Tumor originating in renal sinus (unlike Wilms tumor, which arises from renal cortex) representing 2% of all renal cell tumors (early childhood). Poor prognosis and common metastases to lung, liver, and brain. Associated with primary brain tumors of neuroectodermal origin including medulloblastoma, ependymoma, glioma, and PNET.

Radiographic Features

- Difficult to distinguish from Wilms tumor by imaging alone
- A centrally located renal mass with subcapsular fluid collection and posterior fossa mass will suggest correct diagnosis.
- Peripheral subcapsular fluid collection adjacent to solid tumor lobules is present in 70% of malignant rhabdoid tumors.

NEUROBLASTOMA (Fig. 11-46)

Most common abdominal malignancy in the newborn; rare tumor (incidence 1:30,000). Arises in neural crest tissue (adrenal medulla, sympathetic neural system, Zuckerkandl). Age: 2 years, better prognosis <1 year.

Clinical Findings

- Elevated VMA and HVA
- May cause paraneoplastic syndrome

Radiographic Features

- Solid tumor
- Hyperechoic by US
- Calcification in 85%
- Readily extends across midline
- Frequently encases vessels
- 65% are metastatic at initial presentation; common extensions include:
  - Bone
  - Neural foramina (evaluate)
  - Lymph nodes
  - Liver, lung (uncommon)

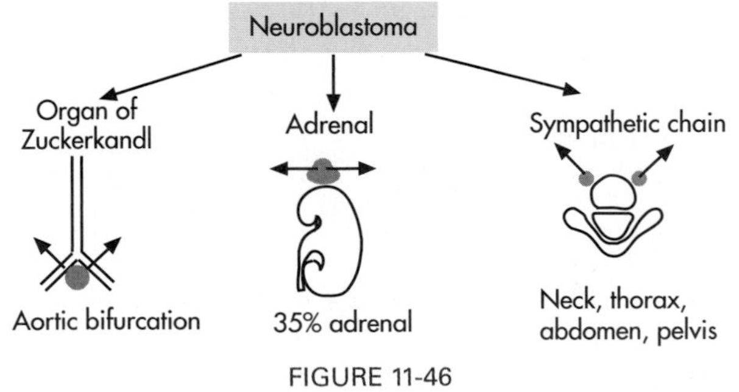

FIGURE 11-46

FEATURES DISTINGUISHING BETWEEN WILMS TUMOR AND NEUROBLASTOMA

Feature	Wilms Tumor	Neuroblastoma
Age	2-3 years	<2 years
Origin	Kidney	Retroperitoneal neural crest
Renal mass effect	Intrinsic mass effect	External compression
Laterality	10% bilateral	Almost always
Calcification	<15%	85%-95%
Vessel involvement	Renal vein invasion in 5%-10%	Frequent encasement

STAGING

- Stage 1: confined to organ of origin
- Stage 2: does not cross midline; homolateral lymph nodes
- Stage 3: crosses midline
- Stage 4: metastases to skeleton, lymph nodes
- Stage 4S: skin liver marrow; <1 year of age; good prognosis

The most important predictors of outcome are age of the patient at diagnosis and INSS disease stage. Children with stages 1, 2, and 4S tumors have a 3-year event-free survival rate of 75%-90%. Children <1 year of age with stages 3 and 4 tumors have a 1-year event-free survival rate of 80%-90% and 60%-75%, respectively. Children >1 year with INSS stages 3 and 4 tumors have a 3-year event-free survival rate of 50% and 15%, respectively.

MESOBLASTIC NEPHROMA (HAMARTOMA)

Most common solid renal mass in the neonate; uncommon in children and rare in adults. The tumor is benign (hamartoma) and is composed primarily of mesenchymal, connective tissue (cut surface looks like leiomyoma of the uterus). It is usually identified within the first 3 months of life, with 90% of cases discovered within the 1st year of life. There is a slight male predominance. Treatment is with surgical resection because of uncertainty that it may contain sarcomatous degeneration.

Radiographic Features

- Solid, very large intrarenal mass in neonate. Imaging studies demonstrate a large solid intrarenal mass that typically involves the renal sinus. The mass replaces a large portion of renal parenchyma and may contain cystic, hemorrhagic, and necrotic regions. Local infiltration of the perinephric tissues is common.
- Often evenly hypoechoic (cystic) regions

ANGIOMYOLIPOMA

- These tumors most often occur sporadically. However, they may occur in 40%-80% of patients with tuberous sclerosis. Angiomyolipoma is also associated with neurofibromatosis and von Hippel-Lindau disease.
- In children, angiomyolipomas are rare in the absence of tuberous sclerosis.
- Lesions <4 cm in diameter are typically asymptomatic; those >4 cm in diameter are more likely to spontaneously hemorrhage. Severe retroperitoneal hemorrhage has been termed *Wunderlich syndrome*.

OSSIFYING RENAL TUMOR OF INFANCY

- Ossifying renal tumor of infancy is a rare benign renal mass.
- Patients have ranged in age from 6 days to 14 months, with 10 of 11 having hematuria as the presenting symptom.
- Boys > girls
- The mass is believed to arise from urothelium and is attached to the renal medulla, specifically the papillary region of the renal pyramids. From this location, it extends in a polypoid fashion into the collecting system.
- At imaging, the renal outline is usually maintained; however, filling defects with partial obstruction of the collecting system are often seen. Because of its location within the collecting system and its characteristic ossification, ossifying renal tumor of infancy may mimic a staghorn calculus, which would be exceedingly rare in the age group in which this lesion occurs.

METANEPHRIC ADENOMA

- Metanephric adenoma, also known as nephrogenic adenofibroma or embryonal adenoma, is a benign renal tumor.
- Presenting features include pain, hypertension, hematoma, a flank mass, hypercalcemia, and polycythemia.
- No age prediction
- By US, the mass is well defined and solid. It can be hypoechoic or hyperechoic or even cystic with a mural nodule.
- By CT performed before IV administration of contrast material, the mass may be isoattenuating or hyperattenuating and small calcifications may be present. The lesion enhances less-than-normal renal parenchyma.

POSTTRANSPLANTATION LYMPHOPROLIFERATIVE DISORDER (PTLD)

- PTLD is a condition in patients who receive transplants in which chronic immunosuppression leads to unregulated expansion of lymphoid cells; the condition ranges from hyperplasia to malignant lymphoid proliferation.
- In most cases, the disorder results from the Epstein-Barr virus (EBV)–induced B-cell lymphoproliferation. The clinical, histopathologic, and imaging features of PTLD differ from those of lymphoma in immunocompetent patients, although they bear some resemblance to the lymphomas that arise in other immunocompromised patients, most notably those with acquired immunodeficiency syndrome (AIDS) or congenital T-cell immunodeficiencies.
- The abdomen is the most common anatomic region involved by PTLD. The abdomen is the only site of involvement in up 50% of patients.

Radiographic Appearance

- Liver: discrete hypoechoic or low-attenuation nodular 1- to 4-cm lesions. May be infiltrative or poorly defined. Hepatomegaly and even liver failure may result. Periportal infiltration or direct extension into the biliary tree is unique to liver transplant recipients and may result in biliary obstruction.
- Spleen: occurring in 28% of allograft recipients with abdominal disease; manifests as discrete hypoechoic or low-attenuation lesions, splenomegaly or both.
- Kidneys: occurs in less than 20% of patients with abdominal disease. Unlike renal lymphoma in the general population, PTLD of the kidney tends to be unilateral and unifocal.
- The small bowel is most frequently involved in the GI tract; colonic and gastric disease are less common. At CT, the typical appearance is circumferential wall thickening of a segment of bowel. Aneurysmal dilatation with luminal excavation, ulceration, or perforation may be an associated finding. Intussusception is another imaging manifestation of bowel involvement.

OVARIAN MASSES

Cyst

- Fairly common
- May cause large abdominal mass
- If >3 cm, need to follow up with US

Teratoma

- Most common ovarian neoplasm in children
- Most occur in adolescents
- Imaging
  - Plain film: abdominal or pelvic mass; calcification, 65%
  - US: mixed echogenicity
  - CT: soft tissue, calcific, and fatty components in tumor

Amputated Ovary

- Secondary to torsion with subsequent infarction
- Produces stippled calcification in atrophied ovary

OTHER

RHABDOMYOSARCOMA

Majority are diagnosed at age <6 years. Location: pelvis/GU tract (e.g., bladder, vagina, prostate), head and neck. Morphology may be "grape-like" (sarcoma botryoides). Pulmonary metastases.

NEONATAL ADRENAL HEMORRHAGE

Common disorder in the perinatal or occasionally prenatal period. Right 70%, left 20%, bilateral 10%. Predisposing conditions:

- Traumatic delivery
- Hypoxia
- Sepsis
- Maternal diabetes mellitus

Radiographic Features

- Initially appears as solid mass, increased density by CT early
- Doppler US may help distinguish from solid mass
- Liquefaction occurs within 10 days to produce a cystlike appearance.
- Wall calcification
- Main differential diagnosis: neuroblastoma

RENAL ARTERY STENOSIS

- Fibromuscular hyperplasia (most common)
- Other less common causes:
  - Neurofibromatosis
  - Williams syndrome (idiopathic hypercalcemia of infancy)
  - Middle aortic syndrome
  - Takayasu arteritis
  - Posttransplant

RENAL VEIN THROMBOSIS

Enlarged echogenic kidneys with loss of corticomedullary differentiation. Causes include:

- Nephrotic syndrome
- Protein C or S deficiency
- Dehydration
- Polycythemia
- Burns
- Left adrenal hemorrhage
- Posttransplant

Musculoskeletal System

TRAUMA

GENERAL

The immature skeleton has growth plates, cartilaginous epiphysis, and a thick, strong periosteum. Pediatric bone is more elastic than adult bone: bowing and bending. Bowing fracture injuries are therefore more common than breaking and splintering. Overall, childhood fractures are less common than adult fractures.

Types of Fractures (Fig. 11-47)

- Elastic deformation (momentary)
- Bowing (permanent)
- Torus (buckle) fractures: buckling of cortex
- Greenstick fracture: incomplete transverse fracture with intact periosteum on the concave side and ruptured periosteum on the convex side. Occurs in patients of elementary school age.
- Complete fracture

Fracture Healing

Fracture healing is rapid in children.

- Periosteal new bone: 1 week
- Loss of fracture line: 2 to 3 weeks
- Hard callus: 2 to 4 weeks
- Remodeling of bone: 12 months

Pearls

- Hyperemia from fracture healing may lead to overgrowth of an extremity.

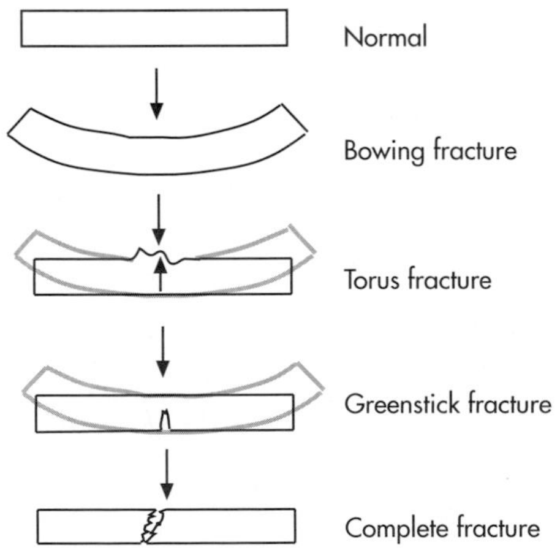

FIGURE 11-47

NORMAL VARIANTS FREQUENTLY CONFUSED WITH DISEASE

- Nutrient foramina: lucencies extending through cortex with straight parallel margins. Usually extend away from joint central to periphery.
- Scalloping of medial distal fibula: this finding may be confused with a buckle fracture or superficial bone destruction.
- Serpentine physes may appear as lucencies suggesting fracture.
- Distal femoral cortical irregularity: posteromedial metaphysis
- Apophyses of the inferior pubic ramus: these apophyses often ossify asymmetrically.
- Dense metaphyseal bands affecting zone of provisional calcification; most common 2 to 6 years of age.
- Calcaneal apophyses: normally denser than adjacent bone; frequently fragmented
- Calcaneal pseudocyst

SALTER-HARRIS FRACTURES (Fig. 11-48)

Epiphyseal plate fractures are analogous to ligamentous injuries in the adult. Growth plate injuries represent 35% of all skeletal injuries in children. Age: 10-15 years (75%). The most common sites for injury are wrist (50%) and ankle (30%). Because the physis is injured in Salter-Harris fractures permanent deformities may occur. Increasing grade correlates with increasing risk of deformity; risk of deformity also varies with joint: distal femur > distal radius. Mnemonic: "SALTR:"

- **S**lipped (type 1)
- **A**bove (type 2)
- **L**ower (type 3)
- **T**ogether (type 4)
- **R**uined (type 5)

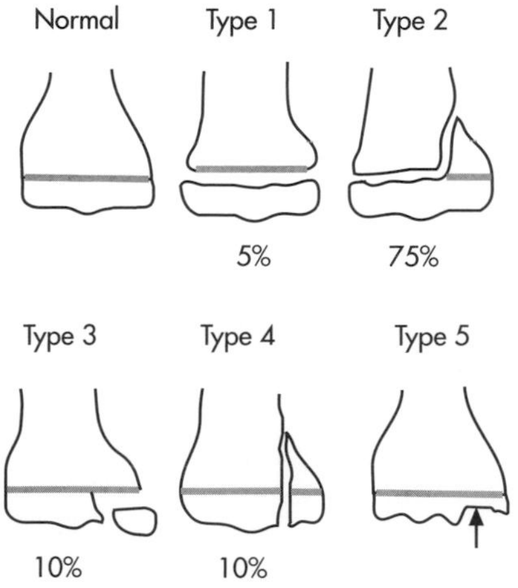

FIGURE 11-48

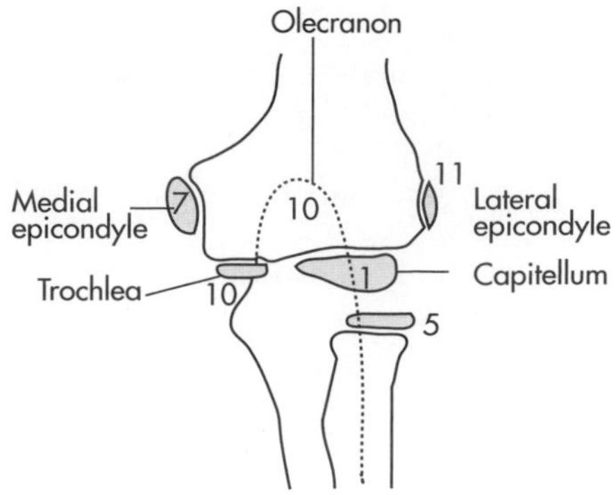

FIGURE 11-49

ELBOW INJURIES

The distal humeral shaft has 4 ossification centers. Ossification sequence (mnemonic: "CRITOE") (Fig. 11-49):

- **C**apitellum, 1 year
- **R**adial head, 5 years
- **I**nternal (medial) epicondyle, 7 years
- **T**rochlea, 10 years
- **O**lecranon, 10 years
- **E**xternal (lateral) epicondyle, 11 years

In females, ossification centers appear 1 to 2 years earlier than in males.

Several radiologic lines and signs are important in evaluating elbow injuries (Fig. 11-50):

- Anterior humeral line passes through the middle third of the capitellum.
- Radiocapitellar line passes through the capitellum on all views and confirms the articulation between radial head and the capitellum.
- Coronoid line projects anterior to the developing capitellum.
- Fat pad sign (posterior pad is normally absent, anterior fat pad is usually present); absence of the posterior fat pad sign virtually excludes a fracture (90% of patients with fat pad sign have a fracture)

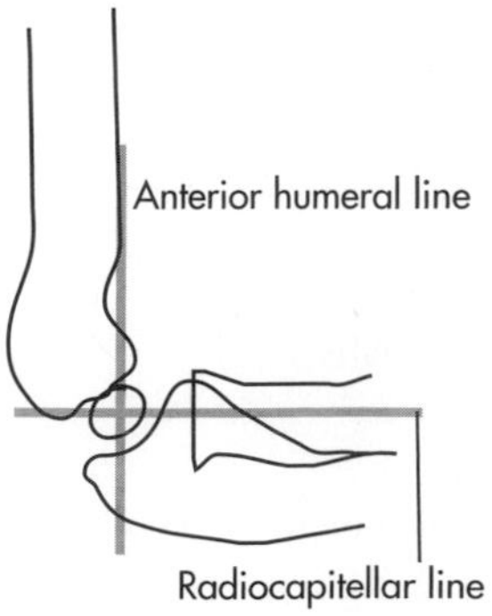

FIGURE 11-50

Common Types (Fig. 11-51)

- Supracondylar fracture, 60%
- Lateral condylar fracture, 15%
- Medial epicondylar fractures, 10%

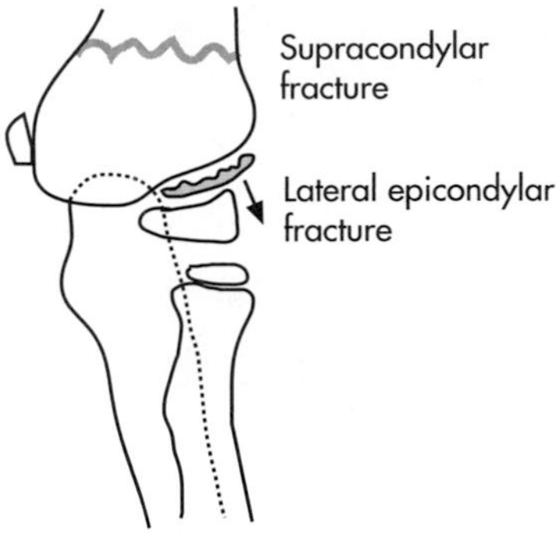

FIGURE 11-51

LITTLE LEAGUE ELBOW

Inflammatory reaction (epiphysitis) of the medial epicondyle as a response to trauma (avulsion tear).

AVULSION FRACTURES (Fig. 11-52)

Abnormal stress on ligaments and tendons. Common sites:

- Iliac spine
  - Superior: sartorius
  - Inferior: rectus femoris
- Pubic ramus: adductors, gracilis
- Lesser trochanter: iliopsoas

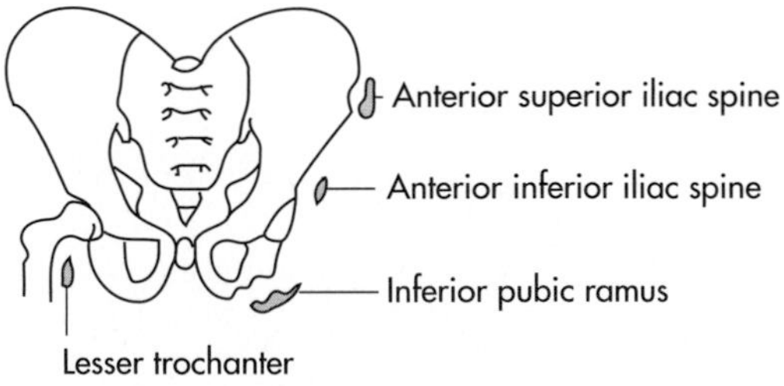

FIGURE 11-52

OSTEOCHONDROSIS DISSECANS (Fig. 11-53)

Marginal fracture of subchondral bone, adjacent cartilage, or both near a joint surface. Male/female = 3:1. Bilateral in 35%. 50% of patients have a history of trauma. In osteochondrosis dissecans of the knee, the medial epicondyle is affected in 90%.

Radiographic Features

- Lucent epicondyle defects, sclerotic edges
- Loose body may be present in joint (but is not seen on plain film unless it is a bony rather than only cartilaginous chip)

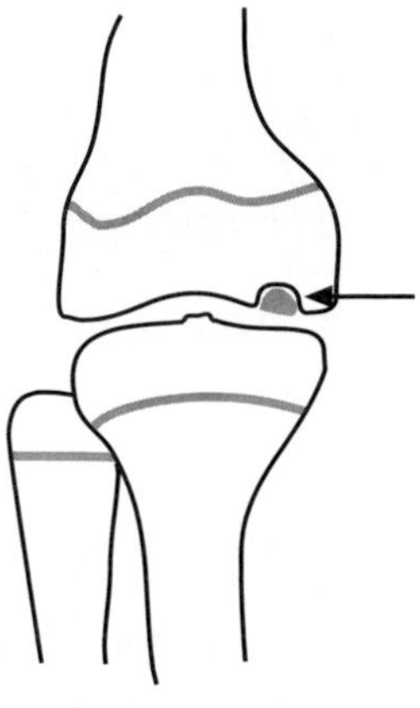

FIGURE 11-53

TODDLER'S FRACTURE

Stress fracture in lower extremity commonly due to fall. Most common fracture sites:

- Isolated spiral fracture of the tibial shaft
- Calcaneal fracture
- Cuboid fracture

STUBBED TOE

Fracture of the distal phalanx of the great toe. May present as an open fracture because of the proximity to the nail matrix and skin damage. Risk of osteomyelitis. Prophylactic antibiotics are recommended.

BATTERED CHILD (TRAUMA X) (Figs. 11-54 and 11-55)

Incidence: 1% of trauma. Injuries:

- Fractures (see below; absence of fractures does not imply absence of abuse)

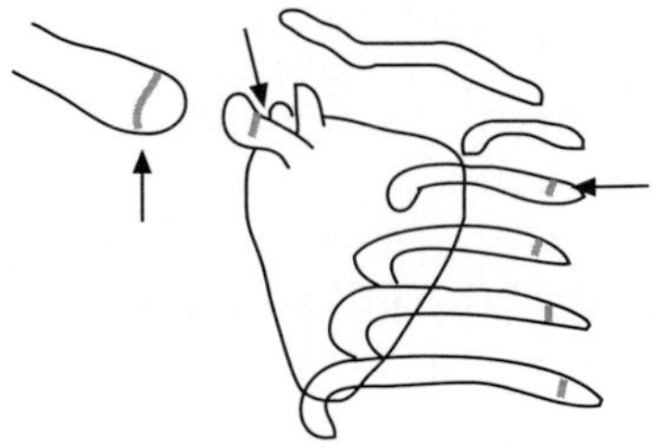

FIGURE 11-54

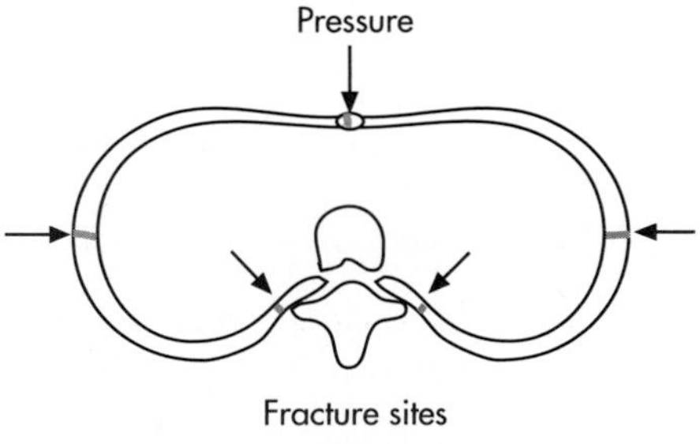

FIGURE 11-55

- CNS
  - Subdural hematoma
  - Retinal hemorrhage
- Chest
  - Pneumothorax, pneumoperitoneum
- Abdomen
  - Retroperitoneal hematoma
  - Pancreatic pseudocysts

Radiographic Features

Typical for battered child:

- Most common child abuse fracture is the diaphyseal fracture, which is indistinguishable from an innocent fracture.
- Highly specific fractures are less common and include metaphyseal fractures of long bones.
- Posterior rib fractures

The "3 Ss"

- Scapular fractures, uncommon
- Spinous process fractures, uncommon
- Sternal fractures, uncommon

Common fractures also often seen in other types of trauma:

- Multiple, bilateral fractures
- Skull fractures
- Fractures of long bones

X-RAY VERSUS SCINTIGRAPHY FOR DETECTION OF CHILD ABUSE

	Skeletal Survey	Bone Scan
Sensitivity	Moderate	High
Specificity	High	Low
Sedation required	Rare	Common
Radiation dose	Very low	Low
Need for additional studies	Occasionally	Always
Cost	Low	High
Utility	Screening	Equivocal cases

INFECTION

HEMATOGENOUS OSTEOMYELITIS

Common hematogenous bacterial osteomyelitis pathogens in children:

- Children (unifocal): *Staphylococcus* (85%), *Streptococcus* (10%)
- Neonates (multifocal): *Streptococcus, Staphylococcus*
- Immunocompromised adults: short bones of hand and feet: *Staphylococcus*
- Drug addicts: *Pseudomonas,* 85%, *Klebsiella, Enterobacter*
- Sickle cell disease: *Salmonella*

In otherwise healthy adults, hematogenous osteomyelitis is very rare; osteomyelitis in adults usually follows direct implantation after surgery or trauma.

Pathogenesis

Bacteria pass through nutrient vessels to metaphyses, where organisms proliferate. Metaphyseal inflammatory reaction progresses to edema, pus, necrosis, thrombosis. In older children, the cartilaginous growth plate becomes avascular and acts as a barrier to epiphyseal extension.

Location (Fig. 11-56)

- Tubular bones with most rapid growth and largest metaphyses are most commonly affected, 75%: femur > tibia > fibula; distal end > proximal end
- Flat bones are less frequently infected, 30%: vertebral bodies, iliac bones

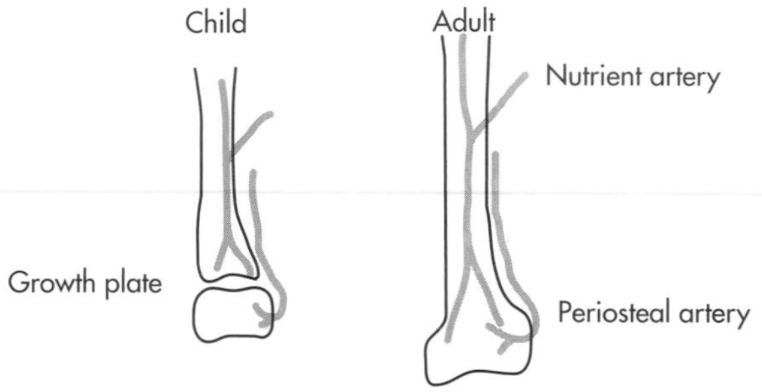

FIGURE 11-56

Radiographic Features

Detection

- Bone scan (^{99m}Tc-MDP > ^{67}Ga imaging) becomes positive within 24 hours after onset of symptoms (90% accuracy).
- Hyperemia on blood pool images
- Hot spot on delayed images
- Plain film
  - Soft tissue swelling, obliteration of fat planes: 3 days
  - Bone destruction, periosteal reaction: 5 to 7 days (children), 10 to 14 days (adults)

Plain film (Fig. 11-57)

- Soft tissue swelling (earliest sign; often in metaphyseal region), blurring of fat planes, sinus tract formation, soft tissue abscess
- Cortical loss (5 to 7 days after infection), bone destruction

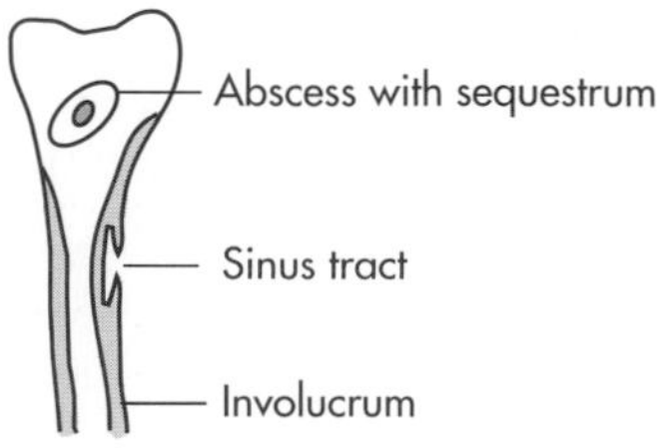

FIGURE 11-57

- Involucrum: shell of periosteum around infected bone (20 days after infection)
- Sequestrum: segmented or necrotic cortical bone separated from living bone by granulation tissue; may be extruded (30 days after infection)
- Periosteal bone formation
- Separation of epiphysis/metaphysis

CHRONIC OSTEOMYELITIS

Chronic osteomyelitis may follow acute osteomyelitis. Often caused by less virulent organism, increased resistance, or partial treatment.

Radiographic Features

- Brodie's abscess:
  - Lucent well-defined lesion with thick sclerotic rim
  - Typically in metaphysis or diaphysis of long bones
- Thick and dense cortex
- Sinus tracts to skin

CONGENITAL INFECTIONS

Rubella

Bone changes in 50% of patients.

Radiographic Features

- "Celery stalking" of metaphysis with vertically oriented, alternating stripes of radiolucency and radiodensity
- Absence of periosteal reaction (unlike congenital syphilis)
- Dense diaphysis
- Delayed appearance of epiphyses

Syphilis

Bone changes may lag infection by 6 to 8 weeks.

Radiographic Features

- Metaphyseal lucent bands
- Symmetrical periosteal reaction
- Wimberger's sign (bilateral destructive lesion on medial aspect proximal tibial metaphysis)
- Should not be confused with Wimberger's ring (dense ring of demineralized epiphysis seen in scurvy)

DEGENERATIVE AND CHRONIC TRAUMATIC DISEASE

OVERVIEW (Fig. 11-58)

Three distinct conditions of the hip occur in children, each of which affects a different age group:

- Neonates, infants: congenital dislocation of the hip (CDH)

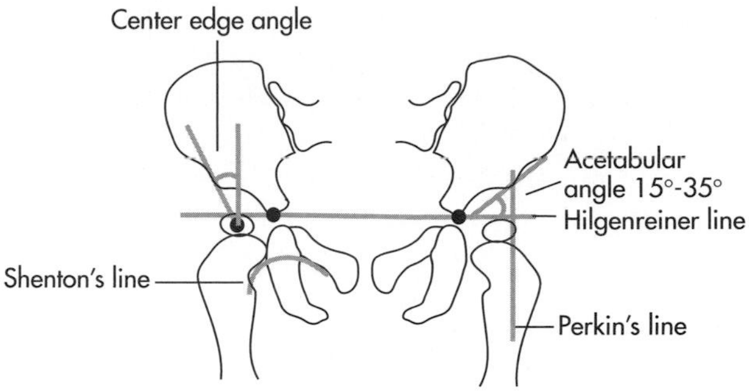

FIGURE 11-58

- School age: Legg-Calvé-Perthes (LCP) disease
- Adolescents: slipped capital femoral epiphysis (SCFE)

OVERVIEW

	CDH	LCP	SCFE
Age	Neonate	5-8 years	Puberty
Sex	Females (estrogen)	Males	Overweight males
Cause	Joint laxity: femoral head falls out of acetabulum	Osteonecrosis	Salter-Harris 1 fracture
Imaging	Putti's triad	Subchondral fissure	Posterior slippage
	US diagnostic	Fragmented epiphysis	Irregular growth plate

DEVELOPMENTAL DYSPLASIA OF THE HIP (DDH) (CONGENITAL DISLOCATION OF THE HIP) (Fig. 11-59)

An abnormally lax joint capsule allows the femoral head to fall out of the acetabulum, leading to deformation. Predisposing factors for the development of DDH are:

- Abnormal ligamentous laxity (effect of estrogen; female:male = 6:1)
- Acetabular dysplasia (there are 2 components to the acetabular dysplasia: increased acetabular angle and shallow acetabular fossae)

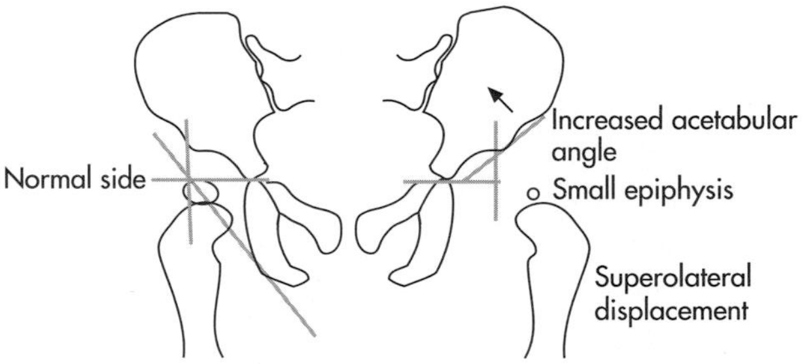

FIGURE 11-59

DDH occurs most commonly (70%) in the left hip. Bilateral involvement is seen in 5%. Treatment:
- Cast: flexion + abduction + external rotation
- Salter osteotomy if chronic

Clinical Findings
- Ortolani's jerk or click sign: relocation click while abducting hip with thumb and placing pressure on greater trochanter
- Barlow's sign: dislocation click while adducting hip with pressure on knee
- Limited abduction of flexed hip
- Shortening of one leg
- Waddling gait

Radiographic Features

US (commonly used today) (Fig. 11-60)
- Normal femoral head is covered at least 50% by acetabulum.
- In DDH, <50% of femoral head is covered by acetabulum.
- Normal alpha angle is >60°.
- In DDH, alpha angle is <60°.

Plain film (rarely used today)
- Radiographic landmarks:
  - Hilgenreiner's line: Drawn through right and left triradiate cartilage
  - Perkin's line: vertical through lateral acetabular margin; should bisect middle third femoral metaphysis
  - Shenton's line: Drawn along medial proximal femur and inferior border of superior pubic ramus

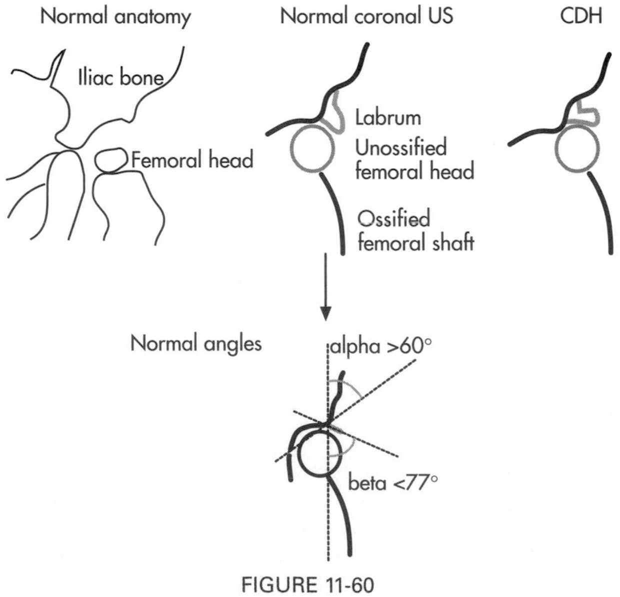

FIGURE 11-60

- Putti's triad:
  - Superolateral displacement of proximal femur
  - Increase in acetabular angle
  - Small capital femoral epiphysis
- Femoral head is located lateral to Perkin's line
- Other features that are sometimes present:
  - Abnormal sclerosis of the acetabulum
  - Formation of a false acetabulum
  - Shallow acetabulum and other deformities
  - Delayed ossification of femoral head

Pearls
- In the neonate, radiographic evaluation of hip dislocation is unreliable because paucity of skeletal ossification and maternal hormones can cause joint laxity; diagnosis becomes more reliable at 1 to 2 months of age.
- AP is the best view to demonstrate abnormalities; the frogleg view is useless because the hip is reduced in this position.
- US may demonstrate fibrofatty tissue (pulvinar) between acetabulum and femoral head

LEGG-CALVÉ-PERTHES (LCP) DISEASE

Avascular necrosis of the femoral head. Age: white males, 5 to 8 years. Bilateral in 15%. Treatment: the femoral head or acetabular component has to be remodeled to achieve acetabular coverage and thus prevent lateral subluxation:
- Abduction bracing (cast)
- Varus derotation osteotomy

Radiographic Features (Fig. 11-61)

Early phase
- Widened joint: may be due to increased cartilage or joint effusion (earliest sign)
- Subchondral fissure fracture, best seen on frogleg view (tangential view of cartilage)
- Increase in bone density

Intermediate phase
- Granular, fragmented appearance of femoral epiphysis due to calcification of avascular cartilage (no fracture of epiphysis)
- Lateralization of ossification center
- Cysts of demineralization (30%)
- Apposition of new bone makes the femoral head appear dense.

Late phase
- Flattened and distorted femoral head
- Osteoarthritis (OA)

MRI
- MRI is useful for the early detection of disease before radiographic or scintigraphic findings become apparent.
- Useful for evaluation of femoral head coverage by acetabulum

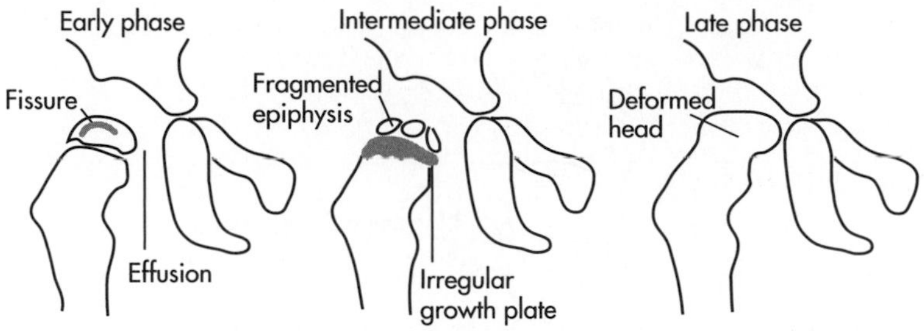

FIGURE 11-61

- Allows assessment of articular cartilage. Thickening of the hyaline cartilage leads to lateral displacement of femoral head.
- In LCP disease the normal high signal intensity of the femoral head epiphysis is low on T1W and T2W images. During the repair phase, fat-containing marrow returns to the epiphysis, and high signal intensity appears.

SLIPPED CAPITAL FEMORAL EPIPHYSIS (SCFE)

Similar appearance as a Salter-Harris type 1 epiphyseal plate fracture of the proximal femur. Cause is unknown. Age: overweight teenagers. Clinical findings: pain, 90%; history of trauma, 50%. Treatment is with fixation of femoral epiphysis (pins, bone pegs).

Radiographic Features (Fig. 11-62)

- 15%-25% are bilateral; subtle changes are difficult to detect.
- Always obtain AP and lateral views.
- Malalignment of epiphysis: femoral neck line (Salter-Harris type 1 fracture)
- Widened growth plate
- Decreased height of epiphysis (slips posterior)
- Decreased angle of femoral neck anteversion by CT

Complications

- Osteonecrosis
- Chondrolysis (cartilage necrosis) from pins
- Varus deformity
- Degenerative OA

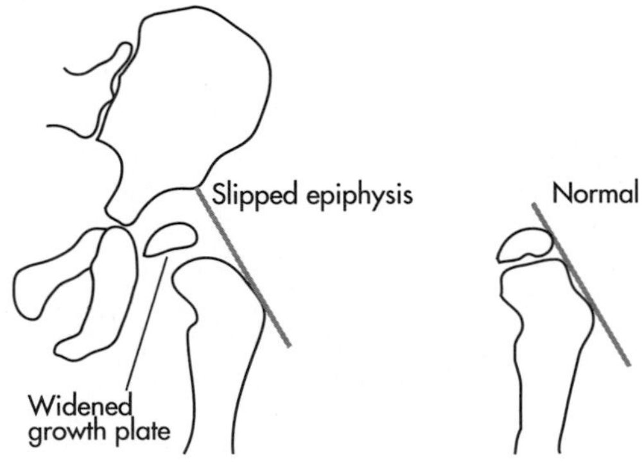

FIGURE 11-62

OSTEOCHONDROSIS

Abnormal bone and cartilage at the end of bone. The term is a catch-all term referring to a spectrum of diseases:

Abnormal endochondral ossification secondary to repeated stress without osteonecrosis
- Scheuermann disease: spine
- Blount disease: tibial epiphysis
- Osgood-Schlatter disease: tibial tubercle

Osteonecrosis disease
- Kienböck disease: lunate
- Freiberg disease: metatarsals
- LCP

SCHEUERMANN DISEASE (ADOLESCENT KYPHOSIS)

Vertebral osteochondrosis refers to the kyphotic deformity of the thoracic (75%) or thoracolumbar (25%) spine in teenagers (13 to 17 years). Diagnostic criteria:

- Kyphosis must be >35°
- Anterior wedging of at least one vertebral body of >5°
- Usually 3 to 5 vertebral bodies are involved.

Schmorl's theory: all pathologic changes in the spine result from herniation of disk material through congenital defects into the vertebral endplates during time of excessive growth in adolescence.

Radiographic Features (Fig. 11-63)

- Progressive narrowing of disk spaces
- Wedging of the anterior portion of vertebral bodies (posterior portion protected by posterior articulation)
- Irregularity of endplates
- Changes seen in >3 vertebral bodies
- Multiple Schmorl's nodes

RADIOULNAR SYNOSTOSIS

Congenital or acquired fusion of the proximal radius and ulna, with cortical and medullary continuation. Usually normal function. May be associated with other abnormalities: Madelung deformity and clubfoot.

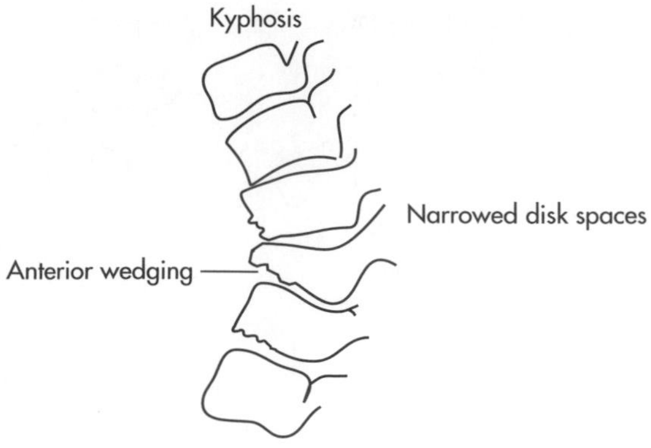

FIGURE 11-63

BLOUNT DISEASE (CONGENITAL TIBIA VARA)

Abnormal endochondral ossification caused by stress and compression. The disease results in deformity of the medial proximal tibial metaphysis and epiphysis. Two forms of Blount disease are distinguished: early onset (infantile, onset 1 to 3 years) and late onset (juvenile, 4 to 10 years; adolescent) forms. Both forms occur more commonly in obese black children.

Clinical Findings

- Bowed legs
- Pain

BLOUNT DISEASE

	Early Onset (Infantile)	Late Onset (Juvenile, Adolescent)
Onset	1-3 years	>4 years
Frequency	Common	Infrequent
Site	Bilateral (80%)	Unilateral (90%)
Recurrence after surgery	Low	High
Course	Progressive deformity	Less deformity

Radiographic Features (Fig. 11-64)

- Fragmentation of medial tibial epiphysis
- Irregular medial physeal line
- Beaking of proximal medial tibial metaphysis
- Bone bridge across the medial physis while the lateral growth plate remains open
- Metaphyseal-diaphyseal angle (MDA) >11°
- Tibiofemoral angle (TFA) >15°, i.e., tibia vara; this finding alone, however, is not diagnostic of Blount disease.

OSGOOD-SCHLATTER DISEASE

Painful irregularity of tibial tuberosity secondary to repeated trauma to deep fibers of patellar tendon. Male:female = 5:1; 25% are bilateral.

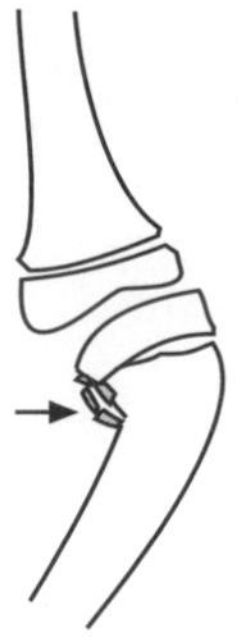

FIGURE 11-64

Radiographic Features

- Irregular tibial tuberosity
- Thickening of patellar tendon; soft tissue swelling around patellar ligament
- Obliteration of infrapatellar fat pad

FREIBERG DISEASE

Osteonecrosis of the distal end of the 2nd (75%) or 3rd (25%) metatarsal. Bilateral in 10% of patients. Occurs between age 11 and 15 years. Freiberg disease is the only osteonecrosis more frequent in females (75%) than in males (25%). Commonly associated with hallux valgus and short 1st metatarsal.

FOOT ANGLES (Figs. 11-65 and 11-66)

Diagnosis of foot abnormalities requires measurement of angles between talus and calcaneus and between forefoot and hindfoot. Films should be obtained while weight bearing.

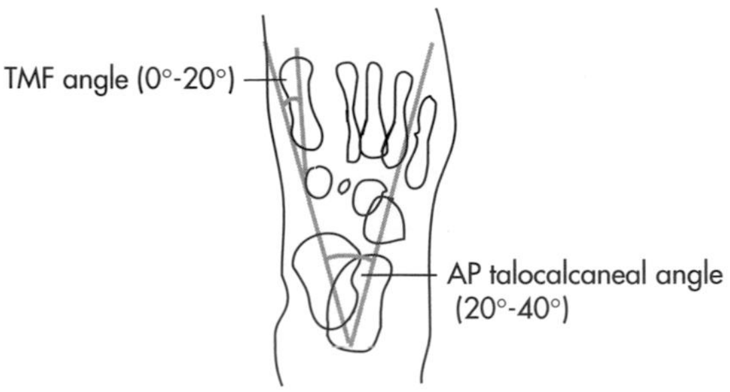

FIGURE 11-65

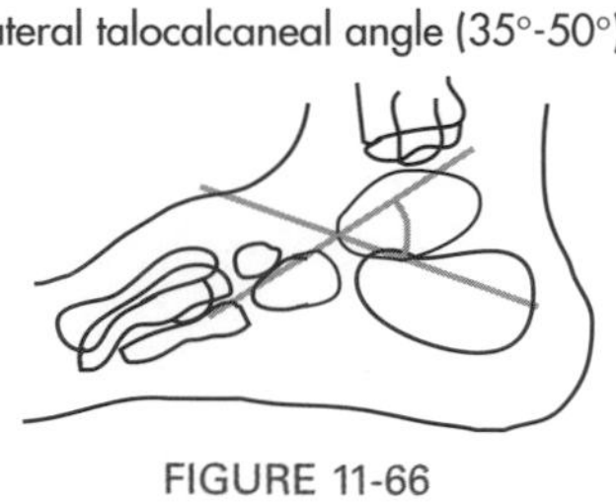

FIGURE 11-66

CLUBFOOT (TALIPES EQUINOVARUS) (Fig. 11-67)

Common abnormality (1:1000); bilateral 50%. The typical clubfoot contains 4 separate components (always need an AP and lateral view):

- Hindfoot varus is the key radiologic finding: AP talocalcaneal angle <20°
- Equinus deformity of the heel: lateral talocalcaneal angle <35°
- Adduction and varus deformity of the forefoot (metatarsus adductus): 1st metatarsal bone is displaced medially with respect to the long axis of the talus.
- Talonavicular subluxation: medial subluxation of the navicular bone; the subluxation is infrequently diagnosed because ossification has not occurred at the time of clubfoot diagnosis.

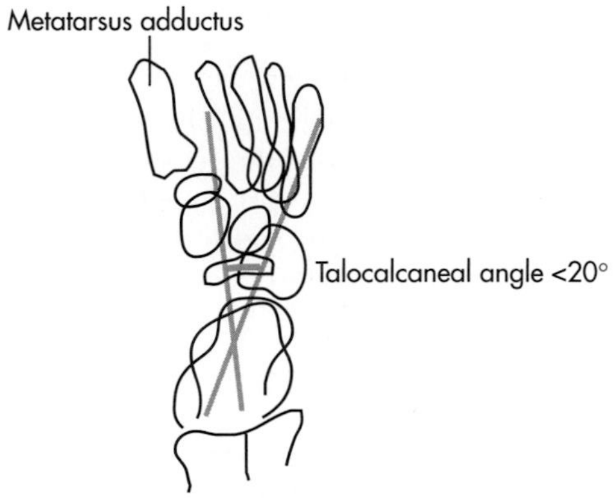

FIGURE 11-67

CONGENITAL VERTICAL TALUS (Fig. 11-68)

Rare deformity characterized by dorsal dislocation of the navicular bone on the talus. Axis of the talus is steep, and a convex plantar surface of the foot may result (rockerbottom feet). Associations include:

- Meningomyelocele
- Arthrogryposis
- Trisomies 13 and 18

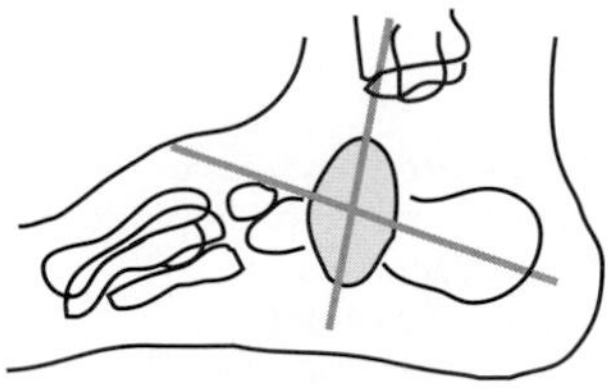

FIGURE 11-68

TARSAL COALITION (Fig. 11-69)

Fusion of 2 or more tarsal bones. Union may be complete, partial, bony, cartilaginous, or fibrous. Present at birth but usually asymptomatic until early adulthood. Location:

- Calcaneonavicular (most common)
- Talocalcaneal (common)

Commonly results in spastic flatfoot. Bilateral. C sign in subtalar bony coalition.

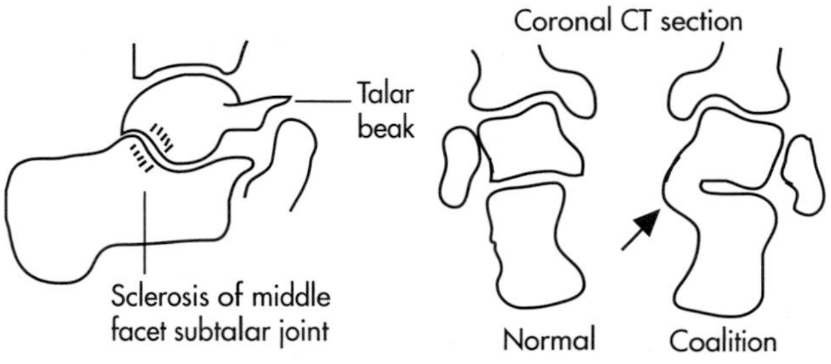

FIGURE 11-69

VARUS AND VALGUS (Fig. 11-70)

Varus and valgus refer to the relationship of a distal part of an extremity to a proximal part (e.g., femur/tibia). Varus refers to an angulation of the distal bone toward the midline. Valgus refers to an angulation of the distal bone away from the midline.

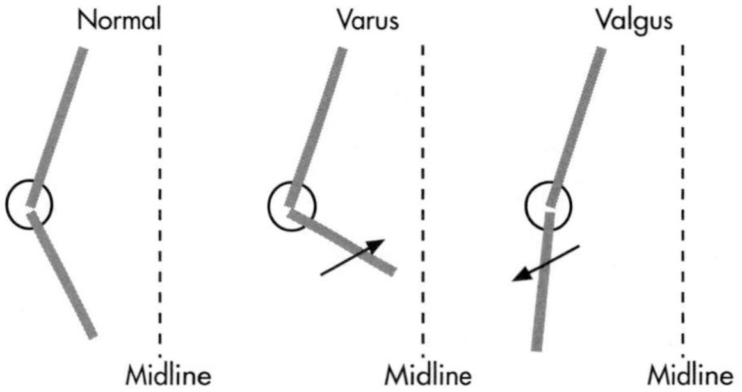

FIGURE 11-70

METABOLIC ABNORMALITIES

RICKETS (Fig. 11-71)

Vitamin D deficiency causes failure of mineralization of bone and cartilage (in adults this is termed *osteomalacia*). Causes of vitamin D deficiency include:

GI tract

- Nutritional deficiency (common)
- Absorption abnormalities

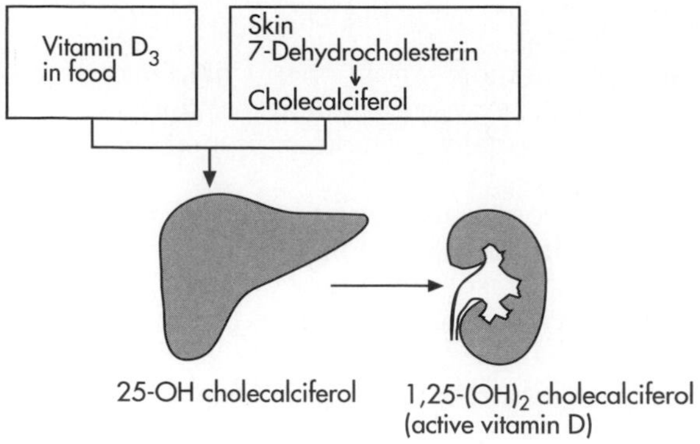

FIGURE 11-71

Skin disease
Liver disease
Renal
- Renal tubular acidosis
- Renal failure (loss of calcium)

Radiographic Features (Fig. 11-72)

Infantile rickets (6 to 18 months of age)
- Growth plate abnormalities (especially long bones)
  - A widened growth plate is due to rickets until proved otherwise.

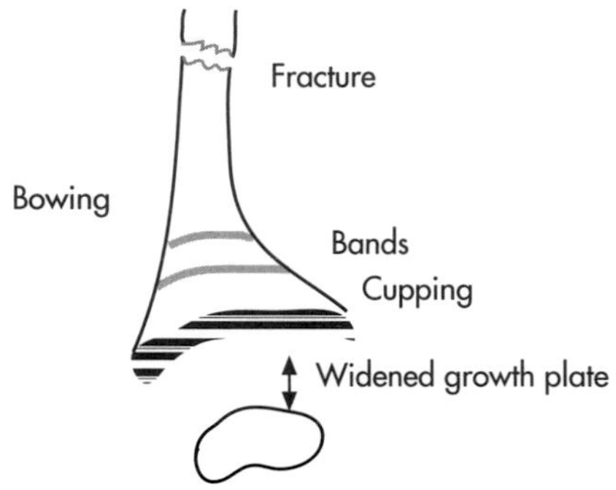

FIGURE 11-72

Cupping of metaphysis
Disorganized (frayed) metaphysis
- Bowing deformities of bones
- Delayed closing of fontanelles
- Softening of cranial vault (craniotabes)
- Rachitic rosary: enlargement of cartilage at costochondral junction

Vitamin D–resistant rickets (>2 years of age)
- Bowing of extremities is marked.
- Bones may appear sclerotic occasionally.

CONGENITAL ANOMALIES

Radiologic parameters used in the description of dysplasias:
- Size of bones
- Pattern of distribution of abnormal bones
- Bone density and structure
- Shape of bones
- Time of onset of abnormality

DWARFISM (Figs. 11-73 and 11-74)

Skeletal dysplasias can be categorized according to the relative shortening of humerus or femur in relation to radius or tibia:
- Rhizomelic dysplasia: shortening of proximal limb (humerus or femur) in relation to distal limb (radius or tibia)

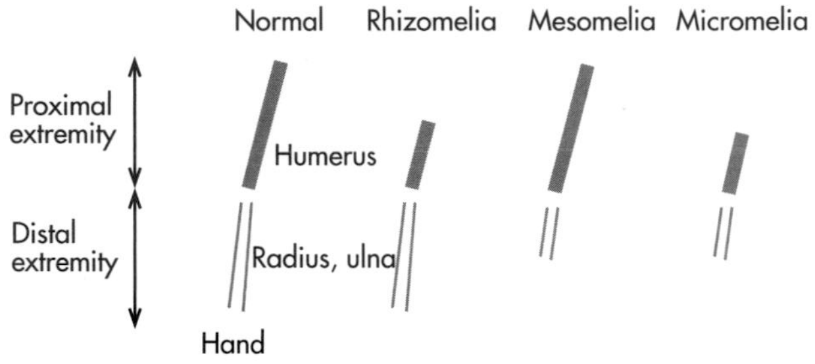

FIGURE 11-73

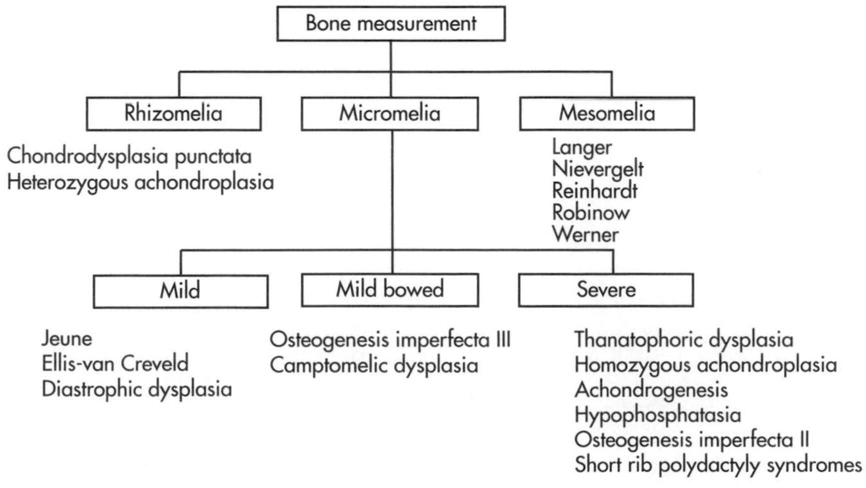

FIGURE 11-74

OVERVIEW OF SYNDROMES

Syndrome	Lethal	In Utero Features (US)	Other Features
Rhizomelia			
Chondrodysplasia punctata	Yes	Hypertelorism, metaphyseal splaying, coronal clefts in vertebra bodies	Stippled epiphyses
Achondroplasia (heterozygous form)	No	Femur length normal until 20 wk; below 95% confidence limits of mean by 27 wk	See p. 618
Mesomelia			
Langer, Nievergelt, Reinhardt, Robinow, Werner syndromes	No	Mesomelic shortening	
Mild Micromelia			
Jeune syndrome (asphyxiating thoracic dysplasia)	Yes	Small thorax; squared iliac wings; polydactyly; ± renal anomalies	Similar to Ellis-van Creveld syndrome
Ellis-van Creveld syndrome	Yes	Similar to Jeune syndrome; ASD 50%	
Diastrophic dysplasia	No	Clubfoot; hitchhiker thumb; scoliosis; joint flexion contractures	
Mild Bowed Micromelia			
Camptomelic dysplasia	Yes	Anterior bowing of the femur and tibia; short fibulae; limbs short due to bowing; ± scoliosis; absent scapulae	
Osteogenesis imperfecta type III	No	Long bones shortened; bowed; ± fractures; humeri less severely involved than femora	See text below
Severe Micromelia			
Thanatophoric dysplasia	Yes	Limb bowing; narrowed thorax; hydramnios; cloverleaf skull (15%); ± ascites or nonimmune hydrops	Both parents of normal stature
Achondroplasia, homozygous form	Yes	Resembles thanatophoric with cloverleaf skull	Rib fractures
Osteogenesis imperfecta type II	Yes	Multiple fractures; hypomineralization; thick long bones	
Hypophosphatasia (congenital lethal)	Yes	Similar to osteogenesis imperfecta; poor mineralization	No rib fracture
Achondrogenesis	Yes	Absent vertebral ossification	
Short rib polydactyly syndromes	Yes	Short ribs; narrow thorax; polydactyly	

- Mesomelic dysplasia: shortening of distal limb (radius or tibia) in relation to proximal limb (humerus or femur)
- Micromelic dysplasia: shortening of proximal and distal limbs

Pearls

- The diagnosis of a specific skeletal dysplasia is based on the best fit of clinical, biochemical, and radiologic data.
- A specific diagnosis is often of no help in management except for determining prognosis and genetic counseling.

OSTEOGENESIS IMPERFECTA (OI)

Inadequate osteoid formation but normal mineralization (thin, osteoporotic fragile bones) causes severe bowing and fractures. Autosomal dominant, 1:40,000 births.

Classification

Type 1: tarda form (OIT, Ekman-Lobstein syndrome), 90%: more benign form with normal life expectancy.
- Blue sclerae, 90%
- Laxity of ligaments
- Dental abnormalities (dentin dysplasia), 30%
- Deafness (otosclerosis), 20%
- Osseous abnormalities

Type 2: congenita (OIC, Vrolik type), 10%: death in utero or neonatal period; detected by prenatal US

Type 3: fractures at birth, progressive limb deformity, occasional fractures, normal sclerae and hearing

Type 4: bone fragility, normal sclerae, normal hearing, discolored teeth

Radiographic Features

General
- Bowing deformities: genu valgum, coxa vara
- Thinning of cortex
- Frequent fractures

Skull
- Wormian bones

Spine
- Vertebral scalloping
- Severe kyphoscoliosis

Pelvis
- Acetabular protrusion is common.

ACHONDROPLASIA

Common dysplasia characterized by abnormal bone formation at growth plate. Autosomal dominant (homozygous forms fatal, patients with heterozygous form have normal life span).

Radiographic Features (Figs. 11-75 and 11-76)
- Rhizomelic dwarfism: short limbs (particularly proximal segments of femurs, humerus)
- Short and stubby fingers (bullet-shaped)
- Trident hand
- Spine
  - Short interpedicular distance (typical)
  - The interpedicular distance narrows distally
  - Spinal stenosis is due to short pedicles.

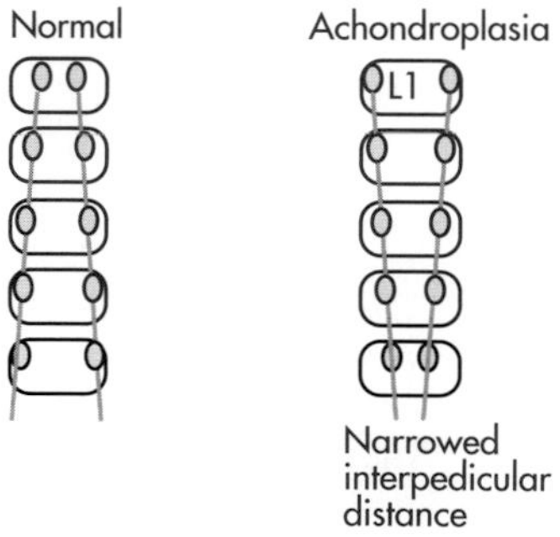

FIGURE 11-75

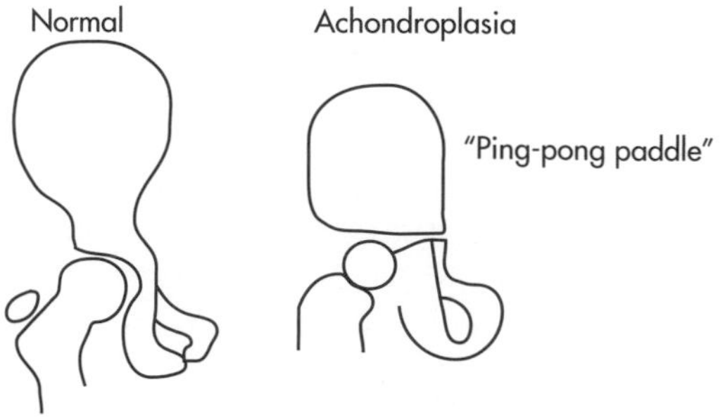

FIGURE 11-76

- "Ping-pong-paddle" pelvis
  - Rounded iliac bones
  - Champagne pelvis
  - Horizontal acetabular roofs
- Skull
  - Small skull base (enchondral ossification) and small foramen magnum
  - Normal-sized calvarium (membranous ossification): frontal bossing
  - Basilar invagination

ASPHYXIATING THORACIC DYSTROPHY (JEUNE SYNDROME)

Jeune syndrome is characterized by distal (acromelic) limb shortening.

Radiographic Features
- Narrow thorax, expanded ribs
- Handlebar clavicles
- Horizontal acetabular roofs with downward-projecting spurs
- Shortened tubular bones with coned-shaped epiphysis

CHONDROECTODERMAL DYSPLASIA (ELLIS-VAN CREVELD SYNDROME)

Ellis-van Creveld syndrome is characterized by distal (acromelic) limb shortening.

Radiographic Features
- Polydactyly (always present)
- Proximal phalanges longer than distal phalanges
- Shortened tubular bones with coned-shaped epiphysis
- Short ribs
- ASD, 50%
- Ectodermal changes (e.g., nails, teeth, hair)

MUCOPOLYSACCHARIDOSIS

Excess of mucopolysaccharide accumulation secondary to enzyme deficiencies. The specific diagnosis is made according to:
- Age
- IQ
- Corneal clouding
- Urinary excretion of heparan, keratin, dermatan
- Other clinical findings

Radiographic Features

Osteoporosis

Spine
- Oval, hook-shaped vertebral bodies
  - Hunter/Hurler: inferior vertebral beaking
  - Morquio: central vertebral beaking
- Severe hyperlordosis, scoliosis

MUCOPOLYSACCHARIDOSIS SYNDROMES

Type	Name	Inheritance	Deficient Enzyme	Prominent Features
1H	Hurler	AR	α-L-Iduronidase	CC, LIQ, HS
1S	Scheie	AR	α-L-Iduronidase	CC, aortic valve disease
2	Hunter	Male recessive	α-L-iduronate-2-sulfatase	LIQ
3	Sanfilippo	AR	Heparan *N*-sulfatase	LIQ, coarse facial features
4	Morquio	AR	Galactosamine-6-sulfate sulfatase	CC, HS, dwarfism
6	Maroteaux-Lamy	AR	Arylsulfatase B	Short stature, HS
7	Sly	AR	Glucuronidase	LIQ, HS, pneumonias
8	DiFerrante	Genetic trait	Glucosamine-6-sulfate sulfatase	Short stature

AR, autosomal recessive; CC, corneal clouding; HS, hepatosplenomegaly; LIQ, low IQ.

Pelvis
- Hypoplastic with some flaring

Extremities
- Shortened bones
- Dysplastic changes at femoral epiphysis
- Short, thick finger bones
- Pointing of bases of metacarpals

CLEIDOCRANIAL DYSOSTOSIS

Defect in ossification of enchondral and intramembranous bones
- Wormian bones
- Clavicle deformity (either absent, partially absent, or unfused)
- Failure of midline ossification (delayed closure of symphysis pubis, fontanelles, mandible, neural arches, sternum, vertebral bodies)
- Supernumerary epiphysis

Osteopetrosis

Osteoclast failure (bone remodels incompletely). Types:
- Autosomal recessive: lethal (anemia, thrombocytopenia, cranial foramina too small → hydrocephalus)
- Autosomal dominant: Albers-Schönberg disease, marble bones

Radiographic Features
- Generalized osteosclerosis
- Erlenmeyer flask deformity of distal femur
- Bone-within-bone appearance
- Alternating dense and lucent metaphyseal lines

Complications
- Frequent fractures
- Anemia (bone marrow replacement)
- Cranial nerve palsies

ARTHRITIS

JUVENILE RHEUMATOID ARTHRITIS (JRA)

RA with onset at <16 years. 70% of JRA is seronegative. Still disease = JRA + lymphadenopathy + splenomegaly.

Radiographic Features
- Spinal involvement is very common (70%) and typically precedes peripheral arthritis:
  - Diffuse ankylosis of posterior articular joints (diagnostic)
  - C2 subluxation (due to destruction of posterior ligament)
  - Odontoid fracture
- Monoarticular in early course in 25%
- Periosteal new bone formation is common (uncommon in adults)
- Soft tissue swelling, edema, synovial congestion
- Growth retardation secondary to premature closure of growth plates: short metacarpals
- Overgrowth of epiphyses (increased perfusion)

OTHER DISORDERS

CAFFEY DISEASE (INFANTILE CORTICAL HYPEROSTOSIS)

Cortical periostitis at multiple sites. The etiology is unknown (viral?). Self-limited and benign condition. Occurs before 6 months of age.

Radiographic Features
- New bone (periostitis) formation along tibia, ulna, mandible

SHORT STATURE

Dwarfism: height is >4 standard deviations below the mean. Human growth hormone (HGH) deficiency: at least two different HGH stimulation tests (hypoglycemia, dopamine, exercise, arginine) have to be abnormal (failure of GH increase >10 mg/mL after stimulation) to establish the diagnosis.

Classification

HGH deficiency (pituitary dwarfism)
- Isolated HGH deficiency
- Craniopharyngioma, infections

Peripheral tissue nonresponsive to HGH
- African pygmies
- Turner syndrome
- Constitutional short stature

Systemic diseases (most common)
- Hypothyroidism (cretinism)
- Cyanotic CHF
- Chronic pulmonary disease

Approach
- Rule out chronic systemic disease (most common cause of short stature).
- Rule out osseous defects.
- If HGH stimulation is normal, measure somatomedins.

FIBROMATOSIS COLLI

Benign fibrous mass of the sternocleidomastoid muscle ("sternocleidomastoid pseudotumor of infancy"). Leading cause of torticollis in infancy. Spontaneous regression.

Radiographic Features
- US: Isoechoic or hypoechoic ill-defined mass in sternocleidomastoid muscle. R > L unilateral.
- CT: Isodense enlargement of the sternocleidomastoid muscle

SACROCOCCYGEAL TERATOMA

Most common tumor in the newborn, F > M. Mature, immature, malignant (10%) varieties. Early diagnosis important as risk of malignant degeneration increases with delay in diagnosis. Tx: Resection of mass and coccyx; chemotherapy for malignant tumors.

Altman Classification
- Type 1: External
- Type 2: Predominantly external with intraabdominal extension
- Type 3: Predominantly intraabdominal
- Type 4: Entirely presacral

Radiographic Features
- Cystic, solid, or mixed
- May contain calcifications
- Widened presacral space, extrinsic compression of rectum on contrast enema
- Hydrops and placentomegaly on prenatal US associated with poor prognosis

KLIPPEL-TRÉNAUNAY SYNDROME

Consists of enlarged extremity, cutaneous vascular lesions, and diffuse venous and lymphatic malformations. Generally involves only one of the lower extremities, although bilateral involvement, upper extremity involvement, or extension into the trunk may occur. Klippel-Trénaunay syndrome must be distinguished from Parkes Weber syndrome (enlarged extremity is due to underlying AVM). The cutaneous vascular lesion is generally a capillary malformation and usually involves the enlarged limb, although involvement of the whole side of the body or of the contralateral limb may be seen. In over two thirds of patients, a characteristic incompetent lateral venous channel arises near the ankle and extends a variable distance up the extremity to the infrainguinal or pelvic deep venous system.

Clinical Findings
- Lymphangitis
- Cutaneous lymphatic vesicles
- Lymphorrhea or mass effect from macrocystic portions of lymphatic malformations
- Extension of venous malformation into the pelvis may result in recurrent rectal bleeding or hematuria.

Radiographic Features
- Bone elongation causing leg-length discrepancy, soft tissue thickening, or calcified phleboliths
- Venography usually demonstrates extensive dilation of superficial veins and enlarged perforating veins. In some patients, segmental absence or hypoplasia of the deep venous system is seen and must be distinguished from incomplete filling with contrast material at venography.
- MRI demonstrates a lack of enlarged high-flow arterial structures. T2W imaging shows malformed venous and lymphatic lesions as areas of high signal intensity. MRI depicts deep extension of low-flow vascular malformations into muscular compartments and the pelvis and their relationship to adjacent organs, as well as bone or soft tissue hypertrophy.

Pediatric Neuroimaging

CRANIAL ULTRASOUND

CORONAL VIEWS (6 SECTIONS) (Fig. 11-77)

1. Frontal lobe view, interhemispheric fissure
2. Circle of Willis view (5-pointed star or bull's head appearance: MCA = horns, sphenoidal sinus = bull's head; thalami = within bull's horns); germinal matrix (echolucent area adjacent to the

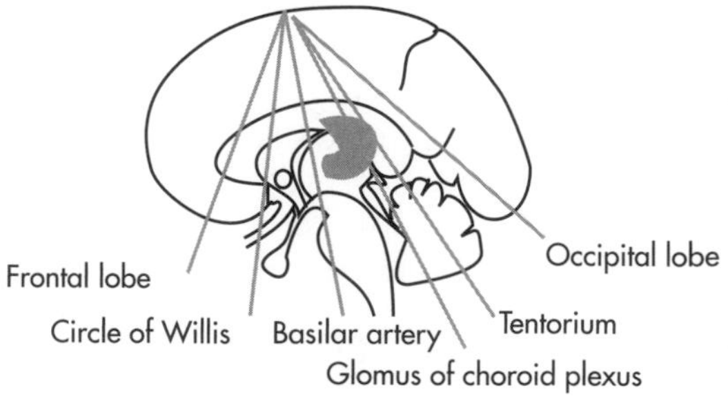

FIGURE 11-77

ventricles), internal capsule, corpus callosum, interhemispheric fissure
3. Basilar artery view (pulsating structure within interpeduncular cistern): 3rd ventricle
4. Glomus view: glomus of choroid plexus is very echogenic
5. Tentorium cerebelli view: cerebellar vermis gives the appearance of a Christmas tree, quadrigeminal plate
6. Occipital lobe view: decussation of fibers of optic tract

SAGITTAL VIEWS (6 SECTIONS) (Fig. 11-78)

1. Two views are taken in the midline; bring into alignment the echogenic vermis of the cerebellum and the corpus callosum; 3rd ventricle and corpus callosum represent the best reference points
2. Parasagittal view of thalamus, choroid plexus
3. Parasagittal view slightly more lateral to first parasagittal view

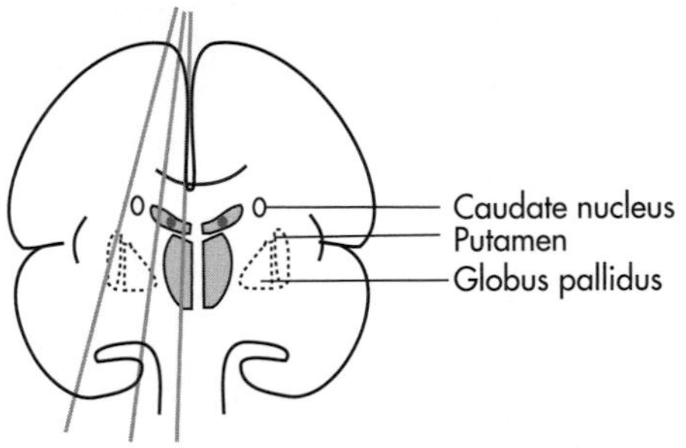

FIGURE 11-78

INDICATIONS FOR CRANIAL US

Screening for ventricular dilatation and hemorrhage
- ECMO patients (ligation of ipsilateral carotid artery; anticoagulation)
- Premature infants (5%-50% incidence of hemorrhage); screen all neonates <1500 g or <32 weeks.
- Low Apgar score

Diagnostic cranial US
- Neurologic changes
- Cranial dysmorphism (Down syndrome, trisomy 18, meningomyelocele)
- Seizures

Follow-up of hemorrhage

Doppler may be useful to distinguish an enlarged subarachnoid space (crossing vessels) from a subdural collection (no crossing vessels)

GERMINAL MATRIX HEMORRHAGE (Fig. 11-79)

Germinal matrix represents highly vascular tissue located near the caudothalamic groove (inferior to lateral ventricles). Germinal matrix exists only during 24th to 32nd week of gestation, and the matrix is highly vulnerable to hypoxemia and ischemia. Later in pregnancy, the mature neuroectodermal cells of the germinal matrix migrate to the cerebral cortex.

Causes of Hemorrhage

- Trauma: birth
- Coagulopathies: e.g., ECMO, Rh incompatibility, drugs

Radiographic Features

General US appearance of hemorrhage
- Acute hemorrhage (<7 days): very hyperechoic, no shadowing
- Aging hemorrhage
  Echogenicity decreases within 2 to 3 weeks.
  Abnormal area decreases in size.

Grading of hemorrhage (Fig. 11-80)
- Grade 1: subependymal hemorrhage; no long-term abnormality

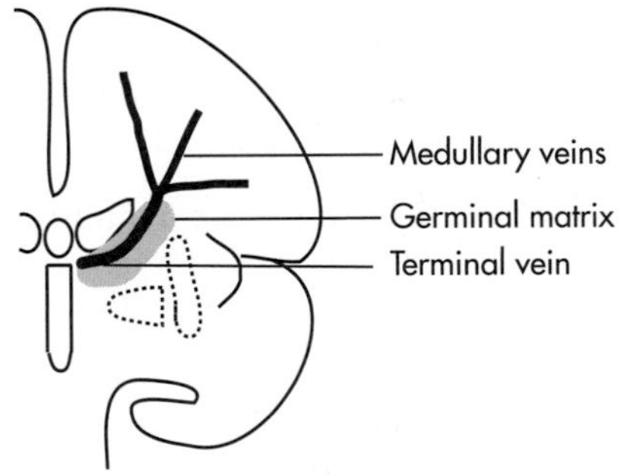

FIGURE 11-79

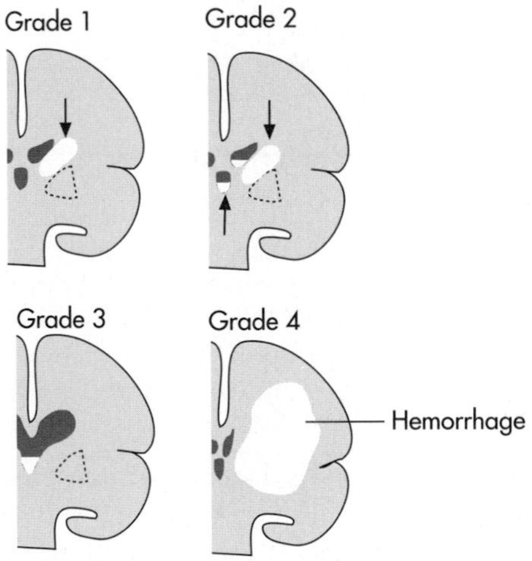

FIGURE 11-80

- Grade 2: intraventricular hemorrhage without ventricular dilatation; 10% mortality
- Grade 3: intraventricular hemorrhage with ventricular dilatation; 20% mortality
- Grade 4: intraparenchymal hemorrhage; >50% mortality

Germinal matrix hemorrhage
- Best seen on sagittal views
- Most frequent location is anterior to caudothalamic groove

Choroid plexus hemorrhage
- Lumpy-bumpy appearance
- Normal choroid plexus pulsates; a blood clot does not.

Intraparenchymal hemorrhage
- May occur as a sequela of germinal matrix hemorrhage, birth trauma, Rh incompatibility, etc.
- Intraparenchymal hemorrhage ultimately results in porencephaly.
- Hematoma becomes hypoechoic within a few days to weeks.

Ventricular dilatation occurs in 75% after hemorrhage.
- Ventricles on the coronal scan should not occupy more than a third of the entire hemisphere.
- Serial qualitative assessment of ventricular size is more useful in practice than quantitative determination of ventricular size.
- Rounding of superolateral angles of frontal horns, dilatation of occipital horns

OTHER TYPES OF HEMORRHAGE (SEE ALSO CHAPTER 6)

Cortical hemorrhage
- AV malformations
- Inflammation
- Trauma
- Tumor

Extracerebral hemorrhage
- Subdural
- Epidural
- Doppler US of ACA: resistive index rises with compression

PERIVENTRICULAR LEUKOMALACIA

Periventricular infarction of cerebral tissue is initially characterized by an increased echogenicity, which on sequential US may transform into cystic areas. Periventricular leukomalacia occurs in 5%-10% of premature infants. Pathogenesis: hypoxemia causes white matter necrosis. Clinical finding: spastic diplegia and intellectual deficits.

Location (in watershed areas of arterial blood flow)

- Adjacent to trigone of the lateral ventricles
- At level of foramen of Monro

Radiographic Features

Acute phase
- Broad zone of increased periventricular echogenicity
- May be symmetrical
- Differential diagnosis:
  - Periventricular echogenic halo from normally dense venous plexus
  - Germinal matrix hemorrhage

Chronic phase (>2 weeks)
- Small cyst formation ("Swiss cheese" appearance)

Differential diagnosis of porencephaly and cysts of periventricular leukomalacia
- Porencephaly seldom disappears over time.
- Porencephaly most often represents an extension of ipsilateral ventricle or subarachnoid space.
- Porencephaly is almost always asymmetrical.

CHOROID PLEXUS CYST

Cysts arise from choroid plexus and occur in 2% to 4% of neonates.
- Small cysts (<10 mm) usually disappear by 28 weeks.
- Large cysts (>10 mm) are frequently associated with trisomy 18; amniocentesis is usually performed once a large cyst is diagnosed.
- Disappearance of the cyst on follow-up does not change association.

VENTRICULOPERITONEAL (VP) SHUNT COMPLICATIONS

- CSFoma: accumulation of fluid collection near intraabdominal catheter tip. Common in patients with abdominal adhesions due to prior surgery.
- Occlusion
- Infection
- Overshunting (collapsed ventricles)
- Disconnection

SKULL

SUTURES (Fig. 11-81)

CRANIOSYNOSTOSIS (Fig. 11-82)

Premature closure of sutures (sagittal suture, 60%; coronal suture, 20%) results in skull shape abnormalities. Treatment is with craniectomy.

Causes

Primary closure

Secondary closure
- Skeletal dysplasia
- Metabolic
- Ventricular shunting
- Hematologic disorders

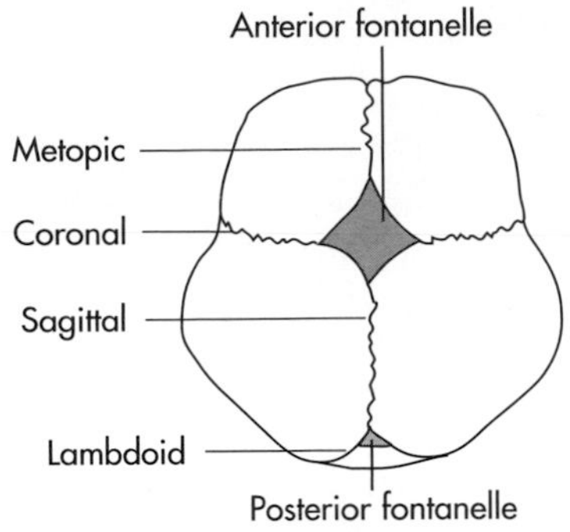

FIGURE 11-81

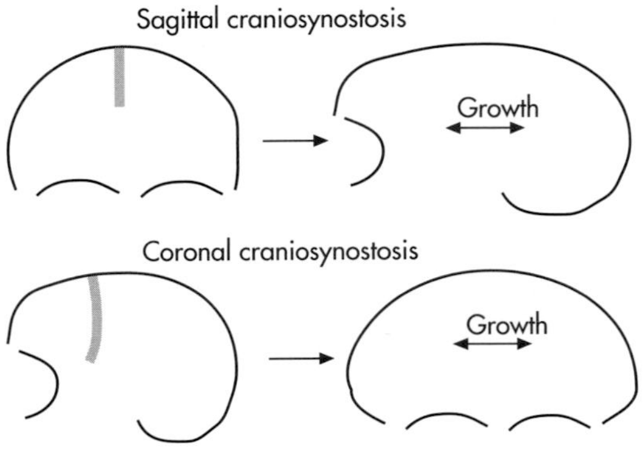

FIGURE 11-82

Types

- Dolichocephaly (scaphocephaly): sagittal suture
- Brachycephaly: coronal suture
- Trigonocephaly: metopic suture
- Oxycephaly: all
- Plagiocephaly: unilateral coronal or lambdoid suture (Harlequin eye if coronal suture)
- Cloverleaf (kleeblattschädel): all except metopic and squamosal sutures

MULTIPLE LACUNAE (Fig. 11-83)

Criteria: prominent depressions in inner table of skull.

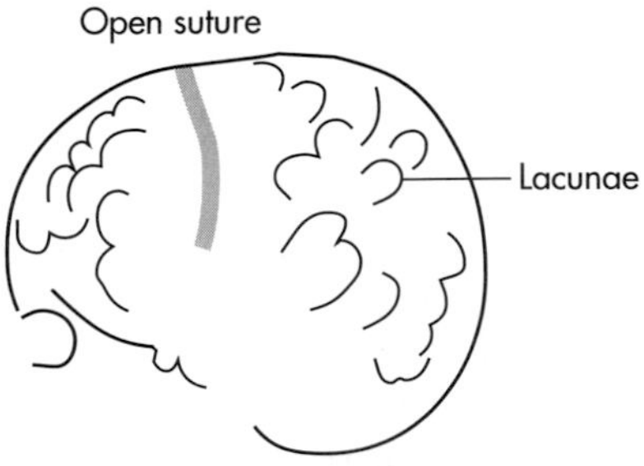

FIGURE 11-83

Causes

- Physiologic up to 6 months
- Increased intracranial pressure
- Mesenchymal dysplasia (lacunar skull, Lückenschädel)
    - Meningoceles
    - Myelomeningoceles
    - Encephaloceles

WORMIAN BONES (Fig. 11-84)

Intrasutural bones (named after Worms, a Danish anatomist), most commonly located in lambdoid suture

Causes

- Normal finding until 1 year of age
- Osteogenesis imperfecta
- Cleidocranial dysplasia
- Hypothyroidism

Mnemonic: "PORKCHOPS":

- **P**yknodysostosis
- **O**steogenesis imperfecta
- **R**ickets in healing
- **K**inky hair syndrome
- **C**leidocranial dysplasia
- **H**ypothyroidism
- **O**topalatodigital syndrome
- **P**achydermoperiostosis
- **S**yndrome of Down

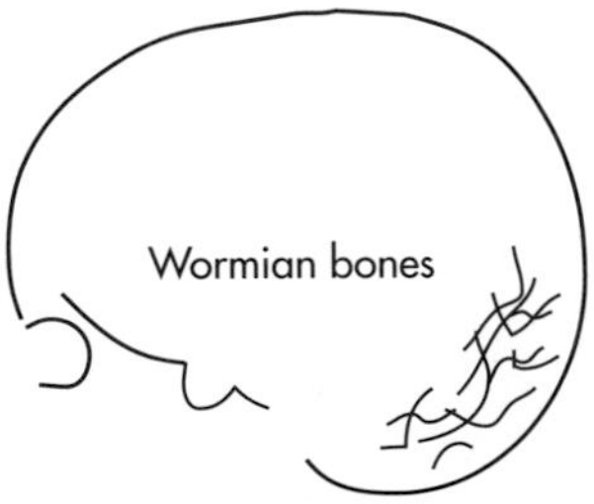

FIGURE 11-84

SKULL FRACTURES

Neonatal skull fractures with torn dura rarely develop into:

- Growing skull fractures
- Leptomeningeal cysts
    - Widely separated skull bone
    - Meninges herniate through torn dura.

CHOANAL ATRESIA

Membranous or bony obstruction of the nasal passage in the newborn. If bilateral, respiratory distress at birth as newborns are obligate nasal breathers.

- Failure to pass small catheter through nasal cavity.
- CT: findings of enlarged vomer and medial bowing of the lateral walls of the nasal cavity are useful to distinguish bony atresia from membranous.

SPINE

DEVELOPMENT (Fig. 11-85)

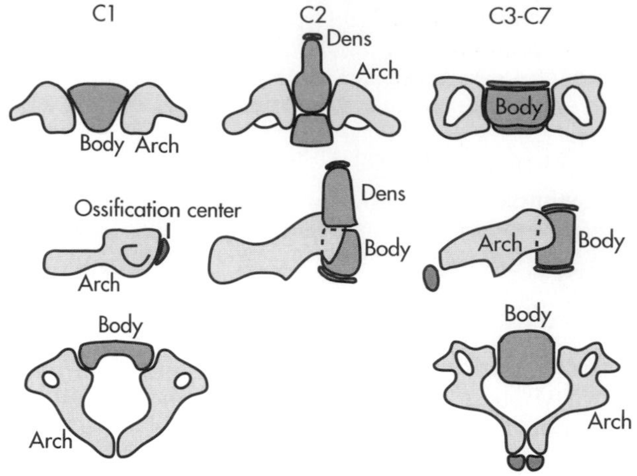

FIGURE 11-85

SCOLIOSIS

Scoliosis refers to lateral curving of the spine with varying degrees of rotation of the vertebral bodies around a vertical axis (Fig. 11-86).

Types

Idiopathic, 90%
- Mild form: 3% prevalence
- Severe form: 0.1% prevalence

Secondary
- Congenital
  - Hemivertebra
  - Trapezoidal vertebra
  - Unilateral neural arch fusions
- Growth asymmetry due to trauma, infection, radiation, neurofibromatosis
- Leg-length discrepancy

Preoperative Radiographic Features (Figs. 11-87 and 11-88)
- Determine type of scoliosis and degree of flexibility of spine.
- Measure the scoliotic curve (Cobb method).

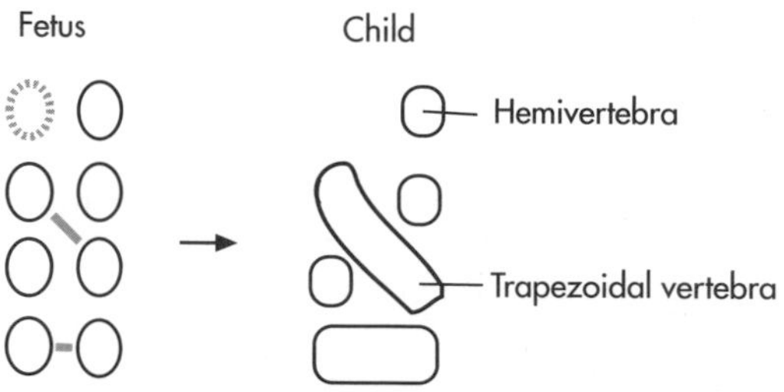

FIGURE 11-86

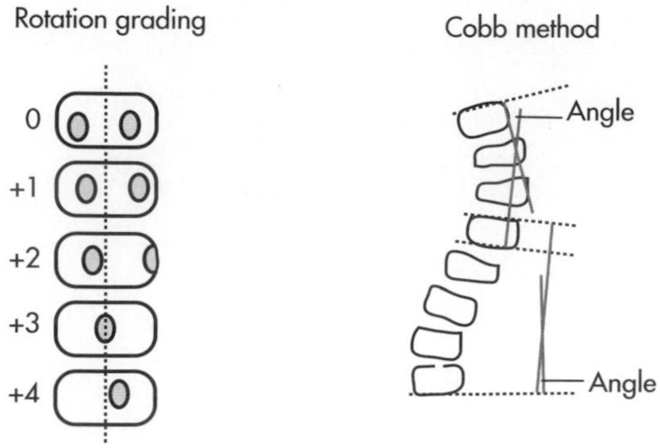

FIGURE 11-87

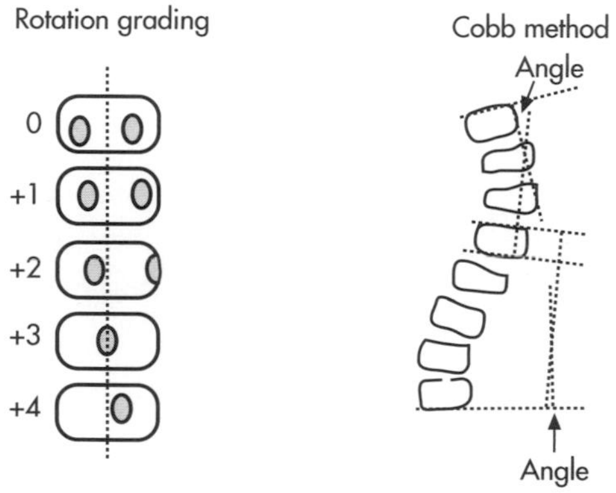

FIGURE 11-88

- Determine the degree of rotation: semiquantitate the midline shift of one of the pedicles toward the midline and score 0 to +4; rotation determines the extent of required bone fusion and the rigidity of the curve.

Postoperative Radiographic Features
- Correction of scoliosis: the general goal is to achieve 50% correction of the scoliotic curve and to maintain normal lung function because scoliosis causes respiratory compromise.
- Bony fusion is complete within 9 months postoperatively; best seen on 60° supine/oblique projections
- Types of surgery
  - Anterior approach: Dwyer cable; screws in lateral vertebral bodies are fastened with cable.
  - Posterior approach: Harrington rod placement is used to achieve fusion of vertebrae.
- Evaluate hardware: slippage or fracture of brackets, Harrington rod, or Dwyer cable

CERVICAL SPINE INJURIES (Fig. 11-89)

Cervical spine injuries are uncommon in children.

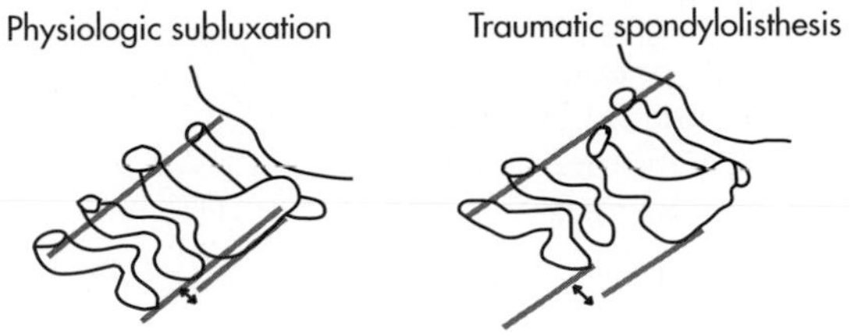

FIGURE 11-89

Pseudosubluxation

Physiologic anterior displacement of C2 or C3 due to normal laxity of ligaments of the cervical spine:

- C2/C3 (25% of children <8 years): normal up to 3 mm (posterior line maintains alignment)
- C3/C4: 15% of children <8 years

Differential Diagnosis

CHEST

STRIDOR, WHEEZING

- Upper airway obstruction
- Tracheal lesions
- Rings and slings
- Foreign bodies
- Asthma

UPPER AIRWAY OBSTRUCTION

Inflammation
- Epiglottitis (*Haemophilus influenzae*)
- Croup (respiratory syncytial virus)
- Retropharyngeal abscess

Exogenous
- Caustic injection
- Foreign body

Extrinsic upper airway compression
- Thyroglossal duct cysts
- Branchial cleft cysts
- Other masses

BUBBLY LUNGS IN NEONATES (Fig. 11-90)

- Bronchopulmonary dysplasia (most common)
- Pulmonary interstitial emphysema
- Cystic fibrosis
- Wilson-Mikity syndrome (form of bronchopulmonary dysplasia)

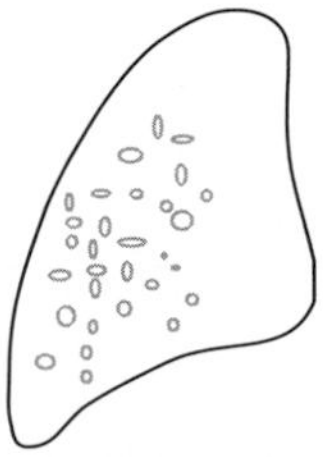

FIGURE 11-90

MASS LESIONS IN THE AIRWAYS

Lymphangioma and hemangioma may occur in any of the 3 locations.

Nasal cavity, nasopharynx
- Antrochoanal polyp
- Meningoencephalocele
- Angiofibroma
- Lymphadenopathy
- Neuroblastoma
- Rhabdomyosarcoma

Oropharynx
- Lymphadenopathy
- Ectopic thyroid tissue

Hypopharynx, larynx, or trachea
- Retention cysts
- Papillomas

NEONATAL LUNG MASSES (Fig. 11-91)

Lung bases; costophrenic angle obliterated
- Sequestration
- Congenital diaphragmatic hernia
- CCAM (first few hours of life)
- Hypoplastic lung (scimitar syndrome)
- Phrenic nerve paralysis: elevation of hemidiaphragm

Other lung zones
- Pulmonary tumor
  - Neuroblastoma
  - Pulmonary blastoma
  - PNET (Askin tumor)
- Congenital lobar emphysema (only early in disease, later lobar emphysema will be partially aerated)

HYPERLUCENT LUNG

- Large anterior pneumothorax (common)
- Congenital lobar emphysema
- Congenital lung cyst
- Bronchiolitis obliterans (Swyer-James syndrome, not until >7 years)
- Obstructive emphysema

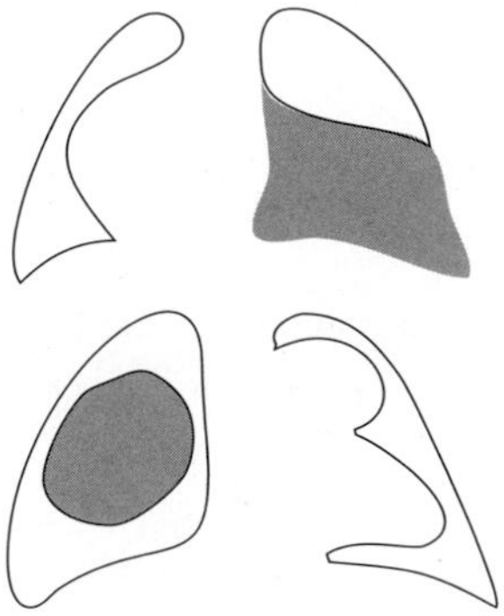

FIGURE 11-91

Obstruction at bronchiolar level: cystic fibrosis, asthma, pneumonia
Foreign body
Extrinsic compression: rings and slings, adenopathy, bronchogenic cyst
- CCAM

NEONATAL PNEUMOTHORAX

- Pressure ventilation
- Interstitial pulmonary emphysema
- Pulmonary hypoplasia (fetal anuria syndrome, Potter sequence, oligohydramnios)

SMALL SOLITARY PULMONARY NODULE (Fig. 11-92)

Congenital
- Bronchogenic cyst (common); 65% arise in lung, 35% from tracheobronchial tree
- Sequestration
- Arteriovenous malformation (AVM), varix
- Bronchial atresia

Infection
- Round pneumonia, most common
- Granuloma
- Abscess cavity

Tumor
- Primary: PNET, pulmonary blastoma
- Neuroblastoma, Wilms tumor metastases

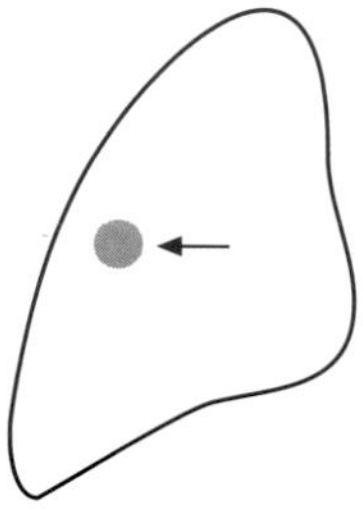

FIGURE 11-92

MULTIPLE PULMONARY NODULES

Tumor
- Metastases: Wilms' tumor, teratoma, rhabdomyosarcoma, osteosarcoma (OSA)
- Laryngeal papillomatosis (pulmonary lesions are rare)

Infection
- Septic emboli
- TB, fungus

Inflammatory
- Wegener disease (sinuses also involved)

PEDIATRIC INTERSTITIAL PATTERN

Congenital
- Storage disease: Gaucher, Niemann-Pick
- Lymphangiectasia (severe disease, usually fatal by 1 to 2 years)

Other common causes
- Viral pneumonia
- Bronchopulmonary dysplasia
- Hyaline membrane disease
- Histiocytosis X

RETICULAR OPACITIES IN A NEWBORN

- Lymphangiectasia
- TAPVR type 3 (edema)
- CHF (vein of Galen malformation, hemangioendothelioma)

PEDIATRIC CHEST WALL TUMORS

Common signs: pleural effusion, rib destruction, soft tissue density
- Eosinophilic granuloma (EG)
- Askin tumor (primitive neuroectodermal tumor [PNET])
- Neuroblastoma
- Metastases
- Ewing sarcoma

ABDOMEN

DILATED STOMACH (Fig. 11-93)

A dilated air-filled stomach may be due to gastric outlet obstruction (no or little distal gas, permanent dilated stomach, contractile waves) but is most commonly due to air swallowing during crying (normal distal gas, temporary distention occurs, no contractile waves). Causes of gastric outlet obstruction include:
- Hypertrophic pyloric stenosis
- Pylorospasm
- Antral web
- Antral gastritis
- Rare
  - Duplication cysts
  - Ectopic pancreatic tissue
  - Polyps, neoplasm

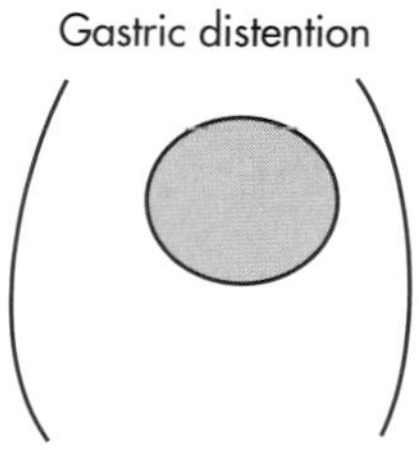

FIGURE 11-93

DOUBLE BUBBLE (Fig. 11-94)

Gas in the stomach and duodenal bulb with no or little gas distally is indicative of duodenal obstruction:
- Duodenal atresia (associated with Down syndrome) or stenosis, most common

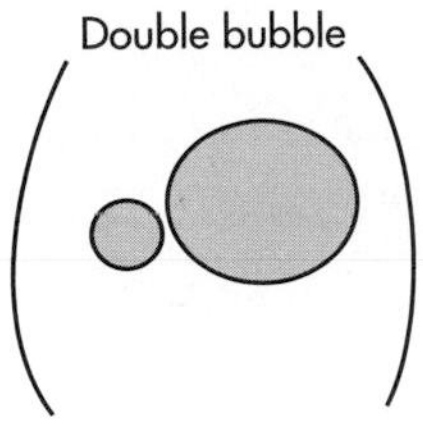

FIGURE 11-94

- Annular pancreas, 2nd most common
- Duodenal diaphragm, bands
- Midgut volvulus, most important entity to diagnose because of high mortality if undiagnosed). Clinical finding of bilious vomiting.
- Vascular
  - Preduodenal vein
  - SMA syndrome
- Rare
  - Duplication cysts
  - Adhesions

PROXIMAL BOWEL OBSTRUCTION (Fig. 11-95)

Neonates (congenital causes)
- Atresia/stenosis of small bowel
- Midgut volvulus
- Ladd's bands

Children (>1 year)
- Intussusception (most common)
- Incarcerated inguinal hernia (6 to 24 months)
- Perforated appendicitis

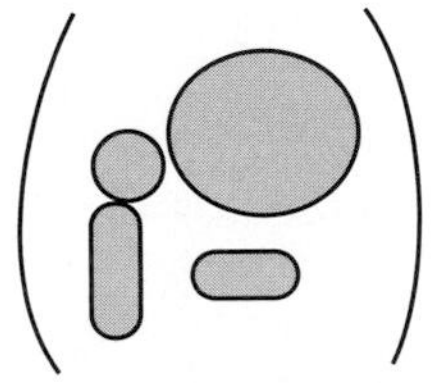

FIGURE 11-95

DISTAL BOWEL OBSTRUCTION (Fig. 11-96)

- Hirschsprung disease
- Meconium plug syndrome
- Colonic atresia/stenosis
- Imperforate anus
- Meconium ileus

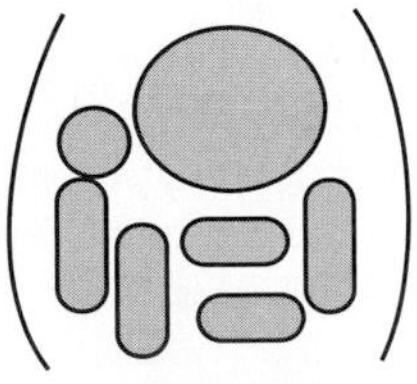

FIGURE 11-96

- Rare causes:
  - Volvulus
  - Presacral tumors
  - Post-NEC strictures

MICROCOLON

Criteria: narrowed (unused) colon. The diagnosis is usually established by barium enema.

Causes

- Diabetic mothers
- Maternal $MgSO_4$ use
- Unused colon (no fecal material or succus has passed through the colon)
  - Ileal atresia
  - Meconium ileus
- Total colonic Hirschsprung disease

Pearls

- Differentiation of small and large bowel in infants is not possible; refer to proximal and distal bowel.
- In patients with low obstructions proceed to enema (water-soluble isoosmolar agents preferred over barium).
- Patients with meconium ileus almost always (98%) have cystic fibrosis. 10%-20% of patients with cystic fibrosis have meconium ileus.

PEDIATRIC PNEUMATOSIS INTESTINALIS

- Necrotizing enterocolitis
- Less common causes (benign pneumatosis; pathogenesis unclear)
  - Cystic fibrosis
  - Collagen vascular disease
  - Leukemia
  - Milk intolerance
  - Immunodeficiency
- Obstruction
- Steroid use

GASLESS ABDOMEN

After birth, air appears normally in the GI tract: stomach, 2 hours; small bowel, 6 hours; rectum, 24 hours.

Causes

Severe vomiting, most common
- Gastroenteritis
- Appendicitis

Impaired swallowing
- Esophageal atresia
- Neurologic impairment
- Mechanical ventilation (paralyzed bowel)

Displaced bowel loops
- Bowel not in abdomen (e.g., hernia, omphalocele)
- Masses
- Ascites

ABDOMINAL CALCIFICATIONS

- Intraabdominal: meconium peritonitis (most common)
- Renal
  - Neuroblastoma, Wilms tumor
  - Nephrocalcinosis
  - Renal cysts
  - Urinary tract calculus
- Bowel: fecalith of appendix, Meckel's diverticulum
- Bladder: hemorrhagic cystitis (cyclophosphamide [Cytoxan] therapy)
- Adrenal: hemorrhage, Wolman disease (very rare)
- Cholelithiasis (sickle cell anemia)
- Liver: hepatoblastoma, granuloma, TORCH

COMMON ABDOMINAL MASS LESIONS

OVERVIEW

Neonates (<1 Month)	Older Infants and Children
Renal, 55% Hydronephrosis MCDK	Renal, 55% Wilms tumor Hydronephrosis
Gastrointestinal, 15% Duplication Meconium pseudocyst Pseudocyst proximal to atresia	Gastrointestinal, 15% Appendiceal abscess Intussusception Neoplasm
Retroperitoneal, 10% Adrenal hemorrhage	Retroperitoneal, 25% Neuroblastoma
Genital, 15% Ovarian cyst Hydrometrocolpos	Genital, 5% Ovarian cyst Hydrometrocolpos
Hepatobiliary, 5% Hemangioendothelioma Choledochal cyst	Hepatobiliary, 5% Hepatoblastoma

GASTRIC FILLING DEFECT

- Foreign bodies, most common
- Lactobezoar (improperly prepared milk), phytobezoars, trichobezoars
- Congenital anomalies
  - Duplications
  - Ectopic pancreatic tissue
- Inflammation, rare
  - Crohn disease
  - Chronic granulomatous diseases (immunodeficiency of the phagocytosis type)
- Tumors, rare
  - Hamartoma
  - Peutz-Jeghers syndrome

THICK FOLDS

Submucosal edema
- Enteritis

Submucosal tumor
- Lymphoma, leukemia

Submucosal hemorrhage
- Henoch-Schönlein purpura
- Hemolytic-uremic syndrome
- Coagulopathies (e.g., hemophilia, vitamin K, anticoagulants)

GI HEMORRHAGE

- Meckel's diverticulum
- Juvenile polyps
- Inflammatory bowel disease
- Portal hypertension

PEDIATRIC LIVER LESIONS

Benign
- Cysts
- Hemangioendothelioma
- Mesenchymal hamartoma

Malignant
- Hepatoblastoma
- Hemangioendothelioma (neonate)
- Hepatocellular carcinoma, if there is underlying liver disease (glycogen storage disorders, portal venous hypertension)
- Metastases from Wilms tumor or neuroblastoma

FATTY LIVER

- Chronic protein malnutrition (most common cause)
- Congenital
  - Cystic fibrosis
  - Glycogen storage disease
  - Wilson disease
  - Galactosemia
  - Fructose intolerance
  - Reye syndrome
- Hepatitis
- Drugs: chemotherapy, steroids, hyperalimentation

PEDIATRIC CHOLELITHIASIS

Hemolysis
- Sickle cell anemia (small spleen)
- Thalassemia (large spleen)
- Spherocystosis

Other
- Cystic fibrosis
- Drugs: furosemide
- Metabolic disorders: hyperparathyroidism (HPT)
- Premature infants with hyaline membrane disease

HYDROPS OF GALLBLADDER

- Sepsis
- Burns
- Leptospirosis
- Kawasaki disease
- Henoch-Schönlein purpura

CHOLECYSTITIS

- Sickle cell
- Hemolytic anemia

BILARY STRICTURES

- Pancreatitis
- Gallstones
- Ascending cholangitis
- Post-Kasai procedure
- Liver transplant

FATTY REPLACEMENT OF PANCREAS

- Cystic fibrosis
- Shwachman-Diamond syndrome:
  - Metaphyseal dysplasia
  - Cyclic neutropenia
  - Pancreatic fatty replacement
  - Flaring of ribs
- Pearson syndrome (mitochondrial)
  - Pediatric pancreatitis
- Trauma
- Viral infection
- Sepsis
- Idiopathic
- Anomaly
- Drugs (steroids, etc.)
- Metabolic
  - Cystic fibrosis
  - Hyperlipidemia

CHRONIC PANCREATITIS

- Repeated acute pancreatitis
- CMV
- Drugs (tetracycline, steroids)
- Pancreatic divisum
- Cystic fibrosis

GENITOURINARY SYSTEM

CYSTIC RENAL MASSES (Fig. 11-97)

Cystic disease (differentiate from hydronephrosis)

- Autosomal recessive kidney disease (infantile polycystic kidney disease)
- Multicystic dysplastic kidney
- Multilocular cystic nephroma
- Cysts associated with phakomatoses
  - von Hippel-Lindau disease
  - Tuberous sclerosis
- Other cystic diseases (see Chapter 4)

Tumors

- Cystic Wilms tumor
- Cystic adenocarcinoma

HYDRONEPHROSIS

Most common abdominal mass in neonates. Causes (in decreasing order of frequency) include:

- Reflux
- UVJ obstruction
- Ureterovesical obstruction
- Ectopic ureterocele
- Posterior urethral valves
- Prune-belly syndrome

SOLID RENAL MASSES

- Wilms tumor: most common solid tumor in children; rare in newborn
- Mesoblastic nephroma: the only solid renal mass lesion in newborns
- Nephroblastomatosis: subcortical masses; associated with Wilms tumor
- Angiomyolipoma: fatty mass; associated with tuberous sclerosis
- Secondary tumors
  - Lymphoma
  - Neuroblastoma
  - Leukemia: diffuse, bilateral enlargement

FIGURE 11-97

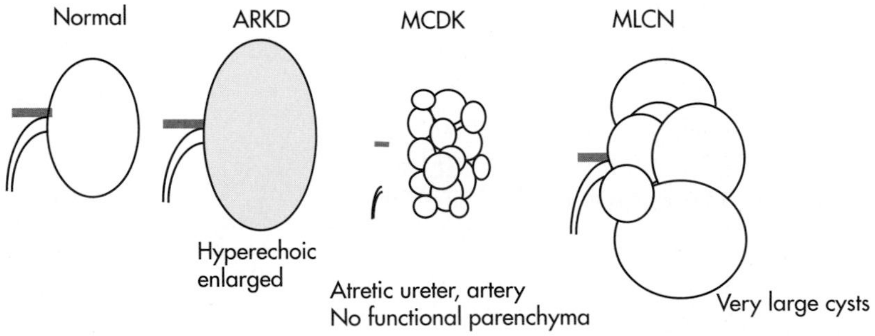

- Rare renal tumors
    - Clear cell sarcoma
    - Malignant rhabdoid
    - Renal cell carcinoma

UNIQUE CLINICAL AND IMAGING FEATURES OF RENAL MASSES

Renal Mass	Clinical and Imaging Features
Wilms tumor	Large solid mass, often vascular invasion Most common solid renal mass of childhood
Nephroblastomatosis	Multiple bilateral subcapsular lesions, associated bilateral solid Wilms tumors
Renal cell carcinoma	von Hippel-Lindau disease
Mesoblastic nephroma	Most common solid renal mass in newborns and infants
Multilocular cystic renal tumor	Multicystic mass with little solid tissue
Clear cell sarcoma	Associated skeletal metastases
Rhabdoid tumor	Associated brain malignancies
Angiomyolipoma	Tuberous sclerosis, neurofibromatosis, von Hippel-Lindau disease
Renal medullary carcinoma	Sickle cell trait or hemoglobin SC disease in adolescents
Ossifying renal tumor of infancy	Mass with calcification in an infant
Metanephric adenoma	Nonspecific features
Lymphoma	Appearance highly variable, frequent associated adenopathy

DIFFUSELY HYPERECHOIC RENAL KIDNEY IN NEWBORN

Increased size
- ARPCKD (bladder is usually empty)
- CMV glomerulonephritis (bladder may have some urine)
- Glomerular cystic disease
- Diffuse cystic dysplasia

Decreased size
- Renal dysplasia from obstructive uropathy or necrosis

ECHOGENIC KIDNEY (CORTEX SIMILAR TO SPLEEN OR LIVER WITH PRESERVED CORTICOMEDULLARY DIFFERENTIATION)

- ATN
- Glomerulonephritis
- Renal infiltration
- Glycogen storage disease
- Diabetes
- Renal vein thrombosis
- Leukemia is the only malignancy causing this appearance
- HIV
- Kawasaki disease

LOSS OF NORMAL CORTICOMEDULLARY DIFFERENTIATION

- Pyelonephritis; focal nephronia
- Infantile polycystic kidney
- Adult polycystic kidney
- Medullary cystic dysplastic kidney
- Late renal vein thrombosis

MEDULLARY NEPHROCALCINOSIS

- Furosemide therapy
- Hyperparathyroidism
- RTA (distal tubular defect)
- Hypercalcemia or hypercalciuria
    - Milk-alkali syndrome
    - Idiopathic hypercalciuria
    - Sarcoidosis
    - Hypervitaminosis D
- Oxalosis
- Medullary sponge kidney

CONGENITAL URETERIC OBSTRUCTION

- Primary megaureter
- Ureterocele (ectopic or orthotopic)
- Distal ureteral stenosis
- Ureteral atresia
- Circumcaval ureter
- Bladder diverticulum

ADRENAL MASS

- Neonatal hemorrhage, common
- Neuroblastoma
- Rare adrenal pediatric tumors
    - Teratoma
    - Adenoma
    - Carcinoma
    - Pheochromocytoma
- Other retroperitoneal masses
    - Wilms tumor
    - Hydronephrotic upper pole
    - Retroperitoneal adenopathy
    - Hepatoblastoma
    - Splenic mass

CYSTIC STRUCTURE IN OR NEAR BLADDER WALL (US)

Bladder
- Hutch diverticulum
- Urachal remnant (dome of the bladder)
- Normal "bladder ears" (incompletely filled bladder extends into femoral/inguinal canal)

Ureter
- Ectopic insertion of ureter
- Ureterocele
- Megaureter

Other
- Ovarian cyst
- Mesenteric, omental cyst

LARGE ABDOMINAL CYSTIC MASS

- Lymphangioma (multiseptated noncalcified)
- Enteric duplication cyst (unilocular noncalcified with bowel signature)
- Meconium pseudocyst (unilocular containing echoes and debris)
- Choledochal cyst
- Adrenal hemorrhage
- Ovarian cyst

PRESACRAL MASS

- Rectal duplication
- Anterior meningocele
- Teratoma
- Neuroblastoma

INTERLABIAL MASS

- Ectopic ureterocele
- Periurethral cysts
- Rhabdomyosarcoma of vagina
- Prolapsed urethra
- Imperforate hymen

CENTRAL NERVOUS SYSTEM

POOR MINERALIZATON OF SKULL

By US this appears as "excellent" visualization of fetal brain.
- Osteogenesis imperfecta
- Hypophosphatasia
- Achondrogenesis

ENLARGED HEAD (MACROCEPHALY)

Hydrocephalus (most common cause of enlargement before closure of sutures)
- Communicating (more common)
- Noncommunicating (less common)

Rare causes
- Subdural hematoma
- Calvarial abnormalities
  - Benign macrocrania
  - Chondrodystrophies
- Brain abnormalities
  - Beckwith-Wiedemann syndrome
  - Hemiatrophy
  - Cerebral gigantism

SMALL HEAD (MICROCEPHALY)

- Absent or atrophic brain (congenital infection, fetal alcohol syndrome)
- Craniosynostosis
- Shunt placement

WIDENED ANTERIOR FONTANELLE

- Cleidocranial dysostosis
- Down syndrome
- Achondroplasia
- Osteogenesis imperfecta
- Rickets
- Hydrocephalus
- Hypothyroidism

THICK SKULL

Metabolic/systemic
- Healing stage of renal osteodystrophy
- Hyperparathyroidism (salt-and-pepper skull)
- Anemias (compensatory hematopoiesis): sickle cell disease, thalassemia

Tumor
- Leukemia, lymphoma

Other
- Chronic decreased intracranial pressure (shunts; most common cause of calvarial thickening)
- Dilantin therapy
- Dysplasia
  - Fibrous dysplasia
  - Engelmann disease

LYTIC SKULL LESIONS

- EG
- Leukemia, lymphoma
- Fibrous dysplasia
- Dermoid, epidermoid
- Hyperparathyroidism

INTRACRANIAL CALCIFICATION

Differentiate abnormal from physiological intracranial calcifications. The latter include:
- Choroid plexus calcification
- Habenula calcification
- Pineal gland calcification
- Falx: dura, pacchionian bodies calcification
- Hemangioblastoma calcification

Abnormal calcifications have a wide differential (mnemonic: "TIC MTV"):
- **T**umor
  - Children: craniopharyngioma > oligodendroglioma > gliomas > other tumors
  - Adults: meningioma > oligodendroglioma > ependymoma
- **I**nfection
  - Children: TORCH
  - Adults: cysticercosis, TB

- **C**ongenital, degenerative, atrophic lesions
  - Congenital atrophy or hypoplasia
  - Tuberous sclerosis (75% have calcifications)
  - Sturge-Weber syndrome (tramtrack gyral calcifications)
- **M**etabolic
  - Idiopathic hypercalcemia
  - Lead poisoning (rare today)
  - Hypoparathyroidism
  - Fahr disease (familial)
- **T**rauma
- **V**ascular lesions
  - AVMs (vein of Galen aneurysm)
  - Hematoma
  - Aneurysms

ENLARGED SELLA TURCICA

- Tumor (most common cause)
  - Most common: craniopharyngioma
  - 2nd most common: optic chiasm, hypothalamic glioma
  - Less common: germ cell tumors, meningioma, pituitary adenoma
- Increased intracranial pressure
- Empty sella
- Nelson disease

MUSCULOSKELETAL SYSTEM

COMMON PEDIATRIC BONE TUMORS

Primary
- EG
- Ewing sarcoma
- OSA
- Bone cysts
  - UBC: single cavity, fallen fragment sign
  - ABC: eccentric

Secondary
- Neuroblastoma metastases
- Lymphoma
- Leukemia

Tumors with Fluid-Fluid Level

- ABC
- Telangiectatic OSA
- Giant cell tumor
- Single cysts with pathologic fracture

WIDENED JOINT SPACE (Fig. 11-98)

Widened joint spaces in pediatric patients are most commonly seen in hip joint or shoulders; other joints have strong capsules. Causes of widened joint space include:

Joint effusion
- Septic arthritis
- Hemarthrosis (intraarticular fracture, hemophiliac)

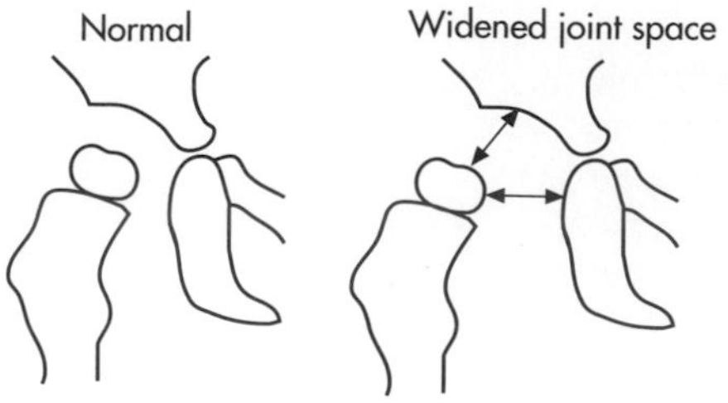

FIGURE 11-98

- Transient toxic synovitis (viral)
- JRA

Synovial thickening without articular cartilage destruction
- JRA
- Hemophiliac arthropathy

BOWED BONES

Anterior and posterior bowing (fetal malposition) is always abnormal. Anterior bowing may be associated with medial and lateral bowing. Isolated medial bowing is usually idiopathic. Common causes of anterior bowing include:

Metabolic
- Rickets (most common)

Dysplasia
- Neurofibromatosis (primary bone dysplasia)
- Osteogenesis imperfecta
- Fibrous dysplasia
- Osteofibrous dysplasia
- Blount disease

Trauma

Physiologic

DIFFUSE PEDIATRIC OSTEOPENIA

- Rickets
- Hyperparathyroidism (secondary to renal disease = renal rickets)
- Immobilization
- JRA
- Uncommon causes
  - Infiltrative disease: gangliosidosis, mucolipidosis
  - Same causes as in adults (see previous sections)

DIFFUSELY DENSE BONES IN CHILDREN

Congenital
- Osteopetrosis
- Pyknodysostosis
- Melorheostosis
- Progressive diaphyseal dysplasia (Engelmann disease)
- Infantile cortical hyperostosis
- Idiopathic hypercalcemia of infancy (Williams syndrome)
- Generalized cortical hyperostosis (van Buchem disease)

- Pachydermoperiostosis
- Tuberous sclerosis

Other
- Hypothyroidism
- Congenital syphilis
- Hypervitaminosis D

ABNORMAL RIB SHAPE

- Pectus excavatum
- Rib notching
- Cerebrocostomandibular syndrome

SLENDER RIBS

- Trisomy 18
- Neurofibromatosis

WIDENED RIBS

- Mucopolysaccharidosis
- Thalassemia major

EXPANSILE RIBS

- Lymphangiomatosis
- Fibrous dysplasia
- Cerebrocostomandibular syndrome

ABNORMAL SIZE OR SHORTENING OF RIBS

- Thanatophoric dysplasia
- Juvenile asphyxiating thoracic dysplasia
- Ellis-van Creveld chondroectodermal dysplasia
- Achondroplasia

SYMMETRICAL PERIOSTEAL REACTION IN CHILDREN (Fig. 11-99)

Symmetrical periosteal reaction can be physiologic during first 6 months of life; thereafter it often is pathologic. Wide differential. Mnemonic: "TIC MTV":

- **T**umor
  Neuroblastoma
  Leukemia, lymphoma
- **I**nfection
  Congenital infection: syphilis, rubella
- **C**ongenital
  Caffey disease (infantile cortical hyperostosis)
  Osteogenesis imperfecta
- **M**etabolic
  Hypervitaminosis A, D
  Prostaglandin E therapy
  Scurvy
- **T**rauma
  Battered child syndrome (subperiosteal hematoma)
- **V**ascular
  Bone infarctions (sickle cell disease)

Mnemonic for periosteal reaction: "SCALP:"
- **S**curvy
- **C**affey disease
- **A**ccident, hypervitaminosis A
- **L**eukemia, lues
- **P**hysiologic, prostaglandin inhibitors

Symmetrical periosteal reaction

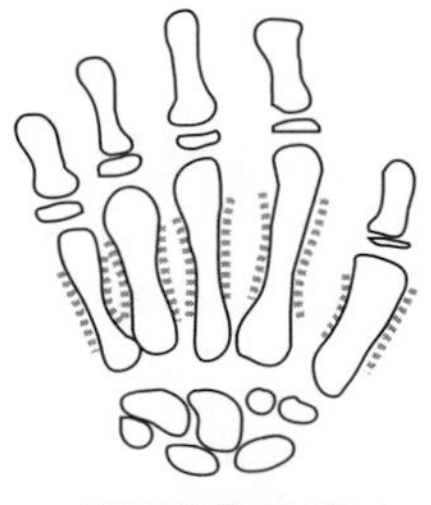

FIGURE 11-99

DEFORMED EPIPHYSIS (Fig. 11-100)

Epiphyseal defect may be solitary (e.g., osteochondritis dissecans), cause complete fragmentation of epiphysis, or affect multiple epiphyses (syndromes).

Acquired (single epiphysis)
- Avascular necrosis:
  LCP disease (most common)
  Steroids
- Trauma (osteochondritis dissecans)
- Infection
- Hypothyroidism

Congenital dysplasia (multiple epiphysis, all rare)
- Multiple epiphyseal dysplasia
- Myer dysplasia
- Morquio syndrome

Fused epiphysis with metaphysis: injury to central growth plate caused by meningococcemia

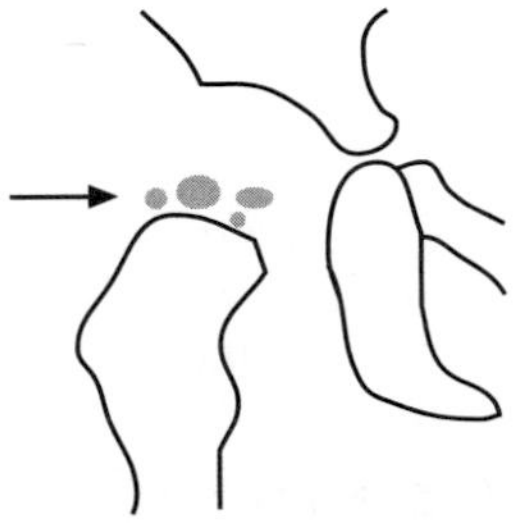

FIGURE 11-100

ENLARGED EPIPHYSIS (Fig. 11-101)

Most commonly caused by hyperemia associated with chronic arthritis.
- Hemophiliac joints

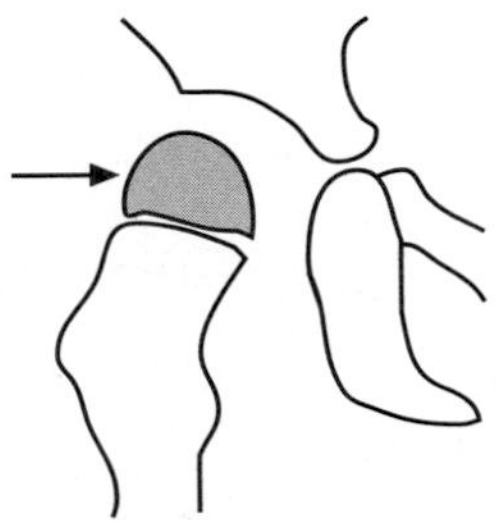

FIGURE 11-101

- JRA
- Chronic infectious arthritis
- Healed LCP disease
- Epiphyseal dysplasia hemimelia (Trevor)

STIPPLED EPIPHYSIS

- Chondrodysplasia punctata
- Warfarin
- Alcohol
- Hypothyroidism

TRANSVERSE METAPHYSEAL LINES

Transverse metaphyseal bands are the result of abnormal enchondral bone growth; undermineralization leads to lucent lines and repair leads to dense metaphyseal lines. In some diseases, dense and lucent lines coexist.

Lucent lines
- Neonates: stress lines (hypoperfusion of rapidly growing metaphyses of long bones) due to fever, congenital heart disease, any severe disease
- >2 years of age consider tumors:
  - Neuroblastoma metastases
  - Lymphoma, leukemia

Dense lines
- Neonates: growth recovery lines
- >2 years of age:
  - Heavy metal poisoning (lead bands)
  - Healing rickets
  - Treated scurvy

WIDENED GROWTH PLATE

Widened growth plate: >1 mm.
- Rickets (most common)
- Salter-Harris fracture, type 1
- Tumor: lymphoma, leukemia, neuroblastoma
- Infection: osteomyelitis

METAPHYSEAL FRAGMENTS (Fig. 11-102)

- Battered child (corner fractures)
- Trauma

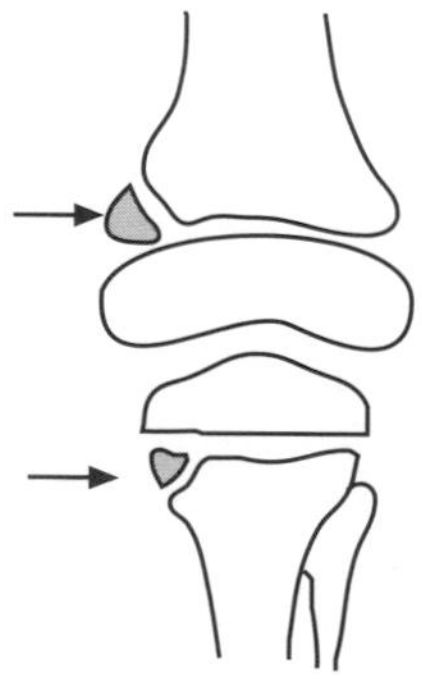

FIGURE 11-102

- Blount disease
- Osteomyelitis

METAPHYSEAL IRREGULARITY

- Rickets
- Syphilis
- Myelodysplasia
- Hypophosphatasia
- Metaphyseal dysplasia

AGGRESSIVE CLAVICULAR LESION

- Langerhans cell histiocytosis
- Infection
- Ewing sarcoma
- Osteosarcoma

VERTEBRAL ABNORMALITIES

Vertebra Plana (Localized Platyspondyly)

- Metastases (neuroblastoma most common)
- EG
- Leukemia, lymphoma
- Infection (less common)
- Trauma

Generalized Platyspondyly (Decreased Height of Vertebral Body) (Fig. 11-103)

- Osteogenesis imperfecta
- Dwarfism (thanatophoric, metatropic)
- Morquio syndrome
- Cushing syndrome

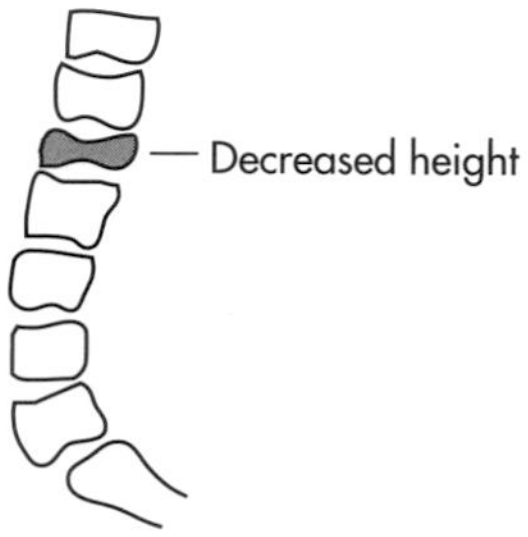

FIGURE 11-103

Fused Vertebrae

- Isolated fusion of vertebral bodies
- Klippel-Feil syndrome (C2-C3 fusion, torticollis, short neck); may be associated with Sprengel deformity (omovertebral bone)
- Posttraumatic

Large Vertebral Body, or Other Abnormal Shapes

- Blood dyscrasia (expansion of red marrow): sickle cell, thalassemia

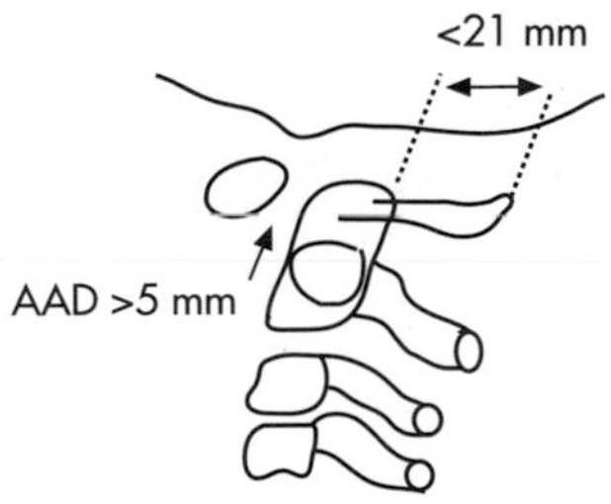

FIGURE 11-104

ALTLANTOAXIAL SUBLUXATION (Fig. 11-104)

- Down syndrome
- Morquio syndrome
- JRA
- Trauma
- Marfan/Ehlers-Danlos syndromes
- Spondyloepiphyseal dysplasia

DISK SPACE NARROWING

Common
- Infection (pyogenic, tuberculous, *Brucella*, typhoid)
- Block vertebra: congenital or acquired
- Scheuermann disease
- Severe kyphosis or scoliosis

Uncommon
- Congenital
- Cockayne syndrome
- Kniest dysplasia
- Morquio syndrome
- Spondyloepiphyseal dysplasia

Acquired
- Inflammatory arthritis (rheumatoid, ankylosing spondylitis)
- Herniated disk
- Neuropathic arthropathy (syrinx)
- Trauma

Enlarged Disk Space

- Osteoporosis
- Biconcave vertebra due to several causes
- Gaucher disease
- Platyspondyly
- Sickle cell anemia
- Trauma

Intervertebral Disk Space Calcification

Common
- Idiopathic (transient in children)
- Posttraumatic

Uncommon
- Spinal fusion
- Ochronosis
- Aarskog syndrome
- Ankylosing spondylitis
- Cockayne syndrome
- Homocystinuria
- Hypercalcemia
- Hyperparathyroidism
- Hypervitaminosis D
- Infection
- Paraplegia
- Juvenile chronic arthritis

PEDIATRIC SACRAL ABNORMALITIES

- Meningocele
- Neurofibromatosis
- Presacral teratoma
- Agenesis

RADIAL RAY DEFICIENCY

Absence of 1st and/or 2nd digits of hand; often involves radius
- Holt-Oram syndrome (triphalangia/hypoplasia/aplasia of thumb, cardiac, chest wall anomalies)
- Poland syndrome
- Fanconi anemia (thumb may be absent or hypoplastic)
- Thrombocytopenia/absent radius syndrome (thumb present)

POLYDACTYLY

- Familial polydactyly
- Chondroectodermal dysplasia (Ellis-van Creveld syndrome)
- Trisomies 13-15
- Laurence-Moon-Bardet-Biedl syndrome

SYNDACTYLY

Usually third and fourth digits are involved. May be isolated, but also associated with:
- Apert syndrome (brachycephaly)
- Poland syndrome
- Constriction band syndrome

ABNORMAL 4TH METACARPAL

Short Metacarpal

- Turner syndrome
- Growth arrest: sickle cell disease, infections

Long Metacarpal

- Macrodystrophia lipomatosa
- Neurofibromatosis

DELAYED BONE AGE

Systemic diseases (most common)
- Hypothyroidism (cretinism; typical: hypoplastic T12 and L1)
- Cyanotic congenital heart failure
- Chronic pulmonary disease

HGH deficiency (pituitary dwarfism)
- Isolated HGH deficiency
- Craniopharyngioma, infections

Peripheral tissue nonresponsive to HGH
- African pygmies
- Turner syndrome
- Constitutional short stature

HEMIHYPERTROPHY

Enlargement of an extremity (rare)
- Intraabdominal tumors (frequently Wilms tumor)
- Arteriovenous fistula
- Lymphangioma
- Klippel-Trénaunay, Parker-Weber syndrome
- Isolated anomaly (idiopathic)

PUBIC SYMPHYSIS DIASTASIS

- Bladder exstrophy
- Cleidocranial dysplasia
- Presacral mass

OTHER

DOWN SYNDROME

- Duodenal atresia
- Tracheoesophageal fistula, esophageal atresia
- Endocardial cushion defect
- Hirschsprung disease
- Multiple sternal ossification centers
- 11 ribs

WILLIAMS SYNDROME (INFANTILE IDIOPATHIC HYPERCALCEMIA)

- Aortic stenosis (supravalvular)
- Peripheral pulmonic stenosis
- Diffuse coarctation of abdominal aorta and stenosis of visceral branches
- Multisystem abnormalities
  - Retardation
  - Dentition abnormalities
  - Elfin facies

BECKWITH-WIEDEMANN SYNDROME

- Macroglossia
- Visceromegaly (e.g., liver, kidneys, pancreas)
- Gigantism
- Omphalocele
- Wilms tumor

PREMATURE INFANTS

- Hyaline membrane disease
- Necrotizing enterocolitis
- Germinal matrix hemorrhage
- Periventricular leukoencephalopathy
- PDA

MALIGNANCY BY AGE

- <5 years: neuroblastoma
- 5 to 10: Ewing sarcoma
- >10: osteosarcoma

Suggested Readings

Blickman JG. *Pediatric Radiology: The Requisites*. St. Louis: Mosby; 1998.

Donnelly LF, Jones B, O'Hara S, et al. *Diagnostic Imaging: Pediatrics*. Salt Lake City: Amirsys; 2005.

Donnelly LF. *Fundamentals of Pediatric Radiology*. Philadelphia: WB Saunders; 2001.

Kirks DR. *Practical Pediatric Imaging: Diagnostic Radiology of Infants and Children*. Philadelphia: Lippincott Williams & Wilkins; 1997.

Kleinman PK. *Diagnostic Imaging of Child Abuse*. Baltimore: Williams & Wilkins; 1987.

Kuhn JP, Slovis TL, Haller JO. *Caffey's Pediatric Diagnostic Imaging*. St. Louis: Mosby; 2003.

Seibert JJ, James CA. *Pediatric Radiology Casebase: The Baby Minnie of Pediatric Radiology*. New York: Thieme Medical; 1998.

Stringer DA. *Pediatric Gastrointestinal Imaging*. Toronto: BC Decker; 2000.

Swischuk LE. *Emergency Radiology of the Acutely Ill or Injured Child*. Philadelphia: Lippincott Williams & Wilkins; 2000.

Swischuk LE. *Imaging of the Newborn, Infant, and Young Child*. Philadelphia: Lippincott Williams & Wilkins; 2003.

CHAPTER 12

Nuclear Imaging

CHAPTER OUTLINE

Pulmonary Imaging

RADIOPHARMACEUTICALS

Pulmonary scintigraphy uses ventilation agents and/or perfusion agents, depending on the specific imaging task.

If both ventilation ($\dot{V}$) and perfusion ($\dot{Q}$) imaging are performed ($\dot{V}/\dot{Q}$ scan), the ventilation imaging part is usually performed first because the 81-keV ^{133}Xe photon energy lies in the range of significant Compton downscatter of the 140 keV^{99m}Tc photon. Examination rooms must have negative internal pressure so that escaped Xe is not recirculated to other

OVERVIEW

Agent	Half-life	Main Energy	Collimator	Comments
Ventilation				
^{133}Xe	5.2 days	81	Low	Inexpensive; washout images helpful
^{127}Xe	36.4 days	203	Medium	Postperfusion imaging possible (high energy)
^{81m}Kr	13 sec	191	Medium	Postperfusion imaging possible; limited availability
^{99m}Tc DTPA aerosol	6 hr	140 keV	Low	Delivery not as good as with gases; multiple projections possible
Perfusion				
^{99m}Tc MAA	6 hr	140 keV	Low	

areas. Exhaled Xe can be vented to the outside atmosphere.

^{133}XENON

^{133}Xe is the most commonly used ventilation agent. It is relatively inexpensive and has a physical half-life of 5.2 days. Xe is an inert gas that is distributed to lung spaces through normally ventilated areas. Three phases of distribution are usually distinguishable although the biologic half-life is less than 1 minute:

- Inspiration (15 to 20 seconds)
- Equilibrium (patient breathes Xe/O_2 mixture in a closed system for 3 to 5 minutes)
- Washout (patient breathes room air and exhales into charcoal trap)

Less than 15% of inhaled gas is absorbed in the body. Since Xe is highly soluble in fat, it localizes to liver and fatty tissues once absorbed. Xe also adsorbs onto plastic syringes (10% at 24 hours), for which reason glass syringes are used for handling. Xe ventilation cannot be performed on a portable basis because negative pressure is required to remove gas. Technetium aerosol can be used for portable scans.

^{127}XENON

^{127}Xe has a similar pharmacologic behavior to ^{133}Xe. However, its physical half-life is longer (36.4 days versus 5.2 days), it is more expensive, and its main photon energy is higher (203 versus 81 keV). Because of the higher photon energy, ventilation imaging can be performed after the ^{99m}Tc MAA scan (140 keV main energy). Thus, the best projection for ventilation imaging can be selected based on the perfusion scan. The high energy of the nuclide requires a medium-energy collimator so that collimators have to be changed between perfusion and ventilation study.

^{81M}KRYPTON

The availability of ^{81m}Kr/^{81}Rb generators is the major limitation of using this nuclide. Because of the short physical half-life (13.4 seconds), washout images cannot be obtained, limiting the sensitivity for detection of obstructive lung disease. As with ^{127}Xe, ventilation imaging can be performed after the ^{99m}Tc MAA scan. A high main photon energy of 191 keV requires the use of a medium-energy collimator (lower resolution, collimators have to be changed during the study). The short half-life of ^{81m}Kr results in images comparable to xenon washin images, even though the images are obtained with continuous breathing of krypton. The higher energy of krypton permits ventilation imaging either before or after perfusion imaging. Because the krypton ventilation images are performed with continuous breathing, it is normal to see some tracer activity in the trachea on the anterior view.

^{99M}TC DTPA AEROSOL

A large amount (1110 to 1850 MBq) of activity is loaded into a specially shielded nebulizer that produces droplets containing the radionuclide. Approximately 18 to 28 MBq of activity reaches the lungs during the 3 to 5 minutes of breathing. Once in the lungs, droplets diffuse through interstitium into capillaries and ^{99m}Tc DTPA is finally excreted renally. Pulmonary clearance usually takes >1 hour (much faster in smokers and those with IPF or ARDS), for which reason the aerosol cannot be used for single breath or washout phase imaging. Slow pulmonary clearance allows multiple projection images to be obtained typically in the same views as in the perfusion study. Because the aerosol delivers only a small amount of activity (20% of activity used for perfusion imaging), ventilation imaging is performed before perfusion imaging. Alternatively, a reduced dose of MAA (1 mCi) can be given first for perfusion imaging. Particle deposition in large central airways occurs in obstructive lung disease.

^{99M}TC MACROAGGREGATED ALBUMIN

The theoretical basis for using macroaggregated albumin particles (MAA) in perfusion imaging is that particles become physically trapped in arterioles, thus allowing one to measure regional perfusion. MAA is prepared by heat and pH denaturation of human serum albumin (HSA). For quality assurance purposes, the size of at least 100 particles has to be determined (optimum from 10 to 90 μm; particles should not be <10 μm or >150 μm). 200,000 to 700,000 MAA particles are injected IV, to occlude precapillary arterioles (20 to 30 μm) and capillaries (8 μm). Injection of <70,000 particles leads to a statistically inaccurate examination (because of quantum mottle). The number of injected particles should be reduced in:

- Pulmonary hypertension
- Neonates, pediatric patients
- Right-to-left shunts

Pharmacokinetics

- >90% of particles are trapped in lung capillaries during 1st pass (particles <10 μm are phagocytosed by liver and spleen).
- Approximately 100,000 of the 280 billion capillaries are occluded during a normal lung perfusion scan.
- Particles are cleared from lungs by enzymatic hydrolysis (biologic half-life: 2 to 10 hours).
- Renal clearance of ^{99m}Tc MAA is 30%-40% at 24 hours.
- Because the particle number/dose must be known at time of administration, all doses must be given within 6 hours of preparation.

TECHNIQUE

INDICATIONS

Common indications for pulmonary imaging include:

- Pulmonary embolism (PE)
  - Elective $\dot{V}/\dot{Q}$ scan
- Clinical suspicion of PE (symptomatic patient and risk factors)
- Baseline posttreatment scan
  - Emergency $\dot{V}/\dot{Q}$ scan (e.g., at night)
- Symptomatic patient and risk factor and normal or abnormal CXR
- Surgical applications
  - Preoperative evaluation of lung function (quantitative)
  - Postsurgical bronchial stump leaks (Xe may show air leak)
  - Transplant rejection (decreased MAA perfusion)
- Right-to left (R-L) shunts

CONTRAINDICATIONS

No absolute contraindications exist. Relative contraindications include:

- Pulmonary arterial hypertension (PAH)
- R-L shunts (particles end up in systemic circulation)
- Hypersensitivity to HSA

PROTOCOL

1. Obtain history and risk factors.
2. Ventilate patient with ^{133}Xe (370 to 740 MBq) and image in posterior projection: The gamma energy of xenon is 81 keV and will be attenuated by 1 cm of inflated lung and overlying breast tissue.
   - Initial breath: single image
   - Equilibrium: 2 × 90-second images
   - Washout: 3 × 45-second images
   - Retention: LPO, posterior, RPO images of 45 seconds each
3. Injection of ^{99m}Tc MAA (150 MBq) in supine position and image:
   - 6-standard views: posterior, RPO, LPO, anterior, RAO, LAO
   - Lateral views (usually not helpful)

Information that should be obtained in all patients includes:

CXR (within 12 hours of assessment)

- Normal or minimal lung abnormality on CXR is typical in PE.
- Normal CXR does not exclude PE but facilitates interpretation of a $\dot{V}/\dot{Q}$ scan (i.e., absence of matched hypoventilated/hypoperfused consolidations).

Arterial blood gases

- Po_2 <80% is seen in 80% of patients with PE.
- An A-a gradient of >14 mm Hg is seen in only 90% of patients.

Lower extremity US (optional)

- Sensitivity for detecting femoropopliteal deep vein thrombosis (DVT), 95%
- Only approximately 30% of patients with PE have documented DVT.

IMAGING

NORMAL IMAGES

Xenon Ventilation

Homogeneous distribution of activity occurs in the 3 phases (Fig. 12-1):

- Washin
- Equilibrium
- Washout; complete clearing should occur within 2 to 3 minutes.

Trapping of Xe on washout is indicative of airway obstruction (e.g., bullae, chronic obstructive pulmonary disease [COPD]). Hallmarks of obstructive disease are decreased washin, slow equilibration, and delayed washout.

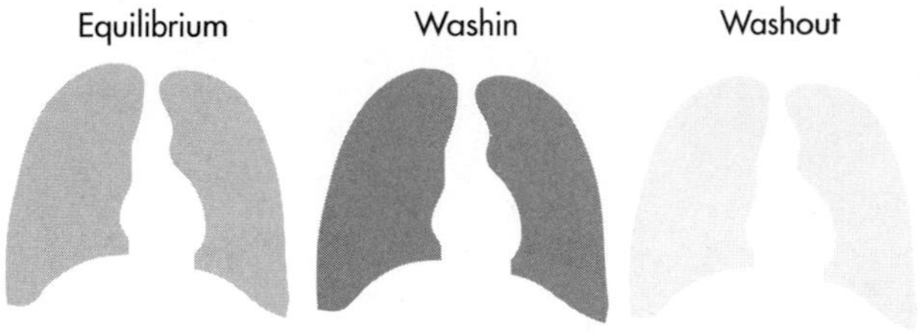

FIGURE 12-1

Perfusion (Fig. 12-2)

- Normal identifiable structures: heart, aortic arch, fissures
- Anterior indentation on lung on LPO represents the heart.
- Slight gradient of activity from posterior to anterior reflects greater perfusion to dependent portions of lung in supine patient.
- Activity at apex is usually less than at bases (less parenchymal volume at apex).
- Subsegmental perfusion defects occur in 7% of normal population.

PULMONARY EMBOLISM

$\dot{V}/\dot{Q}$ imaging requires the use of two sequential tracers: a ventilation (i.e., breathing) agent and a perfusion (i.e., intravascular) agent (Fig. 12-3). Two tracers are used rather than one because altered pulmonary perfusion alone is a nonspecific finding that occurs in many pulmonary diseases, but $\dot{V}/\dot{Q}$ mismatches are fairly specific for PE. $\dot{V}/\dot{Q}$ mismatch refers to regions of decreased perfusion ("cold") that have normal ventilation. If the perfusion part of the study is normal, PE is excluded and ventilation imaging is not required.

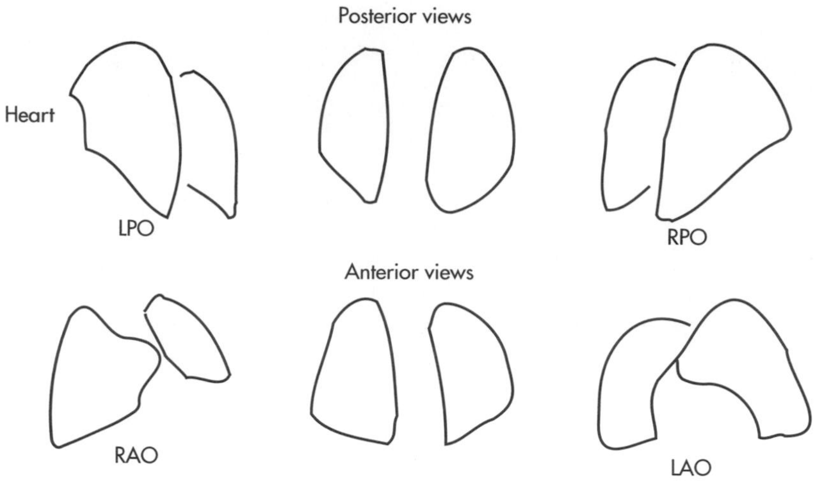

FIGURE 12-2

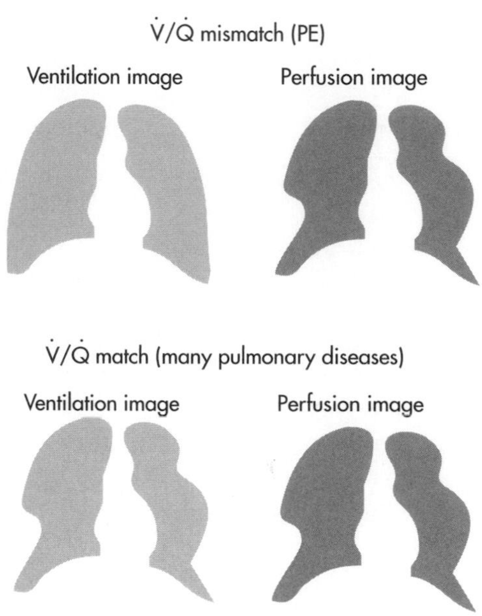

FIGURE 12-3

Recent use of $\dot{V}/\dot{Q}$ scanning with SPECT allows 3-dimensional visualization of segments previously not identified by planar imaging, such as the medial basal segment of the right lower lobe. The lung segments are more clearly defined and can be viewed in any orthogonal plane, resulting in better detection and characterization of defects. SPECT also improves image contrast, thus decreasing the rate of intermediate scan reports.

Scheme for Interpretation (Prospective Investigation of Pulmonary Embolism Diagnosis [PIOPED])

1. Classify perfusion defects by size and segmental anatomy.
   - Small segmental defect: <25% of pulmonary segment affected
   - Moderate segmental defect: 25%-75% of a pulmonary segment affected
   - Large segmental defect: 75% of pulmonary segment affected
   - Lobar defect
   - Nonsegmental defect
2. Correlate perfusion and ventilation images.
3. Cannot interpret study if >75% of a lung zone has obstructive disease

INTERPRETATION OF SCAN RESULTS

Interpretation/Frequency	Pattern	Probability of PE (%)
Normal, 5%	Normal perfusion (ventilation and CXR may be abnormal)	0-5
Low probability, 55%	1. Single segmental perfusion defect (subsegmental)	10-15
	2. Small perfusion defect	
	3. Any perfusion defect with larger corresponding CXR abnormality	
	4. Nonsegmental perfusion abnormalities	
	5. Matched $\dot{V}/\dot{Q}$ abnormalities	
Intermediate probability (indeterminate), 30%	Any scan not falling into high or low probability group	30-40
High probability, 10%	1. 2 segmentals $\dot{V}/\dot{Q}$ mismatches	90-95
	2. 1 segmental and >2 subsegmental $\dot{V}/\dot{Q}$ defects	
	3. 4 subsegmental $\dot{V}/\dot{Q}$ mismatches	

PISAPED (Prospective Investigative Study of Pulmonary Embolism Diagnosis) Criterion for Interpretation of Perfusion Lung Scan

PE present	One or more wedge-shaped perfusion defects
PE absent	1. Normal perfusion
	2. Very low probability
	3. Nonsegmental lesion; e.g., prominent hilum, cardiomegaly, elevated diaphragm, linear atelectasis
	4. Perfusion defect smaller than radiographic lesion
	5. A solitary CXR-Q matched defect in the mid or upper lung confined to a single segment
	6. Stripe sign around the perfusion defect
	7. Pleural effusion ≥ one third of the pleural cavity with no other perfusion defect in either lung
Nondiagnostic	All other findings

Implications of Scan Results

- High probability: treat for PE
- Intermediate/indeterminate probability: pulmonary angiogram
- Low probability: unlikely to be PE. Consider other diagnoses. Obtain pulmonary angiogram if clinical suspicion remains very high.
- Normal perfusion study excludes PE

$\dot{V}/\dot{Q}$ Scan to Monitor Sequelae/Resolution of PE

- Most PE perfusion abnormalities resolve within 3 months. Thus, a baseline posttreatment scan should be obtained several months after initial diagnosis.
- Baseline scans are helpful to diagnose recurrent PE.
- Acute perfusion defects tend to be sharply defined; old or resolving perfusion defects tend to be less well defined.

Modified PIOPED Criteria for Scan Interpretation

High probability >80%

- >2 large (>75% of a segment) segmental perfusion defects without corresponding ventilation or radiographic abnormalities or substantially larger than either matching ventilation or CXR abnormalities
- >2 moderate segmental (>25% and <75% of a segment) perfusion defects without matching ventilation or CXR abnormalities and 1 large mismatched segmental defect
- >4 moderate segmental perfusion defects without ventilation or CXR abnormalities

Intermediate (indeterminate) probability 20%-80%

- Single moderate mismatched segmental perfusion defect with normal CXR
- One large and one moderate mismatched segmental defect with a normal CXR
- Not falling into normal/very low, low, or high probability categories

Low probability, <20%

- Any perfusion defect with a substantially larger CXR abnormality
- Large or moderate segmental perfusion defects involving no more than 50% of the combined lung fields with matching ventilation defects either equal to or larger in size, and CXR either normal or with abnormalities substantially larger than perfusion defects
- Any number of small segmental perfusion defects with a normal CXR

Pearls

- Small perfusion defects ("rat bites") almost never represent PE.
- If ventilation abnormalities occupy >75% of lung, PIOPED criteria classify the abnormality as indeterminate or nondiagnostic for PE.
- If etiology of matched $\dot{V}/\dot{Q}$ abnormalities and CXR abnormality is unknown, then scan is classified as indeterminate.
- Intermediate and indeterminate scans have the same diagnostic significance (i.e., a PE has not been ruled in or ruled out). Some radiologists use the terms interchangeably.
- Right upper quadrant uptake on ventilation images can be seen in fatty liver.
- Injection of Swan-Ganz catheter may lead to accumulation of activity in one lung on perfusion images.
- Heterogeneous perfusion of both lungs with perihilar hot spots may be seen when ^{99m}Tc MAA is allowed to settle and aggregate before injection.
- Right-to-left shunt: uptake in brain, kidneys, spleen
- Free ^{99m}Tc pertechnetate : uptake in thyroid, kidneys, stomach, salivary glands

OTHER PATTERNS

Stripe Sign (Fig. 12-4)

This sign refers to a perfusion abnormality with a zone of preserved peripheral perfusion. Because PE is pleural based, presence of this sign makes PE unlikely.

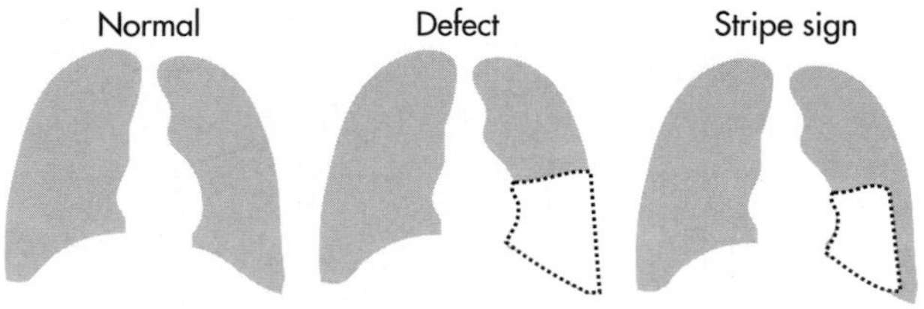

FIGURE 12-4

Reverse Mismatch

Normal perfusion with abnormal ventilation. Most commonly due to atelectasis.

Pulmonary Edema

- Redistribution of blood away from dependent portions of the lung
- Pleural effusions, fissural "highlighting"

Bullae, Emphysema, COPD

- Delayed washout on ventilation images: air trapping
- Matched $\dot{V}/\dot{Q}$ defects

Pulmonary Arterial Hypertension

Diffusely heterogeneous perfusion with many small peripheral perfusion abnormalities, "contour mapping."

Transplant

- Poor perfusion to lung apices may be normal after lung transplant.

EVALUATION OF LUNG FUNCTION (Fig. 12-5)

Commonly performed in patients undergoing lung resection. Using a computer program, the overall ventilation and perfusion of each lung is determined.

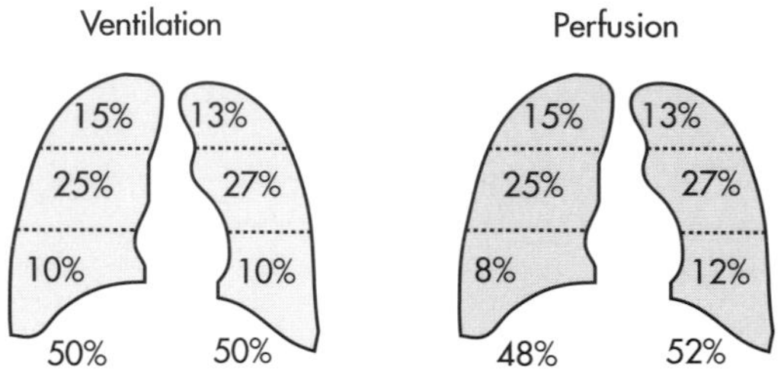

FIGURE 12-5

Cardiac Imaging

RADIOPHARMACEUTICALS

²⁰¹THALLIUM CHLORIDE

^{201}Tl ("perfusion marker") is cyclotron produced. It distributes proportionally to cardiac output in all tissues except brain (because of intact blood-brain barrier) and fat. Cellular uptake occurs in any tissue if the cellular Na^+/K^+ pump is intact.

Pharmacokinetics

- Myocardial extraction: 3%-4% of total dose (at rest). Localization in myocardium occurs in 2 phases:
  - Initial distribution and cellular extraction based on blood flow, which is close to 90%
  - Delayed "redistribution" based on continued extraction of thallium from blood and ongoing washout of previously extracted thallium
  - Unlike the reextraction of thallium by myocardium, the washout component of redistribution strongly depends on coronary perfusion, with ischemic areas demonstrating much slower washout than normal regions
- Blood half-life: ranges from 0.5 minutes (exercise) to 3 minutes (rest)
- Biologic half-life: 10 days ± 2.5 days
- Long biologic and physical half-life (73 hours) limit dose (1 to 2 mCi) that can be given.
- Renal clearance, 4%-8%

Use

- Imaging of myocardial ischemia and infarctions
- Parathyroid adenoma localization

^{99m}TC SESTAMIBI (Fig. 12-6)

^{99m}Tc sestamibi is an isonitrile (hexakis-2-methoxyisobutyl isonitrile) containing 6 isonitrile components. Sestamibi has a high first-pass extraction, a distribution proportional to blood flow, and few or no metabolic side effects. Advantages over ^{201}Tl include:

- Better dosimetry: higher dose can be given, resulting in higher photon flux
- Preferred agent for SPECT imaging (more photons)
- Higher energy than ^{99m}Tc photons: less tissue attenuation
- Preferred for obese patients
- Good correlation between ^{201}Tl and ^{99m}Tc MIBI in terms of imaging characteristics

Pharmacokinetics

- Passive diffusion into myocyte. Myocardial uptake is proportional to diffusion.
- ^{99m}Tc sestamibi is retained in myocardium because of binding to a low molecular weight protein in the cytosol complex.
- Hepatobiliary excretion: prominent liver activity (may interfere with evaluation of inferior wall)
- Wait 30 to 60 minutes before imaging to allow some hepatic clearance.
- There is no myocardial redistribution; thus imaging can be performed 1 to 2 hours after injection.

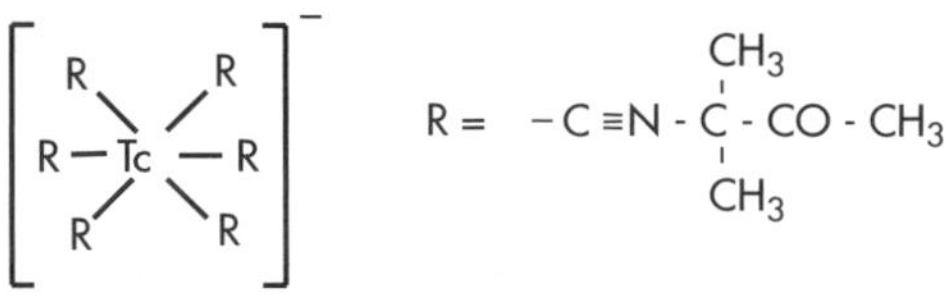

FIGURE 12-6

^{99m}TC TEBOROXIME

^{99m}Tc teboroxime is a neutral lipophilic boronic acid conjugated to technetium dioxime for cardiac imaging. Avidly extracted from blood by myocardium. Myocardial uptake has a linear correlation with blood flow so that regional uptake is a suitable marker of myocardial perfusion. The main disadvantage is rapid myocardial clearance that necessitates imaging immediately after injection and limits its versatility.

Pharmacokinetics

- Cardiac extraction: 3.5% (higher than isonitriles)
- Hepatobiliary excretion (may interfere with inferior wall evaluation)
- Biologic half-life: 10 to 20 minutes
- Very rapid myocardial clearance
- No redistribution

COMPARISON OF AGENTS

	^{201}Thallium	^{99m}Tc Sestamibi	^{99m}Tc Teboroxime
Dose	74-111 MBq	740-1850 MBq	740-850 MBq
Imaging time	Immediate	60 min	1-2 min
Cardiac half-life	3-5 hr	5 hr	5-10 min
Cardiac uptake	3%-4%	2%	3%-4%
Redistribution	Yes	Slight	No

^{99m}TC RBC LABELING

Autologous RBC labeling is best performed by one of three methods of pertechnetate incorporation into RBC. RBC labeling is based on the principle that (+7) TcO_4 crosses the RBC membrane but reduced (+4) Tc does not. TcO_4 can be reduced intracellularly to (+4) Tc with tin (Sn^{2+}); reduced Tc binds to the beta chain of hemoglobin.

Uses

- Cardiac-gated blood-pool studies
- Bleeding studies
- Hemangioma characterization
- Spleen imaging (alternative to sulfur colloid)

Methods of Labeling Autologous RBCs

In vivo labeling
- 1 mg of stannous pyrophosphate injected IV
- After 20 minutes 740 MBq of ^{99m} TcO_4^- is injected.
- Disadvantage: labeling efficiency <85%; low target-to-background ratio

Modified in vivo labeling
- 1 mg of stannous pyrophosphate injected IV
- After 20 minutes, 5 mL of blood is withdrawn and incubated in a syringe with 740 MBq of $^{99m}TcO_4^-$ for 10 minutes
- Incubated RBCs are reinjected.
- Advantage of this method is a higher labeling efficiency: 30 minutes after injection 90% of administered radioactivity remains in the intravascular space.

In vitro labeling
- Entire labeling procedure is performed outside patient
- Requires 30 minutes
- Best labeling efficiency
- Using commercial kit (UltraTag), blood is aspirated in anticoagulant and mixed in vial with stannous ion for 5 minutes
- Subsequently mixed with sodium hypochlorite, then citrate buffer with dextrose
- $^{99m}TcO_4^-$ is added and reinjected after incubation for 20 minutes

Causes of Poor RBC Labeling

- Drug interactions (e.g., heparin, doxorubicin, contrast agents)
- Antibodies: transfusions, transplantation
- Short incubation time
- Too much or too little stannous ion

Pearls

- In vivo methods suffice in clinical practice.
- Heat-damaged RBCs are used for selective spleen imaging.
- ^{99m}Tc-labeled human serum albumin (HSA) is an alternative agent for blood pool imaging but provides less target-to-background due to extracellular diffusion.
- New long circulating polymers are being developed that may obviate the need for RBC labeling.

MYOCARDIAL PERFUSION SCINTIGRAPHY

GENERAL (Figs. 12-7 and 12-8)

Myocardial ischemia is demonstrated only if ^{201}Tl is in circulation while there is myocardial ischemia. For this reason, patients have to be exercised for a few minutes after IV injection of ^{201}Tl ("initial images").

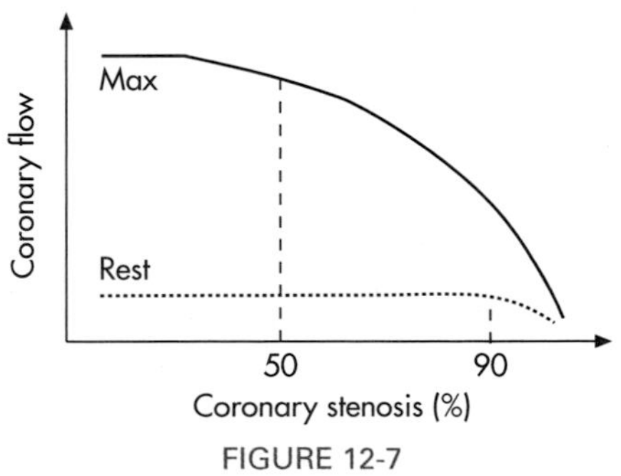

FIGURE 12-7

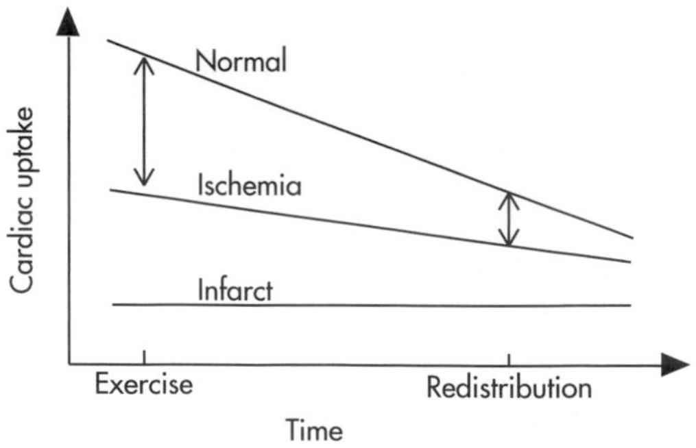

FIGURE 12-8

The sensitivity of ^{201}Tl imaging depends directly on the degree of exercise achieved. A coronary stenosis must exceed 90% of normal diameter before resting blood flow is impaired; with maximum exercise, however, stenosis of >50% is hemodynamically significant.

Images acquired several hours after initial IV injection show a different pattern; areas of initially high activity wash out faster so areas of initially low activity may have relatively higher activity ("redistribution image"). To obtain good-quality redistribution images, a second dose of ^{201}Tl is injected 3 to 4 hours after initial imaging. Reinjection improves differentiation of defects and improves the sensitivity for ischemia as compared with simple redistribution imaging.

TECHNIQUES

There are 3 techniques of nuclear cardiac perfusion imaging:

Physical exercise test (significant increase in myocardial workload). This is the preferred technique:
- Treadmill test (Bruce protocol or modified protocol)
- Bicycling

Pharmacologic "stress" test (no significant increase in myocardial workload)
- Coronary flow increases after administration of vasodilators; stenotic vessels do not respond as much and areas of hypoperfusion are accentuated.
- Workload is not increased; ischemia seldom occurs.
- Agents used: dipyridamole (acts indirectly by reducing the degradation of endogenous adenosine)
- Adenosine (Adenocard): direct vasodilator with short duration
- Dobutamine: chronotropic and inotropic agent

Rest study
- Use: patients for whom exercise or dipyridamole is contraindicated (intraaortic balloon pump, coronary artery bypass graft)
- Not sensitive for detecting ischemia
- Used mainly to determine myocardial viability

Treadmill Test

1. Patient NPO to decrease splanchnic activity
2. Patient is exercised on treadmill to maximum stress (i.e., completion of protocol) or other endpoint
   - 85% predicted maximum heart rate (PMHR = 220 – age in years)
   - Unable to continue secondary to fatigue or dyspnea
   - Cardiovascular signs/symptoms: severe angina, hypotension, arrhythmias, ischemic electrocardiogram (ECG) changes
3. First dose of ^{201}Tl injected at peak exercise (75 MBq). Continue exercise for 1 minute.
4. Image immediately.
5. Second dose of ^{201}Tl (37 MBq) injected at rest after 3 to 4 hours to obtain redistribution images

Factors that limit exercise stress test:
- Inadequate stress decreases diagnostic sensitivity.
- Heart rate should increase to at least 85% of PMHR.
- Drugs that limit heart rate response decrease sensitivity of the stress test (beta-blockers, calcium channel blockers, digoxin).
- Nondiagnostic ECG: left ventricle hypertrophy, left bundle branch block, baseline ST-T abnormalities

Dipyridamole Test

1. Patient NPO (no coffee, caffeine, or other xanthine products for 24 hours)
2. Dipyridamole IV infusion (0.6 mg/kg over 4 minutes): HR increases 20%, BP decreases 10 mm Hg
3. ^{201}Tl (3 mCi) is given 10 minutes after the dipyridamole is started (peak blood dipyridamole level)
4. Image immediately
5. Administer aminophylline (50 to 100 mg) to reverse side effects (flushing, headaches) of dipyridamole
6. Reinject ^{201}Tl (1.5 mCi) for redistribution images.

Adenosine Test

1. Patient NPO (no coffee, caffeine, or other xanthine products for 24 hours)
2. Adenosine IV infusion (0.14 mg/kg/min over 4-6 minutes)
3. ^{201}Tl (3 mCi) is given 3 minutes after the adenosine infusion is started
4. Begin imaging 3 minutes after completion of adenosine infusion.

5. Stop infusion if side effects encountered (AV block) given short half-life (10 seconds)
6. Reinject ^{201}Tl for redistribution images.

Dobutamine Test

1. Hold beta- and calcium-channel blockers
2. Begin dobutamine IV infusion at 0.005 mg/kg/min and increase by 0.005 mg/kg/min every 3 minutes to maximum of 0.04 mg over 4 minutes): HR increases 20%, BP decreases 10 mm Hg
3. ^{201}Tl is given 1 minute after the maximum dose achieved and infusion continued for at least one additional minute
4. Beware of arrhythmias; consider atropine 0.5 mg to raise heart rate and reduce needed dobutamine dose; beta-blocker (esmolol, metoprolol) for reversal

Rest and Redistribution Study

1. Injection of 1st dose of ^{201}Tl (74 MBq)
2. Image immediately
3. No reinjection of 2nd dose

^{99m}TC SESTAMIBI IMAGING

One-day protocol:

1. Rest and stress studies are performed on same day
2. May begin with rest or stress study first
3. Stress-rest: Administer 8-10 mCi ^{99m}Tc sestamibi at peak stress and image in 15-60 min (longer delay is selected in pharmacologic stress due to liver/splanchnic uptake). Wait 2-4 hours and administer a larger dose (25-30 mCi) and image at 30-60 minutes.
4. Rest-stress: Administer 8-10 mCi ^{99m}Tc sestamibi and image 30-60 min. 2-4 hours later, inject larger dose and image 15-60 minutes.

Two-day protocol:

1. Performing rest and stress studies one day apart allows use of full dose (25-30 mCi) of ^{99m}Tc sestamibi.
2. Stress study performed first as if normal, may obviate need for rest study.
3. Stress: Inject 25-30 mCi at peak stress and image 15-60 minutes.
4. Rest: Inject 25-30 mCi and image at 30-60 minutes.

Dual isotope protocol:

1. Rest study with ^{201}Tl (3 mCi) is performed first, followed immediately by stress study with ^{99m}Tc sestamibi (25-30 mCi)
2. Quicker to perform than other protocols

CONTRAINDICATIONS FOR NUCLEAR CARDIOLOGY STRESS TEST

Absolute

- Acute myocardial infarction
- Severe aortic stenosis
- Severe reaction to stress agent
- Severe pulmonary hypertension
- Obstructive hypertrophic cardiomyopathy
- Combination of low ejection fraction (EF) (20%) and documented recent ventricular fibrillation (VF) or ventricular tachycardia (VT)
- Cocaine within 24 hours
- Pregnancy
- Unstable angina

Relative

- Severe mitral stenosis
- Hypertension (>180/100 mm Hg)
- Hypotension (<90 mm Hg, systolic)
- Tachycardia (>120/min)
- Wheezing, bronchospasm
- Inability to communicate
- Acute illness such as pericarditis, pulmonary embolus, infection, fever

NORMAL IMAGES AND VARIANTS (Fig. 12-9)

Uniform distribution of activity should be present in the myocardium.

Variations

- Diaphragmatic attenuation: inferior myocardial wall, especially on anterior and steep LAO views, may be attenuated (Fig. 12-10)
- Thin basal myocardium: decreased activity along the most superior aspect of images (cardiac valve plane)
- Nonuniform activity may be seen in the proximal septum.
- Lung uptake is normal if lung:heart ratio is <50%. A ratio of >0.5% pulmonary activity indicates left ventricular (LV) dysfunction with or without pulmonary edema. Increased lung activity correlates with elevated pulmonary capillary wedge pressure.
- Splanchnic uptake may be seen after a recent meal, with inadequate exercise, and in dipyridamole and sestamibi studies.
- Right ventricular (RV) activity at rest (i.e., on redistribution images but not on stress images) indicates hypertrophy.
- "Hot" papillary muscles may make adjacent myocardium appear hypoperfused.
- Apical thinning refers to decreased activity in the cardiac apex (common in dilated hearts) (Fig. 12-11).

Image Interpretation

1. Adequacy of study
   - Did patient achieve 85% PMHR?
   - Splanchnic uptake (minimal exercise, not NPO)
2. Lung uptake

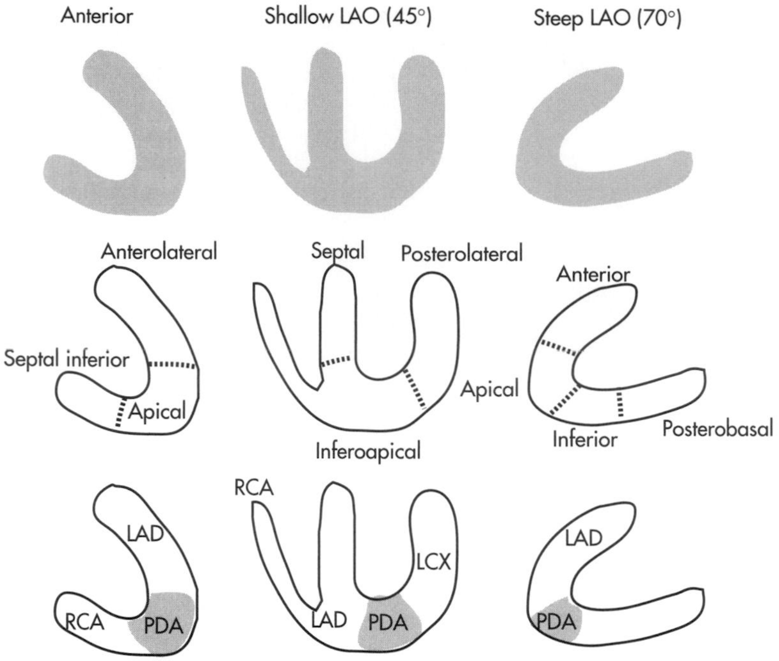

FIGURE 12-09

- Lung/heart ratio >0.5 indicates exercise-induced LV dysfunction.

3. Heart size and wall thickness
   - Subjective assessment
   - Transient cavitary dilatation (dilated cavity on initial but not delayed images) is a sign of LV dysfunction.
4. Distribution defects
   - Full-thickness defect
   - Partial-thickness defects
   - Reversible versus irreversible defects

ABNORMAL PLANAR SCAN PATTERNS

Three patterns (Fig. 12-12):

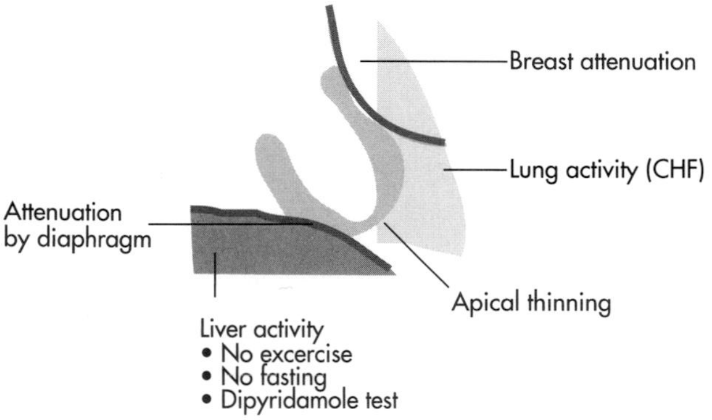

FIGURE 12-10

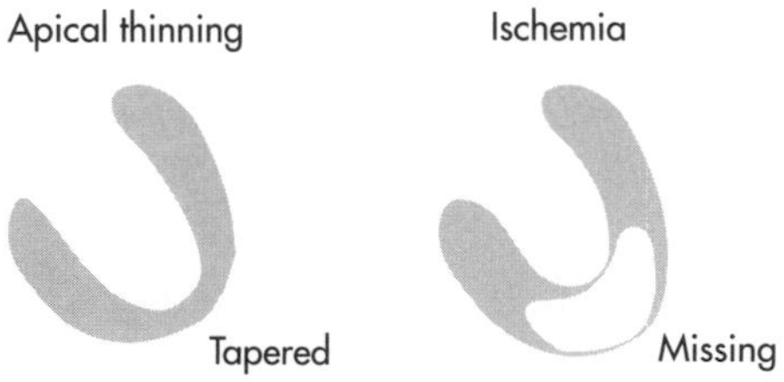

FIGURE 12-11

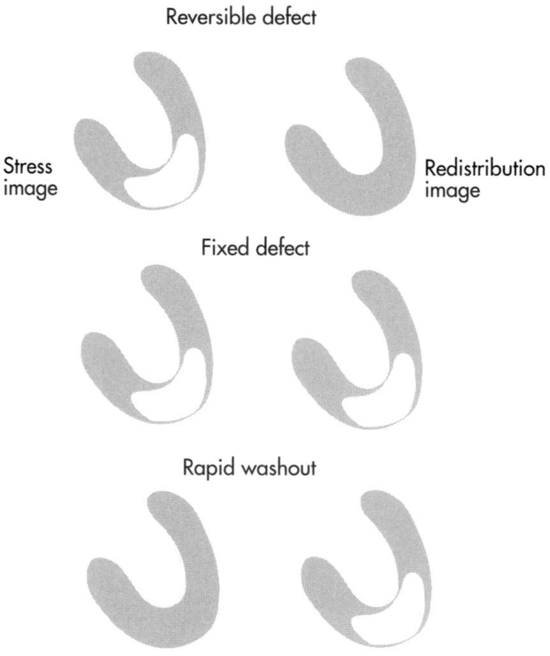

FIGURE 12-12

Reversible perfusion pattern
- Perfusion defect is present in the stress image with partial or complete fill-in on redistribution images.
- Indicative of ischemia
- Rare conditions with this pattern causing false positive results for ischemia: Chagas disease, sarcoid, hypertrophic cardiomyopathy

Irreversible, fixed perfusion pattern
- Perfusion defect persists
- Much less specific for ischemia than reversible defects
- Often seen with scars (old myocardial infarction), cardiomyopathies, idiopathic hypertrophic subaortic stenosis, coronary spasm, infiltrative or metastatic lesions

Rapid washout pattern
- Stress view is normal and redistribution images demonstrate defects.
- Least specific pattern
- May occur in coronary artery disease (CAD), cardiomyopathy, or normal patients

Note that three vessel disease can produce balanced ischemia
- No regional perfusion defect identified
- May see chamber dilatation, wall motion abnormalities, EKG abnormalities on exercise

SENSITIVITY AND SPECIFICITY

	Exercise ECG (%)	^{201}Tl Stress Test (%)	SPECT
Sensitivity	60	85	Marginal improvement over ^{201}Tl
Specificity	85	85	Possibly lower

Sensitivity of ^{201}Tl varies with extent of disease:
- 80% sensitivity for single vessel disease
- 95% sensitivity for triple vessel disease

Dipyridamole ^{201}Tl scan appears to have similar sensitivity/specificity as exercise ^{201}Tl.

SPECT IMAGING

Advantages
- Improved sensitivity for detection of moderate CAD
- More accurate anatomic localization (especially LCx territory)

Technique
- Best performed with multidetector camera
- Images are obtained over a 180° arc at 6° intervals: 45° RAO to 45° LPO
- The slice thickness is approximately 1 cm.
- Total imaging time: single detector 20 to 30 minutes; multidetector 10 to 15 minutes
- Anterior planar images needed to assess lung activity

Interpretation
- 3 standard image reconstruction planes (cardiac axes: short, horizontal, long, and vertical) (Fig. 12-13)
- Compare initial and redistribution images as in planar imaging
- Quantitative polar maps are adjunct to qualitative visual analysis.

HIBERNATING MYOCARDIUM

Refers to chronic ischemia: poorly perfused heart at rest has loss of functional wall motion but is still viable.
- Fixed defects on 4-hour thallium images
- Diminished wall motion
- Requires revascularization procedure
- Reimage at 24 hours after second injection

STUNNED MYOCARDIUM

- Acute event that results from ischemic injury
- Normal or near-normal perfusion with decreased contractility
- Acute coronary artery occlusion

PET IMAGING

^{82}Rubidium
- Myocardial perfusion agent

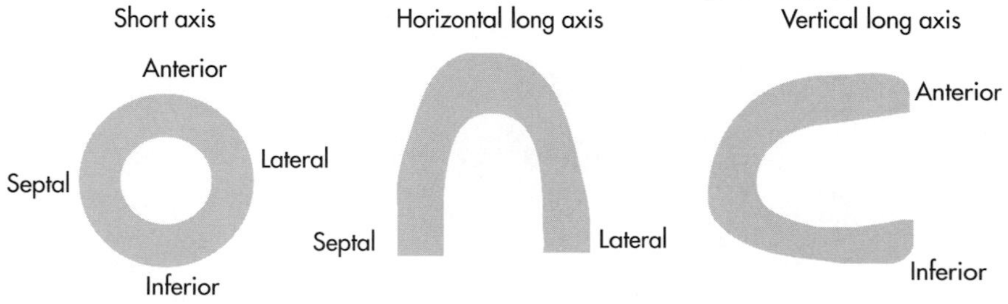

FIGURE 12-13

- Generator produced, potassium analog taken up by myocardium via Na/K pump, half-life 76 seconds
- Imaging within 5 minutes of injection

^{13}N-ammonia

- Myocardial perfusion agent
- ^{13}N is cyclotron produced, diffuses into myocardium and is trapped, half-life 10 minutes

^{18}F-Fluorodeoxyglucose (FDG)

- Myocardial metabolism
- Glucose loading to promote myocardial uptake
- Used in combination with perfusion imaging to assess hibernating myocardium: ^{18}F-FDG uptake in a region of perfusion deficit indicates viable myocardium whereas matched ^{18}F-FDG and perfusion deficit is indicative of infarct

PET IMAGING PATTERNS

Myocardium	Perfusion (NH_3)	Metabolism (FDG)
Normal	+	+
Ischemia	– or decreased	+
Necrosis	–	–

ACUTE MYOCARDIAL INFARCT (AMI) IMAGING

^{99M}TC PYROPHOSPHATE IMAGING (Fig. 12-14)

Indications are limited because AMI is more often diagnosed by ECG and elevated enzymes.

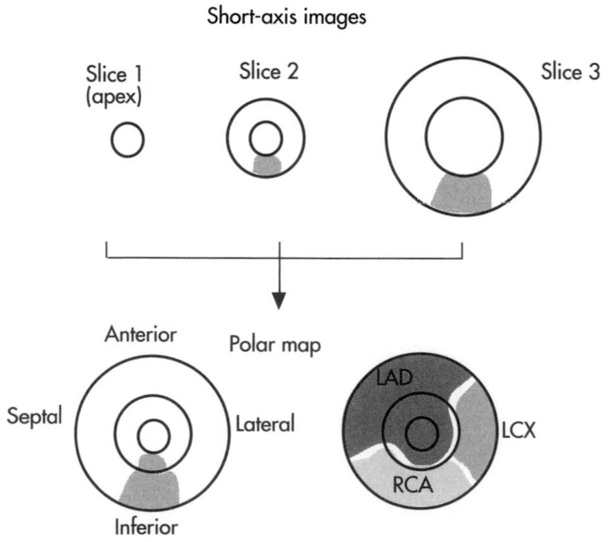

FIGURE 12-14

Technique

- ^{99m}Tc pyrophosphate (370 to 550 MBq) is injected at rest. Pyrophosphate binds to denatured proteins and parallels calcium metabolism.
- Imaging is performed 2 to 4 hours after injection.

Interpretation

- Scans become increasingly positive for 72 hours after infarct. Insensitive within the first 24 hours and 10 days after the MI.
- Focal myocardial activity represents accumulation in damaged myocardium. The severity of uptake may be graded:
  - Grade 0: no uptake, normal
  - Grade 1: less uptake than rib
  - Grade 2: more uptake than rib
  - Grade 3: more uptake than sternum
- A cardiac doughnut pattern may be present: absence of flow to central region of the infarct

Differential diagnosis of thoracic soft tissue uptake of ^{99m}Tc pyrophosphate:

- Infarction
- Direct myocardial injuries (contusion/trauma, cardioversion, myocarditis, cardiac surgery)
- All cardiomyopathies
- Pericarditis, endocarditis
- Unstable angina
- Calcification (dystrophic, valvular, costal cartilage)
- Breast tumors
- Blood pool activity

RESTING ^{201}THALLIUM SCAN

^{201}Tl is injected at rest. The distribution reflects coronary artery perfusion. Very reliable if performed within 12 to 24 hours after Q-wave infarcts (sensitivity 90%). Sensitivity decreases with time after the infarct, possibly related to the resolution of the associated ischemia. The sensitivity is also lower for non-Q-wave infarcts.

Recommended Tests for Intermediate or High Likelihood of CAD

Patient Able To Exercise to 85% of Maximum Predicted HR

- Stress ECG
  - Normal or mildly abnormal ECG
  - No digoxin
- Resting and exercise myocardial perfusion SPECT
  - Ventricular preexcitation
  - >1 mm ST segment depression
  - LV hypertrophy
  - To evaluate physiologic significance of coronary stenosis (25%-75%)
  - Intermediate Duke treadmill score
  - High-risk patients (>20% of 10-year risk of cardiac event)
  - Selected high-risk asymptomatic patients, 3 to 5 years after revascularization

- Resting and adenosine or dipyridamole stress myocardial-perfusion SPECT
  - Cardiac pacemaker
  - Left bundle branch block

Patient Unable to Exercise

- Resting and adenosine or dipyridamole stress myocardial-perfusion SPECT:
  - To evaluate extent, location, and severity of ischemia
  - To evaluate physiologic significance of coronary stenoses (25%-75%)
  - Known CAD: change in symptoms suggests increased likelihood of cardiac event
  - High-risk patients (>20% 10-year risk of cardiac event)
  - Selected high-risk asymptomatic patients, 3 to 5 years after revascularization
- Resting and dobutamine stress myocardial perfusion SPECT:
  - Severe COPD, recent (<1 month) asthma attack
  - 2nd- and 3rd-degree AV block
  - Severe bradycardia of <40 beats/min
  - Adenosine and dipyridamole contraindicated

Indications for PET

- Resting and adenosine or dipyridamole or dobutamine stress myocardial perfusion PET:
  - SPECT study equivocal
  - Obesity (>400 lb)

VENTRICULAR FUNCTION IMAGING

GENERAL

There are two different approaches to studying ventricular function:

1. First-pass studies
   - Immediately after IV injection of a radiotracer (e.g., ^{99m}Tc DTPA) the bolus is imaged as it passes through heart, lungs, and great vessels. The acquisition ends before the agent recirculates.
   - A multidetector camera (multiple crystals and photomultiplier tube) for rapid data acquisition is required.
   - Advantages: fast determination of transit time, intracardiac shunts detectable, RV ejection fraction (RVEF) can be obtained.
   - Disadvantages: imaging time and count density are limited.
2. Equilibrium studies (gated blood pool study [GBPS])
   - The blood pool is currently best imaged with ^{99m}Tc-labeled RBC.
   - Gating to the cardiac cycle (frame mode, list mode)
   - Allows evaluation of segmental wall motion

INDICATIONS

- Assessment of ventricular function in CAD and cardiomyopathies
- Evaluation of cardiac drug toxicity (doxorubicin [Adriamycin] is often discontinued if EF <45%)
- Detection of intracardiac shunts

PROTOCOL

1. Inject ^{99m}Tc RBC (740 MBq).
2. Gated images are triggered to the R-wave. Arrhythmias have R-R interval variability and cause distortion of images. Arrhythmia filtering should therefore be performed.
3. Acquire images in 3 views: anterior, shallow LAO (45°), steep LPO (30°).
4. Calculate ejection fraction and evaluate wall motion.

IMAGE INTERPRETATION

Qualitative Image Assessment

1. Adequacy of study
   - Determine if labeling of RBC is adequate (free TcO_4^- uptake in stomach, thyroid, cardiac-to-background activity)
   - Determine if gating is adequate (jumps, count dropoff at end of cycle)
2. Heart (Fig. 12-15)
   - Size of cardiac chambers
   - Thickness of myocardial walls and septum
   - Ventricular wall motion is graded segmentally. Segments should contract simultaneously; anterior, posterior, lateral walls move to a greater

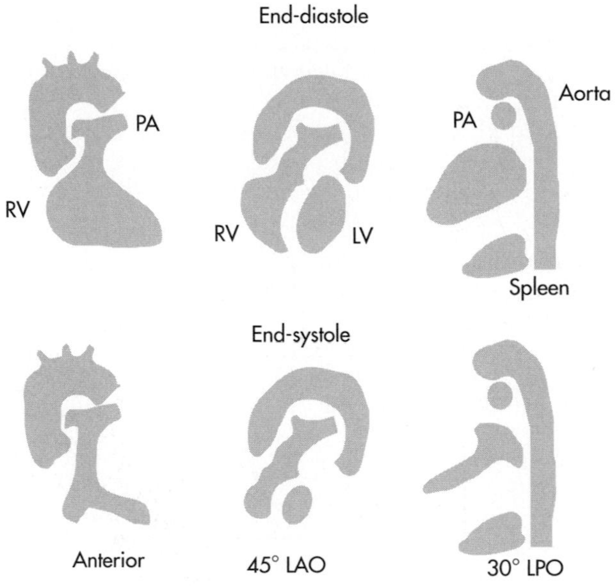

FIGURE 12-15

extent than septum or inferior wall; septum should move toward the LV. Atypical motion:
Hypokinesis: minimal wall movement (e.g., injured myocardium)
Akinesis: no wall movement (e.g., scarred myocardium)
Dyskinesis: paradoxical wall movement (e.g., aneurysm)

3. Lung
   - Lung activity should be similar to liver activity.
   - Evaluate for areas of oligemia.
4. Great vessels
   - Determine course and caliber
   - Aorta should be two thirds of diameter of pulmonary artery

Quantitative Image Assessment

The LV volume is graphed over time by edge tracing algorithms (Fig. 12-16). The most common quantitative parameters are EF and peak filling rate. Stroke volume or index and cardiac index can also be obtained. Quantitative data are obtained from shallow LAO (45°) projection:

EF (systolic function)
- LVEF = [end-diastolic volume (EDV) – end-systolic volume (ESV)]/EDV
- Normal values: LVEF 50%-65%
- Normal variability: 5%

Peak filling rate (diastolic function)
- Index of early ventricular filling
- Abnormalities in peak filling rates may precede EF changes (diastolic dysfunction may be present with normal LV systolic function).

Pearls

- GBPS is the preferred and most accurate imaging technique for LVEF determination.
- The LVEF can be falsely elevated if background ROI includes spleen.
- Motion artifact may be assessed on review of sinogram and unprocessed images.
- LVEF calculations by echocardiography are often less accurate than by nuclear imaging because:
  - Cardiac visualization is incomplete, making quantitation difficult.
  - Sampling error is related to operator differences.
- LVEF determination by contrast ventriculography is limited by geometric assumptions.

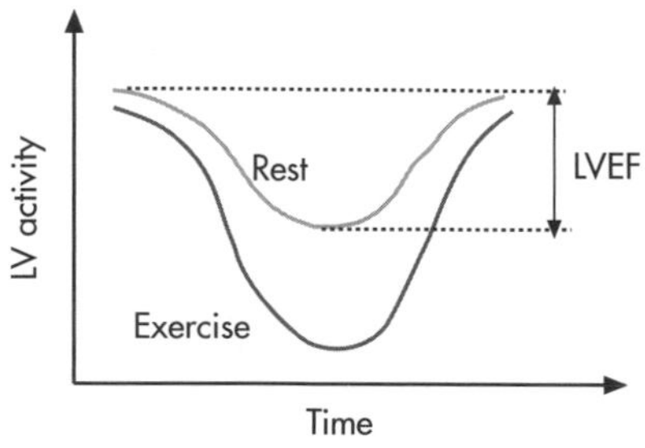

FIGURE 12-16

Gastrointestinal Imaging

RADIOPHARMACEUTICALS

GENERAL

OVERVIEW

Radiopharmaceutical	Target	Main Use
^{99m}Tc sulfur colloid	RES distribution	Atypical splenic tissue, liver lesion
^{99m}Tc HIDA	Biliary excretion	Acute cholecystitis
^{99m}Tc RBC	Blood pool	Hemangioma, bleeding
$^{99m}TcO_4^-$	Mucosal secretion	Meckel scan

^{99M}TECHNETIUM SULFUR COLLOID

Sodium thiosulfate reacts with acid to form sulfur, which reacts to form a colloid. Tc is contained within the colloid in the (+7) valence state. Gelatin stabilizes the colloid sulfide.

$$S_2O_3^{-2} + 2H^+ \rightarrow S + SO_2 + H_2O$$

$$7S_2O_3^{-2} + {}^{99m}TcO_4^- + 4H^+ \rightarrow {}^{99m}Tc_2S_7 + 5SO_4^{-2} + 2HSO_4^- + 2H_2O$$

EDTA is added to bind free TcO_4^-.

Pharmacokinetics

- Blood half-life is 2 to 3 minutes. 90% extraction during first pass.
- Complete clearance by reticuloendothelial system (RES) of liver (80%-90%), spleen (5%-10%), and bone marrow. Localization of the agent in these tissues is flow dependent and requires functional integrity of RES cells.

Pearls

- Sensitivity for detecting hepatic metastases is lower than with CT.
- Overall hepatic function can be assessed by the pattern of uptake.
- Accumulation of ^{99m}Tc sulfur colloid in renal transplants indicates rejection.
- In severe liver dysfunction an increase in activity can be seen in marrow, spleen, lungs, and even kidneys ("colloid shift").

99MTC HEPATOBILIARY AGENTS (Fig. 12-17)

All newer hepatobiliary agents are Tc-labeled iminodiacetic acid derivatives (abbreviated HIDA where *H* stands for hepatic). Commonly used compounds are the diisopropyl derivative (disofenin, DISIDA), which has the highest biliary excretion, and mebrofenin (BROMIDA), which has the fastest hepatobiliary extraction.

Pharmacokinetics

- Blood half-life is short (10 to 20 minutes depending on compound)
- 95%-99% biliary excretion into small bowel
- Urinary excretion may be higher in patients with impaired liver function or CBD obstruction

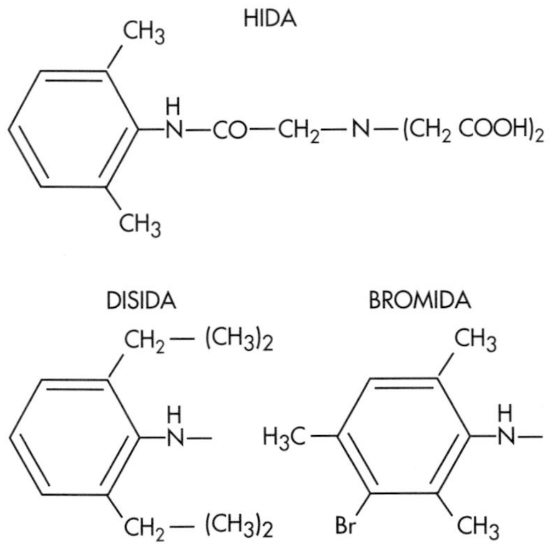

FIGURE 12-17

RES COLLOID IMAGING

INDICATIONS

Define functioning splenic tissue.

- Determine if a primary liver mass has RES activity.
- Bone marrow imaging (rare)

IMAGE INTERPRETATION

- Normal liver uptake > spleen uptake.
- Colloid shift occurs in cirrhosis: spleen, bone marrow uptake > liver uptake.

Other causes:

Hepatic cirrhosis
Alcoholic liver disease
Portal hypertension
Diffuse metastases with severely impaired liver function
Fatty infiltration of liver
Diffuse hepatitis
Hemochromatosis
Amyloidosis
Lymphoma
Leukemia
Sarcoidosis

- All hepatic mass lesions are cold except for focal nodular hyperplasia, which may have RES activity.
  - Causes of pulmonary uptake of ^{99m}Tc colloid include:
    Hepatic cirrhosis
    COPD with superimposed infection
    Estrogen therapy
    Neoplasms (primary and metastatic, including hepatoma)
    Disseminated intravascular coagulation
    Histiocytosis X
    Faulty colloid preparation → excessive aluminum
    Transplant recipient
    Pulmonary trauma
  - Nonvisualization of spleen on colloid scan
    Splenectomy
    Sickle cell disease
    Congenital absence of spleen (Ivemark syndrome)
    Tumor replacement
    Infarction
    Traumatic avulsion or volvulus
    Functional asplenia
      - Postsurgical hypoxia
      - Graft-versus-host disease
      - Chronic hepatitis
      - SLE

HEPATOBILIARY IMAGING

NORMAL SCAN

Protocol

1. Inject 185 to 300 MBq of ^{99m}Tc-labeled IDA (higher dose if bilirubin elevated).
2. Static images every 5 minutes until the gallbladder (GB) and small bowel are identified (usually at <1 hour); when GB and intestines are visualized, the study is completed.
3. Delayed imaging is necessary if GB is not visualized (up to 4 hours).
4. Administer morphine if GB is still not seen.

Interpretation (Fig. 12-18)

1. Hepatic activity can be
   - Normal
   - Delayed (reduced hepatic extraction in hepatocellular disease). With bilirubin levels >20 mg/dL, study results are usually equivocal.

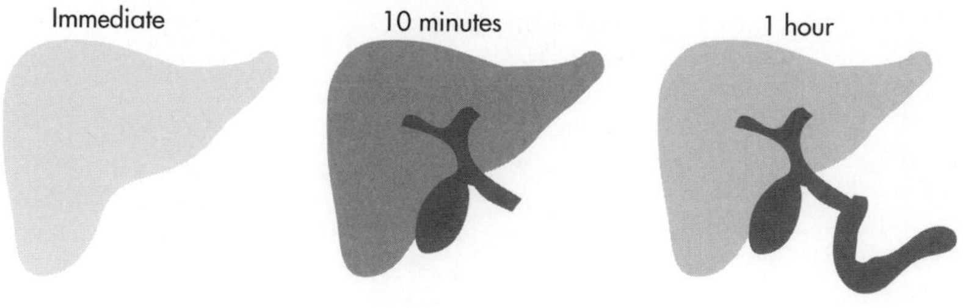

FIGURE 12-18

2. GB activity
   - Present (normal)
   - Nondemonstration of GB at 1 hour after injection may be due to:
     - Prolonged fasting (>24 hours; GB is filled with bile)
     - Recent meal (GB is contracted)
     - Acute cholecystitis
3. Bowel activity
   - Present (normal)
   - Absent (abnormal)
4. Cardiac activity
   - Delayed clearance of cardiac activity: hepatocellular dysfunction, hepatitis

Pharmacologic Intervention If GB Is Not Visualized (Fig. 12-19)

There are two pharmacologic maneuvers that can be performed in an attempt to visualize the GB if it has not become apparent after 1 hour of imaging:

- Sincalide (CCK-8)
  - Used to contract the GB to avoid false-positive results
  - Dose is 0.02 to 0.04 μg/kg in 10 mL of saline; given slowly to avoid discomfort and spasm of GB neck
  - This drug may obscure the diagnosis of chronic cholecystitis by speeding up the visualization of the GB. One way around this it to give CCK only if the GB is not visualized at 30 to 60 minutes; CCK is followed by an injection of IDA 15 to 30 minutes later.
- Morphine is often given before 4 hours to make the diagnosis of acute cholecystitis.
  - Dose is 0.04 mg/kg given slowly.
  - Causes spasm of sphincter of Oddi
  - Can convert true-positive result in case of cystic duct sign to false-negative result

ACUTE CHOLECYSTITIS (Fig. 12-20)

Acute cholecystitis usually results from acute obstruction of the cystic duct. This is commonly due to:

- Cystic duct calculus (most common)
- Other causes (acalculous cholecystitis) usually related to inspissated bile in cystic duct
- Trauma
- Burn
- Diabetes

Indications for Scintigraphic Imaging

- Normal US but high clinical suspicion for cystic duct calculus
- Normal US and suspicion for acalculous cholecystitis

Imaging Findings

- Nonvisualization of GB due to cystic duct obstruction. Prerequisites for establishing the diagnosis:
  - Prolonged imaging (has to be performed for at least 4 hours)
  - Pharmacologic intervention has to be performed: CCK or morphine

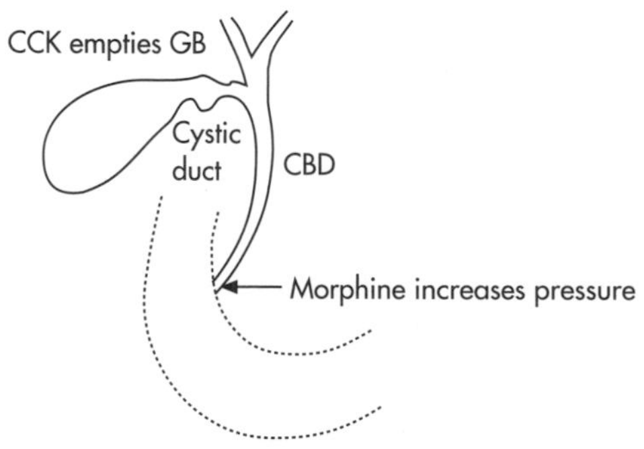

FIGURE 12-19

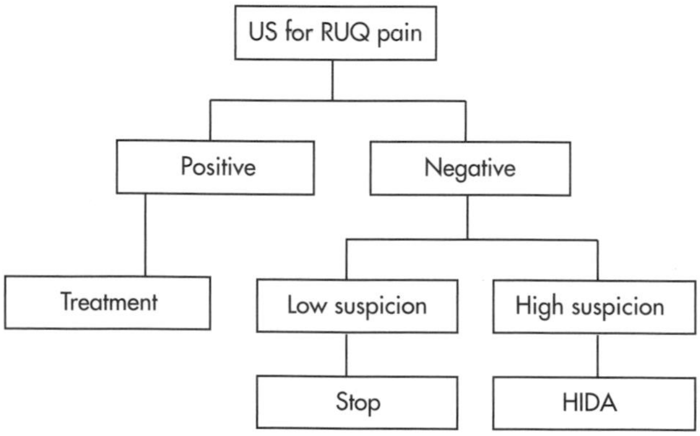

FIGURE 12-20

- Pericholecystic rim of increased activity (hyperemia, local inflammation) in 60%
- Visualization of GB excludes acute cholecystitis
- False-positive results
  - Recent meal within 4 hours of imaging
  - Prolonged fasting for 24 hours of hyperalimentation
  - Alcoholism
  - Pancreatitis
  - Chronic cholecystitis
  - Hepatocellular dysfunction
  - Cholangiocarcinoma of cystic duct
- False-negative results
  - Acalculous cholecystitis
  - Duodenal diverticulum simulating GB
  - Accessory cystic duct
  - Biliary duplication cyst

CHRONIC CHOLECYSTITIS

- Delayed visualization of GB (can occur with acute cholecystitis)
- GB showing a blunted response to CCK is more likely to be chronically inflamed.
- Delayed biliary to bowel time in presence of normal GB

LIVER TUMORS

HIDA IMAGING OF PRIMARY HEPATIC TUMORS

	Flow	Uptake	Clearance
FNH	↑	Immediate	Delayed
Adenoma	Nl	None	—

Nl, normal.

BOWEL IMAGING

HEMORRHAGE

Protocol

1. Tracers:
   - ^{99m}Tc RBC: long half-life, low lesion/background ratio
   - ^{99m}Tc sulfur colloid: short half-life, high lesion/background ratio
2. Sequential imaging for 1 hour
3. Additional delayed or spot images depending on findings

Imaging Findings

Scintigraphic evaluation is usually limited to lower gastrointestinal bleeding.

- Uptake conforming to bowel with no change over time: inflammatory bowel disease, faulty labeling (TcO_4^- excreted into bowel)
- Uptake conforming to bowel with progressive accumulation over time: hemorrhage. Criteria for active bleeding include:
  - Activity appears and conforms to bowel anatomy
  - Activity usually increases with time
  - Activity must move antegrade or retrograde in bowel
- False-positive results:
  - Free pertechnetate
  - Activity in bladder or urinary tract
  - Uterine or penile flush
  - Accessory spleen
  - Hemangioma of liver
  - Varices
  - Aneurysm, other vascular structures
- False-negative results:
  - Bleeding too slow
  - Intermittent bleeding

HEMANGIOMA IMAGING

^{99m}Tc RBC imaging is occasionally performed to diagnose hepatic hemangiomas, although helical CT with contrast and MRI are now used more often. The sensitivity of RBC imaging for detection of hemangiomas depends on lesion size: < 1 cm, 25%; 1 to 2 cm, 65%; >2 cm, 100%.

MECKEL SCAN

Meckel's diverticulum (incidence: 2% of general population) is a remnant of the omphalomesenteric duct. 50% of Meckel's diverticula contain ectopic gastric mucosa, which secretes $^{99m}TcO_4^-$. Meckel's diverticula that do not contain gastric mucosa are not detectable. Most diverticula are asymptomatic, but complications may occur:

- Bleeding (95% of bleeding Meckel's diverticula have gastric mucosa)
- Intestinal obstruction
- Inflammation

Technique

1. Patient NPO
2. H_2 blockers (cimetidine) block secretion of $^{99m}TcO_4^-$ into the bowel lumen and improve the target/background ratio of Meckel's diverticula (300 mg qid for 1 to 3 days before the study)
3. 370 MBq $^{99m}TcO_4^-$ IV
4. Sequential imaging for 1 hour
5. Drugs to enhance the sensitivity detecting Meckel's diverticulum:
   - Cimetidine to block release of pertechnetate from mucosa. Dose: 300 mg 4 times a day; 20 mg/kg/day for 2 days before
   - Pentagastrin to enhance uptake of $^{99m}TcO_4^-$. Note that pentagastrin must be administered before the $^{99m}TcO_4^-$ dose.

Glucagon to decrease small bowel or diverticular motility. Administer IV 10 minutes before study.

Imaging Findings

- Activity in a Meckel's diverticulum increases over time, just like gastric activity. Other causes of increased RLQ activity (e.g., inflammation, tumor) show an initial increase of activity with virtually no changes later on (related to hyperemia and expansion of extracellular space).
- Normal gastric activity quickly enters the lumen and is transported into the small bowel; once the activity reaches the small bowel, it can be confused with Meckel's diverticulum.
- False-positive results:
  - Urinary tract activity
  - Other ectopic gastric mucosa
  - Hyperemic inflammatory lesions
  - Arteriovenous malformations, hemangioma, aneurysm
  - Neoplasms
  - Intussusception
- False-negative results:
  - Minimal amount of gastric mucosa
  - Rapid washout of pertechnetate
  - Meckel's diverticulum with impaired blood supply

GASTRIC EMPTYING (Fig.12-21)

Indications

- Children with gastroesophageal (GE) rcflux
- Adults with diabetic gastroparesis

The stomach handles liquids and solids differently: liquids empty faster and show a monophasic exponential clearance. Solids empty after an initial delay, but emptying is nearly linear.

Liquid-Phase Emptying (Usually In Children, "Milk-Scan")

- 3.7 to 37 MBq of ^{99m}Tc sulfur colloid or ^{111}In DTPA added to formula or milk
- Need to image long enough to determine the emptying half-time (image acquisition at 0, 10, 30, 60, 90 minutes)

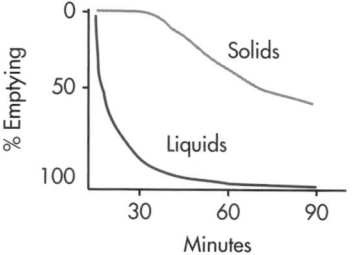

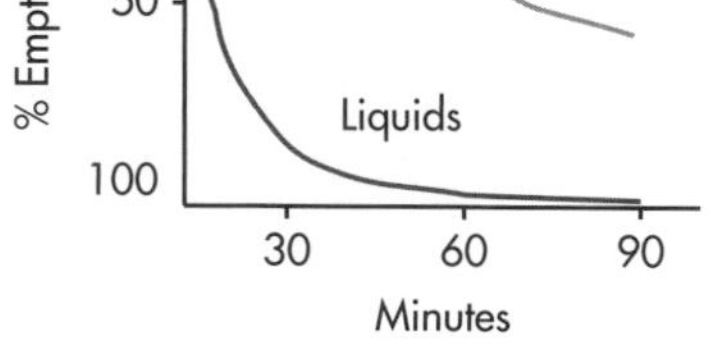

FIGURE 12-21

- Emptying half-time is usually 30 minutes.
- Usually performed in conjunction with a GE reflux study while increasing abdominal pressure with a binder (in adults only)

Solid-Phase Emptying (Usually for Adults)

- 3.7 to 37 MBq of ^{99m}Tc sulfur colloid is added to raw eggs before scrambling them. ^{99m}Tc-labeled resins or iodinated fibers are alternatives.
- Emptying half-time is usually 1 to 2 hours.

Genitourinary Imaging

RADIOPHARMACEUTICALS

OVERVIEW

	Radiopharmaceutical	Comment
Imaging Of Renal Function		
Glomerular filtration rate	^{99m}Tc DTPA	Inexpensive
Effective renal plasma flow	^{99m}Tc MAG_3	Good in renal failure
Imaging Of Renal Mass		
Tubular mass	^{99m}Tc DMSA	40% cortical binding
	^{99m}Tc glucoheptonate	20% cortical binding

The only 2 agents routinely used for renal imaging today are ^{99m}Tc DTPA and ^{99m}Tc MAG_3. The choice of agent depends on the type of information required:

- Quantification of split renal function: DTPA or MAG_3
- Renovascular hypertension: DTPA or MAG_3
- Renal failure, follow-up studies: MAG_3 preferred
- Obstructive uropathy: MAG_3 preferred

DMSA (imaging of renal cortex for scarring in children) and ^{99m}Tc glucoheptonate have limited use. Agents filtered through kidney deliver greatest radiation dose to bladder, whereas tracers bound to renal cortex result in higher renal radiation (i.e., ^{99m}Tc DMSA).

^{99M}TC DTPA

^{99m}Tc DTPA is an inexpensive chelate used primarily for dynamic renal and brain imaging. It has the same biodistribution as gadolinium DTPA used in MRI.

Pharmacokinetics

- Rapid extravascular, extracellular distribution
- Cleared by glomerular filtration (glomerular filtration rate [GFR] agent)
- 5%-10% plasma protein binding; thus, calculated GFR is lower than that obtained by inulin.

- Immediate images provide information about renal perfusion.
- Delayed images provide information about renal function (GFR) and collecting system.
- Target organ: bladder (2.7 rad/370 MBq)
- Hydration and frequent voiding reduce patient radiation dose.

^{99m}Tc MAG$_3$ (Fig. 12-22)

MAG$_3$ is a chelate for ^{99m}Tc. It is physiologically analogous to ^{131}I-ortho iodohippuran but has more favorable dosimetry and results in better images. Administered dose: 185 to 370 MBq. More expensive than DTPA.

Pharmacokinetics

- Cleared mostly by tubular secretion: effective renal plasma flow (ERPF) agent
- Minimal glomerular filtration
- Agent of choice in patients with renal insufficiency. Provides better images because it is not GFR dependent.
- Target organ: bladder (4.8 rad/370 MBq)

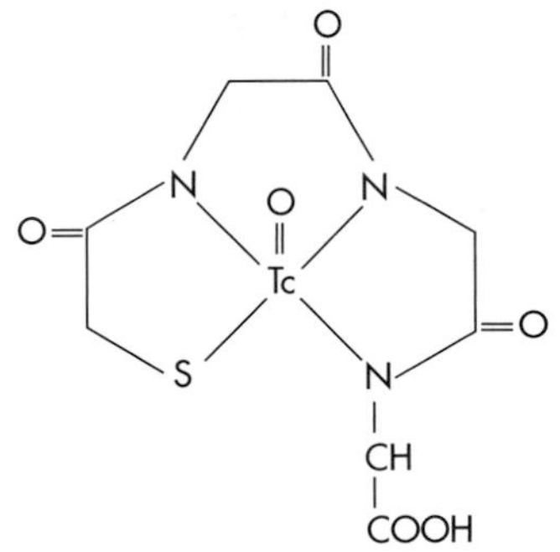

FIGURE 12-22

RENAL IMAGING

INDICATIONS

Renovascular hypertension
- Screening of hypertensive patients with high risk
- Renal flow assessment after revascularization procedure (PTA or surgical)

Renal transplant
- Acute tubular necrosis vs. acute rejection
- Other: cyclosporine toxicity, arterial occlusion, urinary obstruction or urinary leak

Determination of split function
- Prior to nephrectomy
- Radiation therapy planning
- Functional determination before surgical repair (e.g., obstructed kidney)

PROTOCOL

1. Bolus injection of tracer
2. Immediate imaging of sequential flow images: 1- to 3-second frames up to 1 minute to measure perfusion
3. Delayed images obtained at 60 sec/frame for 30 minutes. These images may be summed to obtain 5-minute static images.

NORMAL IMAGES (Figs. 12-23 and 12-24)

Perfusion images (rapid sequential imaging for 1st minute)
- Aorta is seen first.
- Prompt renal activity within 6 seconds of peak aortic activity
- Kidney perfusion should be symmetrical.

Static images (1 to 30 minutes)
- Symmetrical renal uptake, normal renal size
- Peak cortical activity at 3 to 5 minutes
- Peak renal uptake should be higher than spleen uptake.
- Collecting system and ureters begin to fill after 4 to 5 minutes.
- Cortical activity decreases with time.

Quantitative split renal function
- Determined by ROI over each kidney with background correction. Measure activity of both kidneys 2 to 3 minutes after injection (before collecting system fills).
- Split renal function should be 50% on either side.

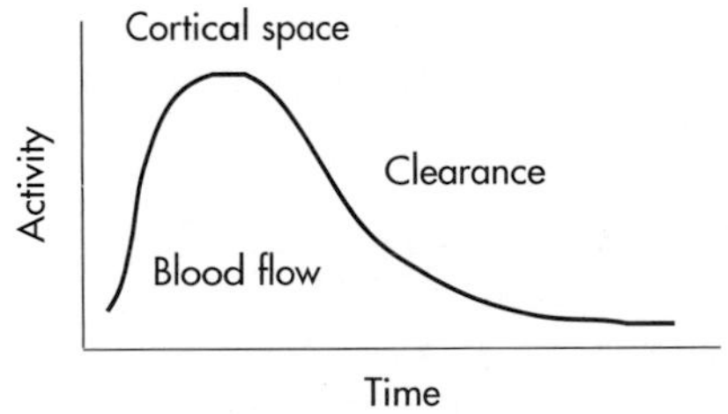

FIGURE 12-23

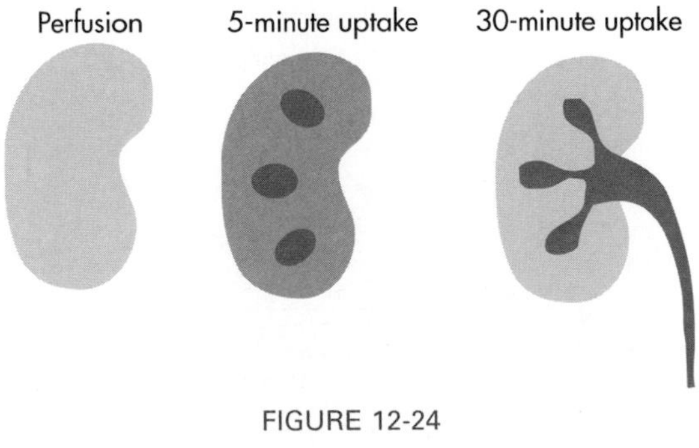

FIGURE 12-24

Interpretation

1. Perfusion images (symmetrical or asymmetrical perfusion? prompt or delayed excretion?)
2. Static images
   - Size and shape of kidney
   - Clearance of tracer through ureters into bladder
3. Quantitative data
   - Determine split renal function in %.
   - Transit time: clearance of half of maximum activity

TRANSPLANT EVALUATION

Acute rejection (2+ weeks)
- Decreased perfusion
- Decreased uptake on static images

Acute tubular necrosis (ATN) reversible (first week to 2 weeks)
- Normal perfusion
- Decreased uptake on static images.
- Cyclosporine toxicity appears similar but appears later

Perinephric collection
- Photopenic halo
- Progressive accumulation of activity outside urinary tract: urinoma

RENOVASCULAR HYPERTENSION (Fig. 12-25)

5% of hypertensive patients have treatable renal artery stenosis. ^{99m}Tc DTPA and ^{99m}Tc MAG_3 studies in these patients may show a unilateral reduction in flow, whereas function is often normal. Captopril (ACE inhibitor) can be used to differentiate normal and dysfunctional stenotic renal arteries; it dilates the efferent arteriole, thus decreasing the GFR of the stenotic kidney.

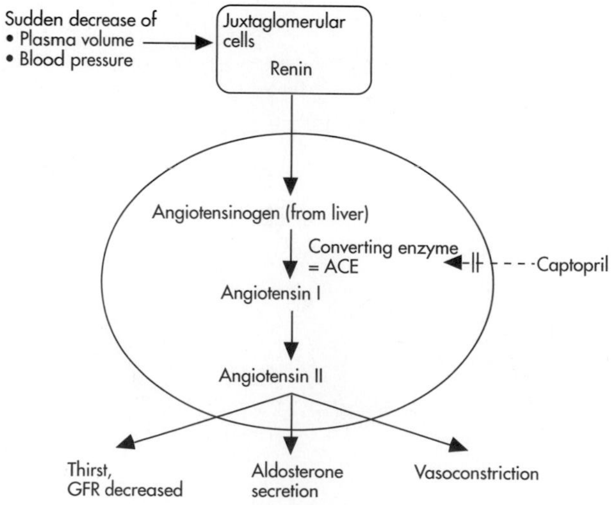

FIGURE 12-25

Technique

1. Withhold diuretics for 48 hours and angiotensin-converting enzyme (ACE) inhibitors for 1 week; hydrate patient to decrease risk of hypotension.
2. Baseline renal scan: low-dose ^{99m}Tc DTPA (37 to 185 MBq) without captopril
3. Wait 4 hours for ^{99m}Tc DTPA to clear.
4. Captopril, 50 mg PO; measure blood pressure every 15 minutes for 1 hour.
5. Repeat renal scan after 1 hour.

Interpretation (Fig. 12-26)

- Bilateral disease is difficult to diagnose.
- A variety of patterns have been described:

  Decreased flow in stenotic kidney (perfusion images)

  Decreased excretion and prolonged cortical transit time (static image)

  Prolonged washout in stenotic kidney (static images)

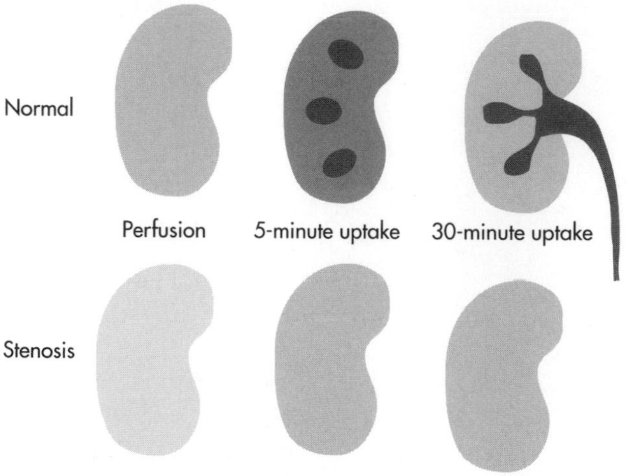

FIGURE 12-26

OBSTRUCTION (Fig. 12-27)

If delayed images and attempts at postural drainage fail, furosemide should be given to differentiate non-obstructive dilated collecting systems from obstructed collecting systems ("diuretic renogram").

Technique

- Proceed with the standard renal scan.
- Administer furosemide IV, 0.3 to 0.5 mg/kg, after dilated pelvis has filled with activity.
- Maximal diuretic response is seen within 15 minutes.

Imaging Findings

- Delayed parenchymal clearance (>20 minutes) in obstructed kidney

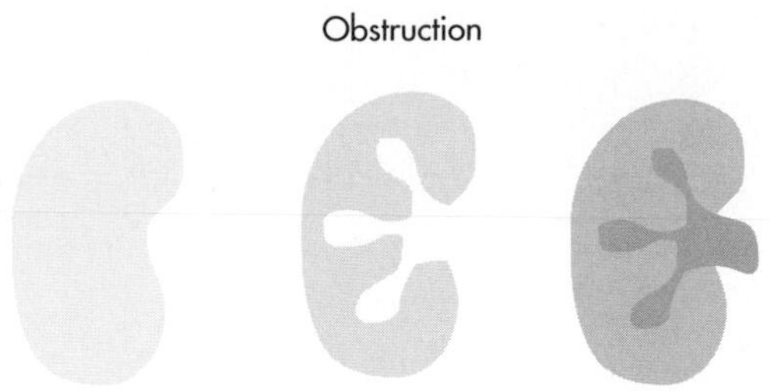

FIGURE 12-27

- Nonvisualization of ureter in obstructed kidney
- Intermediate degrees of washout are of uncertain significance:
  Partial obstruction?
  Patient may require Whitaker test.

False-Positive Furosemide (Lasix) Renal Scans

- Partial obstruction
- Bladder overfilling
- <2 years of age (no response to furosemide)
- Renal insufficiency (no response to furosemide)

RENAL CORTICAL IMAGING

^{99m}Tc DMSA renal scintigraphy may be used to document pyelonephritis in children because management of upper urinary tract infection differs from lower tract infection.

Technique

- 2 hour delayed planar, SPECT imaging after injection of tracer
- Planar imaging: posterior, posterior oblique views, pinhole collimator

Interpretation

- Normal: homogeneous distribution of tracer in cortex; photopenic central collecting system
- Cortical scar, pyelonephritis: Focal cortical photopenic defects
- Column of Bertin demonstrates normal uptake

RETROGRADE RADIONUCLIDE CYSTOGRAM

Useful in the assessment of vesicoureteral reflux and for calculation of postvoid residuals.

Technique

- ^{99m}Tc sulfur colloid, 37 MBq in up to 500 mL normal saline, via Foley
- May also be performed with ^{99m}Tc pertechnetate or DTPA
- Cyclic study in infants
- Dynamic imaging during bladder filling, voiding, and postvoid

Interpretation

- Grade I reflux: ureter
- Grade II reflux: renal pelvis
- Grade III reflux: dilated collecting system

TESTICULAR IMAGING

INDICATION

To identify testicular torsion. Now considered ancillary to testicular US, which can be performed more promptly and is more specific.

PROTOCOL

- Positioning: scrotum on sling, penis taped to anterior abdominal wall
- Inject TcO_4^- intravenously.
- Acquire flow images over 1 minute.
- Delayed static images: mark scrotal raphe for accurate anatomic localization.

NORMAL IMAGES

- Slight uptake of tracer in both testes
- Testes cannot be separated from scrotum.
- Bladder activity is usually seen superior to testes.

Interpretation

Flow images
- Increased (hyperemia) or not increased (no hyperemia)
- Decreased flow cannot be detected.

Static images
- Cold testes
- Ring sign
- Hot testes

TORSION

Imaging Findings (Fig. 12-28)

- Photopenic ("cold") testis indicates torsion.
- "Ring sign" or "bull's eye": peripheral rim of increased activity with central zone of photopenia may represent inflammation of dartos and infarcted/necrotic testis.

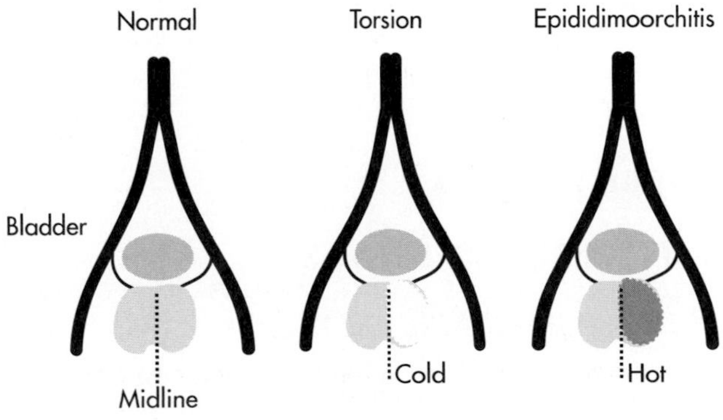

FIGURE 12-28

- "Ring sign": delayed/missed torsion (the more pronounced the rim, the later the torsion or scrotal abscess)
- "Nubbin sign": area of increased activity that extends from the iliac arteries and ends at the torsion. Indicates increased perfusion to the scrotum via the pudendal arteries.
- Torsion of appendix testis cannot be diagnosed (too small).
- Testes in children <2 years old are usually too small to be imaged.

OVERVIEW OF TESTICULAR ABNORMALITIES

Disease	Flow Images	Static Images
Early torsion (<6 hr)	Normal	Cold testis
Late torsion	Variable	Cold testis, hyperemic scrotum (ring sign)
Epididymitis, orchitis	Increased	Increased uptake
Abscess	Increased	Ring sign
Tumor	Variable	Variable
Trauma	Normal or increased	Normal or increased

ADRENAL IMAGING

METAIODOBENZYLGUANIDINE (MIBG)

Adrenal medullary imaging agent MIBG is recognized as a neurotransmitter precursor in:

- Any neuroectodermal tumor: carcinoid (even metastatic), neuroblastoma, pheochromocytoma, paraganglioma (extraadrenal pheochromocytoma)
- Normal activity is also seen in liver, spleen, salivary glands, and myocardium.

Technique

- Block uptake of free iodine into thyroid by administering Lugol's solution
- 18 MBq MIBG IV
- Imaging at 1, 2, and 3 days after administration

Interpretation

- Absent or faint uptake is normal.
- Bilateral increased uptake indicates hyperplasia.
- Unilateral increased adrenal uptake is suggestive of a neuroectodermal tumor.
- Distant metastases are also detectable.

Bone Imaging

RADIOPHARMACEUTICALS

^{99M}TC PHOSPHONATES (Fig. 12-29)

Agents are classified according to the phosphate linkage:

- P-C-P: phosphonates
- P-O-P: polyphosphates

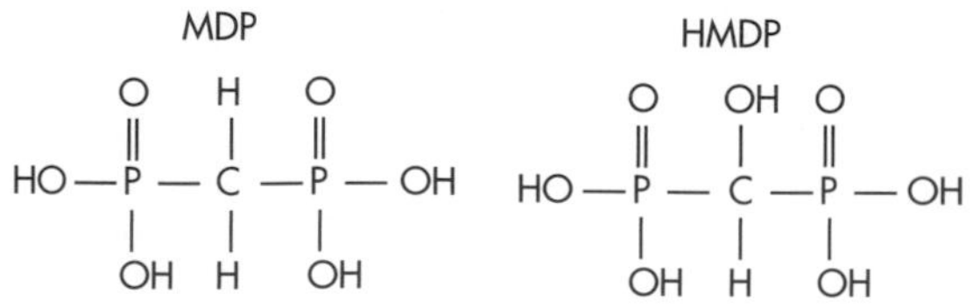

FIGURE 12-29

- P-N-P: imidophosphates
- P-P: pyrophosphates

Methylene diphosphonate (MDP) and hydroxymethylene diphosphonate (HMDP) are the most commonly used agents; both agents resist in vivo hydrolysis by alkaline phosphatase.

Pharmacokinetics

- 50% of injected MDP localizes to bone.
- 70% of dose is excreted renally within 24 hours.
- Biodistribution may be considerably altered by abnormal cardiac output, renal function, and medications.
- MDP is chemiabsorbed onto hydroxyapatite (exact mechanism unknown). 80% of tracer that ultimately localizes in skeleton does so within 5 to 10 minutes. However, one typically waits for 2 to 3 hours for imaging to minimize ECF and blood activity.
- Bone uptake depends on 2 factors:
  - Osteoblastic activity (most important)
  - Blood flow (less important)
- ^{99m}Tc MDP also reacts with mitochondrial calcium crystals. Uptake thus occurs in various types of cell injury:
  - Tissue infarction: myocardial, splenic, cerebral
  - Cardiac contusion, cardiac surgery, unstable angina pectoris, myopathies
- Critical organ is the bladder. Minimize radiation exposure by hydration and frequent voiding (this also helps to detect pelvic lesions).

BONE MARROW AGENTS

^{99m}Tc sulfur colloid is most commonly used for bone marrow imaging. $InCl_2$ is an alternative agent but is not available for clinical use at present. Bone marrow scintigraphy is not important in current practice and has a few limited indications.

Indications

- Determine viability of red marrow
- Localization of marrow before bone marrow aspiration

BONE IMAGING

INDICATIONS

- Detection of metastases
- Staging of malignancies

- Detection of osteomyelitis
- Detection of radiographically occult fractures
- Determine multiplicity of lesions (e.g., fibrous dysplasia, Paget disease)
- Diagnosis of reflex sympathetic dystrophy

TECHNIQUE

1. Inject 740 MBq ^{99m}Tc MDP IV.
2. Take image 2 to 4 hours later.
3. May have to wait longer before imaging patients with renal insufficiency to allow for soft tissue clearance
4. Have patient urinate immediately before imaging to decrease bladder activity.
5. Two image acquisition formats:
   Whole-body single pass (lower resolution)
   Spot views (longer time of acquisition, better resolution)

NORMAL IMAGES

Adults

Locally increased activity may be a normal variant:

Patchy uptake in the skull may be normal.

Common location for degenerative changes (usually at both sides of a joint)

- Sternoclavicular joint, manubriosternal joint
- Lower cervical and lumbar spine (usually at concavity of scoliosis)
- Knees, ankles, wrists, 1st carpometacarpal joint
  Tendon insertions
  Regions of constant stress
  Geometric overlap of bones (ribs)
- Normal, secondary uptake of the label:
  Nasopharynx
  Kidneys
  Soft tissues
- Findings that are always abnormal:
  Strikingly asymmetrical changes
  Very hot spots
- The older the patient, the higher the proportion of poor quality scans.

Children

- Intensive accumulation in growth plates

TUMORS

Indications for Obtaining a Bone Scan

- Diagnosis
- Initial staging
- To follow therapeutic response

Imaging Features

- The majority of bone tumors are "hot" lesions.
- Flare phenomenon: Increased osteoblastic activity at metastatic sites after start of treatment, which may last 6 months.
- Cold lesion (purely osteolytic tumors with no blastic activity): renal cell carcinoma, thyroid cancer, anaplastic tumors, neuroblastoma (uncommon)
- Superscan: diffusely increased bone activity with little to no renal activity. Most commonly due to diffuse osseous metastases (prostate carcinoma).
- Normal distribution: marrow tumors such as lymphoma, leukemia, multiple myeloma
- Soft tissue lesions (tracer uptake in tumor)
- Normal (false negative)

SPECIFIC METASTASES

Tumor	Comment
Prostate cancer	PSA test may be more specific for follow-up
RCC	Osteolytic metastases usually well seen by plain film
Bronchogenic carcinoma	Usually associated with bone pain (especially squamous cell)
Lymphoma	Often false negative (inapparent lesions)
Myeloma	Often false negative (inapparent lesions)
Neuroblastoma	Metastases to metaphyses may mimic normal growth plate

PSA, prostate-specific antigen; RCC, renal cell carcinoma.

Tumors that commonly metastasize to bone:

- Breast
- Prostate (PSA >20)
- Lung
- Renal
- Thyroid

Metastases preferentially localize in bones with red marrow:

- Ribs, 35%
- Spine, 25%
- Pelvis, 5%
- Extremities, 15%
- Skull, 5%

Increased uptake can also be observed in the following conditions:

- Brain infarcts
- Splenic infarcts
- Intramuscular injection sites
- Adrenal neuroblastoma
- Meningioma
- Malignant ascites
- Paget disease of the breast

Bony lesions commonly missed on scan:

- RCC metastases
- Thyroid metastases
- Multiple myeloma
- Neuroblastoma
- Highly anaplastic tumors

Osteomyelitis

Osteomyelitis is commonly evaluated with a 3-phase bone scan: flow ("flow images"), immediate static ("blood pool image"), and delayed static images (metabolic image). Increased activity on flow images suggests hyperemia, often present in inflammation and stress fractures.

3-PHASE BONE SCAN

Disease Process	Flow Images	Blood Pool Images	Delayed Images
Cellulitis	+	+	−
Osteomyelitis	+	+	+
Fracture	+	+	+
Noninflammatory	−	−	+

Pearls

- Bone scan allows detection of osteomyelitis much earlier (24 to 72 hours after onset) than plain radiographs (7 to 14 days).
- Bone scan is sensitive but nonspecific for osteomyelitis.
- Combined ^{99m}Tc MDP/^{111}In WBC scanning maximizes sensitivity and specificity and is the preferred technique for the diagnosis of osteomyelitis. Only modest WBC uptake in fracture, high uptake in infection. Correlation of WBC activity with ^{99m}Tc sulfur colloid may be helpful to distinguish infection from expanded red marrow.
- ^{67}Ga uptake that focally exceeds ^{99m}Tc MDP uptake or differs in distribution increases specificity for diagnosis of infection.
- Sensitivity (95%) and specificity (70%-90%) for detection of osteomyelitis by 3-phase bone scan and MRI are similar.
- Lesions hot on all 3 phases of the bone scan:
  - Osteomyelitis
  - Trauma
  - Hypervascular tumor
  - Reflex sympathetic dystrophy
  - Neuropathic joint

FRACTURES

Indications for Bone Scans

- Stress fractures
- Avulsion injuries
- Radiographically occult fractures
- Shin splints
- Osteochondritis dissecans
- Osteonecrosis
- Hip replacement (loosening)
- Child abuse

Scintigraphic Features

- Time after fracture at which bone scan becomes positive correlates with age of patient:
  - Adult: 24 hours
  - Older patients: 72 hours (i.e., need delayed images if initial images are negative)
- Bone uptake returns to normal within 1 (ribs) to 3 years (elderly patients, long bones)
- Stress fracture: fusiform activity classically in posteromedial tibia
- Shin splints: linear cortical activity on delayed images

REFLEX SYMPATHETIC DYSTROPHY (RSD)

- Bone scan is imaging study of choice for RSD.
- Interpretation requires knowledge of duration of symptomatology.

FINDINGS

	Perfusion/Blood Pool Images	Delayed Images
Very early	Increased	Increased
Within 1 year	Increased/normal	Increased
Late	Decreased	Decreased
Children	Normal/increased	Any appearance

PROSTHESIS

DIFFERENTIATION BETWEEN PROSTHESIS LOOSENING AND INFECTION

	Loosening	Infection
MDP flow image	Normal	Increased
MDP static image	Slight focal increase	Very hot
Ga imaging	Normal	Increased uptake
WBC imaging	Normal	Increased uptake

Total Hip Replacement (THR)

- More accurate in evaluation of femoral component
- Cemented THR MDP scan should be negative within 6 months after THR unless infected or loosened.
- Noncemented THR: may remain hot for up to 24 months
- ^{111}In WBC or ^{67}Ga may help to differentiate infection from loosening.

Bone scan is of little use for evaluating loosening of knee replacements because increased activity is a normal finding.

MARROW IMAGING

TECHNIQUE

1. Inject 370 MBq ^{99m}Tc colloid IV (higher dose than liver/spleen scan).
2. Image entire skeleton.

IMAGING FEATURES

Distribution of activity parallels hematopoietic distribution.

Normal appearance
- Diffuse skeletal activity up to age 8 (diffuse hematopoietic marrow)
- Activity limited to axial skeleton by age 25 (hematopoietic marrow limited to axial skeleton)
- Lower thoracic spine and ribs obscured by intense liver/spleen activity

Abnormal appearance
- Chronic anemias: peripheral marrow expansion with activity in distal extremities
- Lymphoproliferative disorders: bone scan may be useful to localize marrow site for biopsy
- Acute bone infarction (e.g., sickle cell disease): diminished activity, heterogeneous

[18F] SODIUM FLUORIDE PET:

18F fluoride accumulates in the entire skeleton, with somewhat greater deposition in the axial skeleton (e.g., vertebrae and pelvis). 18F also accumulates around primary and metastatic bone malignancy and is useful for their detection. 18F is excreted renally.

Thyroid Imaging

RADIOPHARMACEUTICALS

OVERVIEW (Figs 12-30, 12-31, and 12-32)

- ^{123}I: used for routine imaging. Expensive (cyclotron produced). Imaging should be performed after 24 hours. Organification.

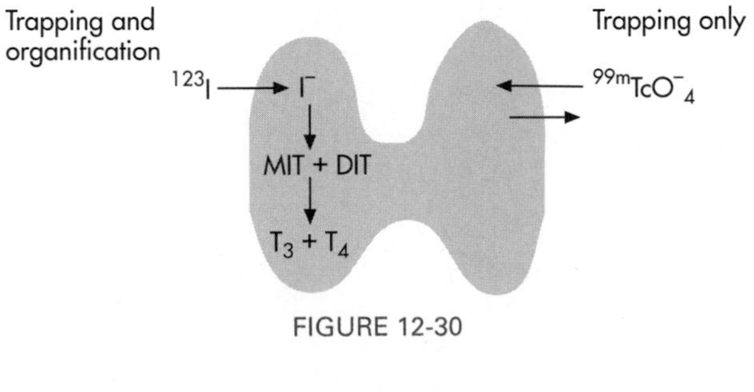

FIGURE 12-30

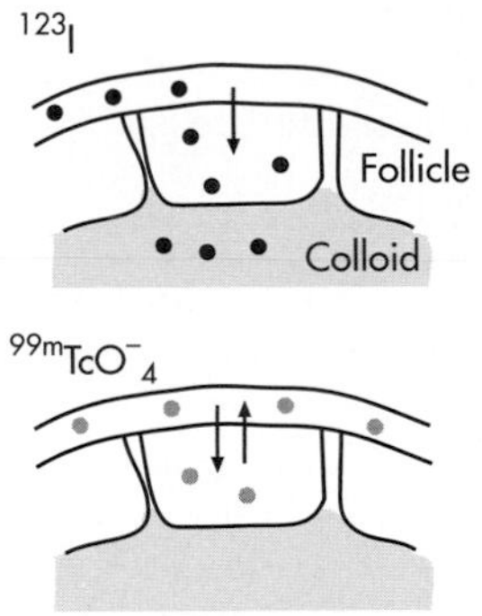

FIGURE 12-31

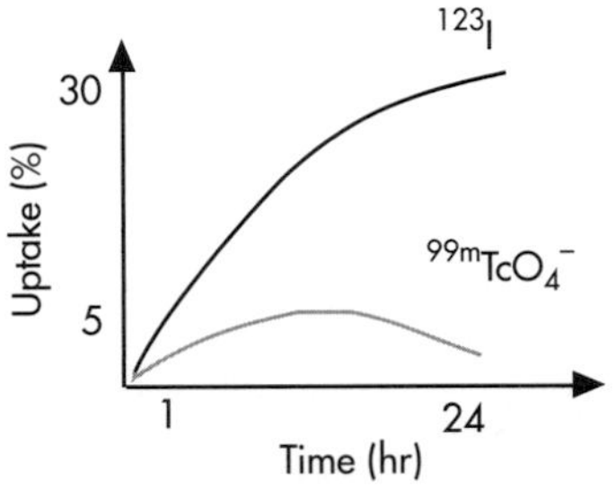

FIGURE 12-32

- $^{99m}TcO_4^-$ used if imaging has to be performed within 1 hour, if patient receives PTU (unlike I, TcO_4^- is not organified), or if patient is not able to ingest I orally. Disadvantage: 5% trapped, no organification.
- ^{131}I: now used only for therapeutic purposes (cancer) because of high energy (364 keV), long half-life (8 days), and beta and gamma decay.

^{123}IODINE

^{123}I is the diagnostic agent of choice for thyroid imaging because of lower patient radiation exposure and higher counting efficiency when compared with ^{131}I. Dose is 4 to 7 MBq sodium iodide orally. Image is taken 24 hours after administration.

Pharmacokinetics
- Readily absorbed from GI tract; primary distribution in extracellular fluid
- Sodium iodide is trapped and organified by the thyroid; there is also trapping by stomach and salivary glands (but no organification).
- Physical half-life: 13 hours
- 35%-70% renal excretion within 24 hours
- Tissue localization:
  - Thyroid and thyroid metastases
  - Nasopharynx
  - Salivary glands
  - Stomach

Colon
Bladder
Rarely in lactating breasts

^{131}IODINE

Indications

- Not for general thyroid imaging because of unfavorable dosimetry
- Detection of thyroid metastases
- Therapeutic thyroid radioablation
- There is no rational basis for using ^{131}I for detection of substernal goiters as suggested in older textbooks.

TYPICAL DOSAGES OF RADIOACTIVE IODINE

Agent*	Typical Dose (mCi)	Average Thyroid Exposure (rad)	Dosage Rate (rad/mCi)
^{123}I	Uptake/thyroid scan: 0.1-0.4 PO; Whole body: 1.5-2 PO	8	11-22
^{131}I	Whole body: 2-4 PO	9.6	1100-1600
$^{99m}TcO_4^-$	1-10 IV	2 (lowest of all)	0.12-0.2
^{125}I	Not for imaging†		

*Tc (140 keV) and ^{123}I (159 keV) have similar photon energies. ^{127}I is stable, nonradioactive iodine.
†^{125}I is a contaminant.

Calculation of ^{131}Iodine Therapeutic Dose

Assumptions for calculation: 80% uptake, desired glandular dose 8000 to 10,000 rad (i.e., 100 μCi/g), gland weight 60 g. To calculate required dose:

Dose (mCi) = (60 g × 100 μCi/g)/(0.8) × 1 mCi/1000 μCi = 7.5 mCi

Complications of ^{131}Iodine Treatment

- Bone marrow depression
- Sterility if pelvic metastases present
- Leukemia

Pertechnetate

$^{99m}TcO_4^-$ distributes similarly to ^{111}In but is not organified when trapped in the thyroid. Also accumulates in salivary glands, stomach, and choroid plexus.

Applications

- Thyroid imaging
- Blood pool imaging (testicular torsion)
- Ectopic gastric mucosa (Meckel's scan)
- Dacryoscintigraphy (nasolacrimal drainage system)
- Brain imaging (passes into brain if there is a blood-brain barrier defect; rarely used)

Pharmacokinetics

- Rapid (30-minute) extraction of $^{99m}TcO_4^-$ by thyroid.
- Thyroid releases $^{99m}TcO_4^-$ over a period of several hours; at 24 hours there is virtually no $^{99m}TcO_4^-$ left in the thyroid

PHARMACOKINETICS OF ^{123}I AND $^{99M}TCO_4^-$

^{123}I	$^{99m}TcO_4^-$
Oral	IV
Organified	Not organified
Image late; 24 hr	Image early; 20 minutes
Maximum uptake at about 24 hr	Maximum uptake at about 20 minutes
Can be incorporated into thyroid hormone	Cannot be incorporated into thyroid hormone

THYROID IMAGING

IODINE UPTAKE TEST

This test determines how much of orally ingested ^{123}I is accumulated in the thyroid at 24 hours. It is thus a measure of I trapping and organification. The test cannot be used as a marker of thyroid function (this is done by measurements of T_3/T_4). Uptake values are classified as hyperthyroid, euthyroid, and hypothyroid states.

Technique

- Measure the dose of ^{123}I to be ingested (8 MBq, 1 to 2 capsules).
- Image thyroid 24 hours after oral administration of capsules; because spatial resolution is not crucial, imaging is performed at 2 cm for 5 minutes without the pinhole insert.
- Thyroid uptake calculation:
  Uptake = (Counts in neck − Background/ Ingested dose) × Decay factor
- Normal values: 5%-15% at 4 hours, 10%-30% at 24 hours of orally ingested dose in thyroid

Increased Uptake

- Hyperthyroidism
- Iodine starvation
- Thyroiditis
- Hypoalbuminemia
- Lithium use

Decreased Uptake

- Hypothyroidism
- Thyroid hormone therapy, Lugol's solution, PTU
- Medications
  - Iodinated contrast agents
  - Certain vitamin preparations
- Thyroiditis

NORMAL IMAGING

Patient Examination

Short medical history

- Hypothyroidism (edema, dry skin, bradycardia, decreased reflexes, hypothermia, loss of lateral eyebrows)

- Hyperthyroidism (diarrhea, sweating, tachycardia, warm and moist skin, ophthalmopathy)
- Enlargement of gland (goiter, nodule)

Current drug history including exposure to iodine contrast agents

Palpation of thyroid

Appearance of Normal Thyroid Scans (Fig. 12-33)

Homogeneous uptake. Each lobe measures 2 to 5 cm; slight asymmetry is common. Variants include:

- Thin pyramidal lobe arising superiorly from isthmus; accentuated in:
  - Graves disease
  - Postsurgical patients
- Lactating breast
- Ectopic thyroid (sublingual, substernal), congenital absence of a lobe (rare)
- $^{99m}TcO_4^-$ scans:
  - Uptake of TcO_4^- in salivary glands
  - Thin, linear band of superimposed activity often represents swallowed $^{99m}TcO_4^-$ activity in the esophagus (have patient drink water).

Interpretation

1. Uptake
   - Homogeneous, heterogeneous
   - Decreased, increased, normal
2. Size, shape
   - Enlarged, normal
   - External compression
3. Nodules
   - Hot, cold
   - Extrathyroid nodules (e.g., metastases)

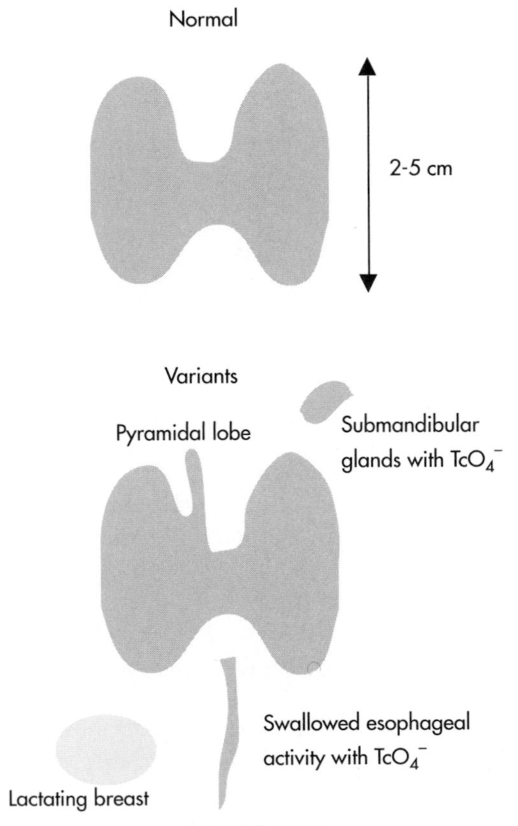

FIGURE 12-33

COLD NODULE (Fig. 12-34)

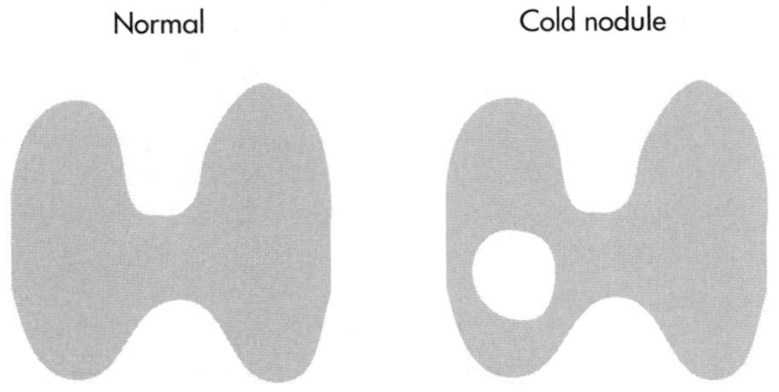

FIGURE 12-34

Of all palpable nodules, 90% are cold, and of these 90% are benign. A cold nodule is nonfunctioning and has to be further worked up to exclude cancer. Cold nodes may represent:

- Adenoma/colloid cyst, 85%
- Carcinoma, 10%
- Focal thyroiditis
- Hemorrhage
- Lymph node
- Abscess
- Parathyroid adenoma

MALIGNANT VERSUS BENIGN COLD NODULES

Benign	Malignant
Older patients	Younger patients
Female	Male
Sudden onset	History of radiation, positive family history
Soft, tender lesion	Hard lesion
Multiple nodules	Other masses in neck
Response to suppression	No response to suppression therapy or iodine therapy

HOT NODULE (Fig. 12-35)

The vast majority of hot nodules represent hyperfunctioning adenomas, half of which are autonomous (i.e., grow without stimulus of thyroid stimulating hormone [TSH]). Autonomous nodules should be suppressed for 5 weeks with T_4 to turn off TSH. If the nodule stays hot, it is a true autonomous nodule that should be treated by surgery, ^{131}I, or alcohol ablation if clinically symptomatic.

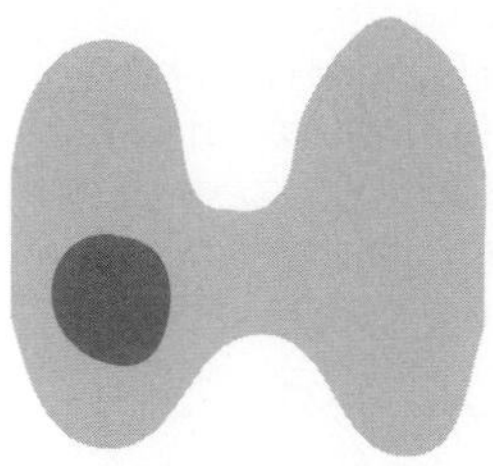

FIGURE 12-35

Discordant Nodules

Refers to a hot nodule by $^{99m}TcO_4^-$ imaging and a cold nodule ^{123}I imaging (i.e., a nonfunctioning nodule). Knowing whether a nodule is discordant is usually of little value per se.

HYPERTHYROIDISM (Fig. 12-36)

- Diffuse toxic goiter (Graves disease): most common form of hyperthyroidism
- Nodular toxic goiter (Plummer disease)
- Functioning adenoma
- Struma ovarii (ovarian teratoma that contains functional thyroid tissue)

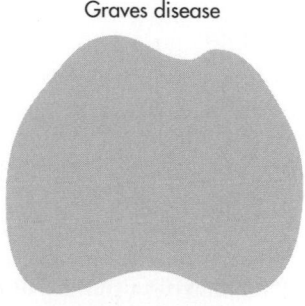

FIGURE 12-36

MULTINODULAR GOITER (Fig. 12-37)

- Enlarged gland
- Multiple cold and hot nodules: spectrum of thyroid adenomas ranging from hyperfunctioning to cystic lesions
- Appearance may be mimicked by Hashimoto thyroiditis

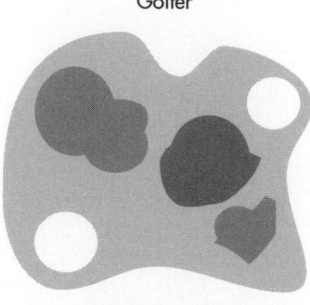

FIGURE 12-37

CONGENITAL ORGANIFICATION DEFECT/ DYSHORMONEGENESIS

- Unable to organify iodine to make thyroid hormone
- High TSH, low T4, hypothyroid
- Perchlorate challenge test
  - Give large dose of potassium perchlorate to wash out radioiodine that is not organified.
  - A decrease of 50% relative RAIU or 5% absolute is positive.

WHOLE BODY THYROID CANCER IMAGING

Whole body radioiodine imaging is used to search for metastatic disease after thyroidectomy. To maximize detection of metastases, TSH stimulation is necessary and is performed in one of two ways:

- Thyroid hormone withdrawal: Off levothyroxine 4-6 weeks, Cytomel 2 weeks
- Recombinant TSH injection: 0.9 mg IM Thyrogen is given on day 1 and day 2; radioiodine is then administered on day 3.

2-4 mCi I-131 is administered and imaging is performed on day 5. A 4 mCi dose is used when Thyrogen stimulation is performed as uptake is generally less compared with TSH stimulation by withdrawal of exogenous thyroid hormone. Pinhole imaging of the neck is helpful to reduce star artifact from septal perforation of the parallel-hole collimator. Doses greater than 5 mCi are generally avoided as "stunning" may render subsequent therapeutic doses less effective. Use of I-123 (2 mCi) is a common alternative, as stunning does not occur and imaging is performed earlier.

PARATHYROID IMAGING

$^{99M}TCO_4^-/^{201}TL$ SUBTRACTION IMAGING

Technique

1. IV injection of 74 to 111 MBq of ^{201}Tl. Imaging for 15 minutes with pinhole collimator. ^{201}Tl localizes in normal thyroid and enlarged parathyroid gland.
2. IV injection of 185 to 370 MBq of $^{99m}TcO_4^-$. Imaging for 15 minutes. $^{99m}TcO_4^-$ localizes in thyroid but not parathyroid.
3. Electronic subtraction of images

Interpretation

- Sensitivity for detecting parathyroid adenomas by scintigraphy: 70%
- Specificity for lesion characterization is only 40% because ^{201}Tl accumulation may also occur in:
  - Benign thyroid adenomas
  - Lymph nodes
  - Carcinomas

- Most authors believe that ^{99m}Tc MIBI is superior to $^{99m}TcO_4^-/^{201}Tl$ subtraction imaging. In ^{99m}Tc MIBI imaging early and late images are compared. Parathyroid adenomas retain ^{99m}Tc MIBI and persist as focal hot spots on delayed images.

^{99M}TC SESTAMIBI IMAGING OF PARATHYROID

Advantages:

- Higher target to background ratios rather than with thallium
- Delay of 2 to 3 hours increases the sensitivity of this technique.
- Parathyroid activity persists while thyroid activity fades away.

^{99m}Tc sestamibi is also used for imaging of thyroid tumors, as well as brain, lung, and bone tumors.

Pet Imaging

^{18}FDG-PET IMAGING

^{18}FDG BASIC MECHANISM (Fig. 12-38)

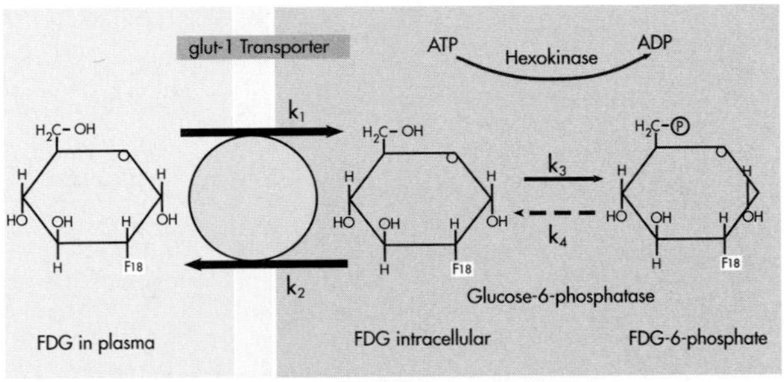

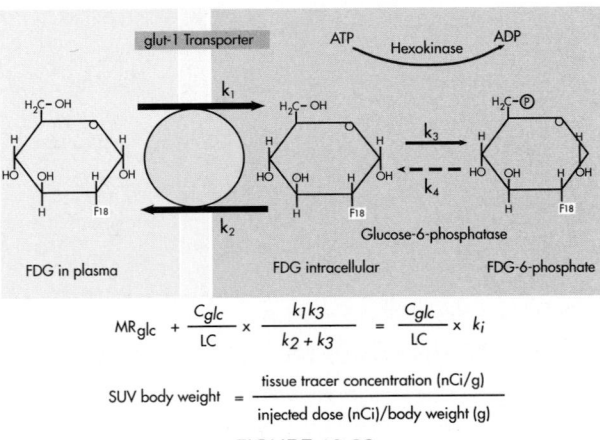

$$MR_{glc} + \frac{C_{glc}}{LC} \times \frac{k_1 k_3}{k_2 + k_3} = \frac{C_{glc}}{LC} \times k_i$$

$$\text{SUV body weight} = \frac{\text{tissue tracer concentration (nCi/g)}}{\text{injected dose (nCi)/body weight (g)}}$$

FIGURE 12-38

- Malignancies often have increased glycolysis (Warburg effect).
- Glucose and ^{18}FDG uptake into malignant cells is facilitated by increased expression of the glucose transporter (glut) in tumor cells.
- ^{18}FDG does not enter the Krebs cycle after phosphorylation (through hexokinase into ^{18}FDG-6 phosphate) and therefore it is effectively trapped in the cells, allowing the measurement of tissue glucose metabolism.
- FDG uptake by neoplastic tumors in vivo depends on numerous physiologic factors such as tissue oxygenation, regional blood flow, peritumoral inflammatory reactions, etc. FDG uptake is not specific for tumors.
- The metabolic rate for glucose (MR_{glc}) can be calculated from the time course of radiotracer concentration in tissue and in arterial blood where C_{glc} is the circulating glucose level, LC is the lumped constant, k_1 and k_2 are the forward and reverse rate constants for FDG capillary transport, k_3 is the FDG phosphorylation rate constant and K_i is the net rate of FDG influx.
- The standardized uptake value (SUV) is a semiquantitative index of tumor uptake normalized to the injected dose and some measure of the total volume of distribution, such as the patient's body weight. The SUV is dependent on patient size, time between injection and scan (uptake period, usually 60 minutes), plasma glucose levels, and method of image reconstruction. Normalizing SUV to body surface area or lean body mass reduces dependency on body weight, which can decrease during cancer therapy.

PRACTICAL ASPECTS OF PET IMAGING

- Most scanners use bismuth germanate (BGO) or NaI crystals.
- Resolution typically varies between 4 and 6 mm FWHM.
- Field of view (FOV) varies between 10 and 16 cm in most scanners, with the largest FOV for single acquisition around 55 cm.
- Patients fast for several hours before the study because elevated serum glucose level can decrease cellular FDG uptake. Water is permitted to promote diuresis.
- In diabetics, insulin is adjusted so that the fasting blood glucose level is below the preferred level of 130 mg/dL.
- FDG is injected intravenously, 100 to 400 MBq.
- Multiple emission images are obtained 30 to 60 minutes after FDG injection.
- Abdominal scanning starts from the inguinal region to minimize bladder activity.
- Data are reviewed in different planes.
- SUV is a simple semiquantitative value that relates the concentration of FDG in the tumor to the average concentration in the body. Higher values indicate likely tumors.

INTEGRATED PET-CT IMAGING

Imaging Systems

- Hybrid PET-CT scanners are composed of two distinct imaging systems integrated into a single gantry with near simultaneous imaging acquisition. PET provides functional, molecular information fused with anatomic localization provided by CT. CT data are reconstructed using filtered back projection, whereas PET data are reconstructed using iterative algorithms such as MLEM, OSEM, or MAP. It has been estimated that there is a 10% advantage of using PET-CT compared with CT or PET examinations alone.

- CT images can be obtained after injection of a PET radiopharmaceutical because CT detectors are insensitive to annihilation radiation.
- Attenuation correction: PET-CT scanners use a set of low dose (130 kVp; 10 to 40 mAs) CT images to derive attenuation correction for PET. This is done by classifying the CT images into two main tissue types (i.e., bone and soft tissues).

Imaging Protocol

- Patients fast 4 to 6 hours and void before scanning; physical activity is restricted to avoid increased muscle activity.
- 60 minutes after the injection of 0.21 mCi/kg of ^{18}FDG, a CT tomogram is obtained. This is followed by helical CT without contrast for attenuation correction. If a contrast-enhanced CT is required, this is done as an additional scan after the standard PET-CT is completed.
- For most whole-body scans (thorax, abdomen, and pelvis) the patient is scanned with arms above head. However, for dedicated head and neck examinations, scanning is performed with the arms in lateral position to avoid beam hardening artifacts.

PET-CT Scanning Artifacts

- Respiratory motion: can result in discrepancy of spatial information from CT and PET leading to artifacts after CT-based attenuation correction. These artifacts can affect the chest wall and regions close to the diaphragm and liver.
- High-density implants and dental fillings may lead to serious artifacts on CT images. These artifacts propagate via CT-based attenuation correction into the corrected PET emission images.
- Positive oral and iodinated intravenous contrast agents

ARTIFACTS AND VARIANTS IN PET-CT IMAGING

Source of Artifact	Cause
Technology-related	System or imaging modality dependent
Patient-related	Motion, moving structures (bowel) or pulsing organs (heart, lung), brown fat (hot), muscle activity, non-fasting (diffuse muscle uptake)
Operator-related	Protocol related, FDG uptake interval
Algorithm-related	Type of image reconstruction, segmentation protocols, attenuation correction methods

NORMAL FDG-PET SCAN

- Normal FDG uptake predominates in brain where gray matter avidly concentrates.
- Myocardial uptake is variable depending on the availability of substrate. About 40% of fasting patients show considerable myocardial uptake.
- FDG is concentrated and eliminated by kidney. Activity seen in the kidney and bladder.
- Activity in GI tract varies. Stomach, colon (flexures and sigmoid colon) can be seen.
- Resting muscle does not show high uptake, but uptake may vary in tensed muscles or with recent muscular activity (diazepam before examination may help).
- Brown fat's high FDG uptake may be minimized by:
    - Warm environment for the patient before FDG injection
    - High-fat, low carbohydrate, protein-permitted diet before the examination
    - Moderate doze of oral diazepam (>0.8 mg/kg, up to 7.5 mg) or IV fentanyl (0.75 μg/kg, up to 50 μg)
    - Low dose (20 mg) oral propranolol 60 min before FDG injection

FALSE-POSITIVE PET SCAN

- Histoplasmosis
- TB
- Benign tumor
- Uterine fibroids

FALSE-NEGATIVE PET SCAN

- BAC
- Carcinoid
- Lesion size <8 mm

FDG-PET IN LUNG CANCER

- Used in the diagnosis/work-up for solitary pulmonary nodules. The negative predictive value is high. In patients with negative results, follow-up at 3- to 6-month intervals for at least 2 years is recommended. The sensitivity of PET declines significantly when solitary nodules are smaller than 8 mm.
- Used in hilar and mediastinal staging. One recommended strategy is to operate on patients with negative PET; patients with positive results should have confirmatory transbronchial biopsy or mediastinoscopy.
- Used for follow-up in patients with small cell carcinoma
- Mucin-producing tumors such as bronchoalveolar carcinomas are frequently false negative by FDG-PET.

- Whole-body PET CT detects unexpected distant metastases in about 10% of all lung cancer patients.
- Neuroendocrine tumors (carcinoid) do not consistently exhibit increased FDG uptake. Absent FDG activity in a suspicious mass does not obviate the need for biopsy.

MELANOMA

- PET can be useful in detecting lymph node and visceral metastases.
- Small subcutaneous lesions can be easily missed.

COLORECTAL CARCINOMA

- PET combined with CT is very useful in detection of recurrence and follow-up staging in colorectal carcinoma.
- PET has been shown to be effective in detecting local and regional recurrence.
- PET can be used in staging patients with suspected or demonstrated recurrence.
- Abnormal FDG uptake in the bowel should be confirmed by endoscopy.

PANCREATIC CARCINOMA

- Differentiation of pancreatic carcinoma from pancreatitis
- Staging of extent of tumor preoperatively

LYMPHOMA AND LEUKEMIA

- PET has been demonstrated in some studies to reveal more lesions than CT and clinical examination. Main value in staging is to provide a baseline for subsequent evaluation of therapy.
- A pattern of diffuse increased bone marrow activity is frequently seen in patients after chemotherapy due to regenerating marrow; other reasons for increased activity include anemia, treatment with granulocyte colony-stimulating factor or erythropoietin, and diffuse bone marrow infiltration from tumor.
- FDG uptake is variable in different types of lymphoma

Lymphoma Type	FDG Uptake
B-cell non-Hodgkin	
Large, Burkitt, anaplastic	High
Follicular (grade 3)	Moderate to high
Follicular (grades 1 and 2), mantle cell	Low to moderate
Marginal zone, MALT	None to high
Small lymphocytic	None to low
Hodgkin	
Nodular sclerosis	High
Mixed, lymphocyte depletion	Moderate to high
Lymphocyte dominant	Low
T-cell	
Extranodal natural-killer/T-cell, peripheral T-cell	High
Adult T-cell leukemia-lymphoma, cutaneous T-cell	Moderate
Mycosis fungoides and Sézary syndrome	Low

BREAST CANCER

- Limited diagnostic value for detecting small primary tumor, well-differentiated breast cancer, or regional lymph node metastasis due to limited resolution at detecting microscopic metastasis.
- Accurate in detecting primary lesions >1 cm. Useful in patients with previous implant surgery or in patients with dense breasts.
- Useful for distant metastasis.
- Suspected recurrence
- Therapy and follow-up
- False positives
  - Fibrocystic change
  - Atypical ductal hyperplasia
  - Ductal ectasia
  - Phyllodes tumor
- Positron emission mammography (PEM)

Emerging technology of dedicated units for breast for detection and depiction of primary breast cancer. Composed of two planar detectors placed opposite the breast. Compared with PET, PEM has increased geometric sensitivity, higher spatial resolution, a shorter imaging time, reduced attenuation, and a small physical footprint.

FDG-PET BRAIN IMAGING

Approximately 5 mCi FDG is administered. Time delay after injection before imaging: 30 min (45 min for body). Brain takes up 6.9% of the injected dose. Primary indications include:

- Refractory seizures: interictal
- Tumor recurrence versus radiation necrosis
- Alzheimer disease
- Neurodegenerative diseases

Hypometabolism in a cerebellar hemisphere may be seen contralateral to a cerebral hemispheric process (e.g., stroke, radiation, tumor), and is known as crossed cerebellar diaschisis.

NORMAL UPTAKE PATTERN

- High uptake in the gray matter (high hexokinase concentration)
- Basal ganglia and thalamus
- Motor strip

- Visual cortex
- Auditory cortex
- Brainstem

REFRACTORY SEIZURE

Indication: focal epilepsy refractory to medical treatment and considered for surgical therapy. Findings:

- Interictal: decreased uptake
- Ictal: increased uptake
- Generalized absence seizure: globally increased uptake

TUMOR RECURRENCE VERSUS RADIATION NECROSIS

Indication: differentiate tumor recurrence from nodular radiation necrosis change; should be interpreted with structural imaging. Findings:

- Areas of radiation injury: decreased uptake
- Tumor: increased uptake

False-negative results:

- Recent radiation treatment
- Low-grade tumor
- Small tumor volume

False-positive results:

- Nonmalignant inflammatory process
- Subclinical seizure activity

Other tumors:

- Lymphoma: high uptake
- Meningioma: variable uptake
- Pilocytic astrocytoma: variable uptake without relation to prognosis

MEMORY LOSS (ALZHEIMER DEMENTIA)

Most common dementia. Patterns:

- Decreased FDG uptake in temporal and parietal cortex
- Most sensitive is posterior cingulated gyrus and precuneus (early), but these areas are not always hypometabolic (normally hypermetabolic) so may be missed.
- Spares basal ganglia, thalamus, motor and visual cortex, and cerebellum
- Unilateral early, symmetrical with disease progression
- Extent of hypometabolism correlates with severity of cognitive decline

OTHER NEURODEGENERATIVE DISORDERS

- Parkinson disease may show similar metabolic impairment as Alzheimer disease, even in the absence of major cognitive deficits. Compare with structural imaging.
- Pick disease: frontal or frontotemporal hypometabolism. Similar pattern also found in:
  Progressive supranuclear palsy
  Spinocerebellar atrophy
  Cocaine abuse
  Some psychiatric disorders
- Huntington chorea: hypometabolism of putamen and caudate; juvenile form: thalamic hypometabolism

OTHER PET TRACERS AND AGENTS

APPROVED AGENTS USED LESS COMMONLY

^{82}Rubidium

- Approved for noninvasive imaging of the perfusion of the heart

^{13}N-ammonia

- Approved for noninvasive imaging of the perfusion of the heart

^{15}O-oxygen

- Useful for cerebral perfusion and oxygen consumption in stroke
- 2-minute half-life

^{18}F-fluoride

- Useful for bone imaging (replacement of ^{99}mTc-MDP planar bone scans)

LIST OF AGENTS IN CLINICAL DEVELOPMENT

- ^{18}FLT (fluorothymidine), ^{11}C-thymidine: proliferation marker (lung cancer, glioma)
- ^{11}C-methionine: proliferation marker (cancer)
- ^{11}C-acetate: lipid synthesis; incorporation into cell membrane lipids (cancer)
- ^{18}F-annexin V: putative apoptosis marker
- ^{64}Cu-ATSM: hypoxia agent
- ^{18}F-MISO, ^{18}F-fluoromisonidazole: hypoxia agent
- ^{18}FACBC: nonmetabolizable amino acid analog
- ^{18}F-Galacto-RGD: integrin marker
- ^{18}FES: estrogen receptor
- ^{18}F-DHT: dihydrotestosterone, androgen receptor
- ^{11}C-acetate: oxidative metabolism, incorporated into membrane lipids
- ^{18}F-choline, ^{11}C-choline: metabolized by choline kinase
- ^{11}C-tyrosine, ^{18}F-fluorotyrosine, ^{18}F-fluoroethyltyrosine: tyrosine amino acid transport (cancer)
- ^{18}F-fluorodihydroxyphenylalanine: response of neuroendocrine and brain tumors
- ^{18}F/^{11}C labeled therapeutic drugs ("minidosing"); example: ^{18}F-fluorouracil (5-FU)
- Labeled cells (lymphocytes, leukocytes, stem cells)

CANCER PATHWAYS RELEVANT TO PET IMAGING (Fig. 12-39)

Figure 12-39 summarizes key pathways in cancer and their effect on proliferation. Shown are also key therapeutic inhibitors whose efficacy can occasionally be assessed by PET imaging.

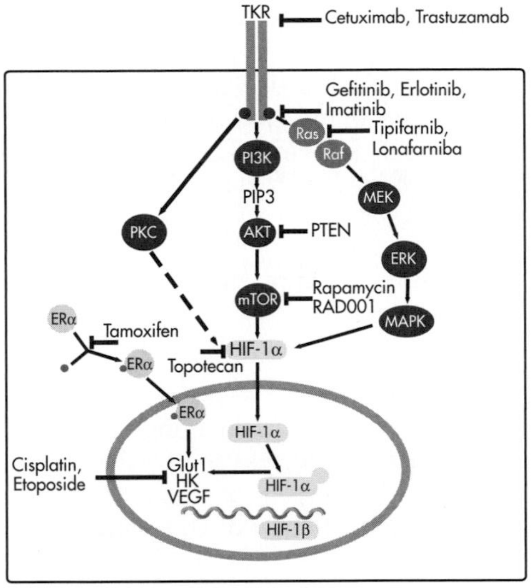

FIGURE 12-39

CENTERS FOR MEDICARE AND MEDICAID SERVICES (CMS) COVERAGE OF PET

Effective Date	Clinical Condition/ Indication	Coverage
March 1995	Myocardial perfusion	Rubidium-82 in coronary artery disease
January 1998	Solitary pulmonary nodule	Characterization
January 1998	Non–small cell lung cancer	Initial staging
July 1999	Colorectal cancer	Suggested recurrence with rising CEA
July 1999	Lymphoma	Staging and restaging as alternative to gallium scan
July 1999	Melanoma	Recurrence before surgery as alternative to gallium scan
July 2001	Non–small cell lung cancer	Diagnosis, staging, and restaging
July 2001	Esophageal cancer	Diagnosis, staging, and restaging
July 2001	Colorectal cancer	Diagnosis, staging, and restaging
July 2001	Lymphoma	Diagnosis, staging, and restaging
July 2001	Melanoma	Diagnosis, staging, and restaging. Not covered for evaluating regional nodes.
July 2001	Head and neck (excluding central nervous system and thyroid)	Diagnosis, staging and restaging
July 2001	Refractory seizures	Presurgical evaluation
July 2001 to September 2002	Myocardial viability	Only following inconclusive SPECT
October 2002	Myocardial viability	Primary or initial diagnosis
October 2002	Breast cancer	Staging, restaging, response to treatment
October 2003	Myocardial perfusion	Ammonia N-13 in coronary artery disease
October 2003	Thyroid cancer	Restaging of recurrent or residual disease
September 2004	Alzheimer disease and dementia	In CMS-approved clinical trial
January 2005	Brain, cervical, ovarian, pancreatic, small cell lung, and testicular cancers	Coverage with evidence development
January 2005	All other cancers and indications not previously specified	Coverage with evidence development

Miscellaneous Imaging Techniques

GALLIUM IMAGING

ISOTOPE (Fig. 12-40)

^{67}Ga citrate is most commonly used for imaging of tumors and inflammation.

Pharmacokinetics

- Physical half-life: 78 hours
- Blood half-life: 12 hours
- ^{67}Ga is bound to iron transport proteins such as transferrin, ferritin, lactoferrin.

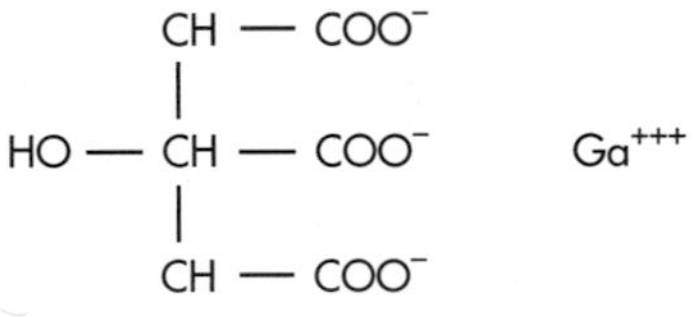

FIGURE 12-40

- ^{67}Ga localizes in infections and tumors because of:
  - Uptake in leukocytes
  - Transferrin and lactoferrin binding at site of infection
  - Abnormal vascular permeability at sites of inflammation and tumors
- Renal and fecal excretion

Radiation

Major radiation is to bone marrow (9 rad), bowel (9 rad), and spleen and liver (7 rad).

Technique

- Usual dosage is 185 to 300 MBq. Higher doses increase lesion detectability.
- Imaging 48 to 72 hours after IV administration
- All 3 major photopeaks (93, 185, 300 keV) are used for imaging to increase signal-to-noise ratio (SNR).

NORMAL IMAGES (Fig. 12-41)

- Low-quality images because:
  - Relatively low dosage
  - Residual blood activity
  - Delayed imaging (days after injection)
  - Need a medium energy collimator that has a lower spatial resolution
- Liver has the most intense uptake.
- Colonic excretion becomes prominent after 48 hours and limits the usefulness of the technique for abdominal imaging.
- Uptake in salivary glands, lacrimal glands, breast
- Epiphyseal plates are prominent in children.
- Lung activity is minimal.
- Renal activity is normal early only; activity after 72 hours is always abnormal.
- Thymus uptake: sail sign.

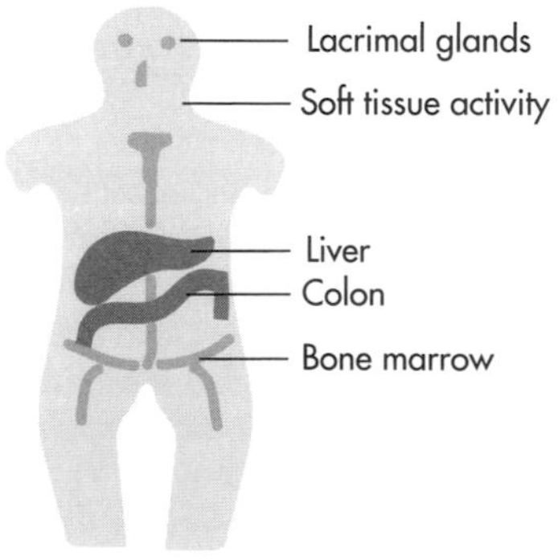

FIGURE 12-41

APPLICATIONS

Chest

Uptake occurs in a wide variety of inflammatory diseases and can be used to determine whether an interstitial process is active or inactive (e.g., interstitial fibrosis is not Ga avid). Most common indications:

- Sarcoid activity
  - Lambda sign: bilateral hilar and paratracheal uptake
  - Panda sign: lacrimal gland uptake
- Detection of early *Pneumocystis carinii* pneumonia (now known as *Pneumocystis jiroveci* [Frenkel 1999])
- Lymphoma imaging (residual disease versus inactive fibrosis)
- Ga-avid tumors: lymphoma > hepatocellular carcinoma > others
- Kaposi sarcoma is not gallium avid.

Other Applications

- Vertebral osteomyelitis imaging (preferred over radiolabeled leukocytes)
- Cardiac amyloidosis
- Increased parotid or lacrimal uptake
  - Sarcoid
  - Sjögren syndrome
  - Radiation

LEUKOCYTE IMAGING

PREPARATION

WBC labeling can be used as a marker of acute inflammation. WBC labeling is performed with ^{111}In oxine, a lipophilic compound that diffuses through cell membranes. Once inside the cell, In and oxine dissociate and In binds to intracellular proteins; oxine diffuses out of cells. Tc HMPAO labeling of WBC is also used. Chronic infection may cause false negative scans.

Indications

- All infectious processes in abdomen (^{67}Ga is less suited because of its bowel excretion)
- Osteomyelitis
- Vascular graft infections

Technique

1. Draw 50 mL blood from patient (anticoagulated with heparin).
2. Separate buffy coat (Ficoll).
3. 37 MBq of ^{111}In oxine or ^{111}In tropolone is incubated (30 minutes) with the separated WBC.
4. Wash cells.
5. Reinject labeled WBC (usually 7.4 to 18 MBq). Labeling procedure takes about 2 hours.
6. Imaging is done at 24 hours after injection.

Radiation

Major radiation is to spleen (20 rad), liver (3 rad), and bone marrow (2 rad). Radiation to other organs is low.

NORMAL IMAGING (Fig. 12-42)

- Images have low SNR
- Spleen very hot (in contrast to Ga images where liver is very hot)
- No bowel activity
- No activity in lacrimal glands

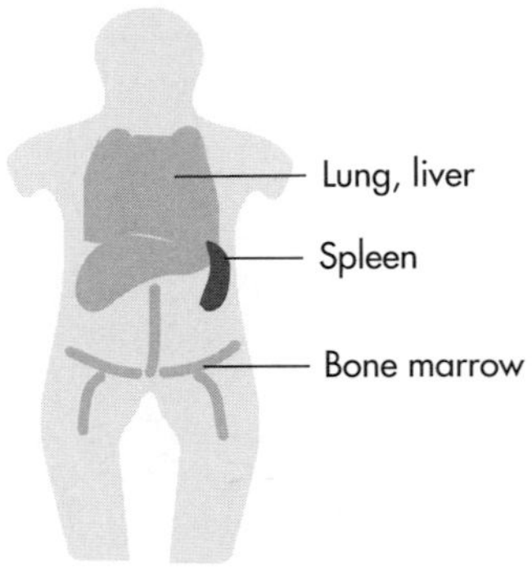

FIGURE 12-42

OTHER INFECTION IMAGING AGENTS

OPTIMAL IMAGING TIME

Agent	Time (hr)
^{67}Ga	48
^{111}In-oxine WBC	24
^{111}In-IgG	12-24
^{99m}Tc HMPAO WBC	2
Chemotactic peptides	1
Long circulating polymers	1-12

BRAIN IMAGING

^{99M}TC HMPAO (Fig. 12-43)

Hexamethylpropyleneamine oxime (HMPAO) is a lipophilic agent that passes through the intact blood-brain barrier, is trapped within neurons, and remains there for several hours after IV administration. The compound is only stable for about 30 minutes after preparation and should therefore be administered immediately, although stabilizers may be added to allow up to a 4 hour window. Quality control is necessary to determine the amount of a less lipophilic complex of HMPAO, which does not accumulate in the brain.

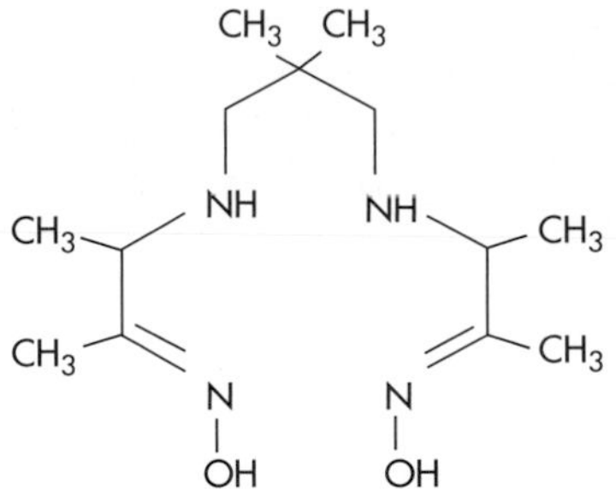

FIGURE 12-43

Pharmacokinetics

- Brain activity is maximum at 1 minute, plateaus at 2 minutes (88% peak activity)
- Brain activity remains constant for 8 hours.
- Organ uptake
  - Brain, 4%
  - Liver, 11%
  - Kidneys, 4%
  - Bladder, urine, 3%
- Gray matter activity > white matter activity

Similarly, ^{99m}Tc ethyl cysteinate dimer (ECD) is a lipophilic radiopharmaceutical which crosses the blood brain barrier and is trapped in neurons; it is stable up to 6 hours after preparation.

BRAIN DEATH STUDY (Fig. 12-44)

Brain death is defined as absent cerebral blood flow despite maintained cardiac and respiratory function. Brain scans are useful to confirm the presence of brain death particularly in barbiturate intoxication and hypothermia (EEG less reliable). There are 2 types of studies:

- ^{99m}Tc DTPA flow study to demonstrate absence of flow
- ^{99m}Tc HMPAO study (preferred method)

Technique

1. Freshly prepare ^{99m}Tc HMPAO.
2. Inject 555 to 740 MBq (high dose).

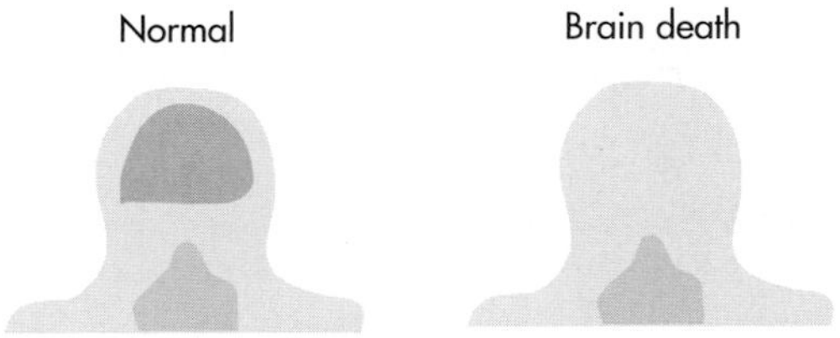

FIGURE 12-44

3. Scalp tourniquet to diminish activity from external carotid circulation (only needed for ^{99m}Tc DTPA but not for ^{99m}Tc HMPAO)
4. Obtain flow images (optional).
5. Obtain delayed images 5 to 15 minutes after injection.

Imaging Findings

- No flow
  - Absent ICA
  - Absent sinuses
- Absent cerebral uptake of HMPAO
- Slight perfusion of scalp veins may be present.
- Hot nose sign: increased intracranial pressure results in increased flow to external carotid system

HMPAO/ECD SPECT IMAGING

Indications

Dementia

- Alzheimer disease: bilateral perfusion defects in temporoparietal regions
- Multiinfarct dementia: asymmetrical perfusion defects

Movement disorders

- Parkinson disease: increased perfusion in basal ganglia
- Huntington disease: decreased striatal metabolism

Tumor

- Residual/recurrent tumor versus radiation necrosis

Technique

1. Freshly prepare ^{99m}Tc HMPAO
2. Inject 555 to 740 MBq
3. Perform imaging 20 minutes after injection
4. Obtain 30- to 40-second acquisitions per view
5. Reconstructions in 3 orthogonal planes

ACETAZOLAMIDE CHALLENGE TEST

Assess cerebral perfusion reserve using ^{99m}Tc ECD or ^{99m}Tc HMPAO with 1 g of acetazolamide, which is a carbonic anhydrase inhibitor. In normal brain, acetazolamide causes an increase in cerebral carbon dioxide, resulting in vasodilation and increased flow. In areas of reduced flow, vessels are already at maximal vasodilation so acetazolamide does not increase flow. Compare with baseline study.

Indications

- CNS territory at risk in patients experiencing transient ischemic attacks
- Patients being considered for carotid ligation surgery

Contraindications

- Cardiovascular instability
- Renal or hepatic disease
- Allergy to sulfa drugs

^{201}THALLIUM BRAIN IMAGING

Used in immunocompromised patients to differentiate between toxoplasmosis and lymphoma:

- Lymphoma: increased uptake
- Toxoplasmosis: decreased uptake

^{111}IN DTPA CISTERNOGRAPHY

- Technique: After intrathecal injection of radiotracer, normal activity is seen in basal cisterns at 2-4 hours (trident sign), over convexities at 24 hours, and there is no reflux into ventricles. Indications: NPH, VP shunts, CSF leaks.
- Normal pressure hydrocephalus: delayed flow over convexities and ventricular reflux.
- VP shunt patency: Injection of radiotracer into reservoir-rapid flow from ventricles, through tubing, and accumulation of activity in peritoneal cavity. ^{99m}Tc TPA may also be used.
- CSF rhinorrhea: 4 hours after intrathecal injection of radiotracer, nasal pledgets are removed. A ratio of radioactivity of pledgets to plasma of at least 2:1 is positive. Scintigraphic imaging may be used to identify other CSF leaks, e.g. otorrhea. Bowel uptake may indicate swallowing of leaked CSF.

LYMPHOSCINTIGRAPHY

AGENTS

Sulfide Colloid

^{99m}Tc sulfide colloid (particle size: 3 to 12 nm) differs from ^{99m}Tc sulfur colloid (particle size: 500 to 1000 nm) used for liver/spleen imaging. Sulfide colloid used for lymphoscintigraphy is prepared by reacting hydrogen sulfide with antimony potassium tartrate to provide Sb_2S_3. Polyvinylpyrrolidone stabilizes the colloid sulfide and limits particle growth.

Human Serum Albumin (HSA) Nanocolloid

Small aggregates of HSA (differs from macroaggregated albumin in size). After SC administration (0.2 mL), particles are cleared by lymphatic vessels (30% at 3 hours); accumulation occurs in normal local lymph nodes. Indications:

- Tumor (unreliable method for detecting lymph node metastases)

- Determination of lymphatic function in lymphedema

^{57}Co flood source is used to produce a transmission image for anatomic delineation.

TUMOR IMAGING

AGENTS

OVERVIEW

Agent	Targets/Tumor Localization
Specific Agents	
^{18}FDG-PET	Glucose metabolism
^{18}F labeled small molecules	Receptors, kinases, drugs
^{111}In OncoScint	TAG-72 (tumor surface antigen)
^{111}In Prostascint	PSMA (tumor surface antigen)
^{99m}Tc CEA-scan	CEA (tumor surface antigen)
^{111}In somatostatin analogues	Somatostatin receptors
^{99m}Tc MDP	Bone metastases, tumor calcification
^{131}I	Thyroid cancer
^{131}MIBG	Adrenal tumors
Nonspecific Agents	
^{67}Ga	Multiple mechanism
^{201}Tl	Multiple mechanism
^{99m}Tc sestamibi	Perfusion imaging, multidrug resistance

ONCOSCINT (^{111}IN DTPA LABELED B72.3 MONOCLONAL ANTIBODY)

Murine immunoglobulin G monoclonal antibody (MAb) directed against a high-molecular-weight glycoprotein (TAG-72) expressed in the majority of colorectal and ovarian tumors (satumomab pendetide). Properties include:

- Biologic half-life: 56 ± 14 hours
- Urine excretion (72 hours): 10%
- Used at 185 MBq; imaging at 48 to 72 hours
- Normal distribution: liver > spleen > bone marrow > other

PROSTASCINT (^{111}IN-LABELED B72.3 MONOCLONAL ANTIBODY)

Murine immunoglobulin G monoclonal antibody 7E11-C5.3 (Capromab pendetide) against prostate-specific membrane antigen (PSMA) expressed on cancers. Properties include:

- Biologic half-life: 67 ± 11 hours
- Urine excretion (72 hours): 10%
- Used at 0.5 mg MAb and 185 MBq
- Imaging on day of injection and 4 to 7 days later (to clear blood pool activity)

CEA-SCAN (^{99M}TC DTPA-LABELED ANTI-CEA)

Fab' fragment generated from IMMU-4, a murine IgG1 monoclonal antibody (arcitumomab). Recognizes CEA on colon adenocarcinoma cells. Labeled with 740 MBq ^{99m}Tc. Properties include:

- Biologic half-life: 13 ± 4 hours
- Urine excretion (24 hours): 30%

SOMATOSTATIN

Human somatostatin (cyclic 14 amino acid peptide) has broad action, usually inhibitory in nature. A large variety of neuroendocrine cells have somatostatin receptors, and imaging may be useful in these cases:

- Paraganglioma
- Pituitary adenoma
- Islet cell tumors
- Pheochromocytoma
- Adrenal neuroblastoma
- Pulmonary oat cell tumors
- Lymphoma
- Medullary thyroid carcinoma
- GI, chest carcinoids

OCTREOTIDE IMAGING (Fig. 12-45)

Octreotide (Phe-Cys-Phe-Trp-Lys-Thr-Cys-Thr), a synthetic cyclic octapeptide, is used for clinical imaging. This agent has pharmacologic action similar to that of somatostatin and can be labeled with either ^{123}I or ^{111}In after certain molecular modification. Blood half-life: 6 hours. Urine excretion: 50% at 6 hours. In the absence of tumors, the main distribution is to the spleen, kidneys, and liver.

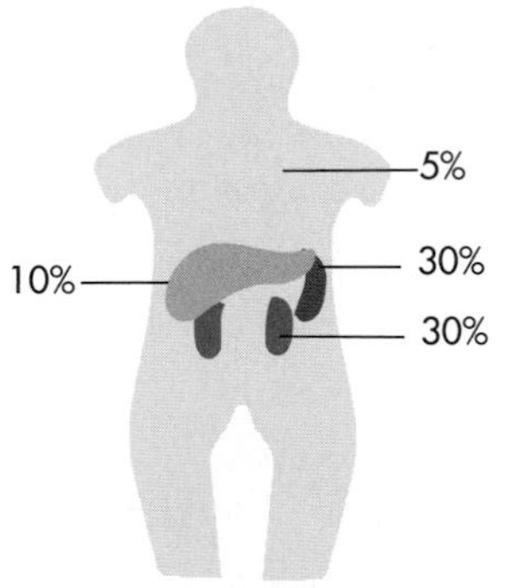

Normal study

FIGURE 12-45

Differential Diagnosis

RADIOPHARMACEUTICALS

OVERVIEW

Organ	Agent	Dose (mCi) *	Mode of Decay	Excretion	Critical Organ (rad/dose)
Bone	^{99m}Tc MDP	20	IT	Renal	2-3/bladder
Lung	^{99m}Tc MAA	4	IT	Renal	1.0/lung
	^{133}Xe	10	β-	Lungs	0.3/lung
Heart	^{201}Tl	2-4	EC	Minimal renal	2.2/kidney
	^{99m}Tc RBC	20	IT	Renal	0.4/body
Thyroid	^{123}I	0.2	EC	GI, renal	5/thyroid
	^{131}I	5-10	β-	GI, renal	500-1000/thyroid
Renal	^{99m}Tc DTPA	10	IT	Renal	2-5/bladder
	^{99m}Tc MAG_3	10	IT	Renal	2-5/bladder
Liver/spleen	^{99m}Tc sulfur colloid	5-8	IT	None	1-2/liver
Hepatobiliary	^{99m}Tc DISIDA	5-8	IT	Biliary	1.6/bowel
Brain	^{99m}Tc DTPA	20	IT	Renal	2-5/bladder
	^{99m}Tc HMPAO	20	IT	Renal, GI	5/lacrimal gland
Infection-tumor	^{67}Ga citrate	5-10	EC	GI, renal	4.5/colon
	^{111}In WBC	0.2-0.5	EC	None	20/spleen
GI hemorrhage	^{99m}Tc RBC	20	IT	Renal	0.4/body
Meckel's diverticulum	^{99m}Tc 04	15	IT	GI	2/stomach
LeVeen shunt	^{99m}Tc MAA	3^-	IT	Renal	Lung/peritoneum
Gastric emptying	^{99m}Tc sulfur colloid	0.5	IT	GI	Colon
Ureteral reflux	^{99m}Tc sulfur colloid	0.5	IT	Urinary	Bladder

*1.0 MBq = 0.027 mCi; 740 MBq = 20 mCi; 1.0 mCi = 37 MBq.

Quality Assurance for Radiopharmaceuticals

Generator
- Aluminum breakthrough: <10 μg/mL
- Molybdenum (Mo) breakthrough: <0.15 μCi/1 mCi of ^{99m}Tc
- Mo breakthrough is determined by counting the eluate in a well counter without (counts ^{99m}Tc + ^{99}Mo) and with a lead shield (count only 600 keV beta (–) radiation).

Radiochemical purity
- Determined with thin layer chromatography
- Free $^{99m}TcO_4^-$ migrates in saline and methanol.
- ^{99m}Tc compounds migrate in saline only.

PULMONARY

V̇/Q̇ MISMATCH (Fig. 12-46)

- Pulmonary embolism
- Vasculitis, radiation therapy, Wegener granulomatosis, autoimmune diseases
- Tumor compression of PA
- Pleural effusion
- Radiation therapy
- Hypoplastic PA

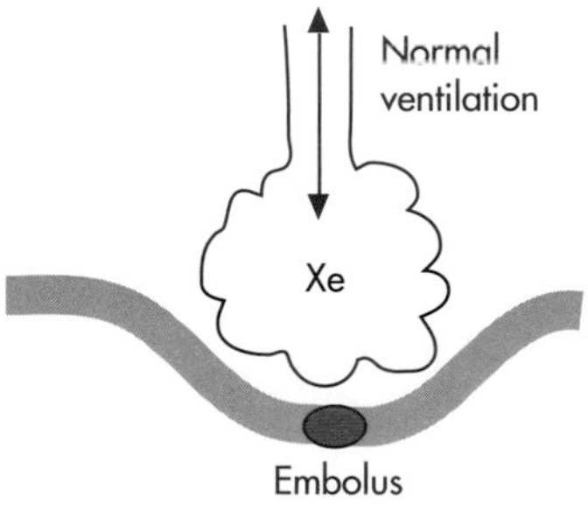

FIGURE 12-46

CAUSES OF PULMONARY EMBOLISM

- Venous thrombus (most common cause)
- Fat embolism; although present in most skeletal trauma, only 1% manifest clinical syndrome.
- Tumor embolism
- Amniotic fluid embolism
- Parasites, especially schistosomiasis
- Talc embolism in intravenous drug abuser (widespread micronodular disease of the lungs)
- Oil embolism from ethiodol after lymphangiogram
- Mercury embolism: thermometer accidents (metallic densities)

- Air embolism: rarely has plain film manifestations

MATCHED $\dot{V}/\dot{Q}$ DEFECT (Fig. 12-47)

Any primary pulmonary parenchymal abnormality may result in secondary arteriolar constriction, thus causing a matched $\dot{V}/\dot{Q}$ defect.

- Consolidation: pneumonia, edema
- COPD
- Atelectasis
- Tumor
- Bullous disease
- Pneumonectomy, surgery
- Pneumonia
- Enlarged hilar nodes
- Edema
- Fibrosis
- Pulmonary infarction
- alpha-1 antitrypsin deficiency, UIP: lower lobes

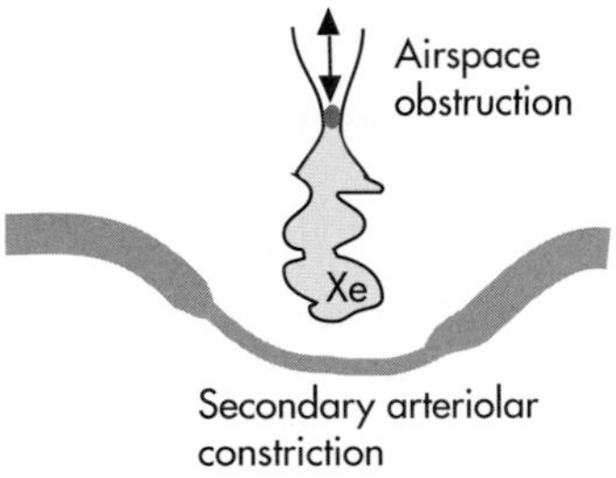

FIGURE 12-47

DECREASED PERFUSION IN ONE LUNG

- Embolus
- Pneumothorax
- Massive effusion
- Tumor
- Pulmonary agenesis or hypoplasia
- Swyer-James syndrome

CARDIOVASCULAR (FIG. 12-48)

FALSE-NEGATIVE THALLIUM STUDIES

- Submaximal exercise (high splanchnic uptake)
- Noncritical stenosis (<40%)
- Small ischemic area
- Coronary collaterals
- Multivessel disease
- Medications:
  - Blunted cardiac response to exercise (beta blockers, calcium channel blockers, digoxin)
  - Altered myocardial extraction (furosemide, lidocaine, dipyridamole, dexamethasone, isoproterenol)

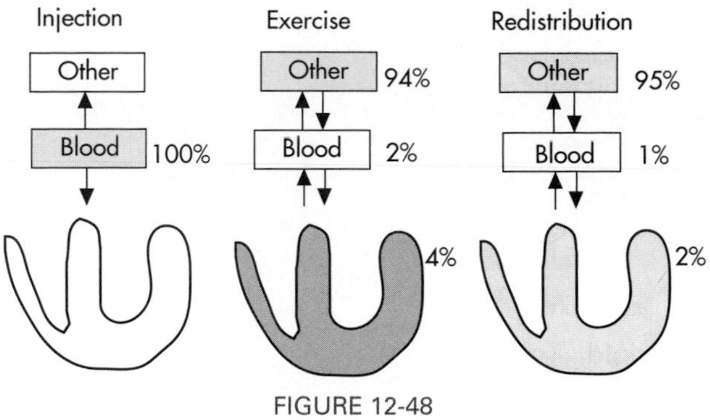

FIGURE 12-48

FALSE-POSITIVE THALLIUM STUDY

- Any cardiomyopathy
- Aortic valve stenosis
- Mitral valve prolapse
- Left bundle branch block (LBBB)
- Infiltrative cardiac disease (sarcoidosis, Chagas disease, amyloidosis)

PARADOXICAL SEPTAL MOVEMENT

- Septal ischemia
- Previous cardiac surgery
- RV overload
- LBBB or pacer placement

FIXED DEFECT

- Infarct
- Attenuation
- Hibernating myocardium
- Apical thinning

PYROPHOSPHATE UPTAKE

- MI
- Unstable angina
- LV aneurysm
- Cardiomyopathy
- Valvular calcification
- Any cause of myocardial injury
  - Contusion or surgery
  - Cardioversion
  - Myocarditis
  - Pericarditis

GASTROINTESTINAL

PATTERNS IN HIDA STUDIES (Fig. 12-49)

GB Not Visualized

Give morphine to increase pressure or cholecystokinin to contract GB. Causes:

- Acute cholecystitis
  - Rim sign: suggestive of gangrenous cholecystitis
- Prolonged fasting
- Recent meal

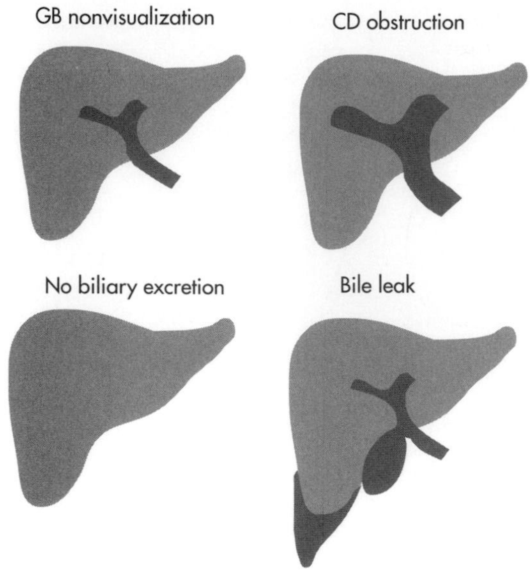

FIGURE 12-49

Biliary System Not Visualized

- Biliary atresia (24-hour delayed images)
- Long-standing bile duct obstruction

Low Hepatic Activity, Renal Activity

- Severe hepatocellular disease
- Neonatal hepatitis; to improve the excretion of tracer in neonatal hepatitis, patients can be pretreated with phenobarbital (5 mg/kg for 5 days).

Bowel Not Visualized

- Choledocholithiasis
- Ampullary stenosis

Abnormal Tracer Collections

- Bile leak (postsurgical, trauma); do delayed imaging to differentiate leak from GB or bowel
- Choledochal cyst
- Caroli disease
- Duodenal diverticulum
- Cystic duct remnant

False-Negative HIDA Study

- Duodenal diverticulum may simulate GB.
- Accessory cystic duct

False-Positive HIDA Study

- Recent meal (within 4 hours)
- Prolonged fasting, intensive care unit patients, parenteral nutrition
- Pancreatitis
- Hepatocellular dysfunction
- Right lower lobe pneumonia
- Cholangiocarcinoma involving cystic duct

Focal Liver Uptake With ^{99m}Tc Sulfur Colloid

- Focal nodular hyperplasia
- Regenerating nodule
- Budd-Chiari syndrome (hot caudate lobe)
- Vena cave obstruction (umbilical vein delivery to segment 1)

Bleeding Studies

- Uptake conforming to bowel with no change over time: inflammatory bowel disease, faulty labeling ($^{99m}TcO_4^-$ excreted into bowel)
- Uptake conforming to bowel with progressive accumulation over time: hemorrhage
- Uptake not conforming to bowel: aneurysm

RLQ ACTIVITY ON MECKEL SCAN

- Meckel's diverticulum or other duplication cysts with ectopic gastric mucosa
- Renal (ectopic kidney, ureteral stenosis)
- Very active bleeding sites
- Tumors
- Inflammatory bowel disease

RAPID GASTRIC EMPTYING

- Postoperative: BI, BII
- Peptic ulcer disease, Zollinger-Ellison syndrome
- Drugs: erythromycin, metoclopramide, domperidone
- Sprue
- Vagotomy with distal partial gastrectomy

DELAYED GASTRIC EMPTYING

- Diabetes
- Hyperglycemia
- Acidosis
- Ileus
- Chronic gastritis
- Chronic ulcer disease
- Drugs: opiates, antacids, gastrin

HOT QUADRATE LOBE

- SVC obstruction with upper extremity injection
- IVC obstruction with lower extremity injection
- Budd-Chiari (sparing of caudate lobe)

GENITOURINARY

PATTERNS

Focal Renal Defects

- Tumor: solid, cystic
- Infection: abscess, cortical scarring
- Congenital: duplex system

- Trauma
- Vascular: complete stenosis

Focal Hot Renal Lesions

- Collecting system
- Urinary leak
- Cross-fused ectopia
- Horseshoe kidney

Dilated Ureter or Collecting System

- Reflux (most common)
- Obstructed ureter

Delayed Uptake and Excretion (Renal Failure)

Prerenal: poor flow and uptake, unilateral
- Arterial stenosis
- Venous thrombosis

Renal (bilateral)
- Acute tubular necrosis: normal flow, poor uptake
- Glomerulonephritis: poor flow and poor uptake
- Chronic renal failure

Postrenal
- Obstruction: dilated calyces

Nonvisualized Kidney

- Nephrectomy
- Ectopic kidney pelvis, fused ectopia
- Renal artery embolus
- Renal artery occlusion

TESTICULAR ANOMALIES

Decreased Uptake

- Torsion
- Orchiectomy

Increased Uptake

- Orchidoepididymitis

Ring Sign

- Late torsion
- Tumor
- Abscess
- Trauma

BONE

FOCAL HOT LESIONS (Fig. 12-50)

Mnemonic: "TIC MTV":
- **T**umor
- **I**nflammation
  - Osteomyelitis
  - Infectious, inflammatory, metabolic arthritis
- **C**ongenital
  - Osteogenesis imperfecta
  - TORCH infections
- **M**etabolic (usually diffuse, multifocal lesions)
  - Marrow hyperplasia
  - Paget disease
  - Fibrous dysplasia
- **T**rauma
  - Stress fracture, avulsion injuries
  - Osteonecrosis
  - Sudeck dystrophy
  - Total hip replacement
  - Child abuse
- **V**ascular
  - Sickle cell (infection versus infarction)

FOCAL COLD BONE LESIONS

Metastases most common cause (80%)
- Multiple myeloma, lymphoma
- Renal
- Thyroid
- Neuroblastoma

Primary bone lesions
- Unicameral bone cyst, ABC, EG, hemangioma

Vascular
- Infarction (acute)
- Aseptic necrosis (early)
- Radiation therapy (endarteritis obliterans)

Artifact
- Overlying pacemaker, barium, jewelry

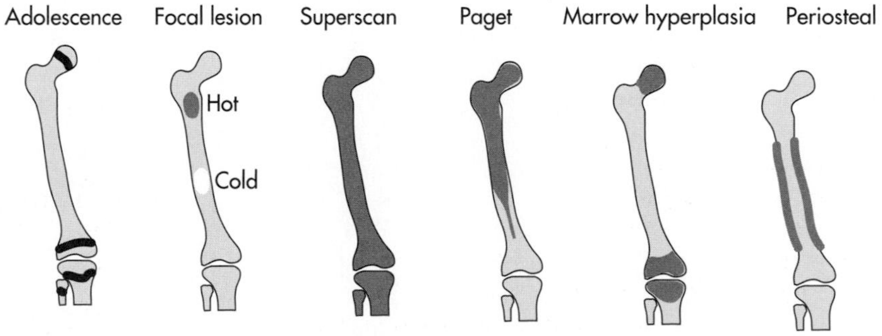

FIGURE 12-50

SUPERSCAN

Criteria: diffuse high bone uptake, diminished soft tissue and renal activity, high sternal uptake (tie sign), increased uptake at costochondral junction (beading).

Metastases (usually also causes focal abnormalities)
- Prostate metastases (most common)
- Lung cancer
- Breast cancer

Metabolic
- Hyperparathyroidism
- Renal osteodystrophy
- Osteomalacia
- Paget disease (hot and cold lesions are typically combined)

Myeloproliferative disease
- Myelofibrosis (large spleen)

DIFFUSE PERIOSTEAL UPTAKE (TRAMTRACK SIGN)

Criteria: bilateral, diffuse periosteal uptake
- Hypertrophic osteoarthropathy (lower extremity > upper extremity)
- Child abuse
- Thyroid acropachy

EXTRAOSSEOUS ACTIVITY

Normally, the kidneys and bladder are the only organs apparent on a bone scan. Causes of increased soft tissue activity:

Soft tissues
- Renal failure
- Radiotherapy ports
- Myositis
  - Myositis ossificans
  - Dermatomyositis
  - Rhabdomyolysis (e.g., ethylene glycol poisoning, alcohol)
- Tumors with calcifications

Kidney
- Focal
  - Obstruction
  - Calcifying metastases
  - Radiation to kidney
  - RCC
- Diffuse
  - Obstruction
  - Dehydration
  - Metastases
  - RCC
  - Chemotherapy
  - Thalassemia
  - Iron overload
  - Pyelonephritis
  - Amyloid

Brain
- Malignancy
- Infarct
- Meningioma

Breast
- Pregnancy, lactation
- Inflammatory breast lesions
- Steroids

Stomach, GI
- Free $^{99m}TcO_4^-$
- Hyperparathyroidism
- Bowel infarction

Liver
- Metastases
- Simultaneous/prior administration of sulfur colloid
- Diffuse hepatic necrosis
- Elevated serum aluminum levels
- Colloid formation
- Hepatoma
- Amyloidosis

Spleen
- Blood dyscrasia (sickle cell, thalassemia: increased intracellular calcium)

Chest
- Cardiac: infarction, myocarditis, pericarditis, amyloidosis
- Lung tumors
- Fibrothorax
- Pleural effusion
- Alveolar microlithiasis
- Metastatic calcification from renal dysfunction

Other
- Urine contamination

DIFFUSE BONE UPTAKE ON PET

- Chemotherapy
- Anemia
- G-CSF/EPO therapy
- Diffuse tumor infiltration

THYROID

DIFFUSELY INCREASED THYROID UPTAKE

Criteria: >30% uptake, enlarged gland, pyramidal lobe
- Graves disease (usually hyperthyroid)
- Early Hashimoto thyroiditis (usually euthyroid)
- Rare causes:
  - Iodine starvation
  - Thyroid metabolism anomalies

DIFFUSELY DECREASED THYROID UPTAKE

Criteria: nonvisualized gland or low uptake, salivary glands may show high uptake because of adjusted windowing. Causes include:

Thyroiditis
- Painful (subacute granulomatous: de Quervain disease)
- Painless (subacute lymphocytic)
- Late Hashimoto disease

Medications
- Thyroid hormone therapy
- Iodine
  - Iodinated contrast agents
  - Vitamin preparations
  - Lugol's solution
- PTU
- Tapazole

Thyroid ablation
- Surgery
- ^{131}I

HETEROGENEOUS THYROID UPTAKE

Criteria: enlarged gland (goiter), hot and cold areas
- Multinodular goiter
- Multiple autonomous nodules
- Hashimoto thyroiditis
- Cancer

Suggested Readings

Delbeke D, Martin WH, Patton JA, et al. *Practical FDG Imaging*. New York: Springer Verlag; 2002.

Habibian RM. *Nuclear Medicine Imaging: A Teaching File*. 2nd ed. Philadelphia: Lippincott Williams & Wilkins; 2008.

Harvey A, Ziessman MD, O'Malley JP, et al. *Nuclear Medicine: The Requisites*. 3rd ed. St. Louis: Mosby; 2005.

Lin E, Alvi A. *PET and PET/CT: A Clinical Guide*. 2nd ed. New York: Thieme; 2009.

Mettler F, Guiberteau M. *Essentials of Nuclear Medicine Imaging*. 5th ed. Philadelphia: WB Saunders; 2005.

Palmer E, Scott J, Strauss H. *Practical Nuclear Medicine*. Philadelphia: WB Saunders; 1992.

Van Heertum RL, Tikofsky RS. *Functional Cerebral SPECT and PET Imaging*. 3rd ed. Philadelphia: Lippincott Williams & Wilkins; 2009.

Wieler HJ, Coleman RE, eds. *PET in Clinical Oncology*. New York: Springer Verlag; 2000.

Workman RB, Coleman RE, eds. *PET/CT: Essentials for Clinical Practice*. New York: Springer; 2000.

CHAPTER 13

Contrast Agents

CHAPTER OUTLINE

X-ray Contrast Agents

GENERAL

COST OF CONTRAST AGENTS

Average Cost Estimates per Patient Dose

- Ionic iodinated IV agent: $10
- Nonionic iodinated agent: $100
- Gastrografin for CT: $1
- Barium: $10
- Gadolinium chelate for MRI: $100

IODINATED CONTRAST AGENTS

CLASSIFICATION

A variety of iodinated contrast agents have been developed and are distributed by different manufacturers. The agents all consist of iodinated benzene ring derivatives, and ionic agents are typically formulated as sodium and/or meglumine salts. Two generic classes of agents include:

- High-osmolar contrast agents (HOCAs, "ionics")
- Low-osmolar contrast agents (LOCAs, "nonionics" and "ionic-LOCAs")

Iodine Content

For nonionic agents, the iodine (I) content is easy to determine because it is written on the label. For example, Omnipaque 300 contains 300 mg I/mL of solution. For ionic agents, the I content has to be calculated because contrast concentrations are expressed

OVERVIEW OF COMMERCIAL AGENTS IN THE UNITED STATES

Manufacturer	HOCA	LOCA	Ionic LOCA
Bayer Healthcare	Urovist Angiovist	Ultravist	
Mallinckrodt	Conray Vascoray	Optiray	Hexabrix
Squibb (Bracco)	Renovue Renografin Renovist	Isovue	
GE Healthcare	Hypaque	Omnipaque Visipaque	
Guerbet		Oxilan	

on a salt weight basis. For example, Conray 60 contains 60% meglumine iothalamate = 600 mg salt/mL = 282 mg I/mL. Because meglumine and sodium have different molecular weights, a 60% (weight/volume) solution of contrast contains different amounts of I, depending on the accompanying cation:

- 60% meglumine diatrizoate: 282 mg I/mL
- 60% sodium diatrizoate: 358 mg I/mL

Meglumine versus Sodium Salts

- All HOCAs are ionic. They are organic acids consisting of an anion (radiodense iodinated benzoic acid derivative) and cation (sodium or meglumine).
- Sodium salts result in better renal opacification than meglumine salts (therefore, sodium salts are used in Urovist).

- Sodium/meglumine diatrizoate mixtures have a lower incidence of ventricular fibrillation than pure meglumine solutions.

HOCAs (Fig. 13-1)

There are 2 major ionic agents on the market, differing in the R-group:

- Diatrizoate (i.e., Hypaque)
- Iothalamate (i.e., Conray)

The osmolarity of ionic agents depends on the concentration, which typically ranges from 30% (550 mOsm/kg H_2O) to 76% (~2000 mOsm/kg H_2O). The ionic agents have been in clinical use since the 1950s.

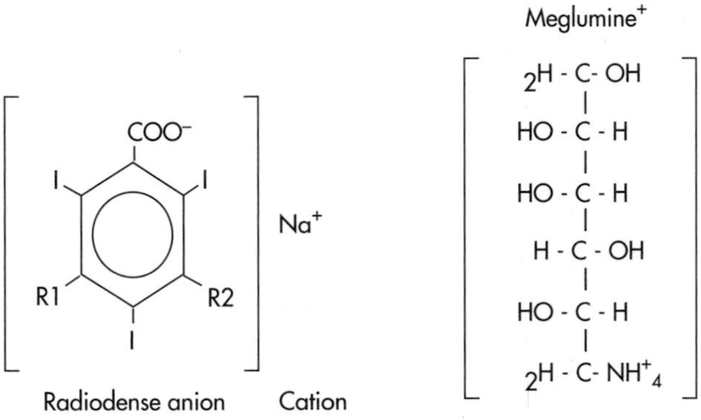

FIGURE 13-1

NONIONIC LOCAS (Fig. 13-2)

Nonionic agents have a lower incidence of adverse reactions (by a factor of 6 for all reactions and a factor of 9 for severe reactions) and are equally effective as imaging agents. They are much higher in cost when compared with HOCA. The main nonionic agents in the market are:

- Gadodiamide (Omniscan)
- Gadoteridol (ProHance)
- Iodixanol (Visipaque)
- Iopamidol (Isovue)
- Ioversol (Optiray)
- Iopromide (Ultravist)

Nonionic agents do not require an accompanying cation and therefore have lower osmolality. The osmolality depends on the concentration, which typically ranges from 300 mg I/mL (= 670 mOsm/kg H_2O) to 370 mg I/mL (= 800 mOsm/kg H_2O). Ionic agents have been in use since 1986. Iodixanol is a new nonionic dimer that is isoosmolar to blood at all concentrations.

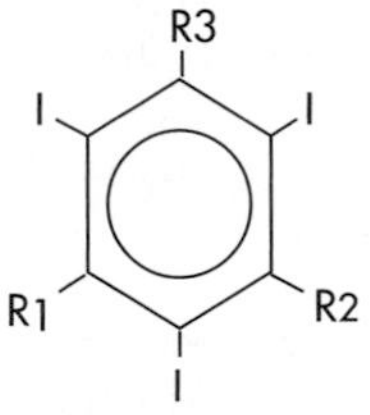

FIGURE 13-2

IONIC LOCA (Fig. 13-3)

There is only one agent on the market in the United States: ioxaglate (Hexabrix). It is a monoacid dimer that is available at a concentration of 320 mg I/mL (600 mOsm/kg H_2O).

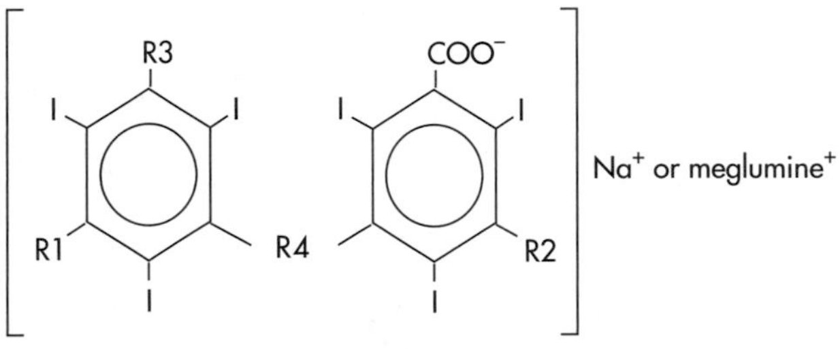

FIGURE 13-3

PHARMACOLOGY (Fig. 13-4)

Plasma levels of iodinated agents depend on:

- Rate of administration (IV bolus, IV drip)
- Blood half-life
- Distribution
  - Rapid exchange between plasma and extracellular space
  - Exclusion from intracellular space
  - Agents do not cross intact blood-brain barrier.
- Excretion
  - Glomerular filtration with no resorption in the tubules
  - Hepatic excretion (vicarious excretion) increases in renal failure.

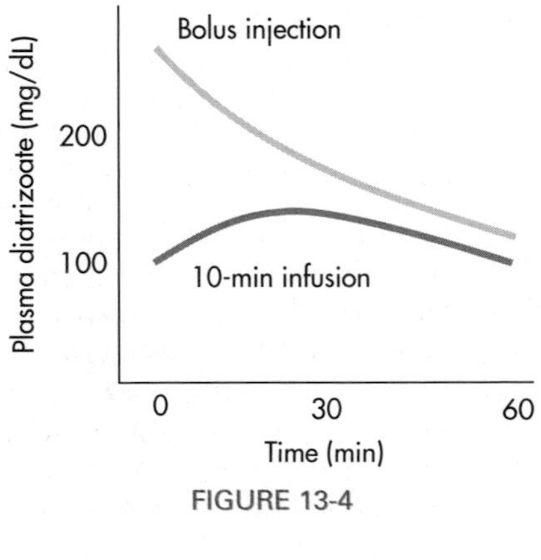

FIGURE 13-4

SIDE EFFECTS

OVERVIEW

Reaction	HOCA	LOCA
Overall	5%	1%-2%
History of allergy, asthma	10%	3%-4%
Severe reaction	0.1%	0.01%
Fatal	1/40,000-170,000	1/200,000-300,000

Types of Reactions

Not caused by iodine or related to shellfish

Idiosyncratic or anaphylactoid

- Urticaria
- Laryngospasm
- Bronchospasm
- Cardiovascular collapse

Nonidiosyncratic

- Vasovagal response
- Pain
- Renal failure
- Cardiac arrhythmias
- Seizures
- Nausea/vomiting

Delayed reactions

- 1 hour to 1 week after contrast agent administration
- Headache, myalgia, skin changes, fever
- Usually self-limiting
- In severe cases, treat with steroids
- Risk factors: prior contrast reaction, interleukin 2 treatment

Risk Factors

High-risk patients should (1) be premedicated with steroids, (2) receive nonionic agents, or (3) be evaluated by MRI/US without contrast agents. Major risk factors are:

- Allergies, asthma, atopy, 10%
- Cardiac disease, 20%
- Previous reaction to contrast agents, 25%

Other Risk Factors

- Pheochromocytoma
- Sickle cell disease
- Hyperproteinemic states (e.g., multiple myeloma)
- Other (e.g., myasthenia gravis, homocystinuria)

All patients now receive LOCAs for contrast CT examinations

Premedication

In patients with prior anaphylactoid reactions, premedication and use of a LOCA are the safest approach. There is no universally accepted premedication regimen.

- Diphenhydramine (Benadryl): 50 mg PO as needed
- Cimetidine: 300 mg PO q6 hours × 3; 1st dose night before
- Prednisone: 50 mg PO q6 hours × 3; 1st dose night before

Contrast-Induced Nephropathy

The overall incidence of contrast-induced renal failure is 0.15%. The mechanism of injury is acute tubular necrosis. Risk factors for development include:

- Creatinine >1.5 mg/dL
- Diabetes, especially insulin dependent
- Multiple myeloma
- Dehydration

Most contrast-induced nephropathies are brief and self-limited with resolution over 2 weeks. LOCA use may be justified in azotemic patients. Prophylactic oral administration of the antioxidant acetylcysteine (600 mg bid for 3 days starting the day before contrast agent administration) together with saline hydration is an effective means of preventing contrast agent—induced renal damage in patients with chronic renal insufficiency.

Breast-Feeding

Express and discard breast milk; no breast-feeding for 24 hours after contrast agent administration.

Contrast Extravasation

- Examine patient, contact referring physician
- Ice pack 3×/day
- Elevate site of injection (usually arm)
- Obtain plastic surgery consultation if:
  - >100 mL (nonionic) or >30 mL (ionic)
  - Skin blistering
  - Altered tissue perfusion/skin discoloration
  - Increased pain
  - Change in sensation distal to site of extravasation

Metformin (Glucophage)

Biguanide oral antihyperglycemic agents used to treat non-insulin-dependent diabetes mellitus (NIDDM). Lactic acidosis is a rare (0 to 0.84 case per 1000) complication with a 50% mortality rate that occurs mainly in patients with concomitant renal failure or hepatic failure. Recommendations regarding use of iodinated contrast in patients on metformin include:

Elective study

- Discontinue metformin for 48 hours before and after the contrast study; control blood glucose level.
- Before restarting metformin, reevaluate renal function.

Urgent contrast study

- Obtain a serum creatinine level. If the patient has normal renal function, the contrast study can be performed. Note that the patient should (1) be well hydrated, (2) receive nonionic agents, (3) not receive metformin for 48 hours after contrast, and (4) have serum creatinine level checked before reinstitution of metformin.

- If the patient has abnormal renal function, metformin has to be stopped for 48 hours before administration of contrast.

OTHER IODINATED AGENTS

GASTROGRAFIN

Gastrografin (Squibb; diatrizoate meglumine and diatrizoate sodium; same as Renografin 76) is an oral contrast medium for opacification of the GI tract. Undiluted or mildly diluted, Gastrografin can be used as a substitute for barium if GI perforation is suspected. A 1:40 dilution results in a CT density of 200 HU. Preparation: 0.25 ounce in 10 ounces of water; 3 cups before CT.

Complications

- Aspiration can cause chemical pneumonitis.
- Diarrhea (systemic dehydration) due to the osmotic activity of the preparation; a 1:4.6 dilution of Gastrografin in water is isotonic.
- Hypovolemic shock has been reported if Gastrografin is used undiluted in pediatric patients.

SINOGRAFIN

Diatrizoate meglumine and iodipamide meglumine 79%. Used for hysterosalpingography.

IOPANOIC ACID (TELEPAQUE)

Iopanoic acid is an oral cholecystographic agent. Oral cholecystographic agents are incompletely substituted benzene derivatives with an amide group at the 3 position to facilitate stable triiodo substitution at 2-, 4-, and 6-. Once in the plasma, these agents bind to albumin and attach to cytoplasmic anion-binding protein in hepatocytes and are excreted after glucuronic acid conjugation. Enterohepatic recirculation occurs. Optimal visualization of these agents occurs after 10 to 20 hours. Standard dose is 3 g as a starting dose for adults; if no visualization occurs after the first administration, the examination should be repeated the next day after a second 3-g dose (double-dose examination). If bilirubin is elevated, opacification of the gallbladder is usually unsuccessful.

Complications:

- Transient hyperbilirubinemia
- Nausea, vomiting, abdominal cramps, and diarrhea in up to 40%
- Renal toxicity

Contraindications:

- Hyperuricemia
- Severe liver disease
- Planned thyroid function tests

BARIUM

COMPOSITION

Micronized barium ($BaSO_4$, particle size 5 to 10 μm) is now commonly used to prepare different barium products such as:

- "Thin barium" (e.g., EZ-Jug) for upper GI studies, small bowel follow-through, barium enema: 40% w/w $BaSO_4$ solution
- "Thick barium" (e.g., EZ-HD) for double contrast studies: 85% w/w $BaSO_4$ solution
- CT barium (e.g., Readicat): 1.2% w/w $BaSO_4$ solution, 450-mL bottles

Typical additives to barium suspensions include:

- Agents to prevent flocculation (clumping)
- Antifoam agents
- Sorbitol
- Sweetening, flavoring, and coloring to improve palatability
- Preservatives: potassium sorbate and sodium benzoate
- Tannic acid, an astringent that precipitates proteins and results in improved mucosal coating; do not use in inflammatory bowel disease

COMPLICATIONS

- Exacerbation of GI obstruction above a preexisting large bowel obstruction (but not small bowel obstruction)
- Intraperitoneal extravasation through esophagus or bowel perforation results in extensive fibrosis.
- Aspiration can cause chemical pneumonitis.
- Hypersensitivity reaction may be caused by latex tip used in barium enema.

MRI Contrast Agents

CLASSES (Fig. 13-5)

There are 4 types of magnetic properties into which MRI contrast agents fall:

- Diamagnetism (generally not used for IV contrast agents)
  - Negative values of susceptibility
  - Diamagnetic materials result in small decreases in magnetization when placed in an external magnetic field.
  - Most tissues are diamagnetic and can cause imaging artifacts at tissue surfaces (e.g., air-bone).

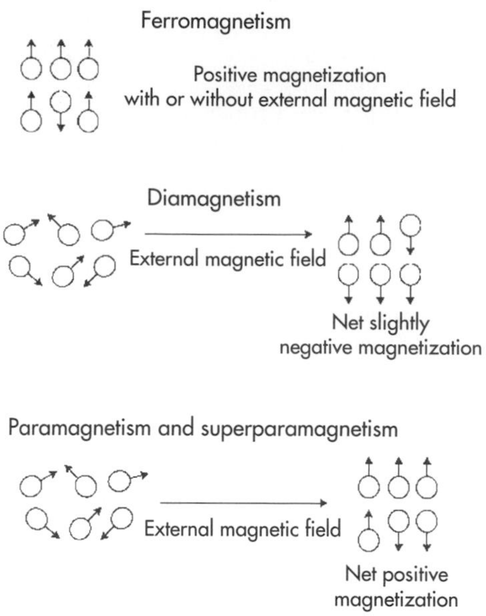

FIGURE 13-5

- Paramagnetism (Gd, Mn agents)
  - Caused by the presence of unpaired electrons in an atom/molecule
  - In the absence of an external magnetic field, the atoms/molecules are randomly aligned with no net magnetization.
  - In the presence of an external magnetic field, these atoms/molecules line up to give a net positive magnetization (positive susceptibility).
  - Much larger effect than for diamagnets, but less than for ferromagnets
  - Materials include Cr, Fe, Mn, Co, Ni, Cu, Gd, and Dy, and deoxyhemoglobin.
- Superparamagnetism (iron oxides)
  - Single domain (nanoparticle) that is not magnetic until placed in an external magnetic field
  - Unlike paramagnets, which are single molecules/atoms that result in net magnetization in an external magnetic field
  - Iron oxide nanoparticles
- Ferromagnetism (not used as IV contrast agents)
  - Strongly coupled unpaired electrons resulting in large magnetic moment and large positive susceptibility
  - Group of atoms in ferromagnetic substance is called a domain; a ferromagnet consists of a large number of domains that have a net particular orientation.
  - Can have residual magnetization even after removal from external magnetic field—permanent magnets
  - Fe, Ni, and Co

Unlike with CT contrast agents, the effect of MRI contrast agents is indirectly visualized via changes in tissue proton behavior or magnetic susceptibility (Fig. 13-6).

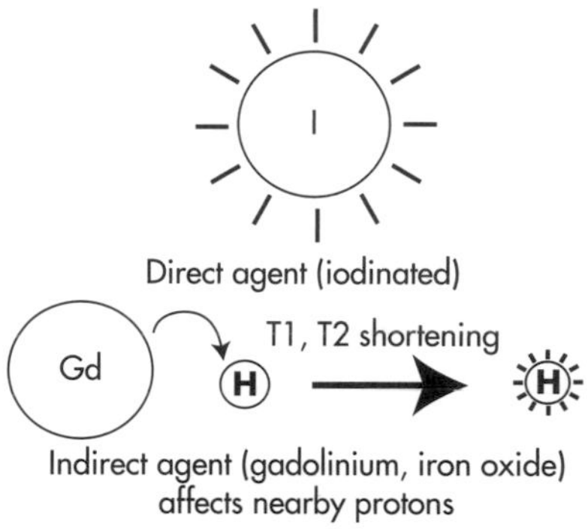

FIGURE 13-6

OVERVIEW OF IMAGING AGENTS

Short Name	Generic Name	Trade Name	Enhancement Pattern
Extracellular Fluid (ECF) Space Agents			
Gd-DTPA	Gadopentetate dimeglumine	Magnevist/ [Magnograf]	Positive
Gd-DOTA	Gadoterate meglumine	Dotarem/ [Artirem]	Positive
Gd-DTPA-BMA	Gadodiamide injection	Omniscan	Positive
Gd-HP-DO3A	Gadoteridol injection	ProHance	Positive
Gd-DTPA-BMEA	Gadoversetamide	Optimark	Positive
Gd-DO3A-butrol	Gadobutrol	Gadovist	Positive
Gd-BOPTA	Gadobenate dimeglumine	MultiHance	Positive
Targeted/Organ-Specific Agents			
Liver Agents			
Mn-DPDP	Mangafodipir trisodium	Teslascan	Positive
Gd-EOB-DTPA	Gadoxetic acid	Primovist/Eovist	Positive

OVERVIEW OF IMAGING AGENTS—cont'd

Targeted/Organ-Specific Agents			
Gd-BOPTA	Gadobenate dimeglumine	MultiHance	Positive
AMI-25*	Ferumoxides (SPIO)	Endorem/Feridex	Negative
SH U 555 A*	Ferucarbotran (SPIO)	Resovist/Cliavist	Negative
Other Targets			
Gadofluorine-M			Positive (lymph nodes)
AMI-227*	Ferumoxtran (USPIO)	Sinerem/Combidex	Negative (lymph nodes)
AMI-25*	Ferumoxides (SPIO)	Endorem/Feridex	Negative (lymph nodes)
EP-2104R*			Positive (visualization of blood clots)
Gd-DTPA mesoporphyrin (gadophrin)			Positive (myocardium, necrosis)
Blood Pool Agents			
NC-100150	PEG-feron (USPIO)	Clariscan	Positive
SH U 555 C	Ferucarbotran (USPIO)	Supravist	Positive
MS-325	Gadofosveset	Formerly, AngioMARK; Vasovist	Positive
Gadomer-17			Positive
Gadofluorine-M			Positive
P792	Macromolecular Gd-DOTA derivate	Vistarem	Positive
MnHa/PEG			
AMI-227*	Ferumoxtran (USPIO)	Sinerem/Combidex	Positive
Feraheme	Ferumoxytol	Feraheme	Positive
Gd-BOPTA	Gadobenate dimeglumine	MultiHance	Positive
Enteral Agents (Orally or Rectally Administered)			
Gd-DTPA	Gadopentetate dimeglumine	Magnevist enteral	Positive
	Ferric ammonium citrate	Ferriseltz	Positive
	Manganese chloride	LumenHance	Positive
	Manganese-loaded zeolite	Gadolite	Positive
OMP	Ferristene	Abdoscan	Negative
AMI-121*	Ferumoxsil (SPIO)	Lumirem/GastroMARK	Negative
PFOB	Perfluorooctylbromide	Imagent-GI	Negative
	Barium sulfate suspensions		Negative
	Clays		Negative
Ventilation Agents			
Perfluorinated gases			
Gadolinium-based aerosols			
Hyperpolarized gases (^{3}He, ^{129}Xe)			
Oxygen			

*Several of the above agents have been discontinued over the years and information is provided for historical purposes.

PARAMAGNETIC AGENTS

GADOLINIUM CHELATES (Fig. 13-7)

Gadolinium ion (Gd^{3+}) is a paramagnetic agent that develops a magnetic moment when placed in a magnetic field (7 unpaired electronic spins). It enhances the relaxation rates ($R1,2 = 1/T1,2$) of protons in its vicinity ($R1 > R2$). Unchelated Gd ion is toxic. The Gd is chelated to diethylenetriamine pentaacetic

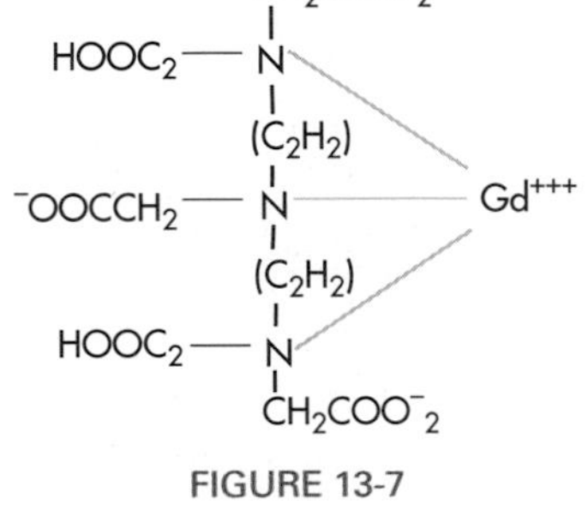

FIGURE 13-7

acid (DTPA). Magnevist (Berlex) is the commercial preparation of Gd-DTPA with meglumine to form a salt. Each milliliter of Magnevist contains 469.01 mg of Gd-DTPA dimeglumine, 0.39 mg of meglumine, 0.15 mg of DTPA, and water for injection. pH = 6.5 to 8.0. Osmolality 1.94 Osm/kg. Dosage: 0.1 mmol/kg.

Pharmacology

- Excretion
  Glomerular filtration, 95%
  Hepatobiliary excretion, 5%
- Half-life, 90 minutes
  83 ± 14% excretion in 6 hours
  91 ± 13% excretion in 24 hours
- In renal failure, there is a slower excretion of Gd-DTPA.
- Exchange between plasma and extracellular fluid space similar to that for iodinated agents

Safety

The safety index (LD_{50} divided by the diagnostic dose) is approximately 10 times higher for Gd-DTPA than for diatrizoate (10 for diatrizoate versus 100 for Gd-DTPA). Gd-related deaths are very rare but have been reported with an incidence of 1:2.5 million. The incidence of minor side effects is 1.5%, the most common ones being:

- Headache, 8%
- Injection site symptoms, 7%
- Nausea, 3%
- Allergic reactions, <0.4%
- Seizure, 0.3%

NEPHROGENIC SYSTEMIC FIBROSIS (NSF)

Rare disease involving fibrosis of skin, joints, eyes, and internal organs. <5% patients with NSF experience rapid and fulminant course that may contribute to death by affecting effective ventilation or mobility

- To date, has only occurred in patients with kidney disease
- Most cases of NSF
  - Have occurred in first 6 months after the last exposure to gadolinium; may occur later
  - Have occurred after single high doses (routine dose is 0.01 mmol/kg) of gadolinium or more commonly after repeated examinations performed in a relatively short period of time
  - Have occurred in patients with end-stage renal disease
  - Have occurred after the administration of gadodiamide (Omniscan)
- Evidence linking gadolinium contrast agents to NSF
  - The earliest cases of NSF coincided with when gadolinium-enhanced MRA was widely used
  - After warnings by the FDA, the incidence of NSF appears to have decreased
  - Most of the cases are associated with Omniscan (lower Kd compared to macrocyclic agents). Animal and cell culture studies suggest that unchelated Gd may cause NSF
- Other possible causes: NSF is also associated with hypercoagulation, recent surgery (especially vascular, including revision of an AV fistula or angioplasty), recent failed kidney transplant, sudden onset of kidney disease.
- Improving renal function can slow or arrest NSF.
- Guidelines
  - Avoid gadolinium agents (especially Omniscan) in patients with estimated GFR <30 mL/min
  - Estimated GFR = 186 × (serum creatinine)$^{-1.154}$ × (Age)$^{-0.203}$ × (0.742 if female) × (1.210 if African American)
- If necessary to use gadolinium contrast agents in these patients, use the lowest possible dose (<½ of standard dose), consider performing additional noncontrast sequences first, and reassess if contrast enhanced sequences are still necessary; hemodialysis should be performed as soon as possible, at least within 2 hours, and then 24 hours after the agent administration
- Caution in patients with GFR between 30 and 60 mL/min
- If gadolinium is administered to patients at risk:
  - Patients on hemodialysis should undergo hemodialysis no later than 2 hours after administration of Gd
  - Follow for 1 year
  - If clinical signs appear, inform FDA and all concerned regulatory bodies
  - Patients with NSF should never be reexposed to gadolinium even if renal function comes back to normal

	Estimated GFR (mL/min)				
Contrast Material	**≥ 60**	**45-59**	**30-44**	**15-29**	**<15 of dialysis**
Iodinated	Safe	Small Risk	Avoid	Avoid, but preferred over Gd if contrast is needed and patient will undergo dialysis	OK if undergoing dialysis
Gadolinium	Safe	Minimal Risk	Preferred	Avoid	Hemodialysis 2 hr and then 24 hr later

- Signs
  - Skin changes
    - Predilection for upper extremity
    - Usually spares the face
    - Begin with brawny hyperpigmentation, tethering of skin
  - Edema
  - Contractures
  - Follicular dimpling

Biochemical abnormalities have also been reported:
- Elevated serum iron levels in 30% of patients
- Elevated bilirubin levels in 3% of patients
- Pregnancy: results of clinical studies have not been reported in pregnant women. In animal studies, however, where Gd chelates have been used at many times the human dose, teratogenic effects have been described.
- Breast-feeding and gadolinium contrast agents

Less than 0.04% of the intravascular dose of gadolinium is excreted into the breast milk in the first 24 hours. Because less than 1% of the contrast medium ingested by the infant is absorbed from its gastrointestinal tract, the expected dose absorbed by the infant from the breast milk is less than 0.0004%. Therefore, the available data suggest that it is safe for the mother and infant to continue breast-feeding after receiving such an agent.

If the mother remains concerned about any potential ill effects, she should be given the opportunity to make an informed decision as to whether to continue or temporarily abstain from breast-feeding after receiving a gadolinium contrast agent. If the mother so desires, she may abstain from breast-feeding for 24 hours with active expression and discarding of breast milk from both breasts during that period. In anticipation of this, she may wish to use a breast pump to obtain milk before the contrast study to feed the infant during the 24-hour period following the examination.

MANGAFODIPIR TRISODIUM (MN-DPDP, TESLASCAN, NYCOMED)

Weak chelate of manganese dissociates into free manganese and DPDP after IV administration. Hepatocytes take up the free manganese, which acts as an intracellular paramagnetic agent and causes marked shortening of the Tl relaxation time. The free DPDP ligand is excreted in the urine. The DPDP ligand does not contribute to the imaging properties of the agent but serves to reduce the toxicity of the manganese ion. After slow intravenous infusion of mangafodipir trisodium at a dose of 5 μmol/kg, near-maximal enhancement of liver parenchyma is observed for 15 minutes to 4 hours. The increased signal intensity of normal liver parenchyma on Tl-weighted (T1W) images results in improved liver-lesion conspicuity with regard to focal hepatic lesions. Malignant and benign liver lesions of hepatocellular origin (focal nodular hyperplasia, adenoma, and well-differentiated HCC) demonstrate uptake of manganese and enhancement on delayed T1W images.

EOVIST (GADOXETATE DISODIUM; BAYER) (Fig. 13-8)

First gadolinium-based, liver-specific MRI contrast agent approved in the United States. It contains the active pharmaceutical ingredient gadoxetate disodium (Gd-EOB-DTPA). Eovist is also known as Primovist(R) and as EOB Primovist.

Indication: detection and characterization of focal liver lesions in adults.

Eovist is equally eliminated via the renal and hepatobiliary routes unlike Magnevist, which is exclusively excreted via the renal route. Because of this, one can perform the dynamic phase imaging, as is currently done with Magnevist, and also "hepatocyte phase" imaging. During this phase the normal liver parenchyma enhances uniformly. Thus the hepatic

OVERVIEW OF PROPERTIES

	Gadopentetate Dimeglumine	Gadodiamide	Gadoteridol
Trade name	Magnevist	Omniscan	ProHance
Chelator type	Linear	Linear	Macrocyclic
Molecular weight (d)	938	574	559
R1 ($mmol^{-1}sec^{-1}$)	3.8 ± 0.1	3.8 ± 0.1	3.7 ± 0.1
Osmolality (mOsm/kg)	1960	789	630
Net charge	− 2	0	0
Elimination half-life (hr)	1.6 ± 0.13	1.3 ± 0.27	1.6 ± 0.08
LD_{50} (mmol/kg)	5-12	15-34	11-14

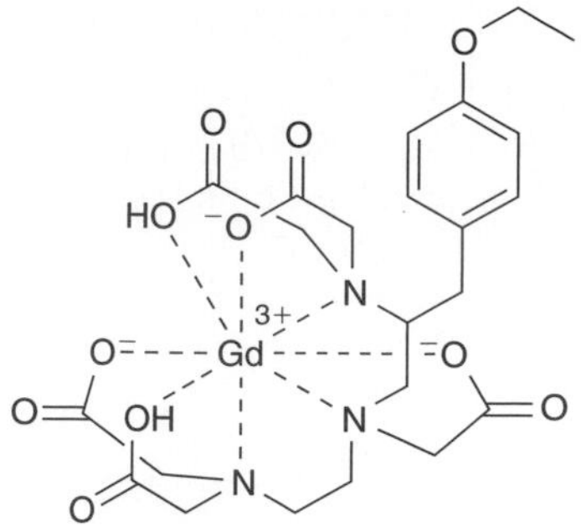

FIGURE 13-8

phase can be used for liver lesion detection (which stand out against background of enhanced normal liver parenchyma) and lesion characterization (which is done during the dynamic phase of contrast). It is not known whether Eovist is excreted in human milk. Based on pharmacokinetics of Eovist, women with normal renal function may resume nursing after 10 hours of administration.

SUPERPARAMAGNETIC AGENTS

A variety of parenteral iron oxides have been developed for contrast-enhanced MRI. Two classes of iron oxides are currently in use:

- Larger superparamagnetic iron oxides (SPIOs), for example, Ferridex (Advanced Magnetics), with a high R2 relaxivity and short blood half-life (minutes)
- Ultrasmall superparamagnetic iron oxides (USPIOs), for example, Ferumoxtran (Advanced Magnetics), with a high Rl relaxivity and long blood half-life (hours)

FERUMOXTRAN-10 (COMBIDEX) AND FERUMOXYTOL (FERAHEME)

These agents have a blood half-life of 10 to 20 hours and thereafter accumulate primarily in lymph nodes, liver, and spleen (SPIOs, on the contrary, are too rapidly cleared by liver to be able to accumulate in lymph nodes). Because these agents have a significant Rl effect, they can also be used as Tl-type blood pool ("brightening") agents for imaging of tumor angiogenesis, MRA, and/or hepatic lesion characterization during the equilibrium phase. Perfused lesions (e.g., hemangioma) increase in signal intensity on T1W, whereas the same lesion decreases in signal intensity on T2W.

Ferumoxtran-10 has been used in clinical trials for lymph node imaging. After intravenous administration, ferumoxtran-10 extravasates slowly from the vascular into the interstitial space and is then transported to lymph nodes through lymphatic vessels. Once within the nodes, these nanoparticles bind to macrophages, producing a decrease in signal intensity (SI) on T2W and T2*W. The degree of signal intensity reduction is dependent on the dose of ferumoxtran-10 and the pulse sequence used for MRI. The recommended optimal dose at this time is 2.6 mg Fe/kg, and the most appropriate pulse sequence for evaluation of signal loss is the gradient-echo (GRE) T2*W sequence. This sequence is more sensitive to the magnetic susceptibility effects of ferumoxtran-10. If part of or the entire node is infiltrated with tumor, there is lack of ferumoxtran-10 uptake, and these areas continue to retain their high signal intensity after administration of the contrast. The spectrum of nodal enhancement patterns after ferumoxtran-10 administration depends on the nodal rumor burden ranging from homogeneous darkening to a complete lack of ferumoxtran-10 uptake.

Ferumoxytol has been FDA approved for iron replacement therapy and is in phase II clinical trial for use in MR angiography.

Treatment of Contrast Reactions

TREATING ADVERSE REACTIONS

TREATING ADVERSE REACTIONS

Clinical Indication	Medication	Dosage*	Comments
Urticaria	Diphenhydramine or hydroxyzine	25-50 mg IV/IM 25-50 mg IM	Treat if symptomatic or progressive
Facial/laryngeal edema	Diphenhydramine or hydroxyzine	25-50 mg IV/IM 25-50 mg IM	Protect the airway, oxygen
	Epinephrine	0.3-0.5 mL SC 1:1000 dilution 1-3 mL slow IV 1:10,000 dilution	Epinephrine may precipitate ischemia in coronary artery disease

TREATING ADVERSE REACTIONS—cont'd

Clinical Indication	Medication	Dosage*	Comments
Bronchospasm	β_2 Agonists	Nebulizer or MDI	Metaproterenol, albuterol
	Epinephrine	0.1-0.3 mg SC (1:1000)	
	Aminophylline	6 mg/kg IV over 20 min	If epinephrine fails
Vasovagal	Isotonic saline	250-500 mL IV	Elevate legs
	Atropine	0.5 mg IV	Up to 3 mg total

*See manufacturer's packet insert for specific rates of administration. Always monitor vital signs and give O_2.
IM, intramuscular; IV, intravenous; SC, subcutaneous.

EMERGENCY TREATMENT

Consult current ACLS guidelines for up-to-date management and drug regimen.

EMERGENCY TREATMENT

Clinical Indication	Medication	Dosage	Comments
Bradycardia	Atropine	0.5 mg IV q5 min up to 3 mg	Doses <0.5 mg may cause paradoxical bradycardia
Ventricular tachyarrhythmia	Cardioversion/ defibrillation/ epinephrine	1-mg bolus IV	
	Lidocaine	1 mg/kg IV bolus	
	Amiodarone	300 mg IV	Give only once
Supraventricular tachycardia	Adenosine	6 mg IV bolus	If fails, give 12 mg IV bolus
	Verapamil	0.1 mg/kg IV slowly (maximum of 10 mg)	Contraindicated with beta blockers
Angina	Nitroglycerin	0.3-0.4 mg SL q5 min; 10-20 mg orally	Obtain ECG and monitor BP
Hypertension	Patient's own HLN meds	1-2 inches q4 hr	Administer oxygen; nifedipine no longer favored
	Nitroglycerin ointment 2%		30 min to see effect
Pheochromocytoma-induced hypertension	Phentolamine	1 mg IV test dose; 5 mg IV as needed	
Hypotension (unresponsive to fluid challenge)	Dopamine	2-5 μg/kg/min (via central venous access)	Significant renal, peripheral, and mesenteric vasoconstriction occurs above 10 mg/kg/min
Seizures	Diazepam	5-10 mg IVP	Lasts 20 minutes
	Phenytoin	18 mg/kg IV at 50 mg/min	ECG monitoring

CHAPTER
14

Imaging Physics

CHAPTER OUTLINE

X-ray Physics

PRODUCTION OF X-RAYS

X-RAY TUBE (Fig 14-1)

An x-ray tube is an energy converter receiving electrical energy and producing heat and x-rays. For a diagnostic x-ray tube operating at 100 kVp, the production of heat and x-rays is:

- Heat, 99%
- X-rays, 1%
  - Electron deceleration (Bremsstrahlung), 0.9%
  - Characteristic radiation through ionization, 0.1%

X-ray tubes are designed to minimize heat production and maximize x-ray output. Tubes consist of 2 main elements: a cathode (for electron production) and an anode (for conversion electron energy into x-rays). During the process of x-ray generation, x-ray beams are generated in all directions; however, the useful beam is composed only of those x-rays leaving the lead-shielded tube. All electrical components in an x-ray tube are in a vacuum. The vacuum prevents dispersion of the electrons and ionization, which could damage the filament.

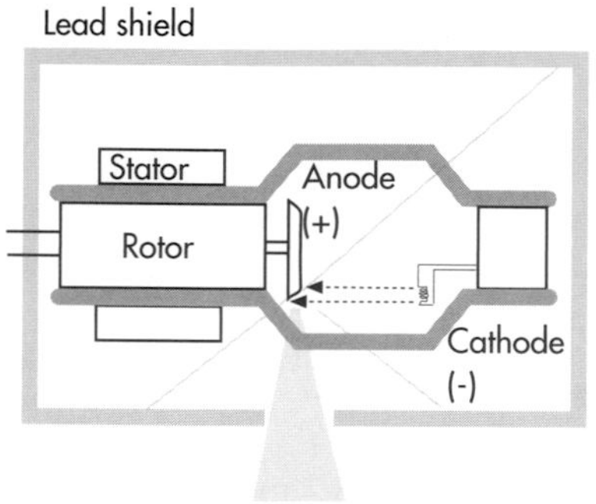

FIGURE 14-1

Cathode

Cathodes produce the electrons necessary for x-ray generation. Cathodes typically consist of a tungsten filament that is heated >2200°C. The filament is surrounded at its cathode end by a negatively charged focusing cup to direct the electrons in a small beam toward the anode.

Anode

The anode has 2 functions: to convert electron energy into x-rays and to dissipate heat. Heat dissipation is achieved by rotating the angulated target (at approximately 3600 rpm, or 60 cycles/sec). The amount of x-rays produced depends on the atomic number (Z) of the anode material and the energy of electrons. Common anode materials include tungsten (W, Z = 74) and W/rhenium (Re) alloys (90%/10%). These materials are used because of their high melting point and the high yield of x-rays. Mammography units frequently use different anode materials (e.g., molybdenum [Mo]).

The focal spot is the small area on the anode in which x-rays are produced. The size of the focal spot is determined by the dimensions of the electron beam and the anode angulation. Typical angles are 12° to 20°; however, smaller angles (6°) are used for neuroangiography. Tubes with smaller focal spot size are used when high image quality is essential.

X-RAY TUBE OUTPUT (Fig. 14-2)

Exposure delivered by an x-ray generator is controlled by selecting appropriate values for mA, kVp, and exposure time. The output of an x-ray tube increases:

- Linearly with mA
- Linearly with Z (number of protons) of the target element
- As the square of kVp

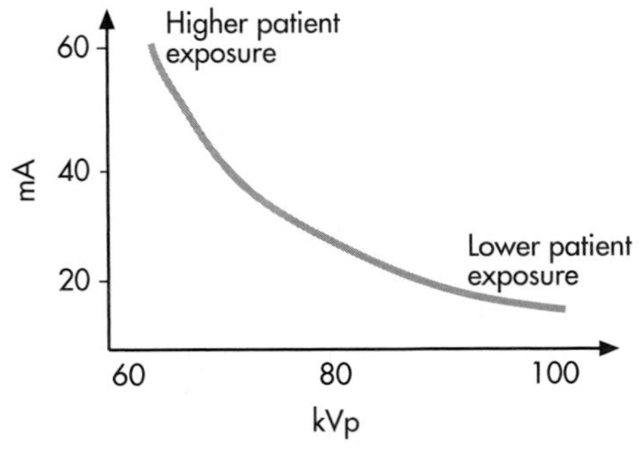

FIGURE 14-2

Milliampere

A milliampere (mA) is a measure of current referring to the number of electrons flowing per second (1 A corresponds to 6.25×10^{18} electrons). The higher the mA, the higher the electron flux and the higher the x-ray production. An increase in mA changes only the amount of x-rays (i.e., the intensity or exposure rate), not the maximum energy of the x-rays produced. Typical mA values range from 25 to 500 on a given x-ray unit. The use of small focal spot sizes (for high resolution) also limits the number of mAs that can be used. General rules for selecting mA include:

- Use lower mA for smaller focal spots when image detail is important.
- Select high mA to reduce exposure time (i.e., to limit motion blurring).
- Select high mA and reduced kVp when high image contrast is desired.

Voltage

The voltage of an x-ray tube is measured in kVp (peak kilovolts). The kVp determines the maximum energy of the x-rays produced. 100 kVp means that the maximum (peak) voltage across the tube causing electron acceleration is 100,000 V. The term keV (kiloelectron volt) refers to the energy of any individual electron in the beam. When an x-ray tube is operated at 100 kVp, only a few electrons will acquire kinetic energy of 100 keV because the applied voltage usually pulsates between lower values and the maximum (peak) selected. The mean energy of an x-ray beam is approximately one third of its peak energy. For 100 kVp, the mean energy would be 33 to 40 keV. An increase in kVp translates into:

- Increased photon frequency
- Increased photon penetration
- Shortening of photon wavelength
- Increased anode heat production
- Decreased skin dose
- Decreased contrast

Film exposure is more sensitive to changes in kVp than to changes in mA or exposure time. General rules for selecting kVp include:

- A 15% increase in kVp doubles exposure at the recording system (e.g., film) and has the same effect on film density as a 100% increase in mA.
- An increase in kVp of 15% will decrease the contrast, so that doubling of mA is usually preferred.
- mA generally needs to be at least doubled when changing from a nongrid to a grid technique (depending on field size and patient thickness).

Exposure Time

Exposure times are set either by the operator (setting of a timer) or by a circuit that terminates the exposure after a selected amount of x-rays have reached the patient. General rules for selecting exposure time include:

- Short exposure time minimizes blurring.
- Long exposure times can be used to reduce either mA or kVp when motion is not a problem.

HEAT UNIT (Fig. 14-3)

Heat is the factor that limits the uninterrupted use of x-ray generators. Heat units (HU) are calculated as:

$$HU = \text{Voltage (kVp)} \times \text{Current (mA)} \times \text{Time (sec)}$$

This formula holds true only for single-phase generators. For 3-phase generators, the HU has to be multiplied by 1.35.

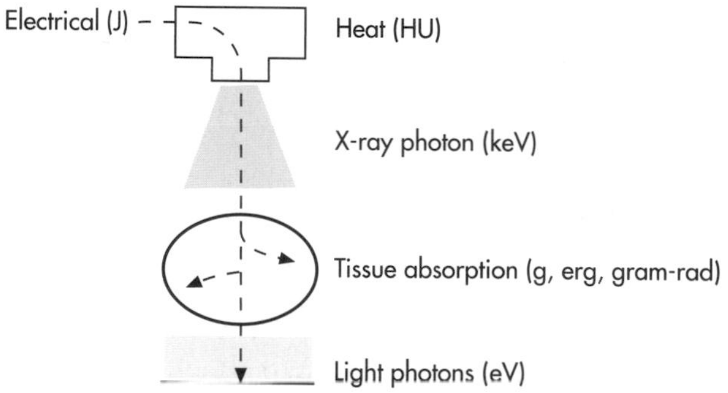

FIGURE 14-3

RATING CHARTS (Fig. 14-4)

The safe limit within which an x-ray tube can be operated for a single exposure can be determined by the tube rating chart. Always convert mA into mA and time before reading the charts.

Example

What is the maximum safe kVp for a 500-mA exposure at 0.1 sec?

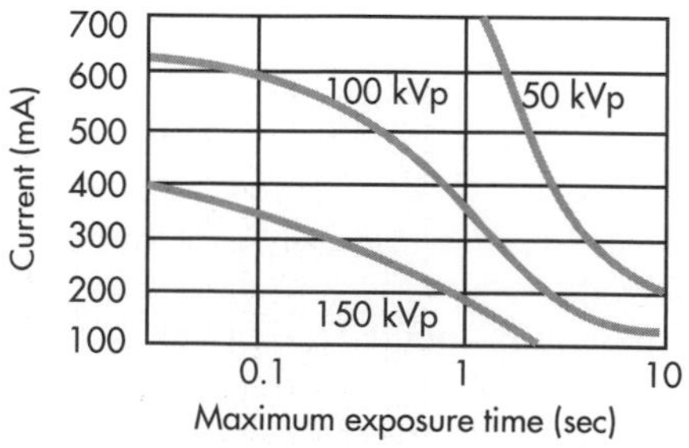

FIGURE 14-4

Answer

Approximately 100 kVp (see chart).

FOCAL SPOT

The focal spot (FS) is the small area on the anode in which x-rays are produced. NEMA specifications require that focal spots of <0.3 mm have to be measured with the line pair resolution test (star pattern) and that larger focal spots can be measured with a pinhole camera. The apparent focal spot increases with:

- Increase in mA ("blooming effect")
- Increase in target angle
- Decrease in kVp

FOCAL SPOT SIZES

FS (mm)	Application
0.1	Magnification x-ray
0.3*	Mammography
0.6	Typical small FS size
1.2	Typical large FS size
1.7 × 2.4	Maximum size of 1.2-mm FS by NEMA standards

* NEMA standards allow a 0.3-mm FS to have a tolerance of -0% and +50% (i.e., a maximum of 0.45 mm).

FOCAL SPOT AND RESOLUTION

Resolution is related to the size of the FS, the FS-object distance (FOD), and the object-detector distance (ODD):

$$\text{Resolution (lines/mm)} = \frac{1.1\text{FOD}}{\text{FS (mm)} \times \text{ODD}}$$

From this equation it is evident that:

- The smaller the FS, the better the resolution.
- The shorter the ODD, the better the resolution.
- The longer the FOD distance, the better the resolution.

MEASUREMENT OF FOCAL SPOT SIZE

Two methods are used to determine the FS size: pinhole method (determines the actual FS size) and star test pattern (determines effective blur size).

Pinhole Method

A pinhole is placed halfway between the FS and the film. The image of the FS on the exposed film will be the same size as the actual physical dimension of the FS.

Pinholes are usually 0.03 mm in diameter.

Star Test Pattern

A star test pattern is positioned midway between FS and film. An image is then obtained in which there is a zone of blurring at some distance from the center of the object. The FS is calculated as:

$$FS = \frac{(\delta \times D \times \pi)}{(180\,(M-1))}$$

where δ = angle of one test pattern segment, D = diameter of the blur circle, and M = magnification factor.

MAGNIFICATION (Fig. 14-5)

The true magnification (M) for a point source is:

$$M = \text{Focus} - \frac{\text{Film distance } (a + b)}{\text{Focus object distance } (a)}$$

In the figure on the right, the magnification would be 36 + 4/36 = 1.11 (equivalent to 11% magnification). However, because FSs are not true point sources, the real magnification of images (including penumbra) depends on the size of the FS and is given by:

$$M = m + (m-1)(f/d)$$

where m = geometric magnification (a + b)/a, f = FS size, and d = object size. For this example, the true magnification would thus be:

M = 1/11 + (1.11 − 1)(0.6/0.2) = 1.44 (equivalent to 44% magnification)

Penumbra: zone of geometric unsharpness (edge gradient) that surrounds the umbra (complete shadow).

Unsharpness

Unsharpness = FS size × (Magnification −1)

Geometric unsharpness is highest with:

- Large FS
- Short focus object distance

Other sources of unsharpness are:

- Intensifying screen (i.e., slow single-screen films)
- Motion

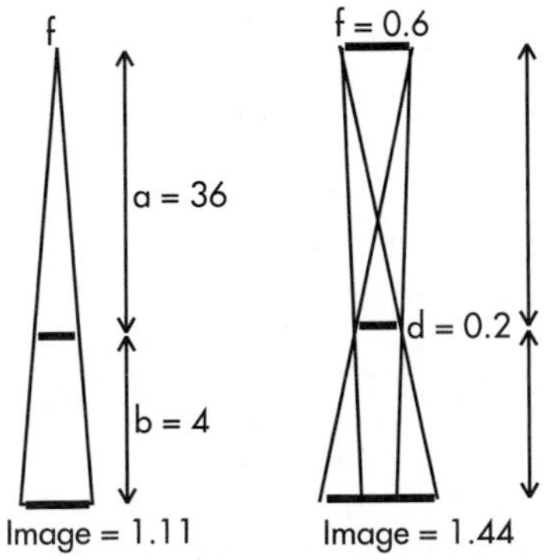

FIGURE 14-5

RADIATION EXPOSURE AND DISTANCE

X-ray exposure to a patient increases as the square of the focus-film distance.

Example

What is the increase in exposure when the focus-film distance is changed from 50 to 75 cm?

Answer

$Exposure_{new}/Exposure_{old} = (Distance_{new}/Distance_{old})^2 = (75/50)^2 = 2.25$-fold increase.

SPECTRUM OF X-RAYS

X-rays are generated by 2 different processes:

- Bremsstrahlung: produces a continuum of photon energy radiation
- Characteristic radiation: produces defined peaks of photon energy

Bremsstrahlung (Fig. 14-6)

Bremsstrahlung refers to the process by which electrons, when slowed down near the nucleus of a target, give off a photon of radiation. The energy of a photon (E) is inversely proportional to its wavelength:

$$E\,(\text{in keV}) = \frac{12.4}{\text{Wavelength (Å)}}$$

For 100 kVp, the maximum energy of an electron would be 100 keV, and its minimum wavelength would therefore be 12.4/100 keV = 0.124 Å. The maximum wavelength of a photon is open ended and only determined by the absorption through glass or filters.

Characteristic Radiation (Fig. 14-7)

Characteristic radiation results when bombarding electrons eject a target electron from the inner orbits of a specific target atom. Characteristic energies from a tungsten target are:

- α_1 peak: 59.3 keV (L shell to K shell)
- α_2 peak: 57.9 keV (L shell to K shell)
- α_1 peak: 67.2 keV (M shell to K shell)
- α_2 peak: 69 keV (N shell to K shell)

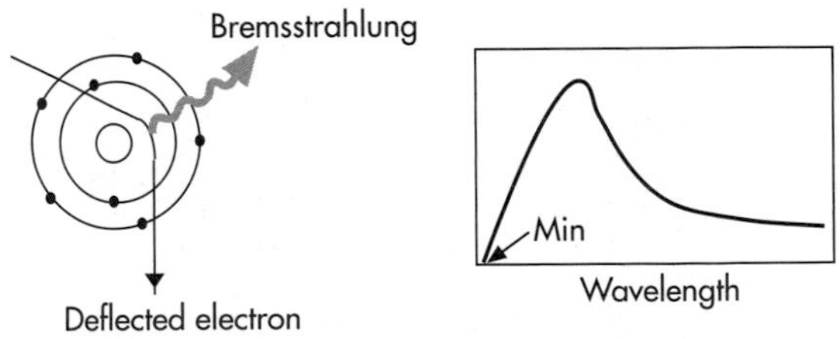

FIGURE 14-6

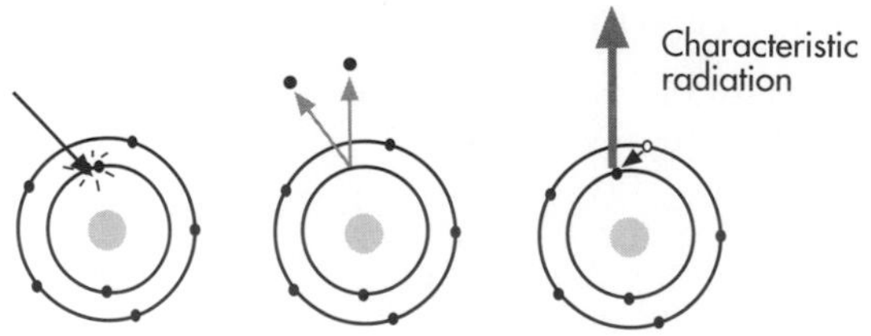

The higher the atomic number of the target atom, the greater the efficiency of x-ray production. The fraction of energy (f) released as x-rays by electrons of energy (E) in a material with atomic number (Z) is given by:

$$f = \frac{Z \times E\ (\text{meV})}{800}$$

For example, in an x-ray tube with a W target (Z = 74) and 100 keV, only 0.92% of total energy is converted into x-rays.

HEEL EFFECT (Fig. 14-8)

The intensity of an x-ray beam that leaves the tube is not uniform across all portions of the beam (heel effect): the intensity on the anode side is always considerably less and is close to zero for x-rays emitted along the inclined surface of the anode (cutoff). Implications of heel effect include:

- Thicker parts of the patient should be placed toward the cathode side of the tube.
- Heel effect is less when large distances are used (see figure).
- Heel effect is less pronounced if smaller films are used.

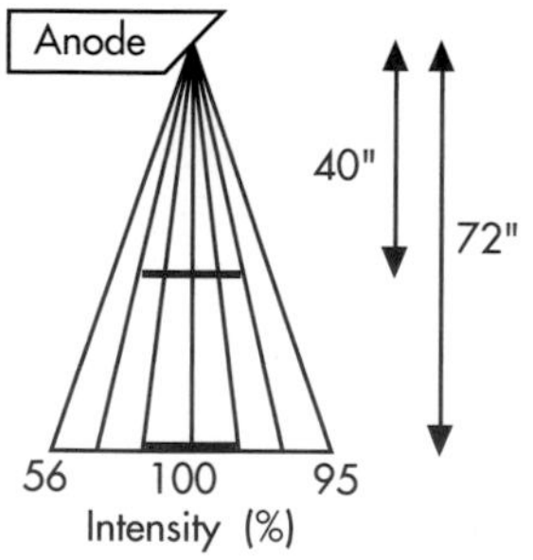

FIGURE 14-8

X-RAY GENERATORS

TRANSFORMER (Fig. 14-9)

A transformer consists of two wire coils wound around an iron ring. When current flows through the primary coil, a magnetic field is created within the

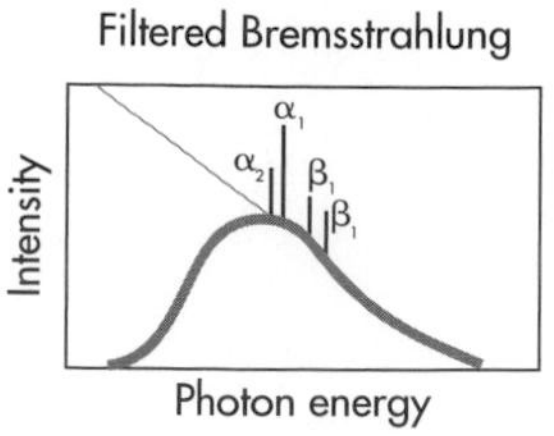

FIGURE 14-7

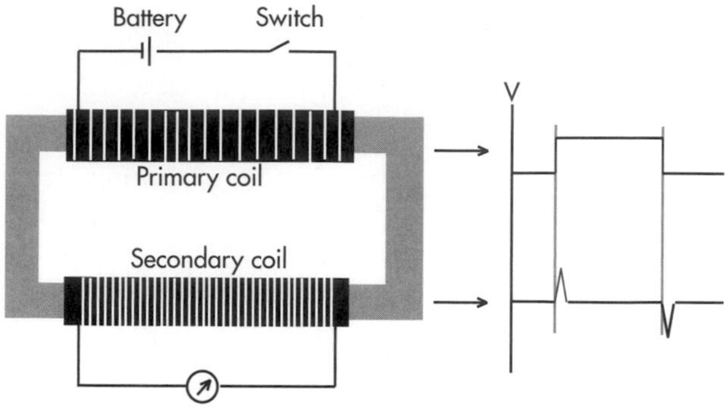

FIGURE 14-9

iron ring. The magnetic field will then create a momentary current in the secondary coil. Current flows through the secondary coil only when the magnetic field is changing (i.e., when it is switched either on or off). For this reason, direct current (DC) cannot be used in the primary coil to create a steady current in the secondary coil. Rather, an alternating current (AC) has to be used in the primary coil. The voltage (V) in the two circuits is proportional to the number of turns (N) in the two coils:

$$N_{primary} / N_{secondary} = V_{primary} / V_{secondary}$$

A transformer with more windings in the primary than in the secondary coil is called a *step-down transformer,* and a transformer with more windings in the secondary coil is called a *step-up transformer.* The product of the voltage (V) and current (I) (which is power [W]: W = V × I) is always equal in both circuits:

$$V_{primary} \times I_{primary} = V_{secondary} \times I_{secondary}$$

CIRCUITS OF X-RAY GENERATORS (Fig. 14-10)

X-ray units have two principal circuits: a high-voltage circuit (consisting of autotransformer, timer, and high-voltage transformer) and a low-voltage filament circuit.

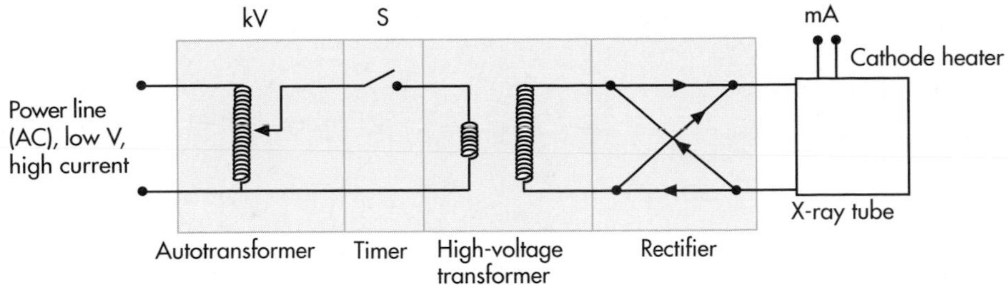

FIGURE 14-10

Autotransformer

This transformer is the kVp selector. The voltage across the primary coil can be varied by changing the number of coils in the autotransformer.

High-Voltage Transformer

This transformer is a step-up transformer, increasing the voltage by a factor of about 600 by having about 600 times more windings in the secondary than in the primary coil. Because the potential of the step-up transformer is up to 150,000 V, the whole transformer is immersed in oil.

Timer

Controls the exposure time.

Rectifier (Fig. 14-11)

The function of the rectifier is to change AC into DC flowing in only one direction at all times. Modern rectifiers use full-wave rectification requiring four rectifiers.

Filament Circuit

Consists of a step-down transformer used to produce approximately 10 V and 3 to 5 Å to heat the x-ray tube filament. The amount of current is controlled by a resistor. The more current, the hotter the filament, and the more electrons are emitted.

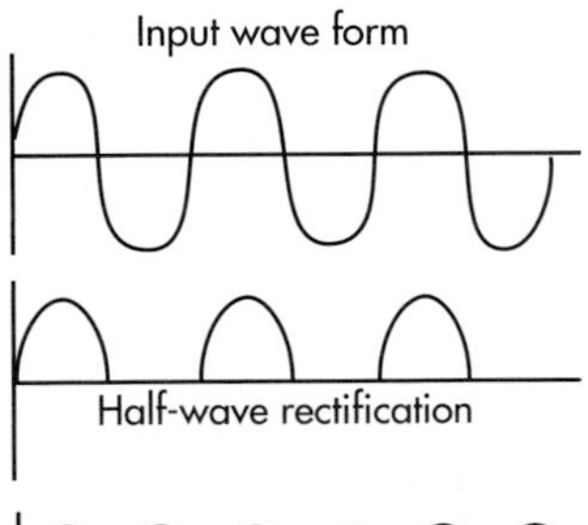

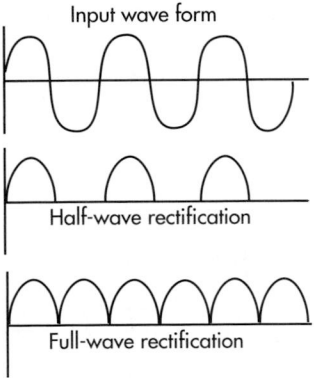

FIGURE 14-11

TYPES OF GENERATORS

Three-Phase Generators (Fig. 14-12)

Three-phase generators produce an almost constant potential difference across an x-ray tube. The three phases lag behind each other by 120°, so there are no deep valleys between the peaks. Ripple refers to the fluctuations of the voltage across the x-ray tube (expressed as a percentage of maximum value). The theoretic ripple factor is:

- Single-phase generator: 100%
- 6-pulse, 3-phase generator: 13%
- 12-pulse, 3-phase generator: 3%

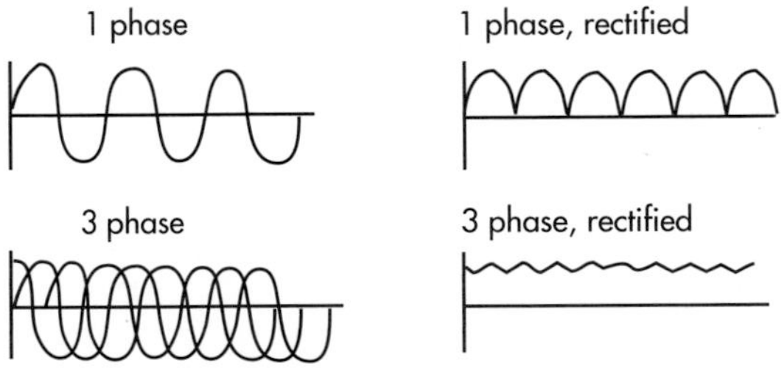

FIGURE 14-12

ADVANTAGES OF 3-PHASE GENERATORS

- Higher average beam energy, less exposure for patient because unnecessary low-level radiation is reduced (higher average dose rate per time unit)
- Shorter exposure time
- Higher tube rating

Mobile Generators (Fig. 14-13)

Most portable x-ray machines are battery powered, whereas others operate directly from a single-phase 60-Hz power outlet. The DC supply in battery-powered units is converted to AC with 60-Hz or higher kilohertz frequency. The high voltage is generated by the usual transformer-rectifier system. A capacitor discharge system is sometimes used for x-ray tube operation.

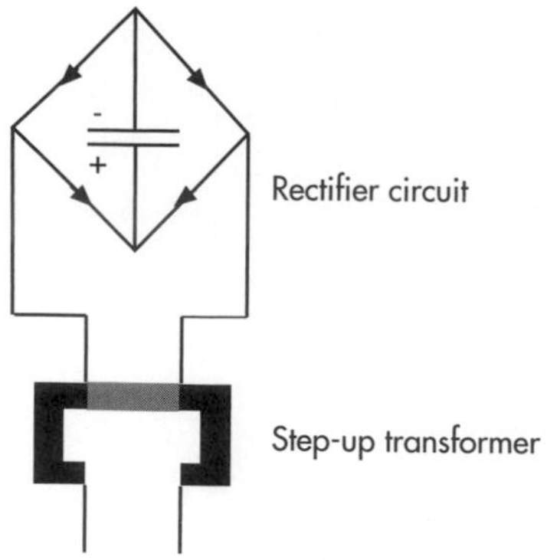

FIGURE 14-13

Capacitor Discharge Generators

The capacitor stores the electrical charge received through rectifiers from a step-up transformer. When a certain potential is achieved, the capacitor is discharged through an x-ray tube. During this discharge both the tube kV and the tube mA fall exponentially.

PHOTOTIMERS

Phototimers are used to terminate unnecessary x-ray generation after optimum exposure has been achieved. In older equipment, photomultiplier tubes were located behind the cassette. Modern x-ray equipment uses radiolucent ionization chambers placed in front of the cassette. Ionization chambers are frequently used in triplets to sample several areas of the radiographic field. A detector then averages the recorded exposure from the three chambers.

INTERACTION BETWEEN X-RAYS AND MATTER

There are five basic ways in which an x-ray or a gamma ray interacts with matter:
- Coherent scattering
- Photoelectric effect
- Compton scattering
- Pair production
- Photodisintegration

COHERENT SCATTERING (Fig. 14-14)

Coherent scattering refers to radiation that undergoes a change in direction without a change in wavelength. It is the only type of interaction that does not cause ionization. Coherent scattering usually represents less than 5% of x-ray matter interaction and does not play a major role in radiology.

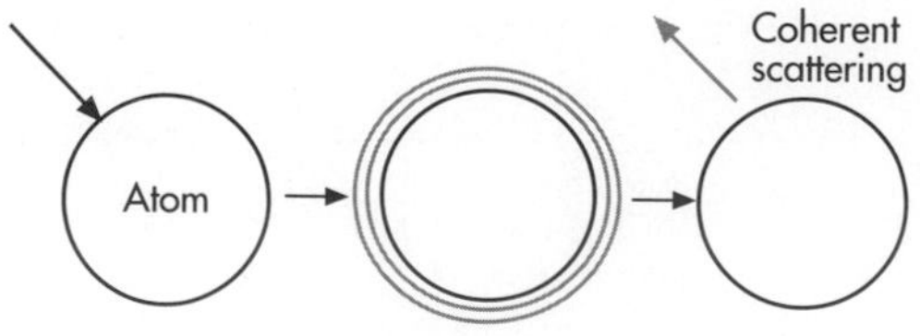

FIGURE 14-14

PHOTOELECTRIC EFFECT (Fig. 14-15)

An incident photon ejects an electron from its orbit. An electron from an outer shell then fills the gap in the K-shell, and characteristic radiation (with wavelength specific for that element) is emitted. For x-ray emission to occur, the orbit must usually be in the K-shell. The end result of the photoelectric effect is:
- Characteristic radiation
- A photoelectron
- A positively charged ion

The probability of the photoelectric effect's occurrence depends on the following:
- The incident photon must have sufficient energy to overcome the binding energy of the electron.
- A photoelectric effect is most likely to occur when the photon energy and electron binding energy are similar.
- The more tightly an electron is bound in its orbit, the more likely it is to be involved in a photoelectric reaction. Electrons are more tightly bound in elements with high atomic numbers.

ELECTRON-BINDING ENERGY

Atomic Number	Atom	K-shell Binding Energy (keV)
6	Carbon	0.28
8	Oxygen	0.53
20	Calcium	4
53	Iodine	33.2
82	Lead	88

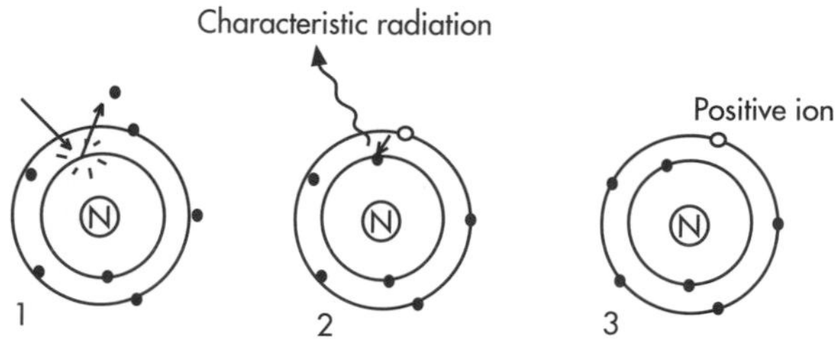

FIGURE 14-15

The statistical probability of the photoelectric effect (PE) occurring per unit mass of a given element is proportional to the atomic number (Z) and inversely proportional to the energy (E) of the x-ray:

$$PE \approx \frac{Z^3}{E^3}$$

Pearls

- More tightly bound electrons are more likely to interact in the photoelectric effect (K > L > M).
- Electrons in the K-shell are at a higher energy level than electrons in the L-shell.
- Characteristic radiation is produced by the photoelectric effect by exactly the same process as discussed in the section on production of x-rays; the only difference is the method of ejecting the inner shell electron.
- Advantages of photoelectric effect:
  - Does not produce scatter radiation
  - Enhances natural tissue contrast by magnifying the difference between tissues composed of different elements
- Disadvantage of photoelectric effect:
  - Patients receive more radiation from each photoelectric reaction than from any other type of interaction.
- If lead (K-shell binding energy of 88 keV) is irradiated with 1-MeV photons, the emitted photoelectrons will have a minimum energy of 912 keV.

COMPTON SCATTERING (Fig. 14-16)

A photon is deflected by an electron so that it assumes a new direction as scattered radiation. The initial photon always retains part of its original energy. Note that the recoil electron is always directed forward, but scatter of x-rays may occur in any direction. Two factors determine the amount of energy that the photon retains:

- Its initial energy
- Angle of deflection from the original photon direction

Calculation of the change in wavelength of a scattered photon:

Δ wavelength = 0.024 (1 − cos angle of deflection)

The maximum energy of a Compton electron in keV is given by:

$$E_{max} = E_{incident} \times \frac{2a}{(1 + 2a)}$$

$$\text{where } a = \frac{E_{incident}}{511\ KeV}.$$

At very high energies (e.g., 1 MeV), most photons are scattered in a forward direction. With lower-energy radiation, fewer photons scatter forward and more scatter at an angle greater than 90°. Therefore, the distribution of scattered photons (e.g., 100 keV) assumes a probability curve as shown in the diagram (gray shading) (Fig. 14-17).

Probability of Compton Scatter

- The higher the atomic number, the higher the probability of Compton scatter per atom.
- The probability relative to the photoelectric effect increases with increasing energy.
- The probability increases with electron density (electrons/cm^3).
- The probability increases with field size and patient thickness.
- The probability does not depend on mA or FS size.

Pearls

- Almost all the scatter in diagnostic radiology is a result of Compton scatter.
- Scatter radiation from Compton reactions is a major safety hazard: a photon that is deflected 90° still retains most of its original energy in the diagnostic range.

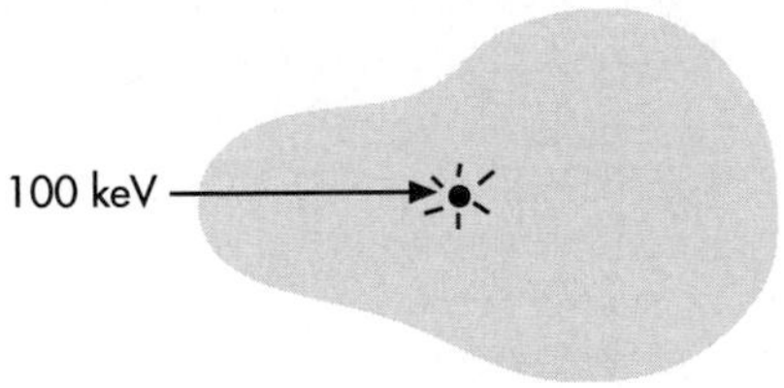

FIGURE 14-17

FIGURE 14-16

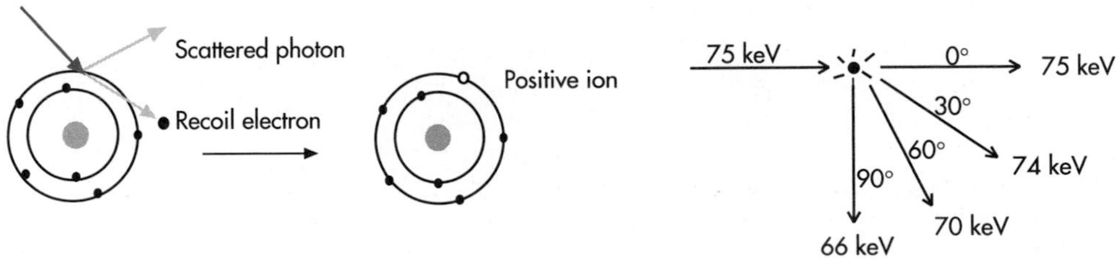

OTHER TYPES OF INTERACTIONS

Pair Production

Occurs only with photons whose energy is >1.02 MeV. The photon interacts with the electric field around the nucleus, and its energy is converted into one electron and one positron. Pair production is the dominant mode of interaction of radiation with tissue >10 MeV.

Photodisintegration

Occurs only with photons whose energy is >7 MeV. In photodisintegration, part of the nucleus is ejected. The ejected portion may be a neutron, a proton, an alpha particle, or a cluster of particles.

COMPARISON OF INTERACTION (Fig. 14-18)

- Only two interactions are important to diagnostic radiology: Compton scatter and the photoelectric effect. Compton scattering is the dominant interaction except at very low energies (20 to 30 keV).

Pearls

- High keV (chest films): Compton effect predominates (determined by electron density), lower bone contrast
- Low keV (mammography): photoelectric effect predominates (determined by Z^3 and E^{-3}), high calcification contrast
- Iodine contrast material: photoelectric effect predominates for photons of energy >33.2 keV

ATTENUATION

Attenuation refers to the reduction in intensity of an x-ray beam as it traverses matter, either by absorption or by deflection. The amount of attenuation depends on:

- Energy of the beam (high energy beams have increased transmission)
- Characteristics of absorber (high Z number material results in decreased transmission)
  - Atomic number (the higher the number, the larger the percentage of photoelectric absorption)
  - Density of absorber
  - Electrons per gram (6×10^{23} × atomic number/atomic weight). The number of electrons per gram of substance is almost the same for all materials except hydrogen (which is approximately twice that of other elements).

ATTENUATION COEFFICIENTS

Linear Attenuation Coefficient (cm^{-1})

This coefficient represents the actual fraction of photons interacting per unit thickness of an absorber and is expressed as the fraction of attenuated photons per centimeter.

Mass Attenuation Coefficient

This coefficient equals the linear attenuation coefficient but is scaled per gram of tissue (cm^2/g) to reflect the attenuation of materials independent of their physical state. For example, the mass attenuation coefficient of ice, water, and vapor is the same, whereas the linear attenuation coefficient is not.

DENSITY

Material	Effective Atomic Number (Z)	Density (g/cm^3)
Water	7.41	1.0
Muscle	7.5	1.0
Fat	5.9	0.9
Air	7.6	0.00129
Calcium	20.0	1.5
Iodine	53.0	4.9
Barium	56.0	3.5

MONOCHROMATIC RADIATION

Monochromatic means that all photons have exactly the same energy (i.e., wavelength). The attenuation of monochromatic radiation is exponential:

$$N = N_o \times e^{-\mu x}$$

where N = number of transmitted photons, N_o = number of incident photons, μ = linear attenuation coefficient, and x = absorber thickness (cm). The linear absorption coefficient is the fractional rate of photon removal from a beam per centimeter of absorber (e.g., $\mu = 0.1\,cm^{-1}$ means 10% absorption per centimeter). The half-value layer (HVL) refers to

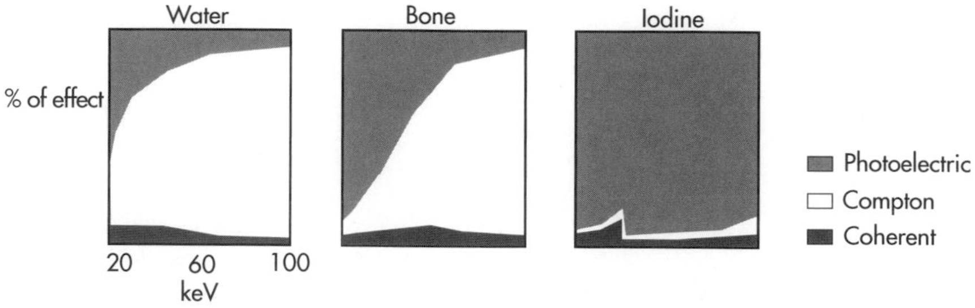

FIGURE 14-18

the absorber thickness required to reduce the intensity of the beam to 50% (n = number of HVL):

HVL = 0.693/ μ

Fraction transmitted = $e^{-0.693n}$ where n = thickness/HVL

Fraction transmitted = $(0.5)^{\text{thickness/HVL}}$

Fraction absorbed = 1-fraction transmitted

The typical HVL in mm of aluminum (Al) for film-screen mammography is approximately kVp/100. For example, if kVp is 27, then the HVL of the beam is roughly 0.27 mm Al.

Example

The HVL of a 140-keV beam through a given material is 0.3 cm. What is the percentage of x-rays transmitted through 1.2 cm?

Answer

Fraction transmitted = $(0.5)^{1.2/0.3}$ = 0.0625 = 6.25%

K-edge (Fig. 14-19)

K-edge refers to a sharp increase in the attenuation coefficient depending on the material and photon energy, which occurs at the binding energy of the K-shell electron being ejected at that specific photon energy (e.g., 29 keV for tin, 88 keV for lead). There are also increases at the binding energy for other shells (e.g., the L-shell), which occur at lower energies. The adjacent graph indicates that on a gram-for-gram basis, tin is a better absorber of x-rays than lead (between 29 and 88 keV).

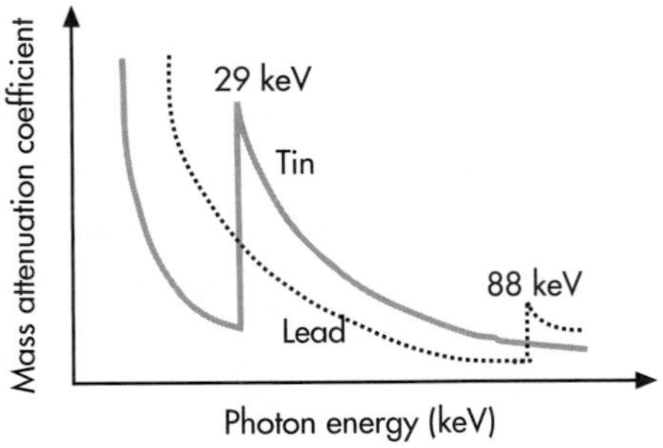

FIGURE 14-19

POLYCHROMATIC (TYPICAL X-RAY) RADIATION (Fig. 14-20)

Polychromatic radiation consists of a spectrum of photons with different energies. Unlike with monochromatic radiation, attenuation of polychromatic radiation is not exponential. In polychromatic radiation, a large percentage of low-energy photons is absorbed throughout the absorber so that the mean energy of remaining photons increases.

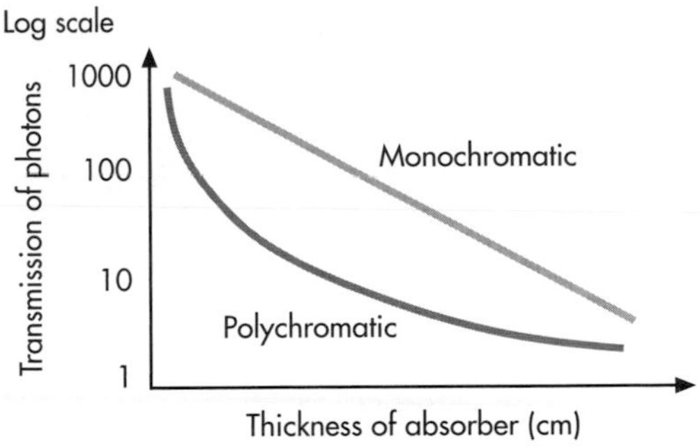

FIGURE 14-20

Factors that affect scatter radiation in radiographic images are:

- Field size (most important): the larger the field size, the more scatter
- Part thickness
- Kilovoltage (not as important as the other 2 factors). At low kV (<30 keV) there is little scatter because the photoelectric effect predominates; as radiation energy increases, the percentage of Compton scatter increases.

Example

Fetus receives the hypothetical x-ray dose of 1 rem. What is the maternal skin entrance dose, assuming μ = 0.2 cm^{-1} and the fetus is 5 cm below the skin surface?

Answer

A μ of 0.2 means that 20% of the beam is attenuated per centimeter and that 80% of the dose is transmitted. For 5 cm, the transmitted dose is 0.8 × 0.8 × 0.8 × 0.8 × 0.8 = 0.33 rem. To obtain 1 rem to the fetus, the incident ray has to be 2.7 rem.

FILTERS

Filters are sheets of metal placed in the path of an x-ray beam near the tube to absorb low-energy radiation before it reaches the patient. The function of a filter is to protect the patient from absorption of unnecessary low-energy radiation, reducing the skin dose by as much as 80%. Use of filters typically has to be compensated for by longer exposure times. Generally, one of two filter types is used:

- Aluminum filter: good filter for low energies. National Council of Radiation Protection (NCRP) recommendations:
  - <50 keV: 0.5 mm Al
  - 50 to 70 keV: 1.5 mm Al
  - >70 keV: 2.5 mm Al
- Copper filter: better filter for high energies. Typically about 0.25 mm thick and backed with 1.0 mm Al to filter out the low-energy scatter and characteristic x-rays from the copper

RESTRICTORS (Fig. 14-21)

The basic function of a restrictor is to regulate the size and shape of the x-ray beam.

Well-collimated beams generate less scatter and thus improve image quality. Three types of x-ray restrictors include:

- Aperture diaphragms
- Cones
- Collimators

The collimator is the best all-round x-ray beam restrictor. Federal regulations require automatic collimators on all new x-ray equipment. To calculate the geometry of the aperture:

$a/b = A/B$

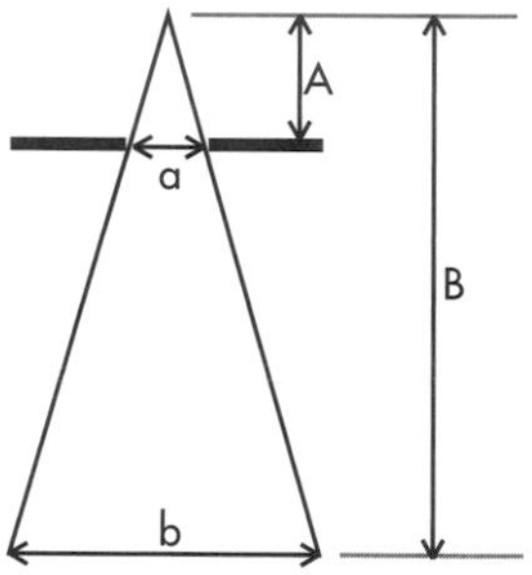

FIGURE 14-21

GRIDS

Grids consist of lead strips separated by plastic spacers. Grids are used to absorb scatter and to improve radiographic image contrast.

GRID RATIO (Fig. 14-22)

The grid ratio is defined as the ratio of the height of the lead strips (H) to the distance between them (D): Grid ratio = H:D

The thickness of the lead strip (d) does not affect the grid ratio, although it does affect the bucky factor. The higher the grid ratio:

- The better the image contrast
- The higher the patient exposure
- The better the grid function (more scatter absorbed)

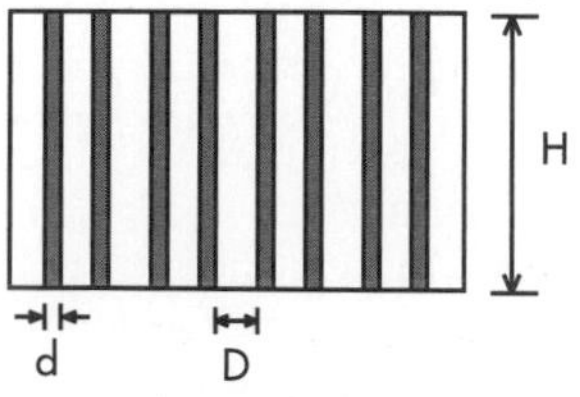

FIGURE 14-22

COMPARISON OF GRIDS

Parameter	12:1 Grid	8:1 Grid
Contrast	Better	Worse
Patient exposure	Higher	Lower
Lateral decentering artifact*	More prominent	Less prominent
Scatter	Lower	Higher

* Loss of density across the image

Rules of thumb regarding grids:

- <90 kVp x-ray: use 8:1 grid
- >90 kVp x-ray: use 12:1 grid
- Mammography: carbon fiber grids, 4:1 ratio, 150 lines/inch (i.e., 60 lines/cm)
- Mobile units: 6:1 ratio grid, 110 lines/inch
- Common reciprocating bucky: 12:1 ratio grid, 80 lines/inch
- High line density for stationary grids

TYPES OF GRIDS (Fig. 14-23)

Linear Grid

Lead strips are parallel to each other. Advantage: angle of x-ray tube can be adjusted along the length of the grid without cutoff.

Crossed Grid

Made up of two superimposed linear grids. Cannot be used with oblique techniques (disadvantage). Only used when there is a great deal of scatter (e.g., in biplane cerebral angiography).

Focused (Convergent) Grid

Lead strips are angulated so that they focus in space (the convergent line). The focal distance is the distance between the grid and the convergent line or point and should be close to the focus-film distance in use.

Moving Grid (Bucky Grid)

If grids are moved during x-ray exposure, the shadow casts produced by lead trips (grid lines) can be blurred out and the image quality can thus be improved. Although it is advantageous to use moving grids, there are certain disadvantages:

- Moving grids increase the patient's radiation dose for two reasons:
  Lateral decentering (see below)

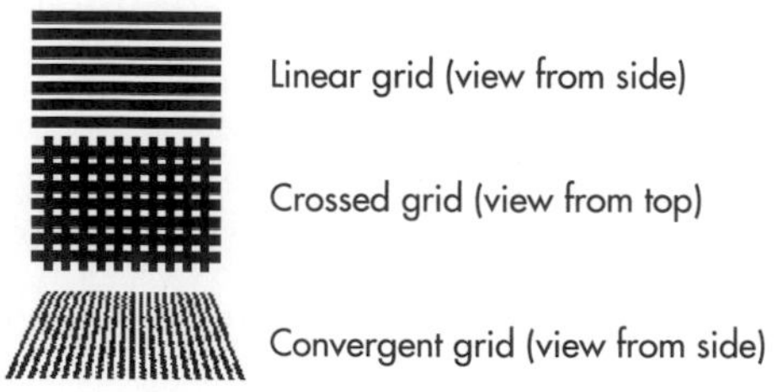

FIGURE 14-23

Exposure is spread out over the entire surface of film

- Longer exposure times are needed (because of lateral decentering)
- Higher cost (because of film advancement mechanism)

A grid-controlled x-ray tube is a tube in which a large negative voltage can be applied to a third electrode near the cathode. This negative voltage repels electrons before they reach the target and prevents x-ray production. Using this method, the x-ray beam can be rapidly switched on and off. When the grid voltage is synchronized with film advancement, this tube is suitable for rapid cinefluoroscopy (e.g., cardiac fluoroscopy).

GRID PERFORMANCE (Fig. 14-24)

Grid performance is usually measured by one of 3 parameters:

- Contrast improvement factor
- Bucky factor
- Primary transmission

Contrast Improvement Factor

Measurement of a grid's ability to improve contrast. High-ratio grids with a high lead content have a high contrast improvement factor (K).

$$K = \frac{\text{Contrast with grid}}{\text{Contrast without grid}}$$

A disadvantage of this parameter is that it depends on kVp, field size, and phantom thickness, the three classic parameters that determine the amount of scatter. The contrast improvement factor is usually determined at 100 kVp with a large field and a phantom thickness of 20 cm.

Bucky Factor

Related to the fraction of the total radiation (primary radiation and scatter) absorbed by a grid. Bucky factors (BFs) usually range from 3 to 7, depending on the grid ratio. The BF indicates:

- How much exposure factor must be increased because of use of a grid
- How much extra radiation the patient receives

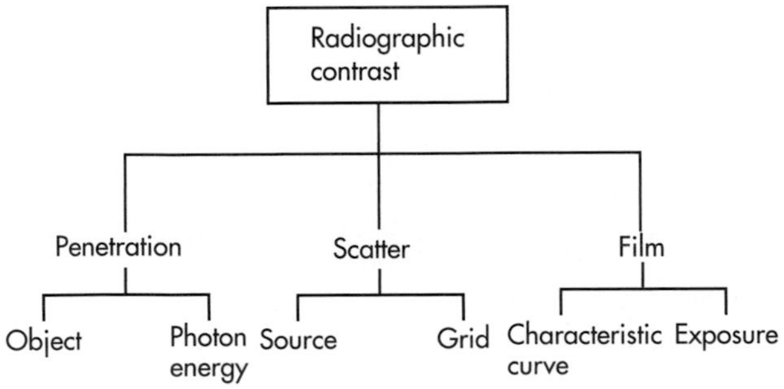

FIGURE 14-24

The BF is calculated as follows:

$$BF = \frac{\text{Incident radiation}}{\text{Transmitted radiation}}$$

BUCKY FACTOR BY GRID RATIO

Grid Ratio	B at 70 kVp	B at 120 kVp
No grid	1	1
5:1	3	3
8:1	3.5	4
12:1	4	5
16:1	4.5	6

Pearls

- The BF increases as the grid ratio increases.
- The BF increases with the thickness of the patient.
- Although a high BF is desirable (good film quality), it has the disadvantage of a higher exposure to the patient.

Primary Transmission

Measurement of the primary radiation (scatter excluded) transmitted through a grid. The scatter is excluded in the experimental setup by the use of a lead diaphragm and placing the phantom a long distance from the grid. The observed transmission is always lower (60%-70%) than calculated transmission (80%-90%) partly because the spacer absorbs some primary beam. The transmission (T) can be calculated by:

$$T_{calc} = (D/D + d) \times 100\%$$

where D = thickness of the spacer and d = thickness of the lead strip.

GRID ARTIFACTS (Fig. 14-25)

Upside-down Focused Grid

All grids have a tube side, which is marked as such. If the grid is inadvertently inserted the other way around, one will see a central area of exposure with peripheral underexposure. One may get the same sort of artifact in two other scenarios:

- A parallel grid is used (i.e., lead strips are not convergent)
- Focus-grid decentering (i.e., x-ray tube is too close or too far from convergent line)

Focus-Grid Distance Decentering

The x-ray tube focus is above (far) or below (near) the convergent line. The artifact is the same as with an upside-down grid.

Lateral Decentering

The more lateral the misalignment of a grid and x-ray focus, the more severe this artifact. The artifact consists of a homogeneous underexposure of the entire

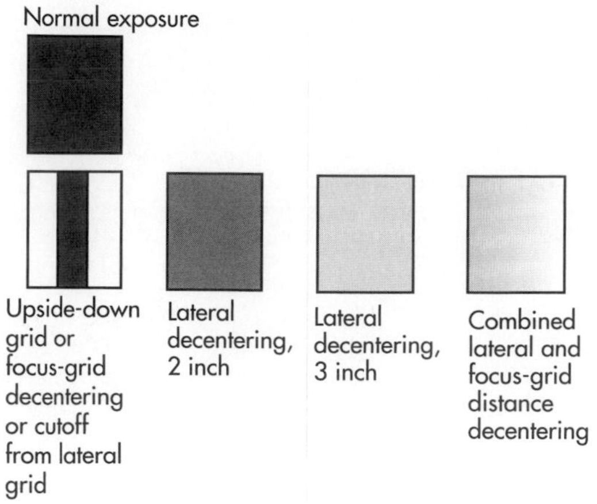

FIGURE 14-25

film. This artifact is probably the most difficult to recognize. The loss of primary radiation (in %) due to lateral decentering is given by:

$$\text{Loss} = \frac{\text{Grid ratio} \times \text{Lateral decentering (cm)}}{\text{Focal distance (cm)}} \times 100$$

When exact centering is not possible (as in portable films), low ratio grids and long focal distances should be used.

Combined Lateral and Focus-Grid Distance Decentering

Probably the most commonly recognized artifact. Causes uneven exposure, resulting in a film that is light on one side and dark on the other side.

AIR GAP TECHNIQUES (Fig. 14-26)

Air gap techniques are an alternative method of eliminating scatter with large radiographic fields. This method is often employed for chest radiographs. Patient exposure is usually lower with this technique than with grids. The intensity of scatter is maximal at the patient's exit surface and diminishes rapidly at increasing distance from the surface. If the film is placed at a distance (gap), most scatter misses the film. Focal film distance is increased in an attempt to maintain image sharpness. As a result, x-ray exposure factors (mAs) are usually greater than with grid techniques.

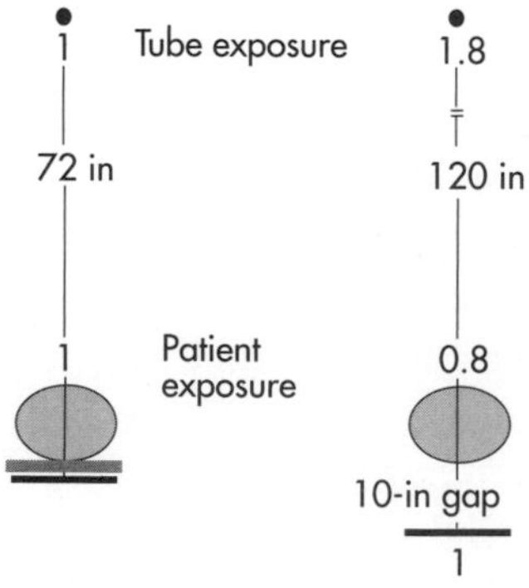

FIGURE 14-26

Screens (Figs. 14-27 and 14-28)

Intensifying screens are thin sheets of fluorescent material that surround radiographic film within the cassette or film changer. Screens are used because light is approximately 100 times more sensitive in exposing film than is radiation. Almost all x-ray absorption in the screen is caused by the photoelectric effect (high atomic number). Implications of using screens include:

- Reduces the x-ray dose to the patient
- Allows lowering of mAs, which results in shorter exposure times and fewer motion artifacts
- Main disadvantage is that they cause blurring of film

A variety of intensification screens are available. Although calcium tungstate ($CaWO_4$) screens were used until the 1970s, only rare earth (such as gadolinium [Ga] and lanthanum [La]) screens are used today because they are faster.

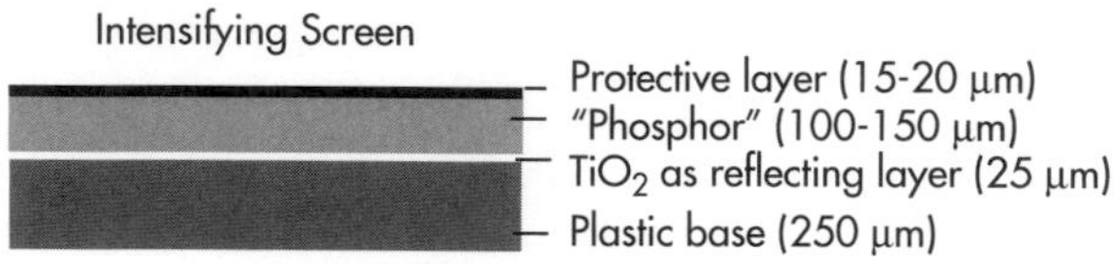

FIGURE 14-27

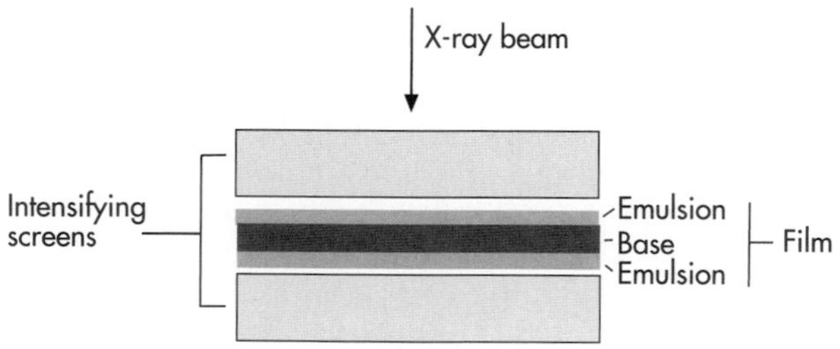

FIGURE 14-28

ABSORPTION EFFICIENCY (Figs. 14-29 and 14-30)

The main function of a screen is to absorb x-rays, and the best screen would be the one that absorbs all radiation leaving the patient's body (100% absorption efficiency). In reality, the absorption efficiency is only 20%-70%. Absorption efficiency depends on:

- Screen thickness: the thicker the screen, the better the absorption (but also the more blur)
- Screen material: absorption efficiency is 5% for $CaWO_4$ screens and 20%-70% for rare earth screens

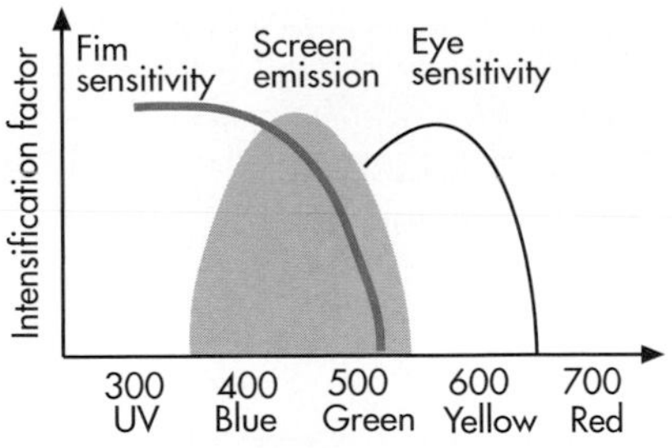

FIGURE 14-29

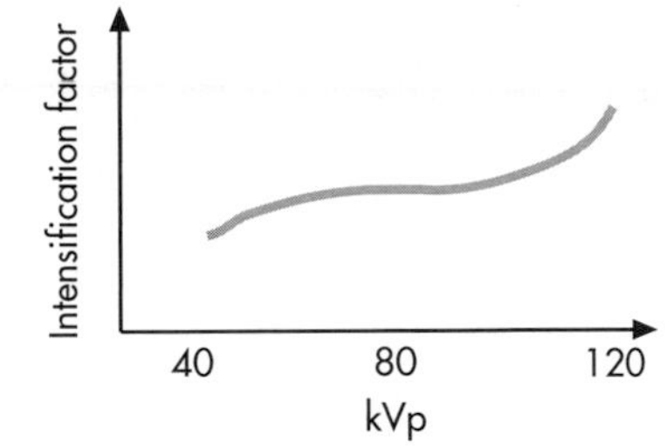

FIGURE 14-30

- Photon energy spectrum
- Intrinsic efficiency: conversion of x-rays to light

To calculate the absorption efficiency:

1. Determine the keV of an x-ray photon (e.g., 100 keV).
2. Determine the keV of a visible light photon: keV = 12.4/wavelength (typically 3 to 5 eV/photon).
3. Compare the keV of x-ray and light photon: 15,000 to 50,000 light photons can theoretically be generated per x-ray photon.

SENSITIVITY AND SPEED

The "speed" of a screen refers to the duration of exposure required to obtain a good image. Speed values are usually provided as 100, 200, 400, etc. by the manufacturer. The relationship between sensitivity (mR) and speed is given by:

Sensitivity (mR) = 128/Speed

Speed of screens ~ Absorption efficiency × Conversion efficiency

Noise of a screen ~ Conversion efficiency

FILM SPEED

Speed	Sensitivity (mR)
12	10
25	5
50	2.56
100	1.28
200	0.64
400	0.32
800	0.16
1200	0.1

The speed of screens can be increased by:

- Increasing the thickness of the phosphor layer
- Increasing the size of the phosphor crystals (grains)
- Adding light-absorbent dyes

IMAGE BLUR (Fig. 14-31)

The selection of an appropriate screen is a compromise between minimizing patient exposure and maximizing image quality. Thinner screens absorb less photons and have better detail, whereas thicker screens absorb more photons but have more blur. Image screens are usually categorized into:

- Mammographic
- Detail (slow)
- Par speed
- Medium speed
- High speed

COMPARISON OF SCREEN PERFORMANCE (ASSUMING THE SAME SCREEN MATERIAL)

Parameter	Medium Screen	Detail Screen
Thickness	Medium	Thin
Screen	Faster	Slower
Resolution	Lower	Higher
Patient dose	Lower	Higher
Noise	Same	Same

COMPARISON OF SCREEN PERFORMANCE (ASSUMING DIFFERENT SCREEN MATERIALS OF SAME THICKNESS)

Parameter	Tungsten Screen	Rare Earth Screen
Speed	Slower	Faster
Resolution	Lower	Higher
Patient dose	Higher	Lower
Noise	Lower	Higher

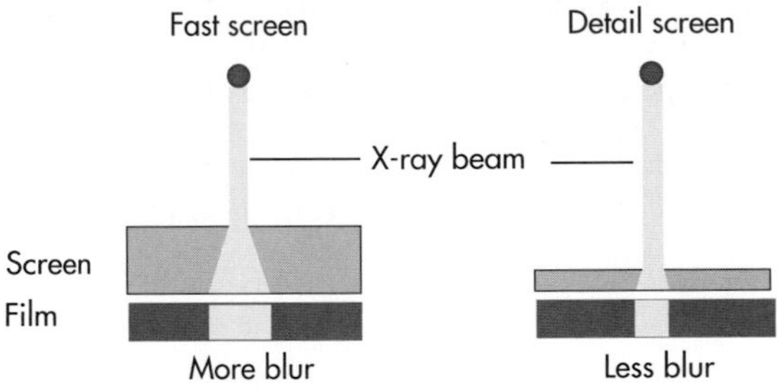

FIGURE 14-31

RARE EARTH SCREENS (Fig. 14-32)

These screens contain:

- Terbium-activated gadolinium oxysulfide (Gd_2O_2S:Tb)
- Thulium-activated lanthanum oxybromide (LaOBr:Tm)

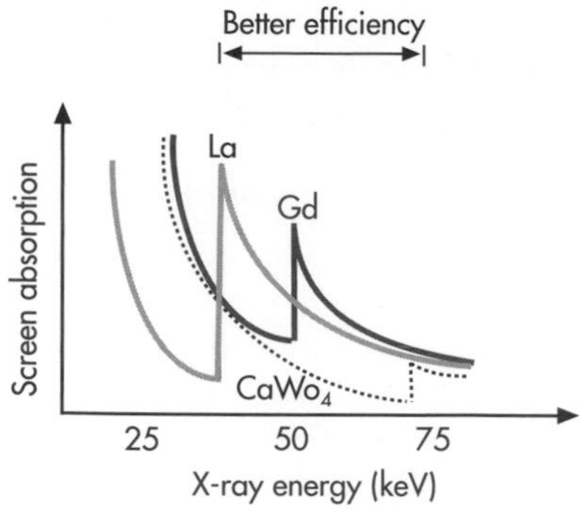

FIGURE 14-32

The reason for the higher efficiency of these screens is the higher absorbance of x-rays because of the lower K-edge of rare earth elements compared with W (La: 39, Gd: 50, W: 70 keV) and the higher light output per photon absorbed. At 40 to 70 keV, the rare earth screens have a significant absorption advantage over $CaWO_4$. Emission spectra of rare earth screens:

- Tb emits green light.
- Tm emits blue light.

QUANTUM MOTTLE

Quantum mottle is due to statistical fluctuation of photons in an x-ray beam. The more photons that are used, the less mottle there is.

QUANTUM MOTTLE

Source of Mottle	Ways to Reduce Quantum Mottle (i.e., Less Noisy Image)
X-ray tube	
mA	Increase the mA (generates more photons)
kVp	Increase the kVp (generates more photons)
Dose	Increase the dose (generates more photons)
Contrast	Decrease the contrast
CT slice thickness	Increase the slice thickness
Screen	
Absorption efficiency	Use thicker screens (capture more photons)
Conversion efficiency	Decrease the conversion efficiency
Speed	Use slower screens
Film speed	Use slower film

FILM

COMPOSITION (Fig. 14-33)

Film Base

- Glass plates were used before 1920, then cellulose (flammable), and now polyester.
- May contain blue tint to produce less eye strain and less crossover for blue light

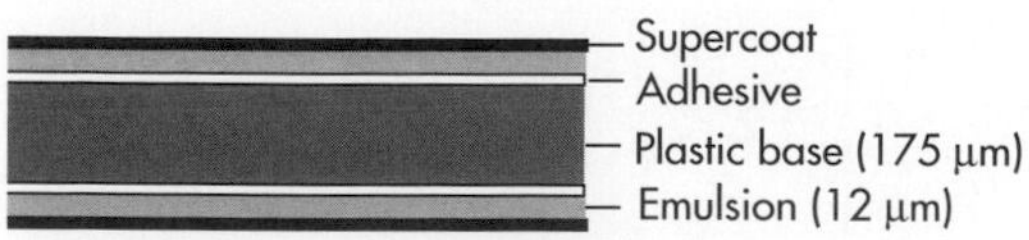

FIGURE 14-33

Emulsion

- Contains silver halide crystals (AgBr 90%-99%, AgI 1%-10%) in gelatin; these crystals have a cubic lattice structure; crystal size = 1 to 2 μm
- Crystals are sensitized by adding allylthiourea to the emulsion. As a result, AgS forms on the surface of the crystal (sensitivity speck).

Supercoating

- Commonly made out of gelatin
- Antistatic protective layer

Processing

Chemical processing of x-ray films amplifies the latent image by a factor of 10^6. This process is necessary because 2 Ag atoms per sensitivity speck would not be enough to be detectable by the eye. Film processing includes three steps:

- Development (reducing Ag), initiated at the site of a latent image speck
- Fixing: removal of nonreduced Ag in emulsion
- Washing, drying

The typical developer temperature is 93° to 95°F. Operating a processor at higher temperatures may result in:

- Increased fog (this will decrease contrast)
- Increased sensitivity and speed
- Increased contrast

Developing solutions:

- Reducers: hydroquinone and phenindone (reduce Ag and produce hydrogen)
- Alkali, buffers at pH 10 to 12
- Preservatives: sodium sulfite

Replenishment solutions have to be added to the developer to maintain its activity.

REPLENISHER

Error	Hydroquinone Concentration	Bromide Concentration	pH
Underreplenishment	Low	High	Low
Overreplenishment	High	Low	High
Oxidized developer	Low	Normal	High

Fixing solutions:

- Thiosulfate to produce water-soluble silver thiosulfate complexes
- Chromium or aluminum to harden the gelatin

FILM DENSITY

Film density refers to film blackening by x-ray exposure. Rules of thumb:

- mA controls film density
- kVp controls image contrast

Optical Density (OD)

$$OD = \log_{10}(I_{in}/I_{out})$$

where I_{in} is the incident light and I_{out} is the transmitted light (in a viewing system or densitometer). A density of 1 indicates that for each 10 photons only 1 will get through the film (log 10/1 = 1). Opacity is defined as: I_{in}/I_{out}. Higher density means a darker film. The densities of x-ray films are additive. Typical densities are:

- Black x-ray film: 2 (1% transmitted light)
- Light film: 0.3 (50% of light transmitted)
- Unexposed film: 0.12 (due to base fog)

PHOTOGRAPHIC DENSITY

Opacity (I_{in}/I_{out})	Density ($\log I_{in}/I_{out}$)	Transmitted Light (%)
1	0	100
2	0.3	50
4	0.6	25
8	0.9	12.5
10	1	10
00	2	1
1000	3	0.1
10,000	4	0.01

Note: log 100 = 2; log 2 = 0.3

To change the density of x-ray film from 2 to 1, one can:

- Decrease kVp 15%
- Decrease mA by 50%
- Change from nongrid to grid technique
- Add one HVL of plastic to collimator

Example

Two films within OD of 1.5 are placed on top of each other. What is the fraction of transmitted light?

Answer

OD = 1.5 + 1.5 = 3. Antilog of 3 is 1000; therefore, 0.001 of incident light is transmitted.

HD CURVE (Fig. 14-34)

HD (**H**urter and **D**riffield) curves provide information about contrast, speed (sensitivity), and latitude of film. The exposure is usually plotted as log on the *x*-axis. Film density is plotted on the *y*-axis.

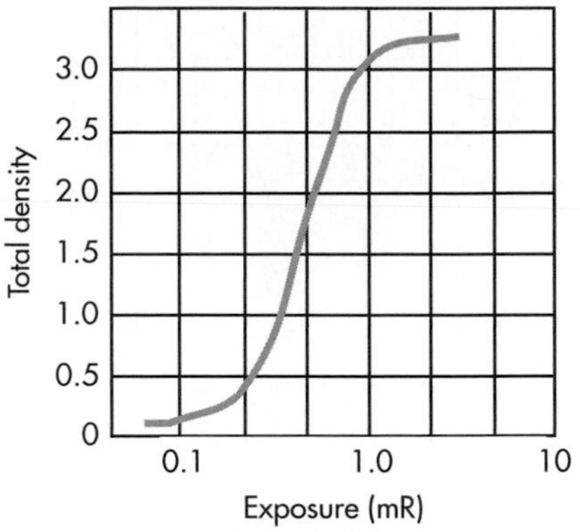

FIGURE 14-34

Film Contrast

Film contrast (best ensured by HD curve) depends on:

- Film density
- Screen or direct x-ray exposure
- Film processing

Shape of HD Curve (Fig. 14-35)

The slope of the curve is given by:

$$\text{Slope (gamma)} = \frac{D2 - D1}{\log E2 - \log E1}$$

Where D = density and E = exposure. The average gradient is measured from D1 = 0.25 to D2 = 2.0 (i.e., D2 – D1 is always 1.75). If the average slope (gradient) is >1 (as in all x-ray films), the film will amplify subject contrast. Usually the gradient ranges from 2 to 3.5.

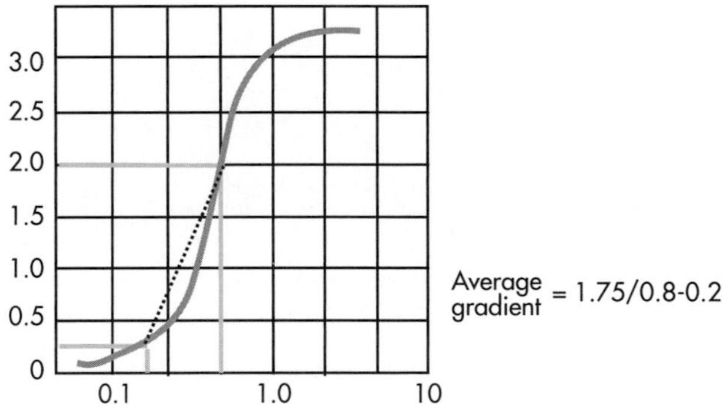

FIGURE 14-35

Example (Fig. 14-36)

Calculate the average gradient if an exposure of 10 gives a density of 1 and an exposure of 100 gives a density of 2.

Answer

$$\text{Gamma} = 2 - 1/(\log 100 - \log 10) = 1/2 - 1 = 1$$

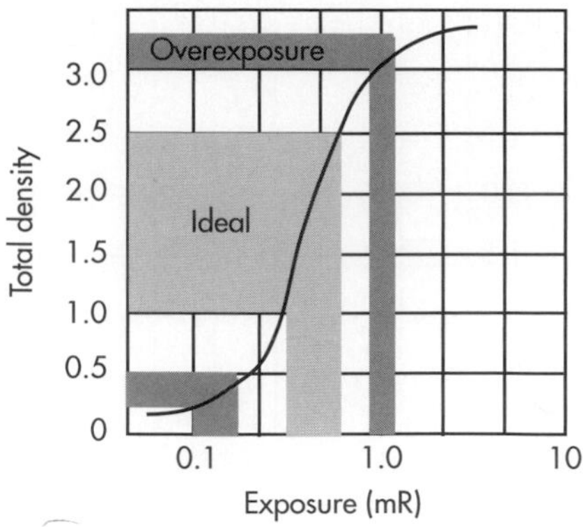

FIGURE 14-36

Density

Proper film exposure should always be made in the linear portion of the HD curve, not at toes or shoulders.

Speed

Film speed refers to the reciprocal value of the exposure (in roentgens) to produce a density of 1.0 above base and fog density:

Speed = 1/roentgens

Latitude (Fig. 14-37)

Latitude refers to the range of log exposure that will produce density within acceptable limits. The more latitude a film has, the less critical the exposure time. Latitude varies inversely with contrast: the more latitude, the less contrast.

Darkroom Safelights

- Infrared laser film: green
- Ortho film: red
- Film for $CaWO_4$ screens: yellow or red

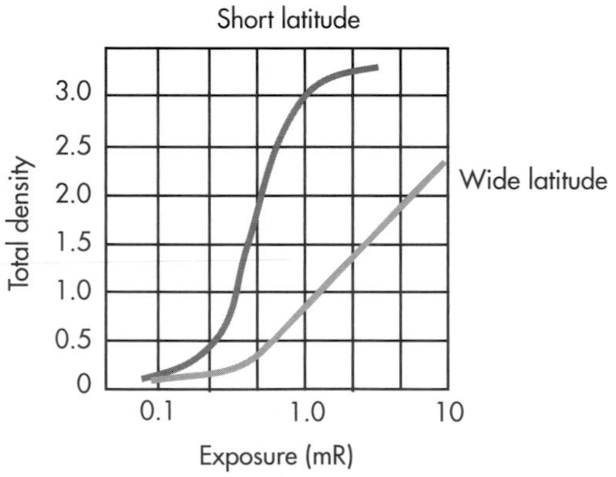

FIGURE 14-37

IMAGE QUALITY

Quality of an x-ray is primarily determined by contrast, resolution, and noise (quantum mottle). The higher the contrast-to-noise ratio, the better the image.

Contrast (Fig. 14-38)

Radiographic contrast depends on three factors:

- Subject contrast
- Film contrast (HD curve)
- Fog and scatter

Subject contrast refers to the difference in x-ray intensity transmitted through one part of the subject as compared with another. Subject contrast depends on:

- Thickness of different portions of the subject (the thicker the subject part, the higher the absorption)
- Density difference (mass per unit volume [i.e., g/cm^3]); the greater the difference, the higher the absorption
- Atomic number difference (photoelectric absorption increases with high atomic numbers)
- Radiation quality (kVp); low kVp will produce high contrast (mammography), provided the kVp is high enough to penetrate the part being examined.

Fog and scatter (especially Compton scatter) are undesirable because they decrease radiographic contrast. Fog is increased by:

- Use of high-speed film (highly sensitive grains)
- Improper film storage
- Contaminated or exhausted development solution
- Excessive time or temperature of development

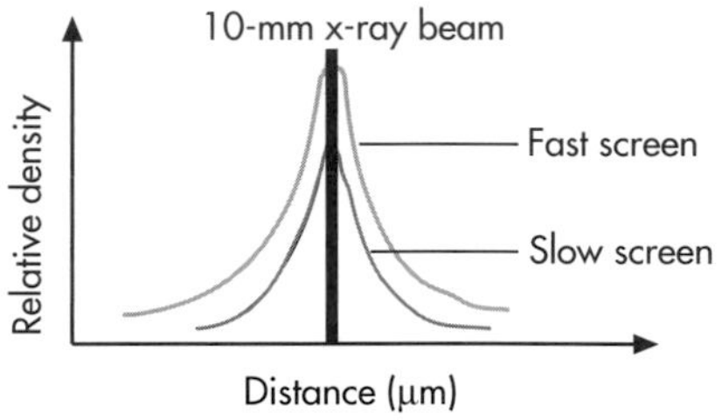

FIGURE 14-38

Line Spread Function

Parameter of image quality. Tested with a vertical 10-μm collimated x-ray beam, which exposes a film-screen combination. The "observed" width of the image (usually the full width at half maximum [FWHM]) is greater than 10 μm and depends on the film-screen combination.

Modulation Transfer Function (MTF) (Figs. 14-39 and 14-40)

Parameter of image quality. The MTF can be expressed as the ratio of the diagnostic information recorded on film divided by the total information available presented as a function of spatial frequency (e.g., line-pairs per millimeter). A ratio of 1 indicates perfect use of information. The lower the ratio, the more information is lost in the recording process.

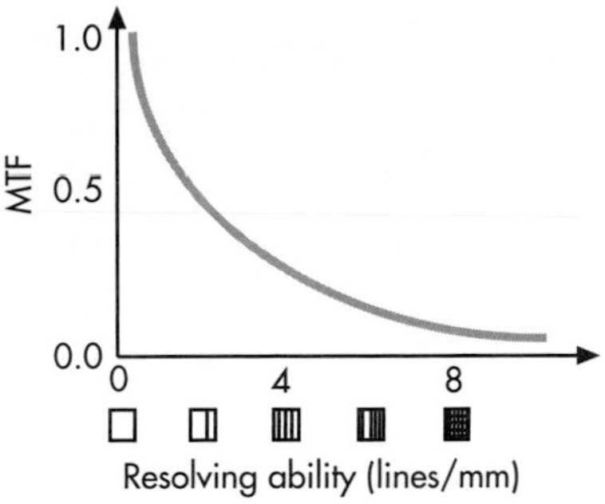

FIGURE 14-39

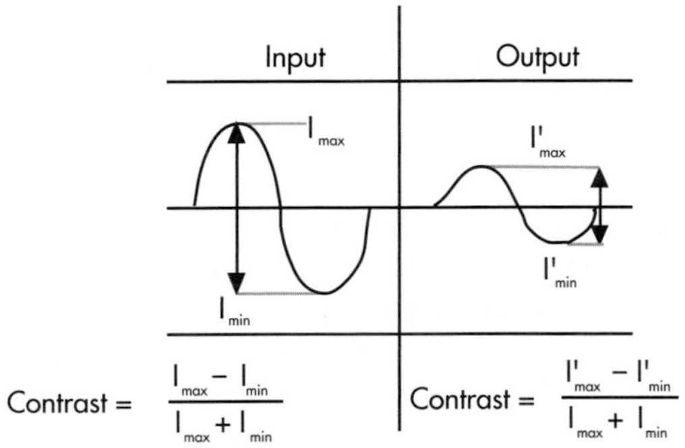

FIGURE 14-40

The individual MTF factors of x-ray film, intensifying screen, and x-ray tube can be multiplied to result in the total MTF of the x-ray system.

$$\text{MTF (at a given line} - \text{pair/mm)} =$$

$$\frac{\text{Contrast output}}{\text{Contrast input}} = \frac{I'_{max} - I'_{min}}{I_{max} - I_{min}}$$

where I = intensity

$$\text{Contrast output} = \frac{I'_{max} - I'_{min}}{I_{max} + I_{min}}$$

$$\text{Contrast input} = \frac{I_{max} - I_{min}}{I_{max} + I_{min}}$$

FLUOROSCOPY

Fluoroscopes produce immediate and continuous images. Historically, flat fluorescent screens were used to intercept and visualize x-ray beams as they left the patient. Today image intensifier tubes are used, which greatly improve image quality by amplifying x-ray beams. TV systems are now also routinely used to transfer the image from the output of the image intensifier tube to a large screen.

IMAGE INTENSIFIER (Fig. 14-41)

An image intensifier is an electronic vacuum tube that converts an incident x-ray image into a light image of small sizc and high brightness.

Image intensifiers are required to amplify the x-ray signal to the light level needed for photopic (cone) vision. The individual components of an image intensifier consist of:

- Input phosphor: absorbs x-ray and converts it to light photons
- Photocathode: light photons strike photocathode, and electrons are emitted.
- Accelerating anode: electron stream is focused by lens system onto a small area (e.g., 1-inch diameter) and accelerated to anode. Anode-cathode potential is 25 kV; because electrons are accelerated, they produce more light on the output phosphor (50-fold increase).
- Output phosphor: converts electron stream to light
- A video camera is usually used to record the small image at the end of the intensifier tube.

Input Phosphor and Photocathode (Fig. 14-42)

- Input phosphor: thin layer of CsI
- Photocathode composed of antimony and cesium compounds
- Output phosphor composed of Ag-activated zinc-cadmium sulfide

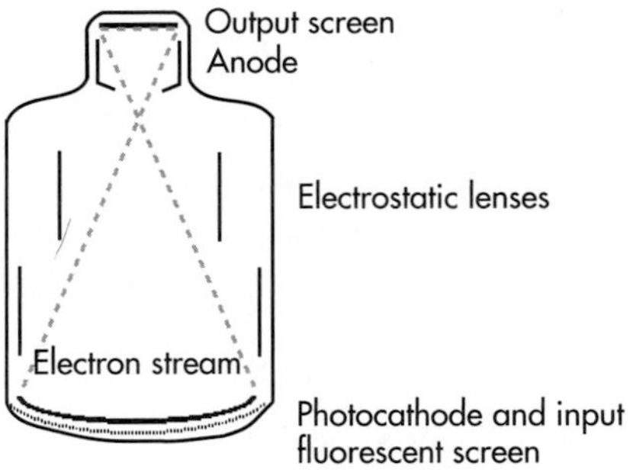

FIGURE 14-41

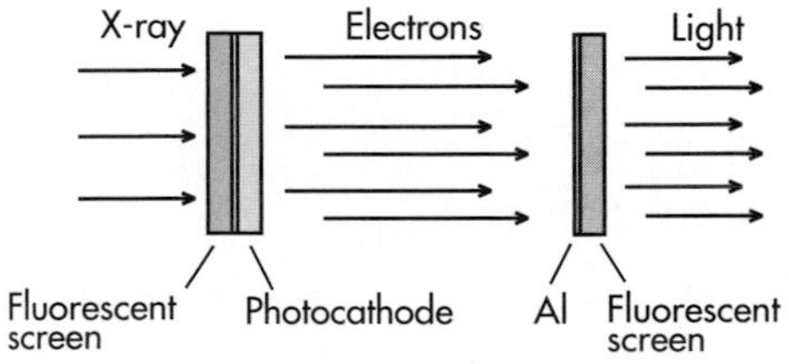

FIGURE 14-42

Brightness Gain

The brightness gain of an image intensifier is measured by the conversion factor: candela per square meter (cd/m^2) at the output phosphor divided by mR/sec input exposure. Brightness gain deteriorates as the image intensifier ages (approximately 10% per year). Flux gain refers to the increase in number of output screen light photons relative to the input screen light photons.

Brightness gain = Minification gain × Flux gain

Example

What is the brightness gain with an input screen of 6 inches, an output screen of 0.5 inch, and a 50-fold light flux gain?

Answer

$$\text{Gain} = (6/0.5)^2 \times 50 = 7200 \text{ times}$$

Minification Gain

$$\text{Minification gain} = \frac{\text{Diameter input screen}^2}{\text{Diameter output screen}^2}$$

Because the output screen is usually 1 inch in diameter, the minification gain is usually the square of the image intensifier diameter (e.g., 81 for a 9-inch intensifier).

Example

What are the consequences when a 9-inch diameter image intensifier is switched to intensify a 6-inch diameter image?

Answer

First, the exposure to the patient will increase to maintain the same image brightness. Second, the new image will be magnified at the ratio of 9:6.

Resolution of Intensifiers

- 1 to 2 line-pairs/mm for old zinc-cadmium intensifiers (similar to old direct fluoroscopic screens with red light adaptation)
- 4 line-pairs/mm for modern CsI intensifiers

Distortion of Intensifiers

- Refers to nonuniform electron beam focusing
- Distortion is most severe at the periphery of the intensifier.
- Distortion is always more severe with large intensifiers.
- Fall-off in brightness toward the periphery of the image is called *vignetting*.

TV RECORDING SYSTEM (Figs. 14-43 and 14-44)

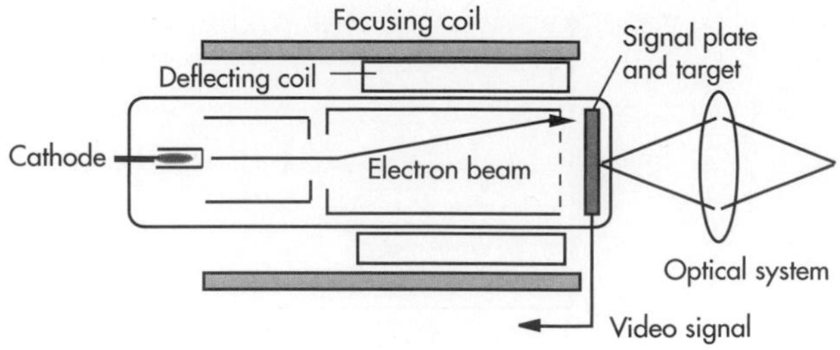

FIGURE 14-43

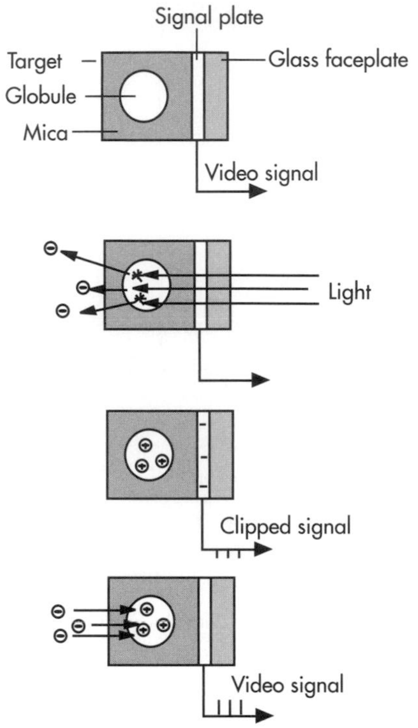

FIGURE 14-44

TV recording systems are usually employed to record the image from the 1-inch screen of the image intensifier. Although different designs of video cameras are available, only the vidicon system is widely used. The camera has the following components:

- Vacuum glass tube
- Target assembly that records the image; this assembly contains 3 structures:
  - Glass faceplate of the tube
  - Signal plate (thin film of graphite, which acts as an electrical conductor)
  - Vidicon target (antimony trisulfide suspended as globules in a mica matrix)
- Cathode electron beam to discharge the vidicon globules once they have been exposed to light. The electron beam is focused and scanned along the target by means of focusing and deflecting coils
- Anode potential: 250 V (electrons fly fast from cathode to anode); signal plate potential: 25 V (electrons flow very slowly from anode to signal plate). Deceleration of the electron beam has 2 functions:

Straightening the final path of the beam
Electrons need to strike the signal plate slowly.

Video Signal

- Photons strike the globule and electrons are emitted.
- Globule becomes positively charged.
- Electron beam from the cathode neutralizes the positively charged globule and a positive signal (video signal) is generated on the signal plate.

TV Monitor

- Electron beam is focused onto a picture tube (fluorescent screen) by means of focusing and deflecting coils.
- The anode-cathode potential is 10 kV (fast electrons emit a lot of photons when they strike the screen).
- *Lag* refers to the "stickiness" of an image when image detail changes rapidly; lag can be reduced with lead monoxide photoconductors (Plumbicon tubes) in the video camera.
- TV resolution (Fig. 14-45)
  - Horizontal resolution depends on bandwidth.
  - Vertical resolution depends on number of scan lines per millimeter.
  - Image resolution can be increased by increasing lines per millimeter or by decreasing field of view (FOV).

Interlaced Horizontal Scanning

TV monitor usually displays 30 frames/second, which is visually perceived as flicker. Instead of scanning all 525 TV lines consecutively, only the even-numbered lines are displayed in one image and the odd-numbered in the 2nd image. The frequency is thus increased to 60 fields/second (no flicker).

Kell Factor

Ratio between the perceived vertical resolution and the number of horizontal scan lines. A resolution of 525 × 370 lines (185 white lines, 185 black lines) is usually maximum for a TV. The Kell factor is thus 0.7 (370/525).

Example

What is the maximum vertical resolution of a 525-line TV system with a 23-cm input?

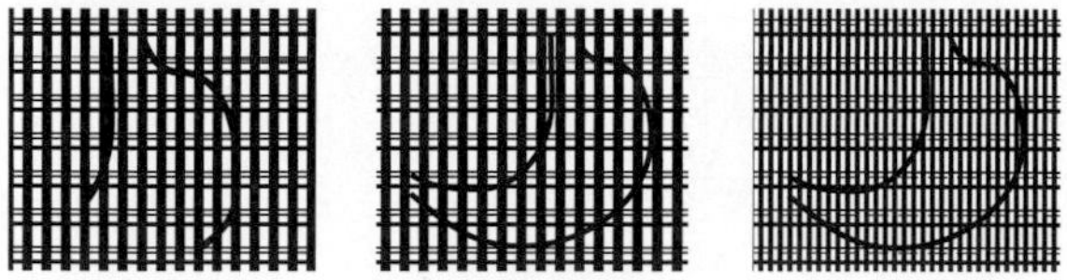

FIGURE 14-45

Answer

Only about 490 lines are used to trace out image. It takes 2 lines to form a line-pair (i.e., 490/2 = 245 line-pairs). Multiply by Kell factor: 245 × 0.7 = 172 line-pairs. If input screen is 23 cm, resolution is 172/230 mm or 0.74 line-pair/mm.

MAMMOGRAPHY

TARGET FILTER COMBINATIONS

Mo is used as anode material for mammography because the characteristic x-rays with energies 17.5 and 19 keV are more desirable for maximum subject contrast. A molybdenum filter with a rhodium target (Rh/Mo) should never be used. Other target/filter combinations for mammography include:

TARGET FILTER COMBINATIONS

Target	Filter
Molybdenum	Molybdenum
Tungsten with beryllium window	Al or carbon fiber (lower glandular dose with the latter)
Tungsten	Palladium (experimental)
Rhodium	Rhodium

TECHNICAL REQUIREMENTS OF FILM SCREEN MAMMOGRAPHY

- A small FS (~0.3 to 0.4 mm) is required for high resolution (the larger the FS, the worse the geometric unsharpness). Mammography units should also have 0.1-mm normal FS for magnification views.
- Low kVp (24 to 25) to obtain good soft tissue contrast
- Long distance of tube to object (65 cm) for high resolution
- Short imaging time (high mA) to reduce motion and dose
- Scatter is best reduced by breast compression and the use of a grid; a grid of 5:1 should be used when compressed breast is >6 cm.
- Compression decreases dose owing to thinner tissue plane, shorter exposure, and separation of overlapping structures.
- Phototiming (automatic exposure control)
- Rare earth screens and single-emulsion film help to decrease dose and cross-talk.
- Processing at 95°C (normal 88° to 92°C) and doubling time in the developer (from 23 to 46 seconds) can be used to increase contrast; this modified processing protocol, however, also increases noise.

TOMOGRAPHY (FIG. 14-46)

Tomography is an x-ray technique in which shadows of superimposed structures are blurred out by a moving x-ray tube. Conventional tomography is now less commonly used because of the availability of cross-sectional imaging techniques such as US, CT, and MRI. There are 2 basic types of tomography: linear and nonlinear. In both techniques, the tube moves in one direction while the film cassette moves in the opposite direction, with both motions centered around a fulcrum.

LINEAR VERSUS NONLINEAR TOMOGRAPHY

Parameter	Linear Tomography	Circular Tomography
Cost	Inexpensive	Expensive
Blur margins	Indistinct	Distinct
Objects outside plane	May be visible (parasite streaks)	No parasite streaks
Phantom images	No	Yes (narrow angle tomography)
Section thickness	Not uniform	Uniform

The amount of blurring depends on the following factors:

- Amplitude of tube travel (more blur with wide-angle motion)
- Distance from focal plane (more blur at long object—focal plane distances)
- Distance from film (more blur at long object-film distances)
- Orientation of tube travel: object needs to be oriented perpendicular to motion
- Blurring is unrelated to size of the object.

The amplitude of tube traveling is measured in degrees (tomographic angle).

- The wider the angle, the thinner the section.
- The narrower the angle, the thicker the section.

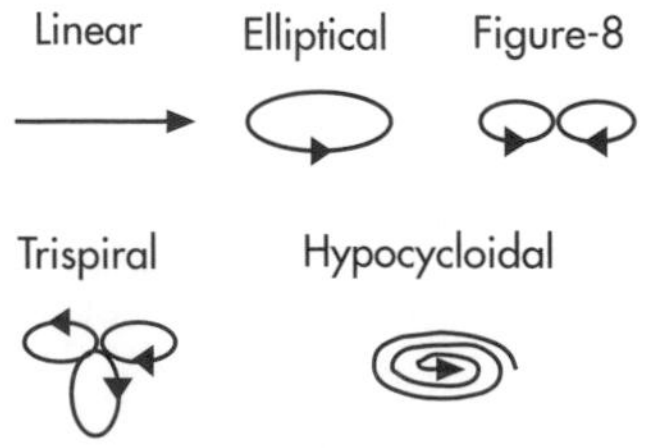

FIGURE 14-46

WIDE-VERSUS NARROW-ANGLE TOMOGRAPHY

Parameter	Wide-Angle Tomography	Narrow-Angle Tomography
Angle	30°-50°	<10°
Section thickness	Thin	Thick
Blurring	Maximum	Minimum
Use	Tissue with high contrast (bone)	Tissue with low contrast (lung)
Type of tomography	Linear or circular	Circular only
Phantom images	Unlikely	Yes
Exposure times	Long	Short

Disadvantages of Tomography

- High patient dose with multiple cuts
- High cost of circular tomography
- Long exposure times (exposure time determined by time it takes to move the tube 3 to 6 seconds)
- Motion artifacts with long exposure times are more common.

STEREOSCOPY (FIG. 14-47)

Stereoscopy is now rarely used. The original advantage of stereoscopy was that confusing shadows could be "untangled" when CT and MRI were not available. However, there are many disadvantages to stereoscopy:

- Twice as much patient exposure
- Patient has to hold absolutely still

Stereoscopic imaging techniques require the exposure of two films (one for each eye), with the x-ray tube minimally shifted between exposures. A good rule of thumb is that the shift should be 10% of the target-film distance (i.e., a 4-inch shift for a 40-inch target-film distance). The 10% shift will produce an angle of approximately 6°.

Pearls

- Best direction of tube shift is along the long axis of a grid (shift across short axis causes cutoff from lateral decentering).

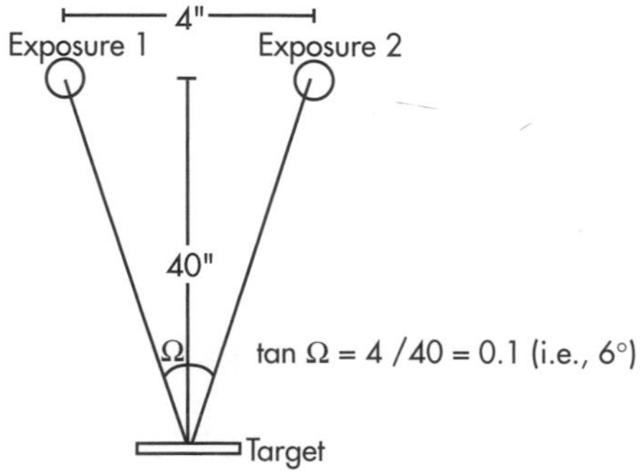

FIGURE 14-47

- It is best to use 8:1 or lower grid ratios.
- To view films stereoscopically, film must be viewed:
  - From the tube side, not the other side (as is usually done on PA films)
  - With the eyes converging along the direction of the tube shift
  - Left film with left eye and right film with right eye

There are a number of viewing systems for stereoscopic films:

- Wheatstone stereoscope: uses mirror to match films
- Binocular prism stereoscope
- Polarized images seen through polarizing glasses
- Green (left) and red (right) images seen through green/red glasses

CT (HELICAL, MULTISLICE) (Fig. 14-48)

OVERVIEW

In CT a thin fan-shaped x-ray beam is projected through a slice of the body to be imaged. Penetrating radiation (or attenuation μ) is then measured by a detector. Images are reconstructed from multiple "views" obtained at different angles as the x-ray beam rotates around the patient.

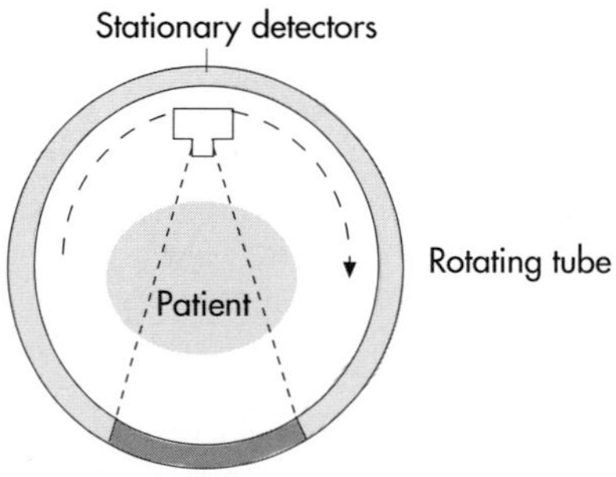

FIGURE 14-48

CT NUMBERS

$$\text{CT number} = \frac{k(\mu\,\text{tissue} - \mu\,\text{water})}{\mu\,\text{water}}$$

where k is a magnifying constant (when k = 1000, the resulting CT number is the Hounsfield unit [HU]). The CT number is a measure of the total absorption coefficient of a tissue element, positive for values higher than water and negative for values less than water (water = zero).

CT NUMBERS OF TISSUES

Tissue	HU
Air	−1000
Lung	−300
Fat	−100
Water	0
White matter	50
Gray matter	40
Muscle	40
Blood	60–80
Bone	1000

CT COMPONENTS

X-ray Tube and Gantry

The x-ray tube is mounted on a gantry that allows rotation of the tube around the patient's body. The x-ray tube typically has a FS size of <0.6 mm. Collimators determine the angular spread of the beam and the slice thickness.

Slip Ring

Allows continuous gantry rotation with table motion.

Filtration

As with other x-ray units, low-energy radiation is attenuated by filtration, typically resulting in an average of 70 keV. Besides reducing radiation, filtration has two specific purposes:

- Results in "hardening" of the beam (increased average photon energy), which reduces beam-hardening artifacts occurring within the patient (e.g., at rib/soft tissue interfaces or around metal clips)
- Compensates for nonuniform thickness of human body

Detectors

Several materials are used for manufacturing CT detectors. Basically there are two types of detectors:

- Scintillation crystals attached to photomultiplier tubes: disadvantage is afterglow
- Gas-filled ionization chambers (25 atm xenon gas): no afterglow

CT SCANNER GENERATIONS

Helical CT

Helical scanners are 3rd or 4th generation scanners. Patient moves horizontally as the x-ray tube rotates around the patient in a helical path.

OVERVIEW OF CT SCANNERS

Generation	Description	Comment
1st	Pencil-like x-ray beam, 1 detector Rotary (1°) motion and linear motion Time: 8-10 min/slice	Historical
2nd	Fan-shaped beam, multiple (30) detectors Rotary (30ldG) motion and linear motion Time: 20-120 sec/slice	Historical
3rd	Wider fan beam and more (300) detectors No linear-type movements Time: 2-10 sec/slice	Rotating detector configuration
4th	Ring of stationary detectors surrounds patient Time: <2 sec/slice	Easy calibration, fast, 3-D (helical)
Electron-beam (5th)	Electron gun deflects and focuses electron beam Time: 50 ms	Fast speed acquisition, minimizes cardiac motion

- "Pitch" = table movement (one rotation of the x-ray tube)/collimation width
- Larger pitch decreases scan time and patient dose but increases slice thickness and slice-sensitivity profile.
- Image reconstruction can occur at any position and any interval, but the smallest slice thickness is equal to collimation width.

Multislice CT

Multislice CT scanners have replaced 4th generation scanners. Multislice CT scanners are 3rd generation scanners with helical capabilities and low voltage slip rings, which acquire up to 16 (or even 32) CT slices per x-ray tube rotation. These scanners can scan large volumes with high z-axis resolution. Multislice CT scanners perform differently from single-slice scanners, especially in the spiral mode. The multislice scanners use a narrow-angle cone beam of x-rays to illuminate the subject and excite the detectors. With cone-beam CT, the relationship between the source and individual detector is variable, with detector elements in the periphery of the array illuminated obliquely while those in the center are not. The concept of pitch, used in helical scanners, is different when applied to multidetector scanners. The two definitions for pitch used in multidetector scanners are "pitch_x" (x-ray beam pitch) and "pitch_d" (detector pitch).

- Pitch = table speed/x-ray beam width
- Pitch_d = table speed/detector width, and varies depending on the number of slices reconstructed. Manufacturers use different terminology to assign pitch values.
- $\text{Pitch}_d = \text{Pitch}_x \times$ number of slices
- For example, the General Electric (GE) multislice system allows the use of two modes: high-quality (HQ) and high-speed (HS) modes. In HQ mode, $\text{pitch}_d = 3$ when four images per rotation are reconstructed. In HS mode, $\text{pitch}_d = 6$ for four reconstructed images. In terms of pitch_x, in HQ mode it is equal to 0.75, and in HS mode it is 1.5, regardless of the number of images reconstructed.

The clinical advantages of multislice scanners can be attributed to the increased speed and volume coverage. The speed can be used for trauma, thoracic, and pediatric examinations. The increased z-axis resolution provides isotropic multiplanar reconstructions and excellent 3-D reconstructions used in CT angiography and virtual endoscopy.

Limitations

- Overbeaming: With >4 slice scanners, the x-ray beam is wider than the total imaged width. Requires slightly higher dose to compensate.
- Cone beam artifact: With an increasing number of slices, the x-ray beam becomes more cone shaped. This increases streak artifacts on objects that are not uniform in the z-axis.

IMAGE RECONSTRUCTION (Fig. 14-49)

Several methods are available for image reconstruction; however, filtered backprojection is used almost exclusively today.

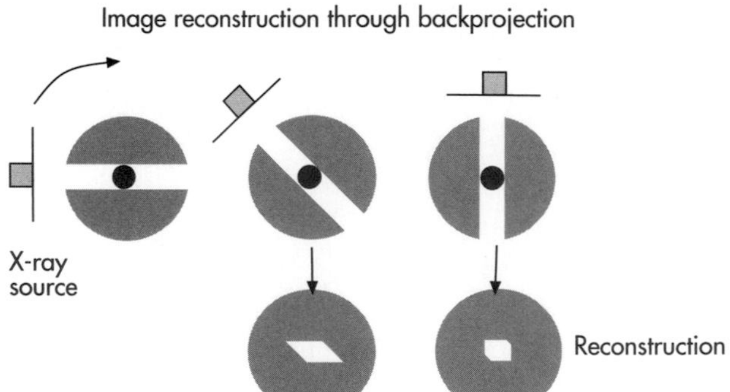

FIGURE 14-49

CT IMAGE QUALITY

Pixel size = FOV/matrix size

Voxel = volume element = pixel size × slice thickness

Factors That Affect Image Quality

OVERVIEW

Parameter	Noise	Heat	Detail	Patient Dose
FS	–	+	+	–
kV	–	+	–	+
mA	+	+	–	+
Slice thickness	+	–	+	–
Matrix size	+	–	+	–
FOV	+	–	+	–
Filter algorithm	+	–	+	–

Example: to decrease the noise on a CT scanner, one could:

- Increase mA
- Increase slice thickness (however, this causes averaging of anatomic structures and partial volume effects)
- Decrease matrix size
- Decrease FOV

Window Width and Level (Fig. 14-50)

Adjustments in window width allow one to expand any segment of the CT number scale to cover the entire gray spectrum. Contrast can therefore be easily controlled. A narrow (small) window produces high contrast (because small differences in CT numbers are viewed with large differences in gray scale). Conversely, a wide (large) window produces low contrast. Window level adjusts the center of the window width.

CT Artifacts

- Patient movement: streak artifacts
- Aliasing: streak artifacts
- Beam hardening (cupping): reduced CT numbers in center of image
- Detector imbalance or miscalibration: ring artifacts

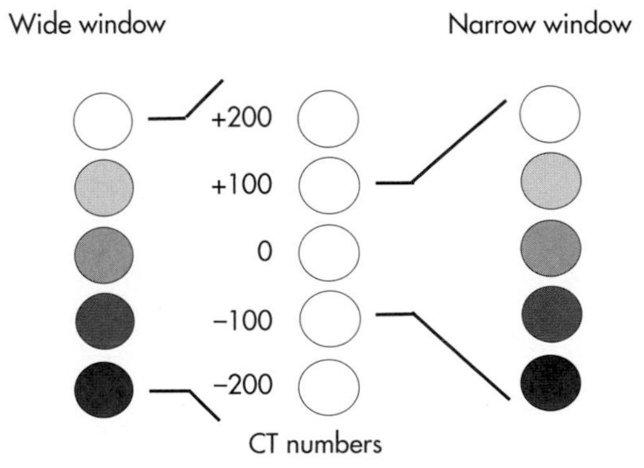

FIGURE 14-50

CT SCANNER-BASED RADIATION DOSE ESTIMATION

Two related measures of CT radiation dose are used:

- CT dose index (CTDI): represents the radiation dose of a single CT slice and is a determined using an acrylic phantom. $CTDI_{vol}$ takes into account the beam pitch factor.
- Dose Length Product (DLP): is the $CTDI_{vol}$ multiplied by the scan length (slice thickness × number of slices) in centimeters. DLP thus takes into account what is actually scanned. The effective dose in mSv is equal to the DLP × conversion factor.

Parameters contributing to CT radiation dose:

- Tube current (mA): direct linear relationship to dose
- Peak kilovoltage (kVp): direct nonlinear relationship to dose
- Pitch: indirect linear relationship to dose
- Gantry cycle time in seconds: direct linear relationship to dose

Risk Estimates for CT scans

A CT examination with an effective dose of 10 mSv has been associated with an increase in the possibility of fatal cancer of approximately 1 in 2000. This value is comparable with the natural incidence of fatal cancer in the U.S. population, about a 1 in 5 chance. The effective dose from diagnostic CT procedures are typically estimated to be in the range of 1 to 10 mSv. This range is similar to the lowest doses of 5 to 20 mSv received by some of the Japanese survivors of the atomic bombs.

Recommendations for Reducing CT Radiation Dose

1. Optimize CT settings. Based on patient weight or diameter and anatomic region of interest, evaluate whether the CT operating conditions are optimally balanced between image quality and radiation exposure.
2. Reduce tube current. With all other factors held constant, patient radiation dose is directly proportional to x-ray tube current
3. Develop and use a chart or table of tube-current settings based on patient weight or diameter and anatomical region of interest. The diameter of the patient is a better predictor than body weight of the tube current required because patient diameter better correlates with the x-ray beam attenuation in the patient.
4. Increase table increment (axial scanning) or pitch (helical scanning). If the pitch is increased, the amount of radiation needed to cover the anatomical area of interest is decreased. Some newer CT scanners automatically suggest or implement an increase in mA if pitch is increased. For these models, increasing the pitch may not result in a lower radiation dose.
5. Reduce the number of multiple scans with contrast. Often, CT scans are done before, during, and after injection of IV contrast material. When

medically appropriate, multiple exposures may be reduced by eliminating precontrast images.
6. Eliminate inappropriate referrals for CT. In some cases, conventional radiography, sonography, or magnetic resonance imaging (MRI) can be just as effective as CT, and with lower radiation exposure.

DIGITAL RADIOGRAPHY (FIG. 14-51)

GENERAL

Digital radiography (computed radiography) replaces the screen/film system of conventional radiographic techniques by processing image data in digital (computer) rather than analog form. The essential parts of a digital radiography system are the image plate and the image reader. Any conventional x-ray system can be used for x-ray generation. For additional information, see *RadioGraphics* 27:675-686, 2007.

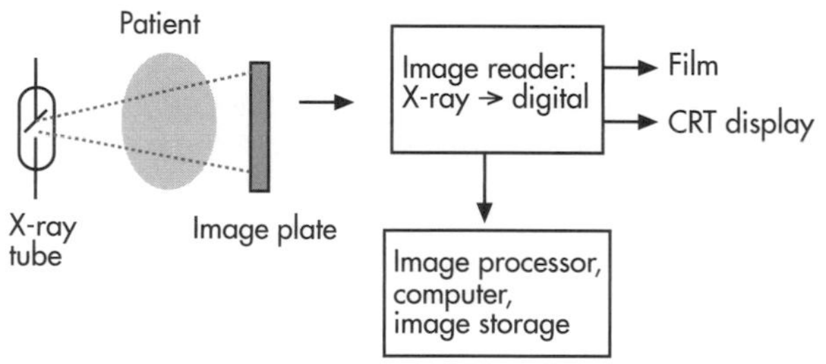

FIGURE 14-51

IMAGE PLATE (Fig. 14-52)

The image plate has features similar to those of a regular screen. However, instead of rare earth elements it contains phosphor, which can be photostimulated. The phosphor consists of europium (Eu)-containing barium (Ba) fluorohalides (Eu^{2+}:BaFX, where X is Cl, Br, I, etc.). This material changes its molecular/ionic structure by exposure to x-ray (primary stimulation), is capable of storing this information, and releases luminescence corresponding to the x-ray image when a 2nd light stimulus (reading light) is applied to the plate. Sequence of events:

1. X-ray strikes the plate
2. Eu^{2+} is ionized to Eu^{3+}

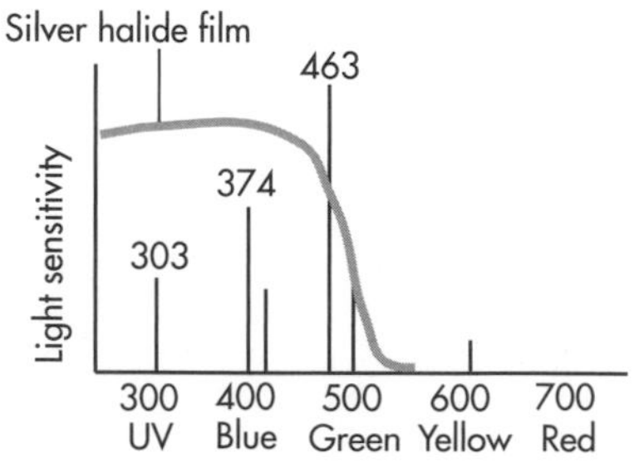

FIGURE 14-52

3. Electron from Eu is captured by the halide, producing a semistable F center (the x-ray is stored in this form)
4. If visible light (>500 nm, usually applied in the form of a scanning helium/neon laser) is now applied to the plate, the electron from the F center is released again.
5. Eu recaptures electron and causes luminescence (emission of blue-purple light at 400 nm).
   - The particle size of the Eu:BaFX in the film is 5 to 10 μm.

   The larger the grain, the greater the light-emitting efficiency. The smaller the grain, the sharper the image.

- The luminescence of Eu:BaFX decays exponentially as soon as the reading light is turned off (half-luminescence time is 0.8 μsec) (Fig. 14-53).
- Fading refers to loss of the stored x-ray information in the image plate with time. As a rule of thumb, light emission will decrease about 25% within 8 hours after acquisition of the x-ray.
- The image plate is also sensitive to other forms of radiation, including gamma rays, alpha rays, beta rays, etc. Therefore, the cassettes should be kept away from other sources of radiation.

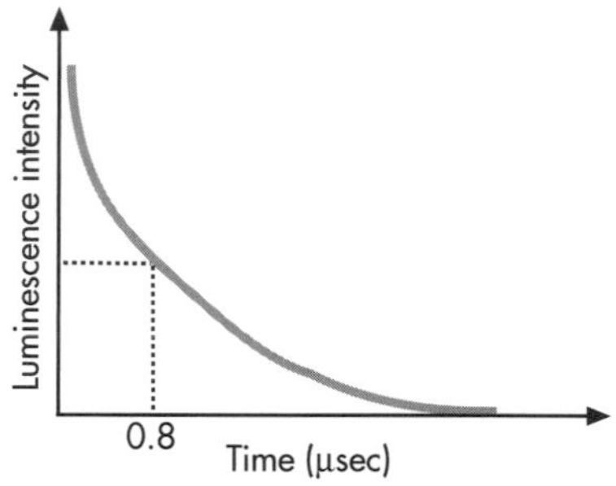

FIGURE 14-53

IMAGE READING (Fig. 14-54)

A laser scanner is used to convert the stored information of the image plate into digital signals. The photostimulated light excited by the laser spots is directed to the photomultiplier tube by high-efficiency light guides.

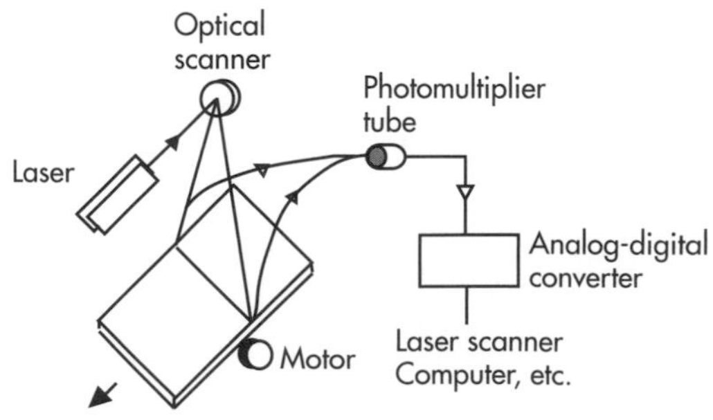

FIGURE 14-54

BINARY CODE

8	7	6	5	4	3	2	1	0
2^8	2^7	2^6	2^5	2^4	2^3	2^2	2^1	2^0
256	128	64	32	16	8	4	2	1
100000000	010000000	001000000	000100000	000010000	000001000	000000100	000000010	000000000

MEMORY

128 shades of gray (or colors) require 2^7 bits of information.

256 shades of gray (or colors) require 2^8 bits of information.

A 256 × 256 matrix image with 256 colors therefore requires 256 × 256 × 1 byte of storage = 65,536 bytes. Since 1 kB ≈ 1024 bytes, approximately 64 kB are needed. Likewise, a 512 × 512 matrix with 64 colors would also require 64 kB.

Example

What is 18 in binary code?

Answer

18 = 16 + 2 = 000010000 + 000000010 = 000010010

Nuclear Physics

ATOMIC STRUCTURE

Atoms consist of protons, neutrons, and electrons.

ATOMS

	Charge (C)	Relative Mass
Proton	$+1.6 \times 10^{-19}$	1820
Neutron	None	1840
Electron	-1.6×10^{-19}	1

Protons and neutrons are approximately 1800 times heavier than electrons. The nucleus is small in comparison to the entire atom (approximately 10^{-5} times smaller, at 10^{-13} cm in size).

Number of electrons per gram of material = Avogadro's number X Z/A

where Z = atomic number and A = atomic mass number (described below).

Electrons are ordered in shells (K < L < M < N) (Fig. 14-55) and subshells (p, q, r, etc.). The binding energy (BE) of electrons in each shell is measured in eV. One eV is the energy acquired by 1 electron accelerated through a potential of 1 volt. Rules:

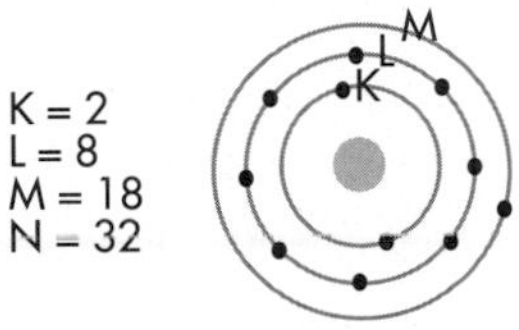

FIGURE 14-55

- BE decreases from inner to outer shell.
- For each shell, BE increases with increasing Z.
- The K-shell binding energy for elements increases roughly proportional to Z^2.

BINDING ENERGY

Element	Z	K-Shell BE (keV)	L-Shell BE (keV)
Hydrogen (H)	1	0.014	–
Carbon (C)	6	0.28	0.007
Oxygen (O)	8	0.53	0.024
Iron (Fe)	26	7.11	0.85
Iodine (I)	53	33.2*	5.19
Indium (In)	69	59.4	10.1
Tungsten (W)	74	69.5	12.1
Lead (Pb)	82	88	15.9

*Ideal keV setting for contrast-enhanced studies.

FORCES (Fig. 14-56)

Four generic types of forces are known:

- Strong (nucleus; relative strength 1)
- Electromagnetic (relative strength 10^{-2})
- Weak (relative strength 10^{-13})
- Gravitational (relative strength 10^{-39})

Charged particles in motion produce electromagnetic forces. Electromagnetic radiation is emitted during interaction of charged matter. The energy (E) of this radiation depends on its wavelength (λ), Planck's

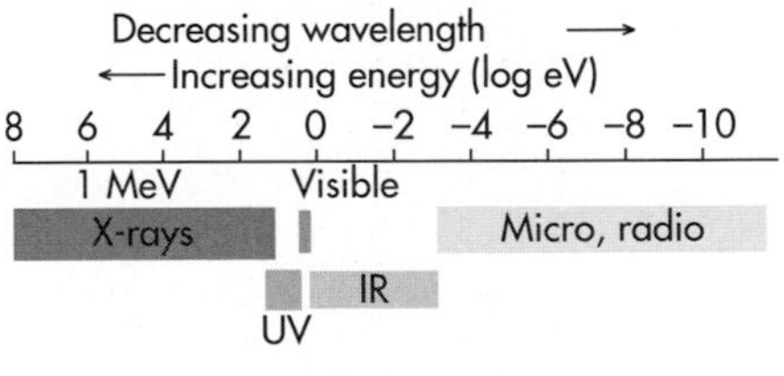

FIGURE 14-56

constant (h), and the velocity (c) of electromagnetic radiation (or light).

$$E = \frac{hc}{\lambda}$$

For the specific case in which wavelength is measured in Å and E expressed in keV, the formula is simplified to:

$$E(\text{keV}) = \frac{12.4}{\lambda(\text{Å})}$$

Energy and mass (m) are related as follows:

$$E = mc^2$$

where c = speed of light. Mass is measured in atomic mass units (amu), 1/12 the mass of a carbon atom. Mass energy is measured in million electron volts (MeV). At high kinetic energies (e.g., 20 MeV) electrons travel near the speed of light. The masses of subatomic structures are:

Electron:	0.000549 amu	0.511 MeV
Proton:	1.00727 amu	937.97 MeV % $1^0$9eV)
Neutron:	1.00866 amu	939.26 MeV

Example

What is the energy required to separate a deuteron (mass = 2.01359 amu) into its components: proton and neutron?

Answer

Mass of deuteron = 2.01359 amu; mass of proton + neutron = 2.01593 amu; difference = 0.00234 amu. This mass is equivalent to 2.18 MeV because 1 amu = 931.2 MeV.

NUCLIDES

An element is defined by the number of protons (Z). There may be multiple isotopes of a given element varying in the number of neutrons (N). The particles (Z + N) within the nucleus are referred to as nucleons. The atomic mass number (A) is given by:

A = 2 + N

NUCLIDES

	Constant	Symbol	Examples
Isotopes	Same number of protons	Z	$^{131}_{53}I$ and $^{125}_{53}I$
Isobars	Same atomic mass	A	$^{131}_{53}I$ and $^{131}_{54}Xe$
Isotones	Same number of neutrons	N	$^{13}_{7}N$ and $^{14}_{8}O$
Isomers	Different energy state	A+Z	^{99}Tc and ^{99m}Tc

An isomer refers to the excited state of a nuclide. The isomer is distinguished from its ground state by placing an asterisk after the symbol of the nuclide. The half-life of the excited state may be fairly long and is then called *metastable*, abbreviated with an *m* (e.g., ^{99m}Tc). Unstable nuclides are called *radionuclides*. Radionuclides try to become stable by emitting radiation or particles. The stability of a nuclide is determined by two opposing forces (Fig. 14-57):

- Strong forces (between a pair of nucleons: proton/proton, proton/neutron) are attractive and act when the distance is very small.
- Electrostatic forces act only between protons and are repulsive.

For a "light" stable nuclide (A <50) the number of protons roughly equals or is slightly less than the number of neutrons. In "heavy" nuclides, the number of neutrons needs to be much higher than the number of protons to maintain stability. Nuclides with neutron excess usually decay by the beta (-) decay route. The binding energy or mass defect of a nucleus is a measure of stability. The stability of a nuclide depends on the number of protons and neutrons.

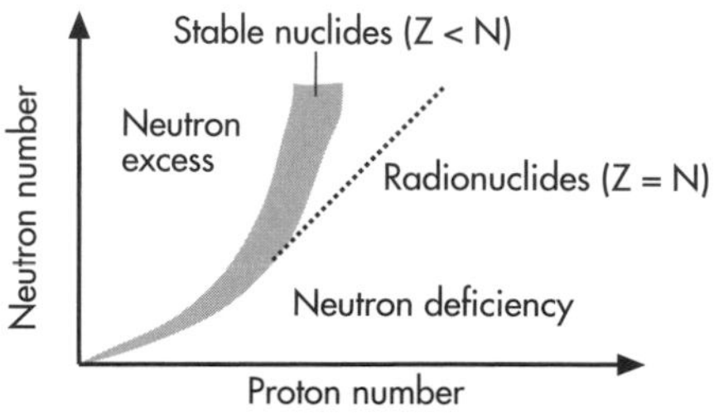

FIGURE 14-57

STABILITY

Z	N	No. of Stable Nuclei
Even	Even	164
Even	Odd	56
Odd	Even	50
Odd	Odd	4

DECAY

The three routes through which a radionuclide can decay and thus attain stability are alpha, beta, and gamma decay.

RADIONUCLIDE DECAY

Decay	Z Change	A Change	Example
Alpha	−2	−4	^{226}RA
Beta (Isobaric Transition)			
Beta (−)	+1	No change	^{131}I, ^{133}Xe
Beta (+)	−1	No change	^{11}C, ^{15}O, ^{18}F, ^{68}Ga
Electron capture	−1	No change	^{123}I, ^{201}TI, ^{111}In, ^{67}GA
Gamma (Isomeric Transition)			
Gamma emission	No change	No change	^{99m}Tc, ^{113m}In, ^{81m}Kr
Internal conversion			

ALPHA DECAY (Fig. 14-58)

An alpha particle (2 protons and 2 neutrons: $^{4}_{2}$He) is released from the nucleus during decay. The mass of alpha particles is great and their velocity relatively low so that they do not even penetrate paper. Alpha emitters are not used for imaging. An example of alpha decay is the decay of $^{222}_{88}$Ra to $^{222}_{88}$Rn. Alpha particle decay occurs most frequently with nuclides of atomic masses >150. The energy of the alpha particles is usually high (e.g., 4.78 MeV from ^{226}Ra).

BETA DECAY

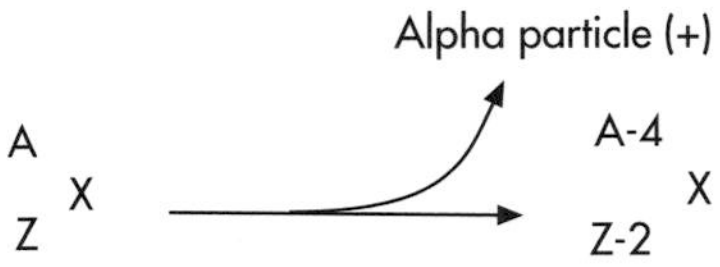

FIGURE 14-58

In this type of decay, a neutron or a proton inside the nucleus is converted to a proton or a neutron, respectively. Beta decay occurs through one of the following processes:

- Beta (–): electron emission
- Beta (+): positron emission
- Electron capture

Beta (–) Electron Emission (Figs. 14-59 and 14-60)

A neutron is transformed into a proton and, as a result, a beta particle (= electron) is released from the nucleus (not the shell) accompanied by an antineutrino (no charge). A 2-MeV beta particle has the

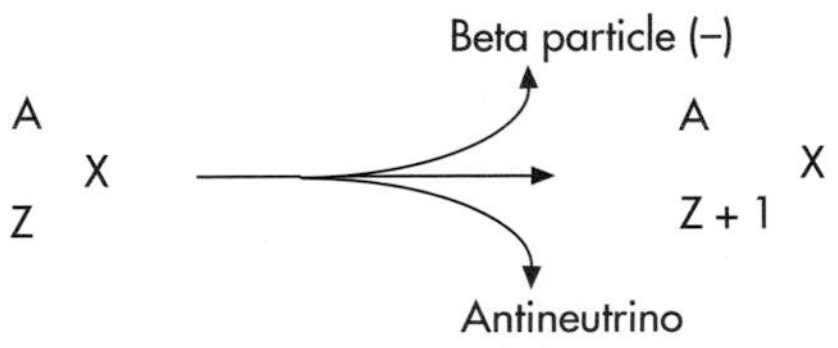

FIGURE 14-59

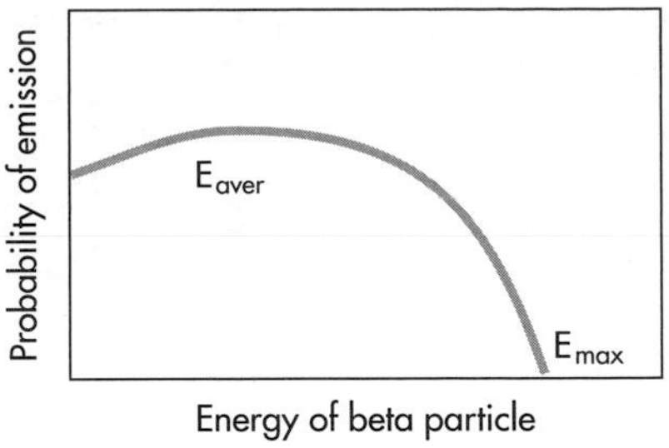

FIGURE 14-60

range of 1 cm in soft tissue and is therefore not used in imaging.

An antineutrino has no rest mass and no electrical charge. It rarely interacts with matter and therefore has little biologic significance. The kinetic energy of the emitted electron is not fixed because the total available energy in the decay is shared between the electron and the antineutrino. Therefore, the spectrum of beta (-) radiation is continuous. The maximum energy (E_{max}) differs for different beta emitters (e.g., ^{3}H decay: 0.018 MeV; ^{32}P decay: 1.71 MeV). The average electron energy (E_{aver}) is approximately one third of E_{max}.

Beta (+) Positron Emission (Fig. 14-61)

A proton is converted into a neutron and the excess energy is emitted as a pair of particles, a positron (beta +) and a neutrino. Positron emission does not occur unless >1.02 MeV (twice the mass of an electron) of energy is available to the nucleus. Positrons travel only short distances and annihilate with electrons. When this occurs, 2 photons of 511 keV are emitted in a process known as pair production. Positron-emitting isotopes (^{11}C, ^{13}N, ^{15}O, ^{18}F, ^{82}Rb) are used in PET imaging.

The emitted energy varies, ranging from 0 to E_{max}, known as the positron spectrum. E_{aver} is approximately one third of E_{max}.

Electron Capture (Positron → Neutron) (Fig. 14-62)

This route of decay is an alternative to positron decay. A proton is converted into a neutron by capturing an electron from one of the shells (K-shell: K-capture). The probability of a capture from the K-shell is generally much higher than that from the

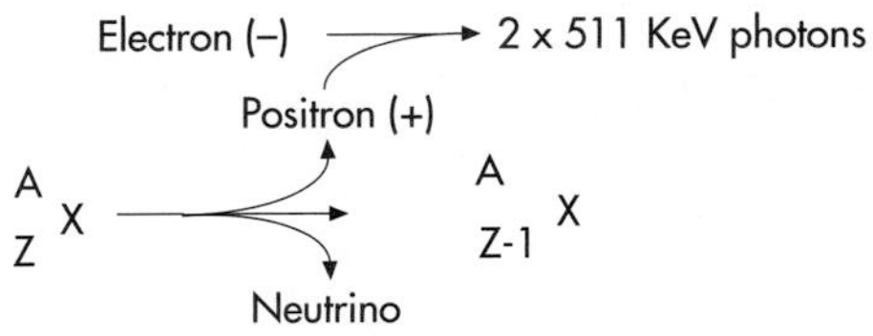

FIGURE 14-61

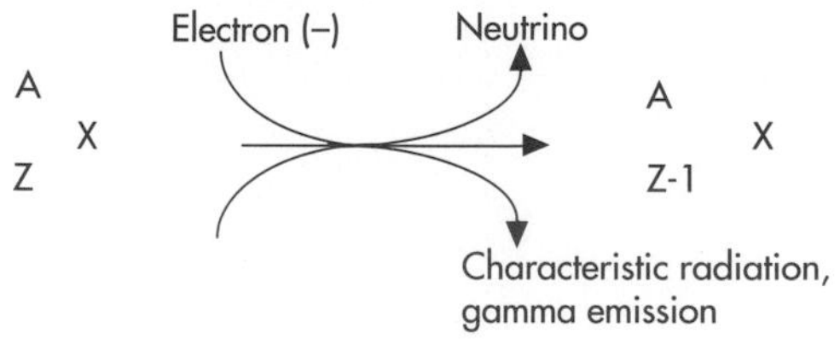

FIGURE 14-62

L- or M-shell. During electron capture a neutrino is emitted.

Electron capture may be accompanied by gamma emission and is always accompanied by characteristic radiation, both of which may be used for imaging.

GAMMA DECAY (Fig. 14-63)

In gamma decay, energy is emitted in the form of gamma rays or as a conversion (Auger) electron without change in neutrons or protons (A and Z remain constant). The decay of an excited state to a lower energy state is known as isomeric transition (as opposed to isobaric transition in the case of beta decay) and proceeds through one of two processes (within the same material):

- Gamma emission of a high-energy photon
- Internal conversion: excess energy is transferred to an orbital electron, which is ejected from its orbit.

The production of characteristic x-rays versus Auger electrons depends mostly on a nuclide's Z. The Auger process occurs most frequently in elements with low Z (<24; e.g., C, N, O), whereas x-ray emission is typical in elements with high Z (>45; e.g., I, Cs, W, Pb). Process:

- Vacancy is created by bombardment of K-shell.
- Vacancy in K-shell is filled by electron from M-shell.

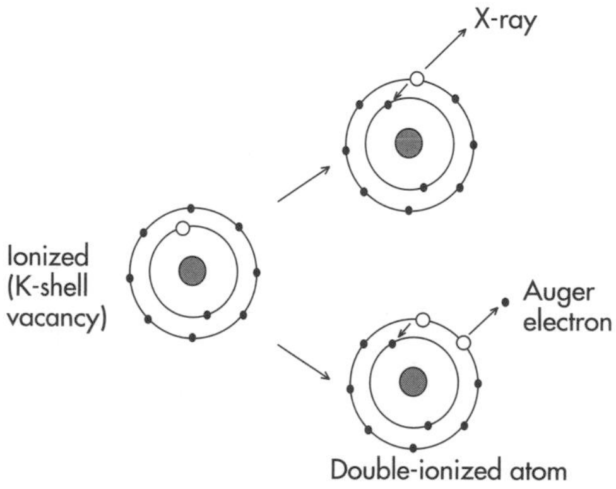

FIGURE 14-63

- Balance of energy can be emitted (x-ray) or transferred to another electron.
- A 2nd electron can be emitted (Auger electron).

Gamma emission and internal conversion usually compete with each other. The conversion ratio (α) is defined as:

α = Number of electrons emitted/Number of gamma rays emitted

A low ratio is always desirable to decrease the dose absorbed by the patient. ^{99m}Tc has a low conversion ratio: 0.1.

Example

The K-shell energy of an electron of W is 69.5 keV and the energy of an L-shell electron is 11 keV. What is the energy of an Auger electron?

Answer

69.5 keV - 11 keV = 58.5 keV is the energy released to fill up the empty K-shell.

58.5 keV - 11 keV = 47.5 keV is the energy of an Auger electron.

SUMMARY OF RADIATION PRODUCTION

Decay	Beta (-) Production	Beta (+) Production	Gamma Radiation	Auger Electron
Beta (–) decay	+	–	+*	–
Beta (+) decay	–	+	511 keV	–
Electron capture	–	–	+	–
Gamma decay	–	–	+	–
Internal conversion	–	–	–	+

*Cascade effect (e.g., ^{131}I decay).

DECAY SCHEMES (Figs. 14-64 and 14-65)

Rules:

- Nuclides are arranged in order of increasing Z from left to right.
- Negative beta decay: arrow to the right
- Positive beta decay: arrow to the left
- Electron capture: arrow to the left
- Isomeric transitions: vertical arrow
- Energy decreases from top to bottom

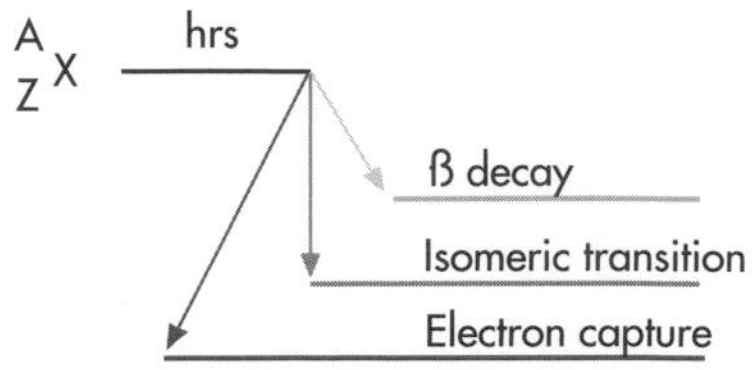

FIGURE 14-64

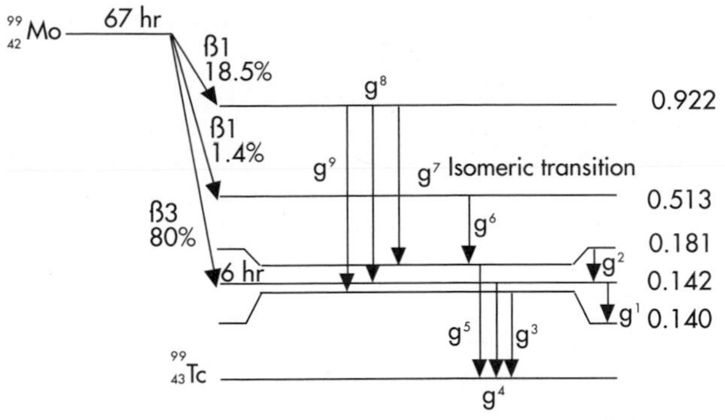

FIGURE 14-65

Decay scheme for ^{99}Mo:

- Except for the 0.142-MeV state (half-life of 6 hours) other excited states are short-lived.
- ^{99}Mo decays via beta emission to the 0.142-, 0.513-, and 0.922-MeV excited state of ^{99m}Tc.
- ^{99m}Tc decays from 0.142 MeV to 0.14 (99%) state (g1); from there it decays to ^{99}Tc via emission of a 0.14-MeV gamma ray or a corresponding conversion electron.

RANGE OF CHARGED PARTICLES

The range (R) that particles travel in matter depends on:

- Energy: the range increases with the energy of the particle; R = aE + b, where a and b are constants.
- Mass: lighter particles have longer ranges (e.g., electron > proton).
- Charge: particles with less charge travel farther; the signs of charge (negative, positive) do not affect the range.
- Density of medium: the denser the medium, the shorter the traveling range.

RADIOACTIVITY

UNITS

1 curie (Ci) = 3.7×10^{10} disintegrations per second
1 becquerel (Bq) = 1 disintegration per second
1 mCi = 37 megabecquerels
1 megabecquerel (MBq) = 27.03 μCi

NUMBER OF NUCLEI

The number of nuclei disintegrating per unit time (activity at a given time, A_t) is the product of the decay constant (c), unique for each nuclide, and the number of radioatoms (N_t) present:

$$A = c \times N$$

Because the constant for each nuclide is unique, 1 mCi of activity of ^{99}Tc and that of ^{131}I differ in the number of atoms. For example:

$$N(^{99m}\text{Tc}) = \frac{3.7 \times 10^{7}}{3.2 \times 10^{-5}} = 1.15 \times 10^{12} \text{ atoms}$$

$$N(^{131}\text{I}) = \frac{3.7 \times 10^{7}}{10^{-6}} = 3.7 \times 10^{13} \text{ atoms}$$

MASS CALCULATION

The mass (M) of a radionuclide sample is calculated from the number of atoms (N_t) and the radionuclide mass number (A):

$$M = \frac{(N_t)}{6 \times 10^{23}} \times \text{Atomic mass number (A)}$$

For example, the M of a 1 mCi ^{99m}Tc sample is:

$$M = \frac{(1.15 \times 10^{12})}{6 \times 10^{23}} \times 99 = 1.8 \times 10^{-10}\,\text{g}$$

SPECIFIC ACTIVITY

Specific activity (SA) refers to the radioactivity per gram of substance (mCi/g) and is simply the inverse of the mass calculation. SA is related to half-life ($T_{½}$):

$$SA \approx 1/(T_{½} \times A)$$

where A is the atomic mass.

HALF-LIFE

The half-life of a radionuclide refers to the time by which half of the original radioactivity (A_o) has decayed. The remaining activity (A_t) can be calculated for any time point (t) if the half-life of the isotope is known:

$$A_t = A_o e^{-(\lambda t)}$$

$$c = \frac{0.693}{T_{½}}$$

$$A_t = A_o (0.5)^{t/T}$$

Example

10 mCi of ^{99m}Tc at 8 am ($T_{½}$ 6 hours). What is the remaining activity at 5 pm?

Answer

Time difference = 9 hours. A_t = 10 mCi $(0.5)^{9/6}$ = 10 × 0.35 mCi = 3.5 mCi.

LOOK-UP TABLE FOR HALF-LIFE

Number of Half-lives	Remaining Activity
0.5	0.707
1.5	0.35
2	0.25
3	0.125
4	0.0625
6	0.0156

Example

If a source decays at 1% per hour, what is the $T_{½}$?

Answer

$$T = 0.693/1\% = 0.693/0.01 = 69.3 \text{ hours.}$$

EFFECTIVE HALF-LIFE

The disappearance of a radionuclide in the human body depends not only on its decay ($T_{phys} - T_{½}$) but also on biologic clearance (T_{bio}). The effective half-life (T_{eff}) is given by:

$$T_{eff} = \frac{T_{phys} \times T_{bio}}{T_{phys} + T_{bio}}$$

Example

^{131}I has a physical half-life of 8 days and biologic half life of 64 days. What is the effective half-life?

Answer

$$T_{eff} = (8 \times 64)/(8 + 64) = 7.1 \text{ days.}$$

CUMULATIVE ACTIVITY

$$A_{cum} = A_o \times \text{Fraction of dose to organ} \times 1.44 \times T_{eff}$$

RADIOACTIVITY STATISTICS

Three types of calculations are frequently performed:

- Confidence and limit calculations
- Count rate calculations
- Count time calculations

Confidence Calculations

For a given sample size N, the standard deviation (SD) of the sample is:

$$SD = \sqrt{N}$$

Therefore:

$$N \pm \sqrt{N} \text{ is 68\% confidence limit}$$

$$N \pm 2\sqrt{N} \text{ is 95\% confidence limit}$$

$$N \pm 3\sqrt{N} \text{ is 99\% confidence limit}$$

The fractional uncertainty for a given confidence level is:

$$\text{Uncertainty} = n\sqrt{N}/N \text{ or } n\,(SD/N)$$

where n is the number of SD (e.g., 1 for 68%, 2 for 95%, 3 for 99% level). The % uncertainty is the fractional uncertainty multiplied by 100. Because the desired uncertainty and confidence levels are usually known, the number of counts to achieve these is given by:

$$N = (n/\text{Uncertainty})^2$$

Example

Calculate the number of counts required to give a 1% uncertainty limit and 95% confidence level.

Answer

$$N = (2/0.01)^2 = 40{,}000 \text{ counts.}$$

Count Rate Calculations

The count rate (R) is obtained by dividing the total number of counts (c) by the time (t):

$$R = \frac{c}{t}$$

A frequently asked question is how to calculate the SD of the net count rate (NR) when the count rate of the sample and the background are given. The NR is simply defined as the difference between two count rates:

$$NR = R_{sample} - R_{background}$$

Example

A sample has 1600 cpm and the background is 900 cpm (each counted for 1 minute). What is the SD of the net count rate?

$$NR = \sqrt{\frac{\text{Sample (cpm)}}{\text{Time (min)}} + \frac{\text{Background (cpm)}}{\text{Time (min)}}}$$

Answer

$$NR = 1600 - 900 = 500 \text{ cpm}$$

$$SD = \sqrt{1600 + 900} = 50 \text{ cpm}$$

$$NR = 500 \pm 50 \text{ cpm}$$

Count Time Calculations

Counting time (t) to achieve a certain accuracy is given by (this formula can be deduced from the above formulas):

$$t\,(\text{min}) = 10{,}000/\text{Activity (cpm)} \times \text{Error (\%)}$$

Example

A sample has 3340 cpm. How long does this sample need to be counted to achieve an accuracy of 1%?

Answer

$t = 10,000/(3340 \times 1) \approx 3\,\text{minutes}.$

RADIONUCLIDE PRODUCTION

Radioactive material can be produced by three methods:

- Irradiation of stable nuclides in a reactor (bombardment with low-energy neutrons)
- Irradiation of stable nuclides in a cyclotron (bombardment with high-energy protons)
- Fission of heavy nuclides

REACTOR (NEUTRAL PARTICLE BOMBARDMENT)

A nuclear reactor is a source of a large number of thermal neutrons of low energy (0.025 eV). At these energies, neutrons can easily be captured by stable nuclides because there are no repulsive Coulomb forces. Note that:

- The mass number during capture increases by 1.
- There is no change in element (i.e., isotopes).
- The resulting nuclide often decays through beta (-) decay.
- Products are usually contaminated with other products (not carrier-free).

Examples (Fig. 14-66)

$^{50}_{24}\text{Cr} + ^{1}_{0}\text{n} \rightarrow ^{51}_{24}\text{Cr}$ + gamma rays

$^{98}_{42}\text{MO} + ^{1}_{0}\text{n} \rightarrow ^{99}_{24}\text{MO}$ + gamma rays

$^{132}_{25}\text{Xe} + ^{1}_{0}\text{n} \rightarrow ^{133}_{54}\text{Xe}$ + gamma rays

$$^{A}_{Z}\text{X} + ^{1}_{0}\text{n} \longrightarrow ^{A+1}_{Z}\text{X} + \text{Gamma rays}$$

FIGURE 14-66

CYCLOTRON (CHARGED PARTICLE BOMBARDMENT)

A cyclotron or accelerator is a source of a large number of high-energy (MeV) charged particles such as protons ($^{1}_{1}$P), deuterons ($^{2}_{1}$D), $^{3}_{2}$He, or alpha particles ($^{4}_{2}$He). For each charged particle, there is an energy threshold below which no interaction occurs because of Coulomb forces. The threshold is usually in the MeV range. Note that:

- There is a change of element during a cyclotron reaction.
- Cyclotron-produced isotopes are neutron deficient and decay by electron capture or positron emission.

Examples (Fig. 14-67)

$^{68}_{30}\text{Zn} + ^{1}_{1}\text{p} \rightarrow ^{67}_{31}\text{Ga} + 2\text{n}$

Indirect formation of radionuclides occurs through decay, for example:

$^{122}_{52}\text{Te} + ^{4}_{2}\text{He} \rightarrow ^{123}_{54}\text{Xe} + 3\text{n} \rightarrow ^{123}_{52}\text{I}$

$^{202}_{81}\text{T1} + \text{p} \rightarrow ^{201}_{82}\text{Pb} + 3\text{n} \rightarrow ^{202}_{81}\text{T1}$

$$^{A}_{Z}\text{X} + ^{1}_{1}\text{p} \longrightarrow ^{A}_{Z+1}\text{Y} + \text{n}$$

$$^{A}_{Z}\text{X} + ^{1}_{1}\text{p} \longrightarrow ^{A-1}_{Z+1}\text{Y} + 2\text{n}$$

FIGURE 14-67

FISSION

Fission refers to the splitting of heavy nuclei into two small nuclei of roughly half the atomic number. Virtually any element with Z = 30 to 60 has been described as the result of fission. One neutron is needed to start the reaction, but 4 neutrons are released per reaction. Fission is a good source of energy (electricity) but, if uncontrolled, causes an uncontrolled chain reaction exploited in the A-bomb. ^{131}I and ^{99}Mo are produced by fission.

Example

$^{235}_{95}\text{U} + \text{n} \rightarrow ^{141}_{56}\text{Ba} + ^{91}_{36}\text{Kr} + 4\text{n}$

COMMON DIAGNOSTIC RADIONUCLIDES

Isotope	Energy (keV)	T½	Production	Best Collimator	Biodistribution	Applications
^{99m}Tc	140	6 hr	Generator	Low	Free pertechnetate: salivary gland, stomach, bowel Sulfur colloid: liver, spleen, RES	Many; see Chapter 12
^{123}I	159, 529	13.2 hr	Accelerator, cyclotron	Low	Thyroid	Diagnostic thyroid
^{131}I	80, 284, 364, 637	8 days	Fission	Medium	Thyroid	Thyroid metastasis, ablation

COMMON DIAGNOSTIC RADIONUCLIDES—cont'd

Isotope	Energy (keV)	T½	Production	Best Collimator	Biodistribution	Applications
^{201}Tl	80, 135, 167	3 days	Cyclotron	Low	"K$^+$"-like; if high splanchnic uptake-submaximal exercise	Cardiac, brain lymphoma vs. toxoplasmosis
^{81m}Kr	191	13 sec	Generator	Medium	Lungs; can use after perfusion; expensive	$\dot{V}/\dot{Q}$ scan
^{133}Xe	80	5.2 days	Fission	Low	Lungs; inexpensive, requires negative-pressure room; use before perfusion because of scatter from ^{99m}Tc at 140 keV	$\dot{V}/\dot{Q}$ scan
^{111}In	172, 247, 392	2.8 days	Cyclotron	Medium	Spleen; use 300-500 μCi	WBC
^{67}Ga	93, 185, 300, 393	3.3 days	Cyclotron	Medium	Soft tissue (wait 3 days to clear), liver, lacrimal gland, colon, marrow	Lymphoma (replaced by PET), myocarditis, *Pneumocystis jiroveci** pneumonia
^{133}Ba	81, 276, 303, 356	10 yr	Fission	—		
^{137}Cs	622	30 yr	Fission	—		

*Now known as *Pneumocystis jiroveci* (Frenkel 1999).

GENERATORS

A radionuclide generator ("cow") is an assembly in which a long-lived radionuclide decays into a daughter nuclide. The most common generator is the ^{99}Mo/^{99m}Tc generator (Figs. 14-68 and 14-69).

The parent nuclide, ^{99}Mo, is currently produced through fission of ^{235}U (the historic production of ^{99}Mo was through neutron activation of ^{98}Mo). After ^{99}Mo production, it is chemically purified and then firmly absorbed onto an anion exchange alumina (Al_2O_3) column. The loaded column is placed in a lead container and sterilized. The daughter product, ^{99m}Tc, can be eluted from the column with saline because it is water soluble, whereas ^{99}Mo is not.

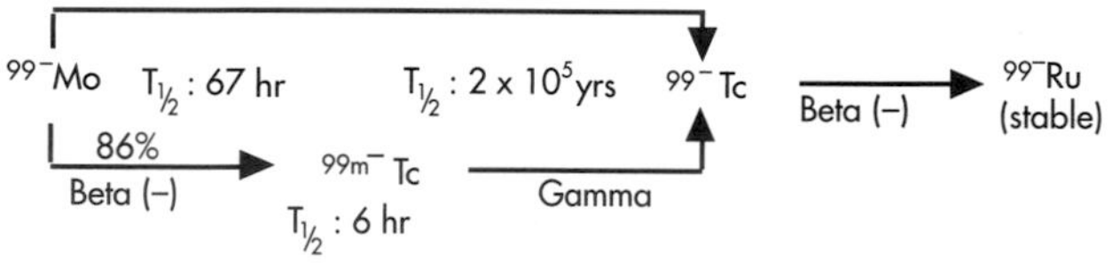

FIGURE 14-68

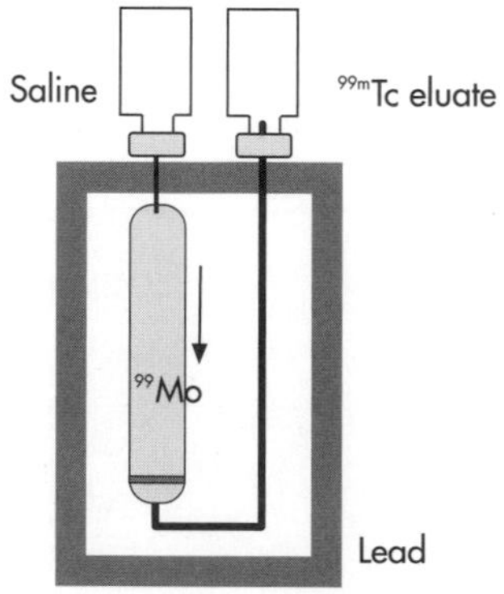

FIGURE 14-69

GENERATOR OPERATION

The adjacent graph shows the decay of ^{99}Mo (half-life of 67 hours) and the ingrowth of ^{99m}Tc (half-life of 6 hours) (Fig. 14-70). Because it takes approximately 4 daughter half-lives to reach equilibrium, this generator can be "milked" daily. If elutions are performed more frequently, less ^{99m}Tc will be available:

- 1 half-life: 44% available
- 2 half-lives: 67% available
- 3 half-lives: 80% available
- 4 half-lives: 87% available

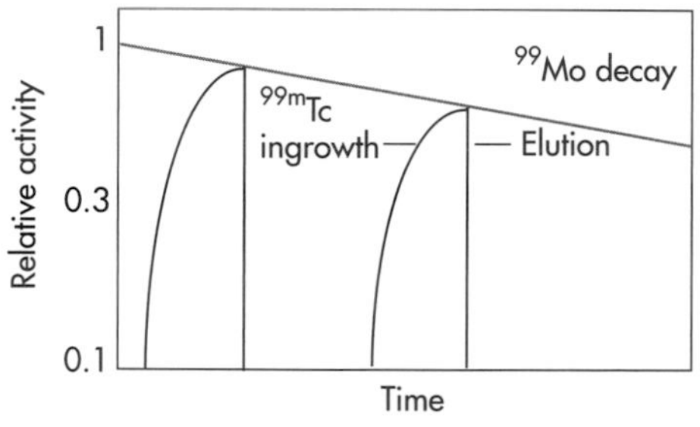

FIGURE 14-70

Equilibrium (Fig. 14-71)

The state of equilibrium between parent and daughter nuclides can be classified into two categories:

- *Transient:* half-life of parent > half-life of daughter (e.g., ^{99}Mo/^{99m}Tc generator). The activity of the daughter nuclide is slightly higher than the activity of the parent nuclide. This is true only if the decay from parent to daughter nuclide is 100% decay. For ^{99}Mo, however, only 86% decays from ^{99}Mo to ^{99m}Tc (14% decays directly to ^{99m}Tc).

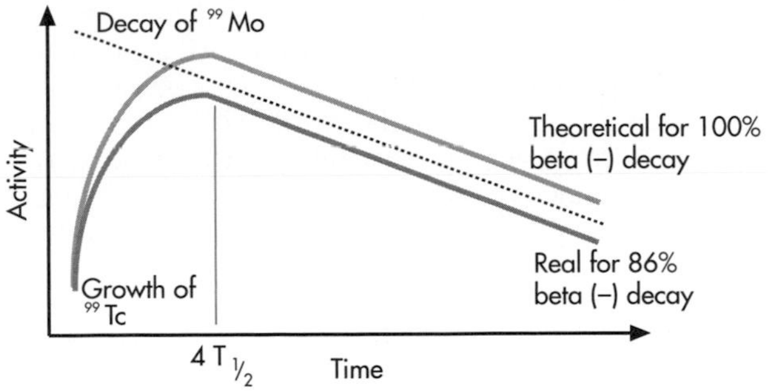

FIGURE 14-71

For this reason, the real activity of ^{99m}Tc is slightly lower than that of ^{99}Mo.

- *Secular:* half-life of parent > half-life of daughter (e.g., ^{113}Sn/^{113m}In, ^{226}Ra/^{222}Rn generators). The activities of parent and daughter nuclides become nearly equal.

Efficiency of a Generator

Efficiency (E) is defined as:

$$E = \frac{\text{Amount of activity eluted}}{\text{Daughter activity in column}}$$

^{99m}Tc generators have an approximate efficiency of 70%-90%.

DOSIMETRY

CUMULATIVE DOSE

The cumulative dose is defined as organ dose (rad) per unit of cumulative activity (μCihr) and is calculated using the S factor. This factor is a single term combining several physical and biologic terms. The S factor is unique for each radionuclide and each organ. The dose (D) in a target (T) organ from a source (S) organ is given by the formula:

$$D(T \leftarrow S) = 1.44 \times \text{Activity in source organ} \times T_{eff} \times \text{S factor}$$

$$D(T \leftarrow S) = A_{cum}\,(\mu\text{Cihr}) \times \text{S factor}$$

Example

What is the radiation dose to liver and testes of 2 mCi of Tc colloid (assuming 90% of activity distributes to the liver and is retained there indefinitely)? S (liver ← liver) = 4.6 × 10^{-5}; S (testes ← liver) = 6.2 × 10^{-8}. T_{eff} = 6 hours.

Answer

$$\text{Activity in source organ (liver)} = 0.9 \times 2.0\ \text{mCi} = 1.8\ \text{mCi}$$

$$D(\text{liver} \leftarrow \text{liver}) = 1.44 \times 1800 \times 6 \times 4.6 \times 10^{-5} = 0.72\ \text{rad}$$

$$D(\text{testes} \leftarrow \text{liver}) = 1.44 \times 1800 \times 6 \times 6.2 \times 10^{-8} = 0.001\ \text{rad}$$

Dose

$$\text{Dose} = 3.07 \times \text{Activity}\ (\mu\text{Ci/g}) \times T_{eff}(h) \times \text{Energy of radiation (MeV)}$$

DETECTORS

TYPES OF DETECTORS

- Gas-filled detectors (ionization chambers, proportional counters, Geiger-Müller counters)
- Scintillation counters (NaI crystal counters)
- Solid state detectors (GeLi counters)

Efficiency (E) of a Detector

OVERVIEW OF DETECTORS

Detector	Efficiency	Dead Time	Energy Discrimination	Use
Ionization chambers	Very low	NA	None	Dose calibration
Proportional counters	Very low	msec	Moderate	Not used
Geiger counters	Moderate	msec	None	Radiation survey
Scintillation counters	High	μsec	Moderate	Universal detector
Solid state counters	Moderate	<1 μsec	Very good	Neutron activation

$$E = \frac{\text{Number of rays detected}}{\text{Number of incident rays}}$$

Dead Time of a Detector (Fig. 14-72)

Refers to the time interval after a count in which a detector is insensitive to radiation. There are 2 types of detectors:

- Paralyzable detector: 2nd ray prolongs the dead time. For example, if the dead time is 100 μsec and ray arrives after 30 μsec, the detector is insensitive for 130 μsec.

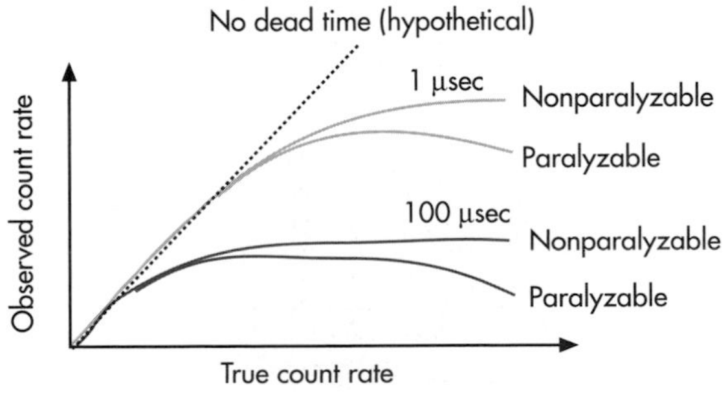

FIGURE 14-72

- Nonparalyzable detector: 2nd ray does not prolong the dead time; if dead time is 100 μsec and the ray arrives after 30 μsec, the detector is still only insensitive for 100 μsec.

GAS-FILLED DETECTORS (Fig. 14-73)

Detectors contain inert gas (argon), usually doped with ether to quench luminescence. Initially an incident beam will create an ion pair, which then produces a current. The amount of current depends on several factors:

- Voltage difference applied (most important)
- Electrodes: separation, shape, geometry
- Gas: type, pressure, temperature

5 distinct responses to increasing voltage exist in detectors (Fig. 14-74):

- Region 1 (<100 V). Voltage is low enough so that ion pairs combine before they reach the electrodes.
- Region 2 (100 to 250 V). Voltage is sufficiently high to attract all ion pairs produced by radiation. Changes in voltage do not increase the current (ionization chambers are therefore stable and reliable). Ionization chambers (i.e., dose calibrators) work in this voltage range.
- Region 3 (250 to 500 V). Voltage is high enough so that secondary ion pairs are produced by collision. Current varies considerably with change in voltage. Proportional detectors operate in this voltage range (rarely used in nuclear medicine).
- Region 4 (750 to 900 V). Voltage is so high that the beam causes a discharge (ionization, excitations, UV light production) in the gas. This region is very sensitive to radiation and is ideal for radiation surveys (Geiger-Müller counters operate in this range). After the discharge, the voltage has to be reduced to zero so that discharge can no longer be sustained. In addition, alcohols, ethers, or halogens are added to the inert gas to quench luminescence. It takes 50 to 200 μsec to quench the discharge (dead time of the detector). Maximum usable count rate is 50,000/minute. Ion recombination may be a problem in this region.
- Region 5 (>900 V). Voltage is so high that radiation is not necessary to produce discharges.

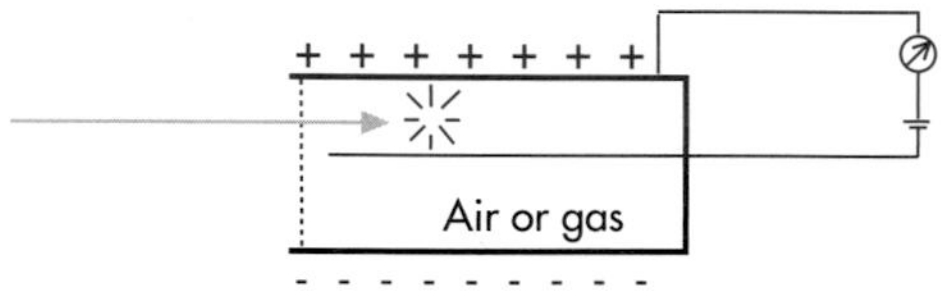

FIGURE 14-73

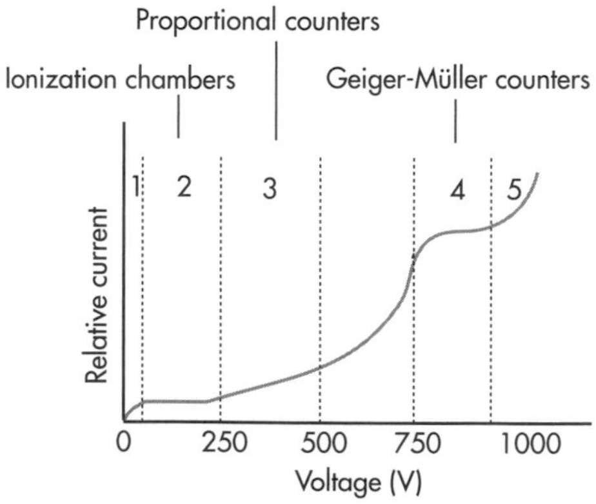

FIGURE 14-74

PHOTOMULTIPLIER (PM) TUBES (Fig. 14-75)

The most common PM tubes contain sodium iodide (NaI) crystals (moderate density, effective atomic number) that are doped with small amounts of thallium, which enhance light output tenfold. NaI crystals are hygroscopic and therefore have to be sealed in aluminum. Dynodes within vacuum PM tubes amplify the primary signal (a photon) by creating secondary electrons. Typically 10^5 to 10^8 electrons are generated for each incident photon.

The amplifier increases the millivolt peaks of the PM tube to volt peaks. The pulse height selector (PHS) is an electronic device that allows the operator to select specific voltage pulses within a preselected range. The PHS is important for:

- Discriminating scatter from characteristic radiation
- Discriminating different peaks (and thus isotopes) in a given spectrum

The response of a PM tube to monochromatic radiation is shown in the graph (Fig. 14-76):

$$\text{Energy resolution (\%)} = \frac{\text{FWHM} \times 100}{\text{Peak voltage}}$$

where FWHM = full width at half maximum. In good detector systems, the energy resolution ranges from 10% to 14% (140 keV of ^{99m}Tc). Besides the photopeak

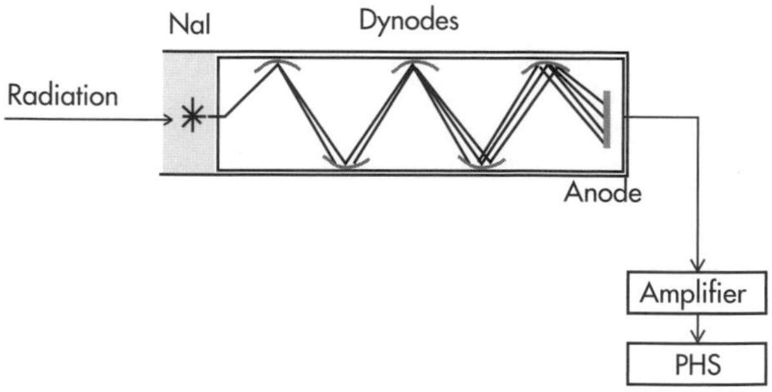

FIGURE 14-75

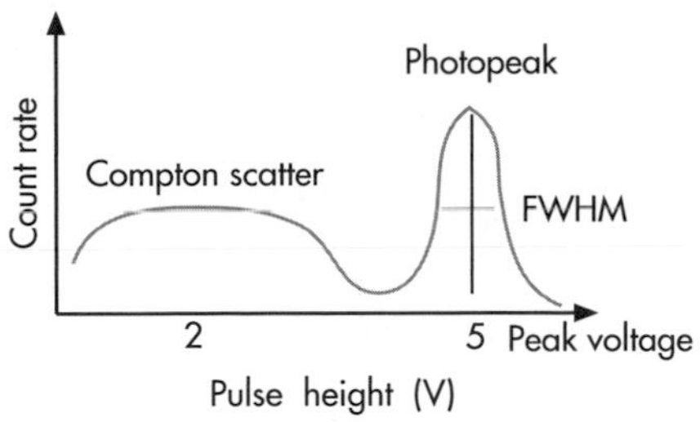

FIGURE 14-76

and the Compton plateau, other peaks that can be detected in PM tubes include:

- K-escape peak: lies 28 keV below the photopeak of the gamma rays (photoelectric interactions of the K-shell of I = 28 keV)
- Summation peak: refers to additional peaks corresponding to the sum of the individual gamma ray energies. Summation peaks are artifactual.
- Back-scattered and lead x-ray peaks result from lead shielding.

WELL COUNTERS

The total efficiency (E_{tot}) of a well counter is given as the product of geometric and intrinsic efficiency:

$$E_{tot} = E_{geom} \times E_{int}$$

where E_{int} = number of rays detected/number of rays incident on detector and E_{geom} = number of rays incident on detector/number of rays emitted by source. The accuracy of a dose calibrator should be better than ± 5%. The geometric efficiency depends on:

- The geometric arrangement of sample in the detector
- The count rate: high count rates (>10^6 cpm) underestimate the true count rate because of the dead time
- Sample volume: high sample volumes (>2 mL) lower the efficiency

Calculation of Photopeak Count Rate

True count rate = Number of rays emitted × E_{tot}

Example

What is the count rate for ^{99m}Tc (140 keV; 1 μCi)?

Answer

Because 1 μCi = 37,000 cps (1 mCi = 37 MBq), the count rate is $3.7 \times 10^4 \times 60$ sec/min $\times 0.84 = 1.86 \times 10^6$.

LIQUID SCINTILLATION DETECTORS

Liquid scintillation counters are mainly used for counting beta-emitting elements (^{3}H, ^{14}C, N, O, P, S) because their radiation (charged particles) has a short range in solids and liquids. Liquid scintillation detectors differ from well counters in that the PM tube is within a light-tight box. The substance to be "counted" (e.g., tissue sample) is incubated with a chemical scintillator (PPO, BBOT) whose purpose is to emit light, which is then detected by the PM tube.

SCANNERS

ANGER CAMERA (FIG. 14-77)

A typical camera consists of a 0.25- to 0.5-inch-thick NaI crystal (total diameter usually 11 to 20 inches) and multiple PM tubes.

- Small FOV, portable cameras: 37 PM tubes
- Large FOV, older cameras: 55 PM tubes
- Large FOV, modern cameras: 55 to 91 PM tubes

Specially designed Anger circuits allow the spatial localization of incident photons. The PM tube closest to the incident light beam will receive the largest amount of signal, and the adjacent PM tube will receive less. Resolution is approximately 1 cm at 10-cm depth. The conversion efficiency to light photons is 10%-15%.

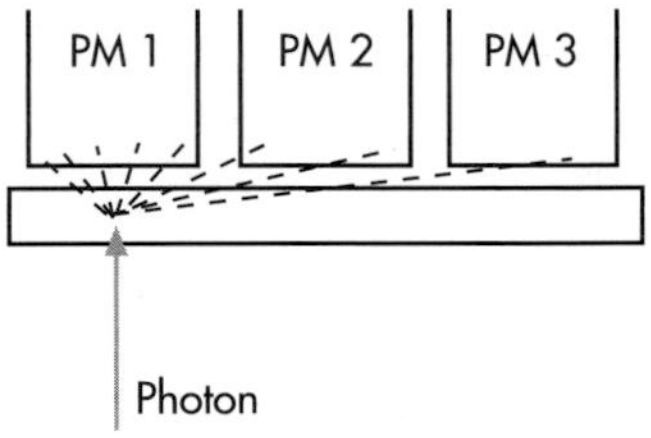

FIGURE 14-77

Information Density

Information density (ID) refers to the number of counts per unit area of crystal surface.

$$ID = \frac{\text{Counts}}{\text{Crystal area (cm}^2\text{)}}$$

Crystal area = $\pi \times$ Radius^2

Image Uniformity

- The most important source of image inhomogeneity is electronic (e.g., response to PM tubes).
- To keep inhomogeneities to a minimum, scintillation cameras must be tuned. Because the PM tube gain may drift (because of fluctuations in voltage), it is important that the uniformity of response be checked routinely.
- Desirable image inhomogeneity should be <3% for conventional imaging and <1% for SPECT and PET.

COLLIMATOR (Fig. 14-78)

A collimator reduces the amount of scattered photons (usually 50% of all photons are scattered) and defines the geometric FOV. For imaging purposes, only primary photons that arise from the object and

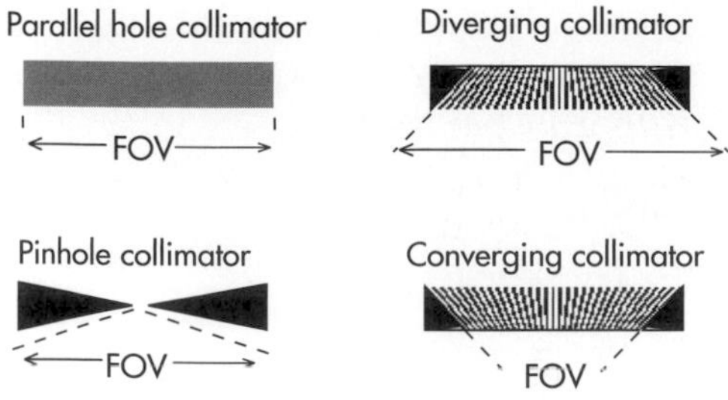

FIGURE 14-78

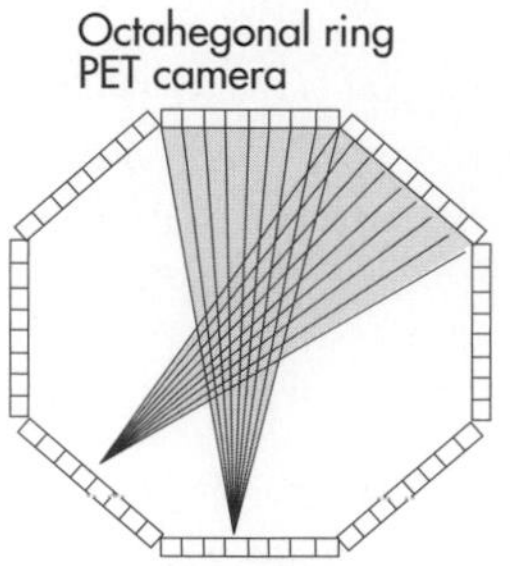

FIGURE 14-79

that travel parallel to the axis of the collimator are useful. A variety of collimators are available. Parallel collimators have the advantage of no distortion and no magnification. Converging collimators are useful for small organs (magnification views), and diverging collimators may be used for organs larger than the size of the crystal. Pinhole collimators have the best resolution; this is the reason why they are used for thyroid imaging. The resolution (R) of a collimator is given by:

$$R = \frac{(F + L + c)}{L}$$

where d is the hole diameter, F the distance of the source from the collimator, L the length, and c the thickness of the crystal. The best resolution is achieved at the face of the collimator.

Pearls

- Parallel collimators are used for most imaging tasks.
- Converging and diverging collimators are no longer in use because the magnification can be done electronically.

SINGLE-PHOTON EMISSION COMPUTED TOMOGRAPHY (SPECT)

SPECT uses parallel hole collimators mounted on a camera head that rotates (32 or 64 stops) around the patient like a CT. Software programs allow reconstruction of slices. Problems inherent in SPECT include:

- Sensitivity for each pixel is not the same.
  - Sensitivity of collimator is depth dependent.
  - Radiation originating from different tissues is attenuated at different degrees.
- Difficult to collect data for a specific column
  - Compton scattering
  - Diverging field of collimator (therefore special collimators with longer holes are used)

POSITRON EMISSION TOMOGRAPHY (PET) (Fig. 14-79)

PET imaging uses the detection of annihilation coincidence. Annihilation is based on the fact that two photons of 511 keV are emitted in opposite directions after the annihilation of a positron with an electron. Positron-emitting radionuclides are ^{11}C, ^{13}N, ^{15}O, ^{18}F, and ^{68}Ga. The two emitted photons can be detected by a pair of detectors. A coincidence circuit records only those events that are detected within a narrow time interval (usually 5 to 20 ns). Photons registered in only 1 detector but not the other are rejected electronically. This mechanism defines a sensitive volume between the detectors; hence, the term *electronic collimation* has been used (no physical collimators are used in PET).

Spatial Resolution

The spatial resolution of PET systems (system resolution is typically 4 to 8 mm) depends on (1) detector resolution and (2) positron range and angular spread of photons. The range of positrons in tissues is determined by their energy and is thus characteristic of a radionuclide (e.g., 2.8 mm for ^{18}F, 3.8 mm for ^{11}C, 9 mm for ^{68}Ga). Deviation from the exact 180° emission of annihilation photons results from the fact that the positron and electron are not completely at rest when annihilation occurs.

Detector Systems (Fig. 14-80)

511-keV annihilation photons require detectors with greater stopping power than is provided by conventional NaI crystals. Bismuth germanate (BGO) is currently the preferred detector material. BaF_2 has the advantage of a shorter decay time but the disadvantage of lower detection efficiency. Gadolinium orthosilicate (GOS) has favorable properties of both detector materials but is expensive.

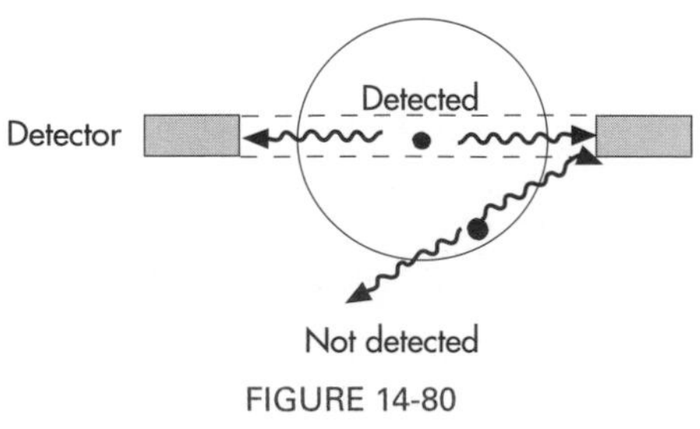

FIGURE 14-80

Sensitivity

To increase sensitivity, multiple pairs of detectors are mounted on a ring or hexagonal array (multiple coincidence detection) where each detector is in coincidence with a large number of detectors on the opposite side. This arrangement provides a 10-fold to 20-fold increase in sensitivity when compared with SPECT.

QUALITY ASSURANCE (QA)

QA FOR PLANAR IMAGING

The three most commonly tested quality parameters are:

- Peaking
- Field uniformity
- Spatial resolution

Peaking

Refers to tuning of the energy window so that it is centered around the photopeak of the isotope:

- Performed daily
- Ensures that the PHS is correctly set on the desired photopeak
- Method
  1 to 2 mCi ^{99m}Tc
  Set 140 keV, 20% window

Field Uniformity (Fig. 14-81)

This test is performed daily with the automatic uniformity correction turned on and turned off.

- Use flood field image; this may be done with a point source (e.g., ^{99m}Tc without collimator) 2 m away from the camera and with the collimator removed. Alternatively this can be achieved with a disk flood source (^{57}Co) with and without collimator.
- If ^{57}Co is used, the photopeak has still to be adjusted with ^{99m}Tc.

The uniformity correction is done on every image according to the flood field as a guide. Field nonuniformity can be due to:

- Crystal: may be damaged
- PM tube: uneven gain, old PM tubes
- Electronics: nonuniform correction, not centered on photopeak window
- Dirt on screen
- Camera: dirt on lens

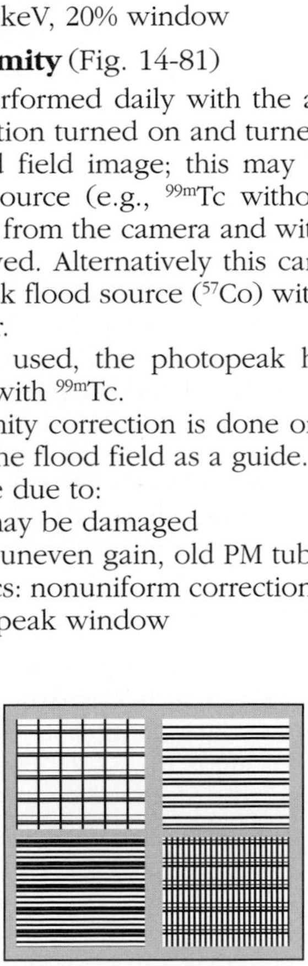

FIGURE 14-81

Resolution and Linearity

Measurements are performed with a bar phantom. The spacing between closest bars is usually 3 mm. Linearity is ensured when lines appear straight.

QA FOR SPECT

- Rotation coordinates calibration. Shift of a few pixels may produce ring artifacts.
- Image uniformity has to be better than 1% (for conventional imaging <3%).
- Uniformity is tested at different angles of tube rotation.

QA FOR DOSE CALIBRATOR

Precision and Accuracy

Measure ^{57}Co (122 keV; near Tc peak) and ^{137}Cs (662 keV; near Mo peak) phantoms daily. Fluctuation should be <5%.

Linearity

Linearity is measured quarterly by repeated measurement of a ^{99m}Tc sample over 48 hours. The decay curve should give a straight line on semilog paper. Accuracy should be <5%.

Radiobiology

GENERAL (Fig. 14-82)

Ionizing radiation consists of either electromagnetic waves, which are indirectly ionizing (x-rays and gamma rays), or particulates, which are directly ionizing (alpha and beta rays, neutrons). Because all

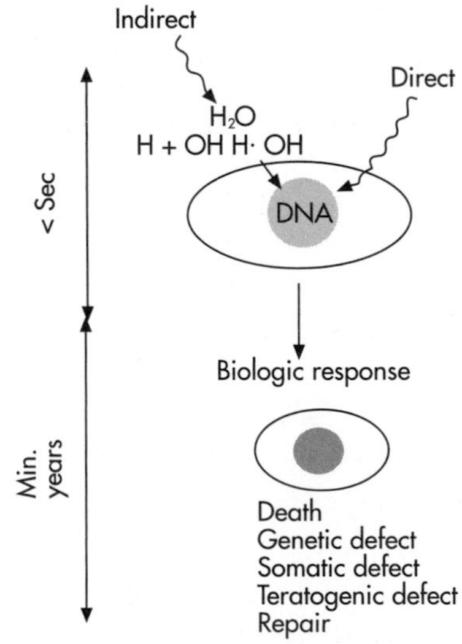

FIGURE 14-82

radiations initiate damage by ionization, differences are quantitative rather than qualitative. In vivo energy deposition occurs by ionization (minimum energy necessary: 13 eV) of cellular molecules:

- Total energy absorbed per gram of tissue is small, but the energy transferred to isolated molecules may be relatively large; a dose of 400 rad/human is severely damaging, but if this energy were to be transferred into heat it would only heat the tissue by 10^{-3}°C.
- Relatively few molecules per gram of water or tissue are ionized by 400 rad, but each ionization is very harmful to molecules.
- Ionization initiates a chain of chemical reactions that may ultimately result in radiation damage.

LINEAR ENERGY TRANSFER (LET) (Fig. 14-83)

LET is defined as the ratio of energy transferred by a charged particle (dE_{local}) to the target atoms along its path through tissue (dx). In other words, LET is a measure of the density of ionizations along a radiation beam.

$$\text{LET}(\text{keV}/\mu\text{m}) = dE_{local}/dx$$

Higher LET radiations (particles: alpha particles, protons, and neutrons) produce greater damage in a biologic system than lower LET radiations (electrons, gamma rays, x-rays). For example, radiation cataracts are 10 times more likely to occur after neutron radiation than after x-ray radiation, with the same amount of absorbed dose. The relationship between relative biologic effectiveness (RBE) and LET is shown in the adjacent graph.

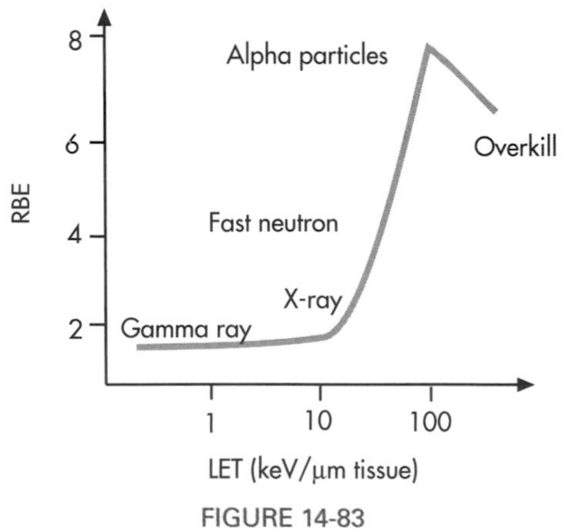

FIGURE 14-83

RADIATION UNITS

Different units and quantities are used to quantify radiation.

OVERVIEW OF UNITS

Quantity	Conventional	SI Unit	Conversions
Exposure	Roentgen (R)	Coulomb/kg of air (C/kg)	1 C/kg = 3876 R 1 R = 258 μCi/kg
Dose	Rad	Gray (Gy)	1 Gy = 100 rad
Dose equivalent	Rem	Sievert (Sv)	1 Sv = 100 rem
Activity	Curie (Ci)	Becquerel (Bq)	1 mCi = 37 MBq

EXPOSURE

This is the most common measure to determine the amount of radiation delivered to an area. The conventional unit is roentgen (R) and the SI unit is coulomb (C) per kilogram. Exposure can be directly measured by quantitating the amount of ionization of air in an ionization chamber placed in an x-ray beam. By definition, one R produces 2.08×10^9 ion pairs per cubic centimeter. Since 1 cm^3 of air has a mass of 0.001293 g, 1 R = 2.58×10^{-4} C (of ionization)/kg of air. The exposure falls inversely to the square of the distance from the radiation source:

$$\text{Exposure at distanced} = \frac{\text{Dose at unit distance} \times 1}{\text{Distance}^2}$$

The exposure rate of a gamma-emitting source rate is determined by:

$$\text{Exposure rate} = \frac{(\text{Activity} \times \text{Rate constant})}{\text{Distance}^2(\text{cm}^2)}$$

Example

What is the exposure rate for hands 5 cm away from 20 mCi of ^{99m}Tc for 2 minutes (typical dose during preparation of a dose for bone scintigraphy)? Rate constant for ^{99m}Tc is 0.7 Rcm^2/mCi/hr.

Answer

$$\text{Rate} = (20\,\text{mCi}) \times (0.7\,\text{Rcm}^2/\text{mCi/hr})/(5\,\text{cm})^2$$
$$= 0.56\,\text{R/hr or } 18.7\,\text{mR in 2 minutes.}$$

ABSORBED DOSE (Fig. 14-84)

The human body absorbs approximately 90% of diagnostic radiation to which it is exposed. Absorbed dose is defined as the quantity of radiation energy absorbed per unit mass of tissue. The conventional unit is the rad and the SI unit is the gray (Gy):

$$1\,\text{Gy} = 100\,\text{rad} = 1\,\text{J/kg} = 10{,}000\,\text{erg/g}$$
$$1\,\text{rad} = 100\,\text{erg/g} = 0.01\,\text{J/kg}$$

For a specific photon energy spectrum and type of tissue, the absorbed dose is proportional to the exposure.

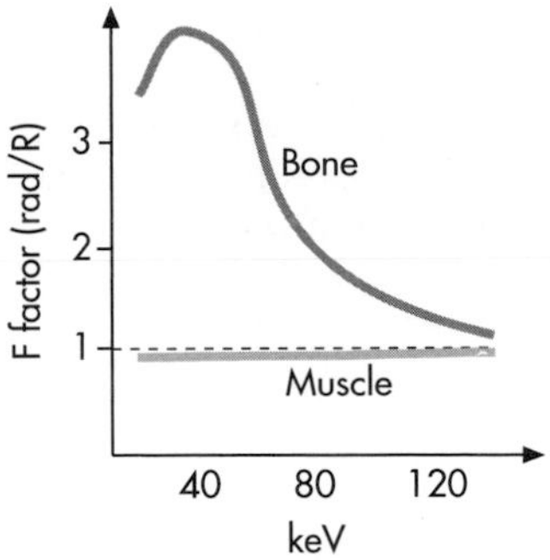

FIGURE 14-84

The F factor is the ratio between absorbed dose (rad) and exposure (R) and thus allows conversion. Rules of thumb for F factor:

- Depends on the energy of radiation
- Different for different materials but constant for air
  - Air: 0.873 rad/R
  - Bone: 3 rad/R for diagnostic x-rays (range is 2.8 to 4+)
  - Soft tissue: 1 rad/R for diagnostic x-rays (range is 2.8 to 4+)
- Greater for high-Z materials and for low-energy photons

The integral dose is the total amount of energy absorbed in the body. It is determined not only by absorbed dose values but also by the total mass of tissue exposed. The conventional unit is the gram-rad (= 100 erg of absorbed energy), and the SI unit is the joule (J):

$$1\,\text{J} = 10^7\,\text{erg} = 10{,}000\,\text{gram-rad}$$

BIOLOGIC IMPACT

Not all types of radiation have the same biologic impact. Two quantities are associated with biologic impact: dose equivalent (H) and RBE. H is the most commonly used measure to record personnel exposure. The conventional unit of H is the rem and the SI unit is the sievert (Sv). 1 Sv = 100 rem.

H (rem) = Dose (rad) × W_R × Dose distribution factor (DF) × Other modifying factors

where W_R is the radiation weighting factor, previously known as the quality factor (NCRP report 91, 1987). The W_R was introduced in 1991 (ICRP report 60, 1991) and updated in 1993 (ICRP report 116, 1993). W_R is defined as an average LET-dependent RBE factor to be used as a common scale in calculating biologically effective doses in humans.

RADIATION WEIGHTING FACTOR (WR)

LET (keV/μm) in Water	W_R	Typical Radiations
≤3.5	1	Beta, gamma, and x-rays
7-23	5-10	Slow neutrons
23-53	20	Fast neutrons
53-175	20	Alpha particles, heavy nuclei

The RBE of a radiation for producing a given biologic effect is defined as:

$$\text{RBE} = \frac{D_{\text{x-ray}}}{D_{\text{radiation}}}$$

where $D_{\text{x-ray}}$ is the dose of standard radiation (250-kVp x-ray) needed to produce a biologic effect and $D_{\text{radiation}}$ is the dose of the test radiation needed to produce the same biologic effect. Because x-rays are used as a reference, the RBE of x-rays is 1.

RADIATION EFFECT

Stages of radiochemical reactions:

- Physical damage (primary event: ionization) takes ~10^{-12} seconds.
- Physiochemical damage (production of free radicals) takes ~10^{-10} seconds.
- Chemical damage (DNA, RNA changes) takes ~10^{-6} seconds.
- Biologic damage lifetime, lasts minutes to years

TARGET THEORY OF RADIATION EFFECT

The target theory assumes that the radiation effect is due to alteration of a sensitive site within a cell (e.g., DNA). According to this theory, the ionizing event must involve this site directly and all other ionizations (those outside the sensitive site) are ineffective. The target theory was originally developed to explain observed dose-response curves (biologic end-effect) purely on the basis of the physical nature of the radiation and the statistical distribution of ionizing events in the cell. This theory is now judged to be outdated because it is known that ionizing radiation produces free radicals in cells (see Indirect Theory section, next).

INDIRECT THEORY OF RADIATION EFFECT

This theory assumes that the effect of radiation on target molecules is mediated through free radicals produced by ionization; radical formation requires the presence of water. Evidence for an indirect effect of radiation comes from Dale's experiments with the enzyme carboxypeptidase. He found that the number of inactivated enzyme molecules in solution was independent of the concentration. Free radical reactions include:

Ionization reactions (primary event)

- $H_2O \rightarrow H_2O^+ + e^-$
- $H_2O + e^- \rightarrow H_2O^-$

Radical reactions (where OH and H are free radicals)

- $H_2O^+ \rightarrow H^+ + OH\cdot$
- $H_2O \rightarrow OH + H\cdot$

Factors modifying aqueous radiochemical reactions:

- LET
  - High LET (i.e., particulate radiation) favors formation of molecular products (forward reactions): $H_2O \rightarrow \cdot H + \rightarrow \cdot OH\ H_2$ or H_2O_2
  - Low LET favors OH and H radical formation and recombination of ·OH and ·H to water
- Oxygen effect
  - High oxygen tension leads to formation of O_2 and HO_2 radicals, increases formation of H_2O_2, and tends to prevent back-reactions
  - Sensitizing effect of oxygen (radiosensitizer) in complex biologic systems is probably due to reaction with organic free radicals leading to peroxidation: ($R\cdot \rightarrow + O_2 \rightarrow RO\cdot_2 \rightarrow$ R-OOH
- Radioprotectors (scavengers of free radicals): cysteine, cystamine, cysteamine (sulfhydryls)

REACTIONS IN MACROMOLECULES

Production of organic free radicals:

- Aqueous radicals usually produce organic radicals by abstraction of hydrogen atoms.
- Free radicals may break up CH, CO, CN, CS, C=C bonds.
- Fate of organic radicals
  - Repair: recombination with hydrogen radical
  - Reaction with another organic radical (on same or different molecule) can lead to rearrangements of molecules, degradation, polymerization, cross-linking, etc.
  - Combination with oxygen results in abnormal (damaged) molecule.
- Effects on DNA
  - Chain breakage at sugar-phosphate bond producing single- or double-strand breaks
  - Specific degradation of bases (pyrimidine or purine)
  - Disruption of sugar-based bond with release of base from polynucleotide chain leading to apurinic or apyrimidinic sites in DNA

Energy transfer:

- Energy from initial ionization may be transferred by several chemical reactions to a target molecule (i.e., different intermediate organic radicals are formed).
- In a large molecule, the energy may be transferred from the point of initial damage to a sensitive site of the molecule.

CELLULAR DAMAGE

Law of Bergonie and Tribondeau: cell radiosensitivity is related to:

- Degree of cell differentiation
- Degree of mitotic activity

Differentiated cells (e.g., hepatocytes, nerve cells) are less sensitive to radiation from undifferentiated cells such as erythroblasts and myeloblasts. Order of radiosensitivity: myeloblasts, erythroblasts > lymphocytes (B > T cells) > granulocytes > intestinal crypt cells > nerve cells.

DNA Repair Processes in Cells

Mammalian cells possess efficient molecular processes for repairing radiation-induced DNA damage. The efficiency and accuracy of these processes may determine in large part the nature and the extent of the ultimate biologic damage (i.e., survival versus mutations). Repair pathways:

- Rejoining of DNA strand breaks
- Excision-resynthesis repair of damaged DNA base (unscheduled DNA synthesis)
- Repair associated with DNA replication (postreplication repair)

Cell Cycle and Radiosensitivity (Fig. 14-85)

Cells are most radiosensitive when they are in mitosis (M phase) or in RNA synthesis phase (G2 phase). Cells are relatively radioresistant in the latter part of the DNA synthesis phase (S phase).

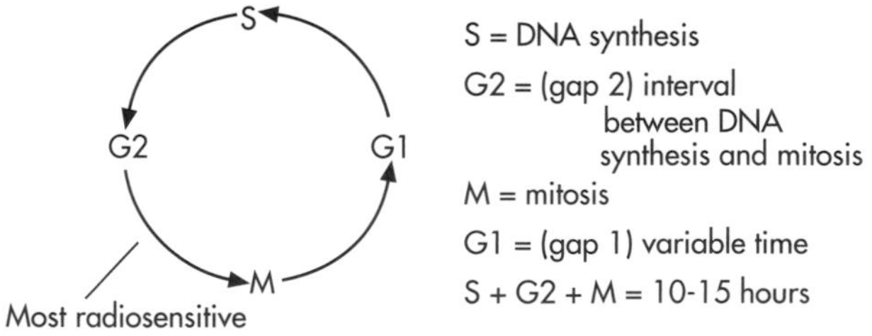

FIGURE 14-85

DOSE-RESPONSE CURVES (Fig. 14-86)

Dose-response models have been developed to predict the risk of cancer in humans. The most relevant dose-response curves are:

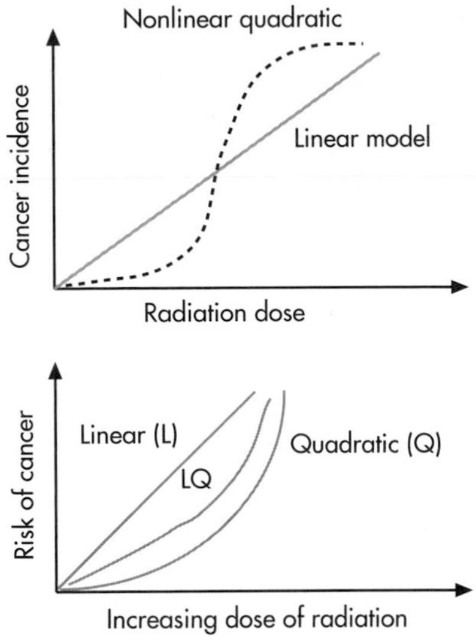

FIGURE 14-86

- Cell culture: linear-quadratic (linear at low dose and quadratic at higher dose)
- In vivo cancer induction: National Academy of Sciences/National Research Council Committee on Biological Effects of Ionizing Radiation (BEIR) published a report in 1990 (BEIR V) indicating that the linear dose-response model was best for all cancers, except for leukemia and bone cancer, for which a linear-quadratic model was suggested.

RISK IN HUMANS (Fig. 14-87)

Biologic effects of radiation are either stochastic or deterministic. A stochastic effect refers to a radiation effect in which the probability, rather than the severity, increases with dose (i.e., there is no threshold). Deterministic (nonstochastic) effects of radiation refer to effects in which the severity rather than the probability increases with dose (e.g., cataract formation in the posterior portion of the lens: minimal dose for cataract formation after x-ray exposure is estimated to be 200 rad; latency period is 6 months to 35 years). High dose rates (high exposure for short time) are more deleterious than low dose rates (low dose for long period of time). The effect of radiation is also less deleterious if the dose is split up into several fractions and if fractions are spaced at >6 hours apart, giving time to repair sublethal damage. Children are twice as sensitive to radiation as adults. Minimal latent period (induction time) is short for leukemia (2 to 5 years) but much longer for most solid tumors (10 to 15 years).

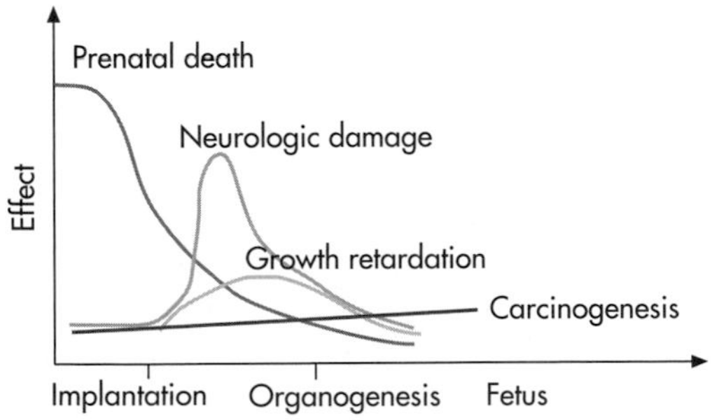

FIGURE 14-87

ACUTE RADIATION EFFECTS

Acute effects occur when the dose and the dose rate are high. There are 4 stages:

ACUTE EFFECTS OF RADIATION EXPOSURE

Stage	Dose (rad)	Target Organ, Symptoms
1	0-200	Subclinical (usually unobservable), transient nausea
2	200-600	Hematopoietic syndrome: survival chance falls to zero at about 600 rad
3	600-1000	Gastrointestinal (GI) syndrome: death in 10 to 24 days
4	>1000	CNS syndrome: shock, burning, death in hours

Pearls

- The minimal erythema dose is 200 to 300 rad for diagnostic x-ray (500 to 1000 rad for high-energy x-rays).
- The lethal dose (LD_{50}) in humans is approximately 450 rad given as a single dose.
- Epilation occurs 2 to 3 weeks after radiation exposure.
- The lowest dose to cause:
  - Depression of sperm count: 15 rad
  - Effect on reproductive capability: 25 rad
  - Sterility: 300 to 500 rad

LATE RADIATION EFFECTS

Precise information about the risk involved with low radiation doses is difficult to obtain because:

- Probability of occurrence is low at low doses
- Latency time is long (on average, 20 to 40 years)
- Late effects also occur from natural (ambient) radiation

The estimations on page 729 are based on NCRP report 115 and are derived from animal experiments and Hiroshima/Nagasaki survivors.

RISK OF RADIATION-INDUCED CANCER

Type of Cancer	Relative Risk* (% Increased/rad)	Absolute Risk† (Incidence/10^6/yr/rad)
Leukemia	2.0	1.0
Thyroid	—	1.0
Bone	0.3	0.1
Skin	<0.3	15
Breast	1.0	0.8
Lung	0.5	1.5
Others	—	1.0

*Relative risk: percentage of increase in cancer risk over that which exists because of natural causes.
†Absolute risk: number of cancer cases per year as a result of 1 rad exposure to 1 million persons.

Rule of thumb: population exposed to 1 rad has an expected incidence of malignancies (leukemia and solid tumors included) of 2 in 10^5 per year. Increased lifetime cancer risk estimate = 0.1% per rad.

Genetically Significant Dose (GSD)

GSD is a parameter of the gonadal radiation exposure to an entire population. In 1970, the GSD in the United States was approximately 20 mrad. Diagnostic radiation contributes much more to the GSD (more people have x-rays) than therapeutic radiation. Recommended average dose limit to gonads of a population: 5 rem in 30 years.

INCREASED CANCER INCIDENCE

Radiation Source, Exposed Population	Increased Cancer Incidence
Radiation for tinea capitis	Thyroid, brain
Hiroshima survivors	Thyroid, leukemia, lung, breast, GI tract
Marshall Islands population	Thyroid
Radium dial painters	Tongue from licking brushes, bone
Radiation for ankylosing spondylitis	Leukemia
Repeated fluoroscopy for TB	Breast

FETUS

For diagnostic levels of radiation (0 to 10 rad) the following figures of malformations and cancers have been reported:

MALFORMATION

Weeks	Gestation	Malformation
<2	Preimplant	Death
2-8	Organogenesis	1% per rad; may have smaller head size above a 5-rad threshold
8-16	CNS development	Mental retardation, likely 10-rad threshold
16-38	Growth	None at diagnostic levels

RISK OF CHILDHOOD CANCER*

Time	0 rad (%)	1 rad (%)	5 rad (%)	10 rad (%)
1st trimester	0.07	0.25	0.88	1.75
2nd and 3rd trimesters	0.07	0.12	0.30	0.52

*These numbers are still controversial.

Pearls

- Children are more susceptible to radiation than adults.
- Most sensitive stage of radiation damage: 2nd to 6th weeks of pregnancy
- Congenital malformations occur with >5 rad.
- 1 rem in 12th week results in 1% of birth defects with likely 5-rad threshold.

DIAGNOSTIC X-RAY DOSES

RADIATION DOSE FOR TYPICAL X-RAY PROCEDURES

Examination	Typical Effective Dose (mSv)	Number of Chest X-rays for Equivalent Effective Dose*	Time Period for Equivalent Effective Dose from Natural Background Radiation[1]
Chest x-ray, PA	0.02	1	2.4 days
Skull x-ray	0.1	5	12 days
Lumbar spine	1.5	75	182 days
IVP	3	150	1 year
Upper GI examination	6	300	2 years
Barium enema	8	400	2.7 years
CT head	2	100	243 days
CT abdomen	8	400	2.7 years

*Based on assumption of an average "effective dose" from chest x-ray of 0.02 mSv.
[1]Based on the assumption of an average "effective dose" from natural background radiation of 3 mSv per year in the United States.

RISK IN MAMMOGRAPHY

- The average glandular dose from mammography is approximately 80 mR/view (no grid) and <200 mR (with grid).
- With a typical 2-view mammography (200 mrad for each view), there is a 0.1% increased cancer risk.
- The mean risk of cancer from mammography is 6 to 8 cancers/rad/million.

RISK IN NUCLEAR MEDICINE

RADIATION DOSE FOR ADULT SCINTIGRAPHY

Study	Activity (mCi)	Target Organ Dose (mrad)	Whole-Body Dose (mrad)
Liver scan (^{99m}Tc)	5	1,400	90
Thyroid (^{123}I)	0.3	10,000	12
Bone scan	2.5	5,000 (bladder)	250
Gallium scan	5	4,500 (colon)	1400

RADIATION DOSE FOR PEDIATRIC SCINTIGRAPHY

Isotope	Activity (mCi)	Whole-Body Dose (mrad)
Cardiac scan (^{201}Tl)	2	800
Renal (^{99m}Tc DTPA)	10	120
Liver (^{99m}Tc)	2.5	100
Bone scan (^{99m}Tc MDP)	10	320

RADIATION PROTECTION

FILM BADGE

Anyone who might receive 10% or more of the maximum permissible dose (MPD) is required to wear film badges. One of the badges should be worn on the front collar above the apron to be close to the lens and thyroid or on the outside of the thyroid shield. A second badge should be worn under the apron or at waist level if high usage of fluoroscopy is intended or if pregnant. The window in the radiation badge is for estimation of beta radiation dose. Peak sensitivity of the emulsion in a film badge is 50 kVp.

APRON

A 0.5-mm lead apron (typical thickness) lets only 1%-3% of diagnostic x-ray radiation pass through (i.e., 30-fold reduction of scattered radiation). When the distance to the x-ray source and collimation are taken into account, radiation exposure from diagnostic x-rays is very low beneath an apron. The recommended minimum thickness of an apron is 0.25 mm lead equivalent, often worn by technologists who are not close to the patient during fluoroscopy.

X-RAY EQUIPMENT

The workload (W) is a measure of how much an x-ray machine is used during a week and reflects the total amount of radiation generated.

W (in mA minutes) = Total exposure in mAs/week × 0.0166 (i.e., total mAs/60)

The total exposure (E) in a radiologic workroom is calculated as:

$$E = (W \times 60) \times k$$

where k = average exposure in R/mAs at a distance of 1 m from the x-ray source, which depends on kVp used. Each R of primary beam exposure of a 20 × 20-cm field produces about 1 mR of scatter at a distance of 1 m from the patient. Because a typical C-arm fluoroscope exposure to a patient is approximately 3 R/minute, the exposure to the radiologist (no apron) at 1 foot from the patient is approximately 27 mR/min; this translates to 270 mR for 10 minutes of fluoroscopy time or to approximately 3 times the MPD for a week.

Pearls

- Maximum permissible leakage from an x-ray tube is 100 mR in 1 hour (when the tube is operated at its highest continuous-rated current [mA] and its maximum-rated kVp).
- The average amount of radiation exposure per frame during cinefluorography is now 30 μR/frame or 27 R/min.
- High kVp with low mA has a lower skin entrance dose than low kVp with high mA.

RADIATION IN WORKING AREAS

A high radiation area must be clearly marked if the exposure rate is >100 mR/hr.

GUIDELINES FOR EXPOSURE LIMITS

Guidelines for exposure limits are recommended by the NCRP. Government agencies such as the NRC establish the regulations and do not always agree with the NCRP. The recommended levels do not represent levels that are absolutely harmless but levels that represent an acceptable risk. For radiation workers the MPD is 5 rem/yr for whole-body exposure. For the lens of the eye and the extremities, the annual limits are 15 rem and 50 rem, respectively. The MPD for nonoccupational persons is 0.1 rem/yr and 0.5 rem for "infrequent" exposure. The MPD for a fetus is 0.5 rem for the entire gestation period.

MAXIMUM PERMISSIBLE DOSES (NCRP)

	Limit*
Radiation workers	
Whole body (prospective)	5 rem/yr
Whole body (retrospective)	10-15 rem in any 1 yr
Whole body (accumulative to age N)	N in rem
Pregnant radiation worker	0.5 rem in gestation period (<0.05/mo)
Skin, extremities	50 rem/yr
Lens, head	15 rem/yr
Life-saving emergency	50 rem
Nonradiation workers	
Whole body	0.1 rem/yr
Whole body, infrequent exposure	0.5 rem/yr
Embryo	0.5 rem/pregnancy

*The dose limits (especially from radioactive materials) are now specified by the NCRP and the ICRP in terms of effective dose (E), which is the weighted sum of the doses to about 10 "critical" organs and not strictly for a "whole-body" dose.
Note: Old NCRP reports (Report 91, 1987) have numbers that differ from the above, taken from NRCP report 116, 1993. ALARA principle: as low as reasonably acceptable.

ENVIRONMENTAL RADIATION

MEAN RADIATION EXPOSURE IN UNITED STATES

Source	Annual Dose (mrem)
Radon (whole body effective)	200
Other natural radiation*	100
Medical procedures	50

*People in high-radiation areas (e.g., Denver) have not been shown to have increased risk of cancer development.

RADON

Radon (Rn) is a radioactive decay product of uranium that has been implicated as a common cause of lung cancer (inhaled alpha-emitting daughter products). Rn is a gas that accumulates in nonventilated basements. It is currently estimated to be the largest contributor to environmental radiation in the United States (200 mrem/yr compared with 100 mrem from all other sources). According to EPA standards, the proportion of lung cancers caused by radon is 10%.

RISK OF DEATH FROM ENVIRONMENTAL SOURCES

EQUIVALENT DEATH RISKS (1:106)

Amount	Activity	Cause of Death
1.2 mrem	CXR	Cancer
3 days	Live in United States	Homicide
1 day	Live in Boston	Air pollution
1	Smoke cigarettes	Cancer
0.5 L	Drink wine	Cirrhosis
10 teaspoons	Eat peanut butter	Liver cancer (aflatoxin)
1 gal	Drink Miami water	Chloroform
6 min	Canoe	Drowning
50 miles	Drive automobile	Accident
5 miles	Drive motorcycle	Accident
1 wk	Visit Denver	Cosmic rays

Ultrasound Physics

CHARACTERISTICS OF SOUND

Unlike x-rays, sound waves are preserved waves (not electromagnetic radiation) that require a medium for transmission (sound waves cannot propagate in a vacuum). Ultrasound (US) waves propagate similarly to other sound waves: an initial US wave hits a molecule, which itself travels for a short distance (μm) and then hits another molecule. Individual molecules move only a few micrometers, whereas a resulting reflected wave travels for a long distance. Clinical US uses frequencies of 1 to 20 MHz (1 hertz = 1 cycle/sec; 1 MHz = 1 million cycles/sec). By timing the period elapsed between emission of the sound and reception of the echo, the distance (D) between the transducer and the echo-producing structure can be calculated:

$$D = \text{Velocity (1540m/sec)} \times \text{Time}$$

VELOCITY OF SOUND

US velocity depends on the physical characteristics of the material the sound wave is traveling through. Most human tissues (except bone) behave like liquids and transmit sound at ~1540 m/sec. The denser the tissue, the faster the sound wave (more molecules to transmit the wave per unit of volume). Sound velocity is determined only by compressibility and/or density of material (not viscosity). Density (g/cm^3) and compressibility are inversely proportional.

VELOCITY OF SOUND WAVES

Medium	Velocity (m/sec)	Acoustic Impedance (rayls)	Absorption Coefficient (dB/MHz/cm)
Air	331	0.0004	12
Fat	1450	1.38	0.63
Soft tissue	1540	1.6	0.94*
Bone	4080	7.8	20

*Rule of thumb: ≈1 dB/MHz/cm.

When the velocity of the US beam increases (e.g., transition from fat to muscle), the wavelength decreases.

ATTENUATION

Sound attenuation refers to loss of sound waves from reflection, scattering, and absorption. Absorption depends mainly on:

- Frequency (therefore the absorption coefficient is expressed in dB/MHz/cm)
- Viscosity of medium
- Acoustic relaxation time of the medium

FREQUENCY (Fig. 14-88)

Refers to the cycles per second with which sound is generated. The higher the frequency, the "shriller" the sound.

$$\text{Velocity of sound} = \text{Frequency (Hz)} \times \text{Wavelength (m)}$$

The frequency of sound is determined by the source. For example, in a piano each string has a certain frequency. In US each transducer has its own frequency (e.g., 2, 3, 5, 7.5 MHz). The only way to change US frequencies is to change the transducer.

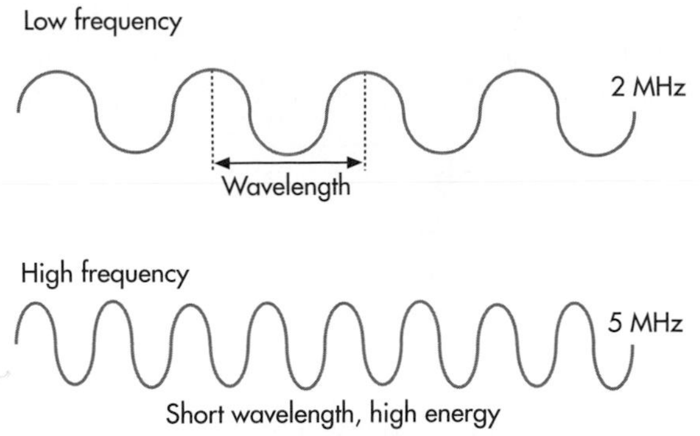

FIGURE 14-88

As sound waves pass from one medium to another, their frequency remains constant but their wavelength changes to accommodate the new velocity in the 2nd medium.

WAVELENGTH (Fig. 14-89)

The distance sound travels during one vibration is known as the wavelength. The wavelength (in meters) is measured from the top of one wave to the next.

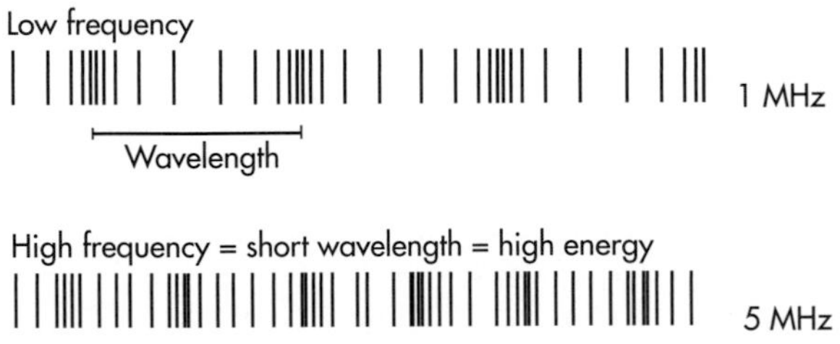

FIGURE 14-89

ACOUSTIC IMPEDANCE (Z)

Acoustic impedance of a tissue is the product of its density and the velocity of sound in that tissue. Since the velocity of sound in tissue is fairly constant over a wide range of frequencies, a tissue's acoustic impedance is proportional to tissue density:

$$Z\ (\text{rayls}) = \text{Density}\ (\text{g/cm}^3) \times \text{Velocity}\ (\text{cm/sec})$$

INTENSITY

Refers to "loudness" of US beam. Loudness is determined by length of oscillation of the particles conducting the waves: the greater the amplitude of oscillation, the more intense the sound. Absolute intensity is measured in watts (W)/cm².

DECIBELS

Relative sound intensity is measured in decibels (dB). Positive dB indicates a gain in power; negative dB indicates a loss in power. One dB is 0.1 ("deci") of 1 bel unit. The definition of dB is:

$$\text{dB} = 10\log\ (\text{Intensity}_{out}/\text{Intensity}_{in})$$

DECIBEL AND INTENSITY

dB	Original Intensity	Attenuated Intensity
0	1	1
−10	10	0.1
−20	100	0.01
−30	1000	0.001

Example

If a US beam has an original intensity of 10 W/cm² and the returning echo is 0.001 W/cm², what is the relative intensity?

Answer

$\text{Log}\ 0.001/10 = \log 0.0001 = -4\text{B} = -40\,\text{dB}$.

Example

A 5-MHz beam passes through 6 cm of soft tissue (1 dB/MHz/cm). How much is the original intensity decreased?

Answer

(1 dB/cm/MHz) × (5 MHz) × (6 cm) = 30 dB. 30 dB = $\log I_{out}/I_{in}$ and therefore $3\text{B} = \log I_{out}/I_{in}$. The original intensity is therefore reduced by a factor of 1000.

Pearls

- The wavelength of clinical US waves is 1.5 to 0.08 mm.
- High-frequency transducers have better resolution.
- High-frequency transducers have lower penetration power.

CHARACTERISTICS OF US BEAM (Fig. 14-90)

Waves traveling in the same direction form a wavefront. The distance at which waves become synchronous depends on their wavelength and marks the so-called point X'. The beam zone proximal to that point is called the Fresnel zone (beam is coherent). The beam zone beyond X' is called the Fraunhofer zone (beam is divergent).

Angle of Divergence (Dispersion)

$$\sin\alpha = 1.22 \times \frac{\text{Wavelength}}{\text{Transducer diameter}}$$

Therefore, lateral resolution is decreased with a small-diameter transducer.

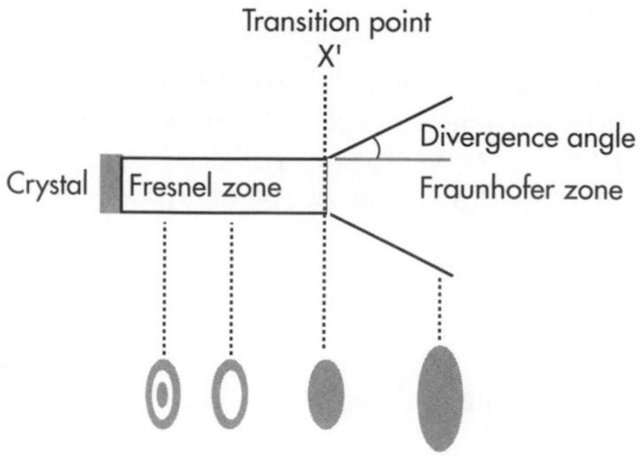

FIGURE 14-90

Fresnel Zone

The length of the Fresnel zone is determined by:

$$\text{Length of zone (cm)} = \frac{\text{Transducer radius}^2(\text{cm}^2)}{\text{Wavelength (cm)}}$$

The Fresnel zone length increases with:

- Increasing diameter of the transducer
- Increasing frequency

REFLECTION

The percentage of beam reflected at a tissue surface depends on:

- Acoustic impedance of tissue
- Angle of incidence into tissue

Reflection (R) can be calculated as:

$$R = \left[(Z2 - Z1)/(Z2 + Z1)\right]^2 \times 100$$

where R is percent of reflected beam, Z1 is acoustic impedance of medium 1, and Z2 is acoustic impedance of medium 2.

Pearls

- Percentage of reflection at tissue/tissue interfaces:
  - Air/lung: 99.9%
  - Water/kidney: 0.64%
  - Skull/brain: 44%
  - Muscle/bone: 80%
- Transmission (%) + reflection (%) = 100%
- The higher the angle of incidence, the lower the amount of reflection.

REFRACTION (Fig. 14-91)

The angle of refraction at media interfaces can be calculated by:

$$\frac{\sin \partial i}{\sin \partial t} = \frac{V1}{V2}$$

where ∂i is the incident angle, ∂t is the transmitted angle, and V1 and V2 are the velocities of sound in the 2 media. In other words, the angle of reflection depends only on the sound velocities in the 2 media. As sound propagates through the parenchyma of an organ that contains microscopic fluctuations in acoustic impedance, small quantities of US are scattered in all directions, an effect that is responsible for the pixelated gray-scale appearance of an organ.

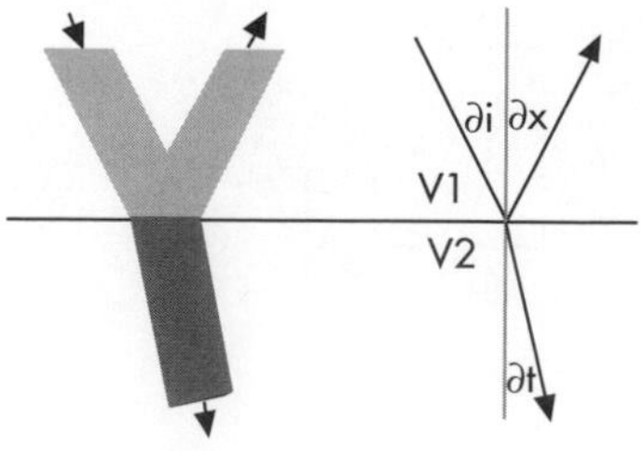

FIGURE 14-91

ABSORPTION

Absorption refers to the energy of an US beam that is converted into heat. Absorption is a result of friction between particles in the medium. The relationship between frequency and absorption is linear: doubling the frequency doubles the absorption.

COMPONENTS

TRANSDUCER

The components of a transducer include:

- Piezoelectric crystal
- Backing block
- Quarter wave matching layer

Piezoelectric Crystal

The crystal consists of many dipoles arranged in a parallel geometric pattern (approximately 0.5 mm thick). Plating electrodes on either side of the crystal produce an electric field, which changes the orientation of the crystals. When an alternating voltage (rapid change in polarity; e.g., 3 MHz) is applied, the crystals vibrate like a cymbal. Piezoelectric crystals are manufactured by heating a ceramic (such as lead zirconium titanate [PZT]) in a strong electric field. As the temperature of the crystal increases, the dipoles are free to move and align themselves in the magnetic field generated by the applied electricity. The crystal is then cooled in the magnetic field so that the dipoles stay aligned in their new parallel orientation. The temperature at which this polarization is lost is called the Curie temperature. Crystals lose their piezoelectric properties above the Curie temperature.

PIEZOELECTRIC MATERIALS

Material	Curie Temperature (°C)	Q Factor
Quartz	573	>25,000
Barium titanate	100	
Lead zirconium titanate (PZT)-4	328	>500
PZT-5	365	75

Resonance Frequency

The resonance frequency of a piezoelectric crystal is determined by the thickness of the crystal. Like a pipe in a church organ—the larger the pipe, the lower the pitch of sound—the thinner the crystal, the higher its frequency.

Crystal thickness = ½ the wavelength of US

Transducer Q Factor (Fig. 14-92)

The Q factor reflects:

- Purity of sound
- Length of time that the sound persists (ring-down time = time for complete stop of vibration)

High-Q crystals are good transmitters; low-Q crystals are good receivers (receiver to a broad spectrum of reflected frequencies).

Backing Block

The backing block is special material at the back of the transducer that quenches the vibration and shortens the sonic pulse. Backing blocks are made of a combination of tungsten, rubber powder, and epoxy.

Quarter Wave Matching Layer

Layer of material located in front of the transducer used to transmit the sonic energy more efficiently to the patient. The thickness of this layer must be equal to ¼ (hence "quarter wave") the wavelength. Layers consist of aluminum in epoxy resin.

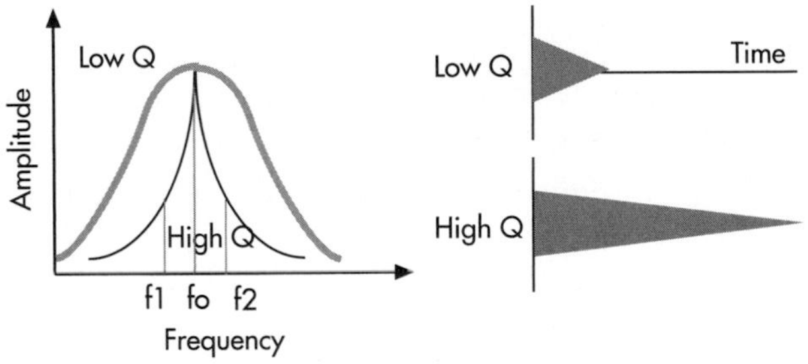

FIGURE 14-92

US EQUIPMENT TYPES

A (Amplitude) Mode

Probe has a single transducer that pulses and displays echo depth and amplitude as a line on an oscilloscope screen. No longer used in medical imaging.

TM (Time Motion) Mode

Spikes from the A mode are converted into dots and displayed on a moving strip. The amplitude of returning pulse is not displayed. Occasionally used in echocardiography to image valve motions.

B (Binary) Mode

Transducer attached to mechanical arm is moved across surface. A series of received echoes form the tomographic image. Gray scale assigns shades of gray to the different amplitudes of returning echoes. No longer used in medical imaging.

Real-Time Mode (Fig. 14-93)

Two types of real-time scanners are commonly used today:

- Mechanical sector scanners: a single transducer oscillates to cover the field; alternatively, 3 or 4 transducers are mounted on a ball that turns in one direction.
- Electronic array scanners that contain 64 to 200 transducers per probe
  - A steered wavefront can be created by sequential simulation of many individual transducers.
  - A beam can be focused by plastic lenses and by the timing of the pulses to the transducers
  - Fresnel zone can be electronically adjusted by determining how many individual transducers are excited at once; decreasing the radius of the transducer decreases the Fresnel zone.

  Real-time US generates images at ~15 frames/sec
- A frame is composed of many vertical lines (~110-220 lines/frame)
- Each line corresponds to a transducer in the probe.
- Relationship between spatial and temporal resolution: high spatial resolution is obtained by increasing the number of lines; high temporal resolution is achieved by increasing the number of frames per second.

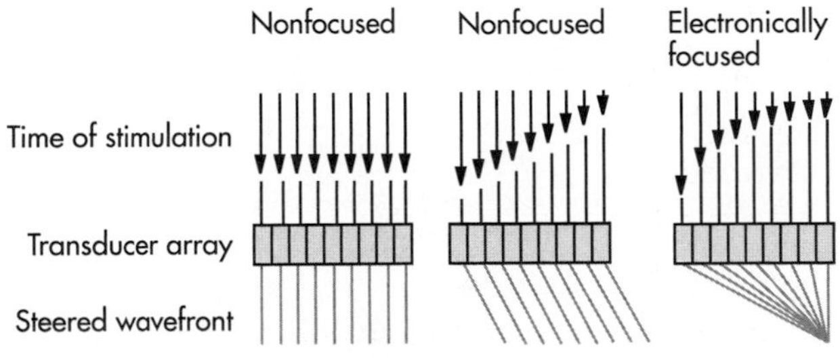

FIGURE 14-93

CONTROLS (Fig. 14-94)

Time-gain compensator (TGC) is an important control function that allows adjustment of attenuated echoes from deep structures.

- Coarse gain: regulates the height of all echoes (amplifier)
- Reject control: rejects unwanted low-level echoes
- Delay control: regulates the depth at which the TGC begins to augment the weaker signals
- Near gain control: diminishes near echoes
- Far gain enhancement: enhances all distant echoes
- Cine mode: computer stores images (frames), which can then be displayed later

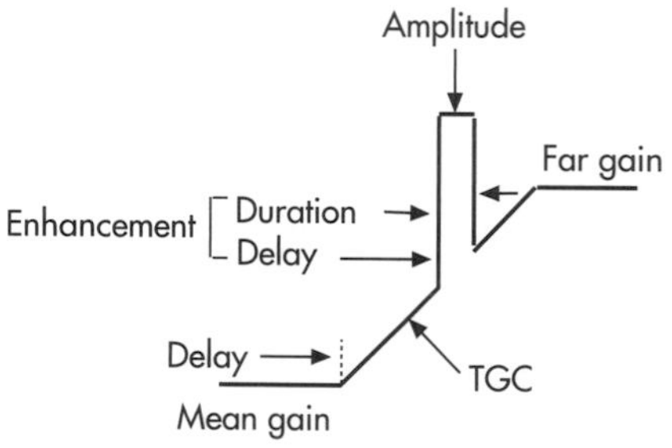

FIGURE 14-94

RESOLUTION (Fig. 14-95)

US allows measurement of distances indirectly by determining time between US waves and then converting them to distance, assuming that velocity in tissues is 1540 m/sec.

Axial Resolution

Axial or depth resolution refers to the ability to separate two objects lying in tandem along the course of the beam. Two objects will be recognized as separate if the spatial pulse length (i.e., the length of each US pulse) is less than twice the distance between the objects. Therefore, axial resolution can be defined as ½ the spatial pulse length.

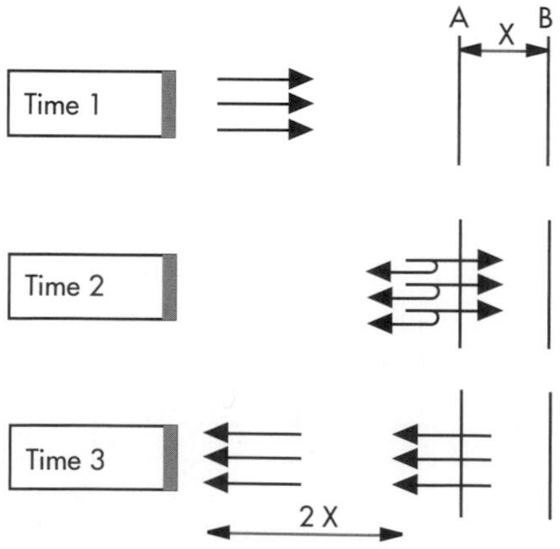

FIGURE 14-95

Pearls

- The higher the frequency, the better the axial resolution.
- Axial resolution is generally better than lateral resolution.
- Axial resolution is the same at all depths.
- Axial resolution is independent of the transducer diameter.

Lateral Resolution (Fig. 14-96)

To resolve two parallel objects next to each other, the US beam has to be narrower than the space separating the two objects. Narrow transducers have a short Fresnel zone, which causes poor resolution of deep structures. Lateral resolution depends on:

- Number of scan lines (the number of scan lines decreases if the frame rate increases)
- Width of US beam: the wider the beam, the less the lateral resolution

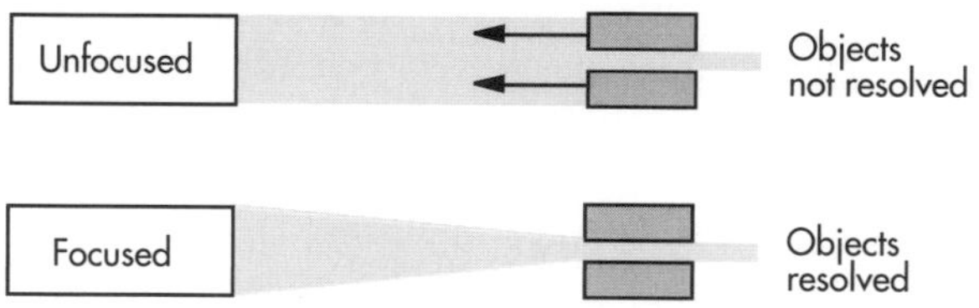

FIGURE 14-96

SCAN TIME

Scan time refers to the time required for a US pulse to be emitted and received by the transducer/receiver. The next pulse cannot be fired before the first one has been received. An image is made up of several scan lines, usually 110 to 220. The frame rate refers to the number of scan lines that can be obtained per second.

$$\text{Time of a scan line} = 2 \times \frac{\text{Imaging depth}}{1540\,\text{m} \times \text{sec}^{-1}}$$

Time of a frame = Time of a scan line × Number of scan lines

Frame rate = Number of scan lines/sec

DOPPLER US (Figs. 14-97 and 14-98)

The Doppler effect refers to a frequency change that occurs in a moving wave. In a stationary wave, wavelengths are equal in all directions. In a moving wave source, however, wavelengths increase and decrease depending on the direction of movement. The Doppler shift refers to the frequency of the

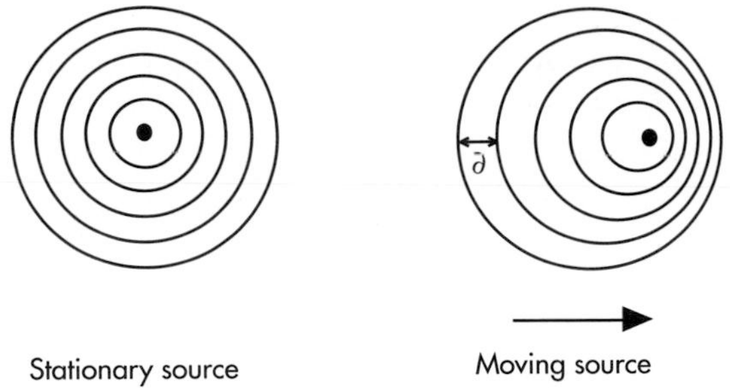

FIGURE 14-97

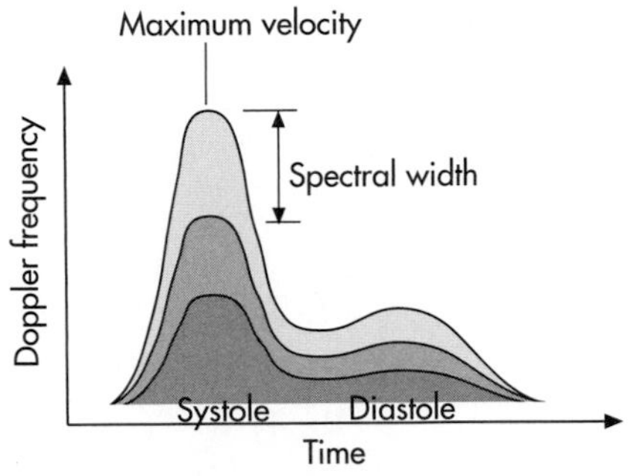

FIGURE 14-98

initial signal, which is subtracted from that of the returning echo. According to the following equation, blood flow can thus be measured:

$$\Delta f = 2f_0 v \cos\theta / C$$

where Δf = Doppler shift, f_o = original frequency transmitted in MHz, v = velocity of moving blood cells, θ = angle of transducer to the moving blood cells (cosine of 90° = 0, and the cosine of 0° = 1), and C = speed of sound in soft tissues. Flow cannot be detected when the angle of a transducer is at 90° relative to the blood vessel. The optimal angle to detect flow would be close to 0° relative to moving blood. A good angle of the transducer in relation to the vessel for imaging is 1° to 60° (relationship between change of frequency and change in velocity of the blood cells is linear). For angles >60°, the relationship is exponential, causing errors in flow measurements.

Pearls

- The higher the US frequency and the lower the angle, the larger the Doppler shift.
- High Q factor is desired for Doppler US.
- Long pulse length is required to increase the Q factor.

Spectral Broadening

Widening of the spectral width, a parameter of flow disturbance. The larger the spectral broadening, the greater the flow disturbance.

CONTINUOUS WAVE DOPPLER

Continuous wave Doppler uses two separate transmitting and receiving transducers within the same transducer, both operating continuously (hence "continuous wave"). The frequency of the initial signal is subtracted from that of returning echoes. The difference is referred to as the Doppler shift and usually falls within the audible frequency range. Continuous wave Doppler is thus used mainly to measure stenosis of vessels.

PULSED DOPPLER

Pulsed Doppler allows measurement of the depth at which a returning signal has originated. This is achieved by emitting a pulse of a sound rather than a continuous sound (hence "pulsed Doppler"). Only echoes received at a precise time (and therefore from a specific depth) are thus sampled. Pulsed Doppler is a more sensitive means to determine flow than color Doppler. The duplex Doppler combines pulsed Doppler and B mode imaging for obtaining real-time images. There are separate transducers within a probe, both of which usually operate at different frequencies (carotids: 7 MHz for the imaging, 5 MHz for the Doppler; abdomen: 5 MHz for the imaging, 3 MHz for the Doppler).

COLOR FLOW DOPPLER

Color flow Doppler US is based on the mean Doppler frequency shift, whereas pulsed Doppler is based on peak Doppler frequency shift. Color Doppler imaging allows one to detect flow throughout the entire image, whereas pulsed Doppler allows measurement in a small area only. The transducer measures the change of frequency over all the lines in the image and assigns a set color to specific frequency ranges (actually it measures changes in phase):

- Blood flowing to transducer = blue
- Blood flowing away from transducer = red
- Velocity determinations (e.g., color assignments) are angle dependent.

Color Doppler imaging has several shortcomings, including a tendency for noise, angle dependence, and aliasing. Power Doppler US has been developed to overcome these shortcomings. Power Doppler US is a color Doppler US method in which the color map displays the integrated power of the Doppler signal, rather than the mean Doppler frequency shift.

Pearls

- As multiple samples are required to measure velocity in the large FOV, the frame is usually reduced; this explains why the temporal resolution of color Doppler is not as good as that with pulsed Doppler.

- Because the sampling rate is slow, there is an increased potential for aliasing when compared with pulsed Doppler. To cut back on this, one can limit color sampling to a defined region.
- Aliasing and turbulent flow on color US are usually encoded by different colors.

ARTIFACTS

REVERBERATION ARTIFACT

Returning echoes are partially reflected at an internal boundary. This produces misregistration and assigns structures to places they do not exist (e.g., a bright line is seen in the bladder).

MIRROR IMAGE ARTIFACT (SPECULAR REFLECTION)

Because of reflection of US waves at acoustic mirrors (e.g., diaphragm), lesions can be projected into locations in which they are not really present. Typical example is that of a liver lesion near the diaphragm that can be projected into the lung because the liver-lung boundary acts as an acoustic mirror.

RING-DOWN ARTIFACT

Occurs when the US beam strikes a structure that is capable of ringing (e.g., metal, cholesterol crystals in the gallbladder wall).

SHADOWING AND ENHANCEMENT

Shadowing refers to absent through-transmission through a lesion (e.g., containing calcium). Enhancement: refers to better through-transmission (e.g., through a fluid-filled structure such as a cyst).

NONSPECULAR REFLECTIONS

Nonspecular reflections occur at objects that are smaller than the wavelength of the US beam. These reflections generally give a weak signal since only a small portion of the beam is reflected back toward the transducer. Particulate US contrast agents exploit this principle.

ALIASING

Aliasing refers to an artifact that may be introduced when converting analog to a digital signal. If the digital sampling is not done frequently enough (too few scan lines), the digital signal may not contain enough information to reproduce the analog signal. In general, one should use twice as many scan lines as expected for resolving described objects without aliasing. In the accompanying diagram (Fig. 14-99):

- A: Digital sampling frequency (black dots) is much greater than analog frequency (sine wave) → no information is lost.

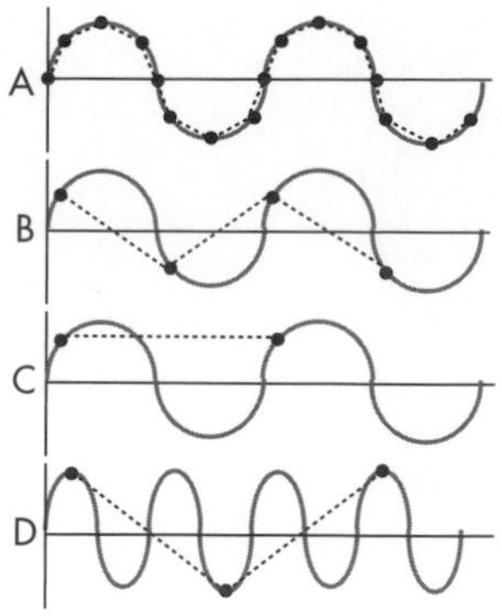

FIGURE 14-99

- B: Digital sampling taken at twice the frequency of the analog signal. This is the minimal sampling rate to preserve all the information, called the Nyquist frequency. To resolve a structure of dimension d, the Nyquist frequency (f_N) must be

$$f_N = 2/d$$

- C: All analog information is lost.
- D: The digital signal has a lower frequency than the analog one. Thus, information not present in the original (analog) signal is produced in the digital signal. This is aliasing.

OTHER ARTIFACTS

- Duplication artifact
- Off-axis artifact
- Section thickness artifact
- Refraction artifact

MRI Physics

GENERAL (Figs. 14-100 and 14-101)

When materials are placed in a magnetic field they can absorb and then reemit electromagnetic radiation of a specific frequency (usually in the form of radio

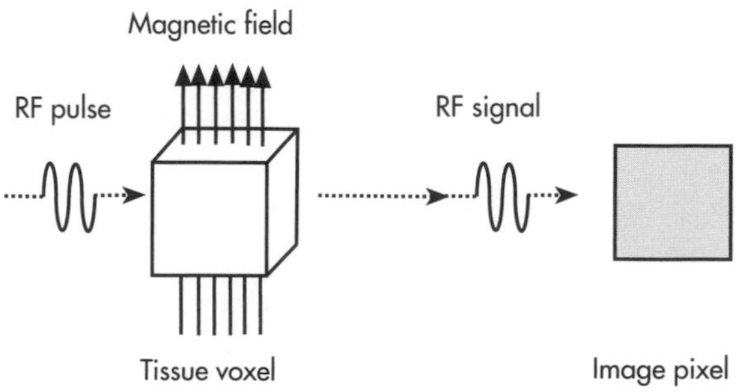

FIGURE 14-100

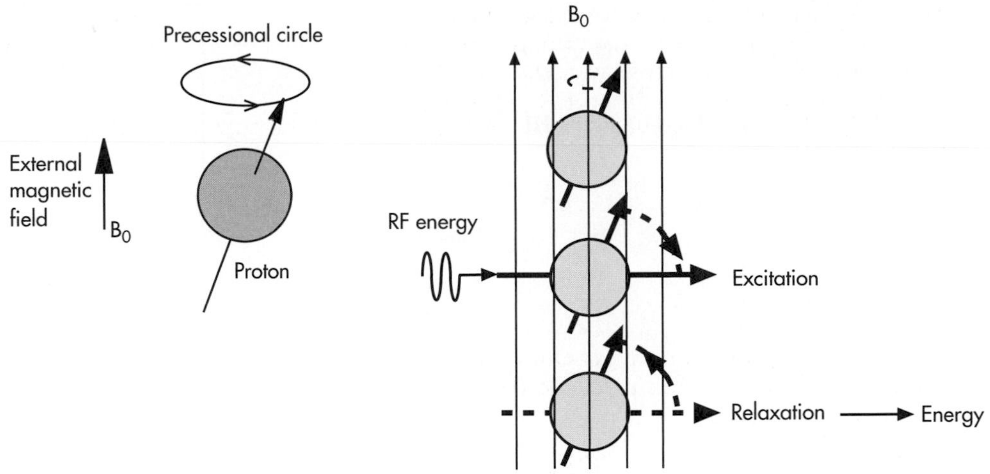

FIGURE 14-101

signals). The signal intensity of a given pixel is determined by:

- Proton (i.e., hydrogen) density ($N_{[H]}$)
- Longitudinal relaxation rate (R_1)
- Transverse relaxation rate (R_2)
- Flow
- Other parameters
  - Diffusion
  - Magnetization exchange rate
  - Magnetic susceptibility
  - Magnetization

MAGNETIZATION

In the absence of a magnetic field, nuclei are randomly oriented and produce no net magnetic effect. When tissue is placed in a magnetic field, some nuclei align with the field, and their combined effect is usually referred to as a magnetization vector (referred to as M_0 when in resting state or as M_z when deflected by radiofrequency). The magnetic field also causes the magnetic moments to precess (a motion similar to that of a gyroscope).

The Larmor frequency (ω_0) is the precession frequency of the nuclei in a magnetic field (B_0) and is related to B_0 by the constant gyromagnetic ratio (γ):

$$\omega_0 = \gamma B_0$$

At 1.5T, the Larmor frequency of protons is 63MHz.

There are two basic directions of tissue magnetization (Figs. 14-102 and 14-103):

- Longitudinal (spin-lattice relaxation) (T1)
- Transverse (spin-spin relaxation) (T2)

Spin-lattice relaxation is a process responsible for the dissipation of energy from radiofrequency-excited protons into their molecular environment or "lattice." T1 relaxation time is a measure of the time required for M_z to return to 63% of its equilibrium magnetization (M_0).

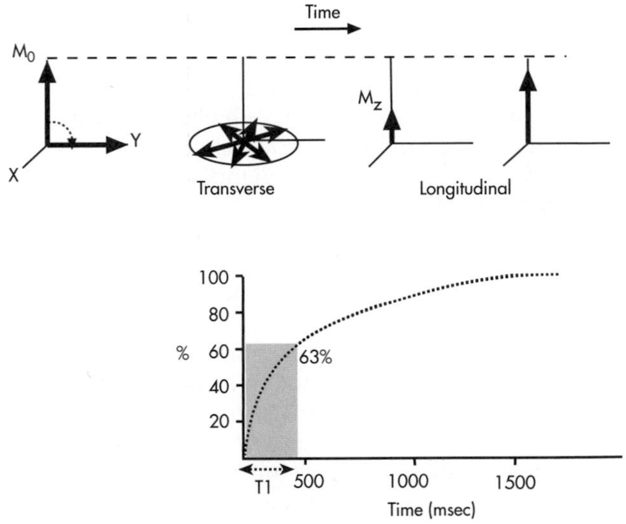

FIGURE 14-102

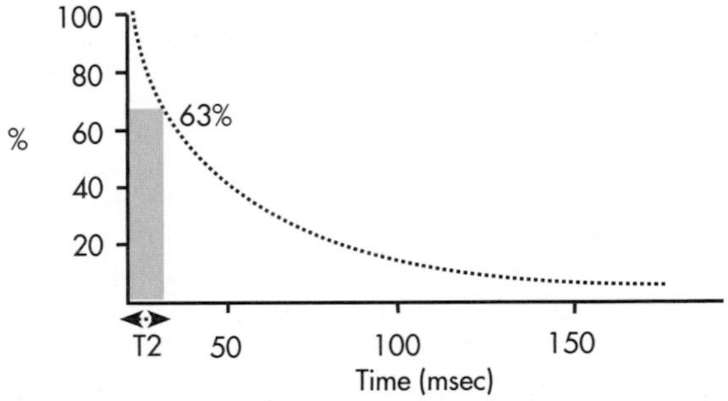

FIGURE 14-103

Spin-spin relaxation is a process that progressively reduces order after an excitation pulse. Individual components of magnetization lose their alignment and rotate at various rates in the transverse plane (dephase). T2 relaxation time is a measure of the time required for 63% of the initial magnetization to dissipate. T2 is usually much shorter than T1.

APPROXIMATE T1 AND T2 VALUES FOR HUMAN TISSUES

Tissue	T1 at 1.5 T (msec)	T1 at 0.5 (msec)	T2 (msec)
Skeletal muscle	870	600	47
Liver	490	323	43
Kidney	650	449	58
Spleen	780	554	62
Fat	260	215	84
Gray matter	920	656	101
White matter	790	539	92
Cerebrospinal fluid	>4,000	>4,000	>2,000
Lung	830	600	79

MR SIGNAL LOCALIZATION

Localization of MR signal is achieved by applying gradients that produce controlled linear variations in the magnetic field. These gradients are used in slice selection (z), phase encoding (y), and frequency encoding (x).

- *Slice selection* gradient determines the amount of tissue that is excited by the RF pulse.
- *Phase encoding* gradient is applied perpendicular to the slice selection gradient and after the initial excitation. Protons will dephase along the gradient.
- *Frequency-encoding* gradient is also referred to as the readout gradient since MR signal is most commonly acquired during the frequency encoding gradient. This gradient is applied to the third perpendicular direction to slice the selection and phase the encoding gradients. The protons are encoded with a different frequency depending on their locations.

K-SPACE

The data obtained from the gradients are stored in a matrix referred to as k-space. High-signal information is concentrated in the center and low-signal information is near the peripheral sections (like edges). This information is then **Fourier** transformed to reconstruct the image.

SPIN-ECHO IMAGING (Fig. 14-104)

Sequence composed of a series of selective 90° to 180° pulses that generate a spin echo at a specified echo time (TE) after the initial 90° pulse. The

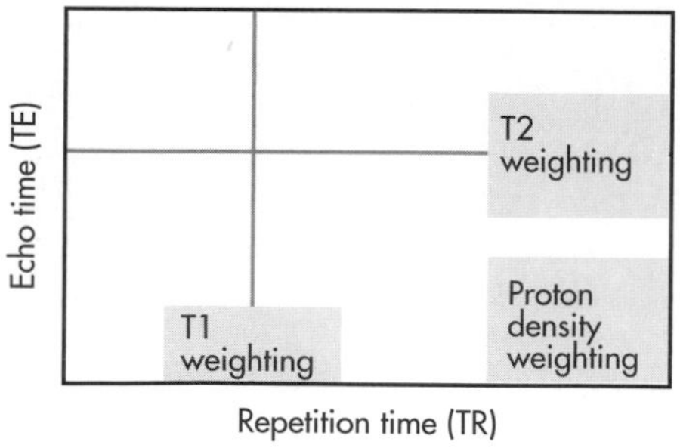

FIGURE 14-104

sequence is repeated at a specified repetition interval (TR). Transverse magnetization is measured in the presence of a read-out gradient (Gx) during which many samples are taken.

$$SI_{SE} = kN_{(H)}\,(1 - e^{-TR/T1})\,e^{-TE/T2}$$

The time (T) required for the acquisition of a pulse sequence is:

T = TR × number of phase-encoding steps (N_{phase}) × number of signal averages (NSA)

Fast Spin-Echo (FSE) Acquisition

Multiple phase-encoding steps are used in conjunction with multiple 180° refocusing pulses for every TR interval, called an echo train. The number of echoes within each TR interval is called echo train length (ETL). This allows for much faster acquisition compared with conventional spin-echo imaging, with acquisition time inversely proportional to the ETL. Increasing ETL decreases acquisition time but decreases SNR. As each echo experiences a different amount of T2 decay, there is some contrast difference from conventional spin-echo sequences. Also it is less susceptible to field inhomogeneity than conventional spin echo. Currently, most T2-weighted imaging is performed with FSE because of the longer TR required.

INVERSION RECOVERY IMAGING (Fig. 14-105)

Sequence composed of a series of 180° pulses to invert the magnetization followed by a 90° pulse. The TR is between the 180° pulses. A time of inversion (TI) may be chosen to selectively null the signal of certain tissue types, such as fat or CSF. Two sequences are commonly used: STIR (short tau inversion recovery, fat) and FLAIR (fluid-attenuated inversion recovery, CSF).

$$SI_{IR} = kN_{(H)}(1 - 2e^{-TI/T1} + e^{-TR/T1})$$

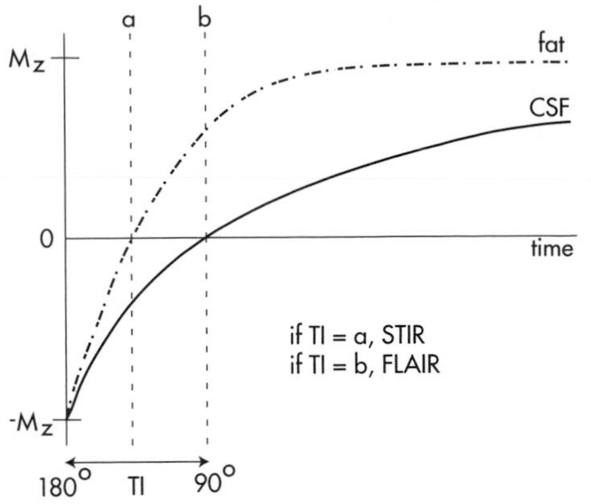

FIGURE 14-105

T2* IMAGING

T2* is used in susceptibility imaging, perfusion imaging, fMRI, and iron oxide imaging. T2* relaxation is the decay of transverse magnetization caused by spin-spin relaxation and magnetic field inhomogeneity:

$1/T2^* = 1/T2 + 1/T2'$, where T2' is field inhomogeneity. T2* is always < T2.

The T2* effect can be seen with gradient-recalled echo (GRE) sequences that have a 90° pulse but no 180° refocusing pulse. A GRE sequence is T2*-weighted with a long TR and long TE (though shorter than for T2-weighted spin echo sequence) and a low flip angle. Susceptibility-weighted sequences also use phase information in addition to T2* effect to examine differences in blood/iron and calcium.

SIGNAL-TO-NOISE RATIO (SNR)

$$\text{SNR} \propto 1 \times \text{voxel} \times \frac{\sqrt{\text{NEX}}}{\sqrt{\text{BW}}} \times f(\text{QF}) \times f(\text{B})$$

$$\text{voxel} = \frac{\text{FOV}_x}{\#\text{ pixels in x}} \times \frac{\text{FOV}_y}{\#\text{ pixels in y}} \times \text{slice thickness(z)}$$

where I = intrinsic signal intensity, f(QF) = coil quality, and f(B) = field strength.

IMAGING PARAMETERS

EFFECTS OF IMAGING PARAMETERS ON SNR AND WEIGHTING

Parameter	Parameter Increased	Parameter Decreased
Slice thickness	Increases SNR	Decreases SNR
	Increases image detail	Decreases image detail
TR	Increases SNR	Decreases SNR
	Longer imaging time	Shorter imaging time
	More sections	Fewer sections
	Less T1W	More T1W
TE	Decreases SNR	Increases SNR
	More T2W	Less T2W
NSA	Increases SNR	Decreases SNR
	Longer imaging time	Shorter imaging time
Matrix size	Decreases SNR	Increases SNR
	Longer imaging time	Shorter imaging time
	Better resolution	Worse resolution

3-D IMAGING

Uses a nonselective RF pulse to excite the entire sample volume simultaneously. Two orthogonal phase-encoding gradients are used. 3-D imaging allows for contiguous sections without section cross-talk and higher resolution imaging but has longer acquisition time, is more susceptible to motion artifacts, and has a lower SNR.

MR ANGIOGRAPHY

Can be performed without (time-of-flight, phase contrast) or with intravenous gadolinium. A maximum-intensity projection (MIP) technique is used to further highlight the vessels.

EFFECTS OF IMAGING PARAMETERS ON SNR, SPATIAL RESOLUTION, AND ACQUISITION TIME

			Spatial Resolution			
Goal	Imaging Parameters	SNR Change*	*Section-Encoding Direction*	*Frequency-Encoding Direction*	*Phase-Encoding Direction*	Time of Acquisition
Higher SNR	NSA × 2	× 1.41	—	—	—	× 2
Higher SNR	BW/2	× 1.41	—	—	—	—
Higher	$\text{FOV}_{phase}/2$	× 0.25	—	× 2	× 2	—
Higher resolution	$N_{freq} \times 2$	× 0.71	—	× 2	—	—
Higher resolution	$N_{phase} \times 2$	× 0.71	—	—	× 2	× 2

*$0.71 = 1/\sqrt{2}$, $1.41 = \sqrt{2}$.

BW, bandwidth in frequency-encoding direction; FOV_{froq} field of view in frequency-encoding direction; FOV_{phase}, field of view in phase-encoding direction; N_{froq}, number of pixels across FOV_{froq} (without interpolation); N_{phase}, number of phase-encoding steps; NSA, number of signals averaged.

Techniques

- *Time-of-flight:* Gradient-echo sequence with short TR, with slices perpendicular to the direction of blood flow. Flowing spins (blood) have higher signal than stationary spins.
- *Phase contrast:* Moving blood produces phase changes while stationary tissues have no net phase change. The amount of change is proportional to velocity and sensitive to direction of flow. Bipolar gradients with opposite polarity are used. Long acquisition time.
- *Gadolinium enhanced:* Gadolinium shortens the T1 value of blood to less than that of surrounding tissues. Performed with short TR (minimize stationary tissue signal) and short TE (decrease T2* effect).

ARTIFACTS

- *Chemical shift:* Caused by slight differences in the frequency between fat and water protons at fat/water interface, resulting in a slight shift in position of fat-containing structures. At 1.5T, fat protons resonate 220Hz downfield from water protons. Seen as dark border on one side of a structure and a light border on the opposite side (e.g., edges of kidneys) in the frequency-encoding direction.
- *Aliasing (wrap-around):* FOV smaller than the body part being imaged so that the part beyond the edge is displayed on the opposite side of the image. Can be corrected with oversampling.
- *Gibbs (truncation):* Dark or light lines parallel to borders of abrupt intensity change. Seen commonly in the spinal cord. It is caused by the finite steps used in the Fourier transformation in reconstructing the image. May be minimized by increasing the resolution.
- *Zipper:* Seen as dotted line across an image. Caused by a hardware or software problem such as a radiofrequency entering the scanning room when the door is open during acquisition.
- *Motion:* Repeated "ghost" structures in the phase direction. Commonly caused by arterial pulsation and patient motion.
- *Moire (fringe):* Field homogeneity degrades over large FOV toward the edge, causing phase differences between the two edges. Aliasing of one side of body to the other side, resulting in superimposition of signals of different phases that alternatively add and cancel. Commonly seen with body coils in the coronal plane.

Statistics

TESTING

MEASUREMENTS

MEASUREMENT SCALES

Type	Example	Appropriate Statistics	Information Content
Nominal	Sex, blood type	Counts, rates, proportions, relative risk, chi-square	Low
Ordinal	Degree of pain	In addition to the above: median, rank correlation	Intermediate
Continuous	Weight, length	In addition to the above: mean, standard deviation, *t*-test, analysis of variance	High

STATISTICAL TESTING

STATISTICAL METHODS TO TEST HYPOTHESES

Type of Data	2 Groups, Different Individuals	≥3 Groups, Different Individuals	Single Treatment, Same Individual	Multiple Treatments, Same Individual	Association Between 2 Variables
Continuous (normally distributed population)	Unpaired *t*-test	Analysis of variance	Paired *t*-test	Repeated measures analysis of variance	Linear regression and Pearson product-moment correlation
Nominal	Chi-square analysis or contingency table	Chi-square analysis or contingency table	McNemar's test	Cochran Q	Contingency coefficient
Ordinal	Mann-Whitney rank-sum test	Kruskal-Wallis statistic	Wilcoxon signed rank test	Friedman statistic	Spearman rank correlation

ACCURACY, PRECISION (Fig. 14-106)

The *accuracy* of a variable is the degree to which it represents what it is supposed to represent. *Precision* is the degree to which a variable can be repeated. The two measures are thus different and not necessarily linked.

PRECISION AND ACCURACY

	Accuracy	Precision
Definition	The degree to which a variable actually represents what it is supposed to represent	The degree to which a variable has nearly the same value when measured several times
Best way to assess	Comparison with a reference standard	Comparison among repeated measures
Threatened by	Systematic error (bias)	Random error (variance)

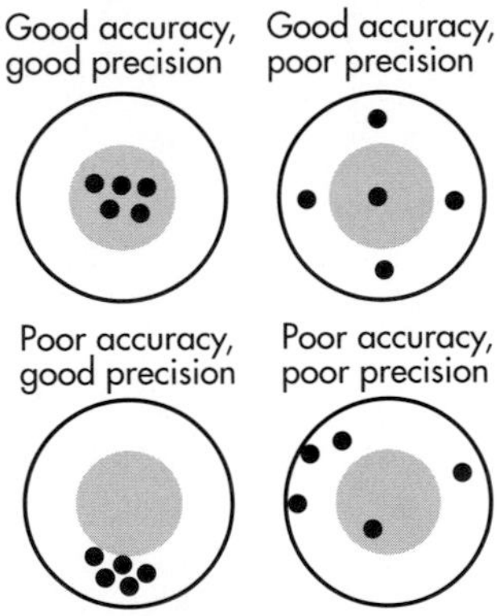

FIGURE 14-106

SENSITIVITY (FIG. 14-107)

Number of patients with disease that have been correctly detected (true positive [TP]) divided by all patients with disease (TP + FN, where FN = false negative):

$$\text{Sensitivity} = \frac{TP}{TP + FN}$$

		Test result: Positive	Negative	
Truth	Positive	TP	FN error type 2	Sensitivity
	Negative	FP error type 1	TN	Specificity
		PPV	NPV	

FIGURE 14-107

SPECIFICITY

Number of patients with no disease that have not been detected (true negative [TN]) divided by all patients without disease (TN + FP, where FP = false positive):

$$\text{Specificity} = \frac{TN}{TN + FP}$$

PREDICTIVE VALUES

The value of a diagnostic test depends not only on its sensitivity and specificity but also on the prevalence of the disease in the population being tested.

Positive Predictive Value (PPV)

This is the probability that a person with a positive test result actually has the disease.

$$PPV = \frac{TP}{TP + FP}$$

Negative Predictive Value (NPV)

This is the probability that a person with a negative test result does not have the disease.

$$NPV = \frac{TN}{TN + FN}$$

ROC ANALYSIS (Fig. 14-108)

The relationship between sensitivity and specificity is usually described by receiver operating characteristic (ROC) curves. An ideal diagnostic test would have 100% sensitivity and 100% specificity. If a diagnostic test has no predictive value, the relationship between sensitivity and specificity is linear. Diagnostic tests typically have a curve shape in between.

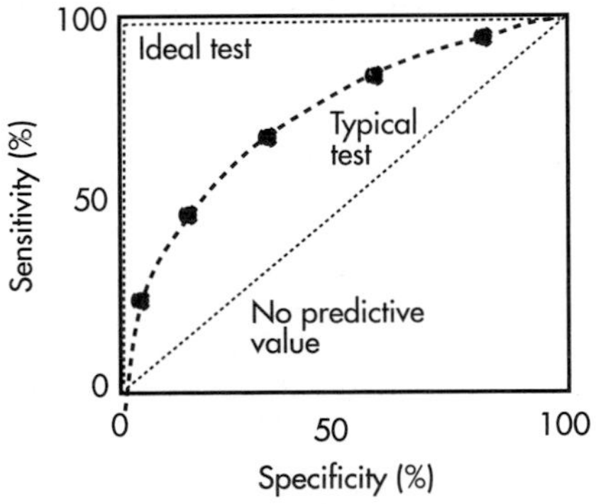

FIGURE 14-108

Suggested Readings

Bushberg JT, Seibert JA, Leidholdt EM, et al. *The Essential Physics of Medical Imaging*. Philadelphia: Lippincott Williams & Wilkins; 2001.

Chandra R. *Introductory Physics of Nuclear Medicine*. Philadelphia: Lippincott Williams & Wilkins; 2004.

Cherry SR, Sorenson JA, Phelps M. *Physics in Nuclear Medicine*. Philadelphia: WB Saunders; 2003.

Curry TS, Dowdey J, Murry RC. *Christensen's Introduction to the Physics of Diagnostic Radiology*. 4th ed. Philadelphia: Lippincott Williams & Wilkins; 1990.

Edelman RR, Hesselink JR, Zlatkin MB. *Clinical Magnetic Resonance Imaging*. Philadelphia: WB Saunders; 2005.

Handee WR, Ritenour ER. *Medical Imaging Physics*. Indianapolis: Wiley-Liss; 2002.

Wolbarst AB. *Physics of Radiology*. Madison: Medical Physics Publishing Corp.; 2005.

Index

Page numbers followed by *f* indicate figures; *t*, tables.

C

D

F

G

H

J

K

L

M

N

Q

R

T

U

V

W

X

Y

Z